Sistema respiratorio
(continued)

ortopnea / dificultad en respirar acostado
respiración poco profunda
taquipnea / respiración muy rápida
respiración jadeante

Sistema cardiovascular

bradicardia / lentitud anormal del pulso
dolor del tórax (pecho)
claudicación intermitente / calambres en la pierna
manchas de Janeway / manchas rojas en las palmas de la mano y plantas del pie
nódulos de Osler / lesiones sensibles, rojas o moradas en las palmas de la mano, yemas de los dedos de la mano y del pie, y plantas del pie
palidez
palpitaciones / pulsación rápida del corazón / sentir en el tórax el latido del corazón o que se salta un latido
disnea nocturna paroxistica / de dificultad en respirar intermitente que ocurre durante la noche y se alivia al sentarse derecho
taquicardia / rápido latido del corazón

Sistema musculosquelético

dolor de brazo
dolor de espalda
contusiones
joroba de búfalo / joroba en la espalda
chichones
edema hinchazón del brazo
edema hinchazón de los dedos
edema hinchazón de la pierna
edema generalizado / hinchazón
nódulos de Heberden / nódulos en las articulaciones de la mano
dolor de pierna
atrofia de músculo / deterioro demúsculo
flacidez de músculo / músculos débiles y laxos
espasticidad de músculo / tonicidad excesiva de músculo
debilidad de músculo

Sistema gastrointestinal

distensión abdominal / hinchazón abdominal
dolor abdominal
rigidez del abdomen
anorexia / pérdida de apetito / no comer / no tener hambre

Gastrointestinal system
(continued)

bloody stools
bowel sounds, hyperactive / stomach growling / gas
breath with fecal odor
constipation / difficulty going to the bathroom
diarrhea
dyspepsia / indigestion / burping / heartburn / gas
dysphagia / difficulty swallowing
eructation / belching
fecal incontinence / uncontrollable passage of bowel movements
fetor hepaticus / musty sweet breath odor
flatulence / gas
halitosis / bad breath
hematemesis / vomiting blood
hematochezia / rectal bleeding
hiccups
jaundice / yellowish tinge to skin or eyes
melena / passing black, tarry stools
nausea
polyphagia / excessive eating before fullness
pyrosis / heartburn
rectal pain
salivation, increased
stool, clay-colored
vomiting

Immune and endocrine systems

breath with ammonia odor
breath with fruity odor
cold intolerance
diaphoresis / sweating / night sweats
fatigue
fever
heat intolerance
lymphadenopathy / enlarged lymph nodes
moon face
pica / craving and eating inedible substances, such as plaster, clay, wool
polydipsia / excessive thirst
salt craving
skin, bronze
skin, clammy
skin, mottled
weight gain
weight loss

Sistema gastrointestinal
(continued)

materia fecal con sangre
ruido hiperactivo en el intestino / gruñidos en el estómago / gas
aliento con olor a materia fecal
estreñimiento / dificultad en evacuar
diarrea
dispepsia / indigestión / eructo / pirosis / gas
disfagia / dificultad en tragar
eructo / expulsion por la boca de aire del estomago
incontinencia fecal / evacuación fecal sin control
fetor hepático / olor dulzón rancio del aliento
flatulencia / gas
halitosis / mal aliento
hematemesis / vómito de sangre
hematoquecia / deposición sanguinolenta
hipo
ictericia / tinte amarillo de la piel y los ojos
melena / evacuar defecación negra y alquitranada
náusea
polifagia / apetito excesivo antes de sentirse lleno(a)
pirosis / acedía
dolor rectal
aumento de salivación
materia fecal de color de arcilla
vomitar

Sistemas immune y endocrino

aliento con olor a amoníaco
aliento con olor a fruta
intolerancia al frío
diaforesis / sudor profuso / sudar por la noche
fatiga
fiebre
intolerancia al calor
linfadenopatía / dilatación de los nódulos linfáticos
carirredondo
pica / deseo y consumo de sustancias incomibles tal como yeso, arcilla, lana
polidipsia / sed excesiva
ansia por sal
piel bronce
piel húmeda y fría
piel abigarrada
aumento de peso
pérdida de peso

(continued on inside back cover)

PROFESSIONAL GUIDE TO SIGNS & SYMPTOMS

SIXTH EDITION

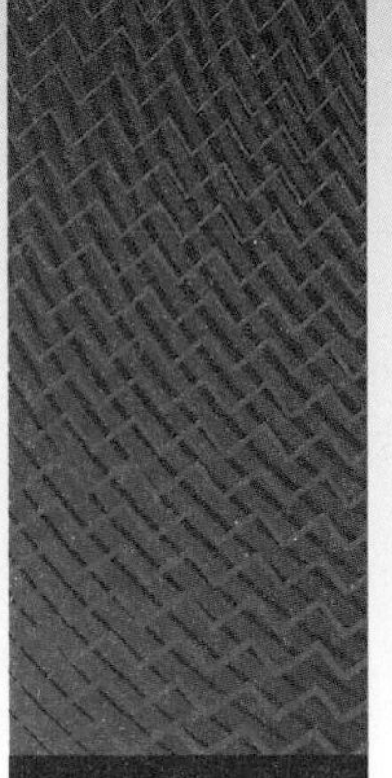

Professional Guide to Signs & Symptoms

Sixth Edition

Wolters Kluwer | Lippincott Williams & Wilkins
Health
Philadelphia • Baltimore • New York • London
Buenos Aires • Hong Kong • Sydney • Tokyo

STAFF

Executive Publisher
Judith A. Schilling McCann, RN, MSN

Clinical Director
Joan M. Robinson, RN, MSN

Clinical Project Manager
Jennifer Meyering, RN, BSN, MS, CCRN

Art Director
Elaine Kasmer

Product Manager
Rosanne Hallowell

Marketing Manager
Kimberly Schonberger

Copy Editor
Amy Furman

Vendor Manager
Beth Martz

Composition Services
Aptara, Inc.

Manufacturing Manager
Beth J. Welsh

The clinical treatments described and recommended in this publication are based on research and consultation with nursing, medical, and legal authorities. To the best of our knowledge, these procedures reflect currently accepted practice. Nevertheless, they can't be considered absolute and universal recommendations. For individual applications, all recommendations must be considered in light of the patient's clinical condition and, before administration of new or infrequently used drugs, in light of the latest package-insert information. The authors and publisher disclaim any responsibility for any adverse effects resulting from the suggested procedures, from any undetected errors, or from the reader's misunderstanding of the text.

Printed in China

PGSS6E010310-020411

Library of Congress Cataloging-in-Publication Data

Professional guide to signs & symptoms. — 6th ed.
p. ; cm.
Includes bibliographical references and index.
ISBN 978-1-60831-098-2 (alk. paper)
1. Symptoms—Handbooks, manuals, etc. I. Lippincott Williams & Wilkins. II. Title: Professional guide to signs and symptoms.
[DNLM: 1. Nursing Assessment—methods—Handbooks. 2. Signs and Symptoms—Handbooks. WY 49 P964 2011]
RC69.P77 2011
616'.047—dc22

2009033038

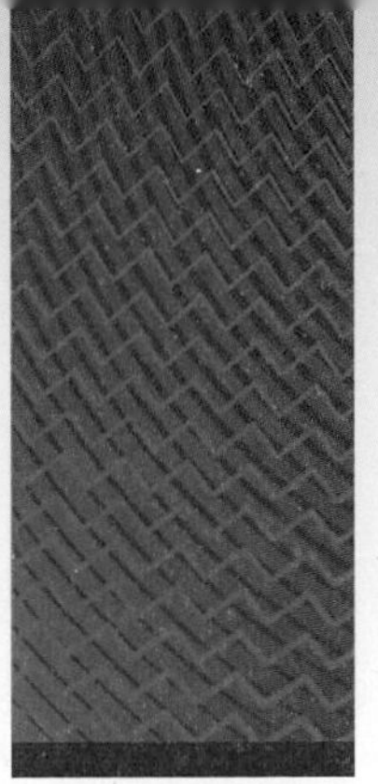

TABLE OF CONTENTS

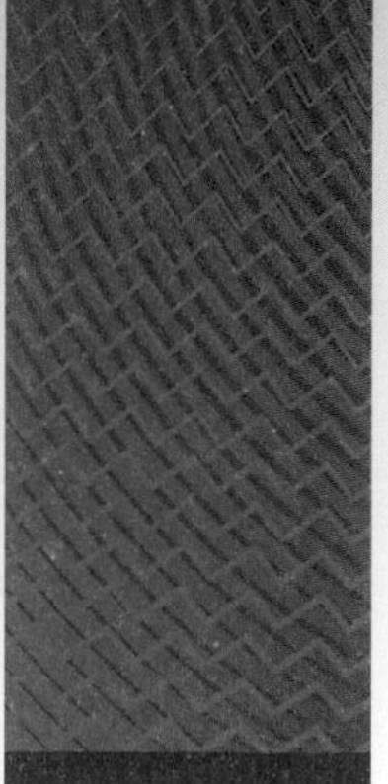

CONTRIBUTORS AND CONSULTANTS

Diane Dixon Abercrombie, MA, MMSc, PhD Candidate, PA-C
Assistant Professor and Academic Coordinator
Department of Physician Assistant Studies
University of South Alabama
Mobile, Alabama

Marylee Bressie, RN, MSN, CCRN, CCNS, CEN
Instructor
Spring Hill College Division of Nursing
Mobile, Alabama

Julie Carman, RN, MS
Instructor
University of Arkansas
Fort Smith, Arkansas

Laura M. Criddle, RN, PhD, CNS-BC, ONC, CCRN, CCNS, CNRN, CEN, CFRN
Clinical Nurse
Oregon Health & Science University
Portland, Oregon

Shelton M. Hisley, RNC, PhD, WHNP-BC
Senior Associate
Coastline Writing Consultants
Assistant Professor (Retired)
University of North Carolina—Wilmington School of Nursing
Wilmington, North Carolina

Julia Anne Isen, RN, MS, FNP-C
Assistant Clinical Professor
University of California
San Francisco, California
Internal Medicine
Uniformed Services University of the Health Sciences
Bethesda, Maryland

Anna Lee Jarrett, PhD, ACNP/ACNS, BC
APN/Program Manager, Rapid Response Team
Central Arkansas Veterans Healthcare System
Little Rock, Arkansas

Cynthia Miculan, RN, MSN, ONC, CE-BC
Clinical Manager
The University Hospital
Cincinnati, Ohio

Steven Noakes, MPAS, PA-C
Division Officer, Acute Care Clinic
Marine Corps Recruit Depot
San Diego, California

Allen Phelps, MPAS, PA-C
Physician Assistant
Naval Medical Center
San Diego, California

Rexann G. Pickering, RN, BSN, MS, MSN, PhD, CIM, CIP
Administrator, Human Protection–Research
Methodist Healthcare
Memphis, Tennessee

Roseanne Hanlon Rafter, RN, MSN, GCNS, BC
Director of Nursing, Professional Practice
Chestnut Hill Hospital
Philadelphia, Pennsylvania

Sundaram V. Ramanan, MD, FRCP
Professor of Medicine
St. Francis Hospital—University of Connecticut
Hartford, Connecticut

Richard R. Roach, MD, FACP
Assistant Professor of Internal Medicine
Michigan State University
Kalamazoo Center for Medical Studies
Kalamazoo, Michigan

Ora V. Robinson, RN, PhD
Assistant Professor
California State University
San Bernardino, California

Phillip Todd Smith, MHS, PA-C
Assistant Professor
Department of Physician Assistant Studies
University of South Alabama
Mobile, Alabama

Allison J. Terry, RN, MSN, PhD
Director, Center for Nursing
Alabama Board of Nursing
Montgomery, Alabama

Daniel T. Vetrosky, PhD, PA-C
Assistant Professor
University of South Alabama
Mobile, Alabama

Gail A. Viergutz, MS, ANP-C
Nurse Practitioner, Emergency Department and Urgent Care
Ministry Corporation
St. Michael's Hospital
Stevens Point, Wisconsin

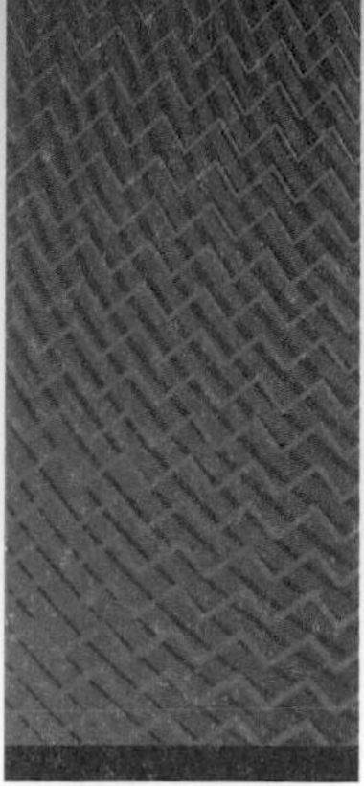

FOREWORD

With continuing advances in medical technology, laboratory studies, and diagnostic testing, clinical diagnosis and physical examination skills are in danger of becoming a lost art. I have seen too many students and novice practitioners become overly dependent on frequently imperfect, unreliable, and expensive tests to diagnose the cause of their patients' illnesses. The sixth edition of *Professional Guide to Signs & Symptoms* will help ensure that this doesn't happen. This fully reviewed and updated edition provides a comprehensive yet easy-to-understand compilation of many important signs and symptoms seen in clinical practice, and can help guide initial interventions and the appropriate use of laboratory and diagnostic studies.

The scope and organization of this sixth edition make it a valuable reference for students, nurses, and practitioners at all levels of training and expertise. More than 500 clinical signs and symptoms are arranged alphabetically and discussed in the body of the text. The new full-color format is appealing and enables quick and easy retrieval of relevant information. Easy-to-read tables, charts, and illustrations make difficult-to-grasp physiologic and clinical concepts understandable. Potentially obscure pathologic signs are clearly explained and should become more readily apparent to the astute clinical observer. New sections examining troublesome infectious diseases (methicillin-resistant *Staphylococcus aureus,* vancomycin-resistant enterococci, and vancomycin-resistant *S. aureus*) and popcorn lung disease (diacetyl exposure) are included.

Each sign and symptom is reviewed in a concise and standard format. Every entry begins with a brief review of the sign or symptom and is followed, where applicable, by a focused discussion of possible emergency interventions. Relevant history and physical findings are then reviewed and possible medical causes are discussed. Special considerations for caregivers provide practical advice, and pointers for pediatric and elderly populations should be particularly helpful for those who care for patients at either end of the age spectrum. Detailed differential diagnosis matrixes and flowcharts interspersed throughout the text aid patient assessment and diagnosis, while patient counseling sections provide helpful recommendations for patients and families once the diagnosis is established.

An additional 250 less frequently encountered selected signs and symptoms are briefly reviewed in the first appendix. Updated sections on the signs and symptoms of bioterrorism agents and the adverse effects of herbal remedies are particularly timely. The guide to obtaining a patient history provides helpful tips for conducting a medical interview, collecting primary clinical data, and performing a thorough review of systems. The index is cross-referenced and thorough, and the inside-the-cover listing of common signs and symptoms in both English and Spanish make this sixth edition a valuable reference for students, nurses, and practitioners living or traveling abroad.

I believe anyone who provides clinical care to patients and who is interested in the focused and appropriate use of medical technology, diagnostic testing, and initial interventions will find this comprehensive text extremely valuable. The standardized format with its easy-to-read tables, charts, and illustrations make this sixth edition an indispensable tool for the inquisitive student, nurse, or clinical practitioner.

Charles W. Mackett III, MD, FAAFP
Associate Professor and Executive Vice Chairman
Department of Family Medicine
University of Pittsburgh (Pa.) Medical Center

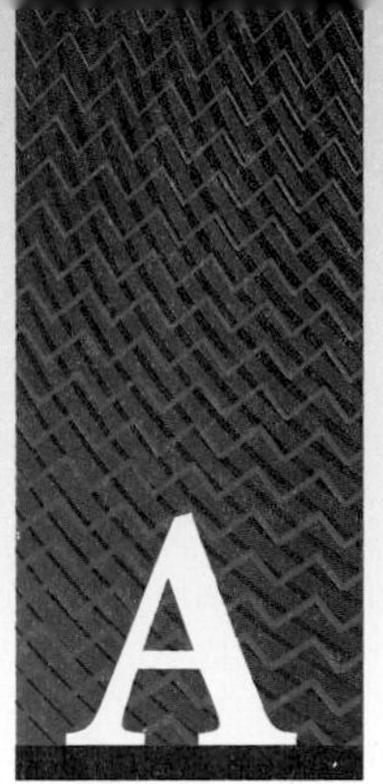

Abdominal distention

Abdominal distention refers to increased abdominal girth—the result of increased intra-abdominal pressure forcing the abdominal wall outward. Distention may be mild or severe, depending on the amount of pressure. It may be localized or diffuse and may occur gradually or suddenly. Acute abdominal distention may signal life-threatening peritonitis or acute bowel obstruction.

Abdominal distention may result from fat, flatus, a fetus (pregnancy or intra-abdominal mass [ectopic pregnancy]), or fluid. Fluid and gas are normally present in the GI tract but not in the peritoneal cavity. However, if fluid and gas are unable to pass freely through the GI tract, abdominal distention occurs. In the peritoneal cavity, distention may reflect acute bleeding, accumulation of ascitic fluid, or air from perforation of an abdominal organ.

Abdominal distention doesn't always signal pathology. For example, in anxious patients or those with digestive distress, localized distention in the left upper quadrant can result from aerophagia—the unconscious swallowing of air. Generalized distention can result from ingestion of fruits or vegetables with large quantities of unabsorbable carbohydrates, such as legumes, or from abnormal food fermentation by microbes. Don't forget to rule out pregnancy in all females with abdominal distention.

EMERGENCY INTERVENTIONS *If the patient displays abdominal distention, quickly check for signs of hypovolemia, such as pallor, diaphoresis, hypotension, rapid and thready pulse, rapid and shallow breathing, decreased urine output, poor capillary refill, and altered mentation. Ask the patient if he's experiencing severe abdominal pain or difficulty breathing. Find out about any recent accidents, and observe the patient for signs of trauma and peritoneal bleeding, such as Cullen's sign or Turner's sign. Then auscultate all abdominal quadrants, noting rapid and high-pitched, diminished, or absent bowel sounds. (If you don't hear bowel sounds immediately, listen for at least 5 minutes.) Gently palpate the abdomen for rigidity. Remember that deep or extensive palpation may increase pain.*

If you detect abdominal distention and rigidity along with abnormal bowel sounds, and the patient complains of pain, begin emergency interventions. Place the patient in the supine position, administer oxygen, and insert an I.V. catheter for fluid replacement. Prepare to insert a nasogastric tube to relieve acute intraluminal distention. Reassure the patient and prepare him for surgery.

History and physical examination

If the patient's abdominal distention isn't acute, ask about its onset and duration and associated signs. A patient with localized distention may report a sensation of pressure, fullness, or tenderness in the affected area. A patient with generalized distention may report a bloated feeling, a pounding heartbeat, and difficulty breathing deeply or breathing when lying flat. The patient may also feel unable to bend at his waist. Be sure to ask about abdominal pain, fever, nausea, vomiting, anorexia, altered bowel habits, and weight gain or loss.

Obtain a medical history, noting GI or biliary disorders that may cause peritonitis or ascites, such as cirrhosis, hepatitis, or inflammatory bowel disease. (See *Detecting ascites*.) Also note chronic constipation. Has the patient recently had abdominal surgery, which can lead to abdominal distention? Ask about recent accidents, even minor ones, like falling off a stepladder.

Perform a complete physical examination. Don't restrict the examination to the abdomen because you could miss important clues to the cause of abdominal distention. Next, stand at the foot of the bed and observe the recumbent patient for abdominal asymmetry to determine if distention is localized or generalized. Then assess abdominal contour by stooping at his side. Inspect for tense, glistening skin and bulging flanks, which may indicate ascites. Observe the umbilicus. An everted umbilicus may indicate ascites or an umbilical hernia. An inverted umbilicus may indicate distention from gas; it's also common in obese individuals. Inspect the abdomen for signs of an inguinal or femoral hernia and for incisions that may point to adhesions; both may lead to intestinal obstruction. Then auscultate for bowel sounds, abdominal friction rubs (indicating peritoneal inflammation), and bruits (indicating an aneurysm). Listen for a succussion splash—a splashing sound normally heard in the stomach when the patient moves or when palpation disturbs the viscera. An abnormally loud splash indicates fluid accumulation, suggesting gastric dilation or obstruction.

Next, percuss and palpate the abdomen to determine if distention results from air, fluid, or both. A tympanic note in the left lower quadrant suggests an air-filled descending or sigmoid colon. A tympanic note throughout a generally distended abdomen suggests an air-filled peritoneal cavity. A dull percussion note throughout a generally distended abdomen suggests a fluid-filled peritoneal cavity. Shifting of dullness laterally when the patient is in the decubitus position also indicates a fluid filled abdominal cavity. A pelvic or intra-abdominal mass causes local dullness upon percussion and should be palpable. Obesity causes a large abdomen with generalized rather then localized dullness and without shifting dullness, prominent tympany, or palpable bowel or other masses.

Palpate the abdomen for tenderness, noting whether it's localized or generalized. Watch for peritoneal signs and symptoms, such as rebound tenderness, guarding, rigidity, McBurney's point, obturator sign, and psoas sign. Female patients should undergo a pelvic examination; males, a genital examination. All patients who report abdominal pain should undergo a digital rectal examination with fecal occult blood testing. Finally, measure abdominal girth for a baseline value. Mark the flanks with a felt-tipped pen as a reference point for subsequent measurements. (See *Abdominal distention: Causes and associated findings,* pages 4 and 5.)

Medical causes

◆ ***Abdominal cancer.*** Generalized abdominal distention may occur when the cancer—most commonly ovarian, hepatic, or pancreatic cancer—produces ascites (usually in a patient with a known tumor). It's an indication of advanced disease. Shifting dullness and a fluid wave accompany distention. Associated signs and symptoms may include severe abdominal pain, an abdominal mass, anorexia, jaundice, GI hemorrhage (hematemesis or melena), dyspepsia, and weight loss that progresses to muscle weakness and atrophy.

◆ ***Abdominal trauma.*** When brisk internal bleeding accompanies trauma, abdominal distention may be acute and dramatic. Associated signs and symptoms of this life-threatening disorder include abdominal rigidity with guarding, decreased or absent bowel sounds, vomiting, tenderness, and abdominal bruising. The patient may feel pain over the trauma site, or over the scapula if abdominal bleeding irritates the phrenic nerve. Signs of hypovolemic shock (such as hypotension and rapid, thready pulse) appear with significant blood loss.

◆ ***Bladder distention.*** Various disorders cause bladder distention, which in turn causes lower abdominal distention. Slight dullness on percussion above the symphysis indicates mild bladder distention. A palpable, smooth, rounded, fluctuant suprapubic mass suggests severe distention; a fluctuant mass extending to the umbilicus indicates extremely severe distention. Urinary dribbling, frequency, or urgency may occur with urinary obstruction. Suprapubic discomfort is also common.

◆ ***Cirrhosis.*** In cirrhosis, ascites causes generalized distention and is confirmed by a fluid wave, shifting dullness, and a puddle sign.

Detecting ascites

To differentiate ascites from other causes of abdominal distention, check for shifting dullness and fluid wave, as described here.

Shifting dullness

Step 1. With the patient in a supine position, percuss from the umbilicus outward to the flank, as shown. Draw a line on the patient's skin to mark the change from tympany to dullness.

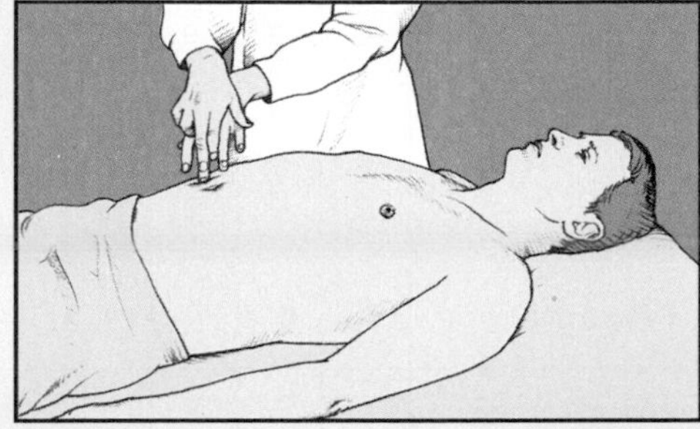

Step 2. Turn the patient onto his side. (Note that this position causes ascitic fluid to shift.) Percuss again and mark the change from tympany to dullness. Any difference between these lines can indicate ascites.

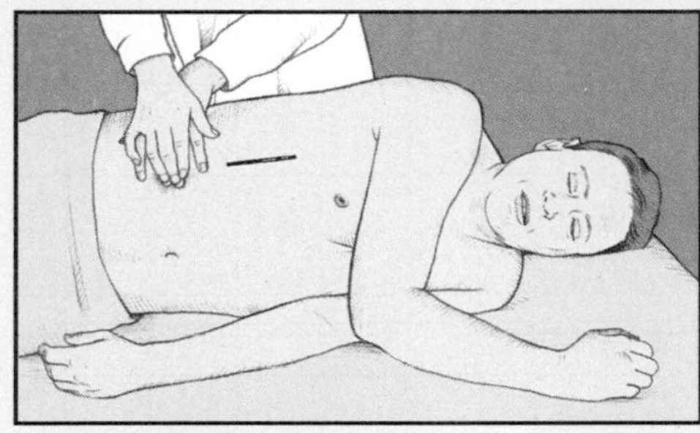

Fluid wave

Have another person press deeply into the patient's midline to prevent vibration from traveling along the abdominal wall. Place one of your palms on one of the patient's flanks, as shown. Strike the opposite flank with your other hand. If you feel the blow in the opposite palm, ascitic fluid is present.

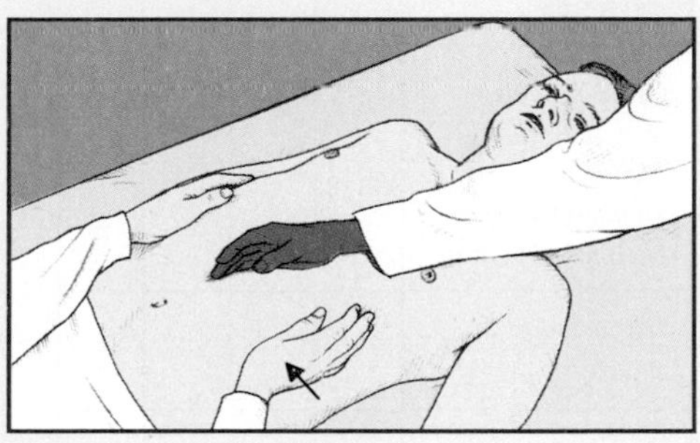

Umbilical eversion and caput medusae (dilated veins around the umbilicus) are common. The patient may report a feeling of fullness or weight gain. Associated findings include vague abdominal pain, fever, anorexia, nausea, vomiting, constipation or diarrhea, bleeding tendencies, severe pruritus, palmar erythema, spider angiomas, leg edema, and possibly splenomegaly. Hematemesis, encephalopathy, gynecomastia, or testicular atrophy may also occur. Jaundice is usually a late sign. Hepatomegaly occurs initially, but the liver may not be palpable in advanced disease.

◆ ***Gastric dilation (acute).*** Left-upper-quadrant distention is characteristic in acute gastric dilation, but the presentation varies. The patient usually complains of epigastric fullness or pain and nausea with or without vomiting. Physical examination reveals tympany, gastric tenderness, and a succussion splash. Initially, peristalsis may be visible. Later, hypoactive or absent bowel sounds confirm ileus. The patient may be pale and diaphoretic and may exhibit tachycardia or bradycardia.

◆ ***Heart failure.*** Generalized abdominal distention due to ascites typically accompanies

(Text continues on page 6.)

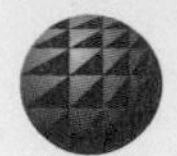

SIGNS & SYMPTOMS

Abdominal distention: Causes and associated findings

Major associated signs and symptoms

Common causes	Abdominal mass	Abdominal pain	Abdominal rigidity	Anorexia	Bowel sounds, absent	Bowel sounds, hyperactive	Bowel sounds, hypoactive	Constipation	Diarrhea	Edema
Abdominal cancer	●	●		●						
Abdominal trauma		●	●		●		●			
Bladder distention	●									
Cirrhosis		●		●				●	●	●
Gastric dilation (acute)		●			●		●			
Heart failure										●
Irritable bowel syndrome		●						●	●	
Large-bowel obstruction		●				●		●		
Mesenteric artery occlusion (acute)		●	●	●	●			●	●	
Nephrotic syndrome				●						●
Ovarian cysts	●	●								
Paralytic ileus		●			●		●	●		
Peritonitis		●	●		●		●			
Small-bowel obstruction		●				●		●		
Toxic megacolon (acute)		●			●		●			

Fever	Hepatomegaly	Hypotension	Jaundice	Jugular vein distention	Nausea	Oliguria	Rebound tenderness	Succussion splash	Tachycardia	Tachypnea	Urinary frequency	Vomiting	Weight change
			●										●
		●										●	
											●		
●	●		●		●							●	●
								●				●	
	●			●	●				●			●	
					●								
												●	
●		●							●	●		●	
						●							
												●	
●		●			●		●		●			●	
					●		●					●	
●							●		●				

severe cardiovascular impairment and is confirmed by shifting dullness and a fluid wave. Signs and symptoms of heart failure are numerous and depend on the disease stage and degree of cardiovascular impairment. Hallmarks include peripheral edema, jugular vein distention, dyspnea, and tachycardia. Common associated signs and symptoms include hepatomegaly (which may cause right-upper-quadrant pain), nausea, vomiting, productive cough, crackles, cool extremities, cyanotic nail beds, nocturia, exercise intolerance, nocturnal wheezing, diastolic hypertension, and cardiomegaly.

◆ ***Irritable bowel syndrome (IBS).*** IBS may produce intermittent, localized distention—the result of periodic intestinal spasms. Lower abdominal pain or cramping typically accompanies these spasms. The pain is usually relieved by defecation or by passage of intestinal gas and is aggravated by stress. Other possible signs and symptoms include diarrhea that may alternate with constipation or normal bowel function; nausea; dyspepsia; straining and urgency at defecation; feeling of incomplete evacuation; and small, mucus-streaked stools.

◆ ***Large-bowel obstruction.*** Dramatic abdominal distention is characteristic in large-bowel obstruction, a life-threatening disorder; in fact, loops of the large bowel may become visible on the abdomen. Constipation precedes distention and may be the only symptom for days. Associated findings include tympany, high-pitched bowel sounds, and sudden onset of colicky lower abdominal pain that becomes persistent. Fecal vomiting and diminished peristaltic waves and bowel sounds are late signs.

◆ ***Mesenteric artery occlusion (acute).*** In mesenteric artery occlusion—a life-threatening disorder—abdominal distention usually occurs several hours after the sudden onset of severe, colicky periumbilical pain accompanied by rapid (even forceful) bowel evacuation. The pain later becomes constant and diffuse. Related signs and symptoms include severe abdominal tenderness with guarding and rigidity, absent bowel sounds and, occasionally, a bruit in the right iliac fossa. The patient may also experience vomiting, anorexia, diarrhea, or constipation. Late signs include fever, tachycardia, tachypnea, hypotension, and cool, clammy skin. Abdominal distention or GI bleeding may be the only clue if pain is absent.

◆ ***Nephrotic syndrome.*** Nephrotic syndrome may produce massive edema, causing generalized abdominal distention with a fluid wave and shifting dullness. It may also produce elevated blood pressure, hematuria or oliguria, fatigue, anorexia, depression, pallor, periorbital edema, scrotal swelling, and skin striae.

◆ ***Ovarian cysts.*** Typically, large ovarian cysts produce lower abdominal distention accompanied by umbilical eversion. Because they're thin walled and fluid filled, these cysts produce a fluid wave and shifting dullness—signs that mimic ascites. Lower abdominal pain and a palpable mass may be present.

◆ ***Paralytic ileus.*** Paralytic ileus, which produces generalized distention with a tympanic percussion note, is accompanied by absent or hypoactive bowel sounds and, occasionally, mild abdominal pain and vomiting. The patient may be severely constipated or may pass flatus and small, liquid stools.

◆ ***Peritonitis.*** In peritonitis—a life-threatening disorder—abdominal distention may be localized or generalized, depending on the extent of peritonitis. Fluid accumulates first within the peritoneal cavity and then within the bowel lumen, causing a fluid wave and shifting dullness. Typically, distention is accompanied by rebound tenderness, abdominal rigidity, and sudden and severe abdominal pain that worsens with movement.

The skin over the patient's abdomen may appear taut. Associated signs and symptoms usually include hypoactive or absent bowel sounds, fever, chills, hyperalgesia, nausea, and vomiting. Signs of shock, such as tachycardia and hypotension, appear with significant fluid loss into the abdomen.

◆ ***Small-bowel obstruction.*** Abdominal distention, which is characteristic in small-bowel obstruction—a life-threatening disorder—is most pronounced during late obstruction, especially in the distal small bowel. Auscultation reveals hypoactive or hyperactive bowel sounds, whereas percussion produces a tympanic note. Accompanying signs and symptoms include colicky periumbilical pain, constipation, nausea, and vomiting; the higher the obstruction, the earlier and more severe the vomiting. Rebound tenderness reflects intestinal strangulation with ischemia. Associated signs and symptoms include drowsiness, malaise, and signs of dehydration. Signs of hypovolemic shock appear with progressive dehydration and plasma loss.

◆ ***Toxic megacolon (acute).*** Toxic megacolon is a life-threatening complication of infectious or ulcerative colitis that produces dramatic abdominal distention. The distention usually develops gradually and is accompanied by a tympanic percussion note, diminished or absent bowel sounds, and mild rebound tenderness. The patient also experiences abdominal pain and tenderness, fever, tachycardia, and dehydration.

SPECIAL CONSIDERATIONS

Position the patient comfortably, using pillows for support. Place him on his left side to help flatus escape or, if he has ascites, elevate the head of the bed to ease his breathing. Administer drugs to relieve pain, and offer emotional support.

Prepare the patient for diagnostic tests, such as abdominal X-rays, endoscopy, laparoscopy, ultrasonography, computed tomography scan, or possibly paracentesis.

PEDIATRIC POINTERS

Because a young child's abdomen is normally rounded, distention may be difficult to observe. However, a child's abdominal wall is less well developed than an adult's, so palpation is easier. When percussing the abdomen, remember that children normally swallow air when eating and crying, resulting in louder-than-normal tympany. Minimal tympany with abdominal distention may result from fluid accumulation or solid masses. To check for abdominal fluid, test for shifting dullness instead of for a fluid wave. (In a child, air swallowing and incomplete abdominal muscle development make the fluid wave difficult to interpret.)

Some children won't cooperate with a physical examination. Try to gain the child's confidence, and consider allowing him to remain in the parent's or caregiver's lap. You can gather clues by observing the child while he's coughing, walking, or even climbing on office furniture. Remove all the child's clothing to avoid missing any diagnostic clues. Also, perform a gentle rectal examination.

In neonates, ascites usually results from GI or urinary perforation; in older children, from heart failure, cirrhosis, or nephrosis. Besides ascites, congenital malformations of the GI tract (such as intussusception and volvulus) may cause abdominal distention. A hernia may cause distention if it produces an intestinal obstruction. In addition, overeating and constipation can cause distention.

GERIATRIC POINTERS

As people age, fat tends to accumulate in the lower abdomen and near the hips, even when body weight is stable. This accumulation, together with weakening abdominal muscles, commonly produces a potbelly, which some elderly patients interpret as fluid collection or evidence of disease.

PATIENT COUNSELING

If the patient's anxiety triggers air swallowing or deep breathing that causes discomfort, advise him to take slow breaths. If the patient has an obstruction or ascites, explain food and fluid restrictions. Stress good oral hygiene to prevent dry mouth.

Abdominal mass

Commonly detected on routine physical examination, an abdominal mass is a localized swelling in one abdominal quadrant. Typically, this sign develops insidiously and may represent an enlarged organ, a neoplasm, an abscess, a vascular defect, or a fecal mass.

Distinguishing an abdominal mass from a normal structure requires skillful palpation. At times, palpation must be repeated with the patient in a different position or performed by a second examiner to verify initial findings. A palpable abdominal mass is an important clinical sign and usually represents a serious—and perhaps life-threatening—disorder.

EMERGENCY INTERVENTIONS *If the patient has a pulsating midabdominal mass and severe abdominal or back pain, suspect an aortic aneurysm. Quickly take his vital signs. Because the patient may require emergency surgery, withhold food or fluids until the patient is examined. Prepare to administer oxygen and to start an I.V. infusion for fluid and blood replacement. Obtain routine preoperative tests, and prepare the patient for angiography. Frequently monitor blood pressure, pulse rate, respirations, and urine output.*

Be alert for signs of shock, such as tachycardia, hypotension, and cool, clammy skin, which may indicate significant blood loss.

HISTORY AND PHYSICAL EXAMINATION

If the patient's abdominal mass doesn't suggest an aortic aneurysm, take a detailed history. Ask the patient if the mass is painful. If so, ask if the pain is constant or if it occurs only on palpation. Is it localized or generalized? Determine if the patient was already aware of the mass. If he was, find out if he noticed any change in its size or location.

Next, review the patient's medical history, paying special attention to GI disorders. Ask the patient about GI symptoms, such as constipation, diarrhea, rectal bleeding, abnormally colored stools, and vomiting. Has the patient noticed a change in appetite? If the patient is female, ask whether her menstrual cycles are regular and when the 1st day of her last menstrual period was.

Perform a complete physical examination. Next, auscultate for bowel sounds in each quadrant. Listen for bruits or friction rubs, and check for enlarged veins. Lightly palpate and then deeply palpate the abdomen, assessing any painful or suspicious areas last. Note the patient's position when you locate the mass. Some masses can be detected only with the patient in a supine position; others require a side-lying position.

Estimate the size of the mass in centimeters. Determine its shape. Is it round or sausage shaped? Describe its contour as smooth, rough, sharply defined, nodular, or irregular. Determine the consistency of the mass. Is it doughy, soft, solid, or hard? Also, percuss the mass. A dull sound indicates a fluid-filled mass; a tympanic sound, an air-filled mass.

Next, determine if the mass moves with your hand or in response to respiration. Is the mass free-floating or attached to intra-abdominal structures? To determine whether the mass is located in the abdominal wall or the abdominal cavity, ask the patient to lift his head and shoulders off the examination table, thereby contracting his abdominal muscles. While these muscles are contracted, try to palpate the mass. If you can, the mass is in the abdominal wall; if you can't, the mass is within the abdominal cavity. (See *Abdominal masses: Locations and causes.*)

After the abdominal examination is complete, perform pelvic, genital, and rectal examinations.

Medical causes

◆ ***Abdominal aortic aneurysm.*** An abdominal aortic aneurysm may persist for years, producing only a pulsating periumbilical mass with a systolic bruit over the aorta. However, it may become life-threatening if the aneurysm expands and its walls weaken. In such cases, the patient initially reports constant upper abdominal pain or, less often, low back or dull abdominal pain. If the aneurysm ruptures, he'll report severe abdominal and back pain. And after rupture, the aneurysm no longer pulsates.

Associated signs and symptoms of rupture include mottled skin below the waist, absent femoral and pedal pulses, lower blood pressure in the legs than in the arms, mild to moderate tenderness with guarding, and abdominal rigidity. Signs of shock—such as tachycardia and cool, clammy skin—appear with significant blood loss.

◆ ***Bladder distention.*** A smooth, rounded, fluctuant suprapubic mass is characteristic. In extreme distention, the mass may extend to the umbilicus. Severe suprapubic pain and urinary frequency and urgency may also occur.

◆ ***Cholecystitis.*** Deep palpation below the liver border may reveal a smooth, firm, sausage-shaped mass. However, in acute inflammation, the gallbladder is usually too tender to be palpated. Cholecystitis can cause severe right-upper-quadrant pain that may radiate to the right shoulder, chest, or back; abdominal rigidity and tenderness; fever; pallor; diaphoresis; anorexia; nausea; and vomiting. Recurrent attacks usually occur 1 to 6 hours after meals. Murphy's sign (inspiratory arrest elicited when the examiner palpates the right upper quadrant as the patient takes a deep breath) is common.

◆ ***Cholelithiasis.*** A stone-filled gallbladder usually produces a painless right-upper-quadrant mass that's smooth and sausage-shaped. However, passage of a stone through the bile or cystic duct may cause severe right-upper-quadrant pain that radiates to the epigastrium, back, or shoulder blades. Accompanying signs and symptoms include anorexia, nausea, vomiting, chills, diaphoresis, restlessness, and low-grade fever. Jaundice may occur with obstruction of the common bile duct. The patient may also experience intolerance of fatty foods and frequent indigestion.

◆ ***Colon cancer.*** A right-lower-quadrant mass may occur in cancer of the right colon, which may also cause occult bleeding with anemia and abdominal aching, pressure, or dull cramps. Associated findings include weakness, fatigue, exertional dyspnea, vertigo, and signs and symptoms of intestinal obstruction, such as obstipation and vomiting.

Abdominal masses: Locations and causes

The location of an abdominal mass provides an important clue to the causative disorder. Below you'll find the disorders responsible for abdominal masses in each of the four abdominal quadrants.

Right upper quadrant
- Aortic aneurysm (epigastric area)
- Cholecystitis or cholelithiasis
- Gallbladder, gastric, or hepatic carcinoma
- Hepatomegaly
- Hydronephrosis
- Pancreatic abscess or pseudocysts
- Renal cell carcinoma

Left upper quadrant
- Aortic aneurysm (epigastric area)
- Gastric carcinoma (epigastric area)
- Hydronephrosis
- Pancreatic abscess (epigastric area)
- Pancreatic pseudocysts (epigastric area)
- Renal cell carcinoma
- Splenomegaly

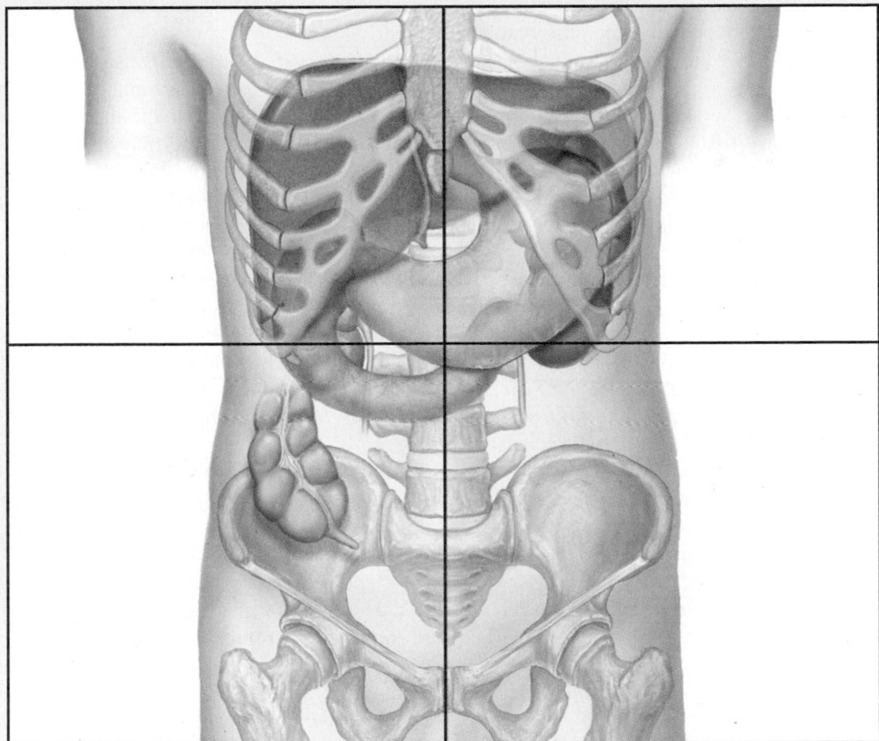

Right lower quadrant
- Bladder distention (suprapubic area)
- Colon cancer
- Crohn's disease
- Ovarian cyst (suprapubic area)
- Uterine leiomyomas (suprapubic area)

Left lower quadrant
- Bladder distention (suprapubic area)
- Colon cancer
- Diverticulitis
- Ovarian cyst (suprapubic area)
- Uterine leiomyomas (suprapubic area)
- Volvulus

Occasionally, cancer of the left colon also causes a palpable mass. Usually though, it produces rectal bleeding, intermittent abdominal fullness or cramping, and rectal pressure. The patient may also report fremitus and pelvic discomfort. Later, he develops obstipation, diarrhea, or pencil-shaped, grossly bloody, or mucus-streaked stools. Typically, defecation relieves pain.

◆ ***Crohn's disease.*** In Crohn's disease, tender, sausage-shaped masses are usually palpable in the right lower quadrant and, at times, in the left lower quadrant. Attacks of colicky right-lower-quadrant pain and diarrhea are common. Associated signs and symptoms include fever, anorexia, weight loss, hyperactive bowel sounds, nausea, abdominal tenderness with guarding, and perirectal, skin, or vaginal fistulas.

◆ ***Diverticulitis.*** Most common in the sigmoid colon, diverticulitis may produce a left-lower-quadrant mass that's usually tender, firm, and fixed. It also produces intermittent abdominal pain that's relieved by defecation or passage of flatus. Other findings may include alternating constipation and diarrhea, nausea, low-grade fever, and a distended and tympanic abdomen.

◆ ***Gallbladder cancer.*** Gallbladder cancer may produce a moderately tender, irregular mass in the right upper quadrant. Accompanying it is chronic, progressively severe epigastric or right-upper-quadrant pain that may radiate to the right shoulder. Associated signs and symptoms include nausea, vomiting, anorexia, weight loss, jaundice, and possibly hepatosplenomegaly.

◆ ***Gastric cancer.*** Advanced gastric cancer may produce an epigastric mass. Early findings include chronic dyspepsia and epigastric discomfort, whereas late findings include weight loss, a feeling of fullness after eating, fatigue, and occasionally coffee-ground vomitus or melena.

◆ ***Hepatic cancer.*** Hepatic cancer produces a tender, nodular mass in the right upper quadrant or right epigastric area accompanied by severe pain that's aggravated by jolting. Other effects include weight loss, weakness, anorexia, nausea, fever, dependent edema, and occasionally jaundice and ascites. A large tumor can also cause a bruit or hum.

◆ ***Hepatomegaly.*** Hepatomegaly produces a firm, blunt, irregular mass in the epigastric region or below the right costal margin. Associated signs and symptoms vary with the causative disorder but commonly include ascites, right-upper-quadrant pain and tenderness, anorexia, nausea, vomiting, leg edema, jaundice, palmar erythema, spider angiomas, gynecomastia, testicular atrophy, and possibly splenomegaly.

◆ ***Hydronephrosis.*** By enlarging one or both kidneys, hydronephrosis produces a smooth, boggy mass in one or both flanks. Other findings vary with the degree of hydronephrosis. The patient may have severe colicky renal pain or dull flank pain that radiates to the groin, vulva, or testes. Hematuria, pyuria, dysuria, alternating oliguria and polyuria, nocturia, accelerated hypertension, nausea, and vomiting may also occur.

◆ ***Ovarian cyst.*** A large ovarian cyst may produce a smooth, rounded, fluctuant mass, resembling a distended bladder, in the suprapubic region. Large or multiple cysts may also cause mild pelvic discomfort, low back pain, menstrual irregularities, and hirsutism. A twisted or ruptured cyst may cause abdominal tenderness, distention, and rigidity.

◆ ***Pancreatic abscess.*** Occasionally, pancreatic abscess may produce a palpable epigastric mass accompanied by epigastric pain and tenderness. The patient's temperature usually rises abruptly but may climb steadily. Nausea, vomiting, diarrhea, tachycardia, and hypotension may also occur.

◆ ***Pancreatic pseudocysts.*** After pancreatitis, pseudocysts may form on the pancreas, causing a palpable nodular mass in the epigastric area. Other findings include nausea, vomiting, diarrhea, abdominal pain and tenderness, low-grade fever, and tachycardia.

◆ ***Renal cell carcinoma.*** Usually occurring in only one kidney, renal cell carcinoma produces a smooth, firm, nontender mass near the affected kidney. Accompanying it are dull, constant abdominal or flank pain and hematuria. Other signs and symptoms include elevated blood pressure, fever, and urine retention. Weight loss, nausea, vomiting, and leg edema occur in late stages.

◆ ***Splenomegaly.*** Lymphomas, leukemias, hemolytic anemias, and inflammatory diseases are among the many disorders that may cause splenomegaly. Typically, the smooth edge of the enlarged spleen is palpable in the left upper quadrant. Associated signs and symptoms vary with the causative disorder but often include a feeling of abdominal fullness, left-upper-quadrant abdominal pain and tenderness, splenic friction rub, splenic bruits, and low-grade fever.

◆ ***Uterine leiomyomas (fibroids).*** If large enough, these common, benign uterine tumors produce a round, multinodular mass in the suprapubic region. The patient's chief complaint is usually menorrhagia; she may also experience a feeling of heaviness in the abdomen, and pressure on surrounding organs may cause back pain, constipation, and urinary frequency or urgency. Edema and varicosities of the lower extremities may develop. Rapid fibroid growth in perimenopausal or postmenopausal women needs further evaluation.

Special considerations

Discovery of an abdominal mass commonly causes anxiety. Offer emotional support to the patient and his family as they await the diagnosis. Position the patient comfortably, and administer drugs for pain or anxiety as needed.

If an abdominal mass causes bowel obstruction, watch for indications of peritonitis—abdominal pain and rebound tenderness—and for signs of shock, such as tachycardia and hypotension.

Pediatric pointers

Detecting an abdominal mass in an infant can be quite a challenge. However, these tips will make palpation easier for you: Allow an infant to suck on his bottle or pacifier to prevent crying, which causes abdominal rigidity and interferes with palpation. Avoid tickling him because laughter also causes abdominal rigidity. Also, reduce his apprehension by distracting him with cheerful conversation. Rest your hand on his abdomen for a few moments before palpation. If he remains sensitive, place his hand under yours as you palpate. Consider allowing the child to remain on the parent's or caregiver's lap. A gentle rectal examination should also be performed.

In neonates, most abdominal masses result from renal disorders, such as polycystic kidney disease or congenital hydronephrosis. In older infants and children, abdominal masses usually are caused by enlarged organs, such as the liver and spleen.

Other common causes include Wilms' tumor, neuroblastoma, intussusception, volvulus, Hirschsprung's disease (congenital megacolon), pyloric stenosis, and abdominal abscess.

Geriatric pointers

Ultrasonography should be used to evaluate a prominent midepigastric mass in thin elderly patients.

Patient counseling

Carefully explain diagnostic tests, which may include blood and urine studies, abdominal X-rays, barium enema, computed tomography scan, ultrasonography, radioisotope scan, and gastroscopy or sigmoidoscopy. A pelvic or rectal examination is usually indicated.

Abdominal pain

Abdominal pain usually results from a GI disorder, but it can also be caused by a reproductive, genitourinary (GU), musculoskeletal, or vascular disorder; drug use; or ingestion of toxins. At times, such pain signals life-threatening complications.

Abdominal pain arises from the abdominopelvic viscera, the parietal peritoneum, or the capsules of the liver, kidney, or spleen. It may be acute or chronic and diffuse or localized. Visceral pain develops slowly into a deep, dull, aching pain that's poorly localized in the epigastric, periumbilical, or lower midabdominal (hypogastric) region. In contrast, somatic (parietal, peritoneal) pain produces a sharp, more intense, and well-localized discomfort that rapidly follows the insult. Movement or coughing aggravates this pain. (See *Abdominal pain: Types and locations,* page 12.)

Pain may also be referred to the abdomen from another site with the same or similar nerve supply. This sharp, well-localized, referred pain is felt in skin or deeper tissues and may coexist with skin hyperesthesia and muscle hyperalgesia.

Mechanisms that produce abdominal pain include stretching or tension of the gut wall, traction on the peritoneum or mesentery, vigorous intestinal contraction, inflammation, ischemia, and sensory nerve irritation.

EMERGENCY INTERVENTIONS *If the patient is experiencing sudden and severe abdominal pain, quickly take his vital signs and palpate pulses below the waist. Be alert for signs of hypovolemic shock, such as tachycardia and hypotension. Obtain I.V. access.*

Emergency surgery may be required if the patient also has mottled skin below the waist and a pulsating epigastric mass or rebound tenderness and rigidity.

Abdominal pain: Types and locations

Affected organ	Visceral pain	Parietal pain	Referred pain
Stomach	Middle epigastrium	Middle epigastrium and left upper quadrant	Shoulders
Small intestine	Periumbilical area	Over affected site	Midback (rare)
Appendix	Periumbilical area	Right lower quadrant	Right lower quadrant
Proximal colon	Periumbilical area and right flank for ascending colon	Over affected site	Right lower quadrant and back (rare)
Distal colon	Hypogastrium and left flank for descending colon	Over affected site	Left lower quadrant and back (rare)
Gallbladder	Middle epigastrium	Right upper quadrant	Right subscapular area
Ureters	Costovertebral angle	Over affected site	Groin; scrotum in men, labia in women (rare)
Pancreas	Middle epigastrium and left upper quadrant	Middle epigastrium and left upper quadrant	Back and left shoulder
Ovaries, fallopian tubes, and uterus	Hypogastrium and groin	Over affected site	Inner thighs

HISTORY AND PHYSICAL EXAMINATION

If the patient has no life-threatening signs or symptoms, take his history. Ask him if he has had this type of pain before. Have him describe the pain—for example, is it dull, sharp, stabbing, or burning? Ask if anything relieves the pain or makes it worse. Ask the patient if the pain is constant or intermittent and when the pain began. Constant, steady abdominal pain suggests organ perforation, ischemia, or inflammation or blood in the peritoneal cavity. Intermittent, cramping abdominal pain suggests the patient may have an obstruction of a hollow organ.

If pain is intermittent, find out the duration of a typical episode. In addition, ask the patient where the pain is located and if it radiates to other areas.

Find out if movement, coughing, exertion, vomiting, eating, elimination, or walking worsens or relieves the pain. The patient may report abdominal pain as indigestion or gas pain, so have him describe it in detail.

Ask the patient about substance abuse and any history of vascular, GI, GU, or reproductive disorders. Ask the female patient the date of her last menses and if she has had changes in her menstrual pattern or dyspareunia.

Also ask about appetite changes and the onset and frequency of nausea or vomiting. Find out about increased flatulence, constipation, diarrhea, and changes in stool consistency. When was his last bowel movement? Ask about urinary frequency, urgency, or pain. Is the urine cloudy or pink?

Perform a physical examination. Take the patient's vital signs, and assess skin turgor and mucous membranes. Inspect his abdomen for distention or visible peristaltic waves and, if indicated, measure his abdominal girth.

Auscultate for bowel sounds and characterize their motility. Percuss all quadrants, noting the percussion sounds. Palpate the entire abdomen for masses, rigidity, and tenderness. Check for costovertebral angle (CVA) tenderness, abdominal tenderness with guarding, and rebound tenderness. (See *Abdominal pain: Causes and associated findings,* pages 14 to 19.)

Medical causes

◆ ***Abdominal aortic aneurysm (dissecting).*** Initially, abdominal aortic aneurysm—a life-threatening disorder—may produce dull lower abdominal, lower back, or severe chest pain. In most cases, however, it produces constant upper abdominal pain, which may worsen when the patient lies down and may abate when he leans forward or sits up. Palpation may reveal an epigastric mass that pulsates before rupture but not after it.

Other findings may include mottled skin below the waist, absent femoral and pedal pulses, blood pressure that's lower in the legs than in the arms, mild to moderate abdominal tenderness with guarding, and abdominal rigidity. Signs of shock, such as tachycardia and tachypnea, may appear.

◆ ***Abdominal cancer.*** Abdominal pain usually occurs late in abdominal cancer. It may be accompanied by anorexia, weight loss, weakness, depression, an abdominal mass, and abdominal distention.

◆ ***Abdominal trauma.*** Generalized or localized abdominal pain occurs with ecchymoses on the abdomen; abdominal tenderness; vomiting; and, with hemorrhage into the peritoneal cavity, abdominal rigidity. Bowel sounds are decreased or absent. The patient may have signs of hypovolemic shock, such as hypotension and a rapid, thready pulse.

◆ ***Adrenal crisis.*** Severe abdominal pain appears early along with nausea, vomiting, dehydration, profound weakness, anorexia, and fever. Later signs are progressive loss of consciousness, hypotension, tachycardia, oliguria, cool and clammy skin, and increased motor activity, which may progress to delirium or seizures.

◆ ***Anthrax, GI.*** Anthrax is an acute infectious disease that's caused by the gram-positive, spore-forming bacterium *Bacillus anthracis.* Although the disease most commonly occurs in wild and domestic grazing animals, such as cattle, sheep, and goats, the spores can live in the soil for many years. The disease can occur in humans exposed to infected animals, tissue from infected animals, or biological agents. Most natural cases occur in agricultural regions worldwide. Anthrax may occur in cutaneous, inhaled, or GI forms.

GI anthrax is caused by eating contaminated meat from an infected animal. Initial signs and symptoms include anorexia, nausea, vomiting, and fever. Late signs and symptoms include abdominal pain, severe bloody diarrhea, and hematemesis.

◆ ***Appendicitis.*** Appendicitis is a life-threatening disorder in which pain initially occurs in the epigastric or umbilical region. Anorexia, nausea, and vomiting may occur after the onset of pain. Pain localizes at McBurney's point in the right lower quadrant and is accompanied by abdominal rigidity, increasing tenderness (especially over McBurney's point), rebound tenderness, and retractive respirations. Later signs and symptoms include malaise, constipation (or diarrhea), low-grade fever, and tachycardia.

◆ ***Cholecystitis.*** Severe pain in the right upper quadrant may arise suddenly or increase gradually over several hours, usually after meals. It may radiate to the right shoulder, chest, or back. Accompanying the pain are anorexia, nausea, vomiting, fever, abdominal rigidity and tenderness, pallor, and diaphoresis. Murphy's sign (inspiratory arrest elicited when the examiner palpates the right upper quadrant as the patient takes a deep breath) is common.

◆ ***Cholelithiasis.*** Patients may suffer sudden, severe, and paroxysmal pain in the right upper quadrant lasting several minutes to several hours. The pain may radiate to the epigastrium, back, or shoulder blades. The pain is accompanied by anorexia, nausea, vomiting (sometimes bilious), diaphoresis, restlessness, and abdominal tenderness with guarding over the gallbladder or biliary duct. The patient may also experience fatty food intolerance and frequent indigestion.

◆ ***Cirrhosis.*** Dull abdominal aching occurs early and is usually accompanied by anorexia, indigestion, nausea, vomiting, and constipation or diarrhea. Subsequent right-upper-quadrant pain worsens when the patient sits up or leans forward. Associated signs include fever, ascites, leg edema, weight gain, hepatomegaly, jaundice, severe pruritus, bleeding tendencies, palmar erythema, and spider angiomas. Gynecomastia and testicular atrophy may also be present.

◆ ***Crohn's disease.*** An acute attack causes severe cramping pain in the lower abdomen, typically preceded by weeks or months of milder cramping pain. Crohn's disease may also cause diarrhea, hyperactive bowel sounds, dehydration, weight loss, fever, abdominal tenderness

(Text continues on page 18.)

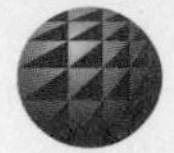

SIGNS & SYMPTOMS

Abdominal pain: Causes and associated findings

Common causes	Abdominal distention	Abdominal mass	Abdominal rigidity	Abdominal tenderness	Amenorrhea	Anorexia	Bowel sounds, absent	Bowel sounds, hyperactive	Bowel sounds, hypoactive	Breath odor, fruity	Chest pain
	Major associated signs and symptoms										
Abdominal aortic aneurysm (dissecting)		●	●	●							●
Abdominal cancer	●	●				●					
Abdominal trauma			●	●			●		●		
Adrenal crisis						●					
Anthrax, GI						●					
Appendicitis			●	●		●					
Cholecystitis			●	●		●					●
Cholelithiasis				●		●					
Cirrhosis	●					●					
Crohn's disease		●		●				●			
Cystitis				●							
Diabetic ketoacidosis										●	
Diverticulitis		●	●								
Duodenal ulcer											●
Ectopic pregnancy		●			●						
Endometriosis				●							
Escherichia coli O157:H7											
Gastric ulcer						●					
Gastritis						●					
Gastroenteritis								●			
Heart failure	●										

	Constipation	Costovertebral angle tenderness	Cough	Diarrhea	Dyspnea	Fever	Kussmaul's respirations	Nausea	Oliguria or anuria	Skin lesions	Skin mottling	Tachycardia	Tachypnea	Urinary frequency	Vomiting	Weakness	Weight change
											●	●	●				
																●	●
												●			●		
						●		●	●			●			●	●	
				●		●		●							●		
	●			●		●		●				●			●		
						●		●							●		
						●		●							●		
	●			●		●		●							●		●
				●		●											●
						●		●					●	●	●		
							●					●					
	●					●		●									
																	●
								●				●		●	●		
	●																
				●		●		●							●		
								●									●
						●		●							●		●
				●				●							●		
			●		●			●				●			●		

(continued)

Abdominal pain: Causes and associated findings *(continued)*

Major associated signs and symptoms

Common causes	Abdominal distention	Abdominal mass	Abdominal rigidity	Abdominal tenderness	Amenorrhea	Anorexia	Bowel sounds, absent	Bowel sounds, hyperactive	Bowel sounds, hypoactive	Breath odor, fruity	Chest pain
Hepatic abscess				●		●					
Hepatic amebiasis				●							
Hepatitis				●		●					
Herpes zoster				●							●
Insect toxins			●								
Intestinal obstruction	●			●			●	●	●		
Irritable bowel syndrome	●			●							
Listeriosis											
Mesenteric artery ischemia			●	●		●					
Myocardial infarction											●
Norovirus infection											
Ovarian cyst	●	●		●	●						
Pancreatitis			●	●					●		
Pelvic inflammatory disease		●		●							
Perforated ulcer			●	●			●				
Peritonitis	●		●	●			●		●		
Pleurisy											●
Pneumonia			●	●							●
Pneumothorax											●
Prostatitis											

	Constipation	Costovertebral angle tenderness	Cough	Diarrhea	Dyspnea	Fever	Kussmaul's respirations	Nausea	Oliguria or anuria	Skin lesions	Skin mottling	Tachycardia	Tachypnea	Urinary frequency	Vomiting	Weakness	Weight change
				●		●		●							●		
						●										●	●
								●							●		
						●				●							
						●		●							●		
	●							●				●			●		
	●			●				●									
				●		●		●							●		
	●			●								●	●		●		
					●			●							●	●	
				●				●							●		
						●		●							●		
						●		●				●			●		
						●		●							●		
						●						●					
						●			●			●	●		●		
													●				
			●		●	●											
					●							●	●				
						●								●			

(continued)

Abdominal pain: Causes and associated findings *(continued)*

Common causes	Major associated signs and symptoms										
	Abdominal distention	Abdominal mass	Abdominal rigidity	Abdominal tenderness	Amenorrhea	Anorexia	Bowel sounds, absent	Bowel sounds, hyperactive	Bowel sounds, hypoactive	Breath odor, fruity	Chest pain
Pyelonephritis (acute)				●							
Renal calculi											
Sickle cell crisis											●
Smallpox (variola major)											
Splenic infarction											●
Systemic lupus erythematosus	●			●		●					●
Ulcerative colitis				●		●			●		
Uremia				●		●					●

with guarding, and possibly a palpable mass in a lower quadrant. Abdominal pain is commonly relieved by defecation. Milder chronic signs and symptoms include right-lower-quadrant pain with diarrhea, steatorrhea, and weight loss. Complications include perirectal or vaginal fistulas.

◆ ***Cystitis.*** Abdominal pain and tenderness usually occur in the suprapubic region. Associated signs and symptoms include malaise, flank pain, low back pain, nausea, vomiting, urinary frequency and urgency, nocturia, dysuria, fever, and chills.

◆ ***Diabetic ketoacidosis.*** Rarely, severe, sharp, shooting, and girdling pain may persist for several days. Fruity breath odor, a weak and rapid pulse, Kussmaul's respirations, poor skin turgor, polyuria, polydipsia, nocturia, hypotension, decreased bowel sounds, and confusion also occur.

◆ ***Diverticulitis.*** Mild cases usually produce intermittent, diffuse left-lower-quadrant pain, which may be relieved by defecation or passage of flatus and worsened by eating. Other signs and symptoms include nausea, constipation or diarrhea, low-grade fever and, in many cases, a palpable abdominal mass that's usually tender, firm, and fixed. Rupture causes severe left-lower-quadrant pain, abdominal rigidity, and possibly signs and symptoms of sepsis and shock (high fever, chills, and hypotension).

◆ ***Duodenal ulcer.*** Localized abdominal pain—described as steady, gnawing, burning, aching, or hungerlike—may occur high in the midepigastrium, slightly off center, usually on the right. The pain usually doesn't radiate unless pancreatic penetration occurs. It typically begins 2 to 4 hours after a meal and may cause nocturnal awakening. Ingestion of food or antacids brings relief until the cycle starts again. Other symptoms include changes in bowel habits and heartburn or retrosternal burning.

◆ ***Ectopic pregnancy.*** Lower abdominal pain may be sharp, dull, or cramping and constant or intermittent in ectopic pregnancy, a potentially life-threatening disorder. Vaginal bleeding, nausea, and vomiting may occur along with urinary frequency, a tender adnexal mass,

	Constipation	Costovertebral angle tenderness	Cough	Diarrhea	Dyspnea	Fever	Kussmaul's respirations	Nausea	Oliguria or anuria	Skin lesions	Skin mottling	Tachycardia	Tachypnea	Urinary frequency	Vomiting	Weakness	Weight change
		●				●		●						●	●	●	
		●				●		●							●		
					●											●	
						●				●							
						●									●		
				●		●		●							●		●
				●				●	●						●		

and a 1- to 2-month history of amenorrhea. Rupture of the fallopian tube produces sharp lower abdominal pain, which may radiate to the shoulders and neck and become extreme with cervical or adnexal palpation. Signs of shock (such as pallor, tachycardia, and hypotension) may also appear.

◆ ***Endometriosis.*** Constant, severe pain in the lower abdomen usually begins 5 to 7 days before the start of menses and may be aggravated by defecation. Depending on the location of the ectopic tissue, abdominal pain may be accompanied by abdominal tenderness, constipation, dysmenorrhea, dyspareunia, and deep sacral pain.

◆ **Escherichia coli *O157:H7.*** *E. coli* O157:H7 is an aerobic, gram-negative bacillus that causes food-borne illness. Most strains of *E. coli* are harmless and are part of the normal intestinal flora of healthy humans and animals. *E. coli* O157:H7, one of hundreds of strains of the bacterium, is capable of producing a powerful toxin and can cause severe illness. Eating undercooked beef or other foods contaminated with the bacterium causes the disease. Signs and symptoms include watery or bloody diarrhea, nausea, vomiting, fever, and abdominal cramps. In children younger than age 5 and the elderly, hemolytic uremic syndrome may develop and ultimately lead to acute renal failure.

◆ ***Gastric ulcer.*** Diffuse, gnawing, burning pain in the left upper quadrant or epigastric area commonly occurs 1 to 2 hours after meals and may be relieved by ingestion of food or antacids. Vague bloating and nausea after eating are common. Indigestion, weight change, anorexia, and episodes of GI bleeding also occur.

◆ ***Gastritis.*** With acute gastritis, the patient experiences rapid onset of abdominal pain that can range from mild epigastric discomfort to burning pain in the left upper quadrant. Other typical features include belching, fever, malaise, anorexia, nausea, bloody or coffee-ground vomitus, and melena. However, significant bleeding is unusual, unless the patient has hemorrhagic gastritis.

◆ ***Gastroenteritis.*** Cramping or colicky abdominal pain, which can be diffuse, originates in the left upper quadrant and radiates or migrates to the other quadrants, usually in a peristaltic manner. It's accompanied by diarrhea, hyperactive bowel sounds, headache, myalgia, nausea, and vomiting.

◆ ***Heart failure.*** Right-upper-quadrant pain commonly accompanies heart failure's hallmarks: jugular vein distention, dyspnea, tachycardia, and peripheral edema. Other findings include nausea, vomiting, ascites, productive cough, crackles, cool extremities, and cyanotic nail beds. Clinical signs are numerous and vary according to the stage of the disease and amount of cardiovascular impairment.

◆ ***Hepatic abscess.*** Steady, severe abdominal pain in the right upper quadrant or midepigastrium commonly accompanies hepatic abscess—a rare disorder—but right-upper-quadrant tenderness is the most important finding. Other signs and symptoms are anorexia, diarrhea, nausea, fever, diaphoresis, elevated right hemidiaphragm and, rarely, vomiting.

◆ ***Hepatic amebiasis.*** Rare in the United States, hepatic amebiasis causes relatively severe right-upper-quadrant pain and tenderness over the liver and possibly the right shoulder. Accompanying signs and symptoms include fever, weakness, weight loss, chills, diaphoresis, and jaundiced or brownish skin.

◆ ***Hepatitis.*** Liver enlargement from any type of hepatitis causes discomfort or dull pain and tenderness in the right upper quadrant. Associated signs and symptoms may include dark urine, clay-colored stools, nausea, vomiting, anorexia, jaundice, malaise, and pruritus.

◆ ***Herpes zoster.*** Herpes zoster of the thoracic, lumbar, or sacral nerves can cause localized abdominal and chest pain in the areas served by these nerves. Pain, tenderness, and fever can precede or accompany erythematous papules, which rapidly evolve into grouped vesicles.

◆ ***Intestinal obstruction.*** Short episodes of intense, colicky, cramping pain alternate with pain-free intervals in intestinal obstruction, a life-threatening disorder. Accompanying signs and symptoms may include abdominal distention, tenderness, and guarding; visible peristaltic waves; high-pitched, tinkling, or hyperactive bowel sounds proximal to the obstruction and hypoactive or absent sounds distally; obstipation; and pain-induced agitation. In jejunal and duodenal obstruction, nausea and bilious vomiting occur early. In distal small- or large-bowel obstruction, nausea and vomiting are commonly feculent. Complete obstruction produces absent bowel sounds. Late-stage obstruction produces signs of hypovolemic shock, such as hypotension and tachycardia.

◆ ***Irritable bowel syndrome.*** Lower abdominal cramping or pain is aggravated by ingestion of coarse or raw foods and may be alleviated by defecation or passage of flatus. Related findings include abdominal tenderness, diurnal diarrhea alternating with constipation or normal bowel function, and small stools with visible mucus. Dyspepsia, nausea, and abdominal distention with a feeling of incomplete evacuation may also occur. Stress, anxiety, and emotional lability intensify the symptoms.

◆ ***Listeriosis.*** Listeriosis is a serious infection that's caused by eating food contaminated with the bacterium *Listeria monocytogenes.* This food-borne illness primarily affects pregnant women, neonates, and those with weakened immune systems. Signs and symptoms include fever, myalgia, abdominal pain, nausea, vomiting, and diarrhea. If the infection spreads to the nervous system, it may cause meningitis, characterized by fever, headache, nuchal rigidity, and altered level of consciousness (LOC).

GENDER CUE *Listeriosis infection during pregnancy may lead to premature delivery, infection of the neonate, or stillbirth.*

◆ ***Mesenteric artery ischemia.*** Always suspect mesenteric artery ischemia in patients older than age 50 with chronic heart failure, cardiac arrhythmias, cardiovascular infarct, or hypotension who develop sudden, severe abdominal pain after 2 to 3 days of colicky periumbilical pain and diarrhea. Initially, the abdomen is soft and tender with decreased bowel sounds. Associated findings include vomiting, anorexia, alternating periods of diarrhea and constipation and, in late stages, extreme abdominal tenderness with rigidity, tachycardia, tachypnea, absent bowel sounds, and cool, clammy skin.

◆ ***Myocardial infarction (MI).*** In MI—a life-threatening disorder—substernal chest pain may radiate to the abdomen. Associated signs and symptoms include weakness, diaphoresis, nausea, vomiting, anxiety, syncope, jugular vein distention, and dyspnea.

◆ ***Norovirus infection.*** Abdominal pain or cramping is a symptom commonly associated with noroviruses. Transmitted by the fecal-oral route and highly contagious, these viruses that cause gastroenteritis may also produce acute-onset vomiting, nausea, and diarrhea. Less common symptoms include low-grade fever, headache, chills, muscle aches, and generalized fatigue. Individuals who are otherwise healthy usually recover in 24 to 60 hours without suffering lasting effects.

◆ ***Ovarian cyst.*** Torsion or hemorrhage causes pain and tenderness in the right or left lower quadrant. Sharp and severe if the patient suddenly stands or stoops, the pain becomes brief and intermittent if the torsion self-corrects or dull and diffuse after several hours if it doesn't. Pain is accompanied by a slight fever, mild nausea and vomiting, abdominal tenderness, a palpable abdominal mass, and possibly amenorrhea. Abdominal distention may occur if the cyst is large. Peritoneal irritation, or rupture and ensuing peritonitis, causes high fever and severe nausea and vomiting.

◆ ***Pancreatitis.*** Life-threatening acute pancreatitis produces fulminating, continuous upper abdominal pain that may radiate to both flanks and to the back. To relieve this pain, the patient may bend forward, draw his knees to his chest, or move about restlessly. Early findings include abdominal tenderness, nausea, vomiting, fever, pallor, tachycardia and, in some patients, abdominal rigidity, rebound tenderness, and hypoactive bowel sounds. Turner's sign (ecchymosis of the abdomen or flank) or Cullen's sign (a bluish tinge around the umbilicus) signals hemorrhagic pancreatitis. Jaundice may occur as inflammation subsides.

Chronic pancreatitis produces severe left-upper-quadrant or epigastric pain that radiates to the back. Abdominal tenderness, a midepigastric mass, jaundice, fever, and splenomegaly may occur. Steatorrhea, weight loss, maldigestion, and diabetes mellitus are common.

◆ ***Pelvic inflammatory disease.*** Pain in the right or left lower quadrant ranges from vague discomfort worsened by movement to deep, severe, and progressive pain. Sometimes, metrorrhagia precedes or accompanies the onset of pain. Extreme pain accompanies cervical or adnexal palpation. Associated findings include abdominal tenderness, a palpable abdominal or pelvic mass, fever, occasional chills, nausea, vomiting, discomfort on urination, and abnormal vaginal bleeding or a purulent vaginal discharge.

◆ ***Perforated ulcer.*** In a life-threatening perforated ulcer, sudden, severe, and prostrating epigastric pain may radiate through the abdomen to the back or right shoulder. Other signs and symptoms include boardlike abdominal rigidity, tenderness with guarding, generalized rebound tenderness, absent bowel sounds, grunting and shallow respirations and, in many cases, fever, tachycardia, hypotension, and syncope.

◆ ***Peritonitis.*** In this life-threatening disorder, sudden and severe pain can be diffuse or localized in the area of the underlying disorder; movement worsens the pain. The degree of abdominal tenderness usually varies according to the extent of disease. Typical findings include fever; chills; nausea; vomiting; hypoactive or absent bowel sounds; abdominal tenderness, distention, and rigidity; rebound tenderness and guarding; hyperalgesia; tachycardia; hypotension; tachypnea; and positive psoas and obturator signs.

◆ ***Pleurisy.*** Pleurisy may produce upper abdominal or costal margin pain referred from the chest. Characteristic sharp, stabbing chest pain increases with inspiration and movement. Many patients have a pleural friction rub and rapid, shallow breathing; some have a low-grade fever.

◆ ***Pneumonia.*** Lower-lobe pneumonia can cause pleuritic chest pain and referred, severe upper abdominal pain, tenderness, and rigidity that diminish with inspiration. It can also cause fever, shaking chills, achiness, headache, blood-tinged or rusty sputum, dyspnea, and a dry, hacking cough. Accompanying signs include crackles, egophony, decreased breath sounds, and dullness on percussion.

◆ ***Pneumothorax.*** Pneumothorax is a potentially life-threatening disorder that can cause referred pain from the chest to the upper abdomen and costal margin. Characteristic chest pain arises suddenly and worsens with deep inspiration or movement. Accompanying signs and symptoms include anxiety, dyspnea, cyanosis, decreased or absent breath sounds over the affected area, tachypnea, and tachycardia. Watch for asymmetrical chest movements on inspiration.

◆ ***Prostatitis.*** Vague abdominal pain or discomfort in the lower abdomen, groin, perineum, or rectum may develop. Other findings include dysuria, urinary frequency and urgency, fever, chills, low back pain, myalgia, arthralgia, and nocturia. Scrotal pain, penile pain, and pain on ejaculation may occur in chronic cases.

◆ ***Pyelonephritis (acute).*** Progressive lower quadrant pain in one or both sides, flank pain, and CVA tenderness characterize pyelonephritis. Pain may radiate to the lower midabdomen or the groin. Additional signs and symptoms include abdominal and back tenderness, high fever, shaking chills, nausea, vomiting, and urinary frequency and urgency.

◆ ***Renal calculi.*** Depending on their location, calculi may cause severe abdominal or back pain. However, the classic symptom is severe, colicky pain that travels from the CVA to the flank, suprapubic region, and external genitalia. The pain may be excruciating or dull and constant and may be accompanied by agitation, nausea, vomiting, abdominal distention, fever, chills, hypertension, and urinary urgency with hematuria and dysuria.

◆ ***Sickle cell crisis.*** Sudden, severe abdominal pain may accompany chest, back, hand, or foot pain. Associated signs and symptoms include weakness, aching joints, dyspnea, and scleral jaundice.

◆ ***Smallpox (variola major).*** Worldwide eradication of smallpox was achieved in 1977; the United States and Russia have the only known storage sites for the virus, which is considered a potential agent for biological warfare. Initial signs and symptoms include high fever, malaise, prostration, severe headache, backache, and abdominal pain. A maculopapular rash develops on the oral mucosa, pharynx, face, and forearms and then spreads to the trunk and legs. Within 2 days, the rash becomes vesicular and later pustular. The lesions develop at the same time, appear identical, and are more prominent on the face and extremities. The pustules are round, firm, and embedded in the skin. After 8 to 9 days, the pustules form a crust, which later separates from the skin, leaving a pitted scar. Death may result from encephalitis, extensive bleeding, or secondary infection.

◆ ***Splenic infarction.*** Fulminating pain in the left upper quadrant occurs with chest pain that may worsen on inspiration. Pain commonly radiates to the left shoulder with splinting of the left diaphragm, abdominal guarding and, occasionally, a splenic friction rub.

◆ ***Systemic lupus erythematosus.*** Generalized abdominal pain is unusual in this disease but may occur after meals. Butterfly rash, photosensitivity, alopecia, mucous membrane ulcers, and nondeforming arthritis are characteristic signs. Other common signs and symptoms include anorexia, vomiting, abdominal tenderness with guarding, abdominal distention after meals, fatigue, fever, and weight loss. Precordial chest pain and a pericardial rub may also occur.

◆ ***Ulcerative colitis.*** Ulcerative colitis may begin with vague abdominal discomfort that leads to cramping lower abdominal pain. As the disorder progresses, pain may become steady and diffuse, increasing with movement and coughing. The most common symptom—recurrent and possibly severe diarrhea with blood, pus, and mucus—may relieve the pain. The abdomen may feel soft and extremely tender. High-pitched, infrequent bowel sounds may accompany nausea, vomiting, anorexia, weight loss, and mild, intermittent fever.

◆ ***Uremia.*** Characterized by generalized or periumbilical pain that shifts and varies in intensity, uremia causes diverse GI signs and symptoms, such as nausea, vomiting, anorexia, and diarrhea. Other findings may include bleeding, abdominal tenderness that changes in location and intensity, visual disturbances, headache, decreased LOC, vertigo, and oliguria or anuria. Chest pain may occur secondary to pericardial effusion. Localized or diffuse pruritus is common.

Other causes

◆ ***Drugs.*** Salicylates and nonsteroidal anti-inflammatories commonly cause burning, gnawing pain in the left upper quadrant or epigastric area as well as nausea and vomiting.

◆ ***Insect toxins.*** Generalized, cramping abdominal pain usually occurs with low-grade fever, nausea, vomiting, abdominal rigidity, tremors, and burning sensations in the hands or feet.

Special considerations

Help the patient find a comfortable position to ease his distress. The patient should lie in a supine position, with his head flat on the table, arms at his sides, and knees slightly flexed to relax the abdominal muscles. Monitor him closely because abdominal pain can signal a life-threatening disorder. Especially important indications include tachycardia, hypotension, clammy skin, abdominal rigidity, rebound tenderness, a change in the pain's location or intensity, or sudden relief from the pain.

Withhold analgesics from the patient because they may mask symptoms. Also withhold food and fluids because surgery may be needed. Prepare for I.V. infusion and insertion of a nasogastric or other intestinal tube. Peritoneal lavage or abdominal paracentesis may be required.

You may have to prepare the patient for a diagnostic procedure, such as a pelvic and rectal examination; blood, urine, and stool tests; X-rays; barium studies; ultrasonography; endoscopy; and biopsy.

Pediatric pointers

Because children commonly have difficulty describing abdominal pain, pay close attention to nonverbal clues, such as wincing, lethargy, or unusual positioning (such as a side-lying position with knees flexed to the abdomen). Observing the child while he coughs, walks, or climbs may offer some diagnostic clues. Also, remember that a parent's description of the child's complaints is a subjective interpretation of what the parent believes is wrong.

Abdominal pain in children may signal a more serious disorder or a disorder that produces different associated signs and symptoms than in adults. For example, appendicitis is more likely to result in rupture and death in children, and vomiting may be its only other sign. Acute pyelonephritis may cause abdominal pain, vomiting, and diarrhea, but not the classic urologic signs found in adults. Peptic ulcer, which is becoming increasingly common in teenagers, causes nocturnal pain and colic that may not be relieved by food, unlike peptic ulcer in adults.

Abdominal pain in children can also result from lactose intolerance, allergic-tension-fatigue syndrome, volvulus, Meckel's diverticulum, intussusception, mesenteric adenitis, diabetes mellitus, juvenile rheumatoid arthritis, and many uncommon disorders, such as heavy metal poisoning. Remember, too, that a child's complaint of abdominal pain may reflect an emotional need, such as a wish to avoid school or to gain adult attention.

Geriatric pointers

Advanced age may decrease the manifestations of acute abdominal disease. Pain may be less severe, fever less pronounced, and signs of peritoneal inflammation diminished or absent.

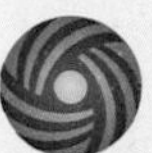

EXAMINATION TIP

Recognizing voluntary rigidity

Distinguishing voluntary from involuntary abdominal rigidity is a must for accurate assessment. Review the comparison below so that you can quickly tell the two apart.

Voluntary rigidity

- Usually symmetrical
- More rigid on inspiration (expiration causes muscle relaxation)
- Eased by relaxation techniques, such as positioning the patient comfortably and talking to him in a calm, soothing manner
- Painless when the patient sits up using his abdominal muscles alone

Involuntary rigidity

- Usually asymmetrical
- Equally rigid on inspiration and expiration
- Unaffected by relaxation techniques
- Painful when the patient sits up using his abdominal muscles alone

Abdominal rigidity

[Abdominal muscle spasm, involuntary guarding]

Detected by palpation, abdominal rigidity refers to abnormal muscle tension or inflexibility of the abdomen. Rigidity may be voluntary or involuntary. Voluntary rigidity reflects the patient's fear or nervousness upon palpation; involuntary rigidity reflects potentially life-threatening peritoneal irritation or inflammation. (See *Recognizing voluntary rigidity.*)

Involuntary rigidity most commonly results from GI disorders but may also result from pulmonary and vascular disorders and from the effects of insect toxins. It's usually accompanied by fever, nausea, vomiting, and abdominal tenderness, distention, and pain.

EMERGENCY INTERVENTIONS *After palpating abdominal rigidity, quickly take the patient's vital signs. Even though the patient may not appear gravely ill or have markedly abnormal vital signs, abdominal rigidity calls for emergency interventions.*

Prepare to administer oxygen and to insert an I.V. catheter for fluid and blood replacement. The patient may require drugs to support blood pressure. Also prepare him for catheterization, and monitor intake and output.

A nasogastric tube may have to be inserted to relieve abdominal distention. Because emergency surgery may be necessary, prepare the patient for laboratory tests and X-rays.

History and physical examination

If the patient's condition allows further assessment, take a brief history. Find out when the abdominal rigidity began. Is it associated with abdominal pain? If so, did the pain begin at the same time? Determine whether the rigidity is localized or generalized. Is it always present? Has its location changed or remained constant? Next, ask about aggravating or alleviating factors, such as position changes, coughing, vomiting, elimination, and walking.

Then explore other signs and symptoms. Inspect the abdomen for peristaltic waves, which may be visible in very thin patients. Also check for a visibly distended bowel loop. Next, auscultate bowel sounds. Perform light palpation to locate the rigidity and to determine its severity. Avoid deep palpation, which may exacerbate abdominal pain. Finally, check for poor skin turgor and dry mucous membranes, which indicate dehydration.

Medical causes

◆ ***Abdominal aortic aneurysm (dissecting).*** Mild to moderate abdominal rigidity occurs in abdominal aortic aneurysm, a life-threatening disorder. It's typically accompanied by constant upper abdominal pain that may radiate to the lower back. The pain may worsen when the patient lies down and may be relieved when he leans forward or sits up. Before rupture, the aneurysm may produce a pulsating mass in the epigastrium, accompanied by a systolic bruit over the aorta. However, the mass stops pulsating after rupture. Associated signs and symptoms include mottled skin below the waist, absent femoral and pedal pulses, blood pressure that's lower in the legs than in the arms, and mild to moderate abdominal tenderness with guarding. Significant blood loss causes signs of shock, such as tachycardia, tachypnea, and cool, clammy skin.

◆ ***Mesenteric artery ischemia.*** This life-threatening disorder is characterized by 2 to 3 days of persistent, low-grade abdominal pain and diarrhea leading to sudden, severe abdominal pain and rigidity. Rigidity occurs in the central or periumbilical region and is accompanied by severe abdominal tenderness, fever, and signs of shock, such as tachycardia and hypotension. Other findings may include vomiting, anorexia, diarrhea, and constipation. Always suspect mesenteric artery ischemia in patients older than age 50 who have a history of heart failure, arrhythmias, cardiovascular infarct, or hypotension.

◆ ***Peritonitis.*** Depending on the cause of peritonitis, abdominal rigidity may be localized or generalized. For example, if an inflamed appendix causes local peritonitis, rigidity may be localized in the right lower quadrant. If a perforated ulcer causes widespread peritonitis, rigidity may be generalized and, in severe cases, boardlike.

Peritonitis also causes sudden and severe abdominal pain that can be localized or generalized. It can also produce abdominal tenderness and distention, rebound tenderness, guarding, hyperalgesia, hypoactive or absent bowel sounds, nausea, and vomiting. Most patients also experience fever, chills, tachycardia, tachypnea, and hypotension.

◆ ***Pneumonia.*** In lower lobe pneumonia, severe upper abdominal pain and tenderness accompany rigidity that diminishes with inspiration. Associated signs and symptoms include blood-tinged or rusty sputum, dyspnea, achiness, headache, fever, sudden onset of chills, crackles, egophony, decreased breath sounds, dullness on percussion, and a dry, hacking cough.

Other causes

◆ ***Insect toxins.*** Insect stings and bites, especially black widow spider bites, release toxins that can produce generalized cramping abdominal pain, usually accompanied by rigidity. These toxins may also cause low-grade fever, nausea, vomiting, tremors, and burning sensations in the hands and feet. Some patients develop increased salivation, hypertension, paresis, and hyperactive reflexes. Children commonly are restless, have an expiratory grunt, and keep their legs flexed.

Special considerations

Continue to monitor the patient closely for signs of shock. Position him as comfortably as possible in a supine position, with his head flat on the table, arms at his sides, and knees slightly flexed to relax the abdominal muscles. Because analgesics may mask symptoms, withhold them until a tentative diagnosis has been made. Also withhold food and fluids and administer an I.V.

antibiotic because emergency surgery may be required. Prepare the patient for diagnostic tests, which may include blood, urine, and stool studies; chest and abdominal X-rays; a computed tomography scan; magnetic resonance imaging; peritoneal lavage; and gastroscopy or colonoscopy. A pelvic or rectal examination may also be done.

Pediatric pointers

Voluntary rigidity may be difficult to distinguish from involuntary rigidity if associated pain makes the child restless, tense, or apprehensive. However, in any child with suspected involuntary rigidity, your priority is early detection of dehydration and shock, which can rapidly become life-threatening.

Abdominal rigidity in children can stem from gastric perforation, hypertrophic pyloric stenosis, duodenal obstruction, meconium ileus, intussusception, cystic fibrosis, celiac disease, and appendicitis.

Geriatric pointers

Advanced age and impaired cognition decrease pain perception and intensity. Weakening of abdominal muscles may decrease muscle spasms and rigidity.

Accessory muscle use

When breathing requires extra effort, the accessory muscles—the sternocleidomastoid, scalene, pectoralis major, trapezius, internal intercostals, and abdominal muscles—stabilize the thorax during respiration. Some accessory muscle use normally takes place during such activities as singing, talking, coughing, defecating, and exercising. (See *Accessory muscles: Locations and functions,* page 26.) However, more pronounced use of these muscles may signal acute respiratory distress, diaphragmatic weakness, or fatigue. It may also result from chronic respiratory disease. Typically, the extent of accessory muscle use reflects the severity of the underlying cause.

EMERGENCY INTERVENTIONS *If the patient displays increased accessory muscle use, immediately look for signs of acute respiratory distress. These include decreased level of consciousness, shortness of breath when speaking, tachypnea, intercostal and sternal retractions, cyanosis, external breath sounds (such as wheezing or stridor), diaphoresis, nasal flaring, and extreme apprehension or agitation. Quickly auscultate for abnormal, diminished, or absent breath sounds. Check for airway obstruction and, if detected, attempt to restore airway patency. Insert an airway or intubate the patient. Then begin suctioning and manual or mechanical ventilation. Assess oxygen saturation using pulse oximetry, if available. Administer oxygen; if the patient has chronic obstructive pulmonary disease (COPD), use only a low flow rate for mild COPD exacerbations. You may need to use a high flow rate initially, but be attentive to the patient's respiratory drive. Giving too much oxygen may decrease the patient's respiratory drive. An I.V. catheter may be required.*

History and physical examination

If the patient's condition allows, examine him more closely. Ask him about the onset, duration, and severity of associated signs and symptoms, such as dyspnea, chest pain, cough, and fever.

Explore his medical history, focusing on respiratory disorders, such as infection or COPD. Ask about cardiac disorders, such as heart failure, which may lead to pulmonary edema; also inquire about neuromuscular disorders, such as amyotrophic lateral sclerosis, which may affect respiratory muscle function. Note a history of allergies or asthma. Because collagen vascular diseases can cause diffuse infiltrative lung disease, ask about such conditions as rheumatoid arthritis and lupus erythematosus.

Ask about recent trauma, especially to the spine or chest. Find out if the patient has recently undergone pulmonary function tests or received respiratory therapy. Ask about smoking and about occupational exposure to chemical fumes or mineral dusts such as asbestos. Explore the family history for such disorders as cystic fibrosis and neurofibromatosis, which can cause diffuse infiltrative lung disease.

Perform a detailed chest examination, noting abnormal respiratory rate, pattern, or depth. Assess the color, temperature, and turgor of the patient's skin, and check for clubbing. (See *Accessory muscle use: Causes and associated findings,* page 27.)

Medical causes

◆ ***Acute respiratory distress syndrome (ARDS).*** In ARDS—a life-threatening disorder—accessory muscle use increases in

Accessory muscles: Locations and functions

Physical exertion and pulmonary disease usually increase the work of breathing, taxing the diaphragm and external intercostal muscles. When this happens, accessory muscles provide the extra effort needed to maintain respirations. The upper accessory muscles assist with inspiration, whereas the upper chest, sternum, internal intercostal, and abdominal muscles assist with expiration.

With inspiration, the scalene muscles elevate, fix, and expand the upper chest. The sternocleidomastoid muscles raise the sternum, expanding the chest's anteroposterior and longitudinal dimensions. The pectoralis major elevates the chest, increasing its anteroposterior size, and the trapezius raises the thoracic cage.

With expiration, the internal intercostals depress the ribs, decreasing the chest size. The abdominal muscles pull the lower chest down, depress the lower ribs, and compress the abdominal contents, which exerts pressure on the chest.

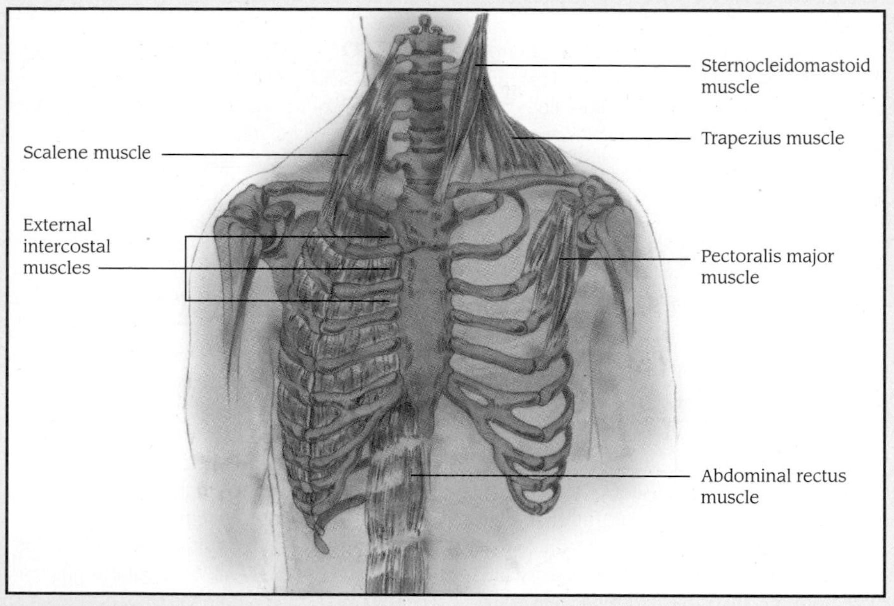

response to hypoxia. It's accompanied by intercostal, supracostal, and sternal retractions on inspiration and by grunting on expiration. Other characteristics include tachypnea, dyspnea, diaphoresis, diffuse crackles, and a cough with pink, frothy sputum. Worsening hypoxia produces anxiety, tachycardia, and mental sluggishness.

◆ ***Airway obstruction.*** An acute upper airway obstruction can be life-threatening; fortunately, most obstructions are subacute or chronic. Typically, this disorder increases accessory muscle use. Its most telling sign, however, is inspiratory stridor. Associated signs and symptoms include dyspnea, tachypnea, gasping, wheezing, coughing, drooling, intercostal retractions, cyanosis, and tachycardia.

◆ ***Amyotrophic lateral sclerosis (ALS).*** Because ALS affects the diaphragm more than the accessory muscles, increased accessory muscle use is characteristic of this disorder. Other signs and symptoms include fasciculations, muscle atrophy and weakness, spasticity, bilateral Babinski's reflex, and hyperactive deep tendon reflexes. Incoordination makes carrying out routine activities difficult for the patient. Associated signs and symptoms include impaired speech; difficulty chewing or swallowing and breathing; urinary frequency and urgency; and, occasionally, choking and

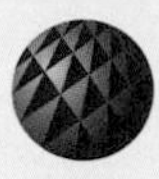

SIGNS & SYMPTOMS

Accessory muscle use: Causes and associated findings

Major associated signs and symptoms

Common causes	Barrel chest	Chest pain	Cough	Crackles	Cyanosis	Diaphoresis	Dyspnea	Fever	Muscle weakness	Paralysis	Stridor	Tachycardia	Tachypnea	Wheezing
Acute respiratory distress syndrome			●	●		●	●					●	●	
Airway obstruction			●		●		●				●	●	●	●
Amyotrophic lateral sclerosis							●		●					
Asthma	●		●	●	●	●	●					●	●	●
Chronic bronchitis	●		●	●	●		●	●					●	●
Diffuse infiltrative (or fibrotic) lung disease		●	●	●			●						●	
Emphysema	●		●		●		●						●	
Pneumonia		●	●	●	●	●	●	●				●	●	
Pulmonary edema			●	●	●		●					●	●	●
Pulmonary embolism		●	●	●	●		●	●				●	●	●
Spinal cord injury									●	●				
Thoracic injury		●			●		●					●		

excessive drooling. (*Note:* Other neuromuscular disorders may produce similar signs and symptoms.) Although the patient's mental status remains intact, his poor prognosis may cause periodic depression.

◆ ***Asthma.*** During acute asthma attacks, the patient usually displays increased accessory muscle use accompanied by severe dyspnea, tachypnea, wheezing, productive cough, nasal flaring, and cyanosis. Auscultation reveals faint or possibly absent breath sounds, musical crackles, and rhonchi. Other signs and symptoms include tachycardia, diaphoresis, and apprehension caused by air hunger. Chronic asthma may also cause barrel chest.

◆ ***Chronic bronchitis.*** In this form of COPD, increased accessory muscle use may be chronic and is preceded by a productive cough and exertional dyspnea. Chronic bronchitis is accompanied by wheezing, basal crackles, tachypnea, jugular vein distention, prolonged expiration, barrel chest, and clubbing. Patients with chronic bronchitis are sometimes called "blue bloaters" because of the cyanosis and weight gain from edema that commonly occur. Low-grade fever may occur with secondary infection.

◆ ***Diffuse infiltrative (or fibrotic) lung disease.*** In diffuse infiltrative lung disease, progressive pulmonary degeneration eventually increases accessory muscle use. Typically, though, the patient reports progressive dyspnea on exertion as his chief complaint. He may also have a cough, anorexia, weakness, fatigue, vague chest pain, tachypnea, and crackles at the base of the lungs.

◆ ***Emphysema.*** Increased accessory muscle use occurs with progressive exertional dyspnea and a minimally productive cough in this form of COPD. These patients are sometimes called "pink puffers" because of their characteristic pursed-lip breathing, tachypnea, and a pink or red complexion. Associated signs and symptoms include peripheral cyanosis, anorexia, weight loss, malaise, barrel chest, and clubbing. Auscultation reveals distant heart sounds; percussion detects hyperresonance.

◆ ***Pneumonia.*** Bacterial pneumonia initially produces sudden high fever with chills. Associated signs and symptoms include increased accessory muscle use, chest pain, productive cough, dyspnea, tachypnea, tachycardia, expiratory grunting, cyanosis, diaphoresis, and fine crackles.

◆ ***Pulmonary edema.*** In acute pulmonary edema, increased accessory muscle use is accompanied by dyspnea, tachypnea, orthopnea, crepitant crackles, wheezing, and a cough with pink, frothy sputum. Other findings include restlessness, tachycardia, ventricular gallop, and cool, clammy, cyanotic skin.

◆ ***Pulmonary embolism.*** Although signs and symptoms vary with the size, number, and location of the emboli, this life-threatening disorder may cause increased accessory muscle use. Common findings include dyspnea and tachypnea that may be accompanied by pleuritic or substernal chest pain. Other signs and symptoms include restlessness, anxiety, tachycardia, productive cough, low-grade fever and, with a large embolus, hemoptysis, cyanosis, syncope, jugular vein distention, scattered crackles, and focal wheezing.

◆ ***Spinal cord injury.*** An injury below L1 typically doesn't affect the diaphragm or accessory muscles, whereas an injury between C3 and C5 affects the upper respiratory muscles and diaphragm, causing increased accessory muscle use.

Associated signs and symptoms of spinal cord injury include unilateral or bilateral Babinski's reflex; hyperactive deep tendon reflexes; spasticity; and variable or total loss of pain and temperature sensation, proprioception, and motor function. Horner's syndrome (unilateral ptosis, pupillary constriction, facial anhidrosis) may occur in lower cervical cord injury.

◆ ***Thoracic injury.*** Increased accessory muscle use may occur, depending on the type and extent of the injury. Associated signs and symptoms of this potentially life-threatening injury include an obvious chest wound or bruising, chest pain, dyspnea, cyanosis, and agitation. Signs of shock, such as tachycardia and hypotension, occur with significant blood loss.

Other causes

◆ ***Diagnostic tests and treatments.*** Pulmonary function tests, incentive spirometry, and intermittent positive-pressure breathing can increase accessory muscle use.

Special considerations

If the patient is alert, elevate the head of the bed to make his breathing as easy as possible. Encourage him to get plenty of rest and to drink plenty of fluids to liquefy secretions. Administer oxygen. Prepare him for such tests as pulmonary function studies, chest X-rays, lung scans, arterial blood gas analysis, complete blood count, and sputum culture.

If appropriate, stress how smoking endangers the patient's health, and refer him to an organized program to stop smoking. Also, teach him how to prevent infection. Explain the purpose of prescribed drugs, such as bronchodilators and mucolytics, and make sure he knows their dosage and schedule.

Pediatric pointers

Because infants and children tire sooner than adults, they can develop respiratory failure from respiratory distress more quickly than adults. Upper airway obstruction—caused by edema, bronchospasm, or a foreign object—usually produces respiratory distress and increased accessory muscle use. Disorders associated with airway obstruction include acute epiglottitis, croup, pertussis, cystic fibrosis, and asthma. Supraventricular, intercostal, or abdominal retractions indicate accessory muscle use.

Geriatric pointers

Because of age-related loss of elasticity in the rib cage, accessory muscle use may be part of an elderly person's normal breathing pattern.

Patient counseling

Because labored breathing can make the patient apprehensive, provide a calm environment and encourage him to perform relaxation techniques while you provide interventions to reduce the work of breathing.

Agitation

Agitation refers to a state of hyperarousal, increased tension, and irritability that can lead to confusion, hyperactivity, and overt hostility. Agitation can result from a toxic (poisons), metabolic, or infectious cause; brain injury; and psychiatric and various other disorders. It can also result from pain, fever, anxiety, drug use or withdrawal, and hypersensitivity reactions. It can arise gradually or suddenly and last for minutes or months. Whether it's mild or severe, agitation worsens with increased fever, pain, stress, or external stimuli.

Agitation alone merely signals a change in the patient's condition, but it can be a useful indicator of a developing disorder. Obtaining a good history is critical to determining the underlying cause of agitation.

History and physical examination

Determine the severity of the patient's agitation by examining the number and quality of agitation-induced behaviors, such as emotional lability, confusion, memory loss, hyperactivity, and hostility. Obtain a history from the patient or a family member, including diet, known allergies, and use of prescribed or over-the-counter drugs, including supplements and herbal medicines.

Ask if the patient is being treated for any illnesses. Has he had any recent infections, trauma, stress, or changes in sleep patterns? Check for signs of drug abuse, such as needle tracks and dilated pupils, and ask about alcohol intake. Obtain baseline vital signs and neurologic status for future comparison.

Medical causes

◆ ***Affective disturbances.*** Agitation may occur in either the depressive or manic phase of affective disturbances and in personality disorders, such as borderline and antisocial personality disorders. The hallmark of the depressive form is depressed mood upon awakening, which eases during the day. Chronic anxiety may be mild or severe. Psychomotor agitation may be characterized by an inability to sit still, hand-wringing, pacing, and irritability. Other findings in the manic state may include decreased sleep, pressured speech, and grandiosity.

◆ ***Alcohol withdrawal syndrome.*** Mild to severe agitation occurs with hyperactivity, tremors, and anxiety. In delirium tremens, the potentially life-threatening stage of alcohol withdrawal, severe agitation accompanies hallucinations, insomnia, diaphoresis, and depressed mood. Pulse rate and temperature rise as withdrawal progresses; status epilepticus, cardiac arrhythmias, and shock can occur.

◆ ***Anxiety.*** Anxiety is a common symptom that produces varying degrees of agitation. The patient may be unaware of his anxiety or may complain of it without knowing its cause. Other findings may include nausea, vomiting, diarrhea, cool and clammy skin, frontal headache, back pain, insomnia, and tremors.

◆ ***Chronic renal failure.*** Moderate to severe agitation occurs in chronic renal failure, which is marked by confusion and memory loss. The agitation is accompanied by diverse signs and symptoms, such as nausea, vomiting, anorexia, mouth ulcers, ammonia breath odor, GI bleeding, pallor, edema, dry skin, and uremic frost.

◆ ***Dementia.*** Mild to severe agitation can result from many common dementia syndromes, such as Alzheimer's and Huntington's diseases. The patient may display a decrease in memory, attention span, problem-solving ability, and alertness. Hypoactivity, wandering behavior, hallucinations, aphasia, and insomnia may also occur.

◆ ***Drug withdrawal syndrome.*** Findings vary with the drug but include mild to severe agitation, anxiety, abdominal cramps, diaphoresis, and anorexia. In opioid or barbiturate withdrawal, a decreased level of consciousness (LOC), seizures, and elevated blood pressure, heart rate, and respiratory rate can also occur.

◆ ***Hepatic encephalopathy.*** Agitation occurs only in fulminating encephalopathy. Other findings include drowsiness, stupor, fetor hepaticus, asterixis, and hyperreflexia.

◆ ***Hypersensitivity reaction.*** Moderate to severe agitation may be the first sign of a hypersensitivity reaction. Depending on the severity of the reaction, agitation may be accompanied by urticaria, pruritus, and facial and dependent edema.

In anaphylactic shock, a potentially life-threatening reaction, agitation occurs rapidly along with apprehension, urticaria or diffuse erythema, warm and moist skin, paresthesia, pruritus, edema, dyspnea, wheezing, stridor, hypotension, and tachycardia. Abdominal cramps, vomiting, and diarrhea can also occur.

◆ ***Hypoxemia.*** Beginning as restlessness, agitation rapidly worsens in hypoxemia. The patient may be confused and have impaired judgment and motor coordination. He may also have tachycardia, tachypnea, dyspnea, and cyanosis.

◆ ***Increased intracranial pressure (ICP).*** Agitation usually precedes other early signs and symptoms, such as headache, nausea, and vomiting. Increased ICP produces respiratory changes, such as Cheyne-Stokes, cluster, ataxic, or apneustic breathing; sluggish, nonreactive, or unequal pupils; widening pulse pressure; tachycardia; decreased LOC; seizures; and motor changes, such as decerebrate or decorticate posture.

◆ ***Organic brain syndrome.*** In organic brain syndrome, agitation is manifested as hyperactivity, emotional lability, confusion, and memory loss. Slurred or incoherent speech and paranoid behavior may also occur.

◆ ***Post-head trauma syndrome.*** Shortly—or even years—after injury, mild to severe agitation develops, characterized by disorientation, loss of concentration, angry outbursts, and emotional lability. Fatigue, wandering behavior, and poor judgment are other findings.

◆ ***Vitamin B_6 deficiency.*** Agitation can range from mild to severe. Other effects include seizures, peripheral paresthesia, and dermatitis. Oculogyric crisis may also occur.

Other causes

◆ ***Drugs.*** Mild to moderate agitation, which is commonly dose related, is an adverse effect of central nervous system stimulants—especially appetite suppressants, such as amphetamines and amphetamine-like drugs; sympathomimetics such as ephedrine; caffeine; and theophylline.

◆ ***Radiographic contrast media.*** Injection of a contrast medium during various diagnostic tests may produce moderate to severe agitation along with other signs of hypersensitivity.

Special considerations

Because agitation can be an early sign of many different disorders, continue to monitor the patient's vital signs and neurologic status while the cause is being determined. Eliminate stressors that can increase agitation. Provide adequate lighting, maintain a calm environment, and allow the patient ample time to sleep. Ensure a balanced diet, and provide vitamin supplements and hydration.

Remain calm, nonjudgmental, and nonargumentative. If appropriate, prepare the patient for diagnostic tests, such as computed tomography scanning, skull X-rays, magnetic resonance imaging, and blood studies.

Pediatric pointers

A common sign in children, agitation accompanies the expected childhood diseases as well as more severe disorders that can lead to brain damage: hyperbilirubinemia, phenylketonuria, vitamin A deficiency, hepatitis, frontal lobe syndrome, increased ICP, and lead poisoning. In neonates, agitation can stem from alcohol or drug withdrawal if the mother abused these substances.

When evaluating an agitated child, remember to use words that he can understand and to look for nonverbal clues. For instance, if you suspect that pain is causing agitation, ask him to tell you where it hurts, but be sure to watch for other indicators, such as wincing, crying, or moving away.

Geriatric pointers

Any deviation from an older person's usual activities or rituals may provoke anxiety or agitation. Any environmental change, such as a transfer to a nursing home or a visit from a stranger in the patient's home, may trigger a need for treatment.

Alopecia

[Hair loss]

Alopecia usually develops gradually and affects the scalp; it may be diffuse or patchy and can be classified as scarring or nonscarring. Scarring alopecia (permanent hair loss) results from hair follicle destruction, which smoothes the skin surface, erasing follicular openings. Nonscarring alopecia (temporary hair loss) results from hair follicle damage that spares follicular openings, allowing future hair growth.

One of the most common causes of alopecia is the use of certain chemotherapeutic drugs. Alopecia may also result from the use of other drugs; radiation therapy; a skin, connective tissue, endocrine, nutritional, or psychological disorder; a neoplasm; an infection; a burn; or exposure to toxins.

Normally, everyone loses about 50 hairs per day, and these hairs are replaced by new ones. However, aging, genetic predisposition, and hormonal changes may contribute to gradual hair thinning and hairline recession. This type of alopecia occurs in about 40% of adult men and may also occur in postmenopausal women.

CULTURAL CUE *People who have fine and relatively scanty hair, such as natives of tropical areas, may not recognize alopecia right away.*

GENDER CUE *In men, hair loss commonly affects the temporal areas, producing an M-shaped hairline. In women, diffuse thinning marks the centrofrontal area.*

In both sexes, hair loss may also occur on the trunk, pubic area, axillae, arms, and legs. Another normal pattern of alopecia occurs 2 to 4 months postpartum. This temporary, diffuse hair loss on the scalp may be scant or dramatic and possibly accentuated at the frontal areas. Anxiety, high fever, and even certain hair styles or grooming methods may also cause alopecia. (See *Recognizing patterns of alopecia*, page 32.)

History and physical examination

If the patient isn't receiving a chemotherapeutic drug or radiation therapy, begin by asking when he first noticed the hair loss or thinning. Does it affect the scalp alone, or does it occur elsewhere on the body? Is it accompanied by itching or rashes? Then carefully explore other signs and symptoms to help distinguish between normal and pathologic hair loss. Ask about recent weight change, anorexia, nausea, vomiting, excessive stress, and altered bowel habits. Also ask about urinary tract changes, such as hematuria or oliguria. Has the patient been especially tired or irritable? Does he have a cough or difficulty breathing? Ask about joint pain or stiffness and about heat or cold intolerance. Inquire about exposure to insecticides. If the patient is female, ask if she has had menstrual irregularities and note her pregnancy history. If the patient is male, ask about sexual dysfunction, such as decreased libido or impotence.

Next, ask about hair care. Does the patient frequently use a hot blow dryer or electric curlers? Does he periodically dye, bleach, or perm his hair? If the patient is black, ask if he uses a hot comb to straighten his hair or a long-toothed comb to achieve an Afro look. Does he ever braid the hair in cornrows? Check for a family history of alopecia, and ask what age relatives were when they started experiencing hair loss. Also ask about nervous habits, such as pulling the hair or twirling it around a finger.

Begin the physical examination by taking vital signs and then assessing the extent and pattern of scalp hair loss. Is it patchy or symmetrical? Is the hair surrounding a bald area brittle or lusterless? Is it a different color than other scalp hair? Does it fall out easily? Inspect the underlying skin for follicular openings, erythema, loss of pigment, scaling, induration, broken hair shafts, and hair regrowth.

Then examine the rest of the skin. Note the size, color, texture, and location of any lesions. Check for jaundice, edema, hyperpigmentation, pallor, or duskiness. Examine nails for vertical or horizontal pitting, thickening, brittleness, or whitening. As you do so, watch for fine tremors in the hands. Observe the patient for muscle weakness and ptosis. Palpate for lymphadenopathy, enlarged thyroid or salivary glands, and masses in the abdomen or chest.

Medical causes

◆ ***Alopecia areata.*** Alopecia areata is usually marked by well-circumscribed patches of nonscarring hair loss on the scalp without skin changes. Occasionally, the patches also appear on the beard, axillae, pubic area, arms, legs, or the entire body (alopecia universalis). "Exclamation point" hairs—loose hairs with rough, brushlike tips on narrow, less-pigmented shafts—typically border expanding patches of alopecia. Although this disorder is recurrent, hair growth usually returns after several months. In about 20% of patients, alopecia areata also causes horizontal or vertical nail pitting.

◆ ***Arsenic poisoning.*** Most common in chronic poisoning, alopecia is diffuse and mainly affects the scalp. Related signs and symptoms include muscle weakness and wasting, areflexia, partial or total vision loss, and bronze skin.

◆ ***Arterial insufficiency.*** Patchy alopecia occurs in arterial insufficiency, typically on the lower extremities, and is accompanied by thin, shiny, atrophic skin and thickened nails. The skin turns pale when the patient's legs are elevated and dusky when they're dependent. Associated findings include weak or absent peripheral pulses, cool extremities, paresthesia, leg ulcers, and intermittent claudication.

Recognizing patterns of alopecia

Distinctive patterns of alopecia result from different causes. The illustrations below show four of the most common patterns.

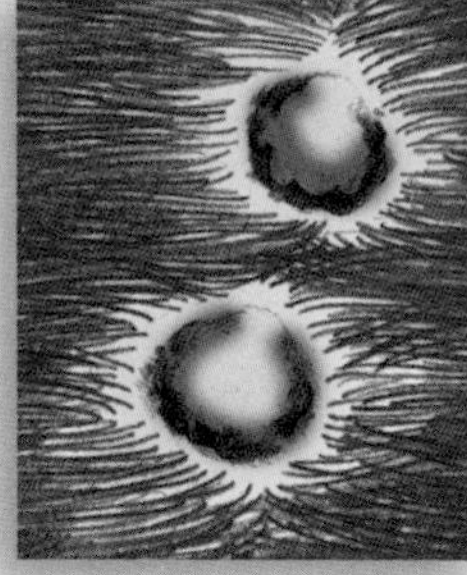

Tinea capitis, a fungal infection, produces irregular bald patches with scaly, red lesions.

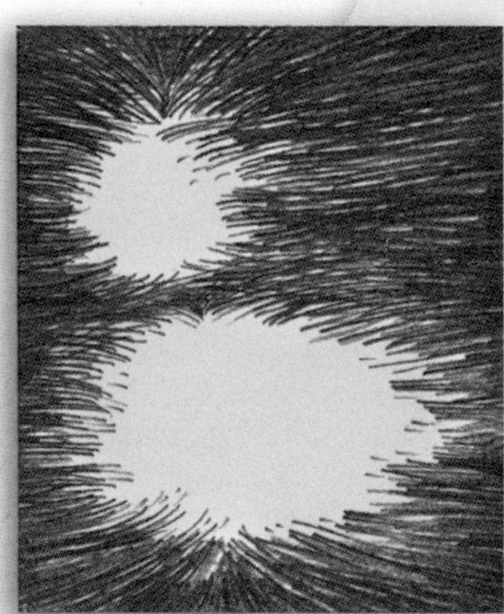

Alopecia areata causes expanding patches of nonscarring hair loss bordered by "exclamation point" hairs.

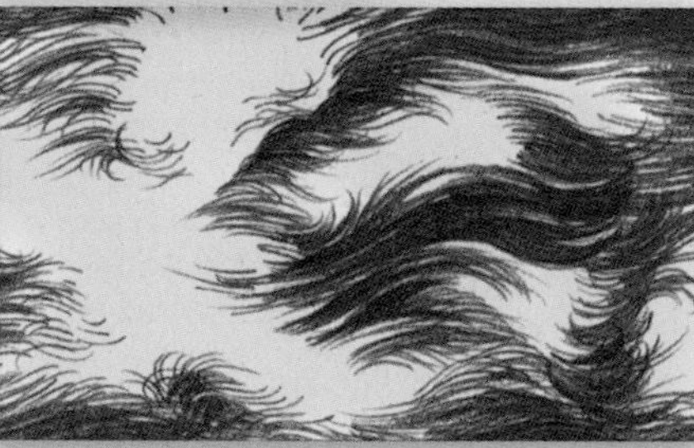

Trauma from habitual hair pulling or injudicious grooming habits may cause permanent peripheral alopecia.

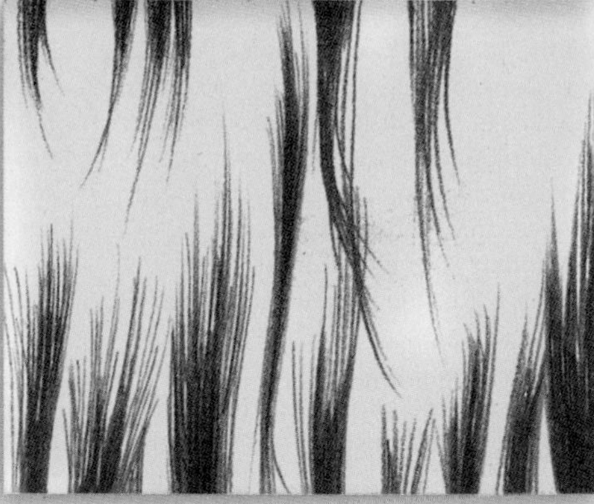

Chemotherapeutic drugs produce diffuse, yet temporary, hair loss.

◆ ***Burns.*** Full-thickness or third-degree burns completely destroy the dermis and epidermis, leaving translucent, charred, or ulcerated skin. Scarring or keloid formation associated with these burns causes permanent alopecia.

◆ ***Cutaneous T-cell lymphoma.*** More common in older patients, cutaneous T-cell lymphoma may be associated with alopecia mucinosa in its first, or premycotic, stage. Scattered papules or plaques may occur on clothed areas, such as breasts and buttocks, or a zebralike pattern of scaly erythema may form on the trunk. Alopecia may persist through the plaque and tumor stages.

◆ ***Dissecting cellulitis of the scalp.*** Resulting from skin infection, dissecting cellulitis of the scalp is characterized by small nodules that eventually rupture and drain. Keloid formation during healing causes permanent alopecia.

◆ ***Exfoliative dermatitis.*** Exfoliative dermatitis is a transient disorder in which loss of scalp and body hair is preceded by several weeks of generalized scaling and erythema. Nail loss commonly occurs along with pruritus, malaise, fever, weight loss, lymphadenopathy, and gynecomastia.

◆ ***Fungal infections.*** Tinea capitis (scalp ringworm), the most common fungal infection, produces irregular balding areas, scaling, and erythematous lesions. As these lesions enlarge, their centers heal, causing the classic ring-shaped appearance. Surrounding the balding areas are broken scalp hairs. When they break off at the scalp surface, hairs resemble black dots. Other findings include pruritus and thick, whitish nails.

◆ ***Hodgkin's disease.*** Permanent alopecia may occur if the lymphoma infiltrates the scalp. It's accompanied by edema, pruritus, and hyperpigmentation. Associated signs vary with the degree and location of lymphadenopathy.

◆ ***Hypopituitarism.*** In adults, hypopituitarism varies greatly, depending on its severity and the number of deficient hormones. Gonadotropin deficiency in the female causes sparse or absent pubic and axillary hair accompanied by infertility, amenorrhea, and breast atrophy. A similar deficiency in the male decreases facial and body hair and causes infertility, decreased libido, impotence, poor muscle development, and undersized testes, penis, and prostate gland. A human growth hormone deficiency at an early age may cause short stature. Deficiency of thyroid-stimulating hormone produces signs of hypothyroidism; deficiency of corticotropin produces signs of adrenocortical insufficiency.

◆ ***Hypothyroidism.*** In hypothyroidism, the hair on the face, scalp, and genitalia thins and becomes dull, coarse, and brittle. Most characteristic, though, is loss of the outer third of the eyebrows. Typically, alopecia is preceded by fatigue, constipation, cold intolerance, and weight gain. Other signs and symptoms include dry, flaky, inelastic skin; puffy face, hands, and feet; hoarseness; thick, brittle nails; slow mental function; bradycardia; menorrhagia; and myalgia.

◆ ***Lichen planus.*** Occasionally, lichen planus disorder produces patchy hair loss on the scalp with skin inflammation. Angular, flat, purple papules typically develop on the lower back, genitalia, arms, and lower legs. Related findings include pruritus and nail changes, ranging from grooves to nail loss. Scarring alopecia may develop with scalp skin atrophy.

◆ ***Lupus erythematosus.*** Hair loss is a chief complaint in patients with either discoid or systemic lupus. Hair tends to become brittle and may fall out in patches; short, broken hairs (known as *lupus hairs)* commonly appear above the forehead. Both types of lupus are characterized by raised, red, scaling plaques with follicular plugging, telangiectasia, and central atrophy. Facial plaques typically assume a distinctive butterfly pattern.

In systemic lupus, however, the rash may vary in severity from malar erythema to discoid lesions. Unlike discoid lupus, systemic lupus affects multiple body systems. It may produce photosensitivity, weight loss, fatigue, lymphadenopathy, arthritis, emotional lability, and other signs and symptoms.

◆ ***Myotonic dystrophy.*** Premature baldness characterizes the adult form of this muscular dystrophy. However, myotonia—the inability to normally relax a muscle after its contraction—is its primary sign. Associated signs include muscle wasting and cataracts.

◆ ***Protein deficiency.*** Protein deficiency produces brittle, fine, dry, and thinning hair and, occasionally, changes in its pigment. Characteristic muscle wasting may be accompanied by edema, hepatomegaly, apathy, irritability, anorexia, diarrhea, and dry, flaky skin.

◆ ***Sarcoidosis.*** Sarcoidosis may produce scarring alopecia if it infiltrates the scalp. Accompanied by various lesions on the face and the oral and nasal mucosa, it may also produce fever, weight loss, fatigue, lymphadenopathy, substernal pain, cough, shortness of breath, visual muscle weakness, arthralgia, myalgia, and cranial nerve palsies.

◆ ***Scleroderma (progressive systemic sclerosis).*** A late sign in scleroderma, permanent alopecia is accompanied by thickening and tightening of the skin, especially on the arms and hands. The skin appears taut and shiny and loses its pigment. Other findings include dysphagia, dyspepsia, abdominal pain, altered bowel habits, cough, dyspnea, and signs of renal failure.

◆ ***Seborrheic dermatitis.*** Erupting in areas with many sebaceous glands and in skin folds, seborrheic dermatitis may produce hair loss on the scalp. Alopecia begins at the vertex and frontal areas and may spread to other scalp areas. The patient's skin is reddened and dry with branlike scales that flake off easily. Pruritus is common.

◆ ***Skin metastasis.*** Occasionally, cancer from an internal site, such as the lung, metastasizes to the skin, causing scarring alopecia that may develop slowly along with scalp induration and atrophy. Related findings include weight loss, fever, altered bowel habits, abdominal pain, and lymphadenopathy.

◆ ***Syphilis, secondary.*** This sexually transmitted disease produces temporary, patchy hair loss that gives the scalp and beard a "moth-eaten" appearance. It also produces loss of eyelashes and eyebrows and a pruritic rash. Associated signs and symptoms include slight fever, weight loss, sore throat, malaise, anorexia, lymphadenopathy, nausea, vomiting, headache, a maculopapular rash, and condyloma latum.

◆ ***Thyrotoxicosis.*** Diffuse hair loss, possibly accentuated at the temples, occurs in this disorder. Hair becomes fine, soft, and friable. The skin becomes uniformly flushed and thickened, marked by red, raised, pruritic patches. Characteristically, this disorder produces fine tremors, nervousness, an enlarged thyroid, sweating, heat intolerance, amenorrhea, palpitations, weight loss despite increased appetite, diarrhea, and possibly exophthalmos.

Other causes

◆ ***Drugs.*** Chemotherapeutic agents—such as bleomycin, cyclophosphamide, dactinomycin, daunorubicin, doxorubicin, fluorouracil, and methotrexate—may cause patchy, reversible alopecia a few weeks after administration. Hair loss is usually limited to the scalp, but with long-term chemotherapy, it may also affect the axillae, arms, legs, face, and pubic area. New hair—which may differ in thickness, texture, and color from the patient's original hair—may begin to grow after the drug is discontinued or between successive treatments.

Other common drugs may cause diffuse hair loss on the scalp a few weeks after administration. These include allopurinol, antithyroid drugs, beta-adrenergic blockers, carbamazepine, gentamicin, heparin, hormonal contraceptives, indomethacin, lithium, trimethadione, valproic acid, excessive doses of vitamin A, and warfarin. Hair growth usually resumes when these drugs are discontinued.

◆ ***Radiation therapy.*** Like certain drugs, radiation therapy produces temporary reversible hair loss a few weeks after exposure. Because X-rays damage hair follicles at the site of therapy, head or scalp X-rays cause the most obvious hair loss.

◆ ***Thallium poisoning.*** Thallium poisoning produces diffuse but temporary hair loss on the scalp. Nausea and vomiting are also common. In acute poisoning, the patient may experience arm and leg pain, bilateral ptosis, ataxia, fever, nasal congestion, conjunctival injection, and abdominal pain. In chronic poisoning, he may experience translucent, thin, and shiny skin and signs of renal damage such as oliguria.

Special considerations

Alopecia can have a devastating impact on the patient's self-image, especially if it's extensive and occurs suddenly, as with chemotherapeutic drugs. Make sure you explain to the patient that this hair loss is reversible. Occasionally, scalp hypothermia methods—such as a cryogen, an ice-filled cap, or a scalp tourniquet—may be used before, during, and after drug administration to cause scalp vasoconstriction, thus decreasing drug delivery to the hair follicles and minimizing hair loss. However, these methods are contraindicated in patients with circulating malignant cancer cells (for example, patients with lymphoma) or scalp metastases.

A skin biopsy may be performed to determine the cause of the alopecia, especially if skin changes are evident. Microscopic examination of a plucked hair may also aid diagnosis.

For patients with partial baldness or alopecia areata, topical application of minoxidil (a common antihypertensive that also produces hair growth) for several months stimulates localized hair growth. However, hair loss may recur if the drug is discontinued.

Pediatric pointers

Alopecia normally occurs during the first 6 months of life, as either a sudden, diffuse hair loss or a gradual thinning that's hardly noticeable. Reassure the infant's parents that this hair loss is normal and temporary. If bald areas result because the infant is left in one position for too long, advise the parents to change his position regularly.

Common causes of alopecia in children include use of chemotherapy or radiation therapy, seborrheic dermatitis (known as *cradle cap*), follicular mucinosis, tinea capitis, and hypopituitarism. Tinea capitis may produce a kerion lesion—a boggy, raised, tender, and hairless lesion. Trichotillomania, a psychological disorder more common in children than adults, may produce patchy baldness with stubby hair growth due to habitual hair pulling. Other causes include progeria and congenital hair shaft defects such as trichorrhexis nodosa.

Patient counseling

Encourage gentle hair care to avoid further hair loss. Also, suggest wearing a wig, cap, or scarf, if appropriate. Remind the patient to cover his head in cold weather to prevent loss of body heat. Encourage patients who are frequently exposed to the sun to use sunblock to decrease the risk of skin cancer.

Amenorrhea

The absence of menstrual flow, amenorrhea can be classified as primary or secondary. In primary amenorrhea, menstruation fails to begin before age 16. In secondary amenorrhea, it begins at an appropriate age but later ceases for 3 or more months in the absence of normal physiologic causes, such as pregnancy, lactation, or menopause.

Pathologic amenorrhea results from anovulation or physical obstruction of menstrual outflow, such as from an imperforate hymen, cervical stenosis, or intrauterine adhesions. Anovulation itself may result from hormonal imbalance, debilitating disease, stress or emotional disturbances, strenuous exercise, malnutrition, obesity, or anatomic abnormalities, such as congenital absence of the ovaries or uterus. Amenorrhea may also result from drug or hormonal treatments. (See *How amenorrhea develops*, pages 36 and 37.)

History and physical examination

Begin by determining whether the amenorrhea is primary or secondary. If it's primary, ask the patient at what age her mother first menstruated because age of menarche is fairly consistent in families. Form an overall impression of the patient's physical, mental, and emotional development because these factors as well as heredity and climate may delay menarche until after age 16.

If menstruation began at an appropriate age but has since ceased, determine the frequency and duration of the patient's previous menstrual cycles. Ask her about the onset and nature of any changes in her normal menstrual pattern, and determine the date of her last menses. Find out if she has noticed any related signs, such as breast swelling or weight changes.

Determine when the patient last had a physical examination. Review her health history, noting especially any long-term illnesses, such as anemia, or use of hormonal contraceptives. Ask about exercise habits, especially running, and whether she experiences stress on the job or at home. Probe the patient's eating habits, including number and size of daily meals and snacks, and ask if she has gained weight recently.

Observe her appearance for secondary sex characteristics or signs of virilization. If you're responsible for performing a pelvic examination, check for anatomic aberrations of the outflow tract, such as cervical adhesions, fibroids, or an imperforate hymen.

Medical causes

- ***Adrenal tumor.*** Amenorrhea may be accompanied by acne, thinning scalp hair, hirsutism, increased blood pressure, truncal obesity, and psychotic changes. Asymmetrical ovarian enlargement in conjunction with rapid onset of virilizing signs is usually indicative.
- ***Adrenocortical hyperplasia.*** Amenorrhea precedes characteristic cushingoid signs, such as truncal obesity, moon face, buffalo hump, bruises, purple striae, hypertension, renal calculi, psychiatric disturbances, and widened pulse pressure. Acne, thinning scalp hair, and hirsutism also typically appear.
- ***Adrenocortical hypofunction.*** Besides amenorrhea, adrenocortical hypofunction may cause fatigue, irritability, weight loss, increased pigmentation (including bluish black discoloration of the areolas and mucous membranes of the lips, mouth, rectum, and vagina), nausea, vomiting, and orthostatic hypotension.

How amenorrhea develops

A disruption at any point in the menstrual cycle can produce amenorrhea, as illustrated in the flowchart below.

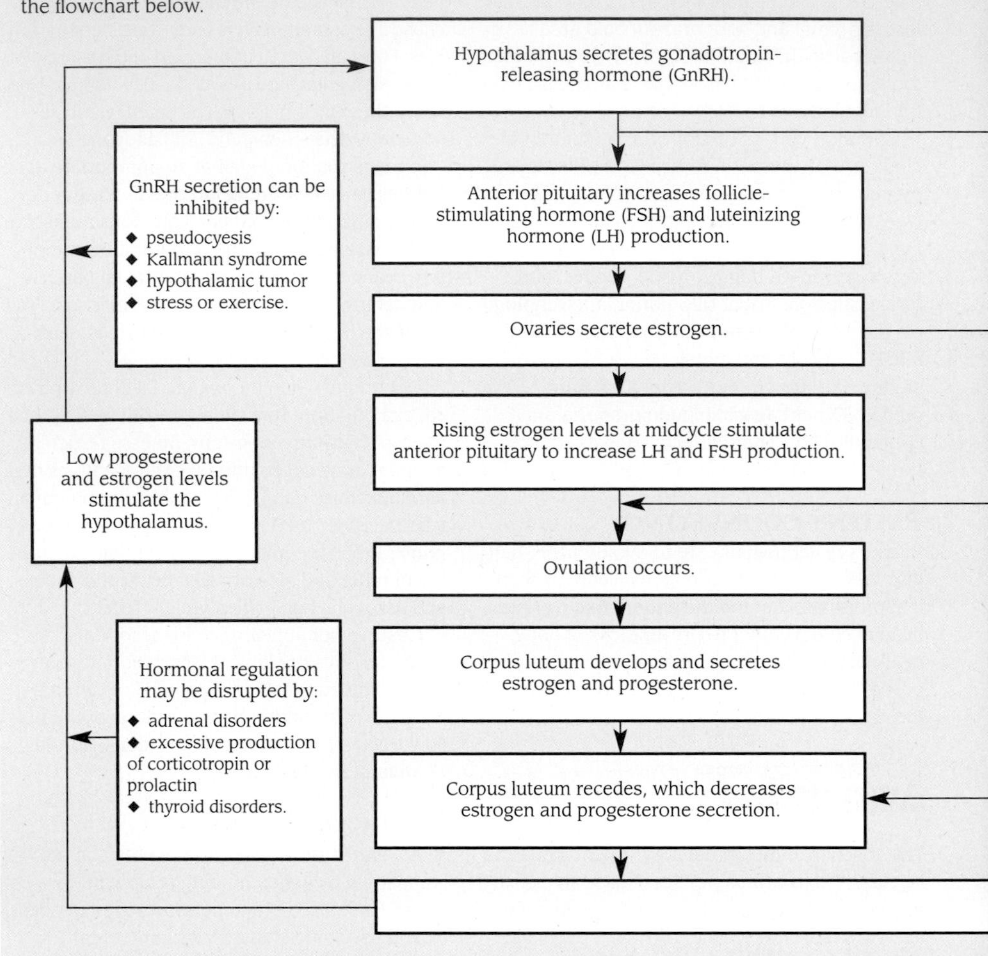

◆ ***Amenorrhea-lactation disorders.*** Amenorrhea-lactation disorders, such as Forbes-Albright and Chiari-Frommel syndromes, produce secondary amenorrhea accompanied by lactation in the absence of breast-feeding. Associated features include hot flashes, dyspareunia, vaginal atrophy, and large, engorged breasts.

◆ ***Anorexia nervosa.*** Anorexia nervosa is a psychological disorder that can cause either primary or secondary amenorrhea. Related findings include significant weight loss, a thin or emaciated appearance, compulsive behavior patterns, blotchy or sallow complexion, constipation, reduced libido, decreased pleasure in once-enjoyable activities, dry skin, loss of scalp hair, lanugo on the face and arms, skeletal muscle atrophy, and sleep disturbances.

◆ ***Congenital absence of the ovaries.*** Congenital absence of the ovaries results in primary amenorrhea and absence of secondary sex characteristics.

◆ ***Congenital absence of the uterus.*** Primary amenorrhea occurs with congenital absence of the uterus. The patient also may fail to develop breasts.

◆ ***Corpus luteum cysts.*** Corpus luteum cysts may cause sudden amenorrhea as well as acute abdominal pain and breast swelling. Examina-

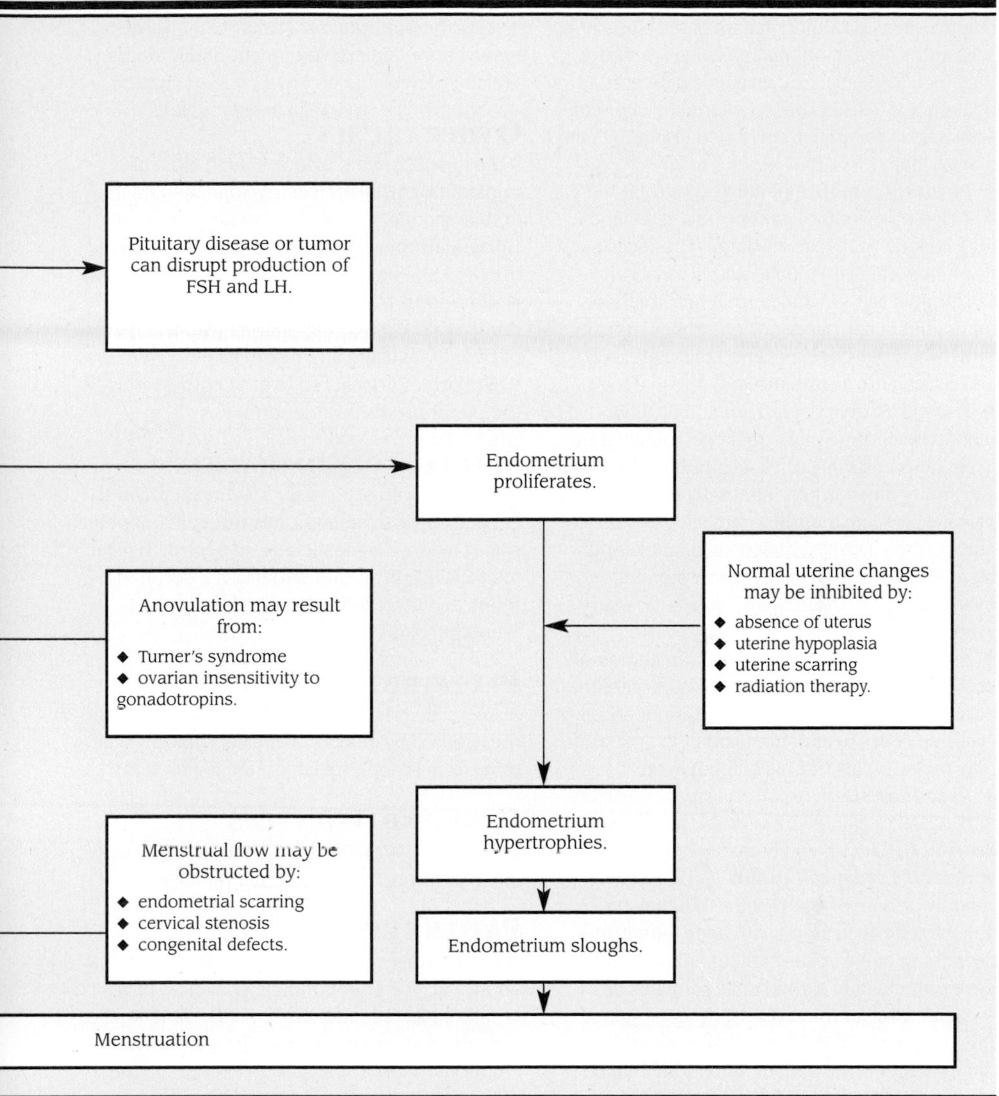
Pituitary disease or tumor can disrupt production of FSH and LH.
Endometrium proliferates.
Normal uterine changes may be inhibited by:
◆ absence of uterus
◆ uterine hypoplasia
◆ uterine scarring
◆ radiation therapy.
Anovulation may result from:
◆ Turner's syndrome
◆ ovarian insensitivity to gonadotropins.
Endometrium hypertrophies.
Menstrual flow may be obstructed by:
◆ endometrial scarring
◆ cervical stenosis
◆ congenital defects.
Endometrium sloughs.
Menstruation

tion may reveal a tender adnexal mass and vaginal and cervical hyperemia.

◆ ***Hypothalamic tumor.*** In addition to amenorrhea, a hypothalamic tumor can cause endocrine and visual field defects, gonadal underdevelopment or dysfunction, and short stature.

◆ ***Hypothyroidism.*** Deficient thyroid hormone levels can cause primary or secondary amenorrhea. Typically vague, early findings include fatigue, forgetfulness, cold intolerance, unexplained weight gain, and constipation. Subsequent signs include bradycardia; decreased mental acuity; dry, flaky, inelastic skin; puffy face, hands, and feet; hoarseness; periorbital edema; ptosis; dry, sparse hair; and thick, brittle nails. Other common findings include anorexia, abdominal distention, decreased libido, ataxia, intention tremor, nystagmus, and delayed reflex relaxation time, especially in the Achilles tendon.

◆ ***Mosaicism.*** Mosaicism is a genetic disorder that results in primary amenorrhea and absence of secondary sex characteristics.

◆ ***Ovarian insensitivity to gonadotropins.*** Ovarian insensitivity to gonadotropins is a hormonal disturbance that leads to amenorrhea and absence of secondary sex characteristics.

◆ ***Pituitary infarction.*** Pituitary infarction usually causes postpartum failure to lactate and to resume menses. Although associated signs and symptoms depend on the infarction's severity, they include headaches, visual field defects, oculomotor palsies, and an altered level of consciousness. The patient may also lose pubic and axillary hair.

◆ ***Pituitary tumor.*** Amenorrhea may be the first sign of a pituitary tumor. Associated findings include headache, visual disturbances such as bitemporal hemianopia, and acromegaly. Cushingoid signs include moon face, buffalo hump, hirsutism, hypertension, truncal obesity, bruises, purple striae, widened pulse pressure, and psychiatric disturbances.

◆ ***Polycystic ovary syndrome.*** Typically, menarche occurs at a normal age, followed by irregular menstrual cycles, oligomenorrhea, and secondary amenorrhea. Alternatively, periods of profuse bleeding may alternate with periods of amenorrhea. Obesity, hirsutism, slight deepening of the voice, and enlarged, "oysterlike" ovaries may also accompany polycystic ovary syndrome.

◆ ***Pseudoamenorrhea.*** An anatomic anomaly, such as imperforate hymen, obstructs menstrual flow, causing primary amenorrhea and, possibly, cyclic episodes of abdominal pain. Examination may reveal a pink or blue bulging hymen.

◆ ***Pseudocyesis.*** In pseudocyesis, amenorrhea may be accompanied by lordosis, abdominal distention, nausea, and breast enlargement.

◆ ***Sertoli-Leydig cell tumor.*** Sertoli-Leydig cell tumor is an ovarian tumor that may produce amenorrhea along with acne, hirsutism, deepening of the voice, balding, muscle mass development, and clitoral enlargement.

◆ ***Testicular feminization.*** Primary amenorrhea may signal this form of male pseudohermaphroditism. The patient, outwardly female but genetically male, exhibits breasts and external genitalia but scant or absent pubic hair.

◆ ***Thyrotoxicosis.*** Thyroid hormone overproduction may result in amenorrhea. Classic signs and symptoms include an enlarged thyroid (goiter), nervousness, heat intolerance, diaphoresis, tremors, palpitations, tachycardia, dyspnea, weakness, and weight loss despite increased appetite.

◆ ***Turner's syndrome.*** Primary amenorrhea and failure to develop secondary sex characteristics may signal this syndrome of genetic ovarian dysgenesis. Typical features include short stature, webbing of the neck, low nuchal hairline, a broad chest with widely spaced nipples and poor breast development, underdeveloped genitalia, and edema of the legs and feet.

◆ ***Uterine hypoplasia.*** Primary amenorrhea results from underdevelopment of the uterus, which is detectable on physical examination.

Other causes

◆ ***Drugs.*** Busulfan, chlorambucil, injectable or implanted contraceptives, cyclophosphamide, and phenothiazines may cause amenorrhea. Hormonal contraceptives may cause anovulation and amenorrhea after they're discontinued.

◆ ***Radiation therapy.*** Irradiation of the abdomen may destroy the endometrium or ovaries, causing amenorrhea.

◆ ***Surgery.*** Surgical removal of both ovaries or the uterus produces amenorrhea.

Special considerations

In patients with secondary amenorrhea, physical and pelvic examinations must rule out pregnancy before diagnostic testing begins. Typical tests include progestin withdrawal, serum hormone and thyroid function studies, and endometrial biopsy.

Pediatric pointers

Adolescent girls are especially prone to amenorrhea caused by emotional upsets, typically stemming from school, social, or family problems.

Geriatric pointers

In women older than age 50, amenorrhea usually represents the onset of menopause.

Patient counseling

After diagnosis, answer the patient's questions about the type of treatment that will be provided and its expected outcome. Because amenorrhea can cause severe emotional distress, provide emotional support. Be sure to encourage the patient to discuss her fears and, if necessary, refer her for psychological counseling.

Amnesia

Amnesia—a disturbance in, or loss of, memory—may be classified as partial or complete and as anterograde or retrograde. Anterograde amnesia denotes memory loss for events that occurred after the onset of the causative trauma or disease; retrograde amnesia, for events that occurred before the onset. Depending on the cause, amnesia may arise suddenly or slowly and may be temporary or permanent.

Organic (or true) amnesia results from temporal lobe dysfunction, and it characteristically spares patches of memory. A common symptom in patients with seizures or head trauma, organic amnesia can also be an early indicator of Alzheimer's disease. Hysterical amnesia has a psychogenic origin and characteristically causes complete memory loss. Treatment-induced amnesia is usually transient.

History and physical examination

Because the patient often isn't aware of his amnesia, you'll usually need help in gathering information from his family or friends. Throughout your assessment, notice the patient's general appearance, behavior, mood, and train of thought. Ask when the amnesia first appeared and what types of things the patient is unable to remember. Can he learn new information? How long does he remember it? Does the amnesia encompass a recent or a remote period?

Test the patient's recent memory by asking him to identify and repeat three items. Retest him after 3 minutes. Test his intermediate memory by asking, "Who was the president before this one?" and "What was the last type of car you bought?" Test remote memory with such questions as "How old are you?" and "Where were you born?"

Take the patient's vital signs and assess his level of consciousness (LOC). Check his pupils: They should be equal in size and should constrict quickly when exposed to direct light. Also, assess his extraocular movements. Test motor function by having the patient move his arms and legs through their range of motion. Evaluate sensory function with pinpricks on the patient's skin. (See *Amnesia: Causes and associated findings,* page 40.)

Medical causes

◆ ***Alzheimer's disease.*** Alzheimer's disease usually begins with retrograde amnesia, which progresses slowly over many months or years to include anterograde amnesia and, eventually, severe and permanent memory loss. Associated findings include agitation, inability to concentrate, disregard for personal hygiene, confusion, irritability, and emotional lability. Later signs include aphasia, incontinence, and muscle rigidity.

◆ ***Cerebral hypoxia.*** After recovery from hypoxia (brought on by such conditions as carbon monoxide poisoning or acute respiratory failure), the patient may experience total amnesia for the event along with sensory disturbances such as numbness and tingling.

◆ ***Head trauma.*** Depending on the trauma's severity, amnesia may last for minutes, hours, or longer. Usually, the patient experiences brief retrograde and longer anterograde amnesia as well as persistent amnesia about the traumatic event. Severe head trauma can cause permanent amnesia or difficulty retaining recent memories. Related findings may include altered respirations and LOC; headache; dizziness; confusion; visual disturbances, such as blurred or double vision; and motor and sensory disturbances, such as hemiparesis and paresthesia, on the side of the body opposite the injury.

◆ ***Herpes simplex encephalitis.*** Recovery from herpes simplex encephalitis commonly leaves the patient with severe and possibly permanent amnesia. Associated findings include signs and symptoms of meningeal irritation, such as headache, fever, and altered LOC; seizures; and various motor and sensory disturbances, such as paresis, numbness, and tingling.

◆ ***Hysteria.*** Hysterical amnesia, a complete and long-lasting memory loss, begins and ends abruptly and is typically accompanied by confusion.

◆ ***Seizures.*** In temporal lobe seizures, amnesia occurs suddenly and lasts for several seconds to minutes. The patient may recall an aura or nothing at all. An irritable focus on the left side of the brain primarily causes amnesia for verbal memories, whereas an irritable focus on the right side of the brain causes graphic and nonverbal amnesia. Associated signs and symptoms may include decreased LOC during the seizure, confusion, abnormal mouth movements, and visual, olfactory, and auditory hallucinations.

◆ ***Vertebrobasilar circulatory disorders.*** Vertebrobasilar ischemia, infarction, embolus, or hemorrhage may cause complete amnesia that begins abruptly, lasts for several hours, and ends abruptly. Associated findings include dizziness, decreased LOC, ataxia, blurred or double vision, vertigo, nausea, and vomiting.

◆ ***Wernicke-Korsakoff syndrome.*** Retrograde and anterograde amnesia can become permanent without treatment in Wernicke-Korsakoff syndrome. Accompanying signs and symptoms include apathy, an inability to concentrate or to put events into sequence, and confabulation to fill memory gaps. The syndrome may also cause

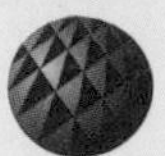

SIGNS & SYMPTOMS

Amnesia: Causes and associated findings

Common causes	Major associated signs and symptoms: Agitation	Ataxia	Confusion	Decreased level of consciousness	Diplopia	Dizziness	Emotional lability	Headache	Nausea	Paresthesia	Vertigo	Visual blurring	Vomiting
Alzheimer's disease	●		●				●						
Cerebral hypoxia	●		●	●			●	●		●			
Head trauma	●		●	●	●	●	●	●	●	●	●	●	●
Herpes simplex encephalitis	●		●	●			●	●		●			
Hysteria			●				●						
Seizures			●	●								●	
Vertebrobasilar circulatory disorders		●		●	●	●	●		●	●	●	●	●
Wernicke-Korsakoff syndrome		●	●	●	●			●		●			

diplopia, decreased LOC, headache, ataxia, and symptoms of peripheral neuropathy such as numbness and tingling.

Other causes

◆ ***Drugs.*** Anterograde amnesia can be precipitated by general anesthetics, especially fentanyl and isoflurane; barbiturates, most commonly pentobarbital; and certain benzodiazepines, especially triazolam.

◆ ***Electroconvulsive therapy.*** Sudden onset of retrograde or anterograde amnesia occurs with electroconvulsive therapy. Typically, the amnesia lasts for several minutes to several hours, but severe, prolonged amnesia occurs with treatments given frequently over a prolonged period.

◆ ***Temporal lobe surgery.*** Usually performed on only one lobe, this surgery causes brief, mild amnesia. However, removal of both lobes results in permanent amnesia.

Special considerations

Prepare the patient for diagnostic tests, such as computed tomography scan, magnetic resonance imaging, EEG, or cerebral angiography.

Provide reality orientation for the patient with retrograde amnesia, and encourage his family to help by supplying familiar photos, objects, and music.

Adjust your patient-teaching techniques for the patient with anterograde amnesia because he can't acquire new information. Include his family in teaching sessions. In addition, write down all instructions—particularly medication dosages and schedules—so the patient won't have to rely on his memory.

If the patient has severe amnesia, consider his basic needs, such as safety, elimination, and nutrition. If necessary, arrange for placement in an extended-care facility.

Pediatric pointers

A child who suffers amnesia during seizures may be mistakenly labeled as "learning disabled." To prevent this mislabeling, stress the importance of adhering to the prescribed drug schedule, and discuss ways that the child, his parents, and his teachers can cope with amnesia.

Analgesia

Analgesia, the absence of sensitivity to pain, is an important sign of central nervous system disease, often indicating a specific type and location of spinal cord lesion. It always occurs with loss of temperature sensation (thermoanesthesia) because these sensory nerve impulses travel together in the spinal cord. It can also occur with other sensory deficits—such as paresthesia, loss of proprioception and vibratory sense, and tactile anesthesia—in various disorders involving the peripheral nerves, spinal cord, and brain. However, when accompanied only by thermoanesthesia, analgesia points to an incomplete lesion of the spinal cord.

Analgesia can be classified as partial or total below the level of the lesion and as unilateral or bilateral, depending on the cause and level of the lesion. Its onset may be slow and progressive with a tumor or abrupt with trauma. Transient in many cases, analgesia may resolve spontaneously.

EMERGENCY INTERVENTIONS *Suspect spinal cord injury if the patient complains of unilateral or bilateral analgesia over a large body area, accompanied by paralysis. Immobilize his spine in proper alignment, using a cervical collar and a long backboard, if possible. If a collar or backboard isn't available, place the patient in a supine position on a flat surface and place sandbags around his head, neck, and torso. Use correct technique and extreme caution when moving him to prevent exacerbating the spinal injury. Continuously monitor respiratory rate and rhythm, and observe him for accessory muscle use because a complete lesion above the T6 level may cause diaphragmatic and intercostal muscle paralysis. Have an artificial airway and a handheld resuscitation bag on hand, and be prepared to initiate emergency resuscitation measures in case of respiratory failure.*

History and physical examination

Once you're satisfied that the patient's spine and respiratory status are stabilized—or if the analgesia isn't severe and isn't accompanied by signs of spinal cord injury—perform a physical examination and baseline neurologic evaluation. First, take the patient's vital signs and assess his level of consciousness. Then test pupillary, corneal, cough, and gag reflexes to rule out brain stem and cranial nerve involvement. If the patient is conscious, evaluate his speech and ability to swallow.

If possible, observe the patient's gait and posture and assess his balance and coordination. Evaluate muscle tone and strength in all extremities. Test for other sensory deficits over all dermatomes (individual skin segments innervated by a specific spinal nerve) by applying light tactile stimulation with a tongue depressor or cotton swab. Perform a more thorough check of pain sensitivity, if necessary, using a pin. (See *Testing for analgesia,* pages 42 and 43.) Also, test temperature sensation over all dermatomes, using two test tubes—one filled with hot water, the other with cold water. In each arm and leg, test vibration sense (using a tuning fork), proprioception, and superficial and deep tendon reflexes (DTRs). Check for increased muscle tone by extending and flexing the patient's elbows and knees as he tries to relax.

Focus your history taking on the onset of analgesia (sudden or gradual) and on any recent trauma, such as a fall, a sports injury, or an automobile accident. Obtain a complete medical history, noting especially any incidence of cancer in the patient or his family.

Medical causes

◆ ***Anterior cord syndrome.*** In anterior cord syndrome, analgesia and thermoanesthesia occur bilaterally below the level of the lesion along with flaccid paralysis and hypoactive DTRs.

◆ ***Central cord syndrome.*** In central cord syndrome, analgesia and thermoanesthesia typically occur bilaterally in several dermatomes and may extend in a capelike fashion over the arms, back, and shoulders. Early weakness in the hands progresses to weakness and muscle spasms in the arms and shoulder girdle. Hyperactive DTRs and spastic weakness of the legs may develop. However, if the lesion affects the

(Text continues on page 44.)

Testing for analgesia

By carefully and systematically testing your patient's sensitivity to pain, you can determine whether his nerve damage has segmental or peripheral distribution and help locate the causative lesion.

Tell the patient to relax, and explain that you're going to lightly touch areas of his skin with a small pin. Have him close his eyes. Apply the pin firmly enough to produce pain without breaking the skin. (Practice on

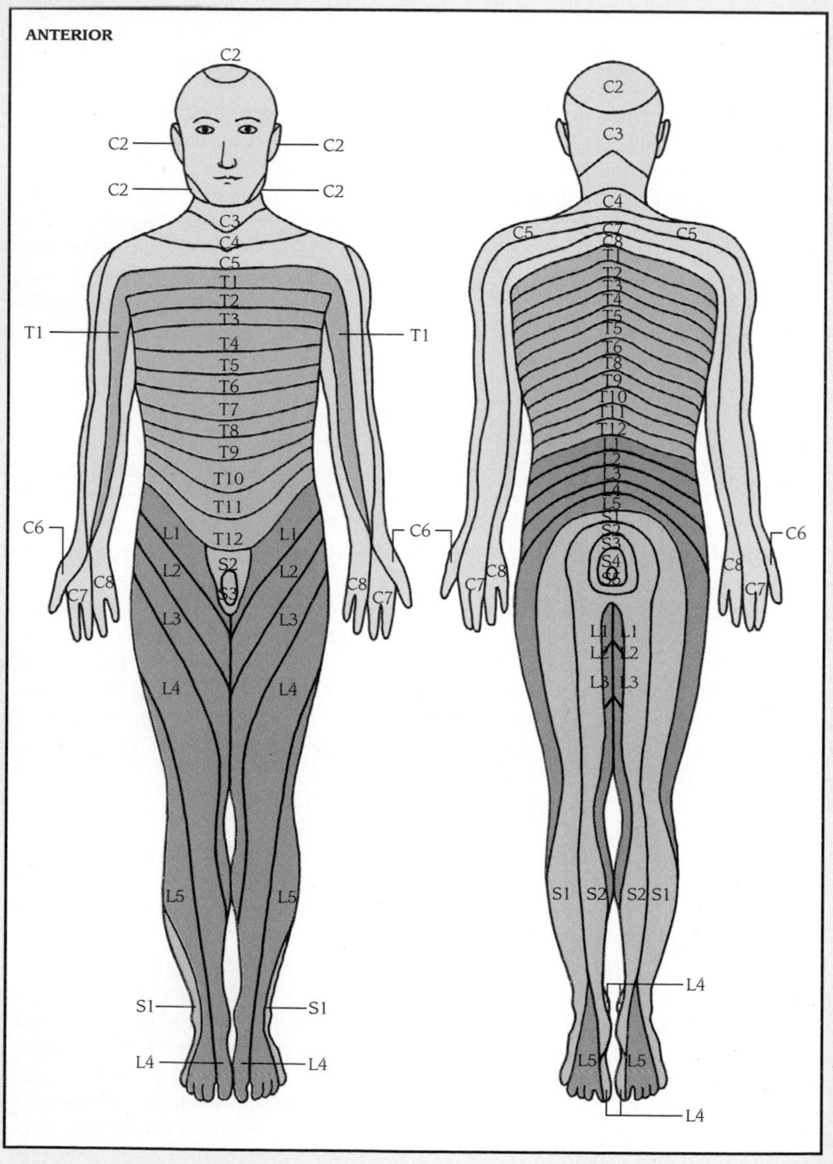

yourself first to learn how to apply the correct pressure.)

Starting with the patient's head and face, move down his body, pricking his skin on alternating sides. Have the patient report when he feels pain. Use the blunt end of the pin occasionally, and vary your test pattern to gauge the accuracy of his response.

Document your findings thoroughly, clearly marking areas of lost pain sensation on a dermatome chart (shown on previous page).

Peripheral nerves

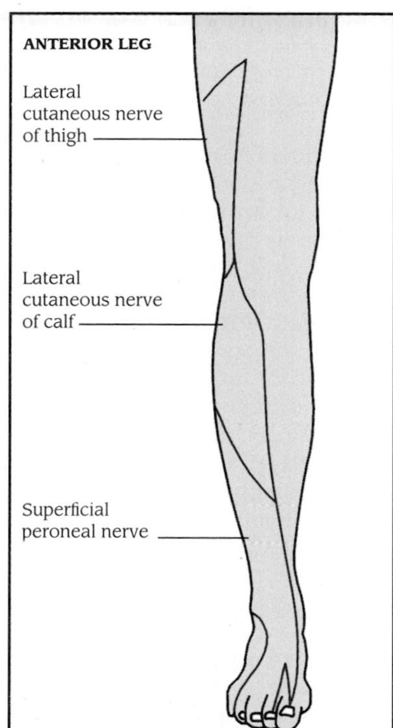

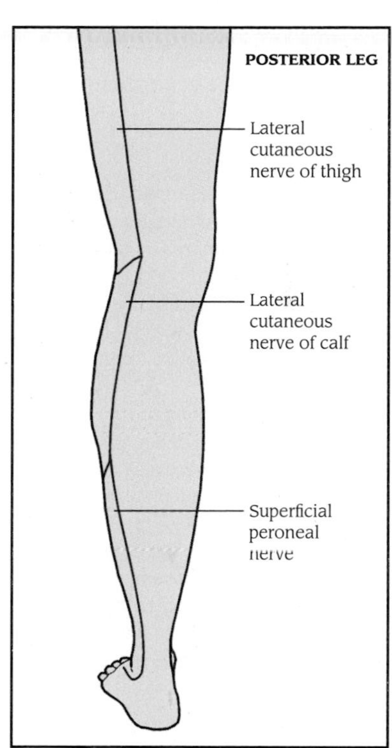

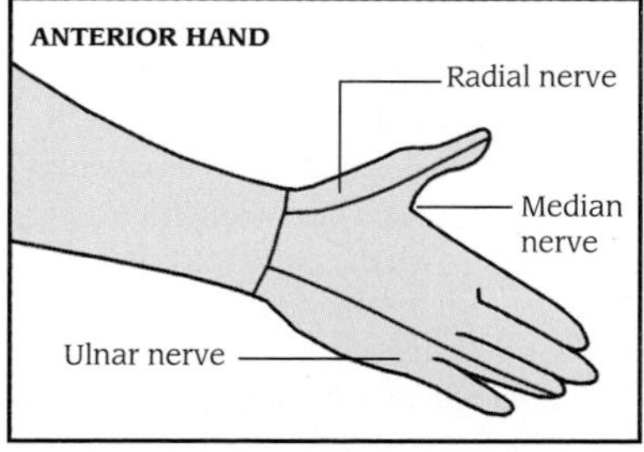

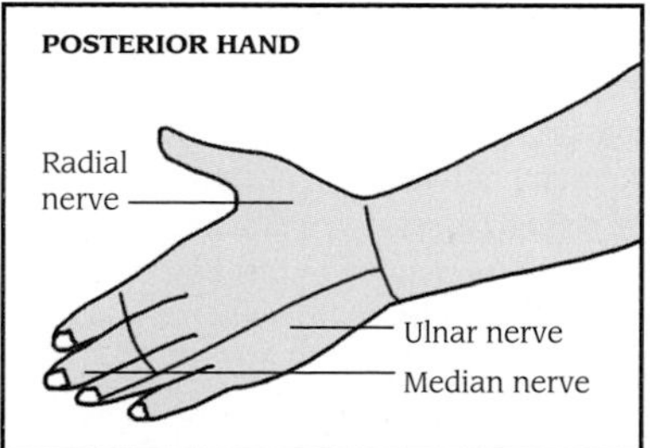

lumbar spine, hypoactive DTRs and flaccid weakness may persist in the legs.

With brain stem involvement, additional findings include facial analgesia and thermoanesthesia, vertigo, nystagmus, atrophy of the tongue, and dysarthria. The patient may also have anhidrosis, dysphagia, urine retention, decreased intestinal motility, and hyperkeratosis.

◆ ***Spinal cord hemisection.*** Contralateral analgesia and thermoanesthesia occur below the level of the lesion. In addition, loss of proprioception, spastic paralysis, and hyperactive deep tendon reflexes develop ipsilaterally. The patient may also experience urine retention with overflow incontinence.

Other causes

◆ ***Drugs.*** Analgesia may occur with use of a topical or local anesthetic, although numbness and tingling are more common.

Special considerations

Prepare the patient for spinal X-rays, and maintain spinal alignment and stability during transport to the laboratory.

Focus your care on preventing further injury to the patient because analgesia can mask injury or developing complications. Prevent formation of pressure ulcers through meticulous skin care, massage, use of lamb's wool pads, and frequent repositioning, especially when significant motor deficits hamper the patient's movement. Guard against scalding by testing the patient's bathwater temperature before he bathes; advise him to test it at home using a thermometer or a body part with intact sensation.

Pediatric pointers

Because a child may have difficulty describing analgesia, observe him carefully during the assessment for nonverbal clues to pain, such as facial expressions, crying, and retraction from stimuli. Remember that pain thresholds are high in infants, so your assessment findings may not be reliable. Also, remember to test bathwater carefully for a child who is too young to test it himself.

Anhidrosis

Anhidrosis, an abnormal deficiency of sweat, can be classified as generalized (complete) or localized (partial). Generalized anhidrosis can lead to life-threatening impairment of thermoregulation. Localized anhidrosis rarely interferes with thermoregulation because it affects only a small percentage of the body's eccrine (sweat) glands.

Anhidrosis results from neurologic and skin disorders; congenital, atrophic, or traumatic changes to sweat glands; and the use of certain drugs. Neurologic disorders disturb central or peripheral nervous pathways that normally activate sweating, causing retention of excess body heat and perspiration. The absence, obstruction, atrophy, or degeneration of sweat glands can produce anhidrosis at the skin surface, even if neurologic stimulation is normal. (See *Eccrine dysfunction in anhidrosis,* pages 46 and 47.)

Anhidrosis may go unrecognized until significant heat or exertion fails to produce sweat. However, localized anhidrosis often provokes compensatory hyperhidrosis in the remaining functional sweat glands, which, in many cases, is the patient's chief complaint.

EMERGENCY INTERVENTIONS *If you detect anhidrosis in a patient whose skin feels hot and flushed, ask if the patient is also experiencing nausea, dizziness, palpitations, and substernal tightness. If he is, quickly take his rectal temperature and other vital signs, and assess his level of consciousness (LOC). If a rectal temperature higher than 102.2° F (39° C) is accompanied by tachycardia, tachypnea, altered blood pressure, and decreased LOC, suspect life-threatening anhidrotic asthenia (heatstroke). Start rapid cooling measures, such as placing the patient on a cooling blanket, and give I.V. fluid replacements. Continue these measures, and frequently check vital signs and neurologic status, until the patient's temperature drops below 102° F (38.9° C). Then place him in an air-conditioned room.*

History and physical examination

If anhidrosis is localized or the patient reports local hyperhidrosis or unexplained fever, take a brief history. Ask the patient to characterize his sweating during heat spells or strenuous activity. Does he usually sweat slightly or profusely? Ask about recent prolonged or extreme exposure to heat and about the onset of anhidrosis or hyperhidrosis. Obtain a complete medical history, focusing on neurologic disorders; skin disorders, such as psoriasis; autoimmune disorders such as scleroderma; systemic diseases that can cause peripheral neuropathies such as diabetes mellitus; and drug use.

Inspect skin color, texture, and turgor. If you detect any skin lesions, document their location, size, color, texture, and pattern.

Medical causes

◆ ***Anhidrotic asthenia (heatstroke).*** Heatstroke is a life-threatening disorder that causes acute, generalized anhidrosis. In early stages, the patient may still sweat and be rational, but his rectal temperature may already exceed 102.2° F (39° C). Associated signs and symptoms include severe headache and muscle cramps, which later disappear; fatigue; nausea and vomiting; dizziness; palpitations; substernal tightness; and elevated blood pressure followed by hypotension. Within minutes, anhidrosis and hot, flushed skin develop, accompanied by tachycardia, tachypnea, and confusion progressing to seizures or loss of consciousness.

◆ ***Burns.*** Depending on their severity, burns may cause permanent anhidrosis in affected areas as well as blistering, edema, and increased pain or loss of sensation.

◆ ***Cerebral lesions.*** Cerebral cortex and brain stem lesions may cause anhidrotic palms and soles along with various motor and sensory disturbances specific to the site of the lesions.

◆ ***Horner's syndrome.*** A supraclavicular spinal cord lesion affecting a cervical nerve produces unilateral facial anhidrosis with compensatory contralateral hyperhidrosis. Other findings include ipsilateral pupillary constriction and ptosis.

◆ ***Miliaria crystallina.*** This usually innocuous form of miliaria causes anhidrosis and tiny, clear, fragile blisters, usually under the arms and breasts.

◆ ***Miliaria profunda.*** If severe and extensive, this form of miliaria can progress to life-threatening anhidrotic asthenia. Typically, it produces localized anhidrosis with compensatory facial hyperhidrosis. Whitish papules appear mostly on the trunk but also on the extremities. Associated signs and symptoms include inguinal and axillary lymphadenopathy, weakness, shortness of breath, palpitations, and fever.

◆ ***Miliaria rubra (prickly heat).*** This common form of miliaria, which typically produces localized anhidrosis, rarely can progress to life-threatening anhidrotic asthenia if it becomes severe and extensive. Small, erythematous papules with centrally placed blisters appear on the trunk and neck and rarely on the face, palms, or soles. Pustules may also appear in extensive and chronic miliaria. Related symptoms include paroxysmal itching and paresthesia.

◆ ***Peripheral neuropathy.*** In this disorder, anhidrosis commonly appears over the legs with compensatory hyperhidrosis over the head and neck. Associated findings mainly involve the extremities and include glossy red skin; paresthesia, hyperesthesia, or anesthesia in the hands and feet; diminished or absent deep tendon reflexes; flaccid paralysis and muscle wasting; footdrop; and burning pain.

◆ ***Shy-Drager syndrome.*** Shy-Drager syndrome is a degenerative neurologic syndrome that causes ascending anhidrosis in the legs. Other signs and symptoms include severe orthostatic hypotension, loss of leg hair, impotence, constipation, urine retention or urinary urgency, decreased salivation and tearing, mydriasis, and impaired visual accommodation. Eventually, focal neurologic signs—such as leg tremors, incoordination, and muscle wasting and fasciculations—may appear.

◆ ***Spinal cord lesions.*** Anhidrosis may occur symmetrically below the level of the lesion, with compensatory hyperhidrosis in adjacent areas. Other findings depend on the site and extent of the lesion but may include partial or total loss of motor and sensory function below the lesion as well as impaired cardiovascular and respiratory function.

Other causes

◆ ***Drugs.*** Anticholinergics, such as atropine and scopolamine, can cause generalized anhidrosis.

Special considerations

Because even a careful evaluation can be inconclusive, you may need to administer specific tests to evaluate anhidrosis. These include wrapping the patient in an electric blanket or placing him in a heated box to observe the skin for sweat patterns, applying a topical agent to detect sweat on the skin, and administering a systemic cholinergic drug to stimulate sweating.

Pediatric pointers

In both infants and children, miliaria rubra and congenital skin disorders, such as ichthyosis and anhidrotic ectodermal dysplasia, are the most common causes of anhidrosis.

Because delayed development of the thermoregulatory center renders an infant—especially a premature one—anhidrotic for several weeks after birth, caution parents against overdressing their infant.

Eccrine dysfunction in anhidrosis

Eccrine glands, located over most of the skin, help regulate body temperature by secreting sweat. Any change or dysfunction in these glands can result in anhidrosis of varying severity. These illustrations show a normal eccrine gland and some common abnormalities.

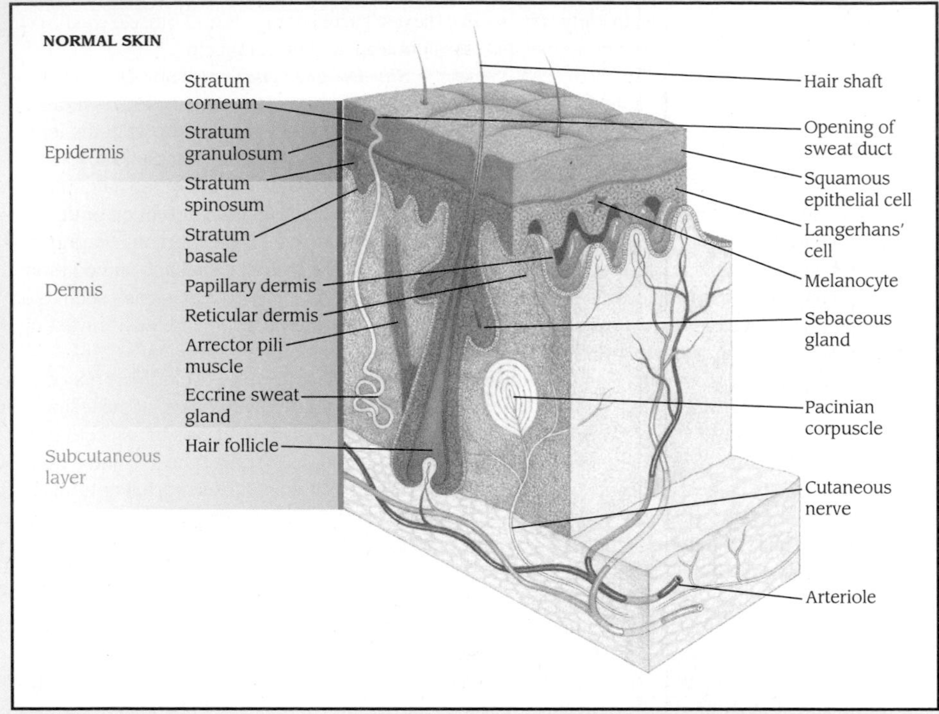

PATIENT COUNSELING

Advise the patient with anhidrosis to remain in cool environments, to move slowly during warm weather, and to avoid strenuous exercise and hot foods. Warn him about the anhidrotic effects of any drugs he's receiving.

Anorexia

Anorexia, a lack of appetite in the presence of a physiologic need for food, is a common symptom of GI and endocrine disorders and is characteristic of certain severe psychological disturbances such as anorexia nervosa. It can also result from such factors as anxiety, chronic pain, poor oral hygiene, increased body temperature due to hot weather or fever, and changes in taste or smell that normally accompany aging. Anorexia also can result from drug therapy or abuse. Short-term anorexia rarely jeopardizes health, but chronic anorexia can lead to life-threatening malnutrition.

HISTORY AND PHYSICAL EXAMINATION

Take the patient's vital signs and weight. Find out previous minimum and maximum weights. Ask about involuntary weight loss greater than 10 lb (4.5 kg) in the last month. Explore dietary habits, including what the patient eats and when. Ask what foods he likes and dislikes and why. The patient may identify tastes and smells that nauseate him and cause loss of appetite. Ask about dental problems that interfere with chewing, including poor-fitting dentures. Ask if he has difficulty or pain when swallowing or if he vomits or has diarrhea after meals. Ask the patient how frequently and intensely he exercises.

OBSTRUCTED ECCRINE GLAND
(occurs in miliaria)

Sweat duct obstruction
Retained sweat

ATROPHY
(occurs with aging)

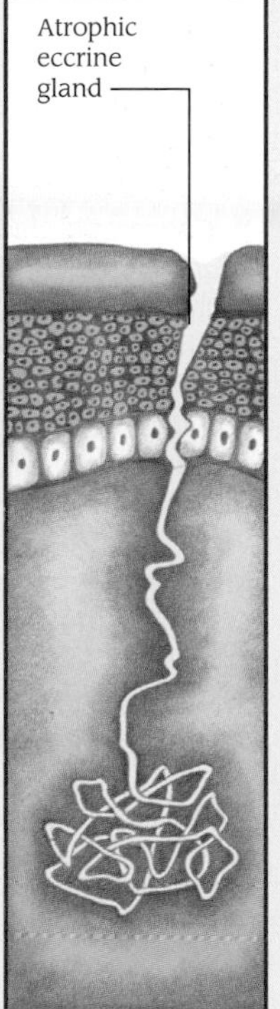

DESTRUCTION
(occurs with burns)

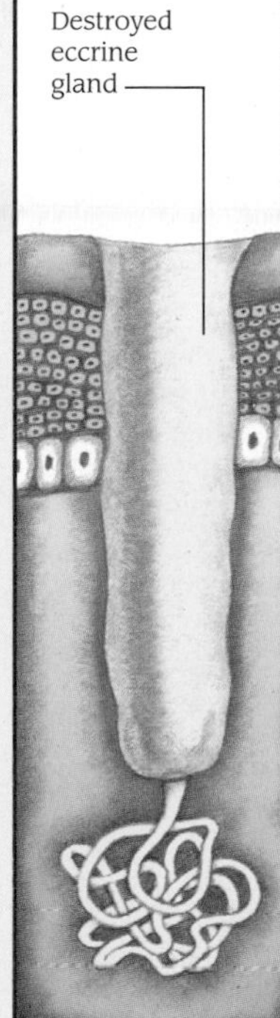

CONGENITAL ABSENCE
(occurs in anhidrotic ectodermal dysplasia)

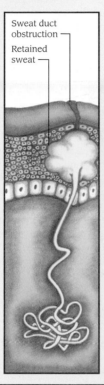

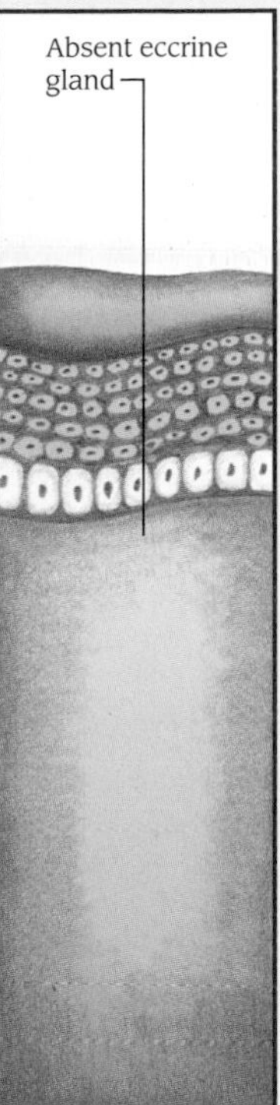

Check for a history of stomach or bowel disorders, which can interfere with the ability to digest, absorb, or metabolize nutrients. Find out about changes in bowel habits. Ask about alcohol use and drug use and dosage.

If the medical history doesn't reveal an organic basis for anorexia, consider psychological factors. Ask the patient if he knows what's causing his decreased appetite. Situational factors—such as a death in the family or problems at school or at work—can lead to depression and subsequent loss of appetite. Be alert for signs of malnutrition, consistent refusal of food, and a 7% to 10% loss of body weight in the preceding month. (See *Is your patient malnourished?* page 48.)

Medical causes

◆ ***Acquired immunodeficiency syndrome (AIDS).*** An infection or Kaposi's sarcoma affecting the GI or respiratory tract may lead to anorexia in a patient with AIDS. Other findings include fatigue, afternoon fevers, night sweats, diarrhea, cough, bleeding, lymphadenopathy, oral thrush, gingivitis, and skin disorders, including persistent herpes zoster and recurrent herpes simplex, herpes labialis, or herpes genitalis.

◆ ***Adrenocortical hypofunction.*** In adrenocortical hypofunction, anorexia may begin slowly and subtly, causing gradual weight loss. Other common signs and symptoms include nausea and vomiting, abdominal pain, diarrhea, weakness, fatigue, malaise, vitiligo, bronze-colored skin, and purple striae on the breasts, abdomen, shoulders, and hips.

◆ ***Alcoholism.*** Chronic anorexia commonly accompanies alcoholism, eventually leading to malnutrition. Other findings include signs of liver damage (jaundice, spider angiomas, ascites,

Is your patient malnourished?

When assessing a patient with anorexia, be sure to check for these common signs of malnutrition.

Hair. Dull, dry, thin, fine, straight, and easily plucked; areas of lighter or darker spots and hair loss

Face. Generalized swelling, dark areas on cheeks and under eyes, lumpy or flaky skin around the nose and mouth, enlarged parotid glands

Eyes. Dull appearance; dry and either pale or red membranes; triangular, shiny gray spots on conjunctivae; red and fissured eyelid corners; bloodshot ring around cornea

Lips. Red and swollen, especially at corners

Tongue. Swollen, purple, and raw-looking, with sores or abnormal papillae

Teeth. Missing or emerging abnormally; visible cavities or dark spots; spongy, bleeding gums

Neck. Swollen thyroid gland

Skin. Dry, flaky, swollen, and dark, with lighter or darker spots, some resembling bruises; tight and drawn, with poor skin turgor

Nails. Spoon-shaped, brittle, and ridged

Musculoskeletal system. Muscle wasting, knock-knee or bowlegs, bumps on ribs, swollen joints, musculoskeletal hemorrhages

Cardiovascular system. Heart rate above 100 beats/minute, arrhythmias, elevated blood pressure

Abdomen. Enlarged liver and spleen

Reproductive system. Decreased libido, amenorrhea

Nervous system. Irritability, confusion, paresthesia in hands and feet, loss of proprioception, decreased ankle and knee reflexes

edema), paresthesia, tremors, increased blood pressure, bruising, GI bleeding, and abdominal pain.

◆ ***Anorexia nervosa.*** Chronic anorexia nervosa is an eating disorder that begins insidiously and eventually leads to life-threatening malnutrition, as evidenced by skeletal muscle atrophy, loss of fatty tissue, constipation, amenorrhea, dry and blotchy or sallow skin, alopecia, sleep disturbances, distorted self-image, anhedonia, and decreased libido. Paradoxically, many patients exhibit extreme restlessness and vigor and may exercise avidly; many also have complicated food preparation and eating rituals.

◆ ***Appendicitis.*** Anorexia closely follows the abrupt onset of generalized or localized epigastric pain, nausea, and vomiting. It can continue as pain localizes in the right lower quadrant (McBurney's point) and other signs and symptoms—abdominal rigidity, rebound tenderness, constipation or diarrhea, slight fever, and tachycardia—appear.

◆ ***Cancer.*** Chronic anorexia may be accompanied by weight loss, weakness, apathy, and cachexia.

◆ ***Chronic renal failure.*** Chronic anorexia is common and develops insidiously in chronic renal failure. It's accompanied by changes in all body systems, such as nausea, vomiting, mouth ulcers, ammonia breath odor, metallic taste, GI bleeding, constipation or diarrhea, drowsiness, confusion, tremors, pallor, dry and scaly skin, pruritus, alopecia, purpuric lesions, and edema.

◆ ***Cirrhosis.*** Anorexia occurs early in cirrhosis and may be accompanied by weakness, nausea, vomiting, constipation or diarrhea, and dull abdominal pain. It continues after these early signs and symptoms subside and is accompanied by lethargy, slurred speech, bleeding tendencies, ascites, severe pruritus, dry skin, poor skin turgor, hepatomegaly, fetor hepaticus, jaundice, edema of the legs, gynecomastia, and right-upper-quadrant pain.

◆ ***Crohn's disease.*** Chronic anorexia causes marked weight loss in Crohn's disease. Associated signs vary according to the site and extent of the lesion but may include diarrhea, abdominal pain, fever, abdominal mass, weakness, perianal or vaginal fistulas and, rarely, clubbing of the fingers. Acute inflammatory signs and symptoms—right-lower-quadrant pain, cramping, tenderness, flatulence, fever, nausea, diarrhea (including nocturnal), and bloody stools—mimic those of appendicitis.

◆ ***Depressive syndrome.*** Anorexia reflects anhedonia in depressive syndrome. Accompanying signs and symptoms include poor concentration, indecisiveness, delusions, menstrual irregularities, decreased libido, insomnia or hypersomnia, fatigue, mood swings, poor self-image, and gradual social withdrawal.

◆ ***Gastritis.*** In acute gastritis, anorexia may have a sudden onset. The patient may experience postprandial epigastric distress accompanied by nausea, vomiting (often with hematemesis), fever, belching, hiccups, and malaise.

◆ ***Hepatitis.*** In viral hepatitis (hepatitis A, B, C, or D), anorexia begins in the preicteric phase and is accompanied by fatigue, malaise, headache, arthralgia, myalgia, photophobia, nausea and vomiting, mild fever, hepatomegaly, and lymphadenopathy. It may continue throughout the icteric phase along with mild weight loss, dark urine, clay-colored stools, jaundice, right-upper-quadrant pain and, possibly, irritability and severe pruritus.

Signs and symptoms of nonviral hepatitis usually resemble those of viral hepatitis but may vary, depending on the cause and the extent of liver damage.

◆ ***Hypopituitarism.*** Anorexia usually develops slowly in hypopituitarism, which usually begins with hypergonadism. Accompanying signs and symptoms vary with the disorder's severity and the number and type of deficient hormones. They may include amenorrhea; decreased libido; lethargy; cold intolerance; pale, thin, and dry skin; dry, brittle hair; and decreased temperature, blood pressure, and pulse rate.

◆ ***Hypothyroidism.*** Anorexia is common and usually insidious in patients with thyroid hormone deficiency. Vague early findings typically include fatigue, forgetfulness, cold intolerance, unexplained weight gain, and constipation. Subsequent findings include decreased mental stability; dry, flaky, and inelastic skin; edema of the face, hands, and feet; ptosis; hoarseness; thick, brittle nails; coarse, broken hair; and signs of decreased cardiac output such as bradycardia. Other common findings include abdominal distention, menstrual irregularities, decreased libido, ataxia, intention tremor, nystagmus, dull facial expression, and slow reflex relaxation time.

◆ ***Ketoacidosis.*** Anorexia usually arises gradually in ketoacidosis and is accompanied by dry, flushed skin; fruity breath odor; polydipsia; polyuria and nocturia; hypotension; weak, rapid pulse; dry mouth; abdominal pain; and vomiting.

◆ ***Pernicious anemia.*** In pernicious anemia, insidious anorexia may cause considerable weight loss. Related findings include the classic triad of burning tongue, general weakness, and numbness and tingling in the extremities; alternating constipation and diarrhea; abdominal pain; nausea and vomiting; bleeding gums; ataxia; positive Babinski's and Romberg's signs; diplopia and blurred vision; irritability, headache, malaise, and fatigue.

OTHER CAUSES

◆ ***Drugs.*** Anorexia may result from the use of amphetamines, chemotherapeutic agents, sympathomimetics such as ephedrine, and some antibiotics. It also may signal digoxin toxicity.

◆ ***Radiation therapy.*** Radiation treatments can cause anorexia, possibly as the result of metabolic disturbances.

◆ ***Total parenteral nutrition.*** Maintenance of blood glucose levels by I.V. therapy may cause anorexia.

SPECIAL CONSIDERATIONS

Because the causes of anorexia are diverse, diagnostic procedures may include thyroid function studies, endoscopy, upper GI series, gallbladder series, barium enema, liver and kidney function tests, hormone assays, computed tomography scans, ultrasonography, and blood studies to assess nutritional status.

Promote adequate protein and caloric intake by providing high-calorie snacks or frequent, small meals. Encourage the patient's family to supply his favorite foods to help stimulate his appetite. Take a 24-hour diet history daily. The patient may consistently exaggerate his food intake (common in patients with anorexia nervosa), so you'll need to maintain strict calorie and nutrient counts for the patient's meals. In severe malnutrition, provide supplemental nutritional support, such as total parenteral nutrition or oral nutritional supplements.

Because anorexia and poor nutrition increase susceptibility to infection, monitor the patient's vital signs and white blood cell count and closely observe any wounds.

PEDIATRIC POINTERS

In children, anorexia commonly accompanies many illnesses but usually resolves promptly. However, be alert for subtle signs of anorexia nervosa in preadolescent and adolescent girls.

Anosmia

Although usually an insignificant consequence of nasal congestion or obstruction, anosmia—absence of the sense of smell—occasionally heralds a serious defect. Temporary anosmia can result from any condition that irritates and causes swelling of the nasal mucosa and obstructs the olfactory area in the nose, such as heavy smoking, rhinitis, or sinusitis. Permanent anosmia usually results when the olfactory neuroepithelium or any part of the olfactory nerve is destroyed. Permanent or temporary anosmia can also result from inhaling irritants that paralyze nasal cilia, such as cocaine and acid fumes. Anosmia may also be reported—without an identifiable organic cause—by patients suffering from hysteria, depression, or schizophrenia.

Anosmia is invariably perceived as bilateral; unilateral anosmia can occur but is seldom recognized by the patient. Because combined stimulation of taste buds and olfactory cells produces the sense of taste, anosmia is usually accompanied by ageusia, loss of the sense of taste. (See *Understanding the sense of smell*.)

History and physical examination

Begin the patient history by asking about the onset and duration of anosmia and related signs and symptoms—stuffy nose, nasal discharge or bleeding, postnasal drip, sneezing, dry or sore mouth and throat, loss of sense of taste or appetite, excessive tearing, and facial or eye pain. Pinpoint any history of nasal disease, allergies, or head trauma. Ask about heavy smoking and the use of prescribed or over-the-counter nose drops or nasal sprays. Be sure to rule out cocaine use.

Inspect and palpate nasal structures for obvious injury, inflammation, deformities, and septal deviation or perforation. Observe the contour and color of the nasal mucosa and the size and color of the turbinates. Check for polyps, which appear as translucent white masses around the middle meatus. Note the source and character of any nasal discharge. Palpate the sinus areas for tenderness and contour.

Assess the patient for nasal obstruction by occluding one nostril at a time with your thumb as the patient breathes quietly; listen for breath sounds and for sounds of moisture or mucus. Test olfactory nerve (cranial nerve I) function by having the patient identify common odors.

Medical causes

◆ ***Anterior cerebral artery occlusion.*** Permanent anosmia may follow vascular damage involving the olfactory nerve. Associated signs and symptoms include contralateral weakness and numbness (especially in the leg), confusion, and impaired motor and sensory functions.

◆ ***Degenerative brain disease.*** Anosmia may accompany Alzheimer's disease, Parkinson's disease, and other degenerative central nervous system disorders. Associated findings include dementia, tremor, rigidity, and gait disturbance.

◆ ***Diabetes mellitus.*** Insidious, permanent anosmia may occur along with fatigue, polyuria, polydipsia, weight loss, polyphagia, and weakness.

◆ ***Head trauma.*** Permanent anosmia may follow damage to the olfactory nerve. Associated findings depend on the type and severity of the trauma but may include epistaxis, headache, nausea and vomiting, altered level of consciousness, blurred or double vision, raccoon eyes, Battle's sign, and otorrhea.

◆ ***Lead poisoning.*** Anosmia due to lead poisoning may be permanent or temporary, depending on the extent of damage to the nasal mucosa. Associated findings include abdominal pain, weakness, headache, nausea, vomiting, constipation, wristdrop or footdrop, lead line on the gums, metallic taste, seizures, delirium, and possibly coma.

◆ ***Lethal midline granuloma.*** Permanent anosmia accompanies lethal midline granuloma—a slowly progressive disease. Examination reveals ulcerative granulation tissue in the nose, sinuses, and palate; widespread crust formation and tissue necrosis; septal cartilage destruction; and possibly purulent rhinorrhea, serous otitis media, and inflammation of the eyelids and lacrimal apparatus.

◆ ***Neoplasms (brain, nasal, or sinus).*** Anosmia may be permanent if the neoplasm destroys or displaces the olfactory nerve. Associated signs and symptoms include unilateral or bilateral epistaxis, swelling and tenderness in the affected area, visual disturbances, decreased tearing, and elevated intracranial pressure.

◆ ***Pernicious anemia.*** Anosmia from pernicious anemia may be temporary or permanent and is accompanied by the classic triad of weakness; sore, pale tongue; and numbness and tingling in the extremities. Related findings include distortion of taste, pallor, headache, irritability, dizziness, nausea, vomiting, diarrhea, and shortness of breath.

Understanding the sense of smell

Our noses can distinguish the odors of thousands of chemicals, thanks to a highly developed complex of sensory cells. The olfactory epithelium contains olfactory receptor cells, along with olfactory glands and sustentacular cells, both of which secrete mucus to keep the epithelial surface moist. The mucus covering the olfactory cells probably traps airborne odorous molecules, which then fit into the appropriate receptors on the cell surface. In response to this stimulus, the receptor cell then transmits an impulse along the olfactory nerve (cranial nerve I) to the olfactory area of the cortex, where it's interpreted. Any disruption along this transmission pathway, or any obstruction of the epithelial surface due to dryness or congestion, can cause anosmia.

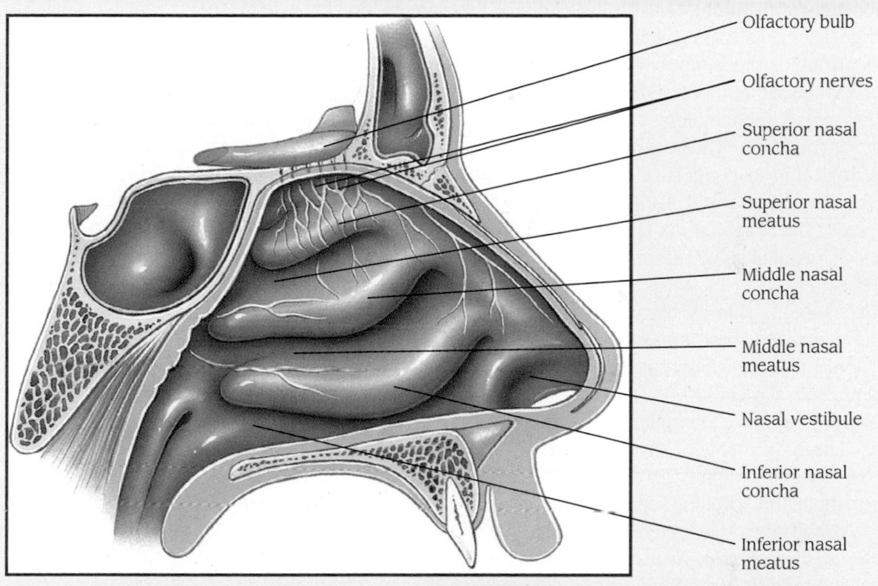

CLOSE-UP OF SENSORY CELLS

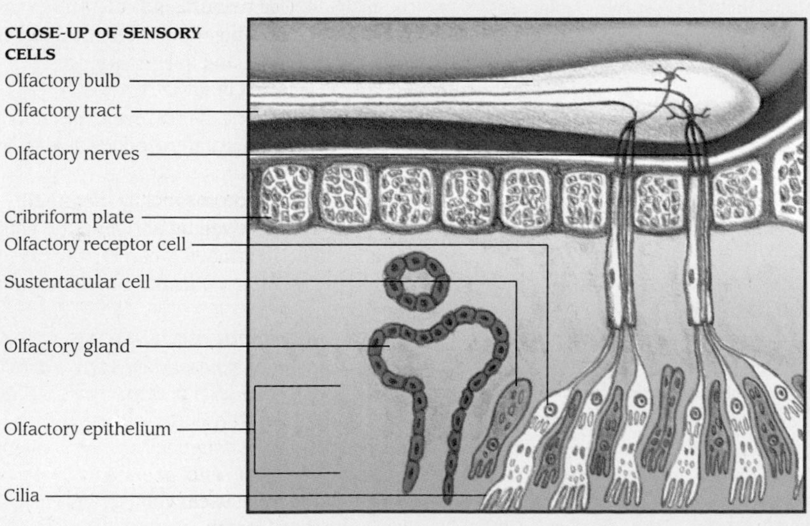

◆ ***Polyps.*** Temporary anosmia occurs when multiple polyps obstruct nasal cavities. Examination reveals the smooth, pale, grapelike polyp clusters.

◆ ***Rhinitis.*** In common acute viral rhinitis, temporary anosmia occurs with nasal congestion; sneezing; watery or purulent nasal discharge; red, swollen nasal mucosa; dryness or a tickling sensation in the nasopharynx; headache; low-grade fever; and chills.

In allergic rhinitis, temporary anosmia accompanies nasal congestion; itching mucosa; pale, edematous turbinates; thin nasal discharge; sneezing; tearing; and headache.

In atrophic rhinitis, anosmia resolves with successful treatment of the disorder. Purulent, yellow-green, foul-smelling crusts on sclerotic mucous membranes are characteristic, with paradoxical nasal congestion in an airway that's more open than normal. Turbinates are thin and atrophic. The nasopharynx and pharynx appear smooth, dry, and shiny rather than pink and moist.

In vasomotor rhinitis, temporary anosmia is accompanied by chronic nasal congestion, watery nasal discharge, postnasal drip, sneezing, and pale nasal mucosa.

◆ ***Septal fracture.*** Anosmia is usually temporary, caused by airflow obstruction, and returns with septal repositioning. Examination reveals septal deviation, swelling, epistaxis, hematoma, nasal congestion, and ecchymoses.

◆ ***Septal hematoma.*** Anosmia is temporary, resolving with repair of the nasal mucosa or absorption of the hematoma. Associated signs and symptoms include epistaxis; dusky red, inflamed nasal mucosa; headache; and mouth breathing.

◆ ***Sinusitis.*** Temporary anosmia may be associated with nasal congestion; sinus pain, tenderness, and swelling; severe headache; watery or purulent nasal discharge; postnasal drip; inflamed throat and nasal mucosa; enlarged, purulent turbinates; malaise; low-grade fever; and chills.

Other causes

◆ ***Drugs.*** Anosmia can result from prolonged use of nasal decongestants, which produces rebound nasal congestion. Occasionally, it results from naphazoline, a local decongestant that may paralyze nasal cilia. It can also result from reserpine and, less commonly, amphetamines, phenothiazines, and estrogen, which cause nasal congestion.

◆ ***Radiation therapy.*** Permanent anosmia may follow radiation damage to the nasal mucosa or olfactory nerve.

◆ ***Surgery.*** Temporary anosmia may result from damage to the olfactory nerve or nasal mucosa during nasal or sinus surgery. Permanent anosmia accompanies a permanent tracheostomy, which disrupts nasal breathing.

Special considerations

If anosmia results from nasal congestion, administer a local decongestant or an antihistamine, and provide a vaporizer or humidifier to prevent mucosal drying and to help thin purulent nasal discharge. Advise the patient to avoid excessive use of local decongestants, which can lead to rebound nasal congestion.

If anosmia doesn't result from simple nasal congestion, prepare the patient for diagnostic tests, such as sinus transillumination, skull X-ray, or computed tomography scan.

Although permanent anosmia usually doesn't respond to treatment, vitamin A given orally or by injection occasionally provides improvement.

Pediatric pointers

Anosmia in children usually results from nasal obstruction by a foreign body or enlarged adenoids.

Anuria

Clinically defined as urine output of less than 100 ml in 24 hours, anuria indicates either urinary tract obstruction or acute renal failure due to various mechanisms. (See *Major causes of acute renal failure*.)

Fortunately, anuria is rare; even with renal failure, the kidneys usually produce at least 75 ml of urine daily.

Because urine output is easily measured, anuria rarely goes undetected. However, without immediate treatment, it can rapidly cause uremia and other complications of urine retention.

EMERGENCY INTERVENTIONS *After detecting anuria, your priorities are to determine if urine formation is occurring and to intervene appropriately. Prepare to catheterize the patient to relieve any lower urinary tract obstruction and to check for residual urine. You may find that an obstruction hinders catheter insertion and* *that urine return is cloudy and foul smelling. If you collect more than 75 ml of urine, suspect lower urinary tract obstruction; if you collect less than 75 ml, suspect renal dysfunction or obstruction higher in the urinary tract.*

History and physical examination

Take the patient's vital signs and obtain a complete history. First ask about any changes in his voiding pattern. Determine the amount of fluid he normally ingests each day, the amount of fluid he ingested in the last 24 to 48 hours, and the time and amount of his last urination. Review his medical history, noting especially previous kidney disease, urinary tract obstruction or infection, prostate enlargement, renal calculi, neurogenic bladder, or congenital abnormalities. Ask about drug use and about any abdominal, renal, or urinary tract surgery.

Inspect and palpate the abdomen for asymmetry, distention, or bulging. Inspect the flank area for edema or erythema, and percuss and palpate the bladder. Palpate the kidneys both anteriorly and posteriorly, and percuss them at the costovertebral angle. Auscultate over the renal arteries, listening for bruits.

Major causes of acute renal failure

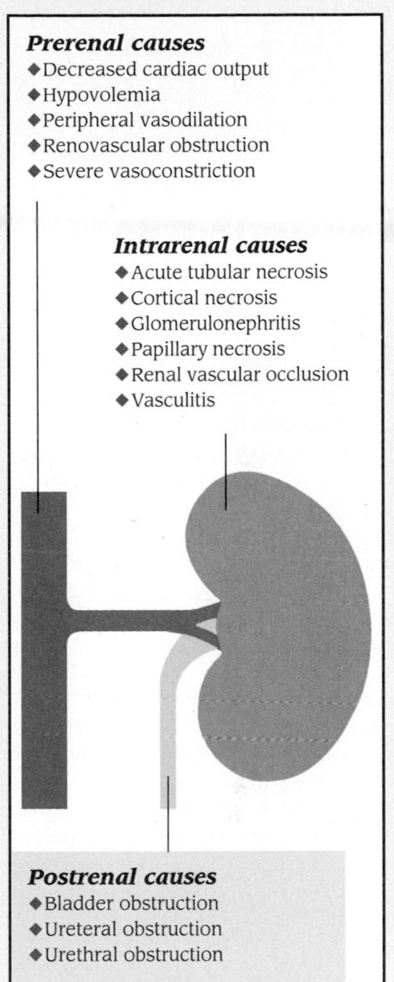

Prerenal causes
◆Decreased cardiac output
◆Hypovolemia
◆Peripheral vasodilation
◆Renovascular obstruction
◆Severe vasoconstriction
Intrarenal causes
◆Acute tubular necrosis
◆Cortical necrosis
◆Glomerulonephritis
◆Papillary necrosis
◆Renal vascular occlusion
◆Vasculitis
Postrenal causes
◆Bladder obstruction
◆Ureteral obstruction
◆Urethral obstruction

Medical causes

◆ ***Acute tubular necrosis.*** Oliguria (occasionally anuria) is a common finding in acute tubular necrosis. It precedes the onset of diuresis, which is heralded by polyuria. Associated findings reflect the underlying cause and may include signs and symptoms of hyperkalemia (muscle weakness, cardiac arrhythmias), uremia (anorexia, nausea, vomiting, confusion, lethargy, twitching, seizures, pruritus, uremic frost, and Kussmaul's respirations), and heart failure (edema, jugular vein distention, crackles, and dyspnea).

◆ ***Cortical necrosis (bilateral).*** Cortical necrosis is characterized by a sudden change from oliguria to anuria along with gross hematuria, flank pain, and fever.

◆ ***Glomerulonephritis (acute).*** Glomerulonephritis produces anuria or oliguria. Related effects include mild fever, malaise, flank pain, gross hematuria, facial and generalized edema, elevated blood pressure, headache, nausea, vomiting, abdominal pain, and signs and symptoms of pulmonary congestion (crackles, dyspnea).

◆ ***Hemolytic-uremic syndrome.*** Anuria commonly occurs in the initial stages of hemolytic-uremic syndrome and may last from 1 to 10 days. The patient may experience vomiting, diarrhea, abdominal pain, hematemesis, melena, purpura, fever, elevated blood pressure, hepatomegaly, ecchymoses, edema, hematuria, and pallor. He may also show signs of upper respiratory tract infection.

◆ ***Papillary necrosis (acute).*** Bilateral papillary necrosis produces anuria or oliguria as well as flank pain, costovertebral angle tenderness, renal colic, abdominal pain and rigidity, fever, vomiting, decreased bowel sounds, hematuria, and pyuria.

◆ ***Renal artery occlusion (bilateral).*** Renal artery occlusion produces anuria or severe oliguria, commonly accompanied by severe, continuous upper abdominal and flank pain; nausea and vomiting; decreased bowel sounds; fever up to 102° F (38.9° C); and diastolic hypertension.

◆ ***Renal vein occlusion (bilateral).*** Renal vein occlusion occasionally causes anuria; more typical signs and symptoms include acute low back pain, fever, flank tenderness, and hematuria. Development of pulmonary emboli—a common complication—produces sudden dyspnea, pleuritic pain, tachypnea, tachycardia, crackles, pleural friction rub, and possibly hemoptysis.

◆ ***Urinary tract obstruction.*** Severe obstruction can produce acute and sometimes total anuria alternating with or preceded by burning and pain on urination, overflow incontinence or dribbling, increased urinary frequency and nocturia, voiding of small amounts, or altered urine stream. Associated findings include bladder distention, pain and a sensation of fullness in the lower abdomen and groin, upper abdominal and flank pain, nausea and vomiting, and signs of secondary infection, such as fever, chills, malaise, and cloudy, foul-smelling urine.

◆ ***Vasculitis.*** Vasculitis occasionally produces anuria. More typical findings include malaise, myalgia, polyarthralgia, fever, elevated blood pressure, hematuria, proteinuria, arrhythmias, pallor, and possibly skin lesions, urticaria, and purpura.

Other causes

◆ ***Diagnostic tests.*** Contrast media used in radiographic studies can cause nephrotoxicity, producing oliguria and, rarely, anuria.

◆ ***Drugs.*** Many classes of drugs can cause anuria or, more commonly, oliguria through their nephrotoxic effects. Antibiotics, especially the aminoglycosides, are the most commonly seen nephrotoxins. Anesthetics, heavy metals, ethyl alcohol, and organic solvents can also be nephrotoxic. Adrenergics and anticholinergics can cause anuria by affecting the nerves and muscles of micturition to produce urine retention.

Special considerations

If catheterization fails to initiate urine flow, prepare the patient for diagnostic studies—such as ultrasonography, cystoscopy, retrograde pyelography, and renal scan—to detect any obstruction higher in the urinary tract. If these tests reveal an obstruction, prepare him for immediate surgery to remove the obstruction, and insert a nephrostomy or ureterostomy tube to drain the urine. If these tests fail to reveal an obstruction, prepare the patient for further kidney function studies.

Carefully monitor the patient's vital signs and intake and output, saving urine for inspection as appropriate. Restrict the daily fluid allowance to 600 ml more than the previous day's total urine output. Restrict foods and juices high in potassium and sodium, and make sure the patient maintains a balanced diet with controlled protein levels. Provide low-sodium hard candy to help decrease thirst. Record fluid intake and output, and weigh the patient daily.

Pediatric pointers

In neonates, anuria is defined as the absence of urine output for 24 hours. It can be classified as primary or secondary. Primary anuria results from bilateral renal agenesis, aplasia, or multicystic dysplasia. Secondary anuria, associated with edema or dehydration, results from renal ischemia, renal vein thrombosis, or congenital anomalies of the genitourinary tract. Anuria in children commonly results from loss of renal function.

Geriatric pointers

In elderly patients, anuria is a gradually occurring sign of underlying pathology. Hospitalized or bedridden elderly patients may be unable to generate the necessary pressure to void if they remain in a supine position.

Anxiety

Anxiety is the most common psychiatric symptom and can result in significant impairment. A subjective reaction to a real or imagined threat, anxiety is a nonspecific feeling of uneasiness or dread. It may be mild, moderate, or severe. Mild anxiety may cause slight physical or psychological discomfort. Severe anxiety may be incapacitating or even life-threatening.

Everyone experiences anxiety from time to time—it's a normal response to actual danger, prompting the body (through stimulation of the sympathetic and parasympathetic nervous systems) to purposeful action. It's also a normal response to physical and emotional stress, which can be produced by virtually any illness. In addition, anxiety can be precipitated or exacerbated by many nonpathologic factors, including lack of sleep, poor diet, and excessive intake of caffeine or other stimulants. However, excessive unwarranted anxiety may indicate an underlying psychological problem.

History and physical examination

If the patient displays acute, severe anxiety, quickly take his vital signs and determine his chief complaint; this will serve as a guide for how to proceed. For example, if the patient's anxiety occurs with chest pain and shortness of breath, you might suspect myocardial infarction and act accordingly. While examining the patient, try to keep him calm. Suggest relaxation techniques, and talk to him in a reassuring, soothing voice. Uncontrolled anxiety can alter vital signs and exacerbate the causative disorder.

If the patient displays mild or moderate anxiety, ask about its duration. Is the anxiety constant or sporadic? Did he notice any precipitating factors? Find out if the anxiety is exacerbated by stress, lack of sleep, or excessive caffeine intake and alleviated by rest, tranquilizers, or exercise.

Obtain a complete medical history, especially noting drug use. Then perform a physical examination, focusing on any complaints that may trigger or be aggravated by anxiety.

If the patient's anxiety isn't accompanied by significant physical signs, suspect a psychological cause. Determine the patient's level of consciousness (LOC) and observe his behavior. If appropriate, refer the patient for psychiatric evaluation.

Medical causes

◆ ***Acute respiratory distress syndrome.*** Acute anxiety occurs along with tachycardia, mental sluggishness and, in severe cases, hypotension. Respiratory signs and symptoms include dyspnea, tachypnea, intercostal and suprasternal retractions, crackles, and rhonchi.

◆ ***Anaphylactic shock.*** Acute anxiety is usually the first sign of anaphylactic shock. It's accompanied by urticaria, angioedema, pruritus, and shortness of breath. Soon, other signs and symptoms develop: light-headedness, hypotension, tachycardia, nasal congestion, sneezing, wheezing, dyspnea, barking cough, abdominal cramps, vomiting, diarrhea, and urinary urgency and incontinence.

◆ ***Angina pectoris.*** Acute anxiety may either precede or follow an attack of angina pectoris. An attack produces sharp and crushing substernal or anterior chest pain that may radiate to the back, neck, arms, or jaw. The pain may be relieved by nitroglycerin or rest, which eases anxiety.

◆ ***Asthma.*** In allergic asthma attacks, acute anxiety occurs with dyspnea, wheezing, productive cough, accessory muscle use, hyperresonant lung fields, diminished breath sounds, coarse crackles, cyanosis, tachycardia, and diaphoresis.

◆ ***Autonomic hyperreflexia.*** The earliest signs of autonomic hyperreflexia may be acute anxiety accompanied by a severe headache and dramatic hypertension. Pallor and motor and sensory deficits occur below the level of the lesion; flushing occurs above it.

◆ ***Cardiogenic shock.*** Acute anxiety is accompanied by cool, pale, clammy skin; tachycardia; weak, thready pulse; tachypnea; ventricular gallop; crackles; jugular vein distention; decreased urine output; hypotension; narrowing pulse pressure; and peripheral edema.

◆ ***Chronic obstructive pulmonary disease (COPD).*** Acute anxiety, exertional dyspnea, cough, wheezing, crackles, hyperresonant lung fields, tachypnea, and accessory muscle use characterize COPD.

◆ ***Heart failure.*** In heart failure, acute anxiety is commonly the first symptom of inadequate oxygenation. Associated findings include restlessness, shortness of breath, tachypnea, decreased LOC, edema, crackles, ventricular gallop, hypotension, diaphoresis, and cyanosis.

◆ ***Hyperthyroidism.*** Acute anxiety may be an early sign of hyperthyroidism. Classic signs and symptoms include heat intolerance, weight loss despite increased appetite, nervousness, tremor, palpitations, diaphoresis, an enlarged thyroid, and diarrhea. Exophthalmos also may occur.

◆ ***Hyperventilation syndrome.*** Hyperventilation syndrome produces acute anxiety, pallor, circumoral and peripheral paresthesia and, occasionally, carpopedal spasms.
◆ ***Hypochondriasis.*** Mild to moderate chronic anxiety occurs in hypochondriasis. The patient focuses more on the belief that he has a specific serious disease rather than on the actual symptoms. Difficulty swallowing, back pain, light-headedness, and upset stomach are common complaints. The patient tends to "physician hop" and isn't reassured by favorable physical examinations and laboratory test results.
◆ ***Hypoglycemia.*** Anxiety resulting from hypoglycemia is usually mild to moderate and associated with hunger, mild headache, palpitations, blurred vision, weakness, and diaphoresis.
◆ ***Mitral valve prolapse.*** Panic may occur in patients with this valvular disorder, also known as *click-murmur syndrome* because its hallmark is a midsystolic click, followed by an apical systolic murmur. Mitral valve prolapse also may cause paroxysmal palpitations accompanied by sharp, stabbing, or aching precordial pain.
◆ ***Mood disorder.*** Anxiety may be the patient's chief complaint in the depressive or manic form of mood disorder. In the depressive form, chronic anxiety of varying severity occurs along with dysphoria; anger; insomnia or hypersomnia; decreased libido, interest, energy, and concentration; appetite disturbance; multiple somatic complaints; and suicidal thoughts. In the manic form, the patient's chief complaint may be a reduced need for sleep, hyperactivity, increased energy, rapid or pressured speech and, in severe cases, paranoid ideas and other psychotic symptoms.
◆ ***Myocardial infarction (MI).*** In this life-threatening disorder, acute anxiety commonly occurs with persistent, crushing substernal pain that may radiate to the left arm, jaw, neck, or shoulder blades. MI may be accompanied by shortness of breath, nausea, vomiting, diaphoresis, and cool, pale skin.
◆ ***Obsessive-compulsive disorder.*** Chronic anxiety occurs in obsessive-compulsive disorder, which is marked by recurrent, unshakable thoughts or impulses to perform ritualistic acts. The patient recognizes these acts as irrational but is unable to control them. Anxiety builds if he can't perform these acts and diminishes after he does.
◆ ***Pheochromocytoma.*** Acute, severe anxiety accompanies pheochromocytoma's cardinal sign: persistent or paroxysmal hypertension. Other common findings include tachycardia, diaphoresis, orthostatic hypotension, tachypnea, flushing, severe headache, palpitations, nausea, vomiting, epigastric pain, and paresthesia.
◆ ***Phobias.*** In phobias, chronic anxiety accompanies persistent fear of an object, an activity, or a situation that results in a compelling desire to avoid it. The patient recognizes the fear as irrational but can't suppress it.
◆ ***Pneumonia.*** Acute anxiety may occur in pneumonia because of hypoxemia. Other findings include productive cough, pleuritic chest pain, fever, chills, crackles, diminished breath sounds, and hyperresonant lung fields.
◆ ***Pneumothorax.*** Acute anxiety occurs in moderate to severe pneumothorax associated with profound respiratory distress. It's accompanied by sharp pleuritic pain, coughing, shortness of breath, cyanosis, asymmetrical chest expansion, pallor, jugular vein distention, and a weak, rapid pulse.
◆ ***Postconcussion syndrome.*** Postconcussion syndrome may produce chronic anxiety or periodic attacks of acute anxiety. The anxiety is usually most pronounced in situations demanding attention, judgment, or comprehension. Associated signs and symptoms include irritability, insomnia, dizziness, and mild headache.
◆ ***Posttraumatic stress disorder.*** Posttraumatic stress disorder occurs in patients who have experienced an extremely traumatic event. It produces chronic anxiety of varying severity and is accompanied by intrusive, vivid memories and thoughts of the traumatic event. The patient also relives the event in dreams and nightmares. Insomnia, depression, and feelings of numbness and detachment are common.
◆ ***Pulmonary edema.*** In pulmonary edema, acute anxiety occurs with dyspnea, orthopnea, cough with frothy sputum, tachycardia, tachypnea, crackles, ventricular gallop, hypotension, and thready pulse. The patient's skin may be cool, clammy, and cyanotic.
◆ ***Pulmonary embolism.*** Acute anxiety is usually accompanied by dyspnea, tachypnea, chest pain, tachycardia, blood-tinged sputum, and low-grade fever.
◆ ***Rabies.*** Anxiety signals the beginning of the acute phase of rabies. This rare disorder is

characterized by painful laryngeal spasms associated with difficulty swallowing and, as a result, hydrophobia.

◆ ***Somatoform disorder.*** Somatoform disorder, which usually begins in young adulthood, is characterized by anxiety and multiple somatic complaints that can't be explained physiologically. The symptoms aren't produced intentionally but are severe enough to significantly impair functioning. Pain disorder, conversion disorder, and hypochondriasis are examples of somatoform disorder.

OTHER CAUSES

◆ ***Drugs.*** Many drugs cause anxiety, especially sympathomimetics and central nervous system stimulants. In addition, many antidepressants may cause paradoxical anxiety.

SPECIAL CONSIDERATIONS

Supportive care can help relieve anxiety in many cases. Provide a calm, quiet atmosphere and make the patient comfortable. Encourage him to express his feelings and concerns freely. If it helps, take a short walk with him while you're talking. Anxiety-reducing measures, such as distraction, relaxation techniques, and biofeedback, may also be helpful.

PEDIATRIC POINTERS

Anxiety in children usually results from painful physical illness or inadequate oxygenation. Its autonomic signs tend to be more common and dramatic than in adults.

GERIATRIC POINTERS

Changes in an elderly patient's routine may provoke anxiety or agitation.

Aphasia

[Dysphasia]

Aphasia, impaired expression or comprehension of written or spoken language, reflects disease or injury of the brain's language centers. (See *Where language originates,* page 58.) Depending on its severity, aphasia may slightly impede communication or may make it impossible. It can be classified as Broca's, Wernicke's, anomic, or global aphasia. Anomic aphasia eventually resolves in more than 50% of patients, but global aphasia is usually irreversible. (See *Identifying types of aphasia,* page 59.)

EMERGENCY INTERVENTIONS *Quickly look for signs and symptoms of increased intracranial pressure (ICP), such as pupillary changes, decreased level of consciousness (LOC), vomiting, seizures, bradycardia, widening pulse pressure, and irregular respirations. If you detect signs of increased ICP, administer mannitol I.V. to decrease cerebral edema. In addition, make sure that emergency resuscitation equipment is readily available to support respiratory and cardiac function, if necessary. You may have to prepare the patient for emergency surgery.*

HISTORY AND PHYSICAL EXAMINATION

If the patient doesn't display signs of increased ICP, or if his aphasia has developed gradually, perform a thorough neurologic examination, starting with the patient history. You'll probably need to obtain this history from the patient's family or companion because of the patient's impairment. Ask if the patient has a history of headaches, hypertension, seizure disorders, or drug use. Also ask about the patient's ability to communicate and perform routine activities before he developed aphasia.

Check for obvious signs of neurologic deficit, such as ptosis or fluid leakage from the nose and ears. Take the patient's vital signs and assess his LOC. Be aware, though, that the patient's verbal responses may be unreliable, making LOC assessment difficult. Also, recognize that dysarthria (impaired articulation due to weakness or paralysis of the muscles necessary for speech) or speech apraxia (inability to voluntarily control the muscles of speech) may accompany aphasia, so speak slowly and distinctly, and allow the patient ample time to respond. Assess the patient's pupillary response, eye movements, and motor function, especially his mouth and tongue movement, swallowing ability, and spontaneous movements and gestures. To best assess motor function, first demonstrate the motions and then have the patient imitate them.

MEDICAL CAUSES

◆ ***Alzheimer's disease.*** In this degenerative disease, anomic aphasia may begin insidiously and then progress to severe global aphasia. Associated signs and symptoms include behavioral changes, loss of memory, poor judgment,

Where language originates

Aphasia reflects damage to one or more of the brain's primary language centers, which, in most people, are located in the left hemisphere. *Broca's area* lies next to the region of the motor cortex that controls the muscles necessary for speech. *Wernicke's area* is the center of auditory, visual, and language comprehension. It lies between *Heschl's gyrus*, the primary receiver of auditory stimuli, and the angular gyrus, a "way station" between the brain's auditory and visual regions. Connecting Wernicke's and Broca's areas is a large nerve bundle, the *arcuate fasciculus*, which allows repetition of speech.

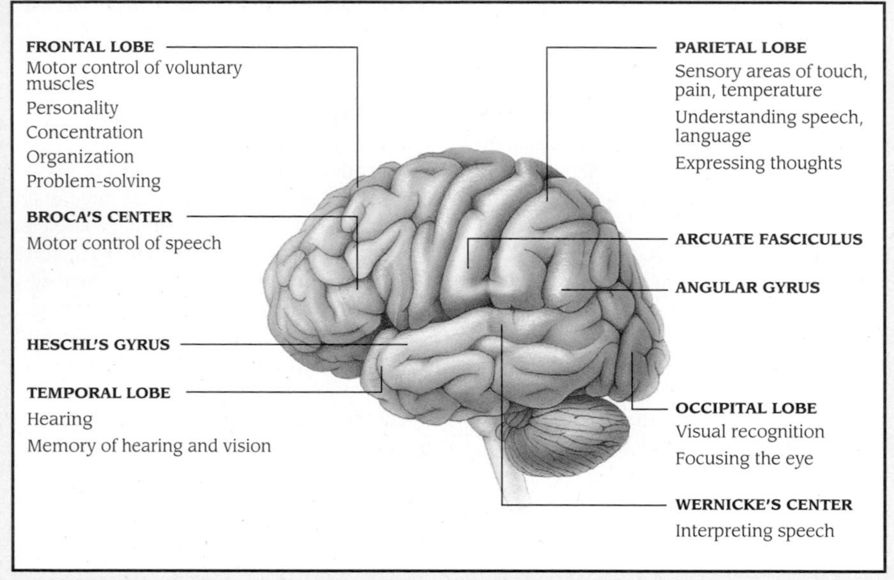

restlessness, myoclonus, and muscle rigidity. Incontinence is usually a late sign.

◆ ***Brain abscess.*** A brain abscess may cause any type of aphasia. Aphasia usually develops insidiously and may be accompanied by hemiparesis, ataxia, facial weakness, and signs of increased ICP.

◆ ***Brain tumor.*** A brain tumor may cause any type of aphasia. As the tumor enlarges, other types of aphasia may occur along with behavioral changes, memory loss, motor weakness, seizures, auditory hallucinations, visual field deficits, and increased ICP.

◆ ***Creutzfeldt-Jakob disease.*** Creutzfeldt-Jakob disease is a rapidly progressive dementia accompanied by neurologic signs and symptoms, such as myoclonic jerking, ataxia, aphasia, visual disturbances, and paralysis. It generally affects adults ages 40 to 65.

◆ ***Encephalitis.*** Encephalitis usually produces transient aphasia. Its early signs and symptoms include fever, headache, and vomiting. Seizures, confusion, stupor or coma, hemiparesis, asymmetrical deep tendon reflexes, positive Babinski's reflex, ataxia, myoclonus, nystagmus, ocular palsies, and facial weakness may accompany aphasia.

◆ ***Head trauma.*** Severe head trauma may cause any type of aphasia, which typically occurs suddenly and may be transient or permanent, depending on the extent of brain damage. Associated signs and symptoms include blurred or double vision, headache, pallor, diaphoresis, numbness and paresis, cerebrospinal otorrhea or rhinorrhea, altered respirations, tachycardia, disorientation, behavioral changes, and signs of increased ICP.

◆ ***Seizures.*** Seizures and the postictal state may cause transient aphasia if the seizures involve the language centers.

◆ ***Stroke.*** The most common cause of aphasia, stroke may produce Wernicke's, Broca's, or

Identifying types of aphasia

Type	Location of lesion	Signs and symptoms
Anomic aphasia	Temporal-parietal area; may extend to angular gyrus, but sometimes poorly localized	Patient's understanding of written and spoken language is relatively unimpaired. His speech, although fluent, lacks meaningful content. Word-finding difficulty and circumlocution are characteristic. Rarely, the patient also displays paraphasias.
Broca's aphasia (expressive aphasia)	Broca's area; usually in third frontal convolution of the left hemisphere	Patient's understanding of written and spoken language is relatively spared, but speech is nonfluent, with word-finding difficulty, jargon, paraphasias, limited vocabulary, and simple sentence construction. The patient can't repeat words and phrases. If Wernicke's area is intact, he recognizes speech errors and shows frustration. Hemiparesis is common.
Global aphasia	Broca's and Wernicke's areas	Patient's receptive and expressive ability is profoundly impaired. He can't repeat words or phrases and can't follow directions. His occasional speech is marked by paraphasias or jargon.
Wernicke's aphasia (receptive aphasia)	Wernicke's area; usually in posterior or superior temporal lobe	Patient has difficulty understanding written and spoken language. He can't repeat words or phrases and can't follow directions. His speech is fluent but may be rapid and rambling, with paraphasias. He has difficulty naming objects (anomia) and is unaware of speech errors.

global aphasia. Associated findings include decreased LOC, right-sided hemiparesis, homonymous hemianopia, paresthesia, and loss of sensation. (These signs and symptoms may appear on the left side if the right hemisphere contains the language centers.)

◆ ***Transient ischemic attack (TIA).*** TIA can produce any type of aphasia, which occurs suddenly and resolves within 24 hours of the attack. Associated signs and symptoms include transient hemiparesis, hemianopia, and paresthesia (all usually right-sided) as well as dizziness and confusion.

Special considerations

Immediately after aphasia develops, the patient may become confused or disoriented. Help to restore a sense of reality by frequently telling him what has happened, where he is and why, and what the date is. Carefully explain diagnostic tests, such as skull X-rays, computed tomography scan or magnetic resonance imaging, angiography, and EEG. Later, expect periods of depression as the patient recognizes his disability. Help him to communicate by providing a relaxed, accepting environment with a minimum of distracting stimuli.

Be alert for sudden outbursts of profanity by the patient. This common behavior usually reflects intense frustration with his impairment. Deal with such outbursts as gently as possible to minimize embarrassment.

When you speak to the patient, don't assume that he understands you. He may simply be interpreting subtle clues to meaning, such as social context, facial expressions, and gestures. To help avoid misunderstanding, use nonverbal techniques, speak to him in simple phrases, and use demonstration to clarify your verbal directions.

Remember that aphasia is a language disorder, not an emotional or auditory one, so speak to the patient in a normal tone of voice. Make sure he has necessary aids, such as eyeglasses or dentures, to facilitate communication. Refer the patient to a speech pathologist early to help him cope with his aphasia.

PEDIATRIC POINTERS

Recognize that the term *childhood aphasia* is sometimes mistakenly applied to children who fail to develop normal language skills but who aren't considered mentally retarded or developmentally delayed. *Aphasia* refers solely to loss of previously developed communication skills.

Brain damage associated with aphasia in children most commonly follows anoxia— the result of near drowning or airway obstruction.

Apnea

Apnea, the cessation of spontaneous respiration, is occasionally temporary and self-limiting, as in Cheyne-Stokes and Biot's respirations. In most cases, though, it's a life-threatening emergency that requires immediate intervention to prevent death.

Apnea usually results from one or more of six pathophysiologic mechanisms, each of which has numerous causes. Its most common causes include trauma, cardiac arrest, neurologic disease, aspiration of foreign objects, bronchospasm, and drug overdose. (See *Causes of apnea.*)

EMERGENCY INTERVENTIONS *If you detect apnea, first establish and maintain a patent airway. Place the patient in a supine position, and open his airway using the head-tilt, chin-lift technique. (*Caution: *If the patient has or may have a head or neck injury, use the jaw-thrust technique to prevent hyperextending the neck.) Next, quickly look, listen, and feel for spontaneous respiration; if it's absent, begin artificial ventilation until it occurs or until mechanical ventilation can be initiated.*

Because apnea may result from (or may cause) cardiac arrest, assess the patient's carotid pulse immediately after you've established a patent airway. Or, if the patient is an infant or small child, assess the brachial pulse instead. If you can't palpate a pulse, begin cardiac compression.

HISTORY AND PHYSICAL EXAMINATION

When the patient's respiratory and cardiac status is stable, investigate the underlying cause of apnea. Ask him (or, if he's unable to answer, anyone who witnessed the episode) about the onset of apnea and events immediately preceding it. The cause may become readily apparent, as in trauma.

Take a patient history, especially noting reports of headache, chest pain, muscle weakness, sore throat, or dyspnea. Ask about a history of respiratory, cardiac, or neurologic disease and about allergies and drug use.

Inspect the head, face, neck, and trunk for soft-tissue injury, hemorrhage, or skeletal deformity. Don't overlook obvious clues, such as oral and nasal secretions (reflecting fluid-filled airways and alveoli) or facial soot and singed nasal hair (suggesting thermal injury to the tracheobronchial tree).

Auscultate over all lung lobes for adventitious breath sounds, particularly crackles and rhonchi, and percuss the lung fields for increased dullness or hyperresonance. Move on to the heart, auscultating for murmurs, pericardial friction rub, and arrhythmias. Check for cyanosis, pallor, jugular vein distention, and edema. If appropriate, perform a neurologic assessment. Evaluate level of consciousness (LOC), orientation, and mental status; test cranial nerve and motor function, sensation, and reflexes in all extremities.

MEDICAL CAUSES

◆ ***Airway obstruction.*** Occlusion or compression of the trachea, central airways, or smaller airways can cause sudden apnea by blocking the patient's airflow and producing acute respiratory failure.

◆ ***Brain stem dysfunction.*** Primary or secondary brain stem dysfunction can cause apnea by destroying the brain stem's ability to initiate respirations. Apnea may arise suddenly (as in trauma, hemorrhage, or infarction) or gradually (as in degenerative disease or tumor). Apnea may be preceded by decreased LOC and various motor and sensory deficits.

◆ ***Neuromuscular failure.*** Trauma or disease can disrupt the mechanics of respiration, causing sudden or gradual apnea. Associated findings include diaphragmatic or intercostal muscle paralysis from injury, or respiratory

Causes of apnea

Various disorders may cause apnea.

Airway obstruction
- Asthma
- Bronchospasm
- Chronic bronchitis
- Chronic obstructive pulmonary disease
- Foreign body aspiration
- Hemothorax or pneumothorax
- Mucus plug
- Obstruction by tongue or tumor
- Obstructive sleep apnea
- Secretion retention
- Tracheal or bronchial rupture

Brain stem dysfunction
- Brain abscess
- Brain stem injury
- Brain tumor
- Central nervous system depressants
- Central sleep apnea
- Cerebral hemorrhage
- Cerebral infarction
- Encephalitis
- Head trauma
- Increased intracranial pressure
- Medullary or pontine hemorrhage or infarction
- Meningitis
- Transtentorial herniation

Neuromuscular failure
- Amyotrophic lateral sclerosis
- Botulism
- Diphtheria
- Guillain-Barré syndrome
- Myasthenia gravis
- Phrenic nerve paralysis
- Rupture of the diaphragm
- Spinal cord injury

Parenchymatous disease
- Acute respiratory distress syndrome
- Diffuse pneumonia
- Emphysema
- Near drowning
- Pulmonary edema
- Pulmonary fibrosis
- Secretion retention

Pleural pressure gradient disruption
- Flail chest
- Open chest wounds

Pulmonary capillary perfusion decrease
- Arrhythmias
- Cardiac arrest
- Myocardial infarction
- Pulmonary embolism
- Pulmonary hypertension
- Shock

weakness or paralysis from acute or degenerative disease.

◆ ***Parenchymatous lung disease.*** An accumulation of fluid within the alveoli produces apnea by interfering with pulmonary gas exchange and producing acute respiratory failure. Apnea may arise suddenly, as in near drowning and acute pulmonary edema, or gradually, as in emphysema. Apnea also may be preceded by crackles and labored respirations with accessory muscle use.

◆ ***Pleural pressure gradient disruption.*** Conversion of normal negative pleural air pressure to positive pressure by chest wall injuries (such as flail chest) causes lung collapse, producing respiratory distress and, if untreated, apnea. Associated signs include an asymmetrical chest wall and asymmetrical or paradoxical respirations.

◆ ***Pulmonary capillary perfusion decrease.*** Apnea can stem from obstructed pulmonary circulation, most commonly due to heart failure or lack of circulatory patency. It occurs suddenly in cardiac arrest, massive pulmonary embolism, and most cases of severe shock; it occurs progressively in septic shock and pulmonary hypertension. Related findings include hypotension, tachycardia, and edema.

OTHER CAUSES

◆ ***Drugs.*** Central nervous system (CNS) depressants may cause hypoventilation and apnea. Benzodiazepines may cause respiratory depression and apnea when given I.V. along with other CNS depressants to elderly or acutely ill patients.

Neuromuscular blockers—such as curariform drugs and anticholinesterases— may produce sudden apnea due to respiratory muscle paralysis.

◆ ***Sleep-related apneas.*** These repetitive apneas occur during sleep from airflow obstruction or brain stem dysfunction.

SPECIAL CONSIDERATIONS

Closely monitor the apneic patient's cardiac and respiratory status to prevent further apneic episodes.

Pediatric pointers
Premature neonates are especially susceptible to periodic apneic episodes because of CNS immaturity. Other common causes of apnea in infants include sepsis, intraventricular and subarachnoid hemorrhage, seizures, bronchiolitis, and sudden infant death syndrome.

In toddlers and older children, the primary cause of apnea is acute airway obstruction from aspiration of foreign objects. Other causes include acute epiglottitis, croup, asthma, and systemic disorders, such as muscular dystrophy and cystic fibrosis.

Geriatric pointers
In elderly patients, increased sensitivity to analgesics, sedative-hypnotics, or any combination of these drugs may produce apnea, even with normal dosage ranges.

Patient counseling
Educate the patient about safety measures related to aspiration of medications. Encourage cardiopulmonary resuscitation training for all adolescents and adults.

Apneustic respirations

Apneustic respirations are characterized by prolonged, gasping inspiration with a pause at full inspiration. This irregular breathing pattern is an important localizing sign of severe brain stem damage.

Involuntary breathing is primarily regulated by groups of neurons located in respiratory centers in the medulla oblongata and the pons. In the medulla, neurons react to impulses from the pons and other areas to regulate respiratory rate and depth. In the pons, two respiratory centers regulate respiratory rhythm by interacting with the medullary respiratory center to smooth the transition from inspiration to expiration and back. The apneustic center in the pons stimulates inspiratory neurons in the medulla to precipitate inspiration. These inspiratory neurons, in turn, stimulate the pneumotaxic center in the pons to precipitate expiration. Destruction of neural pathways by pontine lesions disrupts normal regulation of respiratory rhythm, causing apneustic respirations.

Apneustic respirations must be differentiated from bradypnea and hyperpnea (disturbances in rate and depth, but not in rhythm), Cheyne-Stokes respirations (rhythmic alterations in rate and depth, followed by periods of apnea), and Biot's respirations (irregularly alternating periods of hyperpnea and apnea).

EMERGENCY INTERVENTIONS *Your first priority for a patient with apneustic respirations is to ensure adequate ventilation. You'll need to insert an artificial airway and administer oxygen until mechanical ventilation can begin. Next, thoroughly evaluate the patient's neurologic status, using a standardized tool such as the Glasgow Coma Scale. Finally, obtain a brief patient history from a family member, if possible.*

Medical causes
◆ ***Pontine lesions.*** Apneustic respirations usually result from extensive damage to the upper or lower pons due to infarction, hemorrhage, herniation, severe infection, tumor, or trauma. Typically, these respirations are accompanied by profound stupor or coma; pinpoint midline pupils; ocular bobbing (a spontaneous downward jerk, followed by a slow drift up to midline); quadriplegia or, less commonly, hemiplegia with the eyes pointing toward the weak side; a positive Babinski's reflex; negative oculocephalic and oculovestibular reflexes; and, possibly, decorticate posture.

Special considerations
Constantly monitor the patient's neurologic and respiratory status. Watch for prolonged apneic periods or signs of neurologic deterioration. Monitor the patient's arterial blood gas levels, or use a pulse oximetry device. If appropriate, prepare him for neurologic tests, such as EEG and computed tomography scan or magnetic resonance imaging.

Pediatric pointers
In young children, avoid using the Glasgow Coma Scale because it requires verbal responses and assumes a certain level of language development.

Apraxia

Apraxia is the inability to perform purposeful movements in the absence of significant weakness, sensory loss, poor coordination, or lack of comprehension or motivation. This neurologic

How apraxia interferes with purposeful movement

Type of apraxia	Description	Examination technique
Ideational apraxia	The patient can physically perform the steps required to complete a task but fails to remember the sequence in which they're performed.	Ask the patient to tie his shoelace. Typically, he'll be able to grasp the shoelace, loop it, and pull on it. However, he'll fail to remember the sequence of steps needed to tie a knot.
Ideomotor apraxia	The patient understands and can physically perform the steps required to complete a task but can't formulate a plan to carry them out.	Ask the patient to wave or cross his arms. Typically, he won't respond, but he may be able to spontaneously perform the gesture.
Kinetic apraxia	The patient understands the task and formulates a plan to complete it but fails to set the proper muscles in motion.	Ask the patient to comb his hair. Typically, he'll fail to move his arm and hand correctly to do so. However, he'll be able to state that he needs to pick up the comb and draw it through his hair.

sign usually indicates a lesion in the cerebral hemisphere. Its onset, severity, and duration vary.

Apraxia is classified as ideational, ideomotor, or kinetic, depending on the stage at which voluntary movement is impaired. It can also be classified by type of motor or skill impairment. For example, *facial apraxia* and *gait apraxia* involve specific motor groups and are easily perceived. *Constructional apraxia* refers to the inability to copy simple drawings or patterns. *Dressing apraxia* refers to the inability to correctly dress oneself. *Callosal apraxia* refers to normal motor function on one side of the body accompanied by the inability to reproduce movements on the other side. (See *How apraxia interferes with purposeful movement.*)

History and physical examination

If you detect apraxia, ask about previous neurologic disease. If the patient fails to report such disease, begin a neurologic assessment. First, take the patient's vital signs and assess his level of consciousness. Be alert for any evidence of aphasia or dysarthria. Ask the patient if he has recently experienced headaches or dizziness. Then test the patient's motor function, observing for weakness and tremors. Next, use a small pin or another pointed object to test sensory function. Check deep tendon reflexes for quality and symmetry. Finally, test the patient for visual field deficits.

Be alert for signs and symptoms of increased intracranial pressure (ICP), such as headache and vomiting. If you detect these, elevate the head of the bed 30 degrees and monitor the patient closely for altered pupil size and reactivity, bradycardia, widened pulse pressure, and irregular respirations. Have emergency resuscitation equipment nearby, and be prepared to give mannitol I.V. to decrease cerebral edema.

If the patient is experiencing seizures, stay with him and have another nurse notify the physician immediately. Avoid restraining the patient. Help him to a supine position, loosen tight clothing, and place a pillow or other soft object beneath his head. If the patient's teeth are clenched, don't force anything into his mouth. If his mouth is open, protect the tongue by placing a soft object, such as a washcloth, between his teeth. Turn the patient's head to provide an open airway.

After completing the examination and ensuring the patient's safety, take a history. Ask about previous cerebrovascular disease, atherosclerosis, neoplastic disease, infection, or hepatic disease. Then assess the apraxia further to help determine its type. (See *Apraxia: Causes and associated findings*, page 64.)

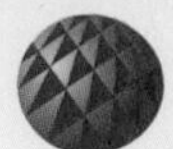

SIGNS & SYMPTOMS

Apraxia: Causes and associated findings

Common causes	Major associated signs and symptoms: Amnesia	Aphasia	Decreased level of consciousness	Decreased mental acuity	Dysarthria	Headache	Hyperreflexia	Incontinence	Seizures	Tremors	Visual field deficits
Alzheimer's disease	●	●						●		●	
Brain abscess		●		●	●	●	●	●	●		●
Brain tumor		●		●	●	●	●	●	●		●
Hepatic encephalopathy		●		●		●		●			●
Stroke		●	●		●	●		●			●

MEDICAL CAUSES

◆ ***Alzheimer's disease.*** Alzheimer's disease sometimes causes gradual and irreversible ideomotor apraxia. It can also cause amnesia, anomia, decreased attention span, apathy, aphasia, restlessness, agitation, paranoid delusions, incontinence, social withdrawal, ataxia, and tremors.

◆ ***Brain abscess.*** Apraxia occasionally results from a large brain abscess but usually resolves spontaneously after the infection subsides. Depending on the location of the abscess, apraxia may be accompanied by headache, fever, drowsiness, decreased mental acuity, aphasia, dysarthria, hemiparesis, hyperreflexia, incontinence, focal or generalized seizures, and ocular disturbances, such as nystagmus, visual field deficits, and unequal pupils.

◆ ***Brain tumor.*** In a brain tumor, progressive apraxia may be preceded by decreased mental acuity, headache, dizziness, and seizures. It may occur with or directly after early signs of increased ICP, such as pupil changes. It may also occur with other localizing signs and symptoms of the tumor, such as aphasia, dysarthria, visual field deficits, weakness, stiffness, and hyperreflexia in the extremities.

◆ ***Hepatic encephalopathy.*** Hepatic encephalopathy may cause gradual onset of constructional apraxia, which may be reversible with treatment. Early associated signs and symptoms include disorientation, amnesia, slurred speech, dysarthria, asterixis, and lethargy. Later signs include hyperreflexia, positive Babinski's reflex, agitation, seizures, fetor hepaticus, stupor, and coma.

◆ ***Stroke.*** Stroke commonly causes sudden onset of apraxia, which typically resolves spontaneously but may persist. Associated signs and symptoms vary according to the affected artery but can include headache, confusion, stupor or coma, hemiplegia, unilateral or bilateral visual field deficits, aphasia, agnosia, dysarthria, and urinary incontinence.

SPECIAL CONSIDERATIONS

Prepare the patient for diagnostic studies, such as computed tomography and radionuclide brain scans. Because weakness, sensory deficits, confusion, and seizures may accompany apraxia, take measures to ensure safety. For example, assist the patient with gait apraxia in walking.

Explain the patient's apraxia to him, and encourage his participation in normal activities. Help him to overcome his frustration at being

Causes of localized arm pain

Various disorders cause hand, wrist, elbow, or shoulder pain. In some disorders, pain may radiate from the injury site to other areas.

Hand pain

- Arthritis
- Buerger's disease
- Carpal tunnel syndrome
- Dupuytren's contracture
- Elbow tunnel syndrome
- Fracture
- Ganglion
- Infection
- Occlusive vascular disease
- Radiculopathy
- Raynaud's disease
- Shoulder-hand syndrome (reflex sympathetic dystrophy)
- Sprain or strain
- Thoracic outlet syndrome
- Trigger finger

Wrist pain

- Arthritis
- Carpal tunnel syndrome
- Fracture
- Ganglion
- Sprain or strain
- Tenosynovitis (de Quervain's disease)

Elbow pain

- Arthritis
- Bursitis
- Dislocation
- Fracture
- Lateral epicondylitis (tennis elbow)
- Tendinitis
- Ulnar neuritis

Shoulder pain

- Acromioclavicular separation
- Acute pancreatitis
- Adhesive capsulitis (frozen shoulder)
- Angina pectoris
- Arthritis
- Bursitis
- Cholecystitis or cholelithiasis
- Clavicle fracture
- Diaphragmatic pleurisy
- Dislocation
- Dissecting aortic aneurysm
- Gastritis
- Humeral neck fracture
- Infection
- Pancoast's syndrome
- Perforated ulcer
- Pneumothorax
- Ruptured spleen (left shoulder)
- Shoulder-hand syndrome
- Subphrenic abscess
- Tendinitis

unable to perform routine tasks by demonstrating each step in these tasks and giving him sufficient time to imitate each step. Avoid giving complex directions, and enlist the help of family members in rehabilitation. Also, refer the patient to a physical or occupational therapist.

Pediatric pointers

Detecting apraxia in children can be difficult. However, any sudden inability to perform a previously accomplished movement warrants prompt neurologic evaluation because a brain tumor—the most common cause of apraxia in children—may be treated effectively if detected early.

Brain damage in a young child may cause developmental apraxia, which interferes with the ability to learn activities that require sequential movement, such as hopping, jumping, dancing, or hitting or kicking a ball. When caring for a child with apraxia, provide an environment that's conducive to rehabilitation while remaining aware of his limitations. Also provide emotional support because playmates may tease a child who can't perform normal physical activities.

Arm pain

Arm pain usually results from musculoskeletal disorders, but it can also stem from neurovascular or cardiovascular disorders. (See *Causes of localized arm pain*.) In some cases, arm pain may be referred from another area, such as the chest, neck, or abdomen. Its location, onset, and character provide clues to its cause. The pain may affect the entire arm or only the upper arm or forearm. It may arise suddenly or gradually and be constant or intermittent. Arm pain can be described as sharp or dull, burning or numbing, and shooting or penetrating. Diffuse arm pain, though, may be difficult to describe, especially if it isn't associated with injury.

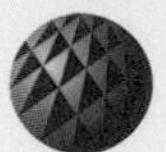

SIGNS & SYMPTOMS

Arm pain: Causes and associated findings

Common causes	Chest pain	Crepitus	Decreased motion	Decreased reflex response	Deformity	Ecchymosis	Edema	Impaired circulation	Muscle weakness	Nausea	Paresthesia	Vomiting
	Major associated signs and symptoms											
Angina	●											
Biceps rupture					●		●		●			
Cellulitis							●					
Cervical nerve root compression				●					●		●	
Compartment syndrome				●			●	●	●		●	
Fractures		●	●		●	●	●	●			●	
Muscle contusion						●	●					
Muscle strain			●						●			
Myocardial infarction	●									●		●
Neoplasm of the arm							●	●			●	
Osteomyelitis			●				●					

History and physical examination

If the patient reports arm pain after an injury, take a brief history of the injury from the patient. Then quickly assess him for severe injuries requiring immediate treatment. If you've ruled out severe injuries, check pulses, capillary refill time, sensation, and movement distal to the affected area because circulatory impairment or nerve injury may require immediate surgery. Inspect the arm for deformities, assess the level of pain, and immobilize the arm to prevent further injury.

If the patient reports continuous or intermittent arm pain, ask him to describe it and to relate when it began. Is the pain associated with repetitive or specific movements or positions? Ask him to point out other painful areas because arm pain may be referred. For example, arm pain commonly accompanies the characteristic chest pain of myocardial infarction, and right shoulder pain may be referred from the right-upper-quadrant abdominal pain of cholecystitis. Ask the patient if the pain worsens in the morning or in the evening, if it prevents him from performing his job, and if it restricts any movements. Also ask if heat, rest, or drugs relieve it. Finally, ask about any preexisting illnesses, a family history of gout or arthritis, and current drug therapy.

Next, perform a focused examination. Observe the way the patient walks, sits, and holds his arm. Inspect the entire arm, comparing it with the opposite arm for symmetry, movement, and muscle atrophy. (It's important to know if the patient is right- or left-handed.) Palpate the entire arm for swelling, nodules, and tender areas. In both arms, compare active range of motion, muscle strength, and reflexes.

If the patient reports numbness or tingling, check his sensation to vibration, temperature, and pinprick. Compare bilateral hand grasps and shoulder strength to detect weakness.

If the patient has a cast, splint, or restrictive dressing, check for circulation, sensation, and mobility distal to the dressing. Ask the patient about edema and if the pain has worsened within the last 24 hours.

Examine the neck for pain on motion, point tenderness, muscle spasms, or arm pain when the neck is extended with the head toward the involved side. (See *Arm pain: Causes and associated findings*.)

MEDICAL CAUSES

◆ ***Angina.*** Angina may cause inner arm pain as well as chest and jaw pain. Typically, the pain follows exertion and persists for a few minutes. Accompanied by dyspnea, diaphoresis, and apprehension, the pain is relieved by rest or vasodilators such as nitroglycerin.

◆ ***Biceps rupture.*** Rupture of the biceps after excessive weight lifting or osteoarthritic degeneration of bicipital tendon insertion at the shoulder can cause pain in the upper arm. Forearm flexion and supination aggravate the pain. Other signs and symptoms include muscle weakness, deformity, and edema.

◆ ***Cellulitis.*** Cellulitis typically affects the legs, but it can also affect the arms. It produces pain as well as redness, tenderness, edema and, at times, fever, chills, tachycardia, headache, and hypotension. Cellulitis usually follows an injury or insect bite.

◆ ***Cervical nerve root compression.*** Compression of the cervical nerves supplying the upper arm produces chronic arm and neck pain, which may worsen with movement or prolonged sitting. The patient may also experience muscle weakness, paresthesia, and decreased reflex response.

◆ ***Compartment syndrome.*** Severe pain with passive muscle stretching is the cardinal symptom of compartment syndrome, which may also impair distal circulation and cause muscle weakness, decreased reflex response, paresthesia, and edema. Ominous signs include paralysis and absent pulse.

◆ ***Fractures.*** In fractures of the cervical vertebrae, humerus, scapula, clavicle, radius, or ulna, pain can occur at the injury site and radiate throughout the entire arm. Pain at a fresh fracture site is intense and worsens with movement. Associated signs and symptoms include crepitus, which is felt and heard from bone ends rubbing together (don't attempt to elicit this sign); deformity if bones are misaligned; local ecchymosis and edema; impaired distal circulation; paresthesia; and decreased sensation distal to the injury site. Fractures of the small wrist bones can manifest with pain and swelling several days after the trauma.

◆ ***Muscle contusion.*** Muscle contusion may cause generalized pain in the injured area as well as local swelling and ecchymosis.

◆ ***Muscle strain.*** Acute or chronic muscle strain causes mild to severe pain with movement. The resultant reduction in arm movement may cause muscle weakness and atrophy.

◆ ***Myocardial infarction.*** In this life-threatening disorder, the patient may complain of left arm pain in addition to the characteristic deep and crushing chest pain. He may display weakness, pallor, nausea, vomiting, diaphoresis, altered blood pressure, tachycardia, dyspnea, and feelings of apprehension or impending doom.

◆ ***Neoplasm of the arm.*** A neoplasm of the arm produces continuous, deep, and penetrating arm pain that worsens at night. Occasionally, redness and swelling accompany arm pain; later, skin breakdown, impaired circulation, and paresthesia may occur.

◆ ***Osteomyelitis.*** Osteomyelitis typically begins with vague and evanescent localized arm pain and fever and is accompanied by local tenderness, painful and restricted movement and, later, swelling. Associated findings include malaise and tachycardia.

SPECIAL CONSIDERATIONS

If you suspect a fracture, apply a sling or a splint to immobilize the arm, and monitor the patient for worsening pain, numbness, or decreased circulation distal to the injury site. Also, monitor vital signs and be alert for tachycardia, hypotension, and diaphoresis. Withhold food, fluids, and

Recognizing asterixis

In asterixis, the patient's wrists and fingers are observed to "flap" because of a brief, rapid relaxation of wrist dorsiflexion.

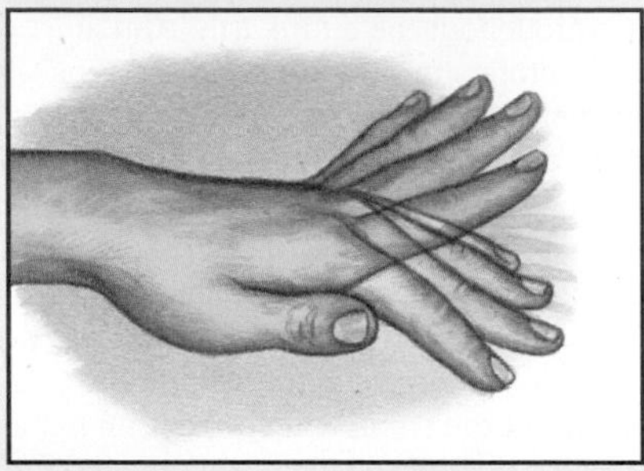

analgesics until potential fractures are evaluated. Promote the patient's comfort by elevating his arm and applying ice. Clean abrasions and lacerations and apply dry, sterile dressings if necessary. Also, prepare the patient for X-rays or other diagnostic tests.

PEDIATRIC POINTERS

In children, arm pain commonly results from fractures, muscle sprain, muscular dystrophy, or rheumatoid arthritis. In young children especially, the exact location of the pain may be difficult to establish. Watch for nonverbal clues, such as wincing or guarding.

If the child has a fracture or sprain, obtain a complete account of the injury. Closely observe interactions between the child and his family, and don't rule out the possibility of child abuse.

GERIATRIC POINTERS

Elderly patients with osteoporosis may experience fractures from simple trauma or even from heavy lifting or unexpected movements. They're also prone to degenerative joint disease that can involve several joints in the arm or neck.

PATIENT COUNSELING

Advise a patient with a cast to notify his physician if he detects worsening swelling, purple discoloration of fingers, or numbness or tingling because these signs may represent vascular compliance due to a tight cast. Also, inform a patient with angina that arm pain, usually left-sided, may represent an ischemic event, especially if accompanied by diaphoresis, nausea, vomiting, and anxiety.

Asterixis

[Liver flap, flapping tremor]

A bilateral, coarse movement, asterixis is characterized by sudden relaxation of muscle groups holding a sustained posture. This elicited sign is most commonly observed in the wrists and fingers but may also appear during any sustained voluntary action. Typically, it signals hepatic, renal, or pulmonary disease.

To elicit asterixis, have the patient extend his arms, dorsiflex his wrists, and spread his fingers (or do this for him, if necessary). Briefly observe him for asterixis. Alternatively, if the patient has a decreased level of consciousness (LOC) but can follow verbal commands, ask him to squeeze two of your fingers. Consider rapid clutching and unclutching indications of asterixis. Or, elevate the patient's leg off the bed and dorsiflex the foot. Briefly check for asterixis in the ankle. If the patient can tightly close his eyes and mouth, watch for irregular tremulous movements of the eyelids and corners of the mouth. If he can stick out his tongue, observe it for continuous quivering. (See *Recognizing asterixis.*)

EMERGENCY INTERVENTIONS *Because asterixis may signal serious metabolic deterioration, quickly evaluate the patient's neurologic status and vital signs. Compare these data with his baseline, and watch carefully for acute changes. Continue to closely monitor neurologic status, vital signs, and urine output.*

Watch for signs of respiratory insufficiency, and be prepared to provide endotracheal intubation and ventilatory support. Also, be alert for complications of end-stage hepatic, renal, or pulmonary disease.

If the patient has hepatic disease, assess him for early indications of hemorrhage, including restlessness, tachypnea, and cool, moist, pale skin. (If the patient is jaundiced, check for pallor in the conjunctivae and mucous membranes of the mouth.) Be aware that hypotension, oliguria, hematemesis, and melena are late signs of hemorrhage. Prepare to insert a large-bore I.V. catheter for fluid and blood replacement. Position the patient flat in bed with his legs elevated 20 degrees. Begin or continue to administer oxygen.

If the patient has renal disease, briefly review the therapy he has received. If he's on dialysis, ask about the frequency of treatments to help gauge the disease's severity. Question a family member if the patient's LOC is significantly decreased.

Then assess the patient for hyperkalemia and metabolic acidosis. Look for tachycardia, nausea, diarrhea, abdominal cramps, muscle weakness, hyperreflexia, and Kussmaul's respirations. Prepare to administer sodium bicarbonate, calcium gluconate, dextrose, insulin, or sodium polystyrene sulfonate (Kayexalate).

If the patient has pulmonary disease, check for labored respirations, tachypnea, accessory muscle use, and cyanosis, which are critical signs. Prepare to provide ventilatory support by nasal cannula, mask, or intubation and mechanical ventilation.

Medical causes

◆ ***Hepatic encephalopathy.*** A life-threatening disorder, hepatic encephalopathy initially causes mild personality changes and a slight tremor. The tremor progresses to asterixis—a hallmark of hepatic encephalopathy—and is accompanied by lethargy, aberrant behavior, and apraxia. Eventually, the patient becomes stuporous and displays hyperventilation. After slipping into a coma, the patient exhibits characteristic hyperactive reflexes, positive Babinski's reflex, and fetor hepaticus. He also may experience bradycardia, decreased respirations, and seizures.

◆ ***Respiratory insufficiency, severe.*** Characterized by life-threatening respiratory acidosis, severe respiratory insufficiency initially produces headache, restlessness, confusion, apprehension, and decreased reflexes. Eventually, the patient becomes somnolent and may demonstrate asterixis before slipping into a coma. Associated signs and symptoms of respiratory insufficiency include difficulty breathing and rapid, shallow respirations. The patient may be hypertensive in early disease but hypotensive later.

◆ ***Uremic syndrome.*** Uremic syndrome is a life-threatening disorder that initially causes lethargy, somnolence, confusion, disorientation, behavior changes, and irritability. Eventually, signs and symptoms appear in diverse body systems. Asterixis is accompanied by stupor, paresthesia, muscle twitching, fasciculations, and footdrop. Other signs and symptoms include polyuria and nocturia followed by oliguria and then anuria, elevated blood pressure, signs of heart failure and pericarditis, Kussmaul's respirations, anorexia, nausea, vomiting diarrhea, GI bleeding, weight loss, ammonia breath odor, and metallic taste (dysgeusia).

Other causes

◆ ***Drugs.*** Certain drugs, such as the anticonvulsant phenytoin, may cause asterixis.

Special considerations

Provide simple comfort measures, such as allowing frequent rest periods to minimize fatigue and elevating the head of the bed to relieve dyspnea and orthopnea. Administer oil baths and avoid soap to relieve itching caused by jaundice and uremia. Provide emotional support to the patient and his family.

If the patient is intubated or has a decreased LOC, provide enteral or parenteral nutrition. Closely monitor serum and urine glucose levels to evaluate hyperalimentation. Because the patient will probably be on bed rest, reposition him at least once every 2 hours to prevent skin breakdown. Also observe strict hand-washing and aseptic techniques when changing dressings and caring for invasive lines because the patient's debilitated state makes him prone to infection.

Pediatric pointers

End-stage hepatic, renal, and pulmonary disease may also cause asterixis in children.

Ataxia

Classified as cerebellar or sensory, ataxia refers to incoordination and irregularity of voluntary, purposeful movements. *Cerebellar ataxia* results from disease of the cerebellum and its pathways to and from the cerebral cortex, brain stem, and spinal cord. It causes gait, trunk, limb, and possibly speech disorders. *Sensory ataxia* results from impaired position sense (proprioception) due to interruption of afferent nerve fibers in the peripheral nerves, posterior roots, posterior columns of the spinal cord, or medial lemnisci or, occasionally, from a lesion in both parietal lobes. It causes gait disorders. (See *Identifying ataxia,* page 70.)

Ataxia occurs in acute and chronic forms. Acute ataxia may result from stroke, hemorrhage, or a large tumor in the posterior fossa. In this life-threatening condition, the cerebellum may herniate downward through the foramen magnum behind the cervical spinal cord, or upward through the tentorium on the cerebral hemispheres. Herniation may also compress the

Identifying ataxia

Ataxia may be observed in the patient's speech, in the movements of his trunk and limbs, or in his gait.

In *speech ataxia*, a form of dysarthria, the patient typically speaks slowly and stresses usually unstressed words and syllables. Speech content is unaffected.

In *truncal ataxia*, a disturbance in equilibrium, the patient can't sit or stand without falling, and his head and trunk may bob and sway (titubation). If he can walk, his gait is reeling.

In *limb ataxia*, the patient loses the ability to gauge distance, speed, and power of movement, resulting in poorly controlled, variable, and inaccurate voluntary movements. He may move too quickly or too slowly, or his movements may break down into component parts, giving him the appearance of a puppet or a robot. Other effects include a coarse, irregular tremor in purposeful movement (but not at rest) and reduced muscle tone.

In *gait ataxia*, the patient's gait is wide based, unsteady, and irregular.

In *cerebellar ataxia*, the patient may stagger or lurch in zigzag fashion, turn with extreme difficulty, and lose his balance when his feet are together.

In *sensory ataxia*, the patient moves abruptly and stomps or taps his feet. This occurs because he throws his feet forward and outward, and then brings them down first on the heels and then on the toes. The patient also fixes his eyes on the ground, watching his steps; if he can't watch his steps, staggering worsens. When he stands with his feet together, he sways or loses balance.

brain stem. Acute ataxia may also result from drug toxicity or poisoning. Chronic ataxia can be progressive and may result from acute disease. It can also occur in metabolic and chronic degenerative neurologic disease.

EMERGENCY INTERVENTIONS *If ataxic movements develop suddenly, examine the patient for signs of increased intracranial pressure and impending herniation. Determine his level of consciousness (LOC), and be alert for pupillary changes, motor weakness or paralysis, neck stiffness or pain, and vomiting. Check vital signs, especially respirations; abnormal respiratory patterns may quickly lead to respiratory arrest. Elevate the head of the bed. Have emergency resuscitation equipment readily available. Prepare the patient for a computed tomography scan or surgery.*

History and physical examination

If the patient isn't in distress, review his history. Ask about multiple sclerosis, diabetes, central nervous system infection, neoplastic disease, previous stroke, and a family history of ataxia. Also ask about chronic alcohol abuse or prolonged exposure to industrial toxins such as mercury. Find out if the ataxia developed suddenly or gradually.

If necessary, perform Romberg's test to help distinguish between cerebellar and sensory ataxia. Instruct the patient to stand with his feet together and his arms at his side. Note his posture and balance, first with his eyes open and then with them closed. Test results may indicate normal posture and balance (minimal swaying), cerebellar ataxia (swaying and inability to maintain balance with eyes open or closed), or sensory ataxia (increased swaying and inability to maintain balance with eyes closed). Stand close to the patient during this test to prevent his falling.

If you test for gait and limb ataxia, be aware that motor weakness may mimic ataxic movements, so check motor strength, too. Gait ataxia may be severe, even when limb ataxia is minimal. Ask the patient with gait ataxia if he tends to fall to one side and if he falls more at night. With truncal ataxia, remember that the patient's inability to walk or stand, combined with the absence of other signs while he's lying down, may give the impression of hysteria or drug or alcohol intoxication.

Medical causes

- ***Cerebellar abscess.*** Cerebellar abscess commonly causes limb ataxia on the same side as the lesion as well as gait and truncal ataxia. Typically, the initial symptom is headache localized behind the ear or in the occipital region, followed by oculomotor palsy, fever, vomiting, altered LOC, and coma.
- ***Cerebellar hemorrhage.*** Cerebellar hemorrhage is a life-threatening disorder in which

ataxia is usually acute but transient. Unilateral or bilateral ataxia affects the trunk, gait, or limbs. The patient initially experiences repeated vomiting, an occipital headache, vertigo, oculomotor palsy, dysphagia, and dysarthria. Later signs, such as decreased LOC or coma, signal impending herniation.

◆ ***Cranial trauma.*** Cranial trauma rarely produces ataxia, but when it does, the ataxia is usually unilateral; bilateral ataxia suggests traumatic hemorrhage. Associated signs and symptoms include vomiting, headache, decreased LOC, irritability, and focal neurologic defects. If the cerebral hemispheres are also affected, focal or generalized seizures may occur.

◆ ***Creutzfeldt-Jakob disease.*** Creutzfeldt-Jakob disease is a rapidly progressive dementia accompanied by neurologic signs and symptoms, such as myoclonic jerking, ataxia, aphasia, visual disturbances, and paralysis. It generally affects adults ages 40 to 65.

◆ ***Diabetic neuropathy.*** Peripheral nerve damage due to diabetes mellitus may cause sensory ataxia, extremity pain, slight leg weakness, skin changes, and bowel and bladder dysfunction.

◆ ***Diphtheria.*** Within 4 to 8 weeks of the onset of symptoms, a life-threatening neuropathy can produce sensory ataxia. Diphtheria can be accompanied by fever, paresthesia, and paralysis of the limbs and possibly the respiratory muscles.

◆ ***Encephalomyelitis.*** Encephalomyelitis is a complication of measles, smallpox, chickenpox, or rubella or of rabies or smallpox vaccine that may damage cerebrospinal white matter. Rarely, it's accompanied by cerebellar ataxia. Other signs and symptoms include headache, fever, vomiting, altered LOC, paralysis, seizures, oculomotor palsy, and pupillary changes.

◆ ***Friedreich's ataxia.*** Friedreich's ataxia is a progressive familial disorder that affects the spinal cord and cerebellum. It causes gait ataxia, followed by truncal, limb, and speech ataxia. Other signs and symptoms include pes cavus, kyphoscoliosis, cranial nerve palsy, and motor and sensory deficits. A positive Babinski's reflex may appear.

◆ ***Guillain-Barré syndrome.*** This syndrome usually begins with a mild viral infection, followed by peripheral nerve involvement and, rarely, sensory ataxia. It may also cause ascending paralysis and respiratory distress.

◆ ***Hepatocerebral degeneration.*** Some patients who survive hepatic coma are left with residual neurologic defects, including mild cerebellar ataxia with a wide-based, unsteady gait. Ataxia may be accompanied by altered LOC, dysarthria, rhythmic arm tremors, and choreoathetosis of the face, neck, and shoulders.

◆ ***Hyperthermia.*** Cerebellar ataxia occurs if the patient survives the coma and seizures characteristic of the acute phase of hyperthermia. Subsequent findings include spastic paralysis, dementia, and slowly resolving confusion.

◆ ***Metastatic cancer.*** Cancer that metastasizes to the cerebellum may cause gait ataxia accompanied by headache, dizziness, nystagmus, decreased LOC, nausea, and vomiting.

◆ ***Multiple sclerosis (MS).*** Nystagmus and cerebellar ataxia commonly occur in MS, but they aren't always accompanied by limb weakness and spasticity. The patient may also have speech ataxia (especially scanning) as well as sensory ataxia from spinal cord involvement. During remissions, ataxia may subside or even disappear. During exacerbations, it may reappear, worsen, or even become permanent. MS also causes optic neuritis, optic atrophy, numbness and weakness, diplopia, dizziness, and bladder dysfunction.

◆ ***Olivopontocerebellar atrophy.*** Olivopontocerebellar atrophy produces gait ataxia and, later, limb and speech ataxia. Rarely, it produces an intention tremor. It's accompanied by choreiform movements, dysphagia, and loss of sphincter tone.

◆ ***Polyarteritis nodosa.*** Acute or subacute polyarteritis may cause sensory ataxia, abdominal and limb pain, hematuria, fever, and elevated blood pressure.

◆ ***Polyneuropathy.*** Carcinomatous and myelomatous polyneuropathy may occur before detection of the primary tumor in cancer, multiple myeloma, or Hodgkin's disease. Signs and symptoms include ataxia, severe motor weakness, muscle atrophy, and sensory loss in the limbs. Pain and skin changes may also occur.

◆ ***Porphyria.*** Porphyria affects the sensory and, more commonly, the motor nerves, possibly leading to ataxia. It also causes abdominal pain, mental disturbances, vomiting, headache, focal neurologic defects, altered LOC, generalized seizures, and skin lesions.

◆ ***Posterior fossa tumor.*** Gait, truncal, or limb ataxia is an early sign and may worsen as the tumor enlarges. It's accompanied by vomiting, headache, papilledema, vertigo, oculomotor palsy, decreased LOC, and motor and sensory impairment on the same side as the lesion.

◆ ***Spinocerebellar ataxia.*** In spinocerebellar ataxia, the patient may initially experience fatigue, followed by stiff-legged gait ataxia. Eventually, limb ataxia, dysarthria, static tremor, nystagmus, cramps, paresthesia, and sensory deficits occur.

◆ ***Stroke.*** In a stroke, occlusions in the vertebrobasilar arteries halt blood flow, causing infarction in the medulla, pons, or cerebellum that may lead to ataxia. Ataxia may occur at the onset of the stroke and remain as a residual deficit. Worsening ataxia during the acute phase may indicate extension of the stroke or severe swelling. Ataxia may be accompanied by unilateral or bilateral motor weakness, altered LOC, sensory loss, vertigo, nausea, vomiting, oculomotor palsy, and dysphagia.

◆ ***Syringomyelia.*** Syringomyelia is a chronic degenerative disorder that may cause a mixed spastic-ataxic gait. It's associated with loss of pain and temperature sensation (but preservation of touch sensation), skin changes, amyotrophy, and thoracic scoliosis.

◆ ***Wernicke's encephalopathy.*** The result of a thiamine deficiency, Wernicke's encephalopathy produces gait ataxia and, rarely, intention tremor or speech ataxia. With severe ataxia, the patient may be unable to stand or walk. Ataxia decreases with thiamine therapy. Associated signs and symptoms include nystagmus, diplopia, ocular palsies, confusion, tachycardia, exertional dyspnea, and orthostatic hypotension.

Other causes

◆ ***Drugs.*** Toxic levels of anticonvulsants, especially phenytoin, may result in gait ataxia. Toxic levels of anticholinergics and tricyclic antidepressants may also result in ataxia.

◆ ***Poisoning.*** Chronic arsenic poisoning may cause sensory ataxia along with headache, seizures, altered LOC, motor deficits, and muscle aching. Chronic mercury poisoning causes gait ataxia and limb ataxia, principally of the arms. Chronic mercury poisoning also causes tremors of the extremities, tongue, and lips; mental confusion; mood changes; and dysarthria.

Special considerations

Prepare the patient for laboratory studies, such as blood tests for toxic drug levels and radiologic tests. Then focus on helping the patient adapt to his condition. Promote rehabilitation goals and help ensure the patient's safety. For example, instruct the patient with sensory ataxia to move slowly, especially when turning or getting up from a chair. Provide a cane or walker for extra support. Ask the patient's family to check his home for hazards, such as uneven surfaces or the absence of handrails on stairs. If appropriate, refer the patient with progressive disease for counseling.

Pediatric pointers

In children, ataxia occurs in acute and chronic forms and results from congenital or acquired disease. Acute ataxia may stem from febrile infection, brain tumors, mumps, and other disorders. Chronic ataxia may stem from Gaucher's disease, Refsum's disease, and other inborn errors of metabolism.

When assessing a child for ataxia, consider his level of motor skills and emotional state. Your examination may be limited to observing the child in spontaneous activity and carefully questioning his parents about changes in his motor activity, such as increased unsteadiness or falling. If you suspect ataxia, refer the child for a neurologic evaluation to rule out a brain tumor.

Athetosis

Athetosis, an extrapyramidal sign, is characterized by slow, continuous, and twisting involuntary movements. Typically, these movements involve the face, neck, and distal extremities, such as the forearm, wrist, and hand. Facial grimaces, jaw and tongue movements, and occasional phonation are associated with neck movements. Athetosis worsens during stress and voluntary activity, may subside during relaxation, and disappears during sleep. Commonly a lifelong affliction, athetosis is sometimes difficult to distinguish from chorea (hence the term *choreoathetosis*). Typically, though, athetoid movements are slower than choreiform movements. (See *Distinguishing athetosis from chorea*.)

Athetosis usually begins during childhood, resulting from hypoxia at birth, kernicterus, or a genetic disorder. In adults, athetosis usually results from vascular or neoplastic lesions, degenerative disease, drug toxicity, or hypoxia.

Distinguishing athetosis from chorea

In *athetosis,* movements are typically slow, twisting, and writhing. They're associated with spasticity and most commonly involve the face, neck, and distal extremities.

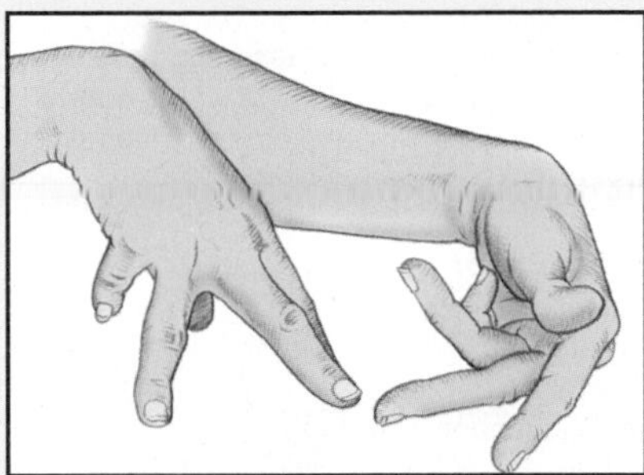

In *chorea,* movements are brief, rapid, jerky, and unpredictable. They can occur at rest or during normal movement and typically involve the hands, lower arm, face, and head.

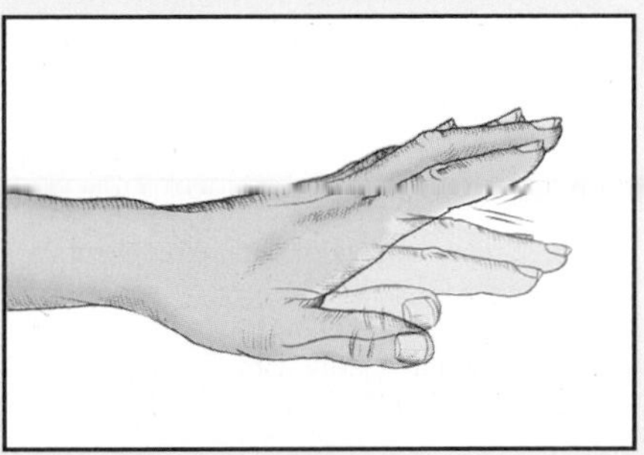

History and physical examination

Begin your neurologic evaluation by taking a comprehensive prenatal and postnatal history, covering maternal and child health, labor and delivery, and possible trauma. Obtain a family health history because many genetic disorders can cause athetosis. Also, ask about current drug therapy.

Ask about the decline in the patient's functional abilities: When was he last able to roll over, sit up, or carry out daily activities? Find out what problem—uncontrollable movements, mental deterioration, or a speech impediment—prompted him to seek medical help. Ask about the effects of rest, stress, and routine activity on his symptoms.

Test the patient's muscle strength and tone, range of motion, fine muscle movements, and ability to perform rapidly alternating movements. Observe the limb muscles during voluntary movements, noting the rhythm and duration of contraction and relaxation.

Medical causes

◆ ***Brain tumor.*** A brain tumor that affects the basal ganglia causes contralateral choreoathetosis and dystonia. Associated signs vary markedly with the type of tumor and its degree of invasion.

◆ ***Calcification of the basal ganglia.*** Calcification of the basal ganglia is a unilateral or bilateral disorder that's characterized by choreoathetosis and rigidity. It usually arises in adolescence or early adulthood.

◆ ***Cerebral infarction.*** In cerebral infarction, contralateral athetosis is accompanied by altered level of consciousness. The patient may also display contralateral paralysis of the face or limbs.

◆ ***Hepatic encephalopathy.*** Episodic or persistent choreoathetosis occurs in the chronic stage of hepatic encephalopathy and is accompanied by cerebellar ataxia, myoclonus of the face and limbs, asterixis, dysarthria, and dementia.

◆ ***Huntington's disease.*** Huntington's disease is a hereditary degenerative disease in which athetosis and chorea develop progressively in middle-aged adults. Accompanying signs and symptoms include dystonia, dysarthria, facial apraxia, rigidity, depression, and progressive mental deterioration leading to dementia.

◆ ***Wilson's disease.*** Wilson's disease is an inherited metabolic disorder in which choreoathetoid movements initially involve the fingers and hands and then spread to the arms, head, trunk, and legs. Associated signs and symptoms include Kayser-Fleischer rings (rusty brown rings around the corneas), arm and hand tremors, facial and muscular rigidity, dysarthria, dysphagia, drooling, and progressive dementia. Hepatomegaly, splenomegaly, jaundice, hematemesis, and spider angiomas may also occur.

Recognizing types of auras

Determining whether an aura marks the patient's thought processes, emotions, or sensory or motor function usually requires keen observation. An aura is typically difficult to describe and is only dimly remembered when associated with seizure activity. Below you'll find the types of auras the patient may experience.

Affective auras

◆ Fear
◆ Paranoia
◆ Other emotions

Cognitive auras

◆ Déjà vu (familiarity with unfamiliar events or environments)
◆ Flashback of past events
◆ *Jamais vu* (unfamiliarity with a known event)
◆ Time standing still

Psychomotor auras

◆ Automatisms (inappropriate, repetitive movements): lip smacking, chewing, swallowing, grimacing, picking at clothes, climbing stairs

Psychosensory auras

◆ Auditory: buzzing or ringing in the ears
◆ Gustatory: acidic, metallic, or bitter tastes
◆ Olfactory: foul odors
◆ Tactile: numbness or tingling
◆ Vertigo
◆ Visual: flashes of light (scintillations)

OTHER CAUSES

◆ ***Levodopa and phenytoin.*** Toxic levels of these drugs may cause athetoid or choreoathetoid movements.

◆ ***Phenothiazines and other antipsychotics.*** The piperazine derivatives, such as meclizine and prochlorperazine, commonly cause athetosis. The aliphatic phenothiazines, such as chlorpromazine, occasionally cause it. A third type of derivative, the piperidine phenothiazines, such as thioridazine and perphenazine, rarely cause it. Other antipsychotics, such as haloperidol, thiothixene, and loxapine, commonly cause athetosis.

SPECIAL CONSIDERATIONS

Prepare the patient for diagnostic tests, such as urine and blood studies, lumbar puncture, EEG, computed tomography scan, and magnetic resonance imaging.

Occasionally, athetosis can be prevented or treated (by decreasing body copper stores in Wilson's disease or by adjusting drug dosages). Typically, though, it has a lifelong impact on the patient's ability to carry out even routine activities. As a result, you'll need to help him adapt to his condition—for example, by supplying him with assistive devices to help him carry out fine-motor tasks.

When appropriate, assist with rehabilitation; some patients can be taught to control erratic movements or convert them into purposeful ones. Also, encourage swimming, stretching, and balance and gait exercises to help maintain coordination, slow deterioration, and minimize antisocial behavior.

Encourage the patient and his family to discuss their feelings about athetosis and its cause. Refer the patient to a self-help group and appropriate support services such as physical therapy.

PEDIATRIC POINTERS

Childhood athetosis may be acquired or inherited. It can result from hypoxia at birth, which causes athetoid cerebral palsy; kernicterus; Sydenham's chorea (in school-age children); and paroxysmal choreoathetosis. Inherited causes of athetosis include Lesch-Nyhan syndrome, Tay-Sachs disease, and phenylketonuria.

Help the child develop self-esteem and a positive self-image. Encourage the child and his family to set realistic goals, tailoring educational plans to the child's level of intelligence.

Refer the child to special education services, rehabilitation centers, and support groups. Provide him with emotional support during the frequent medical evaluations required for athetosis.

Aura

An aura is a sensory or motor phenomenon, idea, or emotion that marks the initial stage of a seizure or the approach of a classic migraine headache. Auras may be classified as cognitive, affective, psychosensory, or psychomotor. (See *Recognizing types of auras*.)

When associated with a seizure, an aura stems from an irritable focus in the brain that spreads throughout the cortex. Although an aura was once considered a sign of an impending seizure, it's now considered the first stage of a seizure. Typically, it occurs seconds to minutes before the ictal phase. Its intensity, duration, and type depend on the origin of the irritable focus. For example, an aura of bitter taste commonly accompanies a frontal lobe lesion. Unfortunately, an aura is difficult to describe because the postictal phase of a seizure temporarily alters the patient's level of consciousness, impairing his memory of the event.

The aura associated with a classic migraine headache results from cranial vasoconstriction and typically involves visual disturbances. Diagnostically important, it helps distinguish a classic migraine from other types of headaches. Typically, the aura develops over 10 to 30 minutes and varies in intensity and duration. If the patient recognizes the aura as a warning sign, he may be able to prevent the headache by taking appropriate drugs.

EMERGENCY INTERVENTIONS *When an aura rapidly progresses to the ictal phase of a seizure, quickly evaluate the seizure and be alert for life-threatening complications such as apnea. When an aura heralds a classic migraine, make the patient as comfortable as possible. Place him in a dark, quiet room and administer drugs to prevent the headache, if necessary.*

History and physical examination

After providing emergency care, obtain a thorough history of the patient's headaches or seizures, asking him to describe any sensory or motor phenomena that precede each headache or seizure. Find out how long each headache or seizure typically lasts. Does anything make it worse, such as bright lights, noise, or caffeine? Does anything make it better? Ask the patient about drugs he takes for pain relief.

Medical causes

◆ ***Migraine headache, classic.*** A classic migraine is preceded by a vague premonition and then, usually, a visual aura involving flashes of light. The aura lasts 10 to 30 minutes and may intensify until it completely obscures the patient's vision. A classic migraine may cause numbness or tingling of the lips, face, or hands; slight confusion; and dizziness before the characteristic unilateral, throbbing headache appears. The headache slowly intensifies; when it peaks, the patient may experience photophobia, nausea, and vomiting.

◆ ***Seizure, generalized tonic-clonic.*** A generalized tonic-clonic seizure may begin with an aura. The patient loses consciousness and falls to the ground. His body stiffens (tonic phase); then he experiences rapid, synchronous muscle jerking and hyperventilation (clonic phase). The seizure usually lasts 2 to 5 minutes.

Special considerations

Advise the patient to keep a diary of factors that precipitate each headache as well as associated symptoms to help you evaluate the effectiveness of drug therapy and recommend lifestyle changes. Stress-reduction measures usually play a role here.

Pediatric pointers

Watch for nonverbal clues that may be associated with an aura, such as rubbing the eyes, coughing, and spitting. When taking the seizure history, recognize that children—like adults—tend to forget the aura. Ask simple, direct questions, such as "Do you see anything funny before the seizure?" and "Do you get a bad taste in your mouth?" Give the child ample time to respond because he may have difficulty describing the aura.

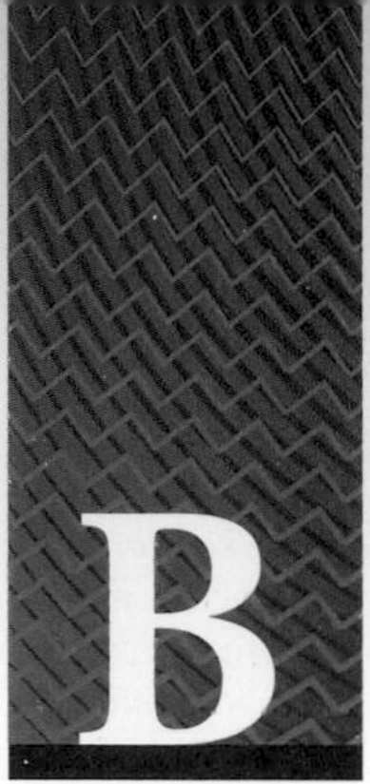

Babinski's reflex

[Extensor plantar reflex]

Babinski's reflex—dorsiflexion of the great toe with extension and fanning of the other toes—is an abnormal reflex elicited by firmly stroking the lateral aspect of the sole of the foot with a blunt object. (See *How to elicit Babinski's reflex.*) In some patients, this reflex can be triggered by noxious stimuli, such as pain, noise, or even bumping of the bed. An indicator of corticospinal damage, Babinski's reflex may occur unilaterally or bilaterally and may be temporary or permanent. A temporary Babinski's reflex commonly occurs during the postictal phase of a seizure, whereas a permanent Babinski's reflex occurs with corticospinal damage. A positive Babinski's reflex is normal in neonates and in infants up to age 24 months.

History and physical examination

After eliciting a positive Babinski's reflex, evaluate the patient for other neurologic signs. Evaluate muscle strength in each extremity by having the patient push or pull against your resistance. Passively flex and extend the extremity to assess muscle tone. Intermittent resistance to flexion and extension indicates spasticity, and a lack of resistance indicates flaccidity.

Next, check for evidence of incoordination by asking the patient to perform a repetitive activity. Test deep tendon reflexes (DTRs) in the patient's elbow, antecubital area, wrist, knee, and ankle by striking the tendon with a reflex hammer. An exaggerated muscle response indicates hyperactive DTRs; little or no muscle response indicates hypoactivity.

Then evaluate pain sensation and proprioception in the feet. As you move the patient's toes up and down, ask him to identify the direction in which the toes have been moved without looking at his feet.

Medical causes

◆ ***Amyotrophic lateral sclerosis (ALS).*** In this progressive motor neuron disorder, bilateral Babinski's reflex may occur with hyperactive DTRs and spasticity. Typically, ALS produces fasciculations accompanied by muscle atrophy and weakness. Incoordination makes carrying out activities of daily living difficult for the patient. Associated signs and symptoms include impaired speech; difficulty chewing, swallowing, and breathing; urinary frequency and urgency; and, occasionally, choking and excessive drooling. Although his mental status remains intact, the patient's poor prognosis may cause periodic depression. Progressive bulbar palsy involves the brain stem and may cause episodes of crying or inappropriate laughter.

◆ ***Brain tumor.*** A brain tumor that involves the corticospinal tract may produce Babinski's reflex. The reflex may be accompanied by hyperactive DTRs (unilateral or bilateral), spasticity, seizures, cranial nerve dysfunction, hemiparesis or hemiplegia, decreased pain sensation, unsteady gait, incoordination, headache, emotional lability, and decreased level of consciousness (LOC).

◆ ***Familial spastic paraparesis.*** Familial spastic paraparesis may produce bilateral Babinski's reflex accompanied by hyperactive DTRs and progressive spasticity with ataxia and weakness.

◆ ***Friedreich's ataxia.*** Friedreich's ataxia is a familial disorder that may produce bilateral Babinski's reflex. Accompanying it are high-arched feet, hypoactive DTRs, hypotonia, ataxia, head tremor, weakness, and paresthesia.

◆ ***Head trauma.*** Unilateral or bilateral Babinski's reflex may occur as the result of primary corticospinal damage or secondary injury associated with increased intracranial pressure. Hyperactive DTRs and spasticity commonly occur with Babinski's reflex. The patient may also have weakness and incoordination. Other signs and symptoms vary with the type of head trauma and include headache, vomiting, behavior changes, altered vital signs, and decreased LOC with abnormal pupillary size and response to light.

◆ ***Hepatic encephalopathy.*** Babinski's reflex occurs late in hepatic encephalopathy when the patient slips into a coma. It's accompanied by hyperactive DTRs and fetor hepaticus.

◆ ***Meningitis.*** In meningitis, bilateral Babinski's reflex commonly follows fever, chills, and malaise and is accompanied by nausea and vomiting. As meningitis progresses, it also causes decreased LOC, nuchal rigidity, positive Brudzinski's and Kernig's signs, hyperactive DTRs, and opisthotonos. Associated signs and symptoms include irritability, photophobia, diplopia, delirium, and deep stupor that may progress to coma.

◆ ***Multiple sclerosis (MS).*** In most patients with MS—a demyelinating disorder—bilateral Babinski's reflex eventually follows initial signs and symptoms of paresthesia, nystagmus, and blurred or double vision. Associated signs and symptoms include scanning speech (clipped speech with some pauses between syllables), dysphagia, intention tremor, weakness, incoordination, spasticity, gait ataxia, seizures, paraparesis or paraplegia, bladder incontinence, and emotional lability. Loss of pain and temperature sensation and proprioception occur occasionally.

◆ ***Pernicious anemia.*** Bilateral Babinski's reflex occurs late in pernicious anemia when vitamin B_{12} deficiency affects the central nervous

How to elicit Babinski's reflex

To elicit Babinski's reflex, stroke the lateral aspect of the sole of the patient's foot with your thumbnail or another moderately sharp object. Normally, this elicits flexion of all toes (a negative Babinski's reflex), as shown in the top illustration. In a positive Babinski's reflex, the great toe dorsiflexes and the other toes fan out, as shown in the bottom illustration.

NORMAL TOE FLEXION

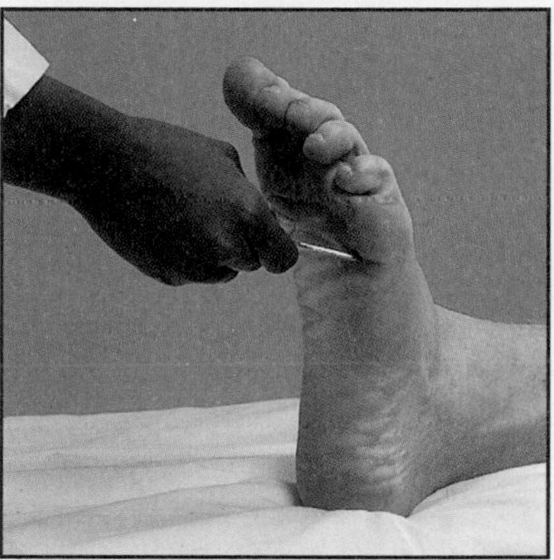

POSITIVE BABINSKI'S REFLEX

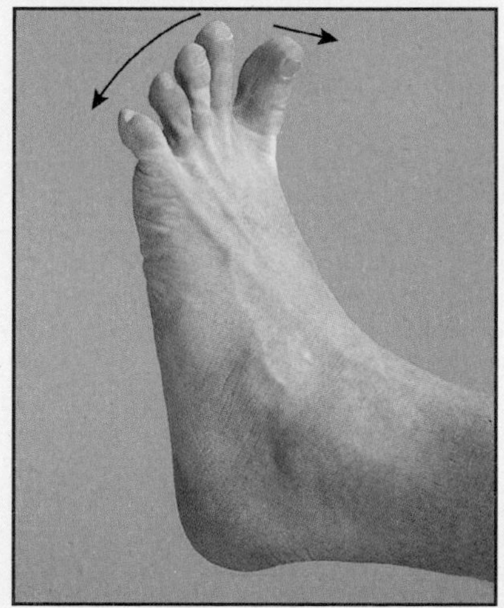

system. Anemia may eventually cause widespread GI, neurologic, and cardiovascular effects. Characteristic GI signs and symptoms include nausea, vomiting, anorexia, weight loss, flatulence, diarrhea, and constipation. Gingival bleeding and a sore, inflamed tongue may make eating painful and intensify anorexia. The lips, gums, and tongue appear markedly pale. Jaundice may cause pale to bright yellow skin.

Characteristic neurologic signs and symptoms include neuritis, weakness, peripheral paresthesia, disturbed position sense, incoordination, ataxia, positive Romberg's sign, lightheadedness, bowel and bladder incontinence, and altered vision (diplopia, blurred vision), taste, and hearing (tinnitus). Pernicious anemia may also produce irritability, poor memory, headache, depression, impotence, and delirium. Characteristic cardiovascular signs and symptoms include palpitations, wide pulse pressure, dyspnea, orthopnea, and tachycardia.

◆ ***Rabies.*** Bilateral Babinski's reflex—possibly elicited by nonspecific noxious stimuli alone—appears in the excitation phase of rabies. This phase occurs 2 to 10 days after the onset of prodromal signs and symptoms, such as fever, malaise, and irritability (which occur 30 to 40 days after a bite from an infected animal). Rabies is characterized by marked restlessness and extremely painful pharyngeal muscle spasms. Difficulty swallowing causes excessive drooling and hydrophobia in about 50% of affected patients. Seizures and hyperactive DTRs may also occur.

◆ ***Spinal cord injury.*** In an acute injury, spinal shock temporarily erases all reflexes. As shock resolves, Babinski's reflex occurs—unilaterally when the injury affects only one side of the spinal cord (Brown-Séquard syndrome) and bilaterally when the injury affects both sides. Rather than signaling the return of neurologic function, this reflex confirms corticospinal damage. It's accompanied by hyperactive DTRs, spasticity, and variable or total loss of pain and temperature sensation, proprioception, and motor function. Horner's syndrome, marked by unilateral ptosis, pupillary constriction, and facial anhidrosis, may occur in a lower cervical cord injury.

◆ ***Spinal cord tumor.*** In a spinal cord tumor, bilateral Babinski's reflex occurs with variable loss of pain and temperature sensation, proprioception, and motor function. Spasticity, hyperactive DTRs, absent abdominal reflexes, and incontinence are also characteristic. Diffuse pain may occur at the level of the tumor.

◆ ***Spinal paralytic poliomyelitis.*** Unilateral or bilateral Babinski's reflex occurs 5 to 7 days after the onset of fever. It's accompanied by progressive weakness, paresthesia, muscle tenderness, spasticity, irritability and, later, atrophy. Resistance to neck flexion is characteristic, as are Hoyne's, Kernig's, and Brudzinski's signs.

◆ ***Spinal tuberculosis.*** Spinal tuberculosis may produce bilateral Babinski's reflex accompanied by variable loss of pain and temperature sensation, proprioception, and motor function. It also causes spasticity, hyperactive DTRs, bladder incontinence, and absent abdominal reflexes.

◆ ***Stroke.*** Babinski's reflex varies with the site of the stroke. A stroke involving the cerebrum produces unilateral Babinski's reflex accompanied by hemiplegia or hemiparesis, unilateral hyperactive DTRs, hemianopsia, and aphasia. A stroke involving the brain stem produces bilateral Babinski's reflex accompanied by bilateral weakness or paralysis, bilateral hyperactive DTRs, cranial nerve dysfunction, incoordination, and unsteady gait. Generalized signs and symptoms of stroke include headache, vomiting, fever, disorientation, nuchal rigidity, seizures, and coma.

◆ ***Syringomyelia.*** In syringomyelia, bilateral Babinski's reflex occurs with muscle atrophy and weakness that may progress to paralysis. It's accompanied by spasticity, ataxia and, occasionally, deep pain. DTRs may be hypoactive or hyperactive. Cranial nerve dysfunction, such as dysphagia and dysarthria, commonly appears late in the disorder.

Special considerations

Babinski's reflex usually occurs with incoordination, weakness, and spasticity, all of which increase the patient's risk of injury. To prevent injury, assist the patient with activities and keep his environment free from obstructions.

Diagnostic tests may include a computed tomography scan or magnetic resonance imaging of the brain or spine, angiography or myelography, and possibly a lumbar puncture to clarify or confirm the cause of Babinski's reflex. Prepare the patient as necessary.

Pediatric pointers

Babinski's reflex occurs normally in infants up to age 24 months, reflecting immaturity of the corticospinal tract. After age 2, Babinski's reflex is pathologic and may result from hydrocephalus or any of the causes commonly seen in adults.

Back pain

Back pain affects an estimated 80% of the population; in fact, it's the second leading reason—after the common cold—for lost time from work. Although this symptom may herald a spondylogenic disorder, it may also result from a genitourinary, GI, cardiovascular, orthopedic, or neoplastic disorder. Postural imbalance associated with pregnancy may also cause back pain.

The onset, location, and distribution of pain and its response to activity and rest provide important clues about the cause. Pain may be acute or chronic and constant or intermittent. It may remain localized in the back or radiate along the spine or down one or both legs. Pain may be exacerbated by activity—usually, bending, stooping, or lifting—and alleviated by rest, or it may be unaffected by either.

Intrinsic back pain results from muscle spasm, nerve root irritation, fracture, or a combination of these mechanisms. It usually occurs in the lower back, or lumbosacral area. Back pain may also be referred from the abdomen or flank, possibly signaling a life-threatening perforated ulcer, acute pancreatitis, or dissecting abdominal aortic aneurysm.

EMERGENCY INTERVENTIONS *If the patient reports acute, severe back pain, quickly take his vital signs; then perform a rapid evaluation to rule out life-threatening causes. Ask him when the pain began. Can he relate it to any causes? For example, did the pain occur after eating? After falling on the ice? Have the patient describe the pain. Is it burning, stabbing, throbbing, or aching? Is it constant or intermittent? Does it radiate to the buttocks or legs? Does he have leg weakness? Does the pain seem to originate in the abdomen and radiate to the back? Has he had a pain like this before? What makes it better or worse? Is it affected by activity or rest? Is it worse in the morning or evening? Does it wake him up? Typically, visceral-referred back pain is unaffected by activity and rest. In contrast, spondylogenic-referred back pain worsens with activity and improves with rest. Pain of neoplastic origin is usually relieved by walking and worsens at night.*

If the patient describes deep lumbar pain unaffected by activity, palpate for a pulsating epigastric mass. If this sign is present, suspect dissecting abdominal aortic aneurysm. Withhold food and fluid in anticipation of emergency surgery. Prepare for I.V. fluid replacement and oxygen administration.

If the patient describes severe epigastric pain that radiates through the abdomen to the back, assess him for absent bowel sounds and for abdominal rigidity and tenderness. If these occur, suspect a perforated ulcer or acute pancreatitis. Start an I.V. catheter for fluids and drugs, administer oxygen, and insert a nasogastric tube while withholding food.

HISTORY AND PHYSICAL EXAMINATION

If life-threatening causes of back pain are ruled out, continue with a complete history and physical examination. Be aware of the patient's expressions of pain as you do so. Obtain a medical history, including past injuries and illnesses, and a family history. Ask about diet and alcohol intake. Also, take a drug history, including past and present prescription and over-the-counter drugs.

Next, perform a thorough physical examination. Observe skin color, especially in the patient's legs, and palpate skin temperature. Palpate femoral, popliteal, posterior tibial, and pedal pulses. Ask about unusual sensations in the legs, such as numbness and tingling. Observe the patient's posture if pain doesn't prohibit standing. Does he stand erect or tend to lean toward one side? Observe the level of the shoulders and pelvis and the curvature of the back. Ask the patient to bend forward, backward, and from side to side while you palpate for paravertebral muscle spasms. Note rotation of the spine on the trunk. Palpate the dorsolumbar spine for point tenderness. Then ask the patient to walk—first on his heels, then on his toes; protect him from falling as he does so. Weakness may reflect a muscular disorder or spinal nerve root irritation. Place the patient in a sitting position to evaluate and compare patellar tendon (knee), Achilles tendon, and Babinski's reflexes. Evaluate the strength of the extensor hallucis longus by asking the patient to hold up his big toe against resistance. Measure leg length and hamstring and quadriceps muscles bilaterally. Note a difference of more than 3/8″ (1 cm) in muscle size, especially in the calf.

To reproduce leg and back pain, place the patient in a supine position on the examining table. Grasp his heel and slowly lift his leg. If he feels pain, note its exact location and the angle between the table and his leg when it occurs. Repeat this maneuver with the opposite leg. Pain along the sciatic nerve may indicate disk herniation or sciatica. Also, note the range of motion of the hip and knee.

Palpate the flanks and percuss with the fingertips or perform fist percussion to elicit costovertebral angle tenderness.

Medical causes

◆ ***Abdominal aortic aneurysm (dissecting).*** Life-threatening dissection of an abdominal aortic aneurysm may initially cause low back pain or dull abdominal pain, but it usually produces constant upper abdominal pain. A pulsating abdominal mass may be palpated in the epigastrium; after rupture, though, it no longer pulsates. Aneurysm dissection can also cause mottled skin below the waist, absent femoral and pedal pulses, blood pressure that's lower in the legs than in the arms, mild to moderate tenderness with guarding, and abdominal rigidity. Signs of shock (such as cool, clammy skin) appear if blood loss is significant.

◆ ***Ankylosing spondylitis.*** Ankylosing spondylitis is a chronic, progressive disorder that causes sacroiliac pain, which radiates up the spine and is aggravated by lateral pressure on the pelvis. The pain is usually most severe in the morning or after a period of inactivity and isn't relieved by rest. Abnormal rigidity of the lumbar spine with forward flexion is also characteristic. This disorder can cause local tenderness, fatigue, fever, anorexia, weight loss, and occasionally iritis.

◆ ***Appendicitis.*** Appendicitis is a life-threatening disorder in which a vague and dull discomfort in the epigastric or umbilical region migrates to McBurney's point in the right lower quadrant. In retrocecal appendicitis, pain may also radiate to the back. The shift in pain is preceded by anorexia and nausea and is accompanied by fever, occasional vomiting, abdominal tenderness (especially over McBurney's point), and rebound tenderness. Some patients also have painful urinary urgency.

◆ ***Cholecystitis.*** Cholecystitis produces severe pain in the right upper quadrant of the abdomen that may radiate to the right shoulder, chest, or back. The pain may arise suddenly or may increase gradually over several hours; many patients have a history of similar pain after a high-fat meal. Accompanying signs and symptoms include anorexia, fever, nausea, vomiting, right-upper-quadrant tenderness, abdominal rigidity, pallor, and sweating.

◆ ***Chordoma.*** A slowly developing malignant tumor, chordoma causes persistent pain in the lower back, sacrum, and coccyx. As the tumor expands, pain may be accompanied by constipation and bowel or bladder incontinence.

◆ ***Endometriosis.*** Endometriosis causes deep sacral pain and severe cramping pain in the lower abdomen. The pain worsens just before or during menstruation and may be aggravated by defecation. It's accompanied by constipation, abdominal tenderness, dysmenorrhea, and dyspareunia.

◆ ***Intervertebral disk rupture.*** Intervertebral disk rupture produces gradual or sudden low back pain with or without leg pain (sciatica). It rarely produces leg pain alone. Pain usually begins in the back and radiates to the buttocks and leg. The pain is exacerbated by activity, coughing, and sneezing and is eased by rest. It's accompanied by paresthesia (most commonly, numbness or tingling in the lower leg and foot), paravertebral muscle spasm, and decreased reflexes on the affected side. This disorder also affects posture and gait. The patient's spine is slightly flexed and he leans toward the painful side. He walks slowly and rises from a sitting to a standing position with extreme difficulty.

◆ ***Lumbosacral sprain.*** Lumbosacral sprain causes localized aching pain and tenderness associated with muscle spasm on lateral motion. The recumbent patient typically flexes his knees and hips to help ease pain. Flexion of the spine and movement intensify the pain, whereas rest helps relieve it.

◆ ***Metastatic tumors.*** Metastatic tumors commonly spread to the spine, causing low back pain in at least 25% of patients. Typically, the pain begins abruptly, is accompanied by cramping muscle pain (usually worse at night), and isn't relieved by rest.

◆ ***Myeloma.*** Back pain caused by myeloma—a primary malignant tumor—usually begins abruptly and worsens with exercise. It may be accompanied by arthritic signs and symptoms, such as achiness, joint swelling, and tenderness. Other signs and symptoms include fever, malaise, peripheral paresthesia, and weight loss.

◆ ***Pancreatitis (acute).*** Pancreatitis is a life-threatening disorder that usually produces fulminating, continuous upper abdominal pain that may radiate to both flanks and to the back. To relieve this pain, the patient may bend forward, draw his knees to his chest, or move about restlessly.

Early associated signs and symptoms include abdominal tenderness, nausea, vomiting, fever, pallor, and tachycardia; some patients experience abdominal guarding and rigidity, rebound tenderness, and hypoactive bowel sounds. Jaundice may be a late sign. Occurring as inflammation subsides, Turner's sign (ecchymosis of the abdomen or flank) or Cullen's sign (bluish discoloration of skin around the umbilicus and in both flanks) signals hemorrhagic pancreatitis.

◆ ***Perforated ulcer.*** In some patients, perforation of a duodenal or gastric ulcer causes sudden, prostrating epigastric pain that may radiate throughout the abdomen and to the back. This life-threatening disorder also causes boardlike abdominal rigidity, tenderness with guarding, generalized rebound tenderness, absence of bowel sounds, and grunting, shallow respirations. Associated signs include fever, tachycardia, and hypotension.

◆ ***Prostate cancer.*** Chronic aching back pain may be the only symptom of prostate cancer. This disorder may also cause hematuria and decreased urine stream.

◆ ***Pyelonephritis (acute).*** Pyelonephritis produces progressive flank and lower abdominal pain accompanied by back pain or tenderness (especially over the costovertebral angle). Other signs and symptoms include high fever and chills, nausea and vomiting, flank and abdominal tenderness, and urinary frequency and urgency.

◆ ***Reiter's syndrome.*** In some patients, sacroiliac pain is the first sign of Reiter's syndrome. Pain is accompanied by the classic triad of conjunctivitis, urethritis, and arthritis.

◆ ***Renal calculi.*** The colicky pain of renal calculi usually results from irritation of the ureteral lining, which increases the frequency and force of peristaltic contractions. The pain travels from the costovertebral angle to the flank, suprapubic region, and external genitalia. It varies in intensity but may become excruciating if calculi travel down a ureter. Calculi in the renal pelvis and calyces may cause dull and constant flank pain. Renal calculi also cause nausea, vomiting, urinary urgency (if a calculus lodges near the bladder), hematuria, and agitation due to pain. Pain resolves or significantly decreases after calculi move to the bladder. Encourage the patient to recover any expelled calculi for analysis.

◆ ***Sacroiliac strain.*** Sacroiliac strain causes sacroiliac pain that may radiate to the buttock, hip, and lateral aspect of the thigh. The pain is aggravated by weight bearing on the affected extremity and by abduction with resistance of the leg. Associated signs and symptoms include tenderness of the symphysis pubis and a limp or a gluteus medius or abductor lurch.

◆ ***Smallpox (variola major).*** Worldwide eradication of smallpox was achieved in 1977; the United States and Russia have the only known storage sites of the virus. The virus is considered a potential agent for biological warfare. Initial signs and symptoms include high fever, malaise, prostration, severe headache, backache, and abdominal pain. A maculopapular rash develops on the oral mucosa, pharynx, face, and forearms and then spreads to the trunk and legs. Within 2 days, the rash becomes vesicular and later pustular. The lesions develop at the same time, appear identical, and are more prominent on the face and extremities. The pustules are round, firm, and deeply embedded in the skin. After 8 to 9 days, the pustules form a crust, which later separates from the skin, leaving a pitted scar. Death may result from encephalitis, extensive bleeding, or secondary infection.

◆ ***Spinal neoplasm (benign).*** Spinal neoplasm typically causes severe localized back pain and scoliosis.

◆ ***Spinal stenosis.*** Resembling a ruptured intervertebral disk, spinal stenosis produces back pain with or without sciatica, which commonly affects both legs. The pain may radiate to the toes and may progress to numbness or weakness unless the patient rests.

◆ ***Spondylolisthesis.*** A major structural disorder characterized by forward slippage of one vertebra onto another, spondylolisthesis may produce no symptoms or may cause low back pain with or without nerve root involvement. Associated symptoms of nerve root involvement include paresthesia, buttock pain, and pain radiating down the leg. Palpation of the lumbar spine may reveal a "step-off" of the spinous process. Flexion of the spine may be limited.

◆ ***Transverse process fracture.*** This type of fracture causes severe localized back pain with muscle spasm and hematoma.

◆ ***Vertebral compression fracture.*** A vertebral compression fracture may be painless

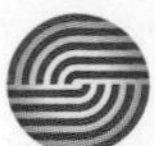

PATIENT-TEACHING AID

Exercises for chronic low back pain

Dear Patient:

If you have chronic low back pain, the exercises illustrated here may help relieve your discomfort and prevent further lumbar deterioration. When you perform these exercises, keep in mind the following points:

- Breathe slowly, inhaling through your nose and exhaling completely through pursed lips.
- Begin gradually, performing each exercise only once per day and progressing to 10 repetitions.
- Exercise moderately; expect mild discomfort, but stop if you experience severe pain.

Back press

Lie on your back, with your arms on your chest or abdomen and your knees bent. Press the small (lower portion) of your back to the floor while tightening your abdominal muscles and buttocks. Count to 10; then slowly relax.

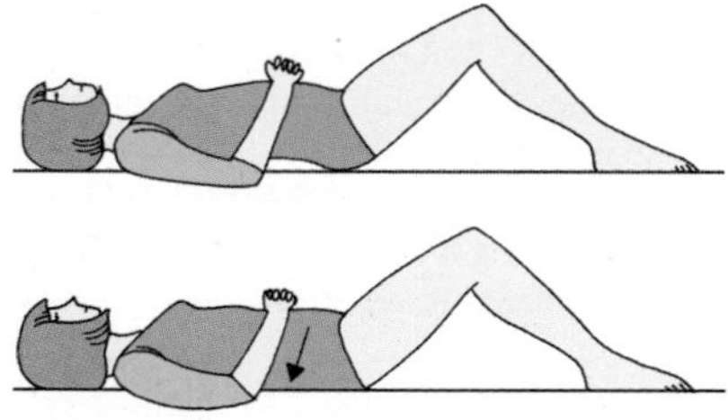

Knee grasp

Lie on your back, with your knees bent. Bring one knee to your chest, grasping it firmly with both hands; lower your knee. Repeat with the other knee—then with *both* knees, as shown here.

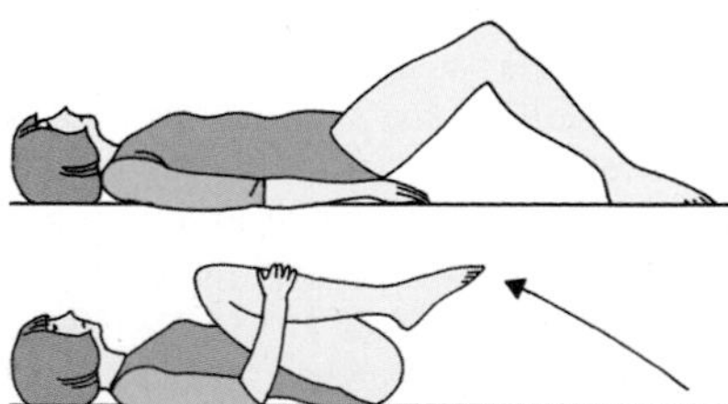

Knee bend

Stand with your hands on the back of a chair for support. Keeping your back straight, slowly bend your knees until you're in a squatting position. Return to your starting position.

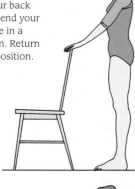

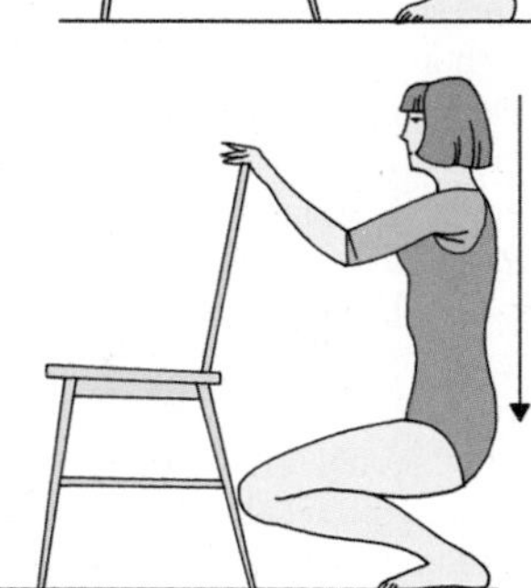

Trunk curl

Lie on your back, with your knees bent and feet flat. Cross your arms on your chest. Lift your head and shoulders off of the floor, and hold for a count of 2. Repeat 10 times. Work up to at least 30, taking brief rests as needed.

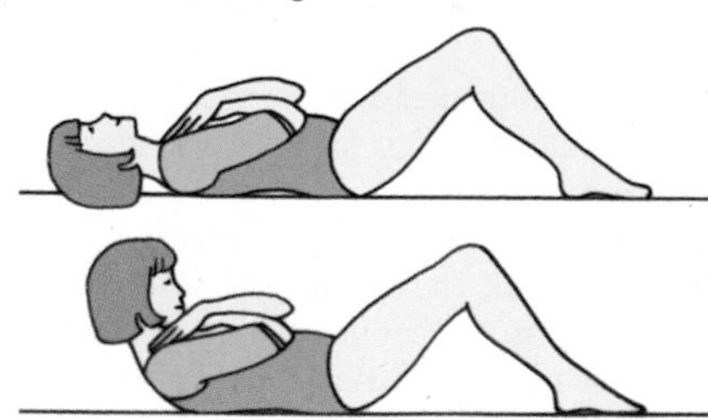

initially. Several weeks later, it causes back pain aggravated by weight bearing and local tenderness. Fracture of a thoracic vertebra may cause referred pain in the lumbar area.

- ***Vertebral osteomyelitis.*** Initially, vertebral osteomyelitis causes insidious back pain. As it progresses, the pain may become constant, more pronounced at night, and aggravated by spinal movement. Accompanying signs and symptoms include vertebral and hamstring spasms, tenderness of the spinous processes, fever, and malaise.
- ***Vertebral osteoporosis.*** Vertebral osteoporosis causes chronic aching back pain that is aggravated by activity and somewhat relieved by rest. Tenderness may also occur.

OTHER CAUSES

- ***Neurologic tests.*** Lumbar puncture and myelography can produce transient back pain.

SPECIAL CONSIDERATIONS

Monitor the patient closely if the back pain suggests a life-threatening cause. Be alert for increasing pain, altered neurovascular status in the legs, loss of bowel or bladder control, altered vital signs, sweating, and cyanosis.

Until a tentative diagnosis is made, withhold analgesics, which may mask symptoms. Also withhold food and fluids in case surgery is necessary. Make the patient as comfortable as possible by elevating the head of the bed and placing a pillow under his knees. Encourage relaxation techniques such as deep breathing. Prepare the patient for a rectal or pelvic examination. He may also require routine blood tests, urinalysis, computed tomography scan, appropriate biopsies, and X-rays of the chest, abdomen, and spine.

Fit the patient for a corset or lumbosacral support, but instruct him not to wear it in bed. He may also require heat or cold therapy, a backboard, a convoluted foam mattress, or pelvic traction. Explain these pain-relief measures to the patient. Teach the patient about alternatives to analgesic drug therapy, such as biofeedback and transcutaneous electrical nerve stimulation.

Be aware that back pain is notoriously associated with malingering. Refer the patient to other professionals, such as a physical therapist, an occupational therapist, or a psychologist, if indicated.

PEDIATRIC POINTERS

Children may have difficulty describing back pain, so be alert for nonverbal clues, such as wincing or refusing to walk. Closely observe the family dynamics during history taking for clues of child abuse.

Back pain in children may stem from intervertebral disk inflammation (diskitis), neoplasms, idiopathic juvenile osteoporosis, and spondylolisthesis. Disk herniation typically doesn't cause back pain. Scoliosis, a common disorder in adolescents, rarely causes back pain.

GERIATRIC POINTERS

Suspect metastatic cancer—especially of the prostate, colon, or breast—in older patients with a recent onset of back pain that usually isn't relieved by rest and worsens at night.

PATIENT COUNSELING

If the patient has chronic back pain, reinforce instructions about bed rest, analgesics, anti-inflammatories, and exercise. (See *Exercises for chronic low back pain*.) Also, suggest that he take daily warm baths to help relieve pain. Help the patient recognize the need to make necessary lifestyle changes, such as losing weight or correcting poor posture. Advise patients with acute back pain secondary to a musculoskeletal problem to continue their daily activities as tolerated, rather than staying on total bed rest.

Barrel chest

In barrel chest, the normal elliptical configuration of the chest is replaced by a rounded one in which the anteroposterior diameter enlarges to approximate the transverse diameter. The diaphragm is depressed and the sternum pushed forward with the ribs attached in a horizontal, not angular, fashion. As a result, the chest appears continuously in the inspiratory position. (See *Recognizing barrel chest,* page 84.)

Typically a late sign of chronic obstructive pulmonary disease (COPD), barrel chest results from augmented lung volumes due to chronic airflow obstruction. The patient may not notice it because it develops gradually.

HISTORY AND PHYSICAL EXAMINATION

Begin by asking about a history of pulmonary disease. Note chronic exposure to environmental

Recognizing barrel chest

In a normal adult chest, the ratio of anteroposterior to transverse (or lateral) diameter is 1:2. In patients with barrel chest, this ratio approaches 1:1 as the anteroposterior diameter enlarges.

NORMAL CHEST

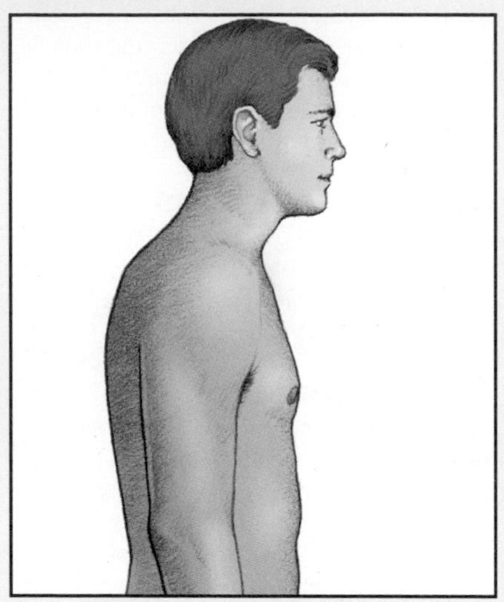

BARREL CHEST

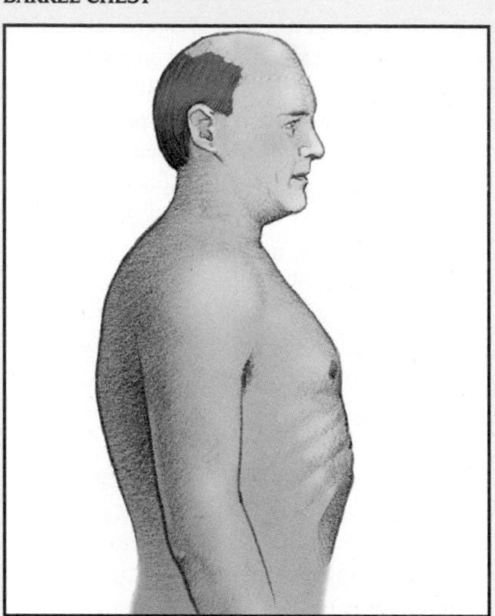

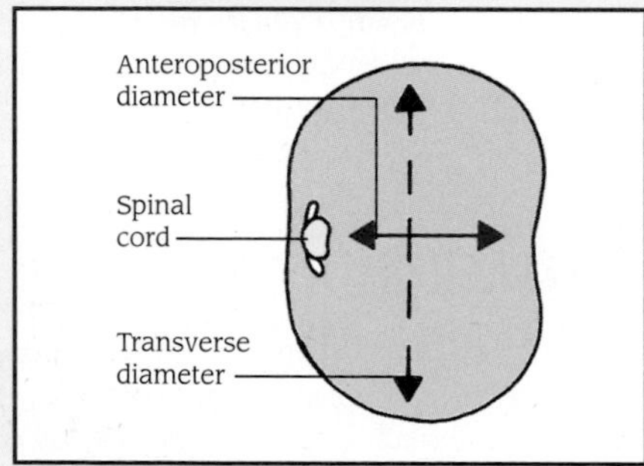

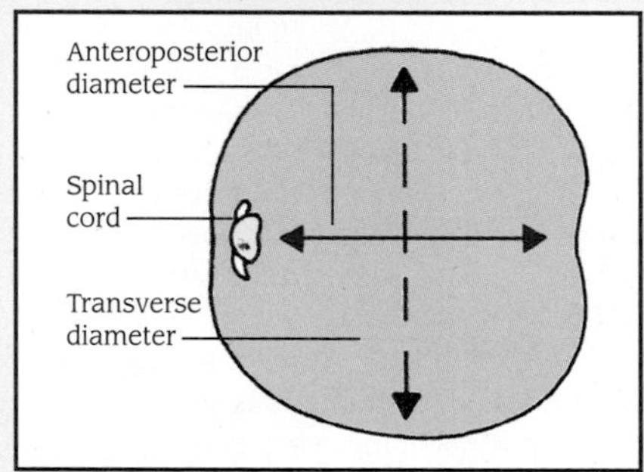

irritants such as asbestos. Also ask about the patient's smoking habits.

Then explore other signs and symptoms of pulmonary disease. Does the patient have a cough? Is it productive or nonproductive? If it's productive, have him describe the sputum's color and consistency. Does the patient experience shortness of breath? Is it related to activity? Although dyspnea is common with COPD, many patients fail to associate it with the disease. Instead, they blame "old age" or "getting out of shape" for causing dyspnea.

Auscultate for abnormal breath sounds, such as crackles and wheezing. Then percuss the chest. Hyperresonant sounds indicate trapped air; dull or flat sounds indicate mucus buildup. Be alert for accessory muscle use, intercostal retractions, and tachypnea, which may signal respiratory distress.

Finally, observe the patient's general appearance. Look for central cyanosis in the cheeks, nose, and mucosa inside the lips. In addition, look for peripheral cyanosis in the nail beds. Also note clubbing, a late sign of COPD.

Medical causes

◆ ***Asthma.*** Typically, barrel chest develops only in chronic asthma. An acute asthma attack causes severe dyspnea, wheezing, and a productive cough. It can also cause prolonged expiratory time, accessory muscle use, tachycardia, tachypnea, perspiration, and flushing.

◆ ***Chronic bronchitis.*** A late sign in chronic bronchitis, barrel chest is characteristically preceded by a productive cough and exertional dyspnea. This form of COPD may also cause cyanosis, tachypnea, wheezing, prolonged expiratory time, and accessory muscle use.

◆ ***Emphysema.*** Barrel chest is a late sign in this form of COPD. Typically, emphysema begins insidiously, with dyspnea the predominant symptom. Eventually, it may also cause chronic cough, anorexia, weight loss, malaise, accessory muscle use, pursed-lip breathing, tachypnea, peripheral cyanosis, and clubbing.

Special considerations

To ease breathing, have the patient sit and lean forward, resting his hands on his knees to support the upper torso (tripod position). This position allows maximum diaphragmatic excursion, facilitating chest expansion.

Pediatric pointers

In infants, the ratio of anteroposterior to transverse diameter is normally 1:1. As the child grows, this ratio gradually changes to 1:2 by age 5 to 6. Cystic fibrosis and chronic asthma may cause barrel chest in children.

Geriatric pointers

In elderly patients, senile kyphosis of the thoracic spine may be mistaken for barrel chest. However, patients with senile kyphosis lack signs of pulmonary disease.

Patient counseling

Advise the patient to avoid bronchial irritants, especially smoking, which may exacerbate COPD. Tell him to report purulent sputum production, which may indicate upper respiratory tract infection. Instruct him to space his activities to help minimize exertional dyspnea.

Battle's sign

Battle's sign—ecchymosis over the mastoid process of the temporal bone—is commonly the only outward sign of a basilar skull fracture. In fact, this type of fracture may go undetected even by X-ray of the skull. If left untreated, a basilar skull fracture can be fatal because of associated injury to the nearby cranial nerves and brain stem as well as to blood vessels and the meninges.

Appearing behind one or both ears, Battle's sign is easily overlooked or hidden by the patient's hair. During emergency care of a trauma victim, it may be overshadowed by imminently life-threatening or more apparent injuries.

A force that's strong enough to fracture the base of the skull causes Battle's sign by damaging supporting tissues of the mastoid area and causing seepage of blood from the fracture site to the mastoid. Battle's sign usually develops 24 to 36 hours after the fracture and may persist for several days to weeks.

History and physical examination

Perform a complete neurologic examination, beginning with the history. Ask the patient about recent trauma to the head. Did he sustain a severe blow to the head? Was he involved in a motor vehicle accident? Note the patient's level of consciousness as he responds. Does he respond quickly or slowly? Are his answers appropriate, or does he appear confused?

Check the patient's vital signs; be alert for widening pulse pressure and bradycardia, signs of increased intracranial pressure. Assess cranial nerve function in nerves II, III, IV, VI, VII, and VIII. Evaluate pupillary size and response to light as well as motor and verbal responses. Relate these data to the Glasgow Coma Scale. Also, note cerebrospinal fluid (CSF) leakage from the nose or ears. Ask about postnasal drip, which may reflect CSF drainage down the throat. Look for the halo sign—a bloodstain encircled by a yellowish ring—on bed linens or dressings. To confirm that drainage is CSF, test it with a Dextrostix; CSF is positive for glucose, whereas mucus isn't. Follow up the neurologic examination with a complete physical examination to detect other injuries associated with a basilar skull fracture.

Medical causes

◆ ***Basilar skull fracture.*** Battle's sign may be the only outward sign of a basilar skull fracture, or it may be accompanied by periorbital ecchymosis (raccoon eyes), conjunctival hemorrhage, nystagmus, ocular deviation, epistaxis, anosmia, a bulging tympanic membrane (from CSF or blood accumulation), visible fracture lines on the external auditory canal, tinnitus, difficulty hearing, facial paralysis, or vertigo.

Identifying Biot's respirations

Biot's respirations, also known as ataxic respirations, have a completely irregular pattern. Shallow and deep breaths occur randomly, with haphazard, irregular pauses. The respiratory rate tends to be slow and may progressively decelerate to apnea.

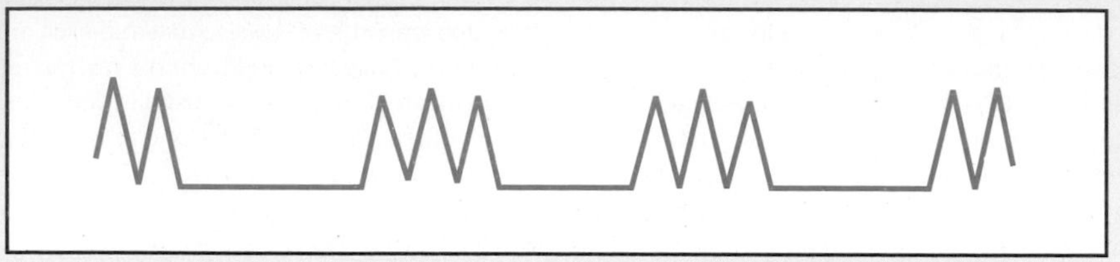

SPECIAL CONSIDERATIONS

Expect a patient with a basilar skull fracture to be on bed rest for several days to weeks. Keep him flat to decrease pressure on dural tears and to minimize CSF leakage. Monitor his neurologic status closely. Avoid nasogastric intubation and nasopharyngeal suction, which may cause cerebral infection. Also, caution the patient against blowing his nose, which may worsen a dural tear.

The patient may need skull X-rays and a computed tomography scan to help confirm a basilar skull fracture and to evaluate the severity of the head injury. Typically, these fractures and any associated dural tears heal spontaneously within several days to weeks. However, if the patient has a large dural tear, a craniotomy may be necessary to repair the tear with a graft patch.

PEDIATRIC POINTERS

Children who are victims of abuse commonly sustain basilar skull fractures from severe blows to the head. As in adults, Battle's sign may be the only outward sign of fracture and, perhaps, the only clue to child abuse. If you suspect child abuse, follow hospital protocol for reporting the incident.

Biot's respirations

[Ataxic respirations]

A late and ominous sign of neurologic deterioration, Biot's respirations are characterized by irregular and unpredictable rate, rhythm, and depth. This rare breathing pattern may appear abruptly and may reflect increased pressure on the medulla coinciding with brain stem compression.

EMERGENCY INTERVENTIONS *Observe the patient's breathing pattern for several minutes to avoid confusing Biot's respirations with other respiratory patterns. (See* Identifying Biot's respirations.*) Prepare to intubate the patient and provide mechanical ventilation. Next, take vital signs, noting especially increased systolic pressure.*

MEDICAL CAUSES

◆ ***Brain stem compression.*** Biot's respirations are characteristic in brain stem compression—a neurologic emergency. Rapidly enlarging lesions may cause ataxic respirations and, eventually, complete respiratory arrest.

SPECIAL CONSIDERATIONS

Monitor vital signs frequently. Elevate the head of the patient's bed 30 degrees to help reduce intracranial pressure. Prepare the patient for emergency surgery to relieve pressure on the brain stem. Computed tomography scans or magnetic resonance imaging may confirm the cause of brain stem compression.

Because Biot's respirations typically reflect a grave prognosis, keep the patient's family informed and provide emotional support.

PEDIATRIC POINTERS

Biot's respirations are rarely seen in children.

Bladder distention

Bladder distention—abnormal enlargement of the bladder—results from an inability to excrete urine, which then accumulates in the bladder. Distention can be caused by a mechanical or anatomic obstruction, a neuromuscular disorder, or the use of certain drugs. Relatively common in all ages and both sexes, it's most common in older men with prostate disorders that cause urine retention.

Distention usually develops gradually, but it occasionally has a sudden onset. Gradual distention usually causes no symptoms until stretching of the bladder produces discomfort. Acute distention produces suprapubic fullness, pressure, and pain. If severe distention isn't corrected promptly by catheterization or massage, the bladder rises within the abdomen, its walls become thin, and renal function can be impaired.

Bladder distention is aggravated by the intake of caffeine, alcohol, large quantities of fluid, and diuretics. (See *Bladder distention: Causes and associated findings,* pages 88 and 89.)

EMERGENCY INTERVENTIONS *If the patient has severe distention, insert an indwelling urinary catheter to help relieve discomfort and prevent bladder rupture. If more than 700 ml is emptied from the bladder, compressed blood vessels dilate, which may make the patient feel faint. Typically, the indwelling urinary catheter is clamped for 30 to 60 minutes to permit vessel compensation.*

HISTORY AND PHYSICAL EXAMINATION

If distention isn't severe, begin by reviewing the patient's voiding patterns. Find out the time and amount of the patient's last voiding and the amount of fluid consumed since then. Ask if he has difficulty urinating. Does he use Valsalva's or Credé's maneuver to initiate urination? Does he urinate with urgency or without warning? Is urination painful or irritating? Ask about the force and continuity of his urine stream and whether he feels that his bladder is empty after voiding.

Explore the patient's history of urinary tract obstruction or infections; venereal disease; neurologic, intestinal, or pelvic surgery; lower abdominal or urinary tract trauma; and systemic or neurologic disorders. Ask about his drug history, including his use of over-the-counter drugs.

Take the patient's vital signs, and percuss and palpate the bladder. (Remember that if the bladder is empty, it can't be palpated through the abdominal wall.) Inspect the urethral meatus, and measure its diameter. Describe the appearance and amount of any discharge. Finally, test for perineal sensation and anal sphincter tone; in male patients, digitally examine the prostate gland.

MEDICAL CAUSES

◆ ***Benign prostatic hyperplasia (BPH).*** In BPH, bladder distention develops gradually as the prostate enlarges. Occasionally, its onset is acute. Initially, the patient experiences urinary hesitancy, straining, and frequency, reduced force of and inability to stop the urine stream; nocturia; and postvoiding dribbling. As the disorder progresses, it produces prostate enlargement, sensations of suprapubic fullness and incomplete bladder emptying, perineal pain, constipation, and hematuria.

◆ ***Bladder calculi.*** Bladder calculi may produce bladder distention, but pain is usually the only symptom. The pain is usually referred to the tip of the penis, the vulvar area, the lower back, or the heel. It worsens during walking or exercise and abates when the patient lies down. It's usually most severe when micturition ceases. The pain may be accompanied by urinary frequency and urgency, terminal hematuria, and dysuria.

◆ ***Bladder cancer.*** By blocking the urethral orifice, neoplasms can cause bladder distention. Associated signs and symptoms include hematuria (most common sign); urinary frequency and urgency; nocturia; dysuria; pyuria; pain in the bladder, rectum, pelvis, flank, back, or legs; vomiting; diarrhea; and sleeplessness. A mass may be palpable on bimanual examination.

CULTURAL CUE *Bladder cancer is twice as common in Whites as in Blacks. It's relatively uncommon among Asians, Hispanics, and Native Americans.*

◆ ***Multiple sclerosis.*** In this neuromuscular disorder, urine retention and bladder distention result from interruption of upper motor neuron control of the bladder. Associated signs and symptoms include optic neuritis, paresthesia, impaired position and vibratory senses, diplopia, nystagmus, dizziness, abnormal reflexes, dysarthria, muscle weakness, emotional lability, Lhermitte's sign (transient, electric-like shocks that spread down the body when the head is flexed), Babinski's sign, and ataxia.

◆ ***Prostate cancer.*** Prostate cancer eventually causes bladder distention in about 25% of

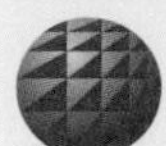

SIGNS & SYMPTOMS

Bladder distention: Causes and associated findings

Common causes	Ataxia	Constipation	Dysuria	Fatigue	Fever	Hematuria	Muscle weakness	Myalgia	Nausea	Nocturia	Pain, buttock and sacral	Pain, flank	Pain, lower back
	Major associated signs and symptoms												
Benign prostatic hyperplasia		●				●				●			
Bladder calculi			●			●							
Bladder cancer			●			●				●	●	●	●
Multiple sclerosis	●						●						
Prostate cancer		●	●	●						●			
Prostatitis (acute)			●	●	●	●		●	●				
Prostatitis (chronic)			●			●					●		●
Spinal neoplasms		●	●			●	●			●			●
Urethral calculi											●		
Urethral strictures			●										

patients. Usual signs and symptoms include dysuria, urinary frequency and urgency, nocturia, weight loss, fatigue, perineal pain, constipation, and induration of the prostate or a rigid, irregular prostate on digital rectal examination. In some patients, urine retention and bladder distention are the only signs.

CULTURAL CUE *Prostate cancer is more common in Blacks than in other ethnic groups.*

◆ ***Prostatitis.*** In acute prostatitis, bladder distention occurs rapidly along with perineal discomfort and a sensation of suprapubic fullness. Other signs and symptoms include perineal pain; tense, boggy, tender, and warm enlarged prostate; decreased libido; impotence; decreased force of the urine stream; dysuria; hematuria; and urinary frequency and urgency. Additional signs and symptoms include fatigue, malaise, myalgia, fever, chills, nausea, and vomiting.

Bladder distention is rare in chronic prostatitis, which may be accompanied by perineal discomfort, a sensation of suprapubic fullness, prostatic tenderness, decreased libido, urinary frequency and urgency, dysuria, pyuria, hematuria, persistent urethral discharge, ejaculatory pain, and dull pain radiating to the lower back, buttocks, penis, or perineum.

◆ ***Spinal neoplasms.*** Disrupting upper neuron control of the bladder, spinal neoplasms cause neurogenic bladder and resultant distention. Associated signs and symptoms include a sense of pelvic fullness, continuous overflow dribbling, back pain that often mimics sciatica pain, constipation, tender vertebral processes, sensory deficits, and muscle weakness, flaccidity, and atrophy. Signs and symptoms of urinary tract infection (dysuria, urinary frequency and

	Pain, pelvic	Pain, penile	Pain, perineal	Pain, vulvar	Prostatic enlargement	Prostatic rigidity	Pyuria	Suprapubic fullness	Urethral discharge	Urinary frequency	Urinary stream changes	Urinary urgency	Vomiting
			●		●			●		●	●		
		●		●						●		●	
	●						●			●		●	●
			●			●				●		●	
			●		●			●		●	●	●	●
					●		●	●	●	●	●	●	
		●	●							●		●	
		●	●	●					●				
							●		●	●	●	●	

urgency, nocturia, tenesmus, hematuria, and weakness) may also occur.

◆ ***Urethral calculi.*** In urethral calculi, urethral obstruction leads to interrupted urine flow and bladder distention. The obstruction causes pain radiating to the penis or vulva and referred to the perineum or rectum. It may also produce a palpable stone and urethral discharge.

◆ ***Urethral stricture.*** Urethral stricture results in urine retention and bladder distention with chronic urethral discharge (most common sign), urinary frequency (also common), dysuria, urgency, decreased force and diameter of the urine stream, and pyuria. Urinoma and urosepsis may also develop.

OTHER CAUSES

◆ ***Catheterization.*** Using an indwelling urinary catheter can result in urine retention and bladder distention. While the catheter is in place, inadequate drainage due to kinked tubing or an occluded lumen may lead to urine retention. In addition, a misplaced urinary catheter or irritation due to catheter removal may cause edema, thereby blocking urine outflow.

◆ ***Drugs.*** Parasympatholytics, anticholinergics, ganglionic blockers, sedatives, anesthetics, and opiates can produce urine retention and bladder distention.

SPECIAL CONSIDERATIONS

Monitor the patient's vital signs and the extent of bladder distention. Encourage the patient to change positions to alleviate discomfort. Provide an analgesic if necessary.

Prepare the patient for diagnostic tests (such as endoscopy and radiologic studies) to determine the cause of bladder distention. You may need to prepare him for surgery if interventions fail to relieve bladder distention and obstruction prevents catheterization.

PEDIATRIC POINTERS

Look for urine retention and bladder distention in any infant who fails to void normal amounts. (In the first 48 hours of life, an infant excretes about 60 ml of urine; during the next week, he excretes about 300 ml of urine daily.) In males, posterior urethral valves, meatal stenosis, phimosis, spinal cord anomalies, bladder diverticula, and other congenital defects may cause urinary obstruction and resultant bladder distention.

PATIENT COUNSELING

If the patient doesn't require immediate urinary catheterization, provide privacy and suggest that he assume the normal voiding position. Teach him to perform Valsalva's maneuver, or gently perform Credé's maneuver. You can also stroke or intermittently apply ice to the inner thigh, or help him relax in a warm tub or sitz bath. Use the power of suggestion to stimulate voiding. For example, run water in the sink, pour warm water over his perineum, place his hands in warm water, or play tapes of aquatic sounds.

Blood pressure decrease

[Hypotension]

Low blood pressure refers to inadequate intravascular pressure to maintain the body's oxygen requirements. Although commonly linked to shock, this sign may also result from cardiovascular, respiratory, neurologic, or metabolic disorders. Hypoperfusion states especially affect the kidneys, brain, and heart, and may lead to renal failure, change in level of consciousness (LOC), or myocardial ischemia. Low blood pressure may also be caused by certain diagnostic tests—most commonly those using contrast media—and the use of certain drugs. It may stem from stress or a change of position—specifically, rising abruptly from a supine or sitting position to a standing position (orthostatic hypotension).

Normal blood pressure varies considerably; what qualifies as low blood pressure for one person may be perfectly normal for another. Consequently, every blood pressure reading must be compared against the patient's baseline. Typically, a reading below 90/60 mm Hg, or a drop of 30 mm Hg from the baseline, is considered low blood pressure.

Low blood pressure can reflect an expanded intravascular space (as in severe infections, allergic reactions, or adrenal insufficiency), reduced intravascular volume (as in dehydration and hemorrhage), or decreased cardiac output (as in impaired cardiac muscle contractility). Because the body's pressure-regulating mechanisms are complex and interrelated, a combination of these factors usually contributes to low blood pressure.

EMERGENCY INTERVENTIONS *If the patient's systolic pressure is less than 80 mm Hg, or 30 mm Hg below his baseline, suspect shock immediately. Quickly evaluate the patient for a decreased LOC. Check his apical pulse for tachycardia and respirations for tachypnea. Also, inspect the patient for cool, clammy skin. Elevate his legs above the level of his heart, or place him in Trendelenburg's position if the bed can be adjusted. Then start an I.V. line using a large-bore catheter to replace fluids and blood or to administer drugs. Prepare to administer oxygen with mechanical ventilation if necessary. Monitor the patient's intake and output, and insert an indwelling urinary catheter for the accurate measurement of urine. The patient may also need a central venous access device or a pulmonary artery catheter to facilitate monitoring of fluid status. Prepare for cardiac monitoring to evaluate cardiac rhythm. Be ready to insert a nasogastric tube to prevent aspiration in the comatose patient. Throughout emergency interventions, keep the patient's spinal column immobile until spinal cord trauma is ruled out.*

HISTORY AND PHYSICAL EXAMINATION

If the patient is conscious, ask him about associated symptoms. For example, does he feel unusually weak or fatigued? Has he had nausea, vomiting, or dark or bloody stools? Is his vision blurred? Gait unsteady? Does he have palpitations, chest or abdominal pain, or difficulty breathing? Has he had episodes of dizziness or fainting? Do these episodes occur when he stands up suddenly? If so, take the patient's blood pressure while he's lying down, sitting, and then standing and compare readings. A drop in systolic or diastolic pressure of 10 mm Hg or more and an increase in heart rate of more than 15 beats/minute between position changes suggest orthostatic hypotension. (See *Ensuring accurate blood pressure measurement,* page 92.)

Next, continue with a physical examination. Inspect the skin for pallor, sweating, and clamminess. Palpate peripheral pulses. Note a paradoxical pulse—an accentuated fall in systolic pressure during inspiration—which suggests pericardial tamponade. Then auscultate for abnormal heart sounds (gallops, murmurs), rate (bradycardia, tachycardia), or rhythm. Auscultate the lungs for abnormal breath sounds (diminished sounds, crackles, wheezing), rate (bradypnea, tachypnea), or rhythm (agonal or Cheyne-Stokes respirations). Look for signs of hemorrhage, including visible bleeding, palpable masses, bruising, and tenderness. Assess the patient for abdominal rigidity and rebound tenderness; auscultate for abnormal bowel sounds. Also, carefully assess the patient for possible sources of infection such as open wounds.

Medical causes

◆ ***Adrenal insufficiency (acute).*** Orthostatic hypotension is characteristic in acute adrenal insufficiency and is accompanied by fatigue, weakness, nausea, vomiting, abdominal discomfort, weight loss, fever, and tachycardia. The patient may also have hyperpigmentation of fingers, nails, nipples, scars, and body folds; pale, cool, clammy skin; restlessness; decreased urine output; tachypnea; and coma.

◆ ***Alcohol toxicity.*** Low blood pressure occurs infrequently in alcohol toxicity; more common signs and symptoms include a distinct alcohol breath odor, tachycardia, bradypnea, hypothermia, decreased LOC, seizures, staggering gait, nausea, vomiting, diuresis, and slow, stertorous breathing.

◆ ***Anaphylactic shock.*** Following exposure to an allergen, such as penicillin or insect venom, a dramatic fall in blood pressure and narrowed pulse pressure signal this severe allergic reaction. Initially, anaphylactic shock causes anxiety, restlessness, a feeling of doom, intense itching (especially of the hands and feet), and a pounding headache. Later, it may also produce weakness, sweating, nasal congestion, coughing, difficulty breathing, nausea, abdominal cramps, involuntary defecation, seizures, flushing, urinary incontinence, tachycardia, and change or loss of voice due to laryngeal edema.

◆ ***Anthrax, inhalation.*** Anthrax is an acute infectious disease that's caused by the gram-positive, spore-forming bacterium *Bacillus anthracis.* Although the disease most commonly occurs in wild and domestic grazing animals, such as cattle, sheep, and goats, the spores can live in the soil for many years. The disease can occur in humans exposed to infected animals, tissue from infected animals, or biological agents. Most natural cases occur in agricultural regions worldwide. Anthrax may occur in cutaneous, inhalation, or GI forms.

Inhalation anthrax is caused by inhalation of aerosolized spores. Initial signs and symptoms are flulike and include fever, chills, weakness, cough, and chest pain. The disease generally occurs in two stages with a period of recovery after the initial signs and symptoms. The second stage develops abruptly with rapid deterioration marked by fever, dyspnea, stridor, and hypotension generally leading to death within 24 hours. Radiologic findings include mediastinitis and symmetrical mediastinal widening.

◆ ***Cardiac arrhythmias.*** In an arrhythmia, blood pressure may fluctuate between normal and low readings. Dizziness, chest pain, difficulty breathing, light-headedness, weakness, fatigue, and palpitations may also occur. Auscultation typically reveals an irregular rhythm and a pulse rate greater than 100 beats/minute or less than 60 beats/minute.

◆ ***Cardiac contusion.*** In a cardiac contusion, low blood pressure occurs along with tachycardia and, at times, anginal pain and dyspnea.

◆ ***Cardiac tamponade.*** An accentuated fall in systolic pressure (more than 10 mm Hg) during inspiration, known as *paradoxical pulse,* is characteristic in patients with cardiac tamponade. This disorder also causes restlessness, cyanosis, tachycardia, jugular vein distention, muffled heart sounds, dyspnea, and Kussmaul's sign (increased venous distention with inspiration).

◆ ***Cardiogenic shock.*** A fall in systolic pressure to less than 80 mm Hg, or to 30 mm Hg less than the patient's baseline, because of decreased cardiac contractility is characteristic in patients with this disorder. Accompanying low blood pressure are tachycardia, narrowed pulse pressure, diminished Korotkoff sounds, peripheral cyanosis, and pale, cool, clammy skin. Cardiogenic shock also causes restlessness and anxiety, which may progress to disorientation and confusion. Associated signs and symptoms include angina, dyspnea, jugular vein distention,

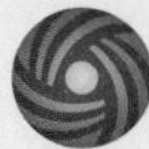

EXAMINATION TIP

Ensuring accurate blood pressure measurement

When taking the patient's blood pressure, begin by applying the cuff properly, as shown here.

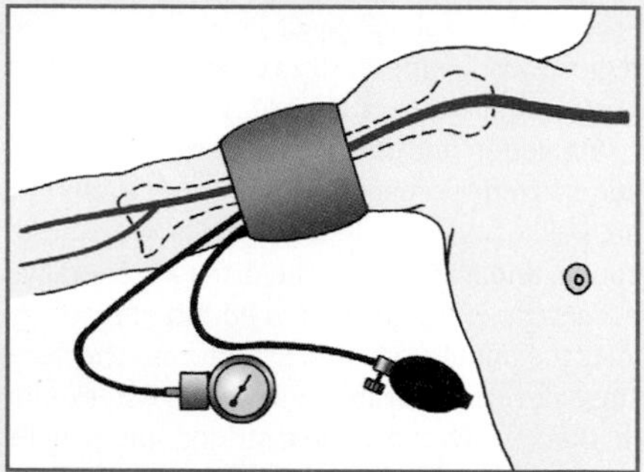

Then be alert for these common pitfalls to avoid recording an inaccurate blood pressure measurement.

◆ *Wrong-sized cuff.* Select the appropriate-sized cuff for the patient. This ensures that adequate pressure is applied to compress the brachial artery during cuff inflation. A cuff bladder that's too narrow will yield a false-high reading; one that's too wide, a false-low reading. The cuff bladder width should be about 40% of the circumference of the midpoint of the limb; bladder length should be twice the width. If the arm circumference is less than 13" (33 cm), select a regular-sized cuff; if it's between 13" and 16" (33 to 40.5 cm), a large-sized cuff; if it's more than 16", a thigh cuff. Pediatric cuffs are also available.

◆ *Slow cuff deflation, causing venous congestion in the extremity.* Don't deflate the cuff more slowly than 2 mm Hg/heartbeat because you'll get a false-high reading.

◆ *Cuff wrapped too loosely, reducing its effective width.* Tighten the cuff to avoid a false-high reading.

◆ *Mercury column not read at eye level.* Read the mercury column at eye level. If the column is below eye level, you may record a false-low reading; if it's above eye level, a false-high reading.

◆ *Tilted mercury column.* Keep the mercury column vertical to avoid a false-high reading.

◆ *Poorly timed measurement.* Don't take the patient's blood pressure if he appears anxious or has just eaten or ambulated; you'll get a false-high reading.

◆ *Incorrect position of the arm.* Keep the patient's arm level with his heart to avoid a false-low reading.

◆ *Cuff overinflation, causing venospasm or pain.* Don't overinflate the cuff because you'll get a false-high reading.

◆ *Failure to notice an auscultatory gap* (sound fades out for 10 to 15 mm Hg, then returns). To avoid missing the top Korotkoff sound, estimate systolic pressure by palpation first. Then inflate the cuff rapidly—at a rate of 2 to 3 mm Hg/second—to about 30 mm Hg above the palpable systolic pressure.

◆ *Inaudibility of feeble sounds.* Before reinflating the cuff, have the patient raise his arm to reduce venous pressure and amplify low-volume sounds. After inflating the cuff, lower the patient's arm; then deflate the cuff and listen. Alternatively, with the patient's arm positioned at heart level, inflate the cuff and have the patient make a fist. Have him rapidly open and close his hand 10 times before you begin to deflate the cuff; then listen. Be sure to document that the blood pressure reading was augmented.

oliguria, ventricular gallop, tachypnea, and weak, rapid pulse.

◆ ***Cholera.*** Cholera is an acute infection caused by the bacterium *Vibrio cholerae* that may be mild with uncomplicated diarrhea or severe and life-threatening. Cholera is spread by ingestion of contaminated water or food, especially shellfish. Signs include abrupt watery diarrhea and vomiting. Severe water and electrolyte loss leads to thirst, weakness, muscle cramps, decreased skin turgor, oliguria, tachycardia, and hypotension. Without treatment, death can occur within hours.

◆ ***Diabetic ketoacidosis.*** Hypovolemia triggered by osmotic diuresis in hyperglycemia is responsible for the low blood pressure associated with diabetic ketoacidosis, which is usually present in patients with type 1 diabetes mellitus. It also commonly produces polydipsia, polyuria, polyphagia, dehydration, weight loss, abdominal pain, nausea, vomiting, breath with fruity odor, Kussmaul's respirations, tachycardia, seizures, confusion, and stupor that may progress to coma.

◆ ***Heart failure.*** In heart failure, blood pressure may fluctuate between normal and low readings, but a precipitous drop in blood pressure may signal cardiogenic shock. Other signs and symptoms of heart failure include exertional dyspnea, dyspnea of abrupt or gradual onset, paroxysmal nocturnal dyspnea or difficulty breathing in the supine position (orthopnea), fatigue, weight gain, pallor or cyanosis, sweating, and anxiety. Auscultation reveals ventricular gallop, tachycardia, bilateral crackles, and tachypnea. Dependent edema, jugular vein distention, increased capillary refill time, and hepatomegaly may also occur.

◆ ***Hyperosmolar hyperglycemic nonketotic syndrome (HHNS).*** HHNS, which is common in persons with type 2 diabetes mellitus, decreases blood pressure—at times dramatically, if the patient loses significant fluid from diuresis due to severe hyperglycemia and hyperosmolarity. It also produces dry mouth, poor skin turgor, tachycardia, confusion progressing to coma and, occasionally, generalized tonic-clonic seizures.

◆ ***Hypovolemic shock.*** A fall in systolic pressure to less than 80 mm Hg, or 30 mm Hg less than the patient's baseline, secondary to acute blood loss or dehydration is characteristic in patients with hypovolemic shock. Accompanying it are diminished Korotkoff sounds, narrowed pulse pressure, and rapid, weak, and irregular pulse. Peripheral vasoconstriction causes cyanosis of the extremities and pale, cool, clammy skin. Other signs and symptoms include oliguria, confusion, disorientation, restlessness, and anxiety.

◆ ***Hypoxemia.*** Initially, blood pressure may be normal or slightly elevated, but as hypoxemia becomes more pronounced blood pressure drops. The patient may also display tachycardia, tachypnea, dyspnea, confusion, and stupor that may progress to coma.

◆ ***Myocardial infarction.*** In this life-threatening disorder, blood pressure may be low or high. However, a precipitous drop in blood pressure may signal cardiogenic shock. Associated signs and symptoms include chest pain that may radiate to the jaw, shoulder, arm, or epigastrium; dyspnea; anxiety; nausea or vomiting; sweating; and cool, pale, or cyanotic skin. Auscultation may reveal an atrial gallop, a murmur and, occasionally, an irregular pulse.

◆ ***Neurogenic shock.*** The result of sympathetic denervation due to cervical injury or anesthesia, neurogenic shock produces low blood pressure and bradycardia. However, the patient's skin remains warm and dry because of cutaneous vasodilation and sweat gland denervation. Depending on the cause of shock, motor weakness of the limbs or diaphragm may also occur.

◆ ***Pulmonary embolism.*** Pulmonary embolism causes sudden, sharp chest pain and dyspnea accompanied by cough and, occasionally, low-grade fever. Low blood pressure occurs with narrowed pulse pressure and diminished Korotkoff sounds. Associated signs include tachycardia, tachypnea, paradoxical pulse, jugular vein distention, and hemoptysis.

◆ ***Septic shock.*** Initially, septic shock produces fever and chills. Low blood pressure, tachycardia, and tachypnea may also develop early, but the patient's skin remains warm. Later, low blood pressure becomes increasingly severe—with systolic pressure less than 80 mm Hg, or 30 mm Hg less than the baseline—and is accompanied by narrowed pulse pressure. Other late signs and symptoms include pale skin, cyanotic extremities, apprehension, thirst, oliguria, and coma.

◆ ***Vasovagal syncope.*** Vasovagal syncope is a transient loss or near-loss of consciousness that's characterized by low blood pressure, pallor, cold sweats, nausea, palpitations or bradycardia, and weakness following stressful, painful, or claustrophobic experiences.

Other causes

◆ ***Diagnostic tests.*** These include the gastric acid stimulation test using histamine and X-ray studies using contrast media. The latter may trigger an allergic reaction, which causes low blood pressure.

◆ ***Drugs.*** Calcium channel blockers, diuretics, vasodilators, alpha- and beta-adrenergic blockers, general anesthetics, opioid analgesics, monoamine oxidase inhibitors, anxiolytics (such as benzodiazepines), tranquilizers, and most I.V. antiarrhythmics (especially bretylium) can cause low blood pressure.

Special considerations

Check the patient's vital signs frequently to determine if low blood pressure is constant or intermittent. If blood pressure is extremely low, an arterial catheter may be inserted to allow close monitoring of pressures. Alternatively, a Doppler flowmeter may be used.

Normal pediatric blood pressure

Age	Normal systolic pressure	Normal diastolic pressure
Birth to 3 months	40 to 80 mm Hg	Not detectable
3 months to 1 year	80 to 100 mm Hg	Not detectable
1 to 4 years	100 to 108 mm Hg	60 mm Hg
4 to 12 years	108 to 124 mm Hg	60 to 70 mm Hg

Place the patient on bed rest. Keep the side rails of the bed up. If the patient is ambulatory, assist him as necessary. To avoid falls, don't leave a dizzy patient unattended when he's sitting or walking.

Prepare the patient for laboratory tests, which may include urinalysis, routine blood studies, an electrocardiogram, and chest, cervical, and abdominal X-rays.

Pediatric pointers

Normal blood pressure is lower in children than in adults. (See *Normal pediatric blood pressure*.)

Because children are prone to accidents, suspect trauma or shock first as a possible cause of low blood pressure. Remember that low blood pressure typically doesn't accompany head injury in adults because intracranial hemorrhage is insufficient to cause hypovolemia. However, it does accompany head injury in infants and young children; their expandable cranial vaults allow significant blood loss into the cranial space, resulting in hypovolemia.

Another common cause of low blood pressure in children is dehydration, which results from failure to thrive or from persistent diarrhea and vomiting for as little as 24 hours.

Geriatric pointers

In elderly patients, low blood pressure commonly results from the use of multiple drugs with this potential adverse effect, a problem that needs to be addressed. Orthostatic hypotension due to autonomic dysfunction is another common cause.

Patient counseling

If the patient has orthostatic hypotension, instruct him to stand up slowly from a sitting or lying position. Advise patients with vasovagal syncope to avoid situations that trigger the episodes. Evaluate the patient's need for a cane or walker.

Blood pressure increase

[Hypertension]

Elevated blood pressure—an intermittent or sustained increase in blood pressure exceeding 140/90 mm Hg—strikes more men than women and twice as many Blacks as Whites. By itself, this common sign is easily ignored by the patient; after all, he can't see or feel it. However, its causes can be life threatening.

GENDER CUE *Hypertension has been reported to be two to three times more common in women taking hormonal contraceptives than those not taking them. Women ages 35 and older who smoke cigarettes should be strongly encouraged to stop; if they continue to smoke, they should be discouraged from using hormonal contraceptives.*

Elevated blood pressure may develop suddenly or gradually. A sudden, severe rise in pressure (exceeding 180/110 mm Hg) may indicate life-threatening hypertensive crisis. However, even a less dramatic rise may be equally significant if it heralds a dissecting aortic aneurysm, increased intracranial pressure, myocardial infarction, eclampsia, or thyrotoxicosis.

Usually associated with essential hypertension, elevated blood pressure may also result from a renal or endocrine disorder, a treatment that affects fluid status (such as dialysis), or from the use of certain drugs. Ingestion of large amounts of certain foods, such as black licorice and cheddar cheese, may temporarily elevate blood pressure. (See *Pathophysiology of elevated blood pressure*.)

Pathophysiology of elevated blood pressure

Blood pressure—the force blood exerts on vessels as it flows through them—depends on cardiac output, peripheral resistance, and blood volume. A brief review of its regulating mechanisms—nervous system control, capillary fluid shifts, kidney excretion, and hormonal changes—will help you understand how elevated blood pressure develops.

- *Nervous system control* involves the sympathetic system, chiefly baroreceptors and chemoreceptors, which promotes moderate vasoconstriction to maintain normal blood pressure. When this system responds inappropriately, increased vasoconstriction enhances peripheral resistance, resulting in elevated blood pressure.
- *Capillary fluid shifts* regulate blood volume by responding to arterial pressure. Increased pressure forces fluid into the interstitial space; decreased pressure allows it to be drawn back into the arteries by osmosis. However, this fluid shift may take several hours to adjust blood pressure.
- *Kidney excretion* also helps regulate blood volume by increasing or decreasing urine formation. Normally, an arterial pressure of about 60 mm Hg maintains urine output. When pressure drops below this reading, urine formation ceases, thereby increasing blood volume. Conversely, when arterial pressure exceeds this reading, urine formation increases, thereby reducing blood volume. Like capillary fluid shifts, this mechanism may take several hours to adjust blood pressure.
- *Hormonal changes* reflect stimulation of the renin-angiotensin-aldosterone system of the kidney in response to low arterial pressure. This system effects vasoconstriction, which increases arterial pressure, and stimulates aldosterone release, which regulates sodium retention—a key determinant of blood volume.

Elevated blood pressure signals the breakdown or inappropriate response of these pressure-regulating mechanisms. Its associated signs and symptoms concentrate in the target organs and tissues illustrated below.

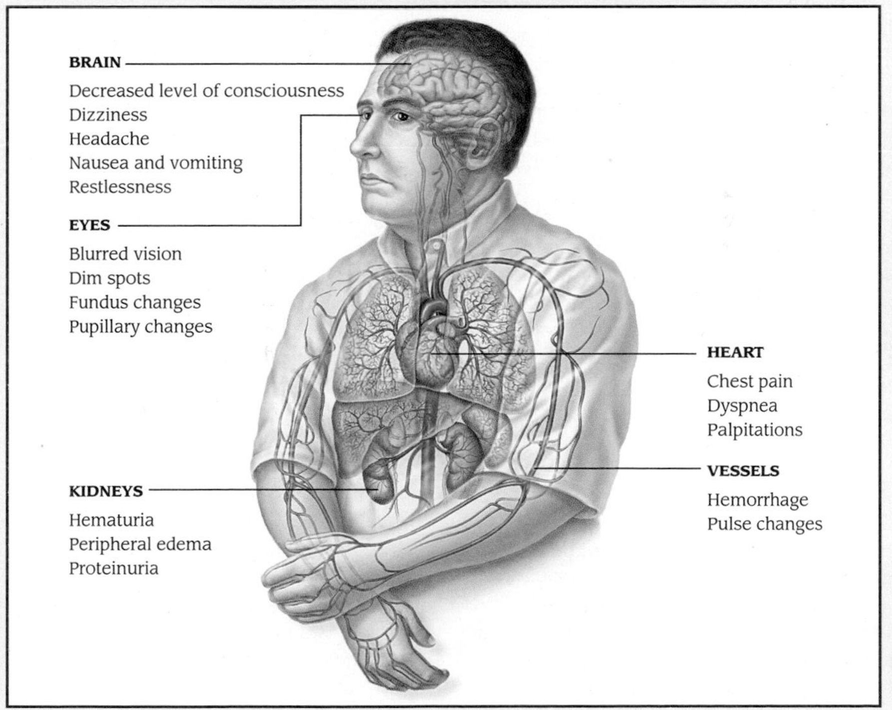

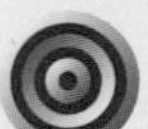

EMERGENCY INTERVENTION

Managing elevated blood pressure

Elevated blood pressure can signal various life-threatening disorders. If pressure exceeds 180/110 mm Hg, the patient may be experiencing hypertensive crisis and may require prompt treatment. Maintain a patent airway in case the patient vomits, and institute seizure precautions. Prepare to administer an I.V. antihypertensive and diuretic. You'll also need to insert an indwelling urinary catheter to accurately monitor urine output.

If blood pressure is less severely elevated, continue to rule out other life-threatening causes. If the patient is pregnant, suspect preeclampsia or eclampsia. Place her on bed rest, and insert an I.V. catheter. Administer magnesium sulfate (to decrease neuromuscular irritability) and an antihypertensive. Monitor vital signs closely for the next 24 hours. If diastolic blood pressure continues to exceed 100 mm Hg despite drug therapy, you may need to prepare the patient for induced labor and delivery or for cesarean birth. Offer emotional support if she must face delivery of a premature neonate.

If the patient isn't pregnant, quickly observe for equally obvious clues. Assess the patient for exophthalmos and an enlarged thyroid gland. If these signs are present, ask about a history of hyperthyroidism. Then look for other associated signs and symptoms, including tachycardia, widened pulse pressure, palpitations, severe weakness, diarrhea, fever exceeding 100° F (37.8° C), and nervousness. Prepare to administer an antithyroid drug orally or by nasogastric tube if necessary. Also, evaluate fluid status; look for signs of dehydration such as poor skin turgor. Prepare for I.V. fluid replacement and temperature control using a cooling blanket if necessary.

If the patient shows signs of increased intracranial pressure (such as decreased level of consciousness and fixed or dilated pupils), ask him or a family member if he has recently experienced head trauma. Then check for an increased respiratory rate and bradycardia. Maintain a patent airway in case the patient vomits. In addition, institute seizure precautions, and prepare to give an I.V. diuretic. Insert an indwelling urinary catheter, and monitor intake and output. Check his vital signs every 15 minutes until stable.

If the patient has absent or weak peripheral pulses, ask about chest pressure or pain, which suggests a dissecting aortic aneurysm. Enforce bed rest until a diagnosis has been established. As appropriate, give the patient an I.V. antihypertensive or prepare him for surgery.

Sometimes, elevated blood pressure may simply reflect inaccurate blood pressure measurement. (See *Ensuring accurate blood pressure measurement,* page 92.) However, careful measurement alone doesn't ensure a clinically useful reading. To be useful, each blood pressure reading must be compared with the patient's baseline. In some cases, serial readings may be necessary to establish elevated blood pressure.

History and Physical Examination

If you detect sharply elevated blood pressure, quickly rule out possible life-threatening causes. (See *Managing elevated blood pressure.*)

After ruling out life-threatening causes, complete a more leisurely history and physical examination. Determine if the patient has a history of cardiovascular or cerebrovascular disease, diabetes, or renal disease. Ask about a family history of high blood pressure—a likely finding in patients with essential hypertension, pheochromocytoma, or polycystic kidney disease. Then ask about its onset. Did high blood pressure appear abruptly? Ask the patient's age. Sudden onset of high blood pressure in middle-aged or elderly patients suggests renovascular stenosis. Although essential hypertension may begin in childhood, it typically isn't diagnosed until near age 35. Pheochromocytoma and primary aldosteronism usually occur between ages 40 and 60. If you suspect either, check for orthostatic hypotension. Take the patient's blood pressure with him supine, sitting, and then standing. Normally, systolic pressure falls and diastolic pressure rises on standing; in orthostatic hypotension, both pressures fall.

Note headache, palpitations, blurred vision, and sweating. Ask about wine-colored urine and decreased urine output; these signs suggest glomerulonephritis, which can cause elevated blood pressure.

Obtain a drug history, including past and present prescription and over-the-counter drugs (especially decongestants) as well as herbal preparations. If the patient is already taking an antihypertensive, determine how well he complies with the regimen. Ask about his perception of elevated blood pressure. How serious does he believe it is? Does he expect drug therapy to help? Explore psychosocial or environmental factors that may impact blood pressure control.

Follow up the history with a thorough physical examination. Using a funduscope, check for intraocular hemorrhage, exudate, and papilledema, which characterize severe hypertension. Perform a thorough cardiovascular assessment. Check for carotid bruits and jugular vein distention. Assess skin color, temperature, and turgor. Palpate peripheral pulses. Auscultate for abnormal heart sounds (gallops, louder second sound, murmurs), rate (bradycardia, tachycardia), or rhythm. Then auscultate for abnormal breath sounds (crackles, wheezing), rate (bradypnea, tachypnea), or rhythm.

Palpate the abdomen for tenderness, masses, or liver enlargement. Auscultate for abdominal bruits. Renal artery stenosis produces bruits over the upper abdomen or in the costovertebral angles. Easily palpable, enlarged kidneys and a large, tender liver suggest polycystic kidney disease. Obtain a urine specimen to check for microscopic hematuria.

Medical causes

◆ ***Aldosteronism (primary).*** In aldosteronism, elevated diastolic pressure may be accompanied by orthostatic hypotension. Other findings include constipation, muscle weakness, polyuria, polydipsia, and personality changes.

◆ ***Anemia.*** Accompanying elevated systolic pressure in anemia are pulsations in the capillary beds, bounding pulse, tachycardia, systolic ejection murmur, pale mucous membranes and, in patients with sickle cell anemia, ventricular gallop and crackles.

◆ ***Aortic aneurysm (dissecting).*** Initially, aortic aneurysm—a life-threatening disorder—causes a sudden rise in systolic pressure (which may be the precipitating event), but no change in diastolic pressure. However, this increase is brief. The body's ability to compensate fails, resulting in hypotension.

Other signs and symptoms vary, depending on the type of aortic aneurysm. An abdominal aneurysm may cause persistent abdominal and back pain, weakness, sweating, tachycardia, dyspnea, a pulsating abdominal mass, restlessness, confusion, and cool, clammy skin. A thoracic aneurysm may cause a ripping or tearing sensation in the chest, which may radiate to the neck, shoulders, lower back, or abdomen; pallor; syncope; blindness; loss of consciousness; sweating; dyspnea; tachycardia; cyanosis; leg weakness; murmur; and absent radial and femoral pulses.

◆ ***Atherosclerosis.*** In atherosclerosis, systolic pressure rises while diastolic pressure commonly remains normal or slightly elevated. The patient may show no other signs, or he may have a weak pulse, flushed skin, tachycardia, angina, and claudication.

◆ ***Cushing's syndrome.*** Twice as common in females as in males, Cushing's syndrome causes elevated blood pressure and widened pulse pressure, as well as truncal obesity, moon face, and other cushingoid signs. It's usually caused by corticosteroid use.

◆ ***Hypertension.*** Essential hypertension develops insidiously and is characterized by a gradual increase in blood pressure from decade to decade. Except for this high blood pressure, the patient may be asymptomatic or (rarely) may complain of suboccipital headache, lightheadedness, tinnitus, and fatigue.

In malignant hypertension, diastolic pressure abruptly rises above 120 mm Hg, and systolic pressure may exceed 200 mm Hg. Typically, the patient has pulmonary edema marked by jugular vein distention, dyspnea, tachypnea, tachycardia, and a cough with pink, frothy sputum. Other characteristic signs and symptoms include severe headache, confusion, blurred vision, tinnitus, epistaxis, muscle twitching, chest pain, nausea, and vomiting.

◆ ***Increased intracranial pressure (ICP).*** Increased ICP causes an increased respiratory rate initially, followed by increased systolic pressure and widened pulse pressure. Increased ICP affects heart rate last, causing bradycardia (Cushing's reflex). Associated signs and symptoms include headache, projectile vomiting, decreased level of consciousness, and fixed or dilated pupils.

◆ ***Metabolic syndrome.*** Blood pressure that exceeds 135/85 mm Hg is one of the conditions associated with metabolic syndrome (previously called *syndrome X*). Other conditions that define this syndrome are obesity, abnormal cholesterol level, and high blood insulin level. Individuals with this combination of risk factors are at a significantly greater risk for developing heart disease, stroke, peripheral vascular disease, and type 2 diabetes. Factors contributing to these conditions include physical inactivity, excessive weight gain, and genetic predisposition. Self-care measures, such as exercising, following a heart-healthy diet, and not smoking, often combined with medical therapy, are essential treatments for this syndrome.

◆ ***Myocardial infarction (MI).*** MI is a life-threatening disorder that may cause high or low blood pressure. The most common symptom is crushing chest pain that may radiate to the jaw, shoulder, arm, or epigastrium. Other findings include dyspnea, anxiety, nausea, vomiting, weakness, diaphoresis, atrial gallop, and murmurs.

◆ ***Pheochromocytoma.*** Paroxysmal or sustained elevated blood pressure characterizes pheochromocytoma and may be accompanied by orthostatic hypotension. Associated signs and symptoms include anxiety, diaphoresis, palpitations, tremors, pallor, nausea, weight loss, and headache.

◆ ***Polycystic kidney disease.*** Elevated blood pressure is typically preceded by flank pain. Other signs and symptoms include enlarged kidneys, an enlarged and tender liver, and intermittent gross hematuria.

◆ ***Preeclampsia-eclampsia.*** Potentially life threatening to the mother and fetus, preeclampsia and eclampsia characteristically increase blood pressure. They're defined as a reading of 140/90 mm Hg or more after 20 weeks' gestation accompanied by proteinuria. Other findings include generalized edema, sudden weight gain of 3 lb (1.4 kg) or more per week during the second or third trimester, severe frontal headache, blurred or double vision, decreased urine output, midabdominal pain, neuromuscular irritability, nausea, and possibly seizures.

◆ ***Renovascular stenosis.*** Renovascular stenosis produces abruptly elevated systolic and diastolic pressures. Other characteristic signs and symptoms include bruits over the upper abdomen or in the costovertebral angles, hematuria, and acute flank pain.

◆ ***Thyrotoxicosis.*** Accompanying the elevated systolic pressure associated with thyrotoxicosis—a potentially life-threatening disorder—are widened pulse pressure, tachycardia, bounding pulse, pulsations in the capillary nail beds, palpitations, weight loss, exophthalmos, an enlarged thyroid gland, weakness, diarrhea, fever over 100° F (37.8° C), and warm, moist skin. The patient may appear nervous and emotionally unstable, displaying occasional outbursts or even psychotic behavior. Heat intolerance, exertional dyspnea and, in females, decreased or absent menses may also occur.

Other causes

◆ ***Drugs.*** Central nervous system stimulants (such as amphetamines), sympathomimetics, corticosteroids, nonsteroidal anti-inflammatory drugs, hormonal contraceptives, monoamine oxidase inhibitors, and over-the-counter cold remedies can increase blood pressure, as can cocaine abuse.

HERB ALERT *Ephedra (ma huang), ginseng, and licorice may cause high blood pressure or an irregular heartbeat. (*Note: *The FDA has banned the sale of dietary supplements containing ephedra on the grounds that they pose an unreasonable risk of injury or illness.) St. John's wort can also raise blood pressure, especially when taken with substances that antagonize hypericin, such as amphetamines, cold and hay fever medications, nasal decongestants, pickled foods, beer, coffee, wine, and chocolate.*

◆ ***Treatments.*** Kidney dialysis and transplantation cause transient elevation of blood pressure.

Special considerations

If routine screening detects elevated blood pressure, stress to the patient the need for follow-up diagnostic tests. Then prepare him for routine blood tests and urinalysis. Depending on the suspected cause of the increased blood pressure, radiographic studies, especially of the kidneys, may be necessary.

If the patient has essential hypertension, explain the importance of long-term control of elevated blood pressure and the purpose, dosage, schedule, route, and adverse effects of prescribed antihypertensives. Reassure him that there are other drugs he can take if the one he's taking isn't effective or causes intolerable adverse reactions. Encourage him to report adverse reactions; the drug dosage or schedule may simply need adjustment.

Be aware that the patient may experience elevated blood pressure only when in the physician's office (known as "white-coat hypertension"). In such cases, 24-hour blood pressure monitoring is indicated to confirm elevated readings in other settings. In addition, other risk factors for coronary artery disease, such as smoking and elevated cholesterol levels, need to be addressed.

PEDIATRIC POINTERS

Normally, blood pressure is lower in children than in adults, an essential point to recognize when assessing a child for elevated blood pressure. (See *Normal pediatric blood pressure,* page 94.)

Elevated blood pressure in children may result from lead or mercury poisoning, essential hypertension, renovascular stenosis, chronic pyelonephritis, coarctation of the aorta, patent ductus arteriosus, glomerulonephritis, adrenogenital syndrome, or neuroblastoma. Treatment typically begins with drug therapy. Surgery may then follow in patients with patent ductus arteriosus, coarctation of the aorta, neuroblastoma, and some cases of renovascular stenosis. Diuretics and antibiotics are used to treat glomerulonephritis and chronic pyelonephritis; hormonal therapy, to treat adrenogenital syndrome.

GERIATRIC POINTERS

Atherosclerosis may produce isolated systolic hypertension in elderly patients. Treatment is warranted to prevent long-term complications.

PATIENT COUNSELING

Encourage the patient to lose weight, if necessary, and to restrict sodium intake. Suggest that he participate in an exercise or stress management program as well. Then teach the patient how to monitor his blood pressure so that he can evaluate the effectiveness of drug therapy and lifestyle changes. Have him record blood pressure readings and symptoms, and ask him to share this information on his return visits.

Bowel sounds, absent

[Silent abdomen]

Absent bowel sounds refers to an inability to hear any bowel sounds through a stethoscope after listening for at least 5 minutes in each abdominal quadrant. Bowel sounds cease when mechanical or vascular obstruction or neurogenic inhibition halts peristalsis. When peristalsis stops, gas from bowel contents and fluid secreted from the intestinal walls accumulate and distend the lumen, leading to life-threatening complications (such as perforation, peritonitis, and sepsis) or hypovolemic shock.

Simple mechanical obstruction, resulting from adhesions, hernia, or tumor, causes loss of fluids and electrolytes and induces dehydration. Vascular obstruction cuts off circulation to the intestinal walls, leading to ischemia, necrosis, and shock. Neurogenic inhibition, affecting innervation of the intestinal wall, may result from infection, bowel distention, or trauma. It may also follow mechanical or vascular obstruction or a metabolic imbalance such as hypokalemia.

Abrupt cessation of bowel sounds, when accompanied by abdominal pain, rigidity, and distention, signals a life-threatening crisis requiring immediate intervention. Absent bowel sounds following a period of hyperactive sounds are equally ominous and may indicate strangulation of a mechanically obstructed bowel.

EMERGENCY INTERVENTIONS *If you fail to detect bowel sounds and the patient reports sudden, severe abdominal pain and cramping or exhibits severe abdominal distention, prepare to insert a nasogastric (NG) or intestinal tube to suction lumen contents and decompress the bowel. (See* Are bowel sounds really absent? page 100.*) Administer I.V. fluids and electrolytes to offset any dehydration and imbalances caused by the dysfunctioning bowel.*

Because the patient may require surgery to relieve an obstruction, withhold oral intake. Take the patient's vital signs, and be alert for signs of shock, such as hypotension, tachycardia, and cool, clammy skin. Measure abdominal girth as a baseline for gauging subsequent changes.

HISTORY AND PHYSICAL EXAMINATION

If the patient's condition permits, proceed with a brief history. Start with abdominal pain: When did it begin? Has it gotten worse? Where does he feel it? Ask about a sensation of bloating and about flatulence. Find out if the patient has had diarrhea or has passed pencil-thin stools—possible signs of a developing luminal obstruction. The patient may have had no bowel movements at all—a possible sign of complete obstruction or paralytic ileus.

Ask about conditions that commonly lead to mechanical obstruction, such as abdominal

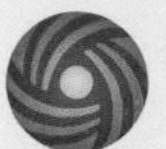

EXAMINATION TIP

Are bowel sounds really absent?

Before concluding that your patient has absent bowel sounds, ask yourself these three questions:

1. *Did you use the diaphragm of your stethoscope to auscultate for the bowel sounds?*
The diaphragm detects high-frequency sounds, such as bowel sounds, whereas the bell detects low-frequency sounds, such as a vascular bruit or a venous hum.

2. *Did you listen in the same spot for at least 5 minutes for the presence of bowel sounds?*
Normally, bowel sounds occur every 5 to 15 seconds, but the duration of a single sound may be less than 1 second.

3. *Did you listen for bowel sounds in all quadrants?*
Bowel sounds may be absent in one quadrant but present in another.

tumors, hernias, and adhesions from past surgery. Determine if the patient was involved in an accident—even a seemingly minor one, such as falling off a stepladder—that may have caused vascular clots. Check for a history of acute pancreatitis, diverticulitis, or gynecologic infection, which may have led to intra-abdominal infection and bowel dysfunction. Be sure to ask about previous toxic conditions, such as uremia, and about spinal cord injury, which can lead to paralytic ileus.

If the patient's pain isn't severe or accompanied by other life-threatening signs or symptoms, obtain a detailed medical and surgical history and perform a complete physical examination followed by an abdominal assessment and a pelvic examination.

Start your assessment by inspecting abdominal contour. Stoop at the recumbent patient's side and then at the foot of his bed to detect localized or generalized distention. Percuss and palpate the abdomen gently. Listen for dullness over fluid-filled areas and tympany over pockets of gas. Palpate for abdominal rigidity and guarding, which suggest peritoneal irritation that can lead to paralytic ileus.

MEDICAL CAUSES

◆ ***Mechanical intestinal obstruction, complete.*** Absent bowel sounds follow a period of hyperactive bowel sounds in complete mechanical intestinal obstruction—a potentially life-threatening disorder. This silence accompanies acute, colicky abdominal pain that arises in the quadrant of obstruction and may radiate to the flank or lumbar regions. Associated signs and symptoms include abdominal distention and bloating, constipation, and nausea and vomiting (the higher the blockage, the earlier and more severe the vomiting). In late stages, signs of shock may occur with fever, rebound tenderness, and abdominal rigidity.

◆ ***Mesenteric artery occlusion.*** In this life-threatening disorder, bowel sounds disappear after a brief period of hyperactive sounds. Sudden, severe midepigastric or periumbilical pain occurs next, followed by abdominal distention, bruits, vomiting, constipation, and signs of shock. Fever is common. Abdominal rigidity may appear later.

◆ ***Paralytic (adynamic) ileus.*** The cardinal sign paralytic ileus is absent bowel sounds. In addition to abdominal distention, associated signs and symptoms of paralytic ileus include generalized discomfort and constipation or passage of small, liquid stools. If paralytic ileus follows acute abdominal infection, the patient may also experience fever and abdominal pain.

OTHER CAUSES

◆ ***Abdominal surgery.*** Bowel sounds are normally absent after abdominal surgery—the result of anesthetic use and surgical manipulation.

SPECIAL CONSIDERATIONS

After you've inserted an NG or intestinal tube, elevate the head of the patient's bed at least 30 degrees, and turn the patient on his right side to facilitate passage of the tube through the GI tract. (Remember not to tape an intestinal tube to the patient's face.) Ensure tube patency by checking for drainage and properly functioning suction devices, and irrigate accordingly.

Continue to administer I.V. fluids and electrolytes, and make sure that you send a serum specimen to the laboratory for electrolyte analysis at least once a day. The patient may need X-ray studies and further blood work to determine the cause of absent bowel sounds.

After mechanical obstruction and intra-abdominal sepsis have been ruled out as the cause of absent bowel sounds, give the patient drugs to control pain and stimulate peristalsis.

Pediatric pointers

Absent bowel sounds in children may result from Hirschsprung's disease or intussusception, both of which can lead to life-threatening obstruction.

Geriatric pointers

Older patients with a bowel obstruction that doesn't respond to decompression should be considered for early surgical intervention to avoid the risk of bowel infarct.

Bowel sounds, hyperactive

Sometimes audible without a stethoscope, hyperactive bowel sounds reflect increased intestinal motility (peristalsis). They're commonly characterized as rapid, rushing, gurgling waves of sounds. (See *Characteristics of bowel sounds*.) They may stem from life-threatening bowel obstruction or GI hemorrhage or from GI infection, inflammatory bowel disease (which usually follows a chronic course), food allergies, or stress. (See *Hyperactive bowel sounds: Causes and associated findings*, page 102.)

Characteristics of bowel sounds

The sounds of swallowed air and fluid moving through the GI tract are known as bowel sounds. These sounds usually occur every 5 to 15 seconds, but their frequency may be irregular. For example, bowel sounds are normally more active just before and after a meal. They may last less than 1 second or up to several seconds.

Normal bowel sounds can be characterized as murmuring, gurgling, or tinkling. *Hyperactive bowel sounds* can be characterized as loud, gurgling, splashing, and rushing; they're higher pitched and occur more frequently than normal sounds. *Hypoactive bowel sounds* are softer or lower in tone and occur less frequently than normal sounds.

EMERGENCY INTERVENTIONS *After detecting hyperactive bowel sounds, quickly check vital signs and ask the patient about associated symptoms, such as abdominal pain, vomiting, and diarrhea. If he reports cramping abdominal pain or vomiting, continue to auscultate for bowel sounds. If bowel sounds stop abruptly, suspect complete bowel obstruction. Prepare to assist with GI suction and decompression and to give I.V. fluids and electrolytes, and prepare the patient for surgery.*

If the patient has diarrhea, record its frequency, amount, color, and consistency. If you detect excessive watery diarrhea or bleeding, prepare to administer an antidiarrheal, I.V. fluids and electrolytes and, possibly, blood transfusions.

GENDER CUE *Homosexual males who report acute diarrhea and who have negative fecal ova and parasite cultures may be infected with chlamydial proctitis not associated with lymphogranuloma venereum. Because rectal cultures will probably be negative, treatment with tetracycline is appropriate.*

History and physical examination

If you've ruled out life-threatening conditions, obtain a detailed medical and surgical history. Ask the patient if he has had a hernia or abdominal surgery because these may cause mechanical intestinal obstruction. Does he have a history of inflammatory bowel disease? Also, ask about recent episodes of gastroenteritis among family members, friends, or coworkers. If the patient has traveled recently, even within the United States, was he aware of any endemic illnesses?

In addition, determine whether stress may have contributed to the patient's problem. Ask about food allergies and recent ingestion of unusual foods or fluids. Check for fever, which suggests infection. Having already auscultated, now gently inspect, percuss, and palpate the abdomen.

Medical causes

◆ ***Crohn's disease.*** Hyperactive bowel sounds usually arise insidiously in Crohn's disease. Associated signs and symptoms include diarrhea, cramping abdominal pain that may be relieved by defecation, anorexia, low-grade fever, abdominal distention and tenderness and, in many cases, a fixed mass in the right lower quadrant. Perianal and vaginal lesions are common. Muscle wasting, weight loss, and signs of dehydration may occur as Crohn's disease progresses.

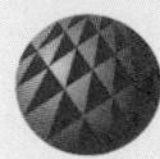

SIGNS & SYMPTOMS

Hyperactive bowel sounds: Causes and associated findings

Common causes	Major associated signs and symptoms: Abdominal distention	Abdominal pain	Anorexia	Constipation	Diarrhea	Fever	Nausea	Perianal lesions	Rectal bleeding	Vomiting	Weight loss
Crohn's disease	●	●	●		●	●		●			●
Food hypersensitivity					●		●			●	
Gastroenteritis		●			●	●	●			●	
GI hemorrhage	●	●			●				●		
Mechanical intestinal obstruction	●	●		●			●			●	
Ulcerative colitis (acute)			●		●	●					●

◆ ***Food hypersensitivity.*** Malabsorption—typically lactose intolerance—may cause hyperactive bowel sounds. Associated signs and symptoms include diarrhea and, possibly, nausea and vomiting, angioedema, and urticaria.

◆ ***Gastroenteritis.*** Hyperactive bowel sounds follow sudden nausea and vomiting and accompany "explosive" diarrhea. Abdominal cramping or pain is common, often after a peristaltic wave. Fever may occur, depending on the causative organism.

◆ ***GI hemorrhage.*** Hyperactive bowel sounds provide the most immediate indication of persistent upper GI bleeding. Other findings include hematemesis, coffee-ground vomitus, abdominal distention, bloody diarrhea, rectal passage of bright red clots and jellylike material or melena, and pain during bleeding. Decreased urine output, tachycardia, and hypotension accompany blood loss.

◆ ***Mechanical intestinal obstruction.*** Hyperactive bowel sounds occur simultaneously with cramping abdominal pain every few minutes in patients with mechanical intestinal obstruction—a potentially life-threatening disorder. Bowel sounds may later become hypoactive and then disappear. Nausea and vomiting occur earlier and with greater severity in small-bowel obstruction than in large-bowel obstruction. In complete bowel obstruction, hyperactive sounds are also accompanied by abdominal distention and constipation, although the part of the bowel distal to the obstruction may continue to empty for up to 3 days.

◆ ***Ulcerative colitis (acute).*** Hyperactive bowel sounds arise abruptly in patients with ulcerative colitis and are accompanied by bloody diarrhea, anorexia, abdominal pain, nausea and vomiting, fever, and tenesmus. Weight loss, arthralgia, and arthritis may occur.

SPECIAL CONSIDERATIONS

Prepare the patient for diagnostic tests, which may include endoscopy to view a suspected lesion, barium X-rays, or stool analysis.

PEDIATRIC POINTERS

Hyperactive bowel sounds in children usually result from gastroenteritis, erratic eating habits, excessive ingestion of certain foods (such as unripened fruit), or food allergy.

PATIENT COUNSELING

Explain prescribed dietary changes to the patient. These may range from complete food and fluid restrictions to a liquid or bland diet. Because stress often precipitates or aggravates bowel hyperactivity, teach the patient relaxation techniques such as deep breathing. Encourage rest and restrict the patient's physical activity.

Bowel sounds, hypoactive

Hypoactive bowel sounds, detected by auscultation, are diminished in regularity, tone, and loudness from normal bowel sounds. In themselves, hypoactive bowel sounds don't herald an emergency; in fact, they're considered normal during sleep. However, they may portend absent bowel sounds, which can indicate a life-threatening disorder.

Hypoactive bowel sounds result from decreased peristalsis, which, in turn, can result from a developing bowel obstruction. The obstruction may be mechanical (as from a hernia, tumor, or twisting), vascular (as from an embolism or thrombosis), or neurogenic (as from mechanical, ischemic, or toxic impairment of bowel innervation). Hypoactive bowel sounds can also result from the use of certain drugs, abdominal surgery, and radiation therapy.

HISTORY AND PHYSICAL EXAMINATION

After detecting hypoactive bowel sounds, look for related symptoms. Ask the patient about the location, onset, duration, frequency, and severity of any pain. Cramping or colicky abdominal pain usually indicates a mechanical bowel obstruction, whereas diffuse abdominal pain usually indicates intestinal distention related to paralytic ileus.

Ask the patient about any recent vomiting: When did it begin? How often does it occur? Does the vomitus look bloody? Also, ask about any changes in bowel habits: Does he have a history of constipation? When was the last time he had a bowel movement or expelled gas?

Obtain a detailed medical and surgical history of any conditions that may cause mechanical bowel obstruction, such as an abdominal tumor or hernia. Does the patient have a history of severe pain; trauma; conditions that can cause paralytic ileus such as pancreatitis; bowel inflammation or gynecologic infection, which may produce peritonitis; or toxic conditions such as uremia? Has he recently had radiation therapy or abdominal surgery, or ingested a drug such as an opiate, which can decrease peristalsis and cause hypoactive bowel sounds?

After the history is complete, perform a careful physical examination. Inspect the abdomen for distention, noting surgical incisions and obvious masses. Gently percuss and palpate the abdomen for masses, gas, fluid, tenderness, and rigidity. Measure abdominal girth to detect any subsequent increase in distention. Also check for poor skin turgor, hypotension, narrowed pulse pressure, and other signs of dehydration and electrolyte imbalance, which may result from paralytic ileus.

MEDICAL CAUSES

◆ ***Mechanical intestinal obstruction.*** Bowel sounds may become hypoactive after a period of hyperactivity. The patient may also have acute colicky abdominal pain in the quadrant of obstruction, possibly radiating to the flank or lumbar region; nausea and vomiting (the higher the obstruction, the earlier and more severe the vomiting); constipation; and abdominal distention and bloating. If the obstruction becomes complete, signs of shock may occur.

◆ ***Mesenteric artery occlusion.*** After a brief period of hyperactivity, bowel sounds become hypoactive and then quickly disappear, signifying a life-threatening crisis. Associated signs and symptoms include fever; a history of colicky abdominal pain leading to sudden and severe midepigastric or periumbilical pain, followed by abdominal distention and possibly bruits; vomiting; constipation; and signs of shock. Abdominal rigidity may appear late.

◆ ***Paralytic (adynamic) ileus.*** Bowel sounds are hypoactive and may become absent in this disorder. Associated signs and symptoms include abdominal distention, generalized discomfort, and constipation or passage of small, liquid stools and flatus. If the disorder follows acute abdominal infection, fever and abdominal pain may occur.

OTHER CAUSES

◆ ***Drugs.*** Certain classes of drugs reduce intestinal motility and thus produce hypoactive bowel sounds. These include opiates such as codeine, anticholinergics such as propantheline bromide, phenothiazines such as chlorpromazine, and vinca alkaloids such as vincristine. General or spinal anesthetics produce transient hypoactive sounds.

◆ ***Radiation therapy.*** Hypoactive bowel sounds and abdominal tenderness may occur after irradiation of the abdomen.

◆ ***Surgery.*** Hypoactive bowel sounds may occur after manipulation of the bowel. Motility and bowel sounds in the small intestine usually resume within 24 hours; colonic bowel sounds, in 3 to 5 days.

Special considerations

Frequently evaluate the patient with hypoactive bowel sounds for indications of shock (thirst; anxiety; restlessness; tachycardia; cool, clammy skin; weak, thready pulse), which can develop if peristalsis continues to diminish and fluid is lost from the circulation.

Be alert for the sudden absence of bowel sounds, especially in postoperative and hypokalemic patients because they're at increased risk for paralytic ileus. Monitor the patient's vital signs and auscultate for bowel sounds every 2 to 4 hours.

Severe pain, abdominal rigidity, guarding, and fever, accompanied by hypoactive bowel sounds, may indicate paralytic ileus from peritonitis. If these signs and symptoms occur, prepare for emergency interventions. (See "Bowel sounds, absent," page 99.)

The patient with hypoactive bowel sounds may require GI suction and decompression, using a nasogastric or intestinal tube. If so, restrict the patient's oral intake. Then elevate the head of the bed at least 30 degrees, and turn the patient on his right side to facilitate passage of the tube through the GI tract.

Remember not to tape an intestinal tube to the patient's face. Ensure tube patency by watching for drainage and properly functioning suction devices. Irrigate the tube and closely monitor drainage.

Continue to administer I.V. fluids and electrolytes, and send a serum specimen to the laboratory for electrolyte analysis at least once a day. Recognize that the patient may need X-ray studies, endoscopic procedures, and further blood work to determine the cause of hypoactive bowel sounds.

Provide comfort measures as needed. Semi-Fowler's position offers the best relief for the patient with paralytic ileus. Sometimes, getting the patient to ambulate can reactivate the sluggish bowel. However, if the patient can't tolerate ambulation, range-of-motion exercises or turning from side to side may stimulate peristalsis. Turning the patient from side to side also helps move gas through the intestines.

Pediatric pointers

Hypoactive bowel sounds in a child may simply be due to bowel distention from excessive swallowing of air while the child was eating or crying. However, be sure to observe the child for further signs of illness. As with an adult, sluggish bowel sounds in a child may signal the onset of paralytic ileus or peritonitis.

Bradycardia

Bradycardia refers to a heart rate of less than 60 beats/minute. It occurs normally in young adults, trained athletes, and elderly people as well as during sleep. It's also a normal response to vagal stimulation caused by coughing, vomiting, or straining during defecation. When bradycardia results from these causes, the heart rate rarely drops below 40 beats/minute. However, when it results from pathologic causes (such as cardiovascular disorders), the heart rate may be slower.

By itself, bradycardia is a nonspecific sign. However, together with such symptoms as chest pain, dizziness, syncope, and shortness of breath, it can signal a life-threatening disorder. (See *Differential diagnosis: Bradycardia,* pages 106 and 107.)

History and physical examination

After detecting bradycardia, check for related signs of life-threatening disorders. (See *Managing severe bradycardia.*) If bradycardia isn't accompanied by untoward signs, ask the patient if he or a family member has a history of a slow pulse rate because this may be inherited. Also, find out if he has an underlying metabolic disorder, such as hypothyroidism, which can precipitate bradycardia. Ask which medications he's taking and if he's complying with the prescribed schedule and dosage. Monitor vital signs, temperature, pulse rate, respirations, blood pressure, and oxygen saturation.

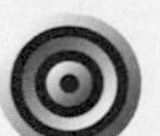

EMERGENCY INTERVENTION

Managing severe bradycardia

Bradycardia can signal prolonged exposure to cold; head or neck trauma; or a life-threatening disorder when accompanied by pain, shortness of breath, dizziness, syncope, or other symptoms. In such patients, quickly take vital signs. Connect the patient to a cardiac monitor, and insert an I.V. catheter. Depending on the cause of bradycardia, you'll need to administer fluids, atropine, steroids, or thyroid medication. If indicated, insert an indwelling urinary catheter. Intubation, mechanical ventilation, or placement of a pacemaker may be necessary if the patient's respiratory rate falls.

If appropriate, perform a focused evaluation to help locate the cause of bradycardia. For example, ask about pain. Viselike pressure or crushing or burning chest pain that radiates to the arms, back, or jaw may indicate an acute myocardial infarction (MI); a severe headache may indicate increased intracranial pressure. Also ask about nausea, vomiting, or shortness of breath—signs and symptoms associated with an acute MI and cardiomyopathy. Observe the patient for peripheral cyanosis, edema, or jugular vein distention, which may indicate cardiomyopathy. Look for a thyroidectomy scar because severe bradycardia may result from hypothyroidism caused by failure to take thyroid hormone replacements.

If the cause of bradycardia is evident, provide supportive care. For example, keep the hypothermic patient warm by applying blankets, and monitor his core temperature until it reaches 99° F (37.2° C); stabilize the head and neck of a trauma patient until cervical spinal injury is ruled out.

Medical causes

◆ ***Cardiac arrhythmias.*** Depending on the type of arrhythmia and the patient's tolerance of it, bradycardia may be transient or sustained and benign or life-threatening. Related findings include hypotension, palpitations, dizziness, weakness, syncope, and fatigue.

◆ ***Cardiomyopathy.*** Cardiomyopathy is a potentially life-threatening disorder that may cause transient or sustained bradycardia. Other findings include dizziness, syncope, edema, fatigue, jugular vein distention, orthopnea, dyspnea, and peripheral cyanosis.

◆ ***Cervical spinal injury.*** Bradycardia may be transient or sustained, depending on the severity of the injury. Its onset coincides with sympathetic denervation. Associated signs and symptoms include hypotension, decreased body temperature, slowed peristalsis, leg paralysis, and partial arm and respiratory muscle paralysis.

◆ ***Hypothermia.*** Bradycardia usually appears when the core temperature drops below 89.6° F (32° C). It's accompanied by shivering, peripheral cyanosis, muscle rigidity, bradypnea, and confusion leading to stupor.

◆ ***Hypothyroidism.*** Hypothyroidism causes severe bradycardia in addition to fatigue, constipation, unexplained weight gain, and sensitivity to cold. Related signs include cool, dry, thick skin; sparse, dry hair; facial swelling; periorbital edema; thick, brittle nails; and confusion leading to stupor.

◆ ***Increased intracranial pressure (ICP).*** Bradycardia occurs as a late sign of increased ICP along with rapid respiratory rate, elevated systolic pressure, decreased diastolic pressure, and widened pulse pressure. Associated signs and symptoms include persistent headache, projectile vomiting, decreased level of consciousness (LOC), and fixed, unequal, and possibly dilated pupils.

◆ ***Myocardial infarction (MI).*** Sinus bradycardia is the most common arrhythmia associated with an acute MI. Accompanying signs and symptoms of an MI include an aching, burning, or viselike pressure in the chest that may radiate to the jaw, shoulder, arm, back, or epigastric area; nausea and vomiting; cool, clammy, and pale or cyanotic skin; anxiety; and dyspnea. Blood pressure may be elevated or depressed. Auscultation may reveal abnormal heart sounds.

Other causes

◆ ***Diagnostic tests.*** Cardiac catheterization and electrophysiologic studies can induce temporary bradycardia.

◆ ***Drugs.*** Beta-adrenergic blockers, some calcium channel blockers, cardiac glycosides, topical miotics (such as pilocarpine), protamine, quinidine and other antiarrhythmics,

(Text continues on page 108.)

Differential diagnosis: Bradycardia

History of present illness

Focused physical examination: Vital signs; thyroid, cardiovascular, neurologic, and pulmonary systems

Cardiac arrhythmia

Signs and symptoms
- Bradycardia (transient or sustained)
- Hypotension
- Palpitations
- Dizziness or syncope
- Nausea
- Weakness or fatigue
- Pallor

Diagnosis: Laboratory tests (arterial blood gas analysis, complete blood count, cardiac enzymes, electrolytes, glucose), electrocardiogram (ECG), 24-hour Holter monitoring

Treatment: Medication (antiarrhythmic, vagolytic), pacemaker

Follow-up: Referral to cardiologist

Cardiomyopathy

Signs and symptoms
- Bradycardia (transient or sustained)
- Dizziness or syncope
- Edema
- Jugular vein distention
- Fatigue
- Orthopnea
- Dyspnea
- Peripheral cyanosis
- Chest pain

Diagnosis: Drug screen, electrolytes, imaging studies (chest X-ray, echocardiogram), ECG, cardiac catheterization

Treatment: Medication (antiarrhythmics, diuretics, angiotensin-converting enzyme inhibitors); oxygen therapy; limited activity; low-fat, low-salt diet

Follow-up: Referral to cardiologist

Cervical spine injury

Signs and symptoms
- Bradycardia (transient or sustained)
- Hypotension
- Hypothermia
- Slowed peristalsis
- Leg paralysis
- Partial arm paralysis

Diagnosis: History of trauma, imaging studies (computed tomography [CT] scan, magnetic resonance imaging [MRI] of spine)

Treatment: Spine stabilization, corticosteroids

Follow-up: Transfer to spinal injury center

Hypothyroidism

Signs and symptoms
- ◆ Fatigue
- ◆ Constipation
- ◆ Weight gain
- ◆ Cold sensitivity
- ◆ Cool, dry, thick skin
- ◆ Sparse, dry hair
- ◆ Alopecia
- ◆ Facial swelling
- ◆ Periorbital edema
- ◆ Thick, brittle nails
- ◆ Neck swelling
- ◆ Goiter

Diagnosis: Thyroid studies, ECG
Treatment: Thyroid hormone replacement
Follow-up: Return visits every 4 to 6 weeks until thyroid-stimulating hormone level is normal, then every 6 months

Myocardial infarction

Signs and symptoms
- ◆ Chest, back, or abdominal pain
- ◆ Shortness of breath
- ◆ Cough
- ◆ Dizziness
- ◆ Nausea and vomiting
- ◆ Diaphoresis
- ◆ Anxiety

Diagnosis: Laboratory tests (isoenzymes, troponin I and T), imaging studies (angiography, echocardiogram), ECG, cardiac catheterization
Treatment: Medication (aspirin, nitrates, analgesics, thrombolytics, anticoagulants, beta-adrenergic blockers, vasopressors), oxygen therapy, angioplasty, coronary artery bypass graft
Follow-up: Referral to cardiologist; return visit 3 to 6 weeks after hospitalization, then every 3 months

Hypothermia

Signs and symptoms
- ◆ Temperature below 89.6° F (32° C)
- ◆ Shivering
- ◆ Peripheral cyanosis
- ◆ Muscle rigidity
- ◆ Bradypnea
- ◆ Confusion and stupor

Diagnosis: Temperature, ECG
Treatment: Establishment of ABCs (airway, breathing, circulation), temperature monitoring, warm I.V. fluids, warming blanket, treatment of underlying cause (if physiologic)
Follow-up: Return visit 2 weeks after hospitalization

Intracranial hypertension

Signs and symptoms
- ◆ Bradypnea or tachypnea
- ◆ Widened pulse pressure
- ◆ Persistent headache
- ◆ Projectile vomiting
- ◆ Fixed, unequal, or dilated pupils
- ◆ Decreased level of consciousness

Diagnosis: Imaging studies (CT scan, MRI)
Treatment: Treatment of underlying cause, medication (osmotic diuretics, barbiturates), ventilatory support
Follow-up: Referral to neurologist or neurosurgeon

Other causes: beta-adrenergic blockers ◆ cardiac glycosides ◆ cardiac surgery ◆ diagnostic tests (cardiac catheterization, electrophysiologic studies) ◆ failure to take thyroid replacements ◆ protamine sulfate ◆ quinidine and other antiarrhythmics ◆ some calcium channel blockers ◆ suctioning ◆ sympatholytics ◆ topical miotics and sympatholytics may cause transient bradycardia. Failure to take thyroid replacements may cause bradycardia.

◆ ***Invasive treatments.*** Suctioning can induce hypoxia and vagal stimulation, causing bradycardia. Cardiac surgery can cause edema or damage to conduction tissues, causing bradycardia.

Special considerations

Continue to monitor vital signs frequently. Be especially alert for changes in cardiac rhythm, respiratory rate, and LOC.

Prepare the patient for laboratory tests, which can include complete blood count; cardiac enzyme, serum electrolyte, blood glucose, blood urea nitrogen, arterial blood gas, and blood drug levels; thyroid function tests; and a 12-lead electrocardiogram. If appropriate, prepare the patient for 24-hour Holter monitoring.

Pediatric pointers

Heart rates are normally higher in children than in adults. Fetal bradycardia—a heart rate of less than 120 beats/minute—may occur during prolonged labor or complications of delivery, such as compression of the umbilical cord, partial abruptio placentae, and placenta previa. Intermittent bradycardia, sometimes accompanied by apnea, commonly occurs in premature infants. Bradycardia rarely occurs in full-term infants or children. However, it can result from congenital heart defects, acute glomerulonephritis, and transient or complete heart block associated with cardiac catheterization or cardiac surgery.

Geriatric pointers

Sinus node dysfunction is the most common bradyarrhythmia in the elderly. Patients with this disorder may cite fatigue, exercise intolerance, dizziness, or syncope as their chief complaint. If the patient is asymptomatic, no intervention is necessary. Symptomatic patients, however, require careful scrutiny of their drug therapy. Beta-adrenergic blockers, verapamil, diazepam, sympatholytics, antihypertensives, and some antiarrhythmics have been implicated; symptoms may clear when these drugs are discontinued. Pacing is usually indicated in patients with symptomatic bradycardia lacking a correctable cause.

Bradypnea

Commonly preceding life-threatening apnea or respiratory arrest, bradypnea is a pattern of regular respirations with a rate of fewer than 10 breaths/minute. This sign may result from neurologic or metabolic disorders or a drug overdose, all of which depress the brain's respiratory control centers. (See *Understanding how the nervous system controls breathing*.)

EMERGENCY INTERVENTIONS *Depending on the degree of central nervous system (CNS) depression, a patient with severe bradypnea may require constant stimulation to breathe. If the patient seems excessively sleepy, try to arouse him by shaking him and instructing him to breathe. Quickly take the patient's vital signs. Assess his neurologic status by checking pupil size and reactions and by evaluating his level of consciousness (LOC) and his ability to move his extremities.*

Connect the patient to an apnea monitor, keep emergency airway equipment available, and be prepared to assist with intubation and mechanical ventilation if spontaneous respirations cease. To prevent aspiration, position the patient on his side or keep his head elevated 30 degrees higher than the rest of the body, and clear his airway with suction if necessary.

History and physical examination

Obtain a brief history from the patient, if possible, or from whoever accompanied him to your facility. Ask if he's experiencing a drug overdose and, if so, try to determine which drugs he took, how much, when, and by what route. Check his arms for needle marks, indicating possible drug abuse. You may need to administer I.V. naloxone, an opioid antagonist.

If you rule out a drug overdose, ask about chronic illnesses, such as diabetes and renal failure. Check for a medical identification bracelet or card that identifies an underlying condition. Also ask whether the patient has a history of head trauma, brain tumor, neurologic infection, or stroke.

Medical causes

◆ ***Diabetic ketoacidosis.*** Bradypnea occurs late in patients with severe, uncontrolled diabetes. Patients with severe ketoacidosis may experience Kussmaul's respirations. Associated signs and symptoms include decreased LOC,

Understanding how the nervous system controls breathing

Stimulation from external sources and from higher brain centers acts on respiratory centers in the pons and medulla. These centers, in turn, send impulses to the various parts of the respiratory system to alter respiratory patterns.

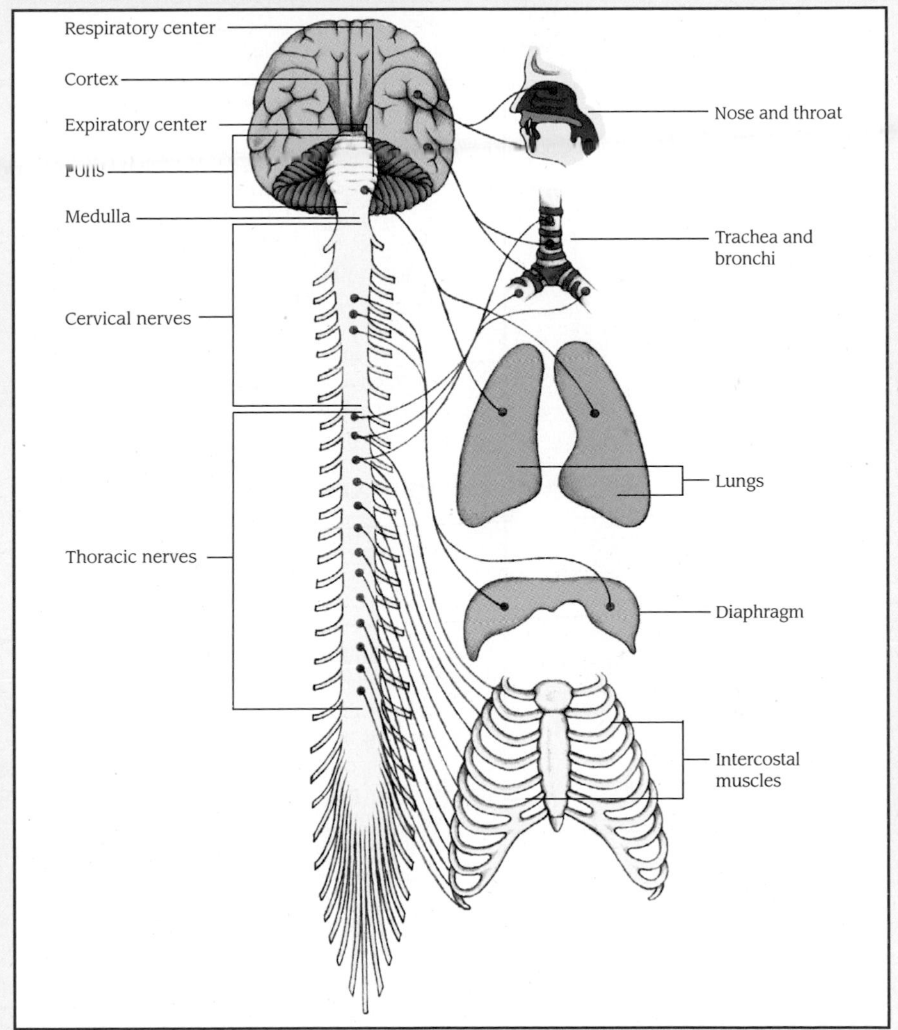

fatigue, weakness, fruity breath odor, and oliguria.

◆ ***Hepatic failure.*** Occurring in end-stage hepatic failure, bradypnea may be accompanied by coma, hyperactive reflexes, asterixis, a positive Babinski's reflex, fetor hepaticus, and other signs.

◆ ***Increased intracranial pressure (ICP).*** A late sign of increased ICP—a life-threatening condition—bradypnea is preceded by decreased LOC, deteriorating motor function, and fixed, dilated pupils. The triad of bradypnea, bradycardia, and hypertension is a classic sign of late medullary strangulation.

Respiratory rates in children

This graph shows normal respiratory rates in children, which are higher than normal rates in adults. Accordingly, bradypnea in children is defined according to age.

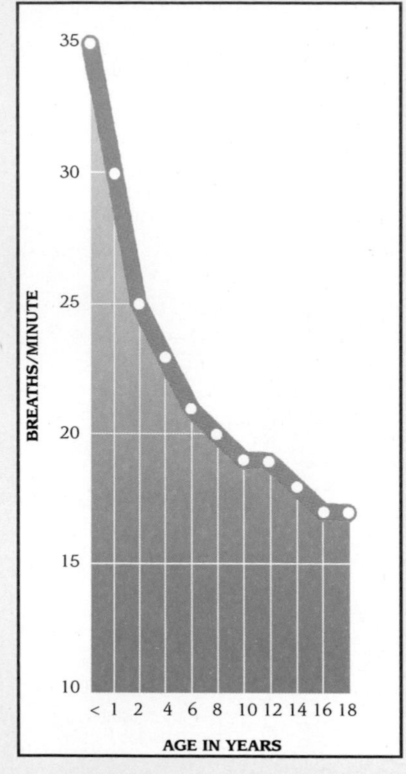

◆ ***Renal failure.*** Occurring in end-stage renal failure, bradypnea may be accompanied by seizures, decreased LOC, GI bleeding, hypotension or hypertension, uremic frost, and diverse other signs.

◆ ***Respiratory failure.*** Bradypnea occurs in end-stage respiratory failure along with cyanosis, diminished breath sounds, tachycardia, mildly increased blood pressure, and decreased LOC.

OTHER CAUSES

◆ ***Drugs.*** An overdose of an opioid analgesic or, less commonly, a sedative, barbiturate, phenothiazine, or another CNS depressant can cause bradypnea. Use of any of these drugs with alcohol can also cause bradypnea.

SPECIAL CONSIDERATIONS

Because a patient with bradypnea may develop apnea, check his respiratory status frequently and be prepared to give ventilatory support if necessary. Don't leave the patient unattended, especially if his LOC is decreased. Keep his bed in the lowest position and raise the side rails. Obtain blood for arterial blood gas analysis, electrolyte studies, and possibly a drug screen. Ready the patient for chest X-rays and possibly a computed tomography scan of the head.

Administer prescribed drugs and oxygen. Avoid giving the patient a CNS depressant because it can exacerbate bradypnea. Similarly, give oxygen judiciously to a patient with chronic carbon dioxide retention, which may occur in chronic obstructive pulmonary disease, because excess oxygen therapy can have a negative effect.

When dealing with slow breathing in hospitalized patients, always review all drugs and dosages given during the last 24 hours.

PEDIATRIC POINTERS

Because respiratory rates are normally higher in children than in adults, bradypnea in children is defined according to age. (See *Respiratory rates in children.*)

GERIATRIC POINTERS

When administering drugs to elderly patients, keep in mind that they have a higher risk of developing bradypnea secondary to drug toxicity. That's because many of them take several drugs that can potentiate this effect or have other conditions that predispose them to it. Warn older patients about this potentially life-threatening complication.

PATIENT COUNSELING

Alert patients who regularly take an opioid—for example, those with advanced cancer or sickle cell anemia—that bradypnea is a serious complication, and teach them to recognize early signs of toxicity, such as nausea and vomiting. Also, try to identify patients who may be abusing these drugs.

Breast dimpling

Breast dimpling—the puckering or retraction of skin on the breast—results from abnormal attachment of the skin to underlying tissue. It suggests an inflammatory or malignant mass beneath the skin surface and usually represents a late sign of breast cancer; benign lesions usually don't produce this effect. Dimpling usually affects women older than age 40, but it also occasionally affects men.

Because breast dimpling occurs over a mass or an induration, the patient usually discovers other signs before becoming aware of the dimpling. A thorough breast examination may reveal dimpling and alert the patient and nurse to a breast problem. (See *How to examine your breasts,* pages 114 and 115.)

History and physical examination

Obtain a medical, reproductive, and family history, noting factors that increase the patient's risk of breast cancer. Also obtain a pregnancy history because women who haven't had a full-term pregnancy before age 30 have a higher risk of developing breast cancer. Has the patient's mother or sister had breast cancer? Has she herself had a previous malignancy, especially cancer in the other breast? Ask about the patient's dietary habits because a high-fat diet predisposes women to breast cancer.

Ask the patient if she has noticed any changes in the shape of her breast. Is any area painful or tender, and is the pain cyclic? If she's breast-feeding, has she recently experienced high fever, chills, malaise, muscle aches, fatigue, or other flulike signs or symptoms? Can she remember sustaining any trauma to the breast?

Carefully inspect the dimpled area. Is it swollen, red, or warm to the touch? Do you see bruises or contusions? Ask the patient to tense her pectoral muscles by pressing her hips with both hands or by raising her hands over her head. Does the puckering increase? Gently pull the skin upward toward the clavicle. Is the dimpling exaggerated?

Observe the breast for nipple retraction. Do both nipples point in the same direction? Is either nipple flattened or inverted? Does the patient report nipple discharge? If so, ask her to describe its color and character. Observe the contour of both breasts. Are they symmetrical?

Examine both breasts with the patient supine, sitting, and then leaning forward. Does the skin move freely over both breasts? If you can palpate a lump, describe its size, location, consistency, mobility, and delineation. What relation does the lump have to the breast dimpling? Gently mold the breast skin around the lump. Is the dimpling exaggerated? Also examine breast and axillary lymph nodes, noting any enlargement.

Medical causes

◆ ***Breast abscess.*** Breast dimpling sometimes accompanies a chronic breast abscess. Associated findings include a firm, irregular, nontender lump and signs of nipple retraction, such as deviation, inversion, or flattening. Axillary lymph nodes may be enlarged.

◆ ***Breast cancer.*** Breast dimpling is an important but somewhat late sign of breast cancer. A neoplasm that causes dimpling is usually close to the skin and at least 1 cm in diameter. It feels irregularly shaped and fixed to underlying tissue, and it's usually painless. Other signs of breast cancer include peau d'orange, changes in breast symmetry or size, nipple retraction, and a unilateral, spontaneous, nonmilky nipple discharge that's serous or bloody. (A bloody nipple discharge in the presence of a lump is a classic sign of breast cancer.) Axillary lymph nodes may be enlarged. Pain may be present but isn't a reliable symptom of breast cancer. A breast ulcer may appear as a late sign.

◆ ***Fat necrosis.*** Breast dimpling due to fat necrosis follows inflammation and trauma to the fatty tissue of the breast (although the patient usually can't remember such trauma). Tenderness, erythema, bruising, and contusions may occur. Other findings include a firm, irregular, fixed mass and skin retraction signs, such as skin dimpling and nipple retraction. Fat necrosis is difficult to differentiate from breast cancer.

◆ ***Mastitis.*** Breast dimpling may signal bacterial mastitis, which usually results from duct obstruction and milk stasis during lactation. Heat, erythema, swelling, induration, pain, and tenderness usually accompany mastitis. Dimpling is more likely to occur with diffuse induration than with a single hard mass. The skin on the breast may feel fixed to underlying tissue. Other possible findings include nipple retraction, nipple cracks, a purulent discharge, and enlarged axillary lymph nodes. Flulike signs and symptoms (such as fever, malaise, fatigue, and aching) are common.

Special considerations

Remember that any breast problem can arouse fears of mutilation, loss of sexuality, and death. Allow the patient to express her feelings.

PEDIATRIC POINTERS

Because breast cancer, the most likely cause of dimpling, is extremely rare in children, consider trauma as a likely cause. As in adults, breast dimpling may occur in adolescents from fatty tissue necrosis due to trauma.

PATIENT COUNSELING

Provide a clear explanation of diagnostic tests that may be ordered, such as mammography, thermography, ultrasonography, cytology of nipple discharge, and biopsy. Discuss breast self-examination, and provide follow-up teaching when the patient expresses a readiness to learn. If a breast-feeding patient has mastitis, advise her to pump her breasts to prevent further milk stasis, to discard the milk, and to substitute formula until the breast infection responds adequately to antibiotic therapy.

Breast nodule

[Breast lump]

A commonly reported gynecologic sign, a breast nodule has two chief causes: benign breast disease and cancer. Benign breast disease, the leading cause of nodules, can stem from cyst formation in obstructed and dilated lactiferous ducts, hypertrophy or tumor formation in the ductal system, inflammation, or infection.

Although fewer than 20% of breast nodules are malignant, the signs and symptoms of breast cancer aren't easily distinguished from those of benign breast disease. Breast cancer is a leading cause of death among women but can occur occasionally in men, with signs and symptoms mimicking those found in women. Thus, breast nodules in both sexes should always be evaluated.

A woman who's familiar with the feel of her breasts and performs monthly breast self-examination can detect a nodule 6.4 mm or less in size, considerably smaller than the 1-cm nodule that's readily detectable by an experienced examiner. However, a woman may fail to report a nodule because of the fear of breast cancer.

HISTORY AND PHYSICAL EXAMINATION

If your patient reports a lump, ask her how and when she discovered it and whether its size and tenderness vary with her menstrual cycle. Has the lump changed since she first noticed it? Has she noticed any other breast signs, such as a change in breast shape, size, or contour; a discharge; or nipple changes?

Is she breast-feeding? If so, does she have fever, chills, fatigue, or other flulike signs or symptoms? Ask her to describe any pain or tenderness associated with the lump. Is the pain in one breast only? Has she sustained recent trauma to the breast?

Explore the patient's medical and family history for factors that increase her risk of breast cancer. These include a high-fat diet, having a mother or sister with breast cancer, or having a history of cancer, especially cancer in the other breast. Other risk factors include nulliparity and a first pregnancy after age 30.

CULTURAL CUE *Breast cancer incidence and mortality are about five times higher in North America and northern Europe than in Asia and Africa.*

Next, perform a thorough breast examination. Pay special attention to the upper outer quadrant of each breast, where one-half of the ductal tissue is located. This is the most common site of malignant breast tumors.

Carefully palpate a suspected breast nodule, noting its location, shape, size, consistency, mobility, and delineation. Does the nodule feel soft, rubbery, and elastic or hard? Is it mobile, slipping away from your fingers as you palpate it, or firmly fixed to adjacent tissue? Does the nodule seem to limit the mobility of the entire breast? Note the nodule's delineation. Are its borders clearly defined or indefinite? Does the area feel more like a hardness or diffuse induration than a nodule with definite borders?

Do you feel one nodule or several small ones? Is the shape round, oval, lobular, or irregular? Inspect and palpate the skin over the nodule for warmth, redness, and edema. Palpate the lymph nodes of the breast and axilla for enlargement.

Observe the contour of the breasts, looking for asymmetry and irregularities. Be alert for signs of retraction, such as skin dimpling and nipple deviation, retraction, or flattening. (To exaggerate dimpling, have your patient raise her arms over her head or press her hands against her hips.) Gently pull the breast skin toward the clavicle. Is dimpling evident? Mold the breast skin and again observe the area for dimpling.

Be alert for a nipple discharge that's spontaneous, unilateral, and nonmilky (serous, bloody, or purulent). Be careful not to confuse it with the grayish discharge that can be elicited from the nipples of a woman who has been pregnant. (See *Breast nodule: Causes and associated findings,* page 116.)

MEDICAL CAUSES

◆ ***Adenofibroma.*** The extremely mobile or "slippery" feel of an adenofibroma—a benign neoplasm—helps distinguish it from other breast nodules. The nodule usually occurs singly and characteristically feels firm, elastic, and round or lobular, with well-defined margins. It doesn't cause pain or tenderness, can vary from pinhead size to very large, often grows rapidly, and usually is located around the nipple or on the lateral side of the upper outer quadrant.

◆ ***Areolar gland abscess.*** A tender, palpable abscess on the periphery of the areola caused by an infection and inflammation of Montgomery's glands. Fever may also be present.

◆ ***Breast abscess.*** A localized, hot, tender, fluctuant mass with erythema and peau d'orange typifies an acute abscess. Associated signs and symptoms include fever, chills, malaise, and generalized discomfort. In a chronic abscess, the nodule is nontender, irregular, and firm and may feel like a thick wall of fibrous tissue. It's commonly accompanied by skin dimpling, peau d'orange, and nipple retraction and sometimes by axillary lymphadenopathy.

◆ ***Breast cancer.*** A hard, poorly delineated nodule that's fixed to the skin or underlying tissue suggests breast cancer. Malignant nodules commonly cause breast dimpling, nipple deviation or retraction, or flattening of the nipple or breast contour. Between 40% and 50% of malignant nodules occur in the upper outer quadrant of the breast.

Malignant nodules are usually nontender and occur singly, although satellite nodules may surround the main one. Nipple discharge may be serous or bloody. (A bloody nipple discharge in the presence of a nodule is a classic sign of breast cancer.) Additional findings may include edema and dimpling (peau d'orange) of the skin overlying the mass, erythema, accentuated veins, and axillary lymphadenopathy. A breast ulcer may occur as a late sign. Breast pain, an unreliable symptom, may be present.

◆ ***Fibrocystic breast disease.*** The most common cause of breast nodules, this condition produces smooth, round, slightly elastic nodules that increase in size and tenderness just before menstruation. The nodules may occur in fine, granular clusters in both breasts or as widespread, well-defined lumps of varying sizes. A thickening of adjacent tissue may be palpable. Cystic nodules are mobile, which helps differentiate them from malignant ones. Because cystic nodules aren't fixed to underlying breast tissue, they don't produce retraction signs, such as nipple deviation or dimpling. A clear, watery (serous), or sticky nipple discharge may appear in one or both breasts. Signs and symptoms of premenstrual syndrome—including headache, irritability, bloating, nausea, vomiting, and abdominal cramping—may also be present.

◆ ***Intraductal papilloma.*** Intraductal papilloma is a small, benign nodule that grows in the lactiferous ducts. A single larger nodule can sometimes be palpated, but multiple diffuse nodules usually resist palpation. Soft and poorly delineated papillomas usually lie in the subareolar margin. The primary sign of this disorder is a serous or bloody nipple discharge, typically from only one duct. Breast pain and tenderness may also occur.

◆ ***Mammary duct ectasia.*** This disorder, which affects menopausal or postmenopausal women, produces a rubbery breast nodule that usually lies under the areola. It's commonly accompanied by transient pain, itching, tenderness, and erythema of the areola; a thick, sticky, multicolored nipple discharge from multiple ducts; nipple retraction; and a bluish green discoloration or peau d'orange on the skin overlying the mass. Axillary lymphadenopathy may also occur.

◆ ***Mastitis.*** In mastitis, breast nodules feel firm and indurated or tender, flocculent, and discrete. Gentle palpation defines the area of maximum purulent accumulation. Skin dimpling and nipple deviation, retraction, or flattening may be present, and the nipple may show a crack or abrasion. Accompanying signs and symptoms include breast warmth, erythema, tenderness, and peau d'orange as well as high fever, chills, malaise, and fatigue.

◆ ***Nipple adenoma.*** Although similar in symptoms to Paget's disease, adenomas rarely produce a deep-seated mass.

◆ ***Paget's disease.*** Paget's disease is a slow-growing intraductal carcinoma that begins as a scaling, eczematoid nipple lesion on one side. The nipple later becomes reddened and excoriated and may eventually be completely destroyed. The process extends along the skin as well as in the ducts, usually progressing to a deep-seated mass.

(Text continues on page 116.)

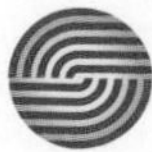

PATIENT-TEACHING AID

How to examine your breasts

Dear Patient:
Examining your breasts may help detect any abnormalities early. Perform this examination 5 to 7 days after the start of your menstrual period. If you're past menopause, choose the same date each month. Follow the steps below, and call your physician if you notice any abnormalities.

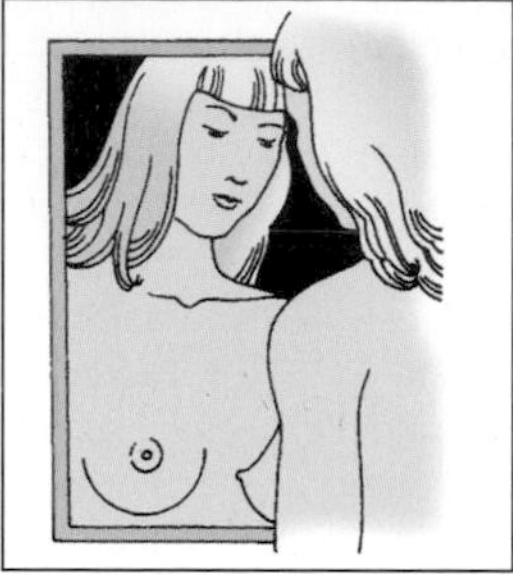

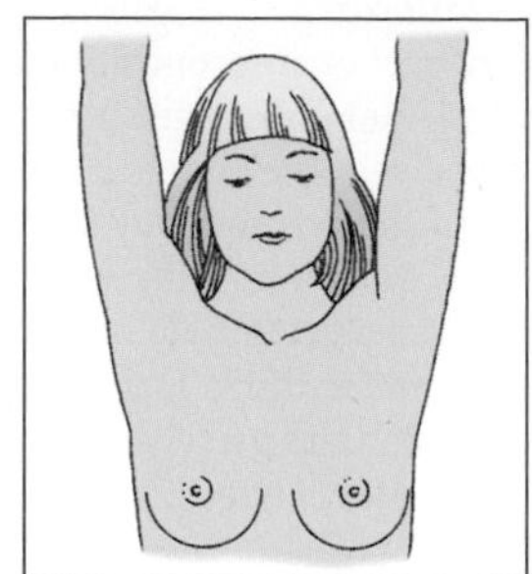

Undress to the waist, and stand in front of a mirror with your arms at your sides. Carefully look for the following: changes in breast shape, size, or symmetry; skin puckering or dimpling; ulceration; lumps; nipple secretions; or retraction of the skin, nipple, or areola. Repeat the inspection with your arms over your head and with your hands on your hips and elbows out to the sides.

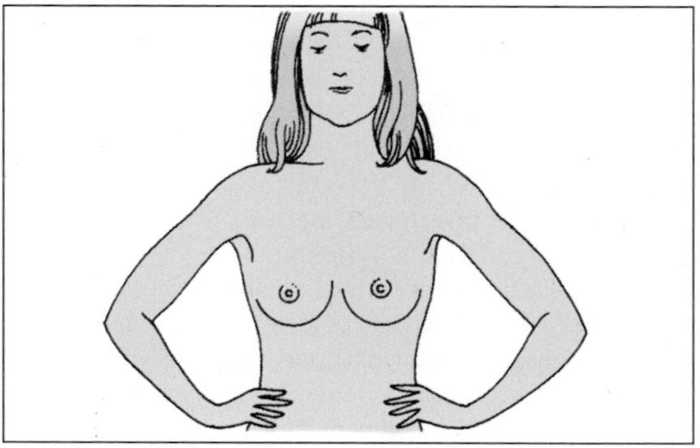

Now, examine your left breast with your right hand. Using the pads of your fingers, move clockwise around your breast to feel for lumps; don't be afraid to press firmly. Start at the outer part of your breast and work inward toward the nipple. You may feel a ridge of firm tissue along the lower part of your breast; this is normal. Repeat the procedure, examining your right breast with your left hand. You may prefer to examine your breasts while standing in the shower, with one hand placed behind your head.

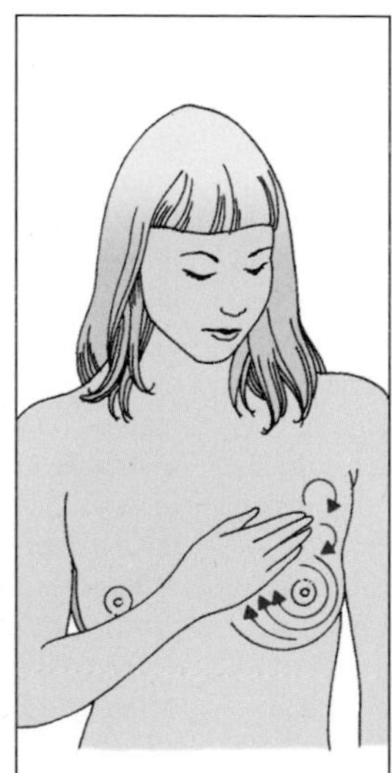

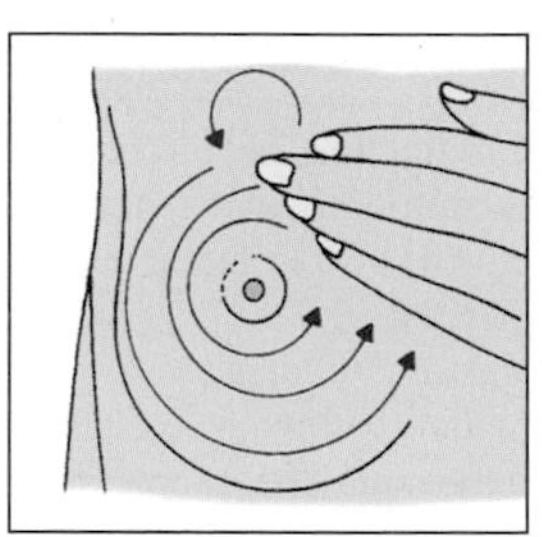

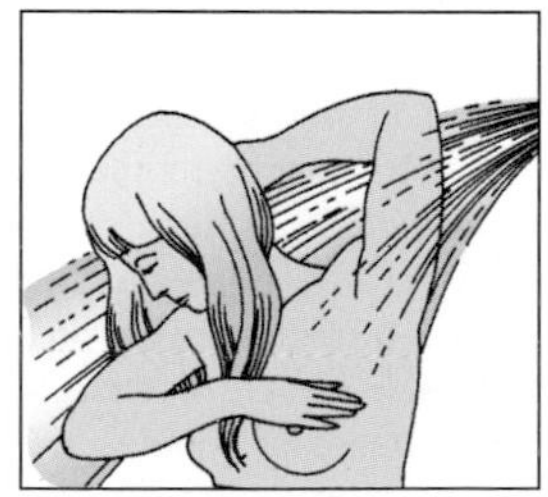

Using the pads of your fingers, feel the opposite armpit. Repeat the examination on the other armpit. Don't be alarmed it you feel a small lump that moves freely; this area contains the lymph glands. However, check the size of the lump daily. If it doesn't go away or if it gets larger, notify your physician.

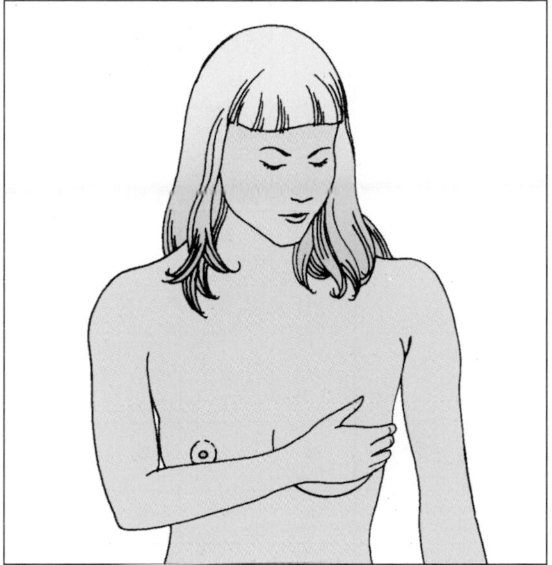

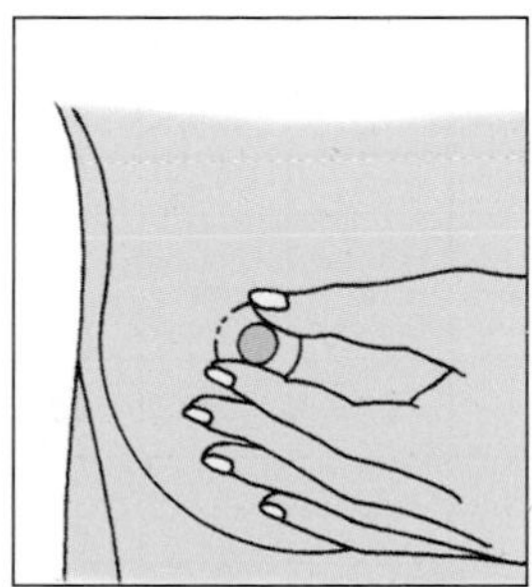

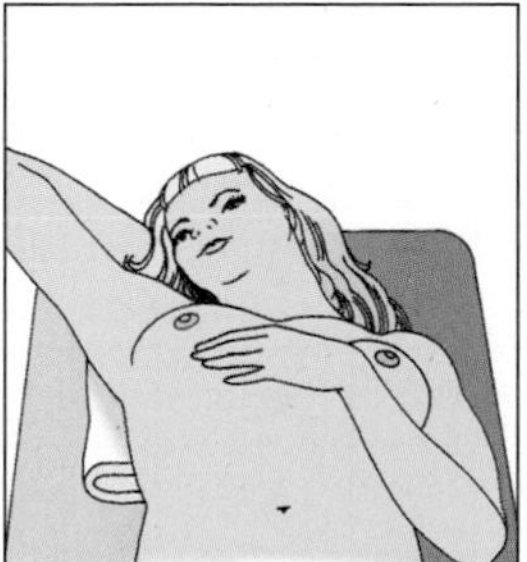

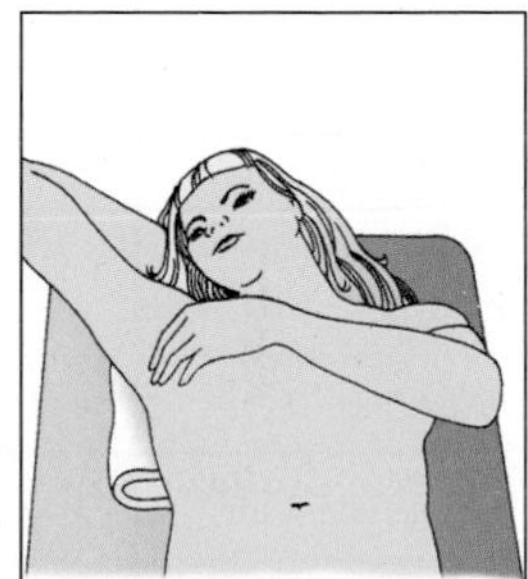

Next, check your nipples for secretions by gently squeezing one nipple between your thumb and forefinger. Check the other nipple the same way. Notify your physician if you see any secretions, and describe the color and amount.

Now, lie down with a rolled-up towel or a small pillow under your right shoulder and your right arm behind your head. Using your left hand, examine your right breast and armpit as you did while standing. Repeat the procedure with your left breast.

If you feel a lump while examining your breasts, note if you can easily lift the skin covering it, if the lump moves under the skin, and if it's soft or hard. Be sure to give your physician this information when you call him.

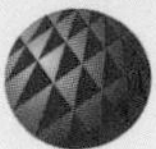

SIGNS & SYMPTOMS

Breast nodule: Causes and associated findings

Common causes	Major associated signs and symptoms: Breast dimpling	Breast pain or tenderness	Erythema	Fever	Lymphadenopathy	Nipple discharge	Nipple retraction	Peau d'orange
Adenofibroma		●						
Areolar gland abscess		●		●				
Breast abscess (acute)		●	●	●				●
Breast abscess (chronic)	●		●		●		●	●
Breast cancer	●	●	●		●	●	●	●
Fibrocystic breast disease		●				●		
Intraductal papilloma		●				●		
Mammary duct ectasia		●	●		●	●	●	●
Mastitis	●	●	●	●			●	●
Nipple adenoma			●			●		
Paget's disease			●			●		

SPECIAL CONSIDERATIONS

Although many women regard a breast lump as a sign of breast cancer, most nodules are benign. As a result, try to avoid alarming your patient further. Provide a simple explanation of your examination, and encourage the patient to express her feelings.

Prepare the patient for diagnostic tests, which may include transillumination, mammography, thermography, needle aspiration or open biopsy of the nodule for tissue examination, and cytologic examination of nipple discharge.

Postpone teaching the patient how to perform breast self-examination until she overcomes her initial anxiety at discovering the nodule. Regular breast self-examination is especially important for women who have had a previous cancer, have a family history of breast cancer, are nulliparous, or had their first child after age 30. (See *How to examine your breasts,* pages 114 and 115.)

Although most nodules occurring in breast-feeding women result from mastitis, the possibility of cancer demands careful evaluation.

Advise the patient with mastitis to pump her breasts to prevent further milk stasis, to discard the milk, and to substitute formula until the infection responds to antibiotics.

PEDIATRIC POINTERS

Most nodules in children and adolescents reflect the normal response of breast tissue to hormonal fluctuations. For instance, the breasts of young teenage girls may normally contain cordlike nodules that become tender just before menstruation.

A transient breast nodule in young boys (as well as women between ages 20 and 30) may result from juvenile mastitis, which usually affects one breast. Signs of inflammation are present in a firm mass beneath the nipple.

GERIATRIC POINTERS

In women age 70 and older, three-quarters of all breast lumps are malignant.

PATIENT COUNSELING

When teaching patients how to perform breast self-examination, advise them to do the examination 5 to 7 days after the first day of their last menstrual period.

Breast pain

[Mastalgia]

An unreliable indicator of cancer, breast pain commonly results from benign breast disease. It may occur during rest or movement and may be aggravated by manipulation or palpation. (Breast tenderness refers to pain elicited by physical contact.) Breast pain may be unilateral or bilateral; cyclic, intermittent, or constant; and dull or sharp. It may result from surface cuts, furuncles, contusions, or similar lesions (superficial pain); nipple fissures or inflammation in the papillary ducts or areolae (severe localized pain); stromal distention in the breast parenchyma; a tumor that affects nerve endings (severe, constant pain); or inflammatory lesions that distend the stroma and irritate sensory nerve endings (severe, constant pain). Breast pain may radiate to the back, the arms, and sometimes the neck.

Breast tenderness in women may occur before menstruation and during pregnancy. Before menstruation, breast pain or tenderness stems from increased mammary blood flow due to hormonal changes. During pregnancy, breast tenderness and throbbing, tingling, or pricking sensations may also occur from hormonal changes. In men, breast pain may stem from gynecomastia (especially during puberty and senescence), reproductive tract anomalies, or organic disease of the liver or pituitary, adrenal cortex, or thyroid glands.

HISTORY AND PHYSICAL EXAMINATION

Begin by asking the patient if breast pain is constant or intermittent. For either type, ask about onset and character. If it's intermittent, determine the relationship of pain to the phase of the menstrual cycle. Is the patient a breast-feeding mother? If not, ask about any nipple discharge and have her describe it. Is she pregnant? Has she reached menopause? Has she recently experienced any flulike symptoms or sustained an injury to the breast? Has she noticed any change in breast shape or contour?

Ask your patient to describe the pain. She may describe it as sticking, stinging, shooting, stabbing, throbbing, or burning. Determine if the pain affects one breast or both, and ask the patient to point to the painful area.

Instruct the patient to place her arms at her sides, and inspect the breasts. Note their size, symmetry, and contour and the appearance of the skin. Remember that breast shape and size vary and that breasts normally change during menses, pregnancy, and lactation and with aging. Are the breasts red or edematous? Are the veins prominent?

Note the size, shape, and symmetry of the nipples and areolae. Do you detect ecchymosis, a rash, ulceration, or a discharge? Do the nipples point in the same direction? Do you see signs of retraction, such as skin dimpling or nipple inversion or flattening? Repeat your inspection, first with the patient's arms raised above her head and then with her hands pressed against her hips.

Palpate the breasts, first with the patient seated and then with her lying down and a pillow placed under her shoulder on the side being examined. Use the pads of your fingers to compress breast tissue against the chest wall. Proceed systematically from the sternum to the midline and from the axilla to the midline, noting any warmth, tenderness, nodules, masses, or irregularities. Palpate the nipple, noting tenderness and nodules, and check for discharge. Palpate axillary lymph nodes, noting any enlargement. (See *Breast pain: Causes and associated findings*, page 118.)

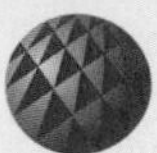

SIGNS & SYMPTOMS

Breast pain: Causes and associated findings

Common causes	Major associated signs and symptoms							
	Breast nodule	Erythema	Fever	Itching	Lymphadenopathy	Nipple discharge	Nipple retraction	Peau d'orange
Areolar gland abscess	●		●					
Breast abscess (acute)	●	●	●					●
Breast cyst	●							
Fat necrosis	●	●					●	
Fibrocystic breast disease	●					●		
Intraductal papilloma	●					●		●
Mammary duct ectasia	●	●		●	●	●	●	●
Mastitis	●	●	●				●	
Sebaceous cyst (infected)	●	●						●

Medical causes

◆ ***Areolar gland abscess.*** A tender, palpable abscess on the periphery of the areola may result from infection and inflammation of Montgomery's glands. Fever may also occur.

◆ ***Breast abscess (acute).*** Local pain, tenderness, erythema, peau d'orange, and warmth are associated with a nodule in the affected breast. Malaise, fever, and chills may also occur.

◆ ***Breast cyst.*** A breast cyst that enlarges rapidly may cause acute, localized, and usually unilateral pain. A breast nodule may be palpable.

◆ ***Fat necrosis.*** Local pain and tenderness may develop in this benign disorder. A history of trauma usually is present. Associated findings include ecchymosis; erythema of the overriding skin; a firm, irregular, fixed mass; and skin retraction signs, such as skin dimpling and nipple retraction. Fat necrosis may be hard to differentiate from breast cancer.

◆ ***Fibrocystic breast disease.*** Fibrocystic breast disease is a common cause of breast pain. Initially, the cysts may cause pain only before menstruation. Later in the course of the disorder, pain and tenderness may persist throughout the cycle. The cysts feel firm, mobile, and well defined. Many occur bilaterally in the upper outer quadrant of the breast, but others are unilateral and generalized. A clear, serous nipple discharge may be present in one or both breasts. Signs and symptoms of premenstrual syndrome—including headache, irritability, bloating, nausea, vomiting, and abdominal cramping—may also be present.

◆ ***Intraductal papilloma.*** Unilateral breast pain or tenderness may accompany intraductal papilloma, although the primary sign is a serous or bloody nipple discharge, usually from only one duct. Intraductal papilloma is the primary cause of nipple discharge in nonpregnant, nonlactating women. Associated signs include a small (usually 1.5- to 3-mm), soft, poorly delineated mass in the ducts beneath the areola.

◆ ***Mammary duct ectasia.*** Burning pain and itching around the areola may occur, although ectasia usually produces no symptoms initially. The history may include one or more episodes of inflammation with pain, tenderness, erythema, and acute fever (or with pain and tenderness alone), which subside spontaneously within 7 to 10 days. Other findings include a rubbery, subareolar breast nodule; areolar swelling and erythema; nipple retraction; a bluish green discoloration or peau d'orange of the skin overlying the nodule; a thick, sticky, multicolored nipple discharge from multiple ducts; and axillary lymphadenopathy. A breast ulcer may occur in late stages.

◆ ***Mastitis.*** Unilateral pain may be severe, particularly when the inflammation occurs near the skin surface. Breast skin is typically red and warm at the inflammation site; peau d'orange may be present. Palpation reveals a firm area of induration. Skin retraction signs—such as breast dimpling and nipple deviation, inversion, or flattening—may be present. Systemic signs and symptoms—such as high fever, chills, malaise, and fatigue—may also occur.

◆ ***Sebaceous cyst (infected).*** Breast pain may be reported with this cutaneous cyst. Associated findings include a small, well-delineated nodule; localized erythema; and induration.

SPECIAL CONSIDERATIONS

Provide emotional support for the patient and, when appropriate, emphasize the importance of monthly breast self-examination. (See *How to examine your breasts,* pages 114 and 115.)

Prepare the patient for diagnostic tests, such as mammography, thermography, cytology of nipple discharge, biopsy, or culture of any aspirate.

PEDIATRIC POINTERS

Transient gynecomastia can cause breast pain in males during puberty.

GERIATRIC POINTERS

Breast pain secondary to benign breast disease is rare in postmenopausal women. Breast pain can also be due to trauma from falls or physical abuse. Because of decreased pain perception and decreased cognitive function, elderly patients may not report breast pain.

PATIENT COUNSELING

Advise the patient to wear a bra that cups and supports the entire breast and has wide shoulder and back straps. Warm or cold compresses may be helpful. Teach the patient how to perform breast self-examination, and instruct her to call the physician immediately if she detects any breast changes.

Breast ulcer

Appearing on the nipple, areola, or the breast itself, an ulcer indicates destruction of the skin and subcutaneous tissue. A breast ulcer is usually a late sign of cancer, appearing well after the confirming diagnosis. However, it may be the presenting sign of breast cancer in men, who are more apt to dismiss earlier breast changes. Breast ulcers can also result from trauma, infection, or radiation.

HISTORY AND PHYSICAL EXAMINATION

Begin the history by asking when the patient first noticed the ulcer and if it was preceded by other breast changes, such as nodules, edema, or nipple discharge, deviation, or retraction. Does the ulcer seem to be getting better or worse? Does it cause pain or produce drainage? Has she noticed any change in breast shape? Has she had a rash? If she has been treating the ulcer at home, find out how.

Review the patient's personal and family history for factors that increase the risk of breast cancer. For example, ask about previous cancer, especially of the breast, and mastectomy. Determine whether the patient's mother or sister has had breast cancer. Ask the patient's age at menarche and menopause because more than 30 years of menstrual activity increases the risk of breast cancer. Also ask about pregnancy because nulliparity or a first pregnancy after age 30 also increases the risk of breast cancer.

If the patient recently gave birth, ask if she breast-feeds her infant or has recently weaned him. Ask if she's currently taking an oral antibiotic and if she's diabetic. All these factors predispose the patient to candidal infections.

Inspect the patient's breast, noting any asymmetry or flattening. Look for a rash, scaling, cracking, or red excoriation on the nipples, areola, and inframammary fold. Check especially for skin changes, such as warmth, erythema, or peau d'orange. Palpate the breast for masses, noting any induration beneath the ulcer. Then carefully palpate for tenderness or nodules around the areola and the axillary lymph nodes.

Medical causes

◆ ***Breast cancer.*** A breast ulcer that doesn't heal within 1 month usually indicates cancer. Ulceration along a mastectomy scar may indicate metastatic cancer; a nodule beneath the ulcer may be a late sign of a fulminating tumor. Other signs include a palpable breast nodule, skin dimpling, nipple retraction, bloody or serous nipple discharge, erythema, peau d'orange, and enlarged axillary lymph nodes.

◆ ***Breast trauma.*** Tissue destruction with inadequate healing may produce breast ulcers. Associated signs depend on the type of trauma but may include ecchymosis, lacerations, abrasions, swelling, and hematoma.

◆ **Candida albicans *infection.*** A severe candidal infection can cause maceration of breast tissue followed by ulceration. Well-defined, bright-red papular patches—usually with scaly borders—characterize the infection, which can develop in the breast folds. Cracked nipples predispose breast-feeding women to this infection, which causes a burning pain that penetrates into the chest wall when the infant sucks.

◆ ***Paget's disease.*** Bright-red nipple excoriation can extend to the areola and ulcerate. A serous or bloody nipple discharge and extreme nipple itching may accompany ulceration. Symptoms are usually unilateral.

Other causes

◆ ***Radiation therapy.*** After radiation, the breasts appear "sunburned." Subsequently, the skin ulcerates and the surrounding area becomes red and tender.

Special considerations

Because breast ulcers become infected easily, teach the patient how to apply topical antifungal ointment or cream. Instruct her to keep the ulcer dry to reduce chafing and to wear loose-fitting undergarments. If breast cancer is suspected, provide emotional support and encourage the patient to express her feelings. Prepare her for diagnostic tests, such as ultrasonography, thermography, mammography, nipple discharge cytology, and breast biopsy. If a candidal infection is suspected, prepare her for skin or blood cultures.

Geriatric pointers

Breast ulcers should be considered cancerous until proven otherwise in elderly women because of their increased breast cancer risk. However, ulcers can also result from normal skin changes in the elderly, such as thinning, decreased vascularity, and loss of elasticity as well as from poor skin hygiene. Pressure ulcers may result from the use of restraints or tight bras; traumatic ulcers, from falls or abuse.

Breath with ammonia odor

[Uremic fetor]

The odor of ammonia on the breath—described as urinous or "fishy" breath—typically occurs in end-stage chronic renal failure. This sign improves slightly after hemodialysis and persists throughout the course of the disorder, but it isn't of great concern.

Ammonia breath odor reflects the long-term metabolic disturbances and biochemical abnormalities associated with uremia and end-stage chronic renal failure. It's produced by metabolic end products blown off by the lungs and the breakdown of urea (to ammonia) in the saliva. However, a specific uremic toxin hasn't been identified. In animals, breath odor analysis has revealed toxic metabolites, such as dimethylamine and trimethylamine, that contribute to the "fishy" odor. The source of these amines, although still unclear, may be intestinal bacteria acting on dietary chlorine.

History and physical examination

When you detect ammonia breath odor, the diagnosis of chronic renal failure will probably be well established. Look for associated GI symptoms so that palliative care and support can be individualized.

Inspect the patient's oral cavity for bleeding, swollen gums or tongue, and ulceration with drainage. Ask the patient if he has experienced a metallic taste, loss of smell, increased thirst, heartburn, difficulty swallowing, loss of appetite at the sight of food, or early morning vomiting. Because GI bleeding is common in patients with chronic renal failure, ask about bowel habits, noting especially melena or constipation.

Take the patient's vital signs. Watch for any indications of hypertension (the patient with end-stage chronic renal failure is usually somewhat hypertensive) or hypotension. Be alert for other signs of shock (such as tachycardia, tachypnea, and cool, clammy skin) and altered mental status. Any significant changes can indicate complications, such as massive GI bleeding or pericarditis with tamponade.

Medical causes

◆ ***End-stage chronic renal failure.*** Ammonia breath odor is a late finding in end-stage chronic renal failure. Accompanying signs and symptoms include anuria, skin pigmentation changes and excoriation, brown arcs under the nail margins, tissue wasting, Kussmaul's respirations, neuropathy, lethargy, somnolence, confusion, disorientation, behavior changes, irritability, and emotional lability. Later neurologic signs that signal impending uremic coma include muscle twitching and fasciculations, asterixis, paresthesia, and footdrop. Cardiovascular findings include hypertension, myocardial infarction, signs of heart failure, pericarditis, and even sudden death and stroke. GI findings include anorexia, weight loss, nausea, heartburn, vomiting, constipation, hiccups, and a metallic taste. Oral signs and symptoms may include stomatitis, gum ulceration and bleeding, and a coated tongue. The patient has an increased risk of peptic ulceration and acute pancreatitis. Uremic frost, pruritus, and signs of hormonal changes, such as impotence or amenorrhea, may also appear.

Special considerations

Ammonia breath odor is offensive to others, but the patient may become accustomed to it. As a result, remind him to perform frequent mouth care, particularly before meals because reducing the foul taste and odor may stimulate his appetite. A half-strength hydrogen peroxide mixture or lemon juice gargle helps neutralize the ammonia; the patient may also want to use commercial lozenges or breath sprays or to suck on hard candy. Advise him to use a soft-bristled toothbrush or sponge to prevent trauma. If he can't perform mouth care, do it for him and teach his family members how to assist him.

Maximize dietary intake by offering the patient frequent small meals of his favorite foods, within dietary limitations.

Pediatric pointers

Ammonia breath odor also occurs in children with end-stage chronic renal failure. Provide hard candy to relieve bad taste and odor. If the child can gargle, try mixing hydrogen peroxide with flavored mouthwashes.

Patient counseling

Involve the patient at an early stage in the various aspects of treatment to help prepare him for any complicated training that may be needed later—for example, if he needs dialysis or transplantation. Explain dietary and drug therapies.

Breath with fecal odor

Fecal breath odor typically accompanies fecal vomiting associated with a long-standing intestinal obstruction or gastrojejunocolic fistula. It represents an important late diagnostic clue to a potentially life-threatening GI disorder because complete obstruction of any part of the bowel, if untreated, can cause death within hours from vascular collapse and shock.

When the obstructed or adynamic intestine attempts self-decompression by regurgitating its contents, vigorous peristaltic waves propel bowel contents backward into the stomach. When the stomach fills with intestinal fluid, further reverse peristalsis results in vomiting. The odor of feculent vomitus lingers in the mouth.

Fecal breath odor may also occur in patients with a nasogastric (NG) or intestinal tube. The odor is detected only while the underlying disorder persists and abates soon after its resolution.

EMERGENCY INTERVENTIONS *Because fecal breath odor signals a potentially life-threatening intestinal obstruction, you'll need to quickly evaluate your patient's condition. Monitor his vital signs, and be alert for signs of shock, such as hypotension, tachycardia, narrowed pulse pressure, and cool, clammy skin. Ask the patient if he's experiencing nausea or has vomited. Find out the frequency of vomiting as well as the color, odor, amount, and consistency of the vomitus. Have an emesis basin nearby to collect and accurately measure the vomitus.*

Anticipate possible surgery to relieve an obstruction or repair a fistula, and withhold all food and fluids. Be prepared to insert an NG or intestinal tube for GI tract decompression. Insert a peripheral I.V. catheter for vascular access, or assist with central venous access device insertion for large-bore access and central venous pressure monitoring. Obtain a blood sample and send it to the laboratory for complete blood count and electrolyte analysis because large fluid losses and shifts can produce electrolyte imbalances. Maintain adequate hydration and support circulatory status with additional fluids. Give a physiologic solution—such as lactated Ringer's or normal saline solution or Plasmanate—to prevent metabolic acidosis from gastric losses and metabolic alkalosis from intestinal fluid losses.

History and physical examination

If the patient's condition permits, ask about previous abdominal surgery because adhesions can cause an obstruction. Also ask about loss of appetite. Is the patient experiencing abdominal pain? If so, have him describe its onset, duration, and location. Ask if the pain is intense, persistent, or spasmodic. Have the patient describe his normal bowel habits, especially noting constipation, diarrhea, or leakage of stool. Ask when the patient's last bowel movement occurred, and have him describe the stool's color and consistency.

Auscultate for bowel sounds; hyperactive, high-pitched sounds may indicate an impending bowel obstruction, whereas hypoactive or absent sounds occur late in obstruction and paralytic ileus. Inspect the abdomen, noting its contour and any surgical scars. Measure abdominal girth to provide baseline data for subsequent assessment of distention. Palpate the abdomen for tenderness, distention, and rigidity. Percuss it for tympany, indicating a gas-filled bowel, and dullness, indicating fluid.

Rectal and pelvic examinations should be performed. All patients with a suspected bowel obstruction should have a flat and upright abdominal X-ray; some will also need a chest X-ray, sigmoidoscopy, and a barium enema.

Medical causes

◆ ***Gastrojejunocolic fistula.*** Symptoms of gastrojejunocolic fistula may be variable and intermittent because of temporary plugging of the fistula. They may include fecal vomiting with resulting fecal breath odor, but the chief complaint is usually diarrhea accompanied by abdominal pain. Related GI findings include anorexia, weight loss, abdominal distention, and possibly marked malabsorption.

◆ ***Large-bowel obstruction.*** Vomiting is usually absent at first, but fecal vomiting with resulting fecal breath odor occurs as a late sign. Typically, symptoms develop more slowly than in small-bowel obstruction. Colicky abdominal pain appears suddenly, followed by continuous hypogastric pain. Marked abdominal distention and tenderness occur, and loops of large bowel may be visible through the abdominal wall. Although constipation develops, defecation may continue for up to 3 days after a complete obstruction because of stool remaining in the bowel below the obstruction. Leakage of stool is common in a partial obstruction.

◆ ***Small-bowel obstruction, distal.*** In late obstruction, nausea is present but vomiting may be delayed. Vomitus initially consists of gastric contents, then changes to bilious contents, followed by fecal contents with resulting fecal breath odor. Accompanying symptoms include achiness, malaise, drowsiness, and polydipsia. Bowel changes (ranging from diarrhea to constipation) are accompanied by abdominal distention, persistent epigastric or periumbilical colicky pain, hyperactive bowel sounds, and borborygmus. As the obstruction becomes complete, bowel sounds become hypoactive or absent. Fever, hypotension, tachycardia, and rebound tenderness may indicate strangulation or perforation.

Special considerations

After an NG or intestinal tube has been inserted, keep the head of the bed elevated at least 30 degrees and turn the patient on his right side to facilitate passage of the intestinal tube through the GI tract. Don't tape the intestinal tube to the patient's face. Ensure tube patency by monitoring drainage and checking that suction devices function properly. Irrigate as required. Monitor GI drainage, and send serum specimens to the laboratory for electrolyte analysis at least once a day. Prepare the patient for diagnostic tests, such as abdominal X-rays, barium enema, and proctoscopy.

Pediatric pointers

Carefully monitor the child's fluid and electrolyte status because dehydration can occur rapidly from persistent vomiting. The absence of tears and dry or parched mucous membranes are important clinical signs of dehydration.

Geriatric pointers

In older patients, early surgical intervention may be necessary for a bowel obstruction that doesn't respond to decompression because of the high risk of bowel infarct.

Patient counseling

Encourage the patient to brush his teeth and gargle with a flavored mouthwash or a half-strength hydrogen peroxide mixture to minimize offensive breath odor. Assure him that the fecal odor is temporary and will abate after treatment of the underlying cause.

Breath with fruity odor

Fruity breath odor results from respiratory elimination of excess acetone. This sign characteristically occurs in ketoacidosis, a potentially life-threatening condition that requires immediate treatment to prevent severe dehydration, irreversible coma, and death.

Ketoacidosis results from the excessive catabolism of fats for cellular energy in the absence of usable carbohydrates. This process begins when insulin levels are insufficient to transport glucose into the cells, as in diabetes mellitus, or when glucose is unavailable and hepatic glycogen stores are depleted, as in low-carbohydrate diets and malnutrition. Lacking glucose, the cells burn fat faster than enzymes can handle the ketones, the acidic end products. As a result, the ketones (acetone, beta-hydroxybutyric acid, and acetoacetic acid) accumulate in the blood and urine. To compensate for increased acidity, Kussmaul's respirations expel carbon dioxide with enough acetone to flavor the breath. Eventually, this compensatory mechanism fails, producing ketoacidosis.

EMERGENCY INTERVENTIONS *When you detect fruity breath odor, check for Kussmaul's respirations and examine the patient's level of consciousness (LOC). Take vital signs and check skin turgor. Be alert for fruity breath odor that accompanies rapid, deep respirations; stupor; and poor skin turgor. Try to obtain a brief history, noting especially diabetes mellitus, nutritional problems such as anorexia nervosa, and fad diets with little or no carbohydrates. Obtain venous and arterial blood samples for complete blood count and glucose, electrolyte, acetone, and arterial blood gas (ABG) levels. Also obtain a urine specimen to test for glucose and acetone. Administer I.V. fluids and electrolytes to maintain hydration and electrolyte balance, and give regular insulin to patients with diabetic ketoacidosis to reduce blood glucose levels.*

If the patient is obtunded, you'll need to insert endotracheal and nasogastric (NG) tubes. Suction as needed. Insert an indwelling urinary catheter, and monitor intake and output. Insert central venous pressure and arterial lines to monitor the patient's fluid status and blood pressure. Connect the patient to a cardiac monitor, monitor vital signs and neurologic status, and draw blood hourly to check glucose, electrolyte, acetone, and ABG levels.

History and physical examination

If the patient isn't in severe distress, obtain a thorough history. Ask about the onset and duration of fruity breath odor. Also ask about any changes in breathing pattern, increased thirst, frequent urination, weight loss, fatigue, and abdominal pain. Ask the female patient if she has had candidal vaginitis or vaginal secretions with itching. If the patient has a history of diabetes mellitus, ask about stress, infections, and noncompliance with therapy—the most common causes of ketoacidosis in known diabetics. If the patient is suspected of having anorexia nervosa, obtain a dietary and weight history.

Medical causes

◆ ***Anorexia nervosa.*** Severe weight loss associated with anorexia nervosa may produce fruity breath odor, usually with nausea, constipation, and cold intolerance. Induced vomiting may cause dental enamel erosion and scars or calluses in the dorsum of the hand.

◆ ***Ketoacidosis.*** Fruity breath odor accompanies alcoholic ketoacidosis, which is usually seen in poorly nourished alcoholics with a history of vomiting, abdominal pain, and only minimal food intake over several days. Kussmaul's respirations begin abruptly and accompany dehydration, abdominal pain and distention, and absent bowel sounds. Blood glucose levels are normal or slightly decreased.

In diabetic ketoacidosis, fruity breath odor commonly acompanies the development of ketoacidosis over 1 to 2 days. Other findings include polydipsia, polyuria, nocturia, weak and rapid pulse, hunger, weight loss, weakness, fatigue, nausea, vomiting, and abdominal pain. Eventually, Kussmaul's respirations, orthostatic hypotension, dehydration, tachycardia, confusion, and stupor occur. Signs and symptoms may lead to coma.

Starvation ketoacidosis is a potentially life-threatening disorder that has a gradual onset. Besides fruity breath odor, typical findings include signs of cachexia and dehydration, decreased LOC, bradycardia, and a history of anorexia nervosa.

Other causes

◆ ***Drugs.*** Any drug known to cause metabolic acidosis, such as nitroprusside and salicylates, can result in fruity breath odor.

◆ ***Low-carbohydrate diets.*** Diets that promote little or no carbohydrate intake may cause ketoacidosis and the resulting fruity breath odor.

Special considerations

Provide emotional support for the patient and his family. Explain tests and treatments clearly. When the patient is more alert and his condition stabilizes, remove the NG tube and start him on an appropriate diet. Switch his insulin from the I.V. to the subcutaneous route.

Pediatric pointers

Fruity breath odor in an infant or a child usually stems from uncontrolled diabetes mellitus. Ketoacidosis develops rapidly in this age-group because of their low glycogen reserves. As a result, prompt administration of insulin and correction of fluid and electrolyte imbalance are necessary to prevent shock and death.

Patient counseling

Patient teaching and referrals should be based on the underlying cause. For example, teach the patient with uncontrolled diabetes mellitus to recognize the signs of hyperglycemia and to wear a medical identification bracelet. Refer the patient with starvation ketoacidosis to a psychologist or a support group, and recognize the need for possible long-term follow-up.

Brudzinski's sign

A positive Brudzinski's sign (flexion of the hips and knees in response to passive flexion of the neck) signals meningeal irritation. Passive flexion of the neck stretches the nerve roots, causing pain and involuntary flexion of the knees and hips.

Brudzinski's sign is a common and important early indicator of life-threatening meningitis and subarachnoid hemorrhage. It can be elicited in children as well as adults, although more reliable indicators of meningeal irritation exist for infants.

Testing for Brudzinski's sign isn't part of a routine physical examination unless meningeal irritation is suspected. (See *Testing for Brudzinski's sign*.)

EMERGENCY INTERVENTIONS *If the patient is alert, ask him about headache, neck pain, nausea, and vision disturbances (blurred or double vision and photophobia)—all indications of increased intracranial pressure (ICP). Next, observe the patient for signs and symptoms of increased ICP, such as an altered level of consciousness (LOC), pupillary changes, bradycardia, widened pulse pressure, irregular respiratory patterns (Cheyne-Stokes or Kussmaul's respirations), vomiting, and moderate fever.*

Keep artificial airways, intubation equipment, a handheld resuscitation bag, and suction equipment on hand because the patient's condition may suddenly deteriorate. Elevate the head of his bed 30 to 60 degrees to promote venous drainage. Administer an osmotic diuretic, such as mannitol, to reduce cerebral edema.

Be alert for further increases in ICP. You may have to provide mechanical ventilation and administer a barbiturate and additional doses of a diuretic. Also, cerebrospinal fluid (CSF) may have to be drained.

History and physical examination

Continue your neurologic examination by evaluating the patient's cranial nerve function and noting any motor or sensory deficits. Be sure to look for Kernig's sign (resistance to knee extension after flexion of the hip), a further indication of meningeal irritation. Also look for signs of central nervous system infection, such as fever and nuchal rigidity.

Ask the patient—or his family if necessary—about a history of hypertension, spinal arthritis, or recent head trauma. Also ask about dental work and abscessed teeth (a possible cause of meningitis), open-head injury, endocarditis, and I.V. drug abuse. Ask about the sudden onset of headaches, which may be associated with subarachnoid hemorrhage.

Medical causes

◆ ***Arthritis.*** A positive Brudzinski's sign can occasionally be elicited in patients with severe spinal arthritis. The patient may also report back pain (especially after weight bearing) and limited mobility.

◆ ***Meningitis.*** A positive Brudzinski's sign can usually be elicited 24 hours after the onset of meningitis, a life-threatening disorder. Accompanying findings may include headache, a positive Kernig's sign, nuchal rigidity, irritability or restlessness, deep stupor or coma, vertigo, fever (high or low, depending on the severity of the infection), chills, malaise, hyperalgesia, muscular hypotonia, opisthotonos, symmetrical deep tendon reflexes, papilledema, ocular and facial palsies, nausea and vomiting, photophobia, diplopia, and unequal, sluggish pupils. As ICP rises, arterial hypertension, bradycardia,

Testing for Brudzinski's sign

Here's how to test for Brudzinski's sign when you suspect meningeal irritation:

With the patient in a supine position, place your hands behind her neck and lift her head toward her chest.

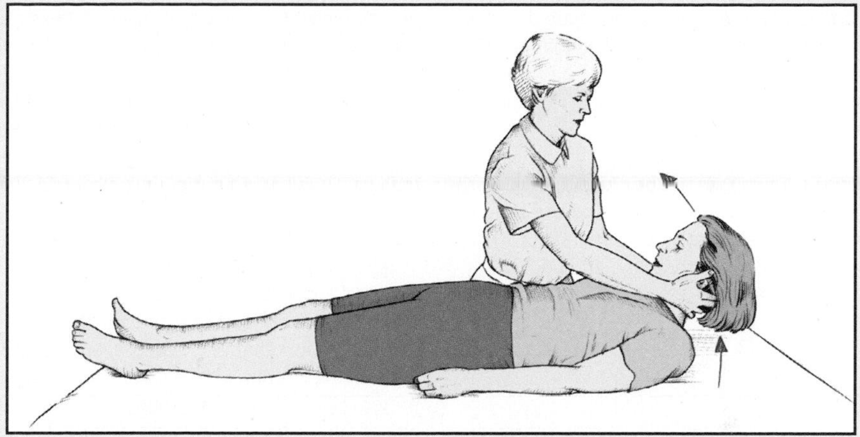

If your patient has meningeal irritation, she'll flex her hips and knees in response to the passive neck flexion.

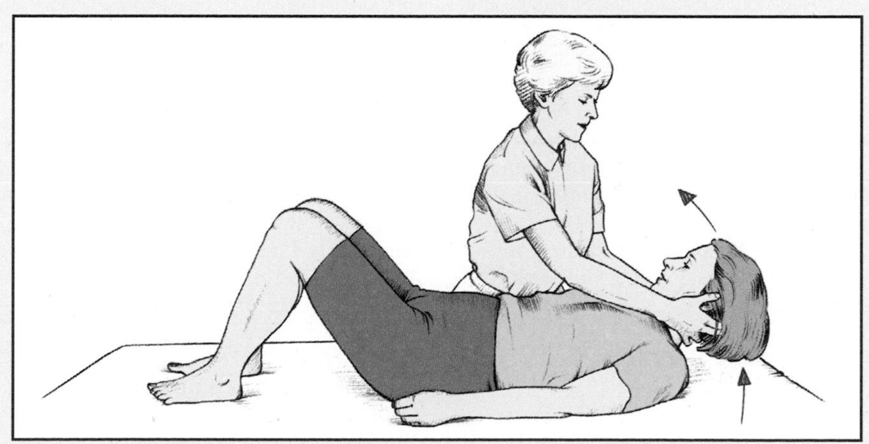

widened pulse pressure, Cheyne-Stokes or Kussmaul's respirations, and coma may develop.

◆ ***Subarachnoid hemorrhage.*** A positive Brudzinski's sign may be elicited within minutes after initial bleeding in subarachnoid hemorrhage, a life-threatening disorder. Accompanying signs and symptoms include sudden onset of a severe headache, nuchal rigidity, altered LOC, dizziness, photophobia, cranial nerve palsies (as evidenced by ptosis, pupil dilation, and limited extraocular muscle movement), nausea and vomiting, fever, and a positive Kernig's sign. Focal signs—such as hemiparesis, vision disturbances, and aphasia—may also occur. As ICP rises, arterial hypertension, bradycardia, widened pulse pressure, Cheyne-Stokes or Kussmaul's respirations, and coma may develop.

Special considerations

Many patients with a positive Brudzinski's sign are critically ill. They need constant ICP monitoring and frequent neurologic checks in addition to intensive assessment and monitoring of vital signs, intake and output, and cardiorespiratory status. To promote patient comfort, maintain low lights and minimal noise and elevate the head of the bed. The patient usually won't receive an opioid analgesic because it may mask signs of increased ICP.

Prepare the patient for diagnostic tests. These may include blood, urine, and sputum cultures to identify bacteria; lumbar puncture to assess CSF and relieve pressure; and computed tomography scan, magnetic resonance imaging, cerebral angiography, or spinal X-rays to locate a hemorrhage.

PEDIATRIC POINTERS

Brudzinski's sign may not be a useful indicator of meningeal irritation in infants because more reliable signs—such as bulging fontanels, a weak cry, fretfulness, vomiting, and poor feeding—appear early.

Bruits

Commonly an indicator of life- or limb-threatening vascular disease, bruits are swishing sounds caused by turbulent blood flow. They're characterized by location, duration, intensity, pitch, and time of onset in the cardiac cycle. Loud bruits produce intense vibration and a palpable thrill. A thrill, however, doesn't provide any further clue to the causative disorder or its severity.

Bruits are most significant when heard over the abdominal aorta; the renal, carotid, femoral, popliteal, or subclavian artery; or the thyroid gland. (See *Preventing false bruits.*) They're also significant when heard consistently despite changes in patient position and when heard during diastole.

HISTORY AND PHYSICAL EXAMINATION

If you detect bruits over the abdominal aorta, check for a pulsating mass or a bluish discoloration around the umbilicus (Cullen's sign). Either of these signs—or severe, tearing pain in the abdomen, flank, or lower back—may signal life-threatening dissection of an aortic aneurysm. Also check peripheral pulses, comparing intensity in the upper and lower extremities.

If you suspect dissection, monitor the patient's vital signs continuously, and withhold food and fluids until a definitive diagnosis is made. Watch for signs and symptoms of hypovolemic shock, such as thirst; hypotension; tachycardia; weak, thready pulse; tachypnea; altered level of consciousness (LOC); mottled knees and elbows; and cool, clammy skin.

If you detect bruits over the thyroid gland, ask the patient if he has a history of hyperthyroidism or signs and symptoms of it, such as nervousness, tremors, weight loss, palpitations, heat intolerance, and (in females) amenorrhea. Watch for signs and symptoms of life-threatening thyroid storm, such as tremor, restlessness, diarrhea, abdominal pain, and hepatomegaly.

If you detect carotid artery bruits, be alert for signs and symptoms of a transient ischemic attack (TIA), including dizziness, diplopia, slurred speech, flashing lights, and syncope. These findings may indicate an impending stroke. Be sure to evaluate the patient frequently for changes in LOC and muscle function.

If you detect bruits over the femoral, popliteal, or subclavian artery, watch for signs and symptoms of decreased or absent peripheral circulation—edema, weakness, and paresthesia. Ask the patient if he has a history of intermittent claudication. Frequently check distal pulses and skin color and temperature. Pallor, coolness, or the sudden absence of a pulse may indicate a threat to the affected limb.

If you detect a bruit, be sure to check for further vascular damage and perform a thorough cardiac assessment.

MEDICAL CAUSES

- ***Abdominal aortic aneurysm.*** A pulsating periumbilical mass accompanied by a systolic bruit over the aorta characterizes an abdominal aortic aneurysm. Associated signs and symptoms include a rigid, tender abdomen; mottled skin; diminished peripheral pulses; and claudication. Sharp, tearing pain in the abdomen, flank, or lower back signals imminent dissection.
- ***Abdominal aortic atherosclerosis.*** Loud systolic bruits in the epigastric and midabdominal areas are common in this disorder. They may be accompanied by leg pain, weakness, numbness, paresthesia, or paralysis or by decreased or absent femoral, popliteal, or pedal pulses. Abdominal pain is rare.
- ***Anemia.*** Increased cardiac output in anemia causes increased blood flow. In patients with severe anemia, short systolic bruits may be heard over both carotid arteries and may be accompanied by headache, fatigue, dizziness, pallor, jaundice, palpitations, mild tachycardia, dyspnea, nausea, anorexia, and glossitis.
- ***Carotid artery stenosis.*** Systolic bruits heard over one or both carotid arteries may be the only sign of this disorder. However, dizziness,

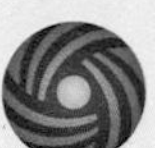

EXAMINATION TIP

Preventing false bruits

Auscultating bruits accurately requires practice and skill. These sounds typically stem from arterial luminal narrowing or arterial dilation, but they can also result from excessive pressure applied to the stethoscope's bell during auscultation. This pressure compresses the artery, creating turbulent blood flow and a false bruit.

To prevent false bruits, place the bell lightly on the patient's skin. Also, if you're auscultating for a popliteal bruit, help the patient to a supine position, place your hand behind his ankle, and lift his leg slightly before placing the bell behind the knee.

NORMAL BLOOD FLOW, NO BRUIT

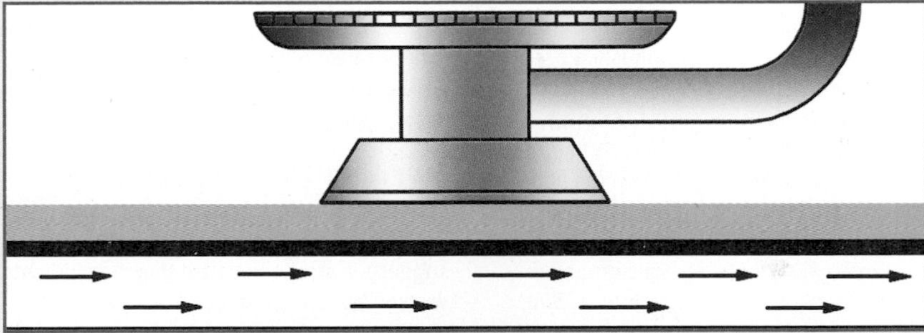

TURBULENT BLOOD FLOW AND RESULTANT BRUIT CAUSED BY ANEURYSM

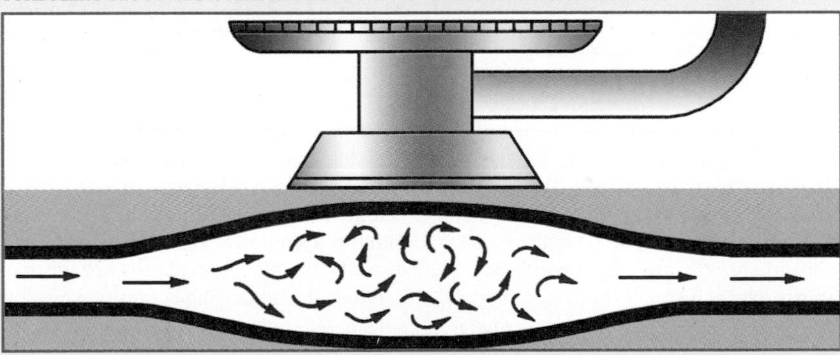

TURBULENT BLOOD FLOW AND FALSE BRUIT CAUSED BY COMPRESSION OF ARTERY

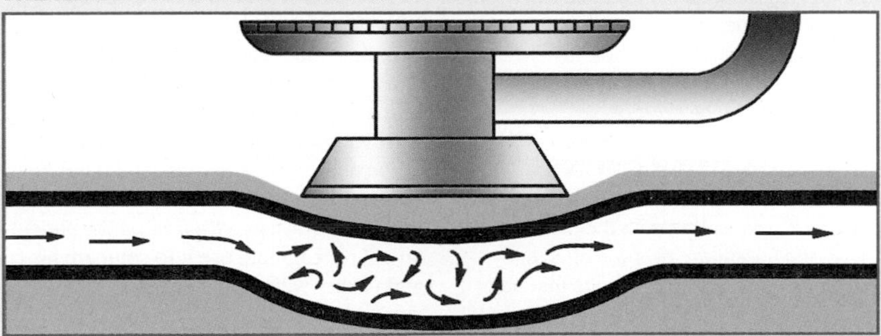

vertigo, headache, syncope, aphasia, dysarthria, sudden vision loss, hemiparesis, or hemiparalysis signals TIA and may herald a stroke.

◆ ***Carotid cavernous fistula.*** Continuous bruits heard over the eyeballs and temples are characteristic, as are vision disturbances and protruding, pulsating eyeballs.

◆ ***Peripheral arteriovenous fistula.*** A rough, continuous bruit with systolic accentuation may be heard over the fistula; a palpable thrill is also common.

◆ ***Peripheral vascular disease.*** Peripheral vascular disease characteristically produces bruits over the femoral artery and other arteries in the legs. It can also cause diminished or absent femoral, popliteal, or pedal pulses; intermittent claudication; numbness, weakness, pain, and cramping in the legs, feet, and hips; and cool, shiny skin and hair loss on the affected extremity. It also predisposes the patient to lower extremity ulcers that heal with difficulty.

◆ ***Renal artery stenosis.*** Systolic bruits are commonly heard over the abdominal midline and flank on the affected side. Hypertension commonly accompanies stenosis. Headache, palpitations, tachycardia, anxiety, dizziness, retinopathy, hematuria, and mental sluggishness may also appear.

◆ ***Subclavian steal syndrome.*** In subclavian steal syndrome, systolic bruits may be heard over one or both subclavian arteries as a result of narrowing of the arterial lumen. They may be accompanied by decreased blood pressure and claudication in the affected arm, hemiparesis, vision disturbances, vertigo, and dysarthria.

◆ ***Thyrotoxicosis.*** A systolic bruit is commonly heard over the thyroid gland. Accompanying signs and symptoms appear in all body systems, but the most characteristic ones include thyroid enlargement, fatigue, nervousness, tachycardia, heat intolerance, sweating, tremor, diarrhea, and weight loss despite increased appetite. Exophthalmos may also be present.

Special considerations

Because bruits can signal a life-threatening vascular disorder, frequently check the patient's vital signs and auscultate over the affected arteries. Be especially alert for bruits that become louder or develop a diastolic component.

As needed, administer prescribed drugs, such as a vasodilator, an anticoagulant, an antiplatelet drug, or an antihypertensive. Prepare the patient for diagnostic tests, such as blood studies, radiography, an electrocardiogram, cardiac catheterization, and ultrasonography.

Pediatric pointers

Bruits are common in young children but are usually of little significance—for example, cranial bruits are normal until age 4. However, certain bruits may be significant. Because birthmarks commonly accompany congenital arteriovenous fistulas, carefully auscultate for bruits in a child with port-wine spots or cavernous or diffuse hemangiomas.

Geriatric pointers

Elderly people with atherosclerosis may experience bruits over several arteries. Those related to carotid artery stenosis are particularly important because of the high incidence of associated stroke. Close follow-up is mandatory as well as prompt surgical referral when indicated.

Patient counseling

Instruct the patient to inform the physician if he develops dizziness, pain, or any symptom that suggests a stroke because this may indicate a worsening of his condition.

Buffalo hump

Buffalo hump, characterized by an accumulation of cervicodorsal fat, may indicate hypercortisolism (Cushing's syndrome). Hypercortisolism itself may result from long-term glucocorticoid therapy, adrenal carcinoma, adrenal adenoma, ectopic corticotropin production, or excessive pituitary secretion of corticotropin (Cushing's disease). Buffalo hump doesn't help distinguish between the underlying causes of hypercortisolism, but it may help direct diagnostic testing.

History and physical examination

Ask the patient about recent weight gain and when he first noticed the buffalo hump. Typically, a history of moderate to extreme obesity, with accumulation of adipose tissue in the nape of the neck, face, and trunk and thinning of the arms and legs, indicates hypercortisolism. (See *Recognizing hypercortisolism*.) If the patient has an old photograph, use it to compare his current and former weight and distribution of adipose tissue. Ask if the patient or any family member has a history of endocrine disorders, cancer, or obesity. If the patient is a female of childbearing age, ask the date of her last menses and about any changes in her normal menstrual pattern. Next, ask about any changes in diet or drug use.

Recognizing hypercortisolism

Buffalo hump, moon face, and truncal obesity are the cardinal signs of hypercortisolism. In addition to these and the other signs shown here, hypertension, osteoporosis, and emotional lability may also occur.

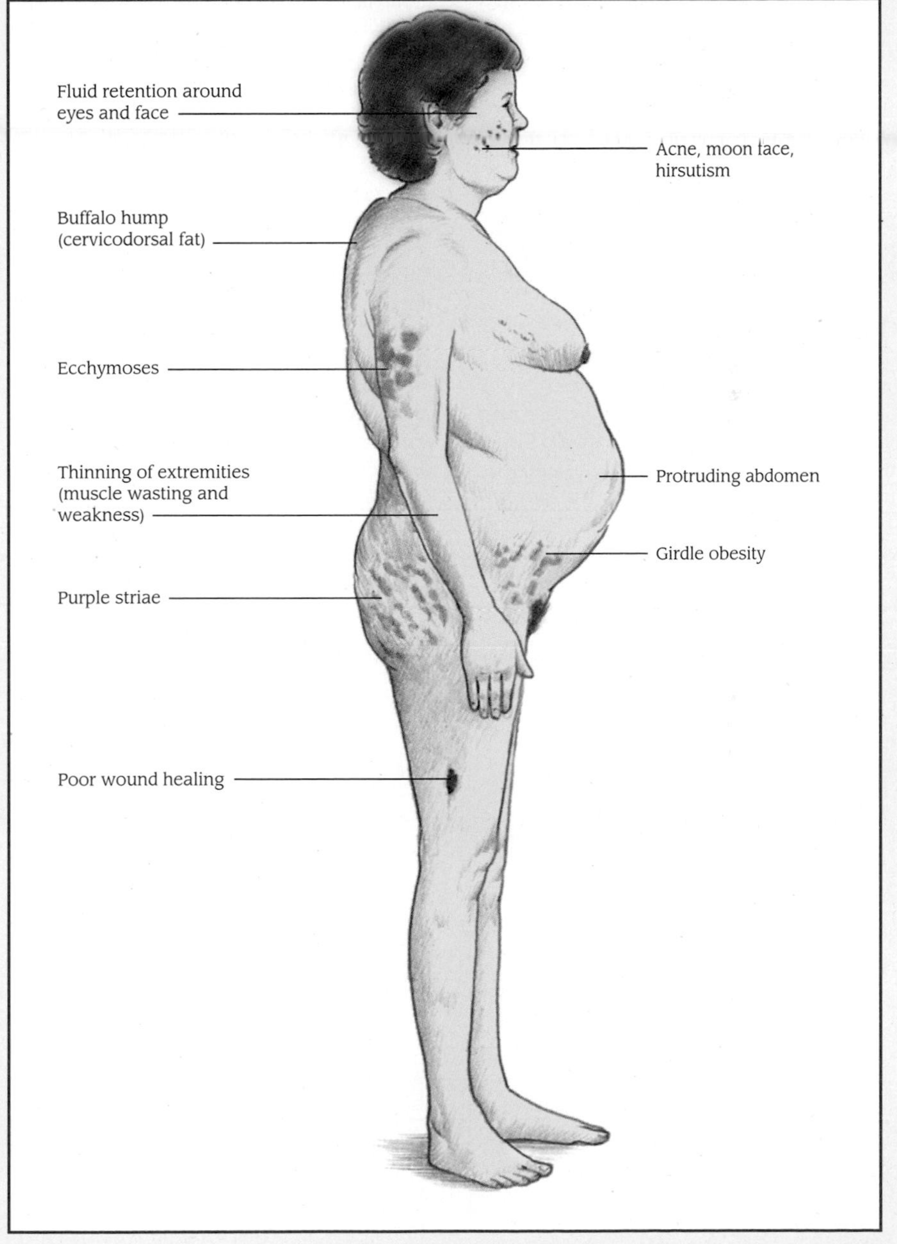

If the patient is receiving glucocorticoid therapy, ask about the dosage, schedule, administration route, and any recent changes in therapy.

Take the patient's vital signs, height, and weight. Form an impression of his appearance, noting obvious signs of hypercortisolism, such as hirsutism, diaphoresis, and moon (roundish) face. Inspect the arms, legs, and trunk for striae, and note skin turgor for thin skin. Assess muscle function by asking the patient to rise from a squatting position; note any difficulty because this may indicate quadriceps muscle weakness. These patients will typically have proximal muscle weakness (for example, limb or girdle weakness).

During your assessment, observe the patient's behavior. Extreme emotional lability along with depression, irritability, or confusion may signal hypercortisolism.

Medical causes

◆ ***Hypercortisolism.*** Buffalo hump varies in size, depending on the severity of hypercortisolism and the amount of weight gain. It's commonly accompanied by hirsutism, moon face, and truncal obesity with slender arms and legs. The skin may appear transparent, with purple striae and ecchymoses. Other findings include acne, muscle weakness and wasting, fatigue, poor wound healing, elevated blood pressure, personality changes, and amenorrhea or oligomenorrhea in women or impotence in men.

◆ ***Morbid obesity.*** The size of the buffalo hump depends on the amount of weight gain and the distribution of adipose tissue. Associated signs and symptoms include generalized adiposity, silver striae, elevated blood pressure, and hypogonadism.

Other causes

◆ ***Drugs.*** Buffalo hump may result from excessive doses of a glucocorticoid, such as cortisone, hydrocortisone, prednisone, or dexamethasone. Long-term glucocorticoid therapy is the most common cause in the United States.

Special considerations

Prepare the patient for diagnostic tests. Blood and urine tests can confirm hypercortisolism; ultrasonography, computed tomography (CT) scan, or arteriography can localize adrenal tumors. Chest X-rays, bronchography, and an

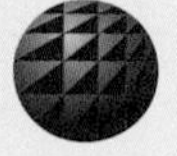

SIGNS & SYMPTOMS

Butterfly rash: Causes and associated findings

Common causes	Major associated signs and symptoms										
	Acne	Alopecia	Anorexia	Cervical adenopathy	Erythema	Fever	Headache	Maculopapular lesions	Malaise	Mucous membrane lesions	Photosensitivity
Discoid lupus erythematosus		●			●					●	●
Erysipelas				●		●	●		●		
Polymorphous light eruption					●			●			●
Rosacea					●			●			
Seborrheic dermatitis	●							●			
Systemic lupus erythematosus		●	●		●	●			●		

abdominal CT scan can determine ectopic involvement. Visual field testing and a skull CT scan can identify pituitary tumors.

Pediatric pointers

Although rare in children, buffalo hump may occur at any age. In children older than age 7, this sign usually results from pituitary oversecretion of corticotropin in bilateral adrenal hyperplasia. In younger children, it commonly results from glucocorticoid therapy—for example, overuse of glucocorticoid eyedrops.

Patient counseling

Advise the patient about proper diet, drug therapy, and exercise. Provide education and intervention for emotional lability.

Butterfly rash

A butterfly rash is typically a sign of systemic lupus erythematosus (SLE), but it can also signal dermatologic disorders. Typically, this rash appears in a malar distribution across the nose and cheeks. (See *Recognizing butterfly rash*.) Similar rashes may appear on the neck, scalp, and other areas. A butterfly rash is sometimes mistaken for sunburn because it can be provoked or aggravated by ultraviolet rays, but it has more substance, is more sharply demarcated, and has a thicker feel in relation to surrounding skin.

History and physical examination

Ask the patient when he first noticed the butterfly rash and if he has recently been exposed to the sun. Has he noticed a rash elsewhere on his body? Also, ask about recent weight or hair loss. Does he have a family history of lupus? Is he taking hydralazine or procainamide (common causes of drug-induced lupus erythematosus)?

Inspect the rash, noting any macules, papules, pustules, or scaling. Is the rash edematous? Are areas of hypopigmentation or hyperpigmentation present? Look for blisters or ulcers in the mouth, and note any inflamed lesions. Check for rashes elsewhere on the body. (See *Butterfly rash: Causes and associated findings*.)

	Plaques	Pruritus	Scaling	Sore throat	Telangiectasia	Vomiting	Weight loss
	●		●		●		
				●		●	
	●	●			●		
					●		
		●					
					●	●	●

Recognizing butterfly rash

In a classic butterfly rash, lesions appear on the cheeks and the bridge of the nose, creating a characteristic butterfly pattern. The rash may vary in severity from malar erythema to discoid lesions (plaques).

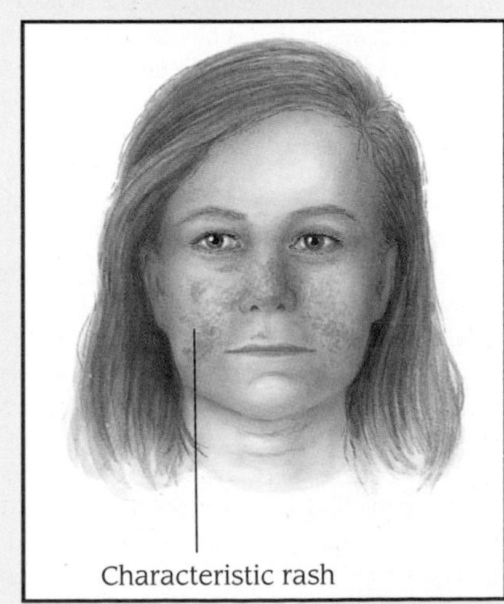

Medical causes

◆ ***Discoid lupus erythematosus.*** Discoid lupus erythematosus is a localized form of lupus erythematosus characterized by a rash on one or both sides of the face that consists of erythematous, raised, sharply demarcated plaques with follicular plugging and central atrophy. The rash may also involve the scalp, ears, chest, and any part of the body exposed to the sun. Telangiectasia, scarring alopecia, and hypopigmentation or hyperpigmentation may occur later. Other accompanying signs include conjunctival redness, dilated capillaries of the nail fold, bilateral parotid gland enlargement, oral lesions, and mottled, reddish blue skin on the legs.

◆ ***Erysipelas.*** Erysipelas causes rosy or crimson swollen lesions, mainly on the neck and head and commonly along the nasolabial fold. It may cause hemorrhagic pus-filled blisters. Other signs and symptoms include fever, chills, cervical lymphadenopathy, and malaise.

◆ ***Polymorphous light eruption.*** A butterfly rash appears as erythema, vesicles, plaques, and multiple small papules that may later become eczematized, lichenified, and excoriated. Provoked by ultraviolet rays, the rash appears on the cheeks and bridge of the nose, the hands and arms, and other areas, beginning a few hours to several days after exposure. It may be accompanied by pruritus.

◆ ***Rosacea.*** Initially, the rash may appear as a prominent, nonscaling, intermittent erythema limited to the lower half of the nose or including the chin, cheeks, and central forehead. As rosacea develops, the duration of the rash increases; instead of disappearing after each episode, the rash varies in intensity and is commonly accompanied by telangiectasia. In advanced rosacea, the skin is oily, with papules, pustules, nodules, and telangiectasia restricted to the central oval of the face. In men with severe rosacea, the butterfly rash may be accompanied by rhinophyma—a thickened, lobulated overgrowth of sebaceous glands and epithelial connective tissue on the lower half of the nose and, possibly, the adjacent cheeks. This is more common in elderly patients.

◆ ***Seborrheic dermatitis.*** In this disorder, greasy, scaling, slightly yellow macules and papules of varying size appear on the cheeks and the bridge of the nose in a butterfly pattern. The scalp, beard, eyebrows, portions of the forehead above the bridge of the nose, nasolabial fold, or trunk may also be involved. Associated signs and symptoms include crusts and fissures (particularly when the external ear and scalp are involved), pruritus, redness, blepharitis, styes, severe acne, and oily skin. Severe seborrheic dermatitis of the face occurs in acquired immunodeficiency syndrome.

◆ ***Systemic lupus erythematosus (SLE).*** Occurring in about 40% of patients with SLE—a connective tissue disorder—a butterfly rash appears as a red, often scaly, sharply demarcated macular eruption. The rash may be transient in patients with acute SLE or may progress slowly to include the forehead, chin, the area around the ears, and other exposed areas. Common associated skin findings include scaling, patchy alopecia, mucous membrane lesions, mottled erythema of the palms and fingers, periungual erythema with edema, reddish purple macular lesions on the volar surfaces of the fingers, telangiectasia of the base of the nails or eyelids, purpura, petechiae, and ecchymoses.

The rash may be accompanied by joint pain, stiffness, and deformities, particularly ulnar deviation of the fingers and subluxation of the proximal interphalangeal joints. Related findings include periorbital and facial edema, dyspnea, low-grade fever, malaise, weakness, fatigue, weight loss, anorexia, nausea, vomiting, lymphadenopathy, photosensitivity, and hepatosplenomegaly.

Other causes

◆ ***Drugs.*** Hydralazine and procainamide can cause a lupuslike syndrome.

Special considerations

Prepare the patient for immunologic studies, complete blood count, and possibly liver studies. Obtain a urine specimen if needed. Withhold photosensitizing drugs, such as phenothiazines, sulfonamides, sulfonylureas, and thiazide diuretics. Instruct the patient to avoid exposure to the sun or to use a sunscreen. Suggest that he use hypoallergenic makeup to help conceal facial lesions.

Pediatric pointers

Rare in pediatric patients, a butterfly rash may occur as part of an infectious disease such as erythema infectiosum ("slapped cheek syndrome").

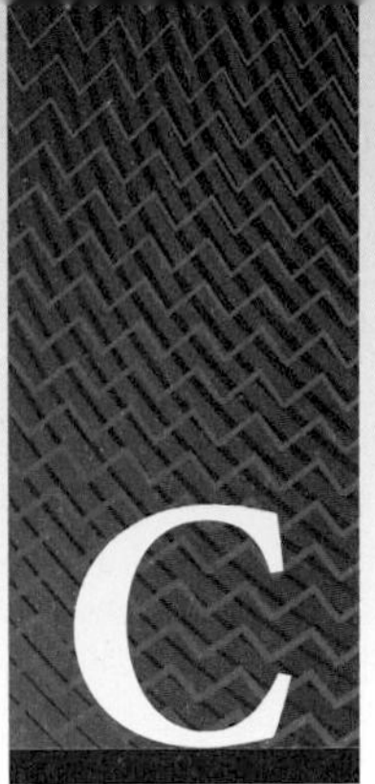

Café-au-lait spots

An important indicator of neurofibromatosis and other congenital melanotic disorders, café-au-lait spots appear as flat, light brown, uniformly hyperpigmented macules or patches on the skin surface. They usually appear during the first 3 years of life but may develop at any age. Café-au-lait spots can be differentiated from freckles and other benign birthmarks by their larger size (a few millimeters to 5/8" [1.6 cm] or larger in diameter) and irregular shape. They usually have no significance; however, six or more café-au-lait spots may be associated with an underlying neurologic disorder.

History and physical examination

Ask the patient or his parents when the café-au-lait spots first appeared. Also ask about a family history of these spots and of neurofibromatosis. Review the patient's history for seizures, frequent fractures, or mental retardation.

Inspect the skin, noting the location and pattern of the spots. Look for distinctive skin lesions, such as axillary freckling, mottling, small spherical patches, and areas of depigmentation. Large lesions should be measured along the longest axis. A wood's light examination may help visualize lesions in pale-skinned individuals. Check for subcutaneous neurofibromas along major nerve branches, especially on the trunk. Also check for bony abnormalities, such as scoliosis or kyphosis.

Medical causes

◆ ***Albright's syndrome.*** In Albright's syndrome, café-au-lait spots are smaller (about 3/8" [1 cm] in diameter) and more irregularly shaped than those in neurofibromatosis. They may stop abruptly at the midline and seem to follow a dermatomal distribution. Usually, fewer than six spots appear, unilaterally on the forehead, neck, and lower back. When they occur on the scalp, the hair overlying them may be more deeply pigmented. Associated signs include skeletal deformities, frequent fractures and, in females, sexual precocity.

◆ ***Neurofibromatosis.*** The most common cause of café-au-lait spots, this disorder (also called von Recklinghausen's disease) is characterized by six or more large, smooth-bordered spots up to 1/4" (6.4 mm) in diameter in prepubertal children and more than 5/8" (15 mm) in diameter in postpubertal children. Associated signs include axillary and inguinal freckling; irregular, hyperpigmented, and mottled skin; and multiple skin-colored pedunculated nodules clustered along nerve sheaths. The nodules develop during childhood, growing larger than 1/4". They proliferate throughout life, affecting all body tissues and causing marked deformity. They grow to 5/8" or larger in adults. Mental impairment, seizures, hearing loss, exophthalmos, decreased visual acuity, and GI bleeding can eventually occur.

◆ ***Tuberous sclerosis.*** Mental retardation and seizures characteristically appear first, followed several years later by cutaneous facial lesions—multiple café-au-lait spots, spherical areas of rough skin, and areas of yellow-red or depigmented nevi.

Special considerations

Although café-au-lait spots require no treatment, you'll need to provide emotional support for the patient and his family. Also, refer them for genetic counseling. Prepare the patient for diagnostic tests, such as tissue biopsy and radiographic studies.

Capillary refill time, increased

Capillary refill time is the duration required for color to return to the nail bed of a finger or toe after application of slight pressure, which causes blanching. This duration reflects the quality of peripheral vasomotor function. Normal capillary refill time is less than 3 seconds.

Increased refill time isn't diagnostic of any disorder but must be evaluated along with other signs and symptoms. However, this sign usually signals obstructive peripheral arterial disease or decreased cardiac output.

Capillary refill time is typically tested during a routine cardiovascular assessment. It isn't tested with suspected life-threatening disorders because other, more characteristic signs and symptoms appear earlier.

History and physical examination

If you detect increased capillary refill time, take the patient's vital signs and check pulses in the affected limb. Does the limb feel cold or look cyanotic? Does the patient report pain or any unusual sensations in his fingers or toes, especially after exposure to cold?

Take a brief medical history, especially noting previous peripheral vascular disease. Find out which medications the patient is taking.

Medical causes

◆ ***Aortic aneurysm (dissecting).*** Capillary refill time is increased in the fingers and toes in a dissecting aneurysm in the thoracic aorta; it's prolonged in just the toes in a dissecting aneurysm in the abdominal aorta. Common accompanying signs and symptoms include a pulsating abdominal mass, a systolic bruit, and substernal back or abdominal pain.

◆ ***Aortic arch syndrome.*** Increased capillary refill time in the fingers is an early sign of aortic arch syndrome. The patient displays absent carotid pulses and possibly unequal radial pulses. Other signs and symptoms usually precede loss of pulses and include fever, night sweats, arthralgia, weight loss, anorexia, nausea, malaise, rash, splenomegaly, and pallor.

◆ ***Aortic bifurcation occlusion (acute).*** Increased capillary refill time in the toes is a late sign in this rare but usually fatal disorder. All lower-extremity pulses are absent, and the patient complains of sudden moderate to severe pain in the legs and, less commonly, in the abdomen, lumbosacral area, or perineum. Both legs are cold, pale, totally numb, and flaccid.

◆ ***Arterial occlusion (acute).*** Increased capillary refill time occurs early in the affected limb. Arterial pulses are usually absent distal to the obstruction; the affected limb appears cool and pale or cyanotic. Intermittent claudication, moderate to severe pain, numbness, and paresthesia or paralysis of the affected limb may occur.

◆ ***Buerger's disease.*** Capillary refill time is increased in the toes in Buerger's disease. Exposure to low temperatures initially turns the feet cold, cyanotic, and numb; later they become red, hot, and tingly. Other findings include intermittent claudication of the instep and weak peripheral pulses; in later stages the patient may experience ulceration, muscle atrophy, and gangrene. If the disease affects the hands, increased capillary refill time may accompany painful fingertip ulcerations.

◆ ***Cardiac tamponade.*** Increased capillary refill time is a late sign of decreased cardiac output. Associated signs include paradoxical pulse, tachycardia, cyanosis, dyspnea, jugular vein distention, and hypotension.

◆ ***Hypothermia.*** Increased capillary refill time may appear early as a compensatory response. Associated signs and symptoms depend on the degree of hypothermia and may include shivering, fatigue, weakness, decreased level of consciousness (LOC), slurred speech, ataxia, muscle stiffness or rigidity, tachycardia or bradycardia, hyporeflexia or areflexia, diuresis, oliguria, bradypnea, decreased blood pressure, and cold, pale skin.

◆ ***Peripheral arterial trauma.*** Any trauma to a peripheral artery that reduces distal blood flow also increases capillary refill time in the affected extremity. Related findings in that extremity include bruising or pulsating bleeding, weakened pulse, cyanosis, paresthesia, sensory loss, and cool, pale skin.

◆ ***Peripheral vascular disease.*** Increased capillary refill time in the affected extremities is a late sign. Peripheral pulses gradually weaken and then disappear. Intermittent claudication, coolness, pallor, and decreased hair growth are associated signs. Impotence may accompany arterial occlusion in the descending aorta or femoral areas.

◆ ***Raynaud's disease.*** Capillary refill time is prolonged in the fingers, the usual site of this disease's characteristic episodic arterial vasospasm. Exposure to cold or stress produces blanching in the fingers, then cyanosis, and then erythema before the fingers return to normal temperature. Warmth relieves the symptoms, which may include paresthesia. Chronic disease may produce trophic changes, such as sclerodactyly, ulcerations, or chronic paronychia.

◆ ***Shock.*** Increased capillary refill time appears late in almost all types of shock. Accompanying signs include hypotension, tachycardia, tachypnea, and cool, clammy skin.

◆ ***Volkmann's contracture.*** Increased capillary refill time results from this contracture's characteristic vasospasm. The affected extremity may also exhibit loss of mobility and strength.

Other causes

◆ ***Diagnostic tests.*** Cardiac catheterization can cause arterial hematoma or clot formation and increased capillary refill time.

◆ ***Drugs.*** Drugs that cause vasoconstriction (particularly alpha-adrenergic blockers) increase capillary refill time.

◆ ***Treatments.*** Increased capillary refill time can result from an arterial line or umbilical line (which can cause arterial hematoma and obstructed distal blood flow) or from an improperly fitting cast (which constricts circulation).

Special considerations

Frequently assess the patient's vital signs, LOC, and affected extremity, and report any changes, such as progressive cyanosis or loss of an existing pulse. Prepare the patient for diagnostic tests, such as arteriography or Doppler ultrasonography, to help confirm or rule out arterial occlusion.

Pediatric pointers

Capillary refill time may be increased in neonates with acrocyanosis; however, this is a normal finding. Typically, increased capillary refill time is associated with the same disorders in children as in adults. However, the most common cause in children is cardiac surgery, such as the repair of congenital heart defects.

Carpopedal spasm

Carpopedal spasm is the violent, painful contraction of the muscles in the hands and feet. (See *Recognizing carpopedal spasm,* page 136.) It's an important sign of tetany, a potentially life-threatening condition that is commonly associated with hypocalcemia and characterized by increased neuromuscular excitation and sustained muscle contraction.

Carpopedal spasm requires prompt evaluation and intervention. If not treated promptly, the patient can also develop laryngospasm, seizures, cardiac arrhythmias, and cardiac and respiratory arrest.

EMERGENCY INTERVENTIONS *If you detect carpopedal spasm, quickly examine the patient for signs of respiratory distress (laryngospasm, stridor, loud crowing noises, cyanosis) or cardiac arrhythmias, which indicate hypocalcemia. Obtain blood samples for electrolyte analysis (especially calcium), and perform an electrocardiogram. Connect the patient to a monitor to watch for the appearance of arrhythmias. Administer an I.V. calcium preparation, and provide emergency respiratory and cardiac support. If a calcium infusion doesn't control seizures, administer a sedative, such as chloral hydrate or phenobarbital.*

History and physical examination

If the patient isn't in distress, obtain a detailed history. Ask about the onset and duration of the spasms and the degree of pain they produce. Also ask about related signs and symptoms of hypocalcemia, such as numbness and tingling of the fingertips and feet, other muscle cramps or spasms, and nausea, vomiting, and abdominal pain. Check for previous neck surgery, calcium or magnesium deficiency, tetanus exposure, and hypoparathyroidism.

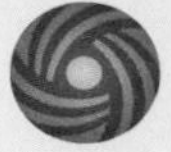

EXAMINATION TIP

Recognizing carpopedal spasm

In the hand, carpopedal spasm involves adduction of the thumb over the palm, followed by flexion of the metacarpophalangeal joints, extension of the interphalangeal joints (fingers together), adduction of the hyperextended fingers, and flexion of the wrist and elbow joints. Similar effects occur in the joints of the feet.

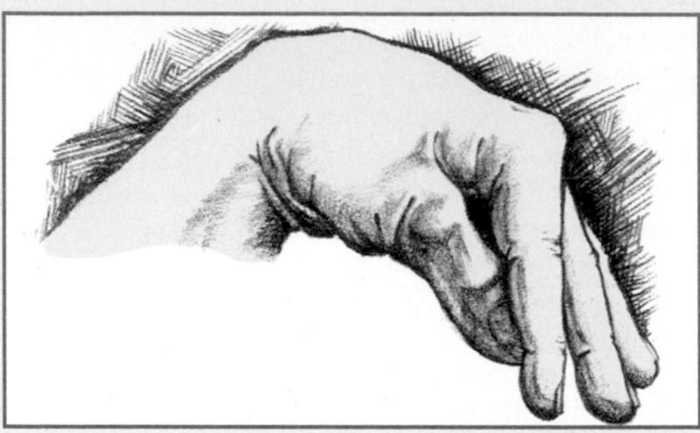

During the history, form a general impression of the patient's mental status and behavior. If possible, ask family members or friends if they've noticed changes in the patient's behavior because hypocalcemia can cause confusion and even personality changes.

Inspect the patient's skin and fingernails, noting any dryness or scaling and ridged, brittle nails.

Medical causes

◆ ***Hypocalcemia.*** Carpopedal spasm is an early sign of hypocalcemia. It's usually accompanied by paresthesia of the fingers, toes, and perioral area; muscle weakness, twitching, and cramping; hyperreflexia; chorea; fatigue; and palpitations. Positive Chvostek's and Trousseau's signs can be elicited. Laryngospasm, stridor, and seizures may appear in severe hypocalcemia.

Chronic hypocalcemia may be accompanied by mental status changes; cramps; dry, scaly skin; brittle nails; and thin, patchy hair and eyebrows.

◆ ***Tetanus.*** Tetanus is an infectious disease that develops when *Clostridium tetani* enters a wound in a nonimmunized individual. The patient develops muscle spasms, painful seizures, difficulty swallowing, and a low-grade fever. Without prompt treatment, mortality is very high.

Other causes

◆ ***Treatments.*** Multiple blood transfusions and parathyroidectomy may cause hypocalcemia, resulting in carpopedal spasm. Surgical procedures that impair calcium absorption, such as ileostomy formation and gastric resection with gastrojejunostomy, may also cause hypocalcemia.

Special considerations

Carpopedal spasm can cause severe pain and anxiety, leading to hyperventilation. If this occurs, help the patient slow his breathing through your relaxing touch, reassuring attitude, and clear directions about what he should do. Provide a quiet, dark environment to reduce his anxiety.

Prepare the patient for laboratory tests, such as complete blood count and serum calcium, phosphorus, and parathyroid hormone studies.

Pediatric pointers

Idiopathic hypoparathyroidism is a common cause of hypocalcemia in children. Carefully monitor children with this condition because carpopedal spasm may herald the onset of epileptiform seizures or generalized tetany followed by prolonged tonic spasms.

Geriatric pointers

Always ask elderly patients about their immunization record. Suspect tetanus in anyone who comes into your facility with carpopedal spasm, difficulty swallowing, and seizures. Such patients may have incomplete immunizations or may not have had a recent booster shot. Always ask about any recent wound, no matter how inconsequential it may seem.

PATIENT COUNSELING

Teach the patient the importance of receiving immunization against tetanus and of keeping a vaccination record. If you have any doubt about his vaccination record, you must give him the vaccine. Tetanus toxoid booster shots must be given every 10 years after the patient has been properly immunized in childhood.

Cat's cry

Occurring during infancy, this mewing, kitten-like sound is the primary indicator of cri du chat (also known as cat's cry) syndrome. This syndrome affects about 1 in 50,000 neonates and causes profound mental retardation and failure to thrive. Most of those affected can have a normal life span, although a small number have serious organ defects and other life-threatening medical conditions.

The chromosomal defect responsible for this disorder (deletion of the short arm of chromosome 5) usually appears spontaneously but may be inherited from a carrier parent. The characteristic cry is thought to result from abnormal laryngeal development.

GENDER CUE *Cri du chat syndrome is more common in females than males.*

EMERGENCY INTERVENTIONS *Suspect cri du chat syndrome if you detect cat's cry in a neonate. Be alert for signs of respiratory distress, such as nasal flaring; irregular, shallow respirations; cyanosis; and a respiratory rate over 60 breaths/minute. Be prepared to suction the neonate and to administer warmed oxygen. Keep emergency resuscitation equipment nearby because bradycardia may develop.*

HISTORY AND PHYSICAL EXAMINATION

Perform a physical examination, and note any abnormalities. If you detect cat's cry in an older infant, ask the parents when it developed. Sudden onset of an abnormal cry in an infant with a previously normal, vigorous cry suggests other disorders. (See "Cry, high-pitched," page 193.)

MEDICAL CAUSES

◆ ***Cri du chat syndrome.*** A kittenlike cry begins at birth or shortly thereafter in this disorder. It's accompanied by profound mental retardation, microcephaly, low birth weight, hypotonia, failure to thrive, and feeding difficulties. Typically, the infant displays a round face with wide-set eyes; strabismus; a broad-based nose with oblique or down-sloping epicanthal folds; abnormally shaped, low-set ears; and an unusually small jaw. He may also have a short neck, webbed fingers, and a simian crease. Other abnormalities may include heart defects and GI abnormalities.

SPECIAL CONSIDERATIONS

Connect the infant to an apnea monitor, and check for signs of respiratory distress. Keep suction equipment and warmed oxygen available. Obtain a blood sample for chromosomal analysis. Prepare the infant for a computed tomography scan to rule out other causes of microcephaly and for an ear, nose, and throat examination to evaluate vocal cords.

Because the infant with cri du chat is usually a poor eater, monitor intake, output, and weight. Instruct the parents to offer the child frequent small feedings. Prepare the parents to work long term with a team of specialists in genetics, neurology, cardiology, and speech and language. Have a counselor or support group available for the parents and family.

Chest expansion, asymmetrical

Asymmetrical chest expansion is the uneven extension of portions of the chest wall during inspiration. During normal respiration, the thorax uniformly expands upward and outward, then contracts downward and inward. When this process is disrupted, breathing becomes uncoordinated, resulting in asymmetrical chest expansion.

Asymmetrical chest expansion may develop suddenly or gradually and may affect one or both sides of the chest wall. It may occur as delayed expiration (chest lag), as abnormal movement during inspiration (for example, intercostal retractions, paradoxical movement, or chest-abdomen asynchrony), or as unilateral absence of movement. This sign usually results from pleural disorders, such as life-threatening hemothorax or tension pneumothorax. (See *Recognizing life-threatening causes of asymmetrical chest expansion,* page 138.) However, it can also result from a musculoskeletal or urologic disorder, airway obstruction, or trauma. Regardless of its

Recognizing life-threatening causes of asymmetrical chest expansion

Asymmetrical chest expansion can result from several life-threatening disorders. Two common causes—bronchial obstruction and flail chest—produce distinctive chest wall movements that provide important clues about the underlying disorder.

In *bronchial obstruction,* only the unaffected portion of the chest wall expands during inspiration. Intercostal bulging during expiration may indicate that the air is trapped in the chest.

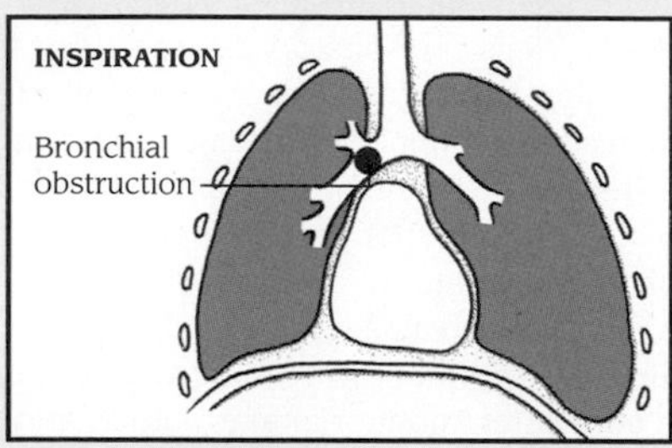

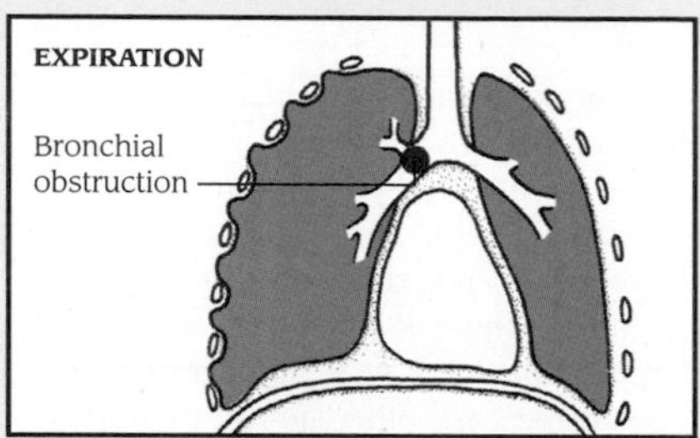

In *flail* chest—a disruption of the thorax due to multiple rib fractures—the unstable portion of the chest wall collapses inward during inspiration and balloons outward during expiration.

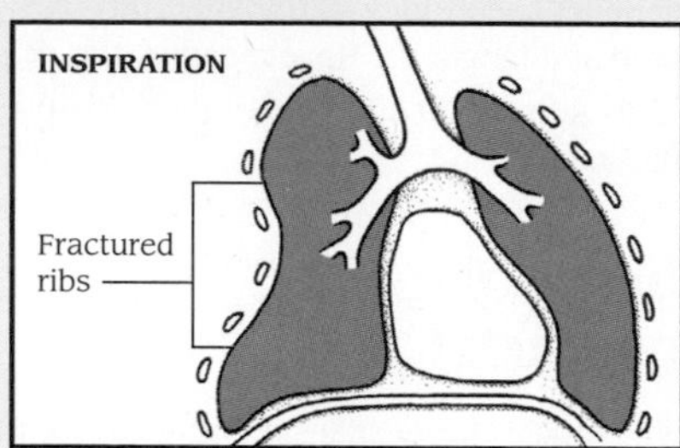

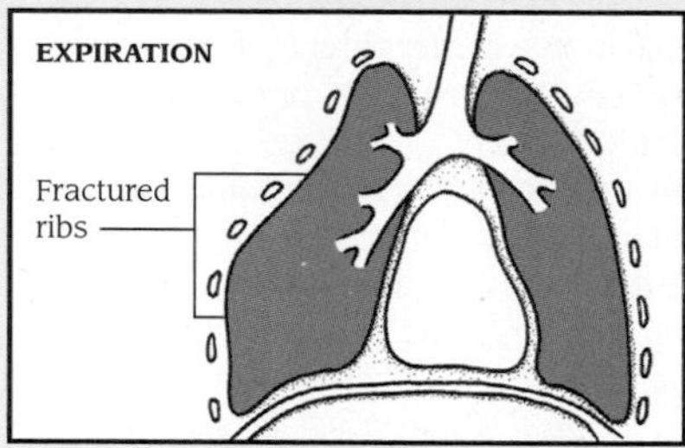

underlying cause, asymmetrical chest expansion produces rapid and shallow or deep respirations that increase the work of breathing.

EMERGENCY INTERVENTIONS *If you detect asymmetrical chest expansion, first consider traumatic injury to the patient's ribs or sternum, which can cause flail chest, a life-threatening emergency characterized by paradoxical chest movement. Quickly take the patient's vital signs and look for signs of acute respiratory distress—rapid and shallow respirations, tachycardia, and cyanosis. Use tape or sandbags to temporarily splint the unstable flail segment.*

Depending on the severity of respiratory distress, administer oxygen by nasal cannula, mask, or mechanical ventilator. Insert an I.V. catheter to allow fluid replacement and administration of pain medication. Draw a blood sample from the patient for arterial blood gas analysis, and connect the patient to a cardiac monitor.

Although asymmetrical chest expansion may result from hemothorax, tension pneumothorax, bronchial obstruction, and other life-threatening causes, it isn't a cardinal sign of these disorders. Because any form of asymmetrical chest expansion can compromise the patient's respiratory status, don't leave the patient unattended, and be alert for signs of respiratory distress.

History and physical examination

If you don't suspect flail chest and if the patient isn't experiencing acute respiratory distress, obtain a brief history. Asymmetrical chest expansion commonly results from mechanical airflow obstruction, so find out if the patient is experiencing dyspnea or pain during breathing. If so, does he feel short of breath constantly or intermittently? Does the pain worsen his feeling of breathlessness? Does repositioning, coughing, or any other activity relieve or worsen the patient's dyspnea or pain? Is the pain more noticeable during inspiration or expiration? Can he inhale deeply?

Ask if the patient has a history of pulmonary or systemic illness, such as frequent upper respiratory tract infections, asthma, tuberculosis, pneumonia, or cancer. Has he had thoracic surgery? (This typically produces asymmetrical chest expansion on the affected side.) Also, ask about blunt or penetrating chest trauma, which may have caused pulmonary injury. Obtain an occupational history to find out if the patient may have inhaled toxic fumes or aspirated a toxic substance.

Next, perform a physical examination. Begin by gently palpating the trachea for midline positioning. (Deviation of the trachea usually indicates an acute problem requiring immediate intervention.) Then examine the posterior chest wall for areas of tenderness or deformity. To evaluate the extent of asymmetrical chest expansion, place your hands—fingers together and thumbs abducted toward the spine—flat on both sections of the lower posterior chest wall. Position your thumbs at the 10th rib, and grasp the lateral rib cage with your hands. As the patient inhales, note the uneven separation of your thumbs, and gauge the distance between them. Then repeat this technique on the upper posterior chest wall. Next, use the ulnar surface of your hand to palpate for vocal or tactile fremitus on both sides of the chest. To check for vocal fremitus, ask the patient to repeat "99" as you proceed. Note any asymmetrical vibrations and areas of enhanced, diminished, or absent fremitus. Then percuss and auscultate to detect air and fluid in the lungs and pleural spaces. Finally, auscultate all lung fields for normal and adventitious breath sounds. Examine the patient's anterior chest wall, using the same assessment techniques.

MEDICAL CAUSES

◆ ***Bronchial obstruction.*** Life-threatening loss of airway patency may occur gradually or suddenly in bronchial obstruction. Typically, lack of chest movement indicates complete obstruction; chest lag signals partial obstruction. If air is trapped in the chest, you may detect intercostal bulging during expiration and hyperresonance on percussion. You may also note dyspnea, accessory muscle use, decreased or absent breath sounds, and suprasternal, substernal, or intercostal retractions.

◆ ***Flail chest.*** In this life-threatening injury to the ribs or sternum, the unstable portion of the chest wall collapses inward during inspiration and balloons outward during expiration (paradoxical movement). The patient may have ecchymoses, severe localized pain, or other signs of traumatic injury to the chest wall. He may also exhibit rapid, shallow respirations, tachycardia, and cyanosis.

◆ ***Hemothorax.*** Hemothorax is life-threatening bleeding into the pleural space that causes chest lag during inspiration. Other findings include signs of traumatic chest injury, stabbing pain at the injury site, anxiety, dullness on percussion, tachypnea, tachycardia, and hypoxemia. If hypovolemia occurs, you'll note signs of shock, such as hypotension and rapid, weak pulse.

◆ ***Kyphoscoliosis.*** Abnormal curvature of the thoracic spine in the anteroposterior direction (kyphosis) and the lateral direction (scoliosis) gradually compresses one lung and distends the other. This produces decreased chest wall movement on the compressed-lung side and expands the intercostal muscles during inspiration on the opposite side. It can also produce ineffective coughing, dyspnea, back pain, and fatigue.

◆ ***Myasthenia gravis.*** Progressive loss of ventilatory muscle function produces asynchrony of the chest and abdomen during inspiration ("abdominal paradox"), which can lead to acute respiratory distress. Typically, the patient's shallow respirations and increased muscle weakness cause severe dyspnea, tachypnea and, possibly, apnea.

◆ ***Phrenic nerve dysfunction.*** In this disorder, the paralyzed hemidiaphragm fails to contract downward, causing asynchrony of the thorax and upper abdomen on the affected side during inspiration ("abdominal paradox"). Its onset may be sudden, as in trauma, or gradual, as in infection or spinal cord disease. If the patient has underlying pulmonary dysfunction that contributes to hyperventilation, his inability to breathe deeply or to cough effectively may cause atelectasis of the affected lung.

◆ ***Pleural effusion.*** Chest lag at end-inspiration occurs gradually in this life-threatening accumulation of fluid, blood, or pus in the pleural space. Usually, some combination of dyspnea, tachypnea, and tachycardia precedes chest lag; the patient may also have pleuritic pain that worsens with coughing or deep breathing. The area of the effusion is delineated by dullness on percussion and by egophony, bronchophony, whispered pectoriloquy, decreased or absent breath sounds, and decreased tactile fremitus. The patient may have a fever if infection caused the effusion.

◆ ***Pneumonia.*** Depending on whether fluid consolidation in the lungs develops unilaterally or bilaterally, asymmetrical chest expansion occurs as inspiratory chest lag or as chest-abdomen asynchrony. The patient typically has fever, chills, tachycardia, tachypnea, and dyspnea along with crackles, rhonchi, and chest pain that worsens during deep breathing. He may also be fatigued and anorexic and have a productive cough with rust-colored sputum.

◆ ***Pneumothorax.*** Entrapment of air in the pleural space can cause chest lag at end-inspiration. This life-threatening condition also causes sudden, stabbing chest pain that may radiate to the arms, face, back, or abdomen and dyspnea unrelated to the chest pain's severity. Other findings include tachypnea, decreased tactile fremitus, tympany on percussion, decreased or absent breath sounds over the trapped air, tachycardia, restlessness, and anxiety.

Tension pneumothorax produces the same signs and symptoms as pneumothorax, but they're much more severe. A tension pneumothorax rapidly compresses the heart and great vessels, causing cyanosis, hypotension, tachycardia, restlessness, and anxiety. The patient may also develop subcutaneous crepitation of the upper trunk, neck, and face and mediastinal and tracheal deviation away from the affected side. Auscultation of a crunching sound over the precordium with each heartbeat indicates pneumomediastinum.

◆ ***Poliomyelitis.*** In this rare disorder, paralysis of the chest wall muscles and diaphragm produces chest-abdomen asynchrony ("abdominal paradox"), fever, muscle pain, and weakness. Other findings include decreased reflex response in the affected muscles and impaired swallowing and speaking.

◆ ***Pulmonary embolism.*** This acute, life-threatening disorder causes chest lag; sudden, stabbing chest pain; and tachycardia. The patient usually has severe dyspnea, blood-tinged sputum, pleural friction rub, and acute anxiety.

OTHER CAUSES

◆ ***Treatments.*** Asymmetrical chest expansion can result from pneumonectomy and surgical removal of several ribs. Chest lag or the absence of chest movement may also result from intubation of a mainstem bronchus, a serious complication typically due to incorrect insertion of an endotracheal tube or movement of the tube while it's in the trachea.

SPECIAL CONSIDERATIONS

If you're caring for an intubated patient, regularly auscultate breath sounds in the lung peripheries to help detect a misplaced tube. If this occurs, prepare the patient for a chest X-ray to allow rapid repositioning of the tube. Because asymmetrical chest expansion increases the work of breathing, supplemental oxygen is usually given during acute events.

PEDIATRIC POINTERS

Children are at greater risk than adults for inadvertent intubation of a mainstem bronchus (especially the left bronchus). Their breath sounds are usually referred from one lung to the other because of the small size of the thoracic cage, so use chest wall expansion as an indicator of correct tube position in children. Children also develop asymmetrical chest expansion, paradoxical breathing, and retractions with acute respiratory illnesses, such as bronchiolitis, asthma, and croup.

Congenital abnormalities, such as cerebral palsy and diaphragmatic hernia, can also cause asymmetrical chest expansion. In cerebral palsy, asymmetrical facial muscles usually accompany chest-abdomen asynchrony. In a life-threatening diaphragmatic hernia, asymmetrical expansion usually occurs on the left side of the chest.

GERIATRIC POINTERS

Asymmetrical chest expansion may be more difficult to determine in elderly patients because of the structural deformities associated with aging.

Chest pain

Chest pain usually results from disorders that affect thoracic or abdominal organs—the heart, pleurae, lungs, esophagus, rib cage, gallbladder, pancreas, or stomach. An important indicator of several acute and life-threatening cardiopulmonary and GI disorders, chest pain can also result from a musculoskeletal or hematologic disorder, anxiety, and drug therapy.

Chest pain may arise suddenly or gradually, and its cause may be difficult to ascertain initially. The pain may radiate to the arms, neck, jaw, or back. It may be steady or intermittent and mild or acute, and it may range in character from a sharp shooting sensation to a feeling of heaviness, fullness, or even indigestion. Chest pain may be provoked or aggravated by stress, anxiety, exertion, deep breathing, or eating certain foods.

EMERGENCY INTERVENTIONS *Ask the patient when his chest pain began. Did it develop suddenly or gradually? Is it more severe or frequent now than when it first started? Does anything relieve the pain? Does anything aggravate it? Ask the patient about associated symptoms. Sudden, severe chest pain requires prompt evaluation and treatment because it may herald a life-threatening disorder. (See* Managing severe chest pain, *pages 142 and 143.)*

History and physical examination

If the chest pain isn't severe, proceed with the history. Ask if the patient feels diffuse pain or can point to the painful area. Sometimes a patient won't perceive the sensation he's feeling as pain, so ask whether he has any discomfort radiating to his neck, jaw, arms, or back. If he does, ask him to describe it. Is it a dull, aching, pressurelike sensation? A sharp, stabbing, knifelike pain? Does he feel it on the surface or deep inside? Find out whether it's constant or intermittent. If it's intermittent, how long does it last? Ask if movement, exertion, breathing, position changes, or eating certain foods worsens or helps relieve the pain. Does anything in particular seem to bring it on?

Review the patient's history for cardiac or pulmonary disease, chest trauma, intestinal disease, or sickle cell anemia. Find out which medications he's taking, if any, and ask about recent dosage or schedule changes.

Take the patient's vital signs, noting tachypnea, fever, tachycardia, oxygen saturation, paradoxical pulse, and hypertension or hypotension. Also, look for jugular vein distention and peripheral edema. Observe the patient's breathing pattern, and inspect his chest for asymmetrical expansion. Auscultate his lungs for pleural friction rub, crackles, rhonchi, wheezing, and diminished or absent breath sounds. Next, auscultate for murmurs, clicks, gallops, and pericardial friction rub. Palpate for lifts, heaves, thrills, gallops, tactile fremitus, and abdominal masses or tenderness. (See *Chest pain: Causes and associated findings,* pages 144 to 147.)

Medical causes

◆ ***Angina pectoris.*** A patient with angina pectoris may experience a feeling of tightness or pressure in the chest that he describes as pain or a sensation of indigestion or expansion. The pain usually occurs in the retrosternal region over a palm-sized or larger area. It may radiate to the neck, jaw, and arms—classically, to the inner aspect of the left arm. Angina tends to begin gradually, build to its maximum, then slowly subside. Provoked by exertion, emotional stress, or a heavy meal, the pain typically lasts 2 to 10 minutes (usually no longer than 20 minutes). Associated findings include dyspnea, nausea, vomiting, tachycardia, dizziness, diaphoresis, belching, and palpitations. You may hear an atrial gallop (a fourth heart sound [S_4]) or a murmur during an anginal episode.

In Prinzmetal's angina, caused by vasospasm of coronary vessels, chest pain typically occurs when the patient is at rest—or it may awaken him. It may be accompanied by dyspnea, nausea, vomiting, dizziness, and palpitations. During an attack, you may hear an atrial gallop.

◆ ***Anthrax (inhalation).*** This acute infectious disease is caused by the gram-positive, spore-forming bacterium *Bacillus anthracis.* Although the disease most commonly occurs in wild and domestic grazing animals, such as cattle, sheep, and goats, the spores can live in the soil for many years. The disease can occur in humans exposed to infected animals, tissue from infected animals, or biological agents. Most natural cases occur in agricultural regions worldwide. Anthrax may occur in cutaneous, inhalation, or GI forms.

Inhalation anthrax is caused by inhalation of aerosolized spores. Initial flulike signs and symptoms include fever, chills, weakness,

(Text continues on page 145.)

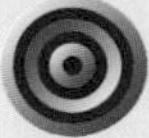

EMERGENCY INTERVENTION

Managing severe chest pain

Sudden, severe chest pain may result from any one of several life-threatening disorders. Your evaluation and interventions will vary, depending on the pain's location and character. The flowchart below will help you establish priorities for managing this emergency successfully.

Ask the patient to characterize his chest pain.

Patient reports sudden onset of pleuritic chest pain, which he characterizes as crushing, shooting, and deep.	Patient reports sudden onset of tearing, ripping, stabbing chest pain, with syncope and hemiplegia.
Assess him for diaphoresis, dyspnea, tachypnea, hemoptysis, and tachycardia.	Assess him for differences in blood pressure between legs and arms as well as weak or absent femoral or pedal pulses.
If you detect these signs and symptoms, suspect pulmonary embolism.	If you detect these signs, suspect dissecting aortic aneurysm.

What to do: Quickly take the patient's vital signs. Obtain a 12-lead electrocardiogram. Insert an I.V. catheter to administer fluids and drugs, and give oxygen. Check the patient's vital signs frequently to detect changes from baseline. Begin cardiac monitoring to detect arrhythmias. As appropriate, prepare the patient for emergency surgery. Prepare patients with pulmonary embolism or myocardial infarction for possible thrombolytic therapy.

Patient reports sudden onset of severe substernal pain that radiates to his left arm, jaw, neck, or shoulder blades; he describes the pain as a squeezing, viselike, burning sensation.

Assess him for pallor, diaphoresis, nausea, vomiting, apprehension, anxiety, weakness, fatigue, and dyspnea.

If you detect these signs and symptoms, suspect myocardial infarction.

Patient reports sudden onset of diffuse chest tightness.

Assess him for wheezing, dry cough, chest tightness, dyspnea, tachycardia, and hyperventilation.

If you detect these signs and symptoms, suspect an acute asthma attack.

What to do: Try to calm the patient to slow his respiratory rate. Ask the patient if he's ever had this pain before and, if so, what (if anything) eased it. Give oxygen and insert an I.V. catheter to administer fluids and drugs. Expect to give epinephrine and a bronchodilator and to begin respiratory therapy.

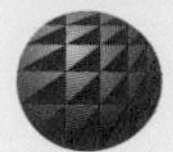

SIGNS & SYMPTOMS

Chest pain: Causes and associated findings

Major associated signs and symptoms

Common causes	Abdominal mass	Abdominal tenderness	Atrial gallop	Breath sounds, decreased	Cough	Crackles	Cyanosis	Diaphoresis	Dizziness	Dyspnea	Fever	Hemoptysis	Murmur
Angina pectoris			●					●	●	●			●
Anthrax (inhalation)					●					●	●		
Anxiety									●	●			
Aortic aneurysm (dissecting)	●	●						●					●
Asthma					●	●	●	●		●			
Blast lung injury							●			●		●	
Blastomycosis					●			●			●		
Bronchitis					●	●					●		
Cardiomyopathy			●		●				●	●			●
Cholecystitis	●	●						●			●		
Coccidioidomycosis					●						●		
Costochondritis										●			
Distention of colon's splenic flexure		●						●					
Esophageal spasm										●			
Herpes zoster (shingles)											●		
Hiatal hernia													
Interstitial lung disease					●	●	●			●			
Legionnaires' disease						●		●		●	●	●	
Lung abscess				●	●	●		●		●	●	●	
Lung cancer						●				●	●	●	
Mediastinitis											●		
Mitral valve prolapse									●	●			●

	Nausea and vomiting	Pericardial friction rub	Pleural friction rub	Skin mottling	Syncope	Tachycardia	Tachypnea	Wheezing
	●					●		
	●					●	●	
				●	●	●		
						●	●	●
								●
						●		●
			●					
	●							
								●
	●							
	●							
	●					●	●	
			●					
								●
						●		

(continued)

cough, and chest pain. The disease generally occurs in two stages with a period of recovery after the initial signs and symptoms. The second stage develops abruptly and causes rapid deterioration marked by fever, dyspnea, stridor, and hypotension; death generally results within 24 hours. Radiologic findings include mediastinitis and symmetrical mediastinal widening.

◆ ***Anxiety.*** Acute anxiety—commonly known as panic attacks—can produce intermittent, sharp, stabbing pain, typically behind the left breast. This pain isn't related to exertion and lasts only a few seconds, but the patient may experience a precordial ache or a sensation of heaviness that lasts for hours or days. Associated signs and symptoms include precordial tenderness, palpitations, fatigue, headache, insomnia, breathlessness, nausea, vomiting, diarrhea, and tremors. Panic attacks may be associated with agoraphobia—fear of leaving home or being in open places with other people.

◆ ***Aortic aneurysm (dissecting).*** The chest pain associated with this life-threatening disorder usually begins suddenly and is most severe at its onset. The patient describes an excruciating tearing, ripping, stabbing pain in his chest and neck that radiates to his upper back, abdomen, and lower back. He may also have abdominal tenderness, a palpable abdominal mass, tachycardia, murmurs, syncope, blindness, loss of consciousness, weakness or transient paralysis of the arms or legs, a systolic bruit, systemic hypotension, asymmetrical brachial pulses, lower blood pressure in the legs than in the arms, and weak or absent femoral or pedal pulses. His skin is pale, cool, diaphoretic, and mottled below the waist. Capillary refill time is increased in the toes, and palpation reveals decreased pulsation in one or both carotid arteries.

◆ ***Asthma.*** In a life-threatening asthma attack, diffuse and painful chest tightness arises suddenly along with a dry cough and mild wheezing, which progress to a productive cough, audible wheezing, and severe dyspnea. Related respiratory findings include rhonchi, crackles, prolonged expirations, intercostal and supraclavicular retractions on inspiration, accessory muscle use, flaring nostrils, and tachypnea. The patient may also experience anxiety, tachycardia, diaphoresis, flushing, and cyanosis.

◆ ***Blast lung injury.*** Caused by a percussive shock wave after an explosion, blast lung injury can cause severe chest pain and possibly tearing, contusion, edema, and hemorrhage of the

Chest pain: Causes and associated findings *(continued)*

Common causes	Abdominal mass	Abdominal tenderness	Atrial gallop	Breath sounds, decreased	Cough	Crackles	Cyanosis	Diaphoresis	Dizziness	Dyspnea	Fever	Hemoptysis	Murmur
	Major associated signs and symptoms												
Muscle strain				●									
Myocardial infarction			●			●		●		●	●		●
Nocardiosis				●	●			●			●		
Pancreatitis		●				●					●		
Peptic ulcer		●											
Pericarditis										●	●		
Plague				●							●	●	●
Pleurisy				●		●	●			●	●		
Pneumonia				●	●	●	●	●		●	●		
Pneumothorax				●	●		●			●			
Psittacosis											●		
Pulmonary actinomycosis					●						●	●	
Pulmonary embolism					●	●	●	●		●	●	●	
Pulmonary hypertension (primary)					●						●		●
Q fever											●		
Rib fracture					●					●			
Sickle cell crisis		●								●	●		
Thoracic outlet syndrome										●			
Tuberculosis					●					●	●	●	
Tularemia				●						●	●		

	Nausea and vomiting	Pericardial friction rub	Pleural friction rub	Skin mottling	Syncope	Tachycardia	Tachypnea	Wheezing
	●							
	●			●		●		
	●							
		●				●		
							●	
			●				●	
						●	●	
							●	
			●			●	●	●
					●			

lungs of affected people. Worldwide terrorist activity has recently increased the incidence of this condition, which may also cause dyspnea, hemoptysis, wheezing, and cyanosis. Chest X-rays, arterial blood gas measurements, and computed tomography scans are common diagnostic tools. Although no definitive guidelines exist for caring for those with blast lung injury, treatment is based on the nature of the explosion, the environment in which it occurred, and any chemical or biological agents involved.

◆ ***Blastomycosis.*** Besides pleuritic chest pain, this disorder initially produces signs and symptoms that mimic those of a viral upper respiratory tract infection: a dry, hacking, or productive cough (and sometimes hemoptysis), fever, chills, anorexia, weight loss, fatigue, night sweats, and malaise.

◆ ***Bronchitis.*** In its acute form, this disorder produces burning chest pain or a sensation of substernal tightness. It also produces a cough, initially dry but later productive, that worsens the chest pain. Other findings include a low-grade fever, chills, sore throat, tachycardia, muscle and back pain, rhonchi, crackles, and wheezing. Severe bronchitis causes a fever of 101° to 102° F (38.3° to 38.9° C) and possibly bronchospasm with increased coughing and wheezing.

◆ ***Cardiomyopathy.*** In hypertrophic cardiomyopathy, angina-like chest pain may occur with dyspnea, a cough, dizziness, syncope, gallops, murmurs, and palpitations.

◆ ***Cholecystitis.*** This disorder typically produces abrupt epigastric or right-upper-quadrant pain, which may be sharp or intensely aching. Steady or intermittent pain may radiate to the back or the right shoulder. Associated findings commonly include nausea, vomiting, fever, diaphoresis, and chills. Palpation of the right upper quadrant may reveal an abdominal mass, rigidity, distention, or tenderness. Murphy's sign—inspiratory arrest elicited when the examiner palpates the right upper quadrant as the patient takes a deep breath—may also occur.

◆ ***Coccidioidomycosis.*** In this disorder, pleuritic chest pain occurs with a dry or slightly productive cough. Other effects include fever, rhonchi, wheezing, occasional chills, sore throat, backache, headache, malaise, marked weakness, anorexia, and a macular rash.

◆ ***Costochondritis.*** Pain and tenderness occur at the costochondral junctions, especially at the second costicartilage. The pain usually can be elicited by palpating the inflamed joint.

◆ ***Distention of colon's splenic flexure.*** Central chest pain may radiate to the left arm in patients with this disorder. The pain may be relieved by defecation or the passage of flatus.

◆ ***Esophageal spasm.*** In this disorder, substernal chest pain may last up to an hour and may radiate to the neck, jaw, arms, or back. It commonly mimics the squeezing or dull sensation associated with angina. Other signs and symptoms include dysphagia for solid foods, bradycardia, and nodal rhythm.

◆ ***Herpes zoster (shingles).*** The pain of preeruptive herpes zoster may mimic that of myocardial infarction (MI). Initially, the pain is characteristically sharp, shooting, and unilateral. About 4 to 5 days after its onset, small, red, nodular lesions erupt on the painful areas—usually the thorax, arms, and legs—and the chest pain becomes burning. Associated findings include fever, malaise, pruritus, and paresthesia or hyperesthesia of the affected areas.

◆ ***Hiatal hernia.*** Typically, this disorder produces an angina-like sternal burning (heartburn), ache, or pressure that may radiate to the left shoulder and arm. The discomfort commonly occurs after a meal when the patient bends over or lies down. Other findings include a bitter taste and pain while eating or drinking, especially spicy foods and hot drinks.

◆ ***Interstitial lung disease.*** As this disease advances, the patient may experience pleuritic chest pain along with progressive dyspnea, cellophane-type crackles, a nonproductive cough, fatigue, weight loss, decreased exercise tolerance, clubbing, and cyanosis.

◆ ***Legionnaires' disease.*** This disorder produces pleuritic chest pain in addition to malaise, headache, and possibly diarrhea, anorexia, diffuse myalgia, and general weakness. Within 12 to 24 hours, the patient suddenly develops a high fever and chills, and an initially nonproductive cough progresses to a productive cough with mucoid and then mucopurulent sputum and possibly hemoptysis. Patients may also experience flushed skin, mild diaphoresis, prostration, nausea and vomiting, mild temporary amnesia, confusion, dyspnea, crackles, tachypnea, and tachycardia.

◆ ***Lung abscess.*** Pleuritic chest pain develops insidiously in a lung abscess along with a pleural friction rub and a cough that produces copious amounts of purulent, foul-smelling, blood-tinged sputum. The affected side is dull on percussion, and decreased breath sounds and crackles may be heard. The patient also displays diaphoresis, anorexia, weight loss, fever, chills, fatigue, weakness, dyspnea, and clubbing.

◆ ***Lung cancer.*** The chest pain associated with lung cancer is commonly described as an intermittent aching felt deep within the chest. If the tumor metastasizes to the ribs or vertebrae, the pain becomes localized, continuous, and gnawing. Associated findings include a cough (sometimes blood-tinged), wheezing, dyspnea, fatigue, anorexia, weight loss, and fever.

◆ ***Mediastinitis.*** This disorder produces severe retrosternal chest pain that radiates to the epigastrium, back, or shoulder and may worsen with breathing, coughing, or sneezing. Accompanying signs and symptoms include chills, fever, and dysphagia.

◆ ***Mitral valve prolapse.*** Most patients with mitral valve prolapse are asymptomatic, but some may experience sharp, stabbing precordial chest pain or precordial ache. The pain can last for seconds or hours and may mimic the pain of ischemic heart disease. The characteristic sign of mitral prolapse is a midsystolic click followed by a systolic murmur at the apex. The patient may experience cardiac awareness, migraine headache, dizziness, weakness, episodic severe fatigue, dyspnea, tachycardia, mood swings, and palpitations.

◆ ***Muscle strain.*** Strained chest, arm, or shoulder muscles may cause a superficial and continuous ache or "pulling" sensation in the chest. Lifting, pulling, or pushing heavy objects may aggravate this discomfort. With acute muscle strain, the patient may experience fatigue, weakness, and rapid swelling of the affected area.

◆ ***Myocardial infarction.*** The crushing substernal chest pain typically associated with an MI lasts from 15 minutes to hours. Typically unrelieved by rest or nitroglycerin, the pain may radiate to the patient's left arm, jaw, neck, or shoulder blades. Other findings include pallor, clammy skin, dyspnea, diaphoresis, nausea, vomiting, anxiety, restlessness, a feeling of impending doom, hypotension or hypertension, an atrial gallop, murmurs, and crackles.

GENDER CUE *An MI may be difficult to diagnose in perimenopausal women because it may produce atypical symptoms, such as* *fatigue, nausea, dyspnea, and shoulder or neck pain, rather than chest pain.*

◆ ***Nocardiosis.*** This disorder causes pleuritic chest pain with a cough that produces thick, tenacious, purulent or mucopurulent, and possibly blood-tinged sputum. Nocardiosis may also cause fever, night sweats, anorexia, malaise, weight loss, and diminished or absent breath sounds.

◆ ***Pancreatitis.*** Acute pancreatitis usually causes intense epigastric pain that radiates to the back and worsens when the patient is in a supine position. Nausea, vomiting, fever, abdominal tenderness and rigidity, diminished bowel sounds, and crackles at the lung bases may also occur. A patient with severe pancreatitis may be extremely restless and have mottled skin, tachycardia, and cold, sweaty extremities. Fulminant pancreatitis causes massive hemorrhage, resulting in shock and coma.

◆ ***Peptic ulcer.*** In this disorder, sharp and burning pain usually arises in the epigastric region. This pain characteristically occurs hours after food intake, commonly during the night. It lasts longer than angina-like pain and is relieved by food or an antacid. Other findings include nausea, vomiting (sometimes with blood), melena, and epigastric tenderness.

◆ ***Pericarditis.*** This disorder produces precordial or retrosternal pain that's aggravated by deep breathing, coughing, position changes, and occasionally by swallowing. The pain is commonly sharp or cutting and radiates to the shoulder and neck. Associated signs and symptoms include pericardial friction rub, fever, tachycardia, and dyspnea. Pericarditis usually follows a viral illness, but several other causes should be considered.

◆ ***Plague.*** Caused by *Yersinia pestis,* plague is one of the most virulent and, if untreated, most lethal bacterial infections known. Most cases are sporadic, but the potential for epidemic spread still exists. Clinical forms include bubonic (the most common), septicemic, and pneumonic plagues. The bubonic form is transmitted to man from the bite of infected fleas. Signs and symptoms include fever, chills, and swollen, inflamed, and tender lymph nodes near the site of the fleabite. Septicemic plague may develop as a complication of untreated bubonic or pneumonic plague and occurs when the plague bacteria enter the bloodstream and multiply. The pneumonic form can be contracted by inhaling respiratory droplets from an infected person or inhaling the organism that has been dispersed in the air through biological warfare. The onset is usually sudden with chills, fever, headache, and myalgia. Pulmonary signs and symptoms include a productive cough, chest pain, tachypnea, dyspnea, hemoptysis, increasing respiratory distress, and cardiopulmonary insufficiency.

◆ ***Pleurisy.*** The sharp, even knifelike chest pain of pleurisy arises abruptly and reaches maximum intensity within a few hours. The pain is usually unilateral and located in the lower and lateral aspects of the chest. Deep breathing, coughing, or thoracic movement characteristically aggravates it. Auscultation over the painful area may reveal decreased breath sounds, inspiratory crackles, and a pleural friction rub. Dyspnea, rapid and shallow breathing, cyanosis, fever, and fatigue may also occur.

◆ ***Pneumonia.*** This disorder produces pleuritic chest pain that increases with deep inspiration and is accompanied by shaking chills and fever. The patient has a dry cough that later becomes productive. Other signs and symptoms include crackles, rhonchi, tachycardia, tachypnea, myalgia, fatigue, headache, dyspnea, abdominal pain, anorexia, cyanosis, decreased breath sounds, and diaphoresis.

◆ ***Pneumothorax.*** Spontaneous pneumothorax, a life-threatening disorder, causes sudden severe, sharp chest pain that increases with chest movement; it's typically unilateral and rarely localized. When the pain is centrally located and radiates to the neck, it may mimic that of an MI. After the pain's onset, dyspnea and cyanosis progressively worsen. Breath sounds are decreased or absent on the affected side with hyperresonance or tympany, subcutaneous crepitation, and decreased vocal fremitus. Asymmetrical chest expansion, accessory muscle use, a nonproductive cough, tachypnea, tachycardia, anxiety, and restlessness also occur.

◆ ***Psittacosis.*** This disorder may produce pleuritic chest pain on rare occasions. It typically begins abruptly with chills, fever, headache, myalgia, epistaxis, and prostration.

◆ ***Pulmonary actinomycosis.*** This disorder causes pleuritic chest pain with a cough that's initially dry but later produces purulent sputum. The patient may also display hemoptysis, fever, weight loss, fatigue, weakness, dyspnea, and night sweats. Multiple sinuses may extend through the chest wall and drain externally.

◆ ***Pulmonary embolism.*** This disorder produces chest pain or a choking sensation. Typically, the patient first experiences sudden dyspnea with intense angina-like or pleuritic pain aggravated by deep breathing and thoracic movement. Other findings include tachycardia, tachypnea, cough (nonproductive or producing blood-tinged sputum), low-grade fever, restlessness, diaphoresis, crackles, pleural friction rub, diffuse wheezing, dullness on percussion, signs of circulatory collapse (weak, rapid pulse; hypotension), paradoxical pulse, signs of cerebral ischemia (transient unconsciousness, coma, seizures), signs of hypoxia (restlessness) and, particularly in the elderly, hemiplegia and other focal neurologic deficits. Less-common signs include massive hemoptysis, chest splinting, and leg edema. A patient with a large embolus may have cyanosis and distended neck veins.

◆ ***Pulmonary hypertension (primary).*** Angina-like pain develops late in patients with this disorder, usually on exertion. The precordial pain may radiate to the neck but doesn't characteristically radiate to the arms. Typical accompanying signs and symptoms include exertional dyspnea, fatigue, syncope, weakness, cough, and hemoptysis.

◆ ***Q fever.*** Q fever is a rickettsial disease caused by *Coxiella burnetii,* an organism found in cattle, sheep, and goats. Human infection usually results from exposure to contaminated milk, urine, feces, or other fluids from infected animals, but it may also result from inhalation of contaminated barnyard dust. *C. burnetii* is highly infectious and is considered a possible airborne agent for biological warfare. Signs and symptoms include fever, chills, severe headache, malaise, chest pain, nausea, vomiting, and diarrhea. The fever may last up to 2 weeks. In severe cases, the patient may develop hepatitis or pneumonia.

◆ ***Rib fracture.*** The chest pain due to fractured ribs is usually sharp, severe, and aggravated by inspiration, coughing, or pressure on the affected area. Besides shallow, splinted respirations, dyspnea, and cough, the patient experiences tenderness and slight edema at the fracture site.

◆ ***Sickle cell crisis.*** Chest pain associated with sickle cell crisis typically has a bizarre distribution. It may start as a vague pain, commonly located in the back, hands, or feet. As the pain worsens, it becomes generalized or localized to the abdomen or chest, causing severe pleuritic pain. The presence of chest pain and difficulty breathing requires prompt intervention. The patient may also have abdominal distention and rigidity, dyspnea, fever, and jaundice.

◆ ***Thoracic outlet syndrome.*** Often causing paresthesia along the ulnar distribution of the arm, this syndrome can be confused with angina, especially when it affects the left arm. The patient usually experiences angina-like pain after lifting his arms above his head, working with his hands above his shoulders, or lifting a weight. The pain disappears as soon as he lowers his arms. Other signs and symptoms include pale skin and a difference in blood pressure between both arms.

◆ ***Tuberculosis.*** Pleuritic chest pain and fine crackles occur after coughing in a patient with tuberculosis. Associated signs and symptoms include night sweats, anorexia, weight loss, fever, malaise, dyspnea, easy fatigability, mild to severe productive cough, occasional hemoptysis, dullness on percussion, increased tactile fremitus, and amphoric breath sounds.

◆ ***Tularemia.*** Also known as "rabbit fever," this infectious disease is caused by the gram-negative, non–spore-forming bacterium *Francisella tularensis.* This organism is found in wild animals, water, and moist soil, typically in rural areas. It's transmitted to humans through the bite of an infected insect or tick, the handling of infected animal carcasses, the drinking of contaminated water, or the inhalation of the bacterium. It's considered a possible airborne agent for biological warfare. Signs and symptoms following inhalation of the organism include the abrupt onset of fever, chills, headache, generalized myalgia, a nonproductive cough, dyspnea, pleuritic chest pain, and empyema.

OTHER CAUSES

◆ ***Chinese restaurant syndrome.*** This benign condition—a reaction to excessive ingestion of monosodium glutamate, an additive in Chinese foods—mimics the signs of an acute MI. The patient may complain of retrosternal burning, ache, or pressure; a burning sensation over his arms, legs, and face; a sensation of facial pressure; headache; shortness of breath, and tachycardia.

◆ ***Drugs.*** Abrupt withdrawal of a beta-adrenergic blocker can cause rebound angina if the patient has coronary artery disease, especially if he has received high doses for a prolonged period.

Special considerations

As needed, prepare the patient for cardiopulmonary studies, such as an electrocardiogram and a lung scan. Perform a venipuncture to collect a serum sample for cardiac enzyme and other studies. Explain the purpose and procedure of each diagnostic test to the patient to help alleviate his anxiety. Also explain the purpose of any prescribed drugs, and make sure that the patient understands the dosage, schedule, and possible adverse effects.

Keep in mind that a patient with chest pain may deny his discomfort, so stress the importance of reporting symptoms to allow adjustment of his treatment.

Pediatric pointers

Even children old enough to talk may have difficulty describing chest pain, so be alert for nonverbal clues, such as restlessness, facial grimaces, or holding of the painful area. Ask the child to point to the painful area and then to where the pain goes (to find out if it's radiating). Determine the pain's severity by asking the parents if the pain interferes with the child's normal activities and behavior. Remember, a child may complain of chest pain in an attempt to get attention or to avoid attending school.

Geriatric pointers

Because older patients have a higher risk of developing life-threatening conditions (such as an MI, angina, and aortic dissection), you must evaluate chest pain carefully in these patients.

Patient counseling

Teach patients with coronary artery disease about the typical features of cardiac ischemia as well as the symptoms that should prompt them to seek medical attention. If the pain fails to disappear after sublingual nitroglycerin, lasts more than 20 minutes, or has a different pattern than the usual angina, the patient must be evaluated immediately.

Cheyne-Stokes respirations

The most common pattern of periodic breathing, Cheyne-Stokes respirations are characterized by a waxing and waning period of hyperpnea that alternates with a shorter period of apnea. This pattern can occur normally in patients with heart or lung disease. It usually indicates increased intracranial pressure (ICP) from a deep cerebral or brain stem lesion, or a metabolic disturbance in the brain. (See *Recognizing Cheyne-Stokes respirations*.)

Cheyne-Stokes respirations may indicate a major change in the patient's condition—usually for the worse. For example, in a patient who has had head trauma or brain surgery, Cheyne-Stokes respirations may signal increasing ICP. Cheyne-Stokes respirations can occur normally in patients who live at high altitudes.

EMERGENCY INTERVENTIONS *If you detect Cheyne-Stokes respirations in a patient with a history of head trauma, recent brain surgery, or another brain insult, quickly take his vital signs. Keep his head elevated 30 degrees, and perform a rapid neurologic examination to obtain baseline data. Reevaluate the patient's neurologic status frequently. If ICP continues to rise, you'll detect changes in the patient's level of consciousness (LOC), pupillary reactions, and ability to move his extremities. ICP monitoring is indicated.*

Time the periods of hyperpnea and apnea for 3 to 4 minutes to evaluate respirations and to obtain baseline data. Be alert for prolonged periods of apnea. Frequently check blood pressure; also check skin color to detect signs of hypoxemia. Maintain airway patency and administer oxygen as needed. If the patient's condition worsens, endotracheal intubation is necessary.

Recognizing Cheyne-Stokes respirations

Cheyne-Stokes respirations are breaths that gradually become faster and deeper than normal, then slower, during a 30- to 170-second period, alternating with 20- to 60-second periods of apnea.

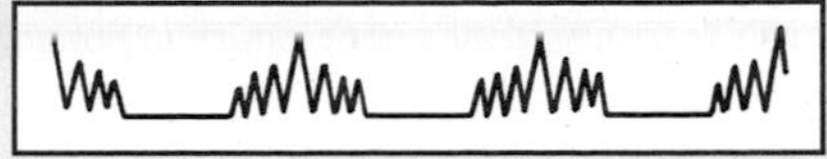

History and physical examination

If the patient's condition permits, obtain a brief history. Ask especially about drug use.

Medical causes

◆ ***Adams-Stokes attacks.*** Cheyne-Stokes respirations may follow an Adams-Stokes attack—a syncopal episode associated with atrioventricular block. The patient is hypotensive, with a heart rate between 20 and 50 beats/minute. He may also appear pale, shaking, and confused.

◆ ***Heart failure.*** In left-sided heart failure, Cheyne-Stokes respirations may occur with exertional dyspnea and orthopnea. Related findings include fatigue, weakness, tachycardia, tachypnea, and crackles. The patient may also have a cough, generally nonproductive but occasionally producing clear or blood-tinged sputum.

◆ ***Hypertensive encephalopathy.*** In this life-threatening disorder, severe hypertension precedes Cheyne-Stokes respirations. The patient's LOC is decreased, and he may experience vomiting, seizures, severe headaches, vision disturbances (including transient blindness), and transient paralysis.

◆ ***Increased ICP.*** As ICP rises, Cheyne-Stokes is the first irregular respiratory pattern to occur. It's preceded by a decreased LOC and accompanied by hypertension, headache, vomiting, impaired or unequal motor movement, and vision disturbances (blurring, diplopia, photophobia, and pupillary changes). In late stages of increased ICP, bradycardia and widened pulse pressure occur.

◆ ***Renal failure.*** End-stage chronic renal failure may produce Cheyne-Stokes respirations, bleeding gums, oral lesions, ammonia breath odor, and marked changes in every body system.

Other causes

◆ ***Drugs.*** Large doses of an opioid, a hypnotic, or a barbiturate can precipitate Cheyne-Stokes respirations.

Special considerations

When evaluating Cheyne-Stokes respirations, be careful not to mistake periods of hypoventilation or decreased tidal volume for complete apnea.

Pediatric pointers

Cheyne-Stokes respirations rarely occur in children, except during late heart failure.

Geriatric pointers

Cheyne-Stokes respirations can occur normally in elderly patients during sleep.

Patient counseling

Inform the patient or his family that sleep apnea and Cheyne-Stokes respirations have different causes and methods of treatment.

Chills

[Rigors]

Chills are extreme, involuntary muscle contractions with characteristic paroxysms of violent shivering and teeth chattering. Commonly caused by an increased body temperature set by the hypothalamic thermostat, chills are usually accompanied by fever and tend to arise suddenly, heralding the onset of infection. Certain diseases, such as pneumococcal pneumonia, produce only a single, shaking chill. Other diseases, such as malaria, produce intermittent chills with recurring high fever. Still others produce continuous chills for up to 1 hour, precipitating a high fever. (See *Why chills accompany fever*.)

Chills can also result from lymphomas, blood transfusion reactions, and the use of certain drugs. Chills without fever are a normal response to exposure to cold. (See *Rare causes of chills*.)

History and physical examination

Ask the patient when the chills began and whether they're continuous or intermittent. Because fever commonly accompanies or follows chills, take his rectal temperature to obtain a baseline reading. Then check his temperature often to monitor fluctuations and to determine his temperature curve. Typically, a localized infection produces a sudden onset of shaking chills, sweats, and high fever, whereas a systemic infection produces intermittent chills with recurring episodes of high fever or continuous chills that may last up to 1 hour and precipitate a high fever.

Ask about related signs and symptoms, such as headache, dysuria, diarrhea, confusion, abdominal pain, cough, sore throat, or nausea. Does the patient have any known allergies, an infection, or a recent history of an infectious disorder? Find out which medications he's taking and whether any drug has improved or worsened his symptoms. Has he received any treatment that may predispose him to an infection (such as chemotherapy)? Ask about recent exposure to farm animals, guinea pigs,

Why chills accompany fever

Fever usually occurs when exogenous pyrogens activate endogenous pyrogens to reset the body's thermostat to a higher level. At this higher thermostatic setpoint, the body feels cold and responds through several compensatory mechanisms, including rhythmic muscle contractions, or chills. These muscle contractions in turn generate body heat and help produce fever. This flowchart outlines the events that link chills to fever.

Exogenous pyrogens (infectious organisms, immune complexes, toxins) enter the body.

▼

Phagocytic leukocytes release endogenous pyrogens.

▼

Endogenous pyrogens — possibly with prostaglandins — stimulate temperature-sensitive receptors in the hypothalamus and raise the thermostatic setpoint to a higher level.

▼

Descending efferent pathways from the hypothalamus innervate effectors, such as skeletal muscles, and stimulate them to rhythmically contract.

▼

Rhythmic muscle contractions, or chills, generate body heat, which helps produce fever.

Rare causes of chills

Chills can result from disorders that are rare in the United States but may be fairly common worldwide. Remember to ask about recent foreign travel when you obtain a patient's history. Among the many rare disorders that produce chills are:
- ◆ brucellosis (undulant fever)
- ◆ dengue fever (breakbone fever)
- ◆ epidemic typhus (louse-borne typhus)
- ◆ leptospirosis
- ◆ lymphocytic choriomeningitis
- ◆ plague
- ◆ pulmonary tularemia
- ◆ rat bite fever
- ◆ relapsing fever.

hamsters, dogs, and such birds as pigeons, parrots, and parakeets. Also ask about recent insect or animal bites, travel to foreign countries, and contact with persons who have an active infection.

Medical causes

◆ ***Acquired immunodeficiency syndrome.*** This commonly fatal disease is caused by infection with human immunodeficiency virus transmitted by blood or semen. The patient usually develops lymphadenopathy and may also experience fatigue, anorexia and weight loss, diarrhea, diaphoresis, skin disorders, and signs of upper respiratory tract infection. Opportunistic infections can cause serious disease in these patients.

◆ ***Anthrax (inhalation).*** This acute infectious disease is caused by the gram-positive, spore-forming bacterium *Bacillus anthracis.* Although the disease most commonly occurs in wild and domestic grazing animals, such as cattle, sheep, and goats, the spores can live in the soil for many years. The disease can occur in humans exposed to infected animals, tissue from infected animals, or biological agents. Most natural cases occur in agricultural regions worldwide. Anthrax may occur in cutaneous, inhalation, or GI forms.

Inhalation anthrax is caused by inhalation of aerosolized spores. Initial signs and symptoms are flulike and include fever, chills, weakness, cough, and chest pain. The disease generally occurs in two stages with a period of recovery after the initial signs and symptoms. The second stage develops abruptly, causing rapid deterioration marked by fever, dyspnea, stridor, and hypotension; death generally results within 24 hours. Radiologic findings include mediastinitis and symmetrical mediastinal widening.

◆ ***Cholangitis.*** Charcot's triad—chills with spiking fever, abdominal pain, and jaundice—characterizes sudden obstruction of the common bile duct. The patient may have associated pruritus, weakness, and fatigue.

◆ ***Gram-negative bacteremia.*** This infection causes sudden chills and fever, nausea, vomiting, diarrhea, and prostration.

◆ ***Hemolytic anemia.*** In acute hemolytic anemia, fulminating chills occur with fever and abdominal pain. The patient rapidly develops jaundice and hepatomegaly; he may develop splenomegaly.

◆ ***Hepatic abscess.*** This infection usually arises abruptly, with chills, fever, nausea, vomiting, diarrhea, anorexia, and severe upper abdominal tenderness and pain that may radiate to the right shoulder.

◆ ***Hodgkin's disease.*** The patient characteristically experiences several days or weeks of fever and chills alternating with periods of no fever and no chills. This disorder commonly produces regional lymphadenopathy that may progress to hepatosplenomegaly. Other findings include diaphoresis, fatigue, and pruritus.

◆ ***Infective endocarditis.*** This infection produces abrupt onset of intermittent shaking chills with fever. In addition to petechiae, the patient may have Janeway lesions on his hands and feet and Osler's nodes on his palms and soles. Associated findings include murmur, hematuria, eye hemorrhage, Roth's spots, and signs of heart failure (dyspnea, peripheral edema).

◆ ***Influenza.*** Initially, this disorder causes an abrupt onset of chills, high fever, malaise, headache, myalgia, and nonproductive cough. Some patients may also suddenly develop rhinitis, rhinorrhea, laryngitis, conjunctivitis, hoarseness, and sore throat. Chills generally subside after the first few days, but intermittent fever, weakness, and cough may persist for up to 1 week.

◆ ***Influenza type A H1N1 virus (Swine flu).*** Influenza type A H1N1, or swine flu, is a respiratory disease of pigs caused by type A influenza virus. Swine flu viruses cause high levels of illness and low death rates in pigs. Swine flu viruses normally don't infect humans. However, sporadic human infections with swine flu have occurred. Most commonly, these cases occur in persons with direct exposure to pigs. The virus has changed slightly and is known as H1N1 flu. Outbreaks of H1N1 flu in 2009 showed that the virus can be transmitted from person to person, causing transmission across the globe. The H1N1 flu is similar to influenza, and causes illness and in some cases death. The symptoms of swine flu include chills, fever, fatigue, myalgia, nonproductive cough, headache, and vomiting. The use of antiviral drugs is recommended to treat H1N1 flu.

◆ ***Legionnaires' disease.*** Within 12 to 48 hours after the onset of this disease, the patient suddenly develops chills and a high fever. Prodromal signs and symptoms characteristically include malaise, headache, and possibly diarrhea, anorexia, diffuse myalgia, and general weakness. An initially nonproductive cough progresses to a productive cough with mucoid or mucopurulent sputum and possibly hemoptysis. Most patients also develop nausea and vomiting, confusion, mild temporary amnesia, pleuritic chest pain, dyspnea, tachypnea, crackles, tachycardia, and flushed and mildly diaphoretic skin.

◆ ***Lung abscess.*** In addition to chills, a lung abscess causes sweating, pleuritic chest pain, dyspnea, clubbing, weakness, headache, malaise, anorexia, weight loss, and a cough that produces large amounts of purulent, foul-smelling and, possibly, bloody sputum.

◆ ***Lyme disease.*** The bite of a tiny deer tick can transmit this infection, which causes a red macule or papule (erythema migrans) to develop at the bite site. It's accompanied by chills, fever, malaise, fatigue, lymphadenopathy, arthralgia, and rash. If untreated, Lyme disease may cause cranial neuritis with facial palsy, heart blocks, arthritis, and a characteristic sclerotic rash.

◆ ***Lymphangitis.*** Acute lymphangitis produces chills and other systemic signs and symptoms, such as fever, malaise, and headache. Its characteristic signs are red streaks radiating from a wound and cellulitis draining toward tender regional lymph nodes.

◆ ***Lymphogranuloma venereum.*** This disorder produces chills, fever, lymphadenopathy, headache, anorexia, myalgia, arthralgia, and weight loss. The primary genital lesion is a papule or small erosion that precedes lymphatic involvement and heals spontaneously within a few days.

◆ ***Malaria.*** The paroxysmal cycle of malaria begins with a period of chills lasting 1 to 2 hours. This is followed by a high fever lasting 3 to 4 hours and then 2 to 4 hours of profuse diaphoresis. Paroxysms occur every 48 to 72 hours when caused by *Plasmodium malariae* and every 42 to 40 hours when caused by *P. vivax* or *P. ovale.* In benign malaria, the paroxysms may be interspersed with periods of well-being. The patient also has a headache, muscle pain, and possibly hepatosplenomegaly.

◆ ***Miliary tuberculosis.*** In the acute form of this disease, the patient suffers intermittent chills, high fever, and night sweats. Epididymal or testicular nodules and splenomegaly may also occur.

◆ ***Monkeypox.*** Many individuals infected with the monkeypox virus experience chills. Other common initial symptoms of this rare virus include fever, lymphadenopathy, sore throat, dyspnea, muscle aches, and rash. Although mon keypox occurs primarily in central and western Africa, it was confirmed in the United States in 2003 when several humans contracted the virus from infected pet prairie dogs. There is no treatment for this virus; however, given its similarity to smallpox, the smallpox vaccine is used in certain circumstances to protect individuals against monkeypox.

◆ ***Otitis media.*** Acute suppurative otitis media produces chills with fever and severe deep, throbbing ear pain. The patient usually displays a mild conductive hearing loss and a bulging, hyperemic tympanic membrane. He may also have dizziness, nausea, and vomiting. When the tympanic membrane ruptures, pus drains externally through the ear canal and the patient feels relief.

◆ ***Pelvic inflammatory disease.*** In this infection, chills and fever are typically accompanied by lower abdominal pain and tenderness; profuse, purulent vaginal discharge; or abnormal menstrual bleeding. The patient may also develop nausea and vomiting, an abdominal mass, and dysuria.

◆ ***Plague.*** Caused by *Yersinia pestis,* plague is one of the most virulent and, if untreated, lethal bacterial infections known. Most cases are sporadic, but the potential for epidemic spread still exists. Clinical forms include bubonic (the most common), septicemic, and pneumonic plagues. The bubonic form is transmitted to man from the bite of infected fleas. Signs and symptoms include fever, chills, and swollen, inflamed, and tender lymph nodes near the site of the fleabite. Septicemic plague may develop as a complication of untreated bubonic or pneumonic plague and occurs when the plague bacteria enter the bloodstream and multiply. The pneumonic form can be contracted by inhaling respiratory droplets from an infected person or inhaling the organism that has been dispersed in the air through biological warfare. The onset is usually sudden with chills, fever, headache, and myalgia. Pulmonary signs and symptoms include a productive cough, chest pain, tachypnea, dyspnea, hemoptysis, increasing respiratory distress, and cardiopulmonary insufficiency.

◆ ***Pneumonia.*** A single shaking chill usually heralds the sudden onset of pneumococcal pneumonia; other pneumonias characteristically cause intermittent chills. In any type of pneumonia, related findings may include fever, productive cough with bloody sputum, pleuritic chest pain, dyspnea, tachypnea, and tachycardia. The patient may be cyanotic and diaphoretic, with bronchial breath sounds and crackles, rhonchi, increased tactile fremitus, and grunting respirations. He may also experience achiness, anorexia, fatigue, and headache.

◆ ***Psittacosis.*** This disease typically begins with the sudden onset of chills, fever, headache, myalgia, epistaxis, and prostration. A dry, hacking cough occurs initially, progressing to pneumonia with a cough that produces small amounts of mucoid, blood-streaked sputum. The patient also experiences tachypnea, fine crackles, photophobia, abdominal distention and tenderness, nausea, vomiting, a faint macular rash and, rarely, chest pain.

◆ ***Pyelonephritis.*** In acute pyelonephritis, the patient develops chills, high fever, and possibly nausea and vomiting over several hours to days. He generally also has anorexia, fatigue, myalgia, flank pain, costovertebral angle tenderness, hematuria or cloudy urine, and urinary frequency, urgency, and burning.

◆ ***Q fever.*** Q fever is a rickettsial disease caused by *Coxiella burnetii,* an organism found in cattle, sheep, and goats. Human infection usually results from exposure to contaminated milk, urine, feces, or other fluids from infected animals, but it may also result from inhalation of contaminated barnyard dust. *C. burnetii* is highly infectious and is considered a possible airborne agent for biological warfare. Signs and symptoms include fever, chills, severe headache, malaise, chest pain, nausea, vomiting, and diarrhea. The fever may last up to 2 weeks. In severe cases, the patient may develop hepatitis or pneumonia.

◆ ***Renal abscess.*** This abscess initially produces sudden chills and fever. Later effects include flank pain, costovertebral angle tenderness, abdominal muscle spasm, and transient hematuria.

◆ ***Rocky Mountain spotted fever.*** This disorder begins suddenly with chills, fever, malaise, an excruciating headache, and muscle, bone, and joint pain. Typically, the patient's tongue is covered with a thick white coating that gradually turns brown. After 2 to 6 days of fever and occasional chills, a macular or maculopapular rash appears on the hands and feet and then becomes generalized; after a few days, the rash becomes petechial.

◆ ***Sepsis, puerperal or postabortal.*** Chills and high fever occur as early as 6 hours or as late as 10 days postpartum or postabortion. The patient may also have a purulent vaginal discharge, an enlarged and tender uterus, abdominal pain, backache and, possibly, nausea, vomiting, and diarrhea.

◆ ***Septic arthritis.*** Chills and fever accompany the characteristic red, swollen, and painful joints caused by this disorder.

◆ ***Septic shock.*** Initially, septic shock produces chills, fever and, possibly, nausea, vomiting, and diarrhea. The patient's skin is typically flushed, warm, and dry; his blood pressure is normal or slightly low; and he has tachycardia and tachypnea. As septic shock progresses, the patient's arms and legs become cool and cyanotic, and he exhibits oliguria, thirst, anxiety, restlessness, confusion, and hypotension. Later, he develops cold and clammy skin, a rapid and thready pulse, severe hypotension, persistent oliguria or anuria, signs of respiratory failure, and coma.

◆ ***Sinusitis.*** In acute sinusitis, chills are accompanied by fever, headache, and pain, tenderness, and swelling over the affected sinuses. Maxillary sinusitis produces pain over the cheeks and upper teeth; ethmoid sinusitis, pain over the eyes; frontal sinusitis, pain over the eyebrows; and sphenoid sinusitis, pain behind the eyes. The primary indicator of sinusitis is nasal discharge, which is commonly bloody for 24 to 48 hours before gradually becoming purulent.

◆ ***Snake bite.*** Most pit viper bites that result in envenomization cause chills, typically with fever. Other systemic signs and symptoms include sweating, weakness, dizziness, fainting, hypotension, nausea, vomiting, diarrhea, and thirst. The area around the snake bite may be marked by immediate swelling and tenderness, pain, ecchymoses, petechiae, blebs, bloody discharge, and local necrosis. The patient may have difficulty speaking, blurred vision, paralysis, bleeding tendencies, and signs of respiratory distress and shock.

◆ ***Tularemia.*** Also known as "rabbit fever," this infectious disease is caused by the gram-negative, non–spore-forming bacterium *Francisella tularensis*. This organism is found in wild animals, water, and moist soil, typically in rural areas. It's transmitted to humans through the bite of an infected insect or tick, the handling of infected animal carcasses, the drinking of contaminated water, or the inhalation of the bacterium. It's considered a possible airborne agent for biological warfare. Signs and symptoms following inhalation of the organism include the abrupt onset of fever, chills, headache, generalized myalgia, a nonproductive cough, dyspnea, pleuritic chest pain, and empyema.

◆ ***Typhoid fever.*** This disorder may initially cause sudden chills and a sharply rising fever. More commonly, though, the patient's body temperature gradually increases for 5 to 7 days with accompanying chilliness or frank chills. Headache, abdominal discomfort, constipation, and demonstrable splenomegaly appear by the end of the first week. A characteristic rash called "rose spots" develops on the upper abdomen and anterior thorax during the second week but lasts only 2 to 3 days. Later, the patient may develop a dry cough, epistaxis, mental dullness or delirium, marked abdominal distention, significant weight loss, profound fatigue, and diarrhea. The heart rate may be unusually slow in relation to the high fever.

◆ ***Typhus.*** Typhus is a rickettsial disease transmitted to humans by fleas, mites, or body louse. Initial signs and symptoms include headache, myalgia, arthralgia, and malaise followed by an abrupt onset of chills, fever, nausea, and vomiting. A maculopapular rash may be present in some cases.

◆ ***Violin spider bite.*** This bite produces chills, fever, malaise, weakness, nausea, vomiting, and joint pain within 24 to 48 hours. The patient may also develop a rash and delirium.

OTHER CAUSES

◆ ***Drugs.*** Amphotericin B is a drug associated with chills. Phenytoin is also a common cause of drug-induced fever that can produce chills.

I.V. bleomycin and intermittent administration of an oral antipyretic can also cause chills.

◆ ***I.V. therapy.*** Infection at the I.V. insertion site (superficial phlebitis) can cause chills, high fever, and local redness, warmth, induration, and tenderness.

◆ ***Transfusion reaction.*** A hemolytic reaction may cause chills during the transfusion or immediately afterward. A nonhemolytic febrile reaction may also cause chills.

Special considerations

Check the patient's vital signs often, especially if his chills result from a known or suspected infection. Be alert for signs of progressive septic shock, such as hypotension, tachycardia, and tachypnea. If appropriate, obtain samples of blood, sputum, or wound drainage for culture tests to determine the causative organism. Give the appropriate antibiotic. Radiographic studies and serum and urine samples may be required.

Because chills are an involuntary response to an increased body temperature, blankets won't stop a patient's chills or shivering. Despite this, keep his room temperature as even as possible. Provide adequate hydration and nutrients, and give an antipyretic to help control fever. Irregular use of an antipyretic can trigger compensatory chills.

Pediatric pointers

Infants don't get chills because they have poorly developed shivering mechanisms. In addition, most classic febrile childhood infections, such as measles and mumps, don't typically produce chills. However, older children and teenagers may have chills with mycoplasma pneumonia and acute pyogenic osteomyelitis.

Geriatric pointers

Chills in an elderly patient usually indicate an underlying infection, such as a urinary tract infection, pneumonia (commonly associated with aspiration of gastric contents), diverticulitis, or skin breakdown in pressure areas. Also, consider an ischemic bowel in an elderly patient who comes into your facility with fever, chills, and abdominal pain.

Patient counseling

Advise the patient to measure his temperature with a thermometer when he experiences chills and to document the exact readings and times. This will help reveal patterns that may point to a specific diagnosis.

Chorea

[Choreiform movements]

Chorea—brief, unpredictable bursts of rapid, jerky motion that interrupt normal coordinated movement—indicates dysfunction of the extrapyramidal system.

Unlike tics, choreiform movements are seldom repetitive but tend to appear purposeful despite their involuntary nature. Although any muscle can be affected, chorea usually involves the face, head, lower arms, and hands. It can affect both sides of the body or only one side; however, when it affects the face, both sides are usually involved. Chorea may be aggravated by excitement or fatigue and may disappear during sleep. In some patients, it may be difficult to distinguish chorea from athetosis (snakelike, writhing movements), although choreiform movements are generally more rapid than athetoid ones. (See *Distinguishing athetosis from chorea,* page 73.)

History and physical examination

Ask the patient and his family when they first noticed the choreiform movements. Do the movements disappear when the patient is asleep? Find out if anyone in the patient's family exhibits the same type of movements, and ask about a family history of such diseases as Huntington's disease. Also ask which medications the patient is taking. Obtain an occupational history, noting especially prolonged exposure to manganese or other metals. As you obtain the history, observe the patient for excessive restlessness and periodic facial grimaces that may interrupt his speech.

Perform a physical examination to evaluate the severity of the patient's chorea. Ask him to stick out his tongue and keep it out. Typically, he'll be unable to do this; instead, his tongue will dart in and out of his mouth. Observe the patient's arms and legs separately for involuntary jerky movements. Ask him to extend and flex his hand as if halting traffic; the choreiform movements will be extremely evident in this position. Also, check for such related signs as athetosis, rigidity, or tremor.

To assess the patient for choreoathetotic gait, ask him to walk. He may change the position of his trunk and upper body parts with each step and jerk and tilt his head to one side. Because of superimposed involuntary movements and postures, the patient's legs may move slowly and awkwardly. (An involuntary movement suspending his leg momentarily with each step may give a dancing quality to his gait.)

Medical causes

◆ ***Cerebral infarction.*** An infarction that involves the thalamic area produces unilateral or bilateral chorea. The patient may also experience dysarthria, tremors, rigidity, weakness, and sensory disturbances such as paresthesia.

◆ ***Encephalitis.*** Chorea may occur in the recovery phase of encephalitis. Low-grade fever and athetosis may also be present, in addition to such focal neurologic signs as hemiparesis, hemiplegia, and facial droop.

◆ ***Huntington's disease.*** In this inherited disease, chorea may be the first sign or it may accompany the intellectual decline that leads to emotional disturbances and dementia. The patient's movements tend to be choreoathetotic and may be accompanied by dysarthria, dystonia, prancing gait, dysphagia, and facial grimacing.

◆ ***Wilson's disease.*** Chorea and dystonia affecting the arms and legs are early indicators of Wilson's disease. The patient typically experiences dysarthria, tremors, hoarseness, dysphagia, and slowed body movements; he may also exhibit emotional and behavioral disturbances, drooling, rigidity, and mental deterioration. The pathognomonic Kayser-Fleischer ring in the cornea appears as the disease progresses.

Other causes

◆ ***Carbon monoxide poisoning.*** A patient who survives severe carbon monoxide poisoning may have neurologic signs and symptoms, such as chorea, rigidity, dementia, impaired sensory function, masklike facies, generalized seizures, and myoclonus.

◆ ***Drugs.*** Phenothiazines (especially the piperazine derivatives), haloperidol, thiothixene, and loxapine commonly produce chorea. Metoclopramide, metyrosine, hormonal contraceptives, levodopa, and phenytoin may also cause this sign.

◆ ***Lead poisoning.*** In the later stages, lead poisoning produces chorea in addition to seizures, headache, memory lapses, and severe mental impairment. The patient may also develop masklike facies, footdrop, wristdrop, dizziness, ataxia, weakness, lethargy, abdominal pain, anorexia, nausea, vomiting, constipation, lead line on the gums, and a metallic taste in his mouth.

◆ ***Manganese poisoning.*** In miners who have been exposed to manganese dioxide for prolonged periods, chorea characteristically occurs with a propulsive gait, dystonia, and rigidity. Initially, the patient may have masklike facies, a resting tremor, and personality changes; later, extreme muscle weakness and lethargy occur.

Special considerations

Because the patient's movements are involuntary and increase his risk of severe injury, pad the side rails of his bed and keep sharp objects out of his environment. Help him minimize physical activity and emotional upset to avoid aggravating the chorea and ensure adequate periods of rest and sleep.

Pediatric pointers

Sydenham's chorea occurs in childhood as a delayed manifestation of rheumatic fever. In Hallervorden-Spatz disease, a rare and inherited degenerative disorder, choreoathetotic movements occur in late childhood or early adolescence. Chorea can also occur in children with athetoid cerebral palsy.

Chvostek's sign

Chvostek's sign is an abnormal spasm of the facial muscles that's elicited by lightly tapping the patient's facial nerve near his lower jaw. (See *Eliciting Chvostek's sign*.) This sign usually suggests hypocalcemia but can occur normally in about 25% of people. Typically, it precedes other signs of hypocalcemia and persists until the onset of tetany. It can't be elicited during tetany because of strong muscle contractions.

Normally, eliciting Chvostek's sign is attempted only in patients with suspected hypocalcemic disorders. However, because the parathyroid gland regulates calcium balance, Chvostek's sign may also be tested in patients before neck surgery to obtain a baseline.

EMERGENCY INTERVENTIONS *Test for Trousseau's sign, a reliable indicator of hypocalcemia. Closely monitor the patient for signs of tetany, such as carpopedal spasms or circumoral and extremity paresthesia.*

Be prepared to act rapidly if a seizure occurs. Perform an electrocardiogram to check for changes associated with hypocalcemia that can predispose the patient to arrhythmias. Place the patient on a cardiac monitor.

Eliciting Chvostek's sign

Begin by telling the patient to relax his facial muscles. Then stand directly in front of him, and tap the facial nerve either just anterior to the earlobe and below the zygomatic arch or between the zygomatic arch and the corner of his mouth. A positive response varies from twitching of the lip at the corner of the mouth to spasm of all facial muscles, depending on the severity of hypocalcemia.

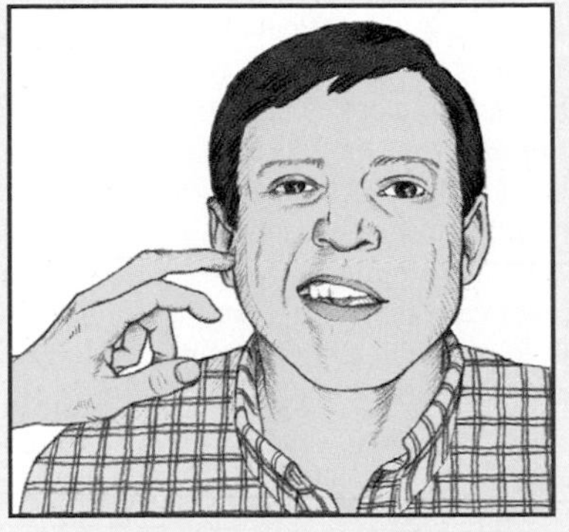

History and physical examination

Obtain a brief history. Find out if the patient has had the parathyroid glands surgically removed or if he has a history of hypoparathyroidism, hypomagnesemia, or malabsorption disorder. Ask him or his family if they have noticed any mental changes, such as depression or slowed responses, which can accompany chronic hypocalcemia.

Medical causes

◆ ***Hypocalcemia.*** The degree of muscle spasm elicited reflects the patient's serum calcium level. Initially, hypocalcemia produces paresthesia in the fingers, toes, and circumoral area that progresses to muscle tension and carpopedal spasms. The patient may also complain of muscle weakness, fatigue, and palpitations. Muscle twitching, hyperactive deep tendon reflexes, choreiform movements, and muscle cramps may also occur. The patient with chronic hypocalcemia may have mental status changes; diplopia; difficulty swallowing; abdominal cramps; dry, scaly skin; brittle nails; and thin, patchy scalp and eyebrow hair.

Other causes

◆ ***Blood transfusion.*** A massive transfusion can lower serum calcium levels and allow Chvostek's sign to be elicited.

Special considerations

Collect blood samples for serial calcium studies to evaluate the severity of hypocalcemia and the effectiveness of therapy, which consists of oral or I.V. calcium supplements. Also, look for Chvostek's sign when evaluating a patient postoperatively.

Pediatric pointers

Because Chvostek's sign may be observed in healthy infants, it isn't elicited to detect neonatal tetany.

Geriatric pointers

Always consider malabsorption and poor nutritional status in an elderly patient with Chvostek's sign and hypocalcemia.

Patient counseling

Inform patients who will be undergoing thyroidectomy or parathyroidectomy about the early signs and symptoms of hypocalcemia, such as numbness, tingling, and muscle cramps, and tell them to seek immediate medical attention if these occur.

Clubbing

A nonspecific sign of pulmonary and cyanotic cardiovascular disorders, clubbing is the painless, usually bilateral increase in soft tissue around the terminal phalanges of the fingers or toes. (See *Rare causes of clubbing,* page 160.) It doesn't involve changes in the underlying bone. In early clubbing, the normal 160-degree angle between the nail and the nail base approximates 180 degrees. As clubbing progresses, this angle widens and the base of the nail becomes visibly swollen. In late clubbing, the angle where the nail meets the now-convex nail base extends more than halfway up the nail.

History and physical examination

You'll probably detect clubbing while evaluating other signs of known pulmonary or cardiovascular disease. Therefore, review the patient's current plan of treatment because clubbing may resolve with correction of the underlying

Rare causes of clubbing

Clubbing is typically a sign of pulmonary or cardiovascular disease, but it can also result from certain hepatic and GI disorders, such as cirrhosis, Crohn's disease, and ulcerative colitis. Clubbing occurs only rarely in these disorders, however, so first check for more common signs and symptoms. For example, a patient with cirrhosis usually experiences right-upper-quadrant pain and hepatomegaly, a patient with Crohn's disease typically has abdominal cramping and tenderness, and a patient with ulcerative colitis may develop diffuse abdominal pain and blood-streaked diarrhea.

disorder. Also, evaluate the extent of clubbing in both the fingers and toes. (See *Checking for clubbed fingers*.)

Medical causes

◆ ***Bronchiectasis.*** Clubbing commonly occurs in the late stage of this disorder. Another classic sign is a cough producing copious, foul-smelling, and mucopurulent sputum. Hemoptysis and coarse crackles heard over the affected area during inspiration are also characteristic. The patient may complain of weight loss, fatigue, weakness, and exertional dyspnea. He may also have rhonchi, fever, malaise, and halitosis.

◆ ***Bronchitis.*** Clubbing may occur as a late sign in chronic bronchitis, but it doesn't reflect the severity of the disease. The patient has a chronic productive cough and may display barrel chest, dyspnea, wheezing, increased use of accessory muscles, cyanosis, tachypnea, crackles, scattered rhonchi, and prolonged expiration.

◆ ***Emphysema.*** Clubbing occurs late in this disease, which may also cause anorexia, malaise, dyspnea, tachypnea, diminished breath sounds, peripheral cyanosis, pursed-lip breathing, accessory muscle use, barrel chest, and a productive cough.

◆ ***Endocarditis.*** In subacute infective endocarditis, clubbing may be accompanied by fever, anorexia, pallor, weakness, night sweats, fatigue, tachycardia, and weight loss. The patient may also develop arthralgia, petechiae, Osler's nodes, splinter hemorrhages, Janeway lesions, splenomegaly, and Roth's spots. Cardiac murmurs are usually present.

◆ ***Heart failure.*** Clubbing is a late sign of heart failure along with wheezing, dyspnea, and fatigue. Other findings include jugular vein distention, hepatomegaly, tachypnea, palpitations, dependent edema, unexplained weight gain, nausea, anorexia, chest tightness, slowed mental response, hypotension, diaphoresis, narrow pulse pressure, pallor, oliguria, a gallop rhythm (a third heart sound), and crackles on inspiration.

◆ ***Interstitial fibrosis.*** Clubbing occurs in almost all patients with advanced interstitial fibrosis. Typically, the patient also develops intermittent chest pain, dyspnea, crackles, fatigue, weight loss and, possibly, cyanosis.

◆ ***Lung abscess.*** Initially, this disorder produces clubbing, which may resolve with resolution of the abscess. It can also cause pleuritic chest pain, dyspnea, crackles, halitosis, and a productive cough with a large amount of purulent, foul-smelling, and commonly bloody sputum. The patient may also experience weakness, fatigue, anorexia, headache, malaise, weight loss, and fever with chills. Auscultation may reveal decreased breath sounds.

◆ ***Lung and pleural cancer.*** Clubbing occurs commonly in these cancers. Associated findings include hemoptysis, dyspnea, wheezing, chest pain, weight loss, anorexia, fatigue, and fever.

Special considerations

Don't mistake curved nails—a normal variation—for clubbing. Remember that the angle between the nail and its base remains normal in curved nails, but not in clubbed nails.

Pediatric pointers

Clubbing usually occurs in children with cyanotic congenital heart disease or cystic fibrosis. Surgical correction of heart defects may reverse clubbing.

Geriatric pointers

Arthritic deformities of the fingers or toes may disguise clubbing in elderly patients.

Patient counseling

Inform the patient that clubbing doesn't always disappear, even if the cause has been resolved.

Checking for clubbed fingers

To assess a patient for chronic tissue hypoxia, check his fingers for clubbing. Normally, the angle between the fingernail and the point where the nail enters the skin is about 160 degrees. Clubbing occurs when that angle increases to 180 degrees or more, as shown below.

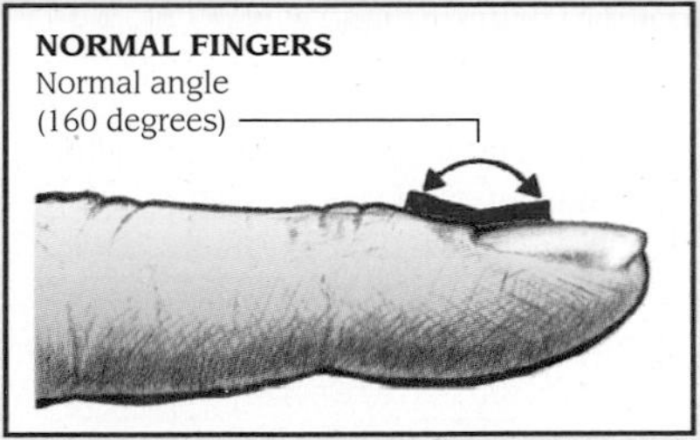

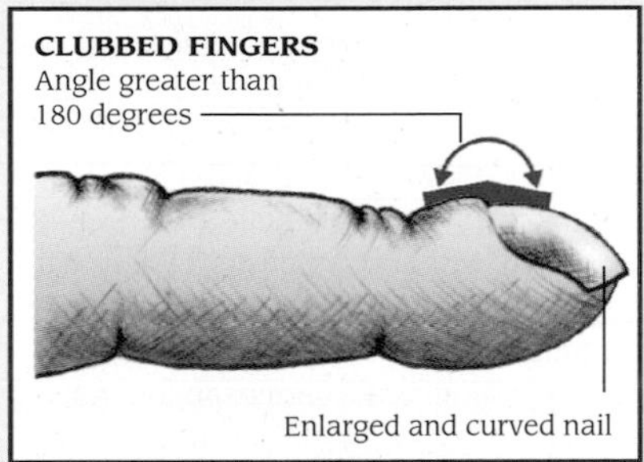

Cogwheel rigidity

Cogwheel rigidity, a cardinal sign of Parkinson's disease, is marked by muscle rigidity that reacts with superimposed ratchetlike movements when the muscle is passively stretched. This sign can be elicited by stabilizing the patient's forearm and then moving his wrist through the range of motion. (Cogwheel rigidity usually appears in the arms but can sometimes be elicited in the ankle.) Both the patient and the examiner can see and feel these characteristic movements, thought to be a combination of rigidity and tremor.

History and physical examination

After you've elicited cogwheel rigidity, take the patient's history to determine when he first noticed associated signs of Parkinson's disease. For example, has he experienced tremors? Did he notice tremors of his hands first? Does he have "pill-rolling" hand movements? When did he first notice that his movements were becoming slower? How long has he been experiencing stiffness in his arms and legs? Has his handwriting gotten smaller? While taking the history, observe the patient for signs of pronounced parkinsonism, such as drooling, masklike facies, dysphagia, monotone speech, and altered gait.

Find out which medications the patient is taking and ask if they've helped relieve some of his symptoms. If he's taking levodopa and his symptoms have worsened, find out if he has exceeded the prescribed dosage. If you suspect an overdose, withhold the drug. If the patient has been taking a phenothiazine or another antipsychotic and has no history of Parkinson's disease, he may be having an adverse reaction. Withhold the drug as appropriate.

Medical causes

- ***Parkinson's disease.*** In this disorder, cogwheel rigidity occurs together with an insidious tremor, which usually begins in the fingers (unilateral pill-roll tremor), increases during stress or anxiety, and decreases with purposeful movement and sleep.

  Bradykinesia (slowness of voluntary movements and speech) also occurs. The patient walks with short, shuffling steps; his gait lacks normal parallel motion and may be retropulsive or propulsive. He has a monotonal way of speaking and a masklike facial expression. He may also experience drooling, dysphagia, dysarthria, and loss of posture control, causing him to walk with his body bent forward. An oculogyric crisis (eyes fixed upward and involuntary tonic movements) or blepharospasm (complete eyelid closure) may also occur.

Other causes

- ***Drugs.*** Phenothiazines and other antipsychotics (such as haloperidol, thiothixene, and loxapine) can cause cogwheel rigidity. Metoclopramide causes it infrequently.

Special considerations

If the patient has associated muscular dysfunction, assist him with ambulation, feeding, and other activities of daily living, as needed. Provide symptomatic care as appropriate. For example, if the patient develops constipation, administer a stool softener; if he experiences dysphagia, offer a soft diet with frequent small feedings. Refer the patient to the National Parkinson Foundation or the American Parkinson Disease Association, both of which provide educational materials and support.

Pediatric pointers

Cogwheel rigidity doesn't occur in children.

Cold intolerance

Usually developing gradually, this increased sensitivity to cold temperatures reflects damage to the body's temperature-regulating mechanism, based on interactions between the hypothalamus and the thyroid gland. Typically, the symptom results from a tumor or a hormonal deficiency. In elderly patients, cold intolerance reflects normal age-related physiologic changes.

History and physical examination

Find out when the patient first noticed cold intolerance by asking when he began using more blankets or wearing heavier clothing. A person may suffer transitory cold intolerance when moving from a tropical to a temperate climate; ask if the patient has recently made such a move. Ask about associated signs and symptoms, such as changes in vision or in the texture or amount of body hair. If the patient is female, ask about changes in her normal menstrual pattern.

Before proceeding with the physical examination, obtain a brief history. Does the patient have a history of hypothyroidism or hypothalamic disease? Is he taking any medications? If so, is he complying with the prescribed schedule and dosage? Has the regimen been changed recently?

Begin the physical examination by taking the patient's vital signs and checking for hypothermia, dry skin, and hair loss. Then ask the patient to straighten and extend his arms. Are his hands shaking? During the examination, note if the patient shivers or complains of chills. Provide a blanket if necessary.

Medical causes

◆ ***Hypopituitarism.*** Signs and symptoms of hypopituitarism usually develop slowly and vary with the disorder's severity. Cold intolerance and shivering typically accompany cold, dry, thin skin with a waxy pallor and fine wrinkles around the mouth. Other findings include fatigue, lethargy, menstrual disturbances, impotence, decreased libido, nervousness, irritability, headache, and hunger. If hypopituitarism results from a pituitary tumor, expect neurologic signs and symptoms, such as headache, bilateral temporal hemianopsia, loss of visual acuity, and possibly blindness.

◆ ***Hypothalamic lesion.*** A patient with hypothalamic damage may alternate from cold intolerance to heat intolerance. Cold intolerance develops suddenly; the patient typically complains of feeling chilled, shivering, and wearing extra clothes to keep warm. Related findings include amenorrhea, disturbed sleep pattern, increased thirst and urination, vigorous appetite with weight gain, impaired vision, headache, and personality changes, such as attacks of rage, laughing, and crying.

◆ ***Hypothyroidism.*** Cold intolerance develops early and worsens progressively in patients with this disorder. Other early findings include fatigue, anorexia with weight gain, constipation, and menorrhagia. As hypothyroidism progresses, the patient experiences loss of libido and slowed intellectual and motor activity. His hair becomes dry and sparse; nails, thick and brittle; and skin, dry, pale, cool, and doughy. Eventually, the patient displays a dull expression with periorbital and facial edema and puffy hands and feet. Relaxation is delayed after deep tendon reflex testing. Bradycardia, abdominal distention, and ataxia may also occur.

Special considerations

Help increase the patient's comfort by regulating his room temperature and providing extra clothing and blankets. Prepare him for diagnostic tests to determine the cause of cold intolerance.

Pediatric pointers

Some degree of cold intolerance is normal in infants because fat distribution is decreased and the temperature-regulating mechanism is immature at birth. Make sure parents understand that their infant will quickly lose body heat if he's exposed to cold temperatures. Instruct them to dress the infant warmly before sleep and going outdoors and to avoid chilling him during his bath.

An infant with cold intolerance due to hypothyroidism may have subtle, nonspecific signs of the underlying disorder or none at all. Typically, the infant shivers and has a temperature below 86° F (30° C), blue lips, and cold, mottled skin, especially on the extremities.

GERIATRIC POINTERS

Cold intolerance is common in older people because of metabolic changes associated with aging.

PATIENT COUNSELING

Allow the patient to openly express his concerns about body image changes related to his cold intolerance. Instruct him and his family to adapt the patient's environment to meet his needs. After the cause of cold intolerance is known, explain the disease process to the patient and his family to help alleviate their anxiety. Also explain that, with proper treatment, he can expect relief from his symptoms.

Confusion

An umbrella term for puzzling or inappropriate behavior or responses, confusion is the inability to think quickly and coherently. Depending on its cause, confusion may arise suddenly or gradually and may be temporary or irreversible. Aggravated by stress and sensory deprivation, confusion commonly occurs in hospitalized patients—especially the elderly, in whom it may be mistaken for senility.

Sudden severe confusion combined with hallucinations and psychomotor hyperactivity is classified as *delirium*. Long-term, progressive confusion with deterioration of all cognitive functions is classified as *dementia*.

Confusion can result from fluid and electrolyte imbalance or from hypoxemia due to pulmonary disorders. It can also stem from metabolic, neurologic, cardiovascular, cerebrovascular, or nutritional disorders; a severe systemic infection; or the effects of toxins, drugs, or alcohol. Confusion also may signal worsening of an underlying and perhaps irreversible disease.

HISTORY AND PHYSICAL EXAMINATION

When you take his history, ask the patient to describe what's bothering him. He may not report confusion as his chief complaint but may complain of memory loss, persistent apprehension, or the inability to concentrate. He may be unable to respond logically to direct questions. Check with a family member or friend about the onset and frequency of the patient's confusion. Find out, too, if the patient has a history of head trauma or a cardiopulmonary, metabolic, cerebrovascular, or neurologic disorder. Which medications is he taking, if any? Ask about any changes in eating or sleeping habits and in drug or alcohol use.

Perform an assessment to determine the presence of systemic disorders. Check vital signs, and assess the patient for changes in blood pressure, temperature, and pulse.

Next, perform a neurologic assessment to establish the patient's level of consciousness.

MEDICAL CAUSES

◆ ***Brain tumor.*** In the early stages of a brain tumor, confusion is usually mild and difficult to detect. As the tumor impinges on cerebral structures, however, confusion worsens and the patient may exhibit personality changes, bizarre behavior, sensory and motor deficits, visual field deficits, and aphasia.

◆ ***Cerebrovascular disorders.*** These disorders produce confusion due to tissue hypoxia and ischemia. Confusion may be insidious and fleeting, as in a transient ischemic attack, or acute and permanent, as in a stroke.

◆ ***Decreased cerebral perfusion.*** Mild confusion is an early symptom of decreased cerebral perfusion. Associated findings usually include hypotension, tachycardia or bradycardia, irregular pulse, ventricular gallop, edema, and cyanosis.

◆ ***Fluid and electrolyte imbalance.*** The extent of the imbalance determines the severity of the patient's confusion. Typically, he'll show signs of dehydration, such as lassitude, poor skin turgor, dry skin and mucous membranes, and oliguria. He may also develop hypotension and a low-grade fever.

◆ ***Head trauma.*** Concussion, contusion, and brain hemorrhage may produce confusion at the time of injury, shortly afterward, or months or even years afterward. The patient may be delirious, with periodic loss of consciousness. Vomiting, severe headache, pupillary changes, and sensory and motor deficits are also common.

◆ ***Heatstroke.*** This disorder causes pronounced confusion that gradually worsens as body temperature rises. Initially, the patient may be irritable and dizzy; later, he may become delirious, have seizures, and lose consciousness.

◆ ***Hypothermia.*** Confusion may be an early sign of this disorder. Typically, the patient displays slurred speech, cold and pale skin, hyperactive deep tendon reflexes, rapid pulse, and decreased blood pressure and respiratory rate. As his body temperature continues to drop, his confusion progresses to stupor and coma, his muscles become rigid, and his respiratory rate decreases.

◆ ***Hypoxemia.*** Acute pulmonary disorders that result in hypoxemia produce confusion that can range from mild disorientation to delirium. Chronic pulmonary disorders produce persistent confusion.

◆ ***Infection.*** A severe generalized infection, such as sepsis, commonly produces delirium. Central nervous system (CNS) infections, such as meningitis, cause varying degrees of confusion along with headache and nuchal rigidity.

◆ ***Metabolic encephalopathy.*** Both hyperglycemia and hypoglycemia can produce sudden confusion. A patient with hypoglycemia may also experience transient delirium and seizures. Uremic and hepatic encephalopathies produce gradual confusion that may progress to seizures and coma. Usually, the patient also experiences tremors and restlessness.

◆ ***Nutritional deficiencies.*** Inadequate dietary intake of thiamine, niacin, or vitamin B_{12} produces insidious, progressive confusion and possibly mental deterioration.

◆ ***Seizure disorders.*** Mild to moderate confusion may immediately follow any type of seizure. The confusion usually disappears within several hours.

◆ ***Thyroid hormone disorders.*** Hyperthyroidism produces mild to moderate confusion along with nervousness, inability to concentrate, weight loss, flushed skin, and tachycardia. Hypothyroidism produces mild, insidious confusion and memory loss; weight gain; bradycardia; and fatigue.

OTHER CAUSES

◆ ***Alcohol.*** Intoxication causes confusion and stupor, and alcohol withdrawal may cause delirium and seizures.

◆ ***Drugs.*** Large doses of CNS depressants produce confusion that can persist for several days after the drug is discontinued. Opioid and barbiturate withdrawal also causes acute confusion, possibly with delirium. Other drugs that commonly cause confusion include lidocaine, cardiac glycosides, indomethacin, cycloserine, chloroquine, atropine, and cimetidine.

◆ ***Heavy metal poisoning.*** Chronic ingestion or inhalation of heavy metals (such as lead, arsenic, mercury, and manganese) eventually produces confusion and, typically, weakness and drowsiness. The patient may also experience headache, vomiting, seizures, tremors, gait disturbances, and mental deterioration.

HERB ALERT *Herbal medicines, such as St. John's wort, can cause confusion, especially when taken in conjunction with an antidepressant or another serotonergic drug.*

SPECIAL CONSIDERATIONS

Never leave a confused patient unattended to prevent injury to himself and others. Keep the patient calm and quiet, and plan uninterrupted rest periods. To help him stay oriented, keep a large calendar and a clock visible, and make a list of his activities with specific dates and times. Reintroduce yourself to the patient each time you enter his room.

PEDIATRIC POINTERS

Confusion can't be determined in infants and very young children. However, older children with acute febrile illnesses commonly experience transient delirium or acute confusion.

Conjunctival injection

A common ocular sign associated with inflammation, conjunctival injection is nonuniform redness of the conjunctiva from hyperemia. This redness can be diffuse, localized, or peripheral, or it may encircle a clear cornea.

Conjunctival injection usually results from bacterial or viral conjunctivitis, but it can also signal a severe ocular disorder that, if untreated, may lead to permanent blindness. Conjunctival injection can also result from minor eye irritation due to inadequate sleep, overuse of contact lenses, environmental irritants, and excessive eye rubbing.

EMERGENCY INTERVENTIONS *If the patient with conjunctival injection reports a chemical splash to the eye, quickly irrigate the eye with copious amounts of normal saline solution. (First, remove contact lenses.) Evert the lids and wipe the fornices with a cotton-tipped applicator to remove any foreign body particles and as much of the chemical as possible.*

History and physical examination

When you take the patient's history, always ask if he has associated pain. If so, when did the pain begin, and where is it located? Is it constant or intermittent? Also, ask about itching, burning, photophobia, blurred vision, halo vision, excessive tearing, or a foreign body sensation in his eye. Does the patient have a history of eye disease or trauma? If he has suffered ocular trauma, avoid touching the affected eye. Test his visual acuity and intraocular pressure (IOP) only if his eyelids can be opened without applying pressure. Place a metal shield over the affected eye to protect it, if necessary.

If the patient's condition permits, examine the affected eye. First, determine the location and severity of conjunctival injection. Is it circumcorneal or localized? Peripheral or diffuse? Note any conjunctival or lid edema, ocular deviation, conjunctival follicles, ptosis, or exophthalmos. Also note the type and amount of any discharge.

Test the patient's visual acuity to establish a baseline. Note if the patient has had vision changes: Is his vision blurred or his visual acuity markedly decreased? Next, test pupillary reaction to light.

Perform IOP measurements. To gauge increased IOP without a tonometer, gently place your index finger over the closed eyelid; if the globe feels rock-hard, IOP is elevated.

Medical causes

◆ ***Blepharitis.*** This disorder produces diffuse conjunctival injection. Ulcerations appear on the eyelids, which burn, itch, and have no lashes.

◆ ***Chemical burns.*** Diffuse conjunctival injection occurs in this ocular emergency, but severe pain is the main symptom. The patient also displays photophobia, blepharospasm, and decreased visual acuity in the affected eye; the cornea may appear gray, and the pupil may be unilaterally smaller.

◆ ***Conjunctival foreign bodies and abrasions.*** These conditions feature localized conjunctival injection with sudden, severe eye pain. The patient may have increased tearing and photophobia, but his visual acuity usually isn't impaired.

◆ ***Conjunctivitis.*** Allergic conjunctivitis produces milky, diffuse peripheral conjunctival injection. Related findings include a watery, stringy eye discharge; increased tearing; itching; palpebral conjunctival follicles; and (with hay fever) conjunctival edema, photophobia, and a feeling of fullness around the eyes.

Bacterial conjunctivitis causes diffuse peripheral conjunctival injection along with a thick, purulent eye discharge that contains mucous threads. The patient's lids and lashes stick together, and he has excessive tearing, photophobia, burning, and itching. He may have pain and a foreign body sensation if the cornea is involved.

Besides diffuse peripheral conjunctival injection, the patient with fungal conjunctivitis complains of photophobia and increased tearing, itching, and burning. The discharge is thick and purulent, making his eyelids crusted, sticky, and swollen. Corneal involvement causes pain.

In viral conjunctivitis, the conjunctival injection is bright red, diffuse, and peripheral. The patient may also have conjunctival edema, follicles on the palpebral conjunctiva, and lid edema; a local viral rash; and signs of upper respiratory tract infection. He complains of itching, increased tearing and, possibly, a foreign body sensation.

◆ ***Corneal abrasion.*** Diffuse conjunctival injection is extremely painful in this disorder, especially when the eyelids move over the abrasion. The patient may also report photophobia, excessive tearing, blurred vision, and a foreign body sensation.

◆ ***Corneal erosion.*** Recurrent corneal erosion produces diffuse conjunctival injection; severe, continuous pain from rubbing of the eyelid over the eroded area of the cornea; and photophobia.

◆ ***Corneal ulcer.*** Bacterial, viral, and fungal corneal ulcers produce diffuse conjunctival injection that increases in the circumcorneal area. Accompanying findings include severe photophobia, severe pain in and around the eye, markedly decreased visual acuity, and a copious amount of purulent eye discharge and crusting. If the patient develops associated iritis, a physical examination will also reveal corneal opacities and an abnormal pupillary response to light.

◆ ***Dacryoadenitis.*** This disorder produces diffuse conjunctival injection, pain over the temporal part of the eye, considerable lid swelling and, possibly, a purulent eye discharge.

◆ ***Episcleritis.*** Conjunctival injection is localized and raised and may be violet or purplish pink in patients with episcleritis. Associated signs and symptoms include an inflamed sclera, deep pain, photophobia, increased tearing, and conjunctival edema.

◆ ***Glaucoma.*** In acute angle-closure glaucoma, conjunctival injection is typically circumcorneal. Other signs and symptoms include severe eye pain, nausea and vomiting, severely elevated IOP, blurred vision, and the perception of rainbow-colored halos around lights. Corneas appear steamy because of corneal edema. The pupil of the affected eye is moderately dilated and completely unresponsive to light.

◆ ***Hyphema.*** Depending on the type and extent of traumatic injury, a hyphema may produce diffuse conjunctival injection, possibly with lid and orbital edema. The patient may complain of pain in and around the eye. The extent of visual impairment depends on the hyphema's size and location.

◆ ***Iritis.*** In acute iritis, marked conjunctival injection is found mainly around the cornea. Other findings include moderate to severe pain, photophobia, blurred vision, constricted pupils, and poor pupillary response to light.

◆ ***Kawasaki syndrome.*** Conjunctival injection is a characteristic sign of Kawasaki syndrome and usually occurs bilaterally. This febrile illness, which primarily affects children under age 5, also causes erythema, lymphadenopathy, and swelling in the peripheral extremities. Treatment with I.V. gamma globulin is extremely effective if given immediately, so early detection is essential. Delaying treatment may cause coronary artery dilation and aneurysm, resulting in ischemic heart disease and, possibly, sudden death.

◆ ***Keratoconjunctivitis sicca.*** This disorder produces severe diffuse conjunctival injection. The patient reports generalized eye pain along with burning, itching, a foreign body sensation, excessive mucus secretion from the eye, absence of tears, and photophobia.

◆ ***Lyme disease.*** Spread by tick bites, Lyme disease may cause conjunctival injection, diffuse urticaria, malaise, fatigue, headache, fever, chills, aches, and lymphadenopathy.

◆ ***Ocular lacerations and intraocular foreign bodies.*** Diffuse conjunctival injection may be increased in the area of injury. The patient experiences impaired visual acuity and moderate to severe pain that varies with the type and extent of injury. He may also develop lid edema, photophobia, excessive tearing, and an abnormal pupillary response to light.

◆ ***Ocular tumors.*** A tumor located in the orbit behind the globe may produce conjunctival injection together with exophthalmos. Conjunctival edema, ocular deviation, and diplopia usually occur if muscles are involved.

◆ ***Refractive error.*** An uncorrected or poorly corrected refractive error can produce conjunctival injection. The patient may complain of headache, eye pain, and eye fatigue.

◆ ***Scleritis.*** In this relatively rare disorder, conjunctival injection can be diffuse or localized over the area of the scleritis nodule. The patient has severe pain on moving the eye, photophobia, tenderness, and tearing.

◆ ***Stevens-Johnson syndrome.*** This disorder produces diffuse conjunctival injection, a purulent eye discharge, severe eye pain, photophobia, decreased tearing, entropion, and trichiasis.

◆ ***Trachoma.*** Conjunctival injection is an early sign of trachoma, a leading cause of blindness in Third World countries and among Native Americans in the southwestern United States. Caused by a bacterial infection, trachoma may also produce eyelid swelling and corneal cloudiness.

◆ ***Uveitis.*** Diffuse conjunctival injection, which may be increased in the circumcorneal area, characterizes this disorder. Accompanying signs and symptoms include constricted, irregularly shaped pupils; blurred vision; tenderness; photophobia; and possibly sudden, severe ocular pain.

Special considerations

As indicated, prepare the patient for such diagnostic tests as orbital X-rays, ocular ultrasonography, and fluorescein staining. Obtain cultures of any eye discharge, and record its appearance, consistency, and amount.

Most forms of conjunctivitis are contagious and can easily spread to the other eye or to family members. Stress the importance of frequent hand washing and of not touching the affected eye to prevent contagion.

Pediatric pointers

An infant can develop self-limiting chemical conjunctivitis at birth from the ocular instillation of silver nitrate. He may also develop bacterial conjunctivitis 2 to 5 days after birth from contamination of the birth canal. An infant with congenital syphilis has prominent conjunctival injection and grayish pink corneas.

Patient counseling

If the patient complains of photophobia, darken the room or suggest that he wear sunglasses. If the patient's visual acuity is markedly decreased, orient him to his environment to ensure his comfort and safety.

Constipation

Constipation is defined as small, infrequent, or difficult bowel movements. Because normal bowel movements can vary in frequency and from individual to individual, constipation must be determined in relation to the patient's normal elimination pattern. Constipation may be a minor annoyance or, occasionally, a sign of a life-threatening disorder such as acute intestinal obstruction. Untreated, constipation can lead to headache, anorexia, and abdominal discomfort and can adversely affect the patient's lifestyle and well-being.

Constipation usually occurs when the urge to defecate is suppressed and the muscles associated with bowel movements remain contracted. Because the autonomic nervous system controls bowel movements—by sensing rectal distention from fecal contents and by stimulating the external sphincter—any factor that influences this system may cause bowel dysfunction. (See *How habits and stress cause constipation,* page 168.)

History and physical examination

Ask the patient to describe the frequency of his bowel movements and the size and consistency of his stools. How long has he had constipation? Acute constipation usually has an organic cause, such as an anal or rectal disorder. In a patient over age 45, a recent onset of constipation may be an early sign of colorectal cancer. Conversely, chronic constipation typically has a functional cause and may be related to stress.

Does the patient have pain related to constipation? If so, when did he first notice the pain, and where is it located? Cramping abdominal pain and distention suggest obstipation—extreme, persistent constipation due to intestinal tract obstruction. Ask the patient if defecation worsens or helps relieve the pain. Defecation usually worsens the pain, but in disorders such as irritable bowel syndrome, it may relieve it.

Ask the patient to describe a typical day's menu; estimate his daily fiber and fluid intake. Ask him, too, about any changes in eating habits, medication or alcohol use, or physical activity. Has he experienced recent emotional distress? Has constipation affected his family life or social contacts? Also, ask about his job. A sedentary or stressful job can contribute to constipation.

Find out whether the patient has a history of GI, rectoanal, neurologic, or metabolic disorders; abdominal surgery; or radiation therapy. Then ask about the medications he's taking, including over-the-counter preparations, such as laxatives, mineral oil, stool softeners, and enemas.

Inspect the abdomen for distention or scars from previous surgery. Then auscultate for bowel sounds, and characterize their motility. Percuss all four quadrants, and gently palpate for abdominal tenderness, a palpable mass, and hepatomegaly. Next, examine the patient's rectum. Spread his buttocks to expose the anus, and inspect for inflammation, lesions, scars, fissures, and external hemorrhoids. Use a disposable glove and lubricant to palpate the anal sphincter for laxity or stricture. Also palpate for rectal masses and fecal impaction. Finally, obtain a stool specimen and test it for occult blood.

As you assess the patient, remember that constipation can result from several life-threatening disorders, such as acute intestinal obstruction and mesenteric artery ischemia, but it doesn't herald these conditions.

Medical causes

◆ ***Anal fissure.*** A crack or laceration in the lining of the anal wall can cause acute constipation, usually due to the patient's fear of the severe tearing or burning pain associated with bowel movements. He may notice a few drops of blood streaking toilet tissue or his underwear.

◆ ***Anorectal abscess.*** In this disorder, constipation occurs together with severe, throbbing, localized pain and tenderness at the abscess site. The patient may also have localized inflammation, swelling, and purulent drainage and may complain of fever and malaise.

◆ ***Cirrhosis.*** In the early stages of cirrhosis, the patient experiences constipation along with nausea and vomiting, and a dull pain in the right upper quadrant. Other early findings include indigestion, anorexia, fatigue, malaise,

How habits and stress cause constipation

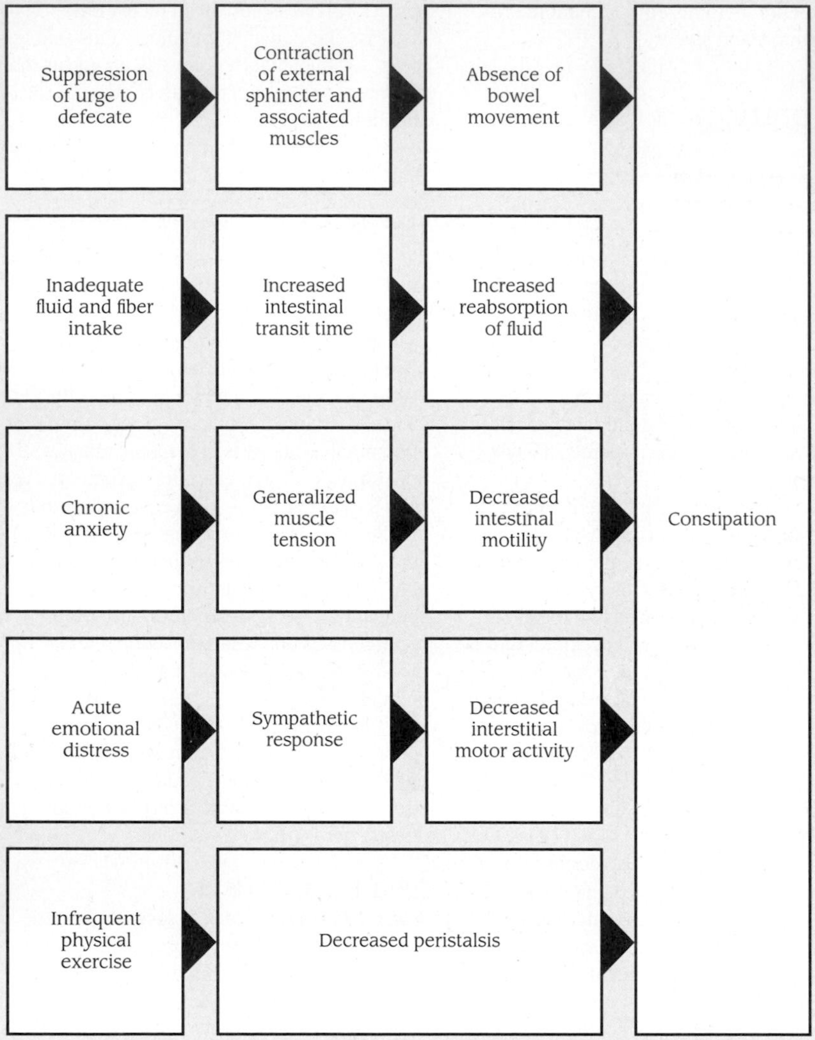

Suppression of urge to defecate	Contraction of external sphincter and associated muscles	Absence of bowel movement	Constipation
Inadequate fluid and fiber intake	Increased intestinal transit time	Increased reabsorption of fluid	Constipation
Chronic anxiety	Generalized muscle tension	Decreased intestinal motility	Constipation
Acute emotional distress	Sympathetic response	Decreased interstitial motor activity	Constipation
Infrequent physical exercise	Decreased peristalsis		Constipation

flatulence, hepatomegaly and, possibly, splenomegaly and diarrhea.

◆ ***Diabetic neuropathy.*** This type of neuropathy produces episodic constipation or diarrhea. Other signs and symptoms include dysphagia, orthostatic hypotension, syncope, and painless bladder distention with overflow incontinence. A male patient may also experience impotence and retrograde ejaculation.

◆ ***Diverticulitis.*** In this disorder, constipation or diarrhea occurs with left-lower-quadrant pain and tenderness and possibly a palpable, tender, firm, fixed abdominal mass. The patient may develop mild nausea, flatulence, or a low-grade fever.

◆ ***Hemorrhoids.*** Thrombosed hemorrhoids cause constipation as the patient tries to avoid the severe pain of defecation. The hemorrhoids may bleed during defecation.

◆ ***Hepatic porphyria.*** Abdominal pain, which may be severe, colicky, and localized or generalized, precedes constipation in hepatic porphyria. The patient may also have a fever, sinus tachycardia, labile hypertension, diaphoresis, severe vomiting, photophobia, urine retention, nervousness or restlessness, disorientation and, possibly, visual hallucinations. Deep tendon reflexes may be diminished or absent. Some patients have skin lesions causing itching, burning, erythema, altered pigmentation, and edema in areas exposed to light. Severe hepatic porphyria can produce delirium, coma, seizures, paraplegia, or complete flaccid quadriplegia.

◆ ***Hypercalcemia.*** In hypercalcemia, constipation usually is accompanied by anorexia, nausea, vomiting, polyuria, and polydipsia. The patient may also display arrhythmias, bone pain, muscle weakness and atrophy, hypoactive deep tendon reflexes, and personality changes.

◆ ***Hypothyroidism.*** Constipation occurs early and insidiously in patients with hypothyroidism; it may be accompanied by fatigue, sensitivity to cold, anorexia with weight gain, menorrhagia, decreased memory, hearing impairment, muscle cramps, and paresthesia.

◆ ***Intestinal obstruction.*** Constipation associated with this disorder varies in severity and onset, depending on the location and extent of the obstruction. In a partial obstruction, constipation may alternate with leakage of liquid stools. In a complete obstruction, obstipation may occur. Constipation can be the earliest sign of partial colon obstruction, but it usually occurs later if the level of the obstruction is more proximal. Associated findings include episodes of colicky abdominal pain, abdominal distention, nausea, and vomiting. The patient may also develop hyperactive bowel sounds, visible peristaltic waves, a palpable abdominal mass, and abdominal tenderness.

◆ ***Irritable bowel syndrome.*** This common syndrome usually produces intermittent watery diarrhea, although some patients have chronic constipation and others complain of alternating constipation and diarrhea. Stress may trigger nausea and abdominal distention and tenderness, but defecation usually relieves these signs and symptoms. Many patients have an intense urge to defecate and feelings of incomplete evacuation. Typically, the stools are scybalous and contain visible mucus.

◆ ***Mesenteric artery ischemia.*** This life-threatening disorder produces sudden constipation with failure to expel stool or flatus. Initially, the abdomen is soft and nontender but soon severe abdominal pain, tenderness, vomiting, and anorexia occur. Later, the patient may develop abdominal guarding, rigidity, and distention; tachycardia; syncope; tachypnea; fever; and signs of shock, such as cool, clammy skin and hypotension. A bruit may be heard.

◆ ***Multiple sclerosis (MS).*** This disorder can produce constipation in addition to ocular disturbances, such as nystagmus, blurred vision, and diplopia; vertigo; and sensory disturbances. The patient may also have motor weakness, seizures, paralysis, muscle spasticity, gait ataxia, intention tremor, hyperreflexia, dysarthria, or dysphagia. MS can also produce urinary urgency, frequency, and incontinence as well as emotional instability. A male patient may experience impotence.

◆ ***Spinal cord lesion.*** Constipation may occur in this disorder along with urine retention, sexual dysfunction, pain, and possibly motor weakness, paralysis, or sensory impairment below the level of the lesion.

◆ ***Tabes dorsalis.*** In tabes dorsalis, constipation is accompanied by an ataxic gait; paresthesia; loss of sensation of body position, deep pain, and temperature; Charcot's joints; Argyll Robertson pupils; diminished deep tendon reflexes; and possibly impotence.

◆ ***Ulcerative colitis.*** Constipation may occur in patients with chronic ulcerative colitis, but bloody diarrhea with pus, mucus, or both is the hallmark of this disorder. Other signs and symptoms include cramping lower abdominal pain, tenesmus, anorexia, low-grade fever and, occasionally, nausea and vomiting. Bowel sounds may be hyperactive. Later, weight loss, weakness, and arthralgias occur.

◆ ***Ulcerative proctitis.*** This disorder produces acute constipation with tenesmus. The patient feels an intense urge to defecate but is unable to do so. Instead, he may eliminate mucus, pus, or blood.

OTHER CAUSES

◆ ***Diagnostic tests.*** Constipation can result from the retention of barium given during certain GI studies.

◆ ***Drugs.*** Many patients experience constipation when taking an opioid analgesic or other drugs, including vinca alkaloids, calcium channel blockers, antacids containing aluminum or calcium, anticholinergics, and drugs with anticholinergic effects (such as tricyclic antidepressants). Patients may also experience constipation from excessive use of laxatives or enemas.

◆ ***Surgery and radiation therapy.*** Constipation can result from rectoanal surgery, which may traumatize nerves, and abdominal irradiation, which may cause intestinal stricture.

Special considerations

As indicated, prepare the patient for diagnostic tests, such as proctosigmoidoscopy, colonoscopy, barium enema, plain abdominal films, and an upper GI series. If the patient is on bed rest, reposition him frequently, and help him perform active or passive exercises as indicated. Teach him abdominal toning exercises if his abdominal muscles are weak and relaxation techniques to help him reduce stress related to constipation.

Pediatric pointers

The high content of casein and calcium in cow's milk can produce hard stools and possibly constipation in bottle-fed infants. Other causes of constipation in infants include Hirschsprung's disease, inadequate fluid intake, and anal fissures. In older children, constipation usually results from inadequate fiber intake and excessive intake of milk; it can also result from bowel spasm, mechanical obstruction, hypothyroidism, reluctance to stop playing for bathroom breaks, and the lack of privacy in some school bathrooms.

Geriatric pointers

Acute constipation in elderly patients is usually associated with underlying structural abnormalities. Chronic constipation, however, is chiefly caused by lifelong bowel elimination and dietary habits and laxative use.

Patient counseling

Caution the patient not to strain during defecation to prevent injuring rectoanal tissue. Instruct him to avoid using laxatives or enemas. If he has been abusing these products, begin to wean him from them. Use a disposable glove and lubricant to remove impacted fecal contents. (Check if an oil-retention enema can be given first to soften the fecal mass.)

Stress the importance of a high-fiber diet, and encourage the patient to drink plenty of fluids. (Explain that he may experience temporary bloating or flatulence after adding fiber to his diet.) Also, encourage him to exercise at least 1 1/2 hours each week, if possible.

Corneal reflex, absent

The corneal reflex is tested bilaterally by drawing a fine-pointed wisp of sterile cotton from a corner of each eye to the cornea. Normally, even though only one eye is tested at a time, the patient blinks bilaterally each time either cornea is touched—this is the corneal reflex. When this reflex is absent, neither eyelid closes when the cornea of one is touched. (See *Eliciting the corneal reflex.*)

The afferent fibers for this reflex are located in the ophthalmic branch of the trigeminal nerve (cranial nerve V); the efferent fibers are located in the facial nerve (cranial nerve VII). Unilateral or bilateral absence of the corneal reflex may result from damage to these nerves.

History and physical examination

If you can't elicit the corneal reflex, look for other signs of trigeminal nerve dysfunction. To test the three sensory portions of the nerve, touch each side of the patient's face on the brow, cheek, and jaw with a cotton wisp, and ask him to compare the sensations.

If you suspect facial nerve involvement, determine whether both the upper face (brow and eyes) and lower face (cheek, mouth, and chin) are weak bilaterally. Lower-motor-neuron facial weakness affects the face on the same side as the lesion, whereas upper-motor-neuron weakness affects the side opposite the lesion—predominantly the lower facial muscles.

Because an absent corneal reflex may signify such progressive neurologic disorders as Guillain-Barré syndrome, ask the patient about associated symptoms, such as facial pain, dysphagia, and limb weakness.

Medical causes

◆ ***Acoustic neuroma.*** This tumor affects the trigeminal nerve, causing a diminished or absent corneal reflex, tinnitus, and unilateral hearing impairment. Facial palsy and anesthesia, palate weakness, and signs of cerebellar dysfunction (ataxia, nystagmus) may result if the tumor impinges on the adjacent cranial nerves, brain stem, and cerebellum.

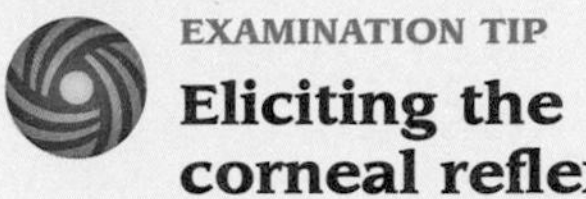

EXAMINATION TIP

Eliciting the corneal reflex

To elicit the corneal reflex, have the patient turn his eyes away from you to avoid blinking involuntarily during the procedure. Then approach the patient from the opposite side, out of his line of vision, and brush the cornea lightly with a fine wisp of sterile cotton. Repeat the procedure on the other eye.

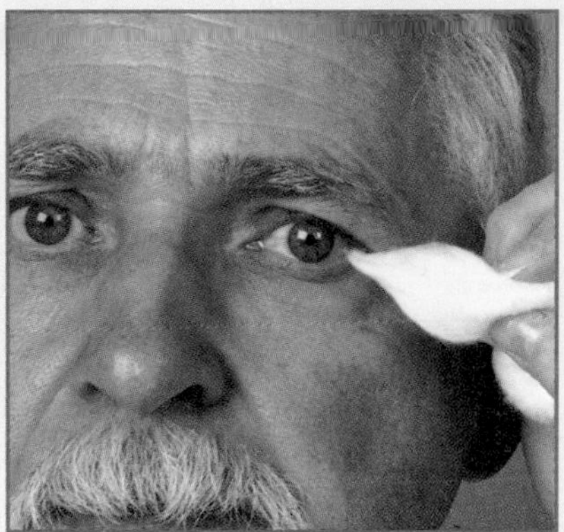

◆ ***Bell's palsy.*** A common cause of diminished or absent corneal reflex, Bell's palsy causes paralysis of cranial nerve VII. It can also produce complete hemifacial weakness or paralysis and drooling on the affected side. The affected side also sags and appears masklike. The eye on this side can't be shut and tears constantly.

◆ ***Brain stem infarction or injury.*** An absent corneal reflex can occur on the side opposite the lesion when a brain stem infarction or injury affects cranial nerve V or VII or their connection in the central trigeminal tract. Associated findings include decreased level of consciousness, dysphagia, dysarthria, contralateral limb weakness, and early signs and symptoms of increased intracranial pressure, such as headache and vomiting.

In a massive brain stem infarction or injury, the patient also displays respiratory changes, such as apneustic breathing or periods of apnea; bilateral pupillary dilation or constriction with decreased responsiveness to light; rising systolic blood pressure; widening pulse pressure; bradycardia; and coma.

◆ ***Guillain-Barré syndrome.*** In this polyneuropathic disorder, a diminished or absent corneal reflex accompanies ipsilateral loss of facial muscle control. Muscle weakness, the primary neurologic sign of this disorder, typically starts in the legs, then extends to the arms and facial nerves within 72 hours. Other findings include dysarthria, dysphagia, paresthesia, respiratory muscle paralysis, respiratory insufficiency, orthostatic hypotension, incontinence, diaphoresis, and tachycardia.

◆ ***Herpetic keratoconjunctivitis.*** This disorder may cause corneal anesthesia, usually unilaterally. Other findings include regional adenopathy, blepharitis, and vesicles on the eyelid.

◆ ***Trigeminal neuralgia (tic douloureux).*** A diminished or absent corneal reflex may stem from a superior maxillary lesion that affects the ophthalmic branch. The patient with trigeminal neuralgia characteristically experiences sudden bursts of intense pain or shooting sensations, lasting from 1 to 15 minutes, in one of the divisions of the trigeminal nerve, primarily the superior mandibular or maxillary division. An attack may be triggered by local stimulation, such as a light touch to the cheeks, exposure to hot or cold temperatures, or eating or drinking hot or cold food or beverages. Areas around the patient's nose and mouth may be hypersensitive.

SPECIAL CONSIDERATIONS

When the corneal reflex is absent, you'll need to take measures to protect the patient's affected eye from injury, such as lubricating the eye with artificial tears to prevent drying. Cover the cornea with a shield and avoid excessive corneal reflex testing. Prepare the patient for a computed tomography scan or cranial X-rays.

PEDIATRIC POINTERS

Brain stem lesions and injuries are the most common causes of an absent corneal reflex in children; Guillain-Barré syndrome and trigeminal neuralgia are less common causes. Infants, especially those born prematurely, may have an absent corneal reflex due to anoxic damage to the brain stem.

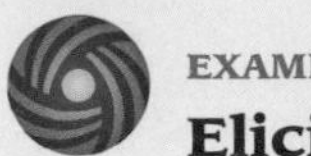

EXAMINATION TIP

Eliciting CVA tenderness

To elicit costovertebral angle (CVA) tenderness, have the patient sit upright facing away from you or have him lie in a prone position. Place the palm of your left hand over the left CVA; then strike the back of your left hand with the ulnar surface of your right fist (as shown). Repeat this percussion technique over the right CVA. A patient with CVA tenderness will experience intense pain.

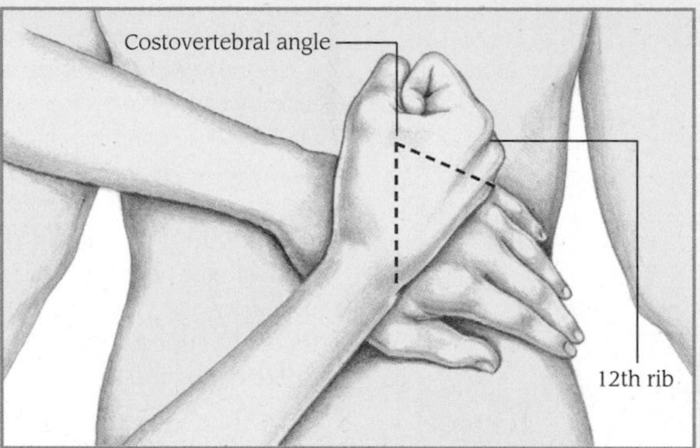

Costovertebral angle tenderness

Costovertebral angle (CVA) tenderness indicates sudden distention of the renal capsule. It almost always accompanies unelicited, dull, constant flank pain in the CVA just lateral to the sacrospinal muscle and below the 12th rib. This associated pain typically travels anteriorly in the subcostal region toward the umbilicus.

Percussing the CVA elicits tenderness, if present. (See *Eliciting CVA tenderness.*) A patient who doesn't have this symptom will perceive a thudding, jarring, or pressurelike sensation—but no pain—when tested. A patient with a disorder that distends the renal capsule will experience intense pain as the renal capsule stretches and stimulates the afferent nerves that emanate from the spinal cord at levels T11 through L2 and innervate the kidney.

History and physical examination

After detecting CVA tenderness, determine the possible extent of renal damage. First, find out if the patient has other symptoms of renal or urologic dysfunction. Ask about voiding habits: How frequently does he urinate and in what amounts? Has he noticed any change in intake or output? If so, when did he notice it? (Ask about fluid intake before judging his output as abnormal.) Does he have nocturia, pain or burning during urination, or difficulty starting a stream? Does the patient strain to urinate without being able to do so (tenesmus)? Ask about urine color; brown or bright red urine may contain blood.

Explore other signs and symptoms. For example, if the patient is experiencing pain in his flank, abdomen, or back, when did he first notice it? How severe is it, and where is it located? Find out if the patient or a family member has a history of urinary tract infections, congenital anomalies, calculi, or other obstructive nephropathies or uropathies. Also, ask about a history of renovascular disorders, such as occlusion of the renal arteries or veins.

Perform a brief physical examination. Begin by taking the patient's vital signs. Fever and chills in a patient with CVA tenderness may indicate acute pyelonephritis. If the patient has hypertension and bradycardia, be alert for other autonomic effects of renal pain, such as diaphoresis and pallor. Inspect, auscultate, and gently palpate the abdomen for clues to the underlying cause of CVA tenderness. Be alert for abdominal distention, hypoactive bowel sounds, and palpable masses.

Medical causes

◆ ***Calculi.*** Infundibular and ureteropelvic or ureteral calculi produce CVA tenderness and waves of waxing and waning flank pain that may radiate to the groin, testicles, suprapubic area, or labia. The patient may also develop nausea, vomiting, severe abdominal pain, abdominal distention, and decreased bowel sounds.

◆ ***Perirenal abscess.*** Causing exquisite CVA tenderness, this disorder may also produce severe unilateral flank pain, dysuria, persistent high fever, chills, erythema of the skin, and sometimes a palpable abdominal mass.

◆ ***Pyelonephritis (acute).*** Perhaps the most common cause of CVA tenderness, acute pyelonephritis is commonly accompanied by persistent high fever, chills, flank pain, anorexia, nausea and vomiting, weakness, dysuria, hematuria, nocturia, urinary urgency and frequency, and tenesmus.

◆ ***Renal artery occlusion.*** In this disorder, the patient experiences flank pain as well as CVA tenderness. Other findings include severe, continuous upper abdominal pain; nausea; vomiting; decreased bowel sounds; and high fever.

◆ ***Renal vein occlusion.*** The patient with this disorder has CVA tenderness and flank pain. He may also have sudden, severe back pain; fever; oliguria; edema; and hematuria.

Special considerations

Administer pain medication, and continue to monitor the patient's vital signs and intake and output. Collect blood and urine samples, and then prepare the patient for radiologic studies, such as excretory urography, renal arteriography, and computed tomography scan.

Pediatric pointers

An infant with a disorder that distends the renal capsule won't exhibit CVA tenderness. Instead, he'll display nonspecific signs and symptoms, such as vomiting, diarrhea, fever, irritability, poor skin perfusion, and yellow to gray skin color. In older children, however, CVA tenderness has the same diagnostic significance as in adults. Vaginal discharge, vulval soreness, and pruritus may occur in girls.

Geriatric pointers

Advanced age and cognitive impairment reduce an elderly patient's ability to perceive pain or to describe its intensity.

Cough, barking

Resonant, brassy, and harsh, a barking cough is part of a complex of signs and symptoms that characterize croup syndrome, a group of pediatric disorders marked by varying degrees of respiratory distress. Croup syndrome is most common in boys and most prevalent in the fall; it may recur in the same child.

A barking cough indicates edema of the larynx and surrounding tissue. Because children's airways are smaller in diameter than those of adults, edema can rapidly lead to airway occlusion, a life-threatening emergency.

EMERGENCY INTERVENTIONS *Quickly evaluate the child's respiratory status. Then take his vital signs. Be particularly alert for tachycardia and signs of hypoxemia. Also, check for a decreased level of consciousness. Try to determine if the child was playing with a small object that he may have aspirated.*

Check for cyanosis in the lips and nail beds. Observe the patient for sternal or intercostal retractions or nasal flaring. Next, note the depth and rate of his respirations; they may become increasingly shallow as respiratory distress increases. Observe the child's body position. Is he sitting up, leaning forward, and struggling to breathe? Observe his activity level and facial expression. As respiratory distress increases from airway edema, the child will become restless and have a frightened, wide-eyed expression. As air hunger continues, the child will become lethargic and difficult to arouse.

If the child shows signs of severe respiratory distress, try to calm him, maintain airway patency, and provide oxygen. Endotracheal intubation or a tracheotomy may be necessary.

History and physical examination

Ask the child's parents when the barking cough began and what other signs and symptoms accompanied it. When did the child first appear to be ill? Has he had previous episodes of croup syndrome? Did his condition improve upon exposure to cold air?

Spasmodic croup and epiglottiditis typically occur in the middle of the night. The child with spasmodic croup has no fever, but the child with epiglottiditis has a high fever of sudden onset. An upper respiratory tract infection typically is followed by laryngotracheobronchitis.

Medical causes

◆ ***Aspiration of foreign body.*** Partial obstruction of the upper airway first produces sudden hoarseness, then a barking cough and inspiratory stridor. Other effects of this life-threatening condition include gagging, tachycardia, dyspnea, decreased breath sounds, wheezing, and possibly cyanosis.

◆ ***Epiglottiditis.*** This life-threatening disorder has become less common since the use of influenza vaccines. It occurs nocturnally, heralded by a barking cough and a high fever. The child is hoarse, dysphagic, dyspneic, and restless and appears extremely ill and panicky. The cough may progress to severe respiratory distress with sternal and intercostal retractions, nasal flaring, cyanosis, and tachycardia. The child will struggle to get sufficient air as epiglottic edema increases. Epiglottiditis is a true medical emergency.

◆ ***Laryngotracheobronchitis (acute).*** Also known as viral croup, this infection is most common in children between ages 9 and 18 months and usually occurs in the fall and early winter. It initially produces low to moderate fever, runny nose, poor appetite, and infrequent cough. When the infection descends into the laryngotracheal area, a barking cough, hoarseness, and inspiratory stridor occur.

As respiratory distress progresses, substernal and intercostal retractions occur along with tachycardia and shallow, rapid respirations. Sleeping in a dry room worsens these signs. The patient becomes restless, irritable, pale, and cyanotic.

◆ ***Spasmodic croup.*** Acute spasmodic croup usually occurs during sleep with the abrupt onset of a barking cough that awakens the child. Typically, he doesn't have a fever but may be hoarse, restless, and dyspneic. As his respiratory distress worsens, the child may exhibit sternal and intercostal retractions, nasal flaring, tachycardia, cyanosis, and an anxious, frantic appearance. The signs usually subside within a few hours, but attacks tend to recur.

Special considerations

Don't attempt to inspect the throat of a child with a barking cough unless intubation equipment is available. If the child isn't in severe respiratory distress, a lateral neck X-ray may be done to visualize epiglottal edema; however, a negative X-ray doesn't completely rule out epiglottal edema. A chest X-ray may also be done to rule out lower respiratory tract infection. Depending on the child's age and the degree of respiratory distress, oxygen may be administered. Rapid-acting epinephrine and a steroid should be considered.

Be sure to observe the child frequently, and monitor the oxygen level if used. Provide the child with periods of rest with minimal interruptions. Maintain a calm, quiet environment and offer reassurance. Encourage the parents to stay with the child to help alleviate stress.

Teach the parents how to evaluate and treat recurrent episodes of croup syndrome. For example, creating steam by running hot water in a sink or shower and sitting with the child in the closed bathroom may help relieve subsequent attacks. The child may also benefit from being brought outside (properly dressed) to breathe cold night air.

Cough, nonproductive

A nonproductive cough is a noisy, forceful expulsion of air from the lungs that doesn't yield sputum or blood. It's one of the most common complaints of patients with respiratory disorders.

Coughing is a necessary protective mechanism that clears airway passages. However, a nonproductive cough is ineffective and can cause damage, such as airway collapse or rupture of alveoli or blebs. A nonproductive cough that later becomes productive is a classic sign of progressive respiratory disease.

The cough reflex generally occurs when mechanical, chemical, thermal, inflammatory, or psychogenic stimuli activate cough receptors. (See *Reviewing the cough mechanism*.) However, external pressure—for example, from subdiaphragmatic irritation or a mediastinal tumor—can also induce it, as can voluntary expiration of air, which occasionally occurs as a nervous habit.

A nonproductive cough may occur in paroxysms and can worsen by becoming more frequent. An acute cough has a sudden

Reviewing the cough mechanism

Cough receptors are thought to be located in the nose, sinuses, auditory canals, nasopharynx, larynx, trachea, bronchi, pleurae, diaphragm and, possibly, the pericardium and GI tract. Once a cough receptor is stimulated, the vagus and glossopharyngeal nerves transmit the impulse to the "cough center" in the medulla. From there, the impulse is transmitted to the larynx and to the intercostal and abdominal muscles. Deep inspiration (1) is followed by closure of the glottis (2), relaxation of the diaphragm, and contraction of the abdominal and intercostal muscles. The resulting increased pressure in the lungs opens the glottis to release the forceful, noisy expiration known as a cough (3).

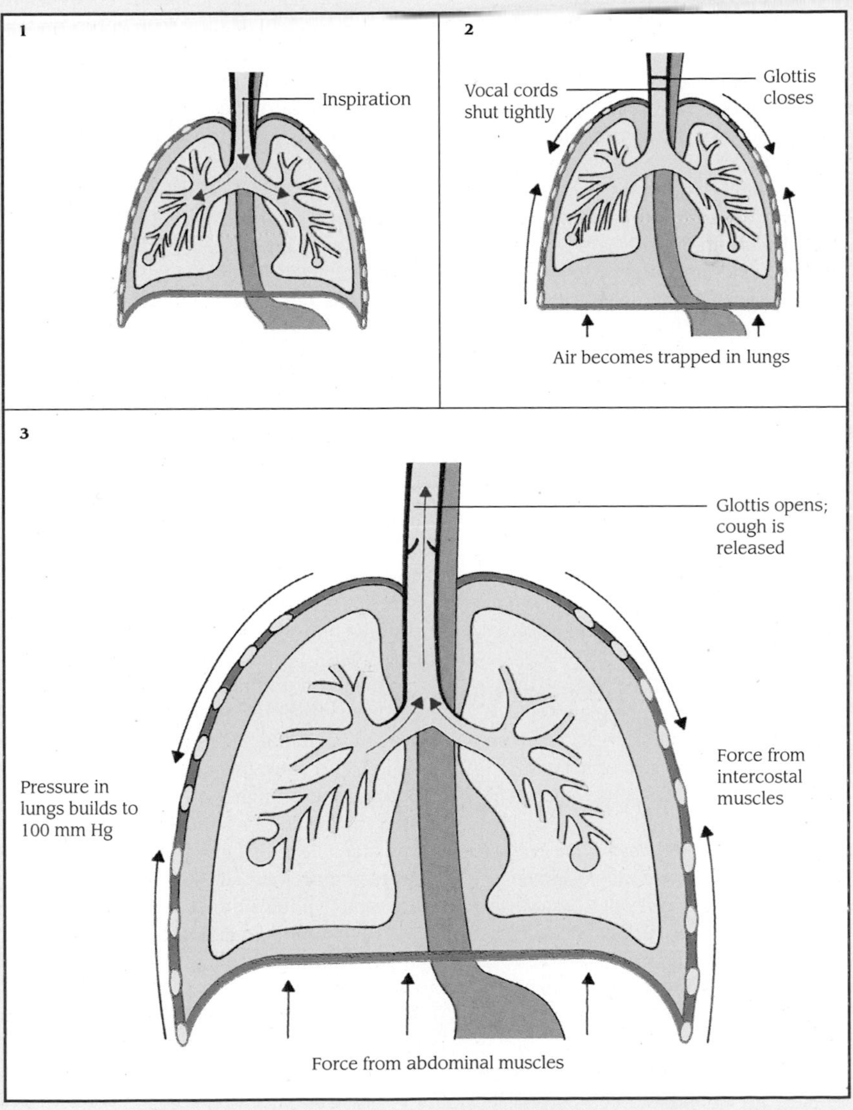
1
Inspiration
2
Vocal cords shut tightly
Glottis closes
Air becomes trapped in lungs
3
Glottis opens; cough is released
Pressure in lungs builds to 100 mm Hg
Force from intercostal muscles
Force from abdominal muscles

onset and may be self-limiting; a cough that persists beyond 1 month is considered chronic and commonly results from cigarette smoking.

Someone with a chronic nonproductive cough may downplay or overlook it or accept it as normal. In fact, he generally won't seek medical attention unless he has other symptoms. A foreign body in a child's external auditory canal may result in a cough. Always examine the child's ears.

History and physical examination

Ask the patient when his cough began and whether any body position, time of day, or specific activity affects it. How does the cough sound—harsh, brassy, dry, or hacking? Try to determine if the cough is related to smoking or a chemical irritant. If the patient smokes or has smoked, note the number of packs smoked daily multiplied by years ("pack-years"). Next, ask about the frequency and intensity of the coughing. If he has any pain associated with coughing, breathing, or activity, when did it begin and where is it located?

Ask the patient about recent illness (especially a cardiovascular or pulmonary disorder), surgery, or trauma. Also ask about hypersensitivity to drugs, foods, pets, dust, or pollen. Find out which medications the patient takes, if any, and ask about recent changes in schedule or dosages. Also ask about recent changes in his appetite, weight, exercise tolerance, or energy level; recent exposure to irritating fumes, chemicals, or smoke; and recent travel to foreign countries.

As you're taking his history, observe the patient's general appearance and manner: Is he agitated, restless, or lethargic; pale, diaphoretic, or flushed; anxious, confused, or nervous? Also, note whether he's cyanotic or has clubbed fingers or peripheral edema.

CULTURAL CUE *Because of the fear of being known as someone with tuberculosis (TB), the patient may be reluctant to provide information about his signs and symptoms such as cough. Ask the patient at risk for TB—those born in another country, those in contact with acute TB, and those with high-risk behaviors—about potential TB exposure.*

Next, perform a physical examination. Start by taking the patient's vital signs. Check the depth and rhythm of his respirations, and note wheezing or "crowing" noises that occur with breathing. Feel the patient's skin: Is it cold or warm; clammy or dry? Check his nose and mouth for congestion, inflammation, drainage, or signs of infection. Inspect his neck for distended veins and tracheal deviation, and palpate for masses or enlarged lymph nodes.

Examine his chest, observing its configuration and looking for abnormal chest wall motion. Do you note any retractions or use of accessory muscles? Percuss for dullness, tympany, or flatness. Auscultate for wheezing, crackles, rhonchi, pleural friction rub, and decreased or absent breath sounds. Finally, examine his abdomen for distention, tenderness, or masses, and auscultate it for abnormal bowel sounds.

Medical causes

◆ ***Airway occlusion.*** Partial occlusion of the upper airway produces a sudden onset of dry, paroxysmal coughing. The patient exhibits gagging, wheezing, hoarseness, stridor, tachycardia, and decreased breath sounds.

◆ ***Anthrax (inhalation).*** This acute infectious disease is caused by the gram-positive, spore-forming bacterium *Bacillus anthracis.* Although the disease most commonly occurs in wild and domestic grazing animals, such as cattle, sheep, and goats, the spores can live in the soil for many years. The disease can occur in humans exposed to infected animals, tissue from infected animals, or biological agents. Most natural cases occur in agricultural regions worldwide. Anthrax may occur in cutaneous, inhalation, or GI forms.

Inhalation anthrax is caused by inhalation of aerosolized spores. Initial signs and symptoms are flulike and include fever, chills, weakness, cough, and chest pain. The disease generally occurs in two stages with a period of recovery after the initial signs and symptoms. The second stage develops abruptly and causes rapid deterioration marked by fever, dyspnea, stridor, and hypotension; death generally results within 24 hours. Radiologic findings include mediastinitis and symmetrical mediastinal widening.

◆ ***Aortic aneurysm (thoracic).*** This disorder causes a brassy cough with dyspnea, hoarseness, wheezing, and a substernal ache in the shoulders, lower back, or abdomen. The patient may also have facial or neck edema, jugular vein distention, dysphagia, prominent veins over his chest, stridor, and possibly paresthesia or neuralgia.

◆ ***Asthma.*** Asthma attacks commonly occur at night, starting with a nonproductive cough and mild wheezing and progressing to severe dyspnea, audible wheezing, chest tightness, and a cough that produces thick mucus. Other signs include apprehension, rhonchi, prolonged expirations, intercostal and supraclavicular retractions on inspiration, accessory muscle use, flaring nostrils, tachypnea, tachycardia, diaphoresis, and flushing or cyanosis.

◆ ***Atelectasis.*** As lung tissue deflates in atelectasis, it stimulates cough receptors, causing a nonproductive cough. The patient may also have pleuritic chest pain, anxiety, dyspnea, tachypnea, tachycardia, decreased breath sounds, cyanotic skin, and diaphoresis. His chest may be dull on percussion, and he may exhibit inspiratory lag, substernal or intercostal retractions, decreased vocal fremitus, and tracheal deviation toward the affected side.

◆ ***Avian influenza.*** These potentially life-threatening viruses are spread to humans through infected poultry and surfaces contaminated with infected bird excretions. Infected individuals may initially have symptoms of conventional influenza, including a nonproductive cough, fever, sore throat, and muscle aches. The most virulent avian virus, influenza A (H5N1), may lead to severe and life-threatening complications, such as acute respiratory distress and pneumonia. To date this strain of the virus has not surfaced in the United States; however, a recent outbreak in Asian and European countries has caused worldwide concern that the virus may spread through both infected humans and birds. Treatment with two of the four FDA-approved antiviral medications has proven effective with some virus strains, and an experimental vaccine is currently under investigation.

◆ ***Bronchitis (chronic).*** This disorder starts with a nonproductive, hacking cough that later becomes productive. Other findings include prolonged expiration, wheezing, dyspnea, accessory muscle use, barrel chest, cyanosis, tachypnea, crackles, and scattered rhonchi. Clubbing can occur in late stages.

◆ ***Bronchogenic carcinoma.*** The earliest indicators of this disease can be a chronic nonproductive cough, dyspnea, and vague chest pain. The patient may also be wheezing.

◆ ***Common cold.*** Most colds start with a nonproductive, hacking cough and progress to some mix of sneezing, rhinorrhea, nasal congestion, sore throat, headache, malaise, fatigue, myalgia, and arthralgia.

◆ ***Esophageal achalasia.*** In this disorder, regurgitation and aspiration produce a dry cough and, possibly, recurrent pulmonary infections and dysphagia.

◆ ***Esophageal diverticula.*** The patient with this disorder has a nocturnal nonproductive cough, regurgitation and aspiration, dyspepsia, and dysphagia. His neck may appear swollen and have a gurgling sound. He may also exhibit halitosis and weight loss.

◆ ***Esophageal occlusion.*** This disorder is marked by sudden nonproductive coughing and gagging with a sensation of something stuck in the throat. Other findings include neck or chest pain and dysphagia.

◆ ***Esophagitis with reflux.*** This disorder commonly causes a nonproductive nocturnal cough due to regurgitation and aspiration. The patient may also experience chest pain that mimics angina pectoris, heartburn that worsens if he lies down after eating, increased salivation, dysphagia, hematemesis, and melena.

◆ **Hantavirus *pulmonary syndrome.*** A nonproductive cough is common in patients with this disorder, which is marked by noncardiogenic pulmonary edema. Other findings include headache, myalgia, fever, nausea, and vomiting.

◆ ***Hodgkin's disease.*** This disease may cause a crowing nonproductive cough. However, the earliest sign is usually painless swelling of one of the cervical lymph nodes or, occasionally, of the axillary, mediastinal, or inguinal lymph nodes. Another early sign is pruritus. Other findings depend on the degree and location of systemic involvement and include dyspnea, dysphagia, hepatosplenomegaly, edema, jaundice, nerve pain, and hyperpigmentation.

◆ ***Hypersensitivity pneumonitis.*** In this disorder, an acute nonproductive cough, fever, dyspnea, and malaise usually occur 5 to 6 hours after exposure to an antigen.

◆ ***Influenza type A H1N1 virus (Swine flu).*** Influenza type A H1N1, or swine flu, is a respiratory disease of pigs caused by type A influenza virus. Swine flu viruses cause high levels of illness and low death rates in pigs. Swine flu viruses normally don't infect humans. However, sporadic human infections with swine flu have occurred. Most commonly, these cases occur in persons with direct exposure to pigs. The virus has changed slightly and is known as H1N1 flu. Outbreaks of H1N1 flu in 2009 showed that the virus is able to be transmitted from person to person, causing transmission across the globe. The H1N1 flu is similar to influenza, and causes illness and in some cases death. The symptoms of swine flu include nonproductive cough, fever, fatigue, myalgia, chills, headache, and vomiting. The use of antiviral drugs is recommended to treat H1N1 flu.

◆ ***Interstitial lung disease.*** A patient with this disorder has a nonproductive cough and progressive dyspnea. He may also be cyanotic and have clubbing, fine crackles, fatigue, variable chest pain, and weight loss.

◆ ***Laryngeal tumor.*** A mild nonproductive cough, minor throat discomfort, and hoarseness are early signs of this disorder. Later, dysphagia, dyspnea, cervical lymphadenopathy, stridor, and earache may occur.

◆ ***Laryngitis.*** Acute laryngitis causes a nonproductive cough with localized pain (especially when the patient swallows or speaks) as well as fever and malaise. His hoarseness can range from mild to complete loss of voice.

◆ ***Legionnaires' disease.*** After a prodrome of malaise, headache and, possibly, diarrhea, anorexia, diffuse myalgia, and general weakness, legionnaires' disease causes a nonproductive cough that later produces mucoid, nonpurulent and, possibly, blood-tinged sputum.

◆ ***Lung abscess.*** This disorder typically begins with a nonproductive cough, weakness, dyspnea, and pleuritic chest pain. The patient may also exhibit diaphoresis, fever, headache, malaise, fatigue, crackles, decreased breath sounds, anorexia, and weight loss. Later, his cough produces large amounts of purulent, foul-smelling and, possibly, blood-tinged sputum.

◆ ***Mediastinal tumor.*** A large mediastinal tumor produces a nonproductive cough, dyspnea, and retrosternal pain. The patient may also develop stertorous respirations with suprasternal retraction on inspiration, hoarseness, dysphagia, tracheal shift or tug, jugular vein distention, and facial or neck edema.

◆ ***Pericardial effusion.*** The most common signs and symptoms of this disorder are dysphagia, fever, pleuritic chest pain, and pericardial friction rub. A severe nonproductive cough occurs rarely.

◆ ***Pleural effusion.*** A nonproductive cough, dyspnea, pleuritic chest pain, and decreased chest motion are characteristic of pleural effusion. Other findings include pleural friction rub, tachycardia, tachypnea, egophony, flatness on percussion, decreased or absent breath sounds, and decreased tactile fremitus.

◆ ***Pneumonia.*** Bacterial pneumonia usually starts with a nonproductive, hacking, painful cough that rapidly becomes productive. Other findings include shaking chills, headache, high fever, dyspnea, pleuritic chest pain, tachypnea, tachycardia, grunting respirations, nasal flaring, decreased breath sounds, fine crackles, rhonchi, and cyanosis. The patient's chest may be dull on percussion.

In mycoplasmal pneumonia, a nonproductive cough develops 2 to 3 days after the onset of malaise, headache, and sore throat. The cough may be paroxysmal, causing substernal chest pain. The patient commonly has a fever but doesn't appear seriously ill.

Viral pneumonia causes a nonproductive, hacking cough and the gradual onset of malaise, headache, anorexia, and low-grade fever.

◆ ***Pneumothorax.*** This life-threatening disorder causes a dry cough and signs of respiratory distress, such as severe dyspnea, tachycardia, tachypnea, and cyanosis. The patient experiences sudden, sharp chest pain that worsens with chest movement as well as subcutaneous crepitation, hyperresonance or tympany, decreased vocal fremitus, and decreased or absent breath sounds on the affected side.

◆ ***Popcorn lung disease.*** Popcorn lung disease occurs in factory workers who experience respiratory symptoms after inhaling butter flavoring chemicals such as diacetyl, used in the manufacture of microwave popcorn. The patient typically complains of gradual onset of a nonproductive cough that worsens over time, progressive shortness of breath, and unusual fatigue. Clinical findings include wheezing, chest pain, fever, night sweats, and weight loss. Bronchiolitis fibrosa obliterans, an irreversible fixed airway obstructive lung disorder, is the most severe condition reported.

◆ ***Psittacosis.*** In this disorder, an initially dry, hacking cough later produces small amounts of blood-streaked, mucoid sputum. Psittacosis may begin abruptly with chills, fever, headache, myalgia, and prostration. The patient may also have tachypnea, fine crackles, epistaxis and, rarely, chest pain.

◆ ***Pulmonary edema.*** This disorder initially causes a dry cough, exertional dyspnea, paroxysmal nocturnal dyspnea, orthopnea, tachycardia, tachypnea, dependent crackles, and ventricular gallop. If pulmonary edema is severe, the patient's respirations become more rapid and labored, with diffuse crackles and a cough that produces frothy, blood-streaked sputum.

◆ ***Pulmonary embolism.*** A life-threatening pulmonary embolism may suddenly produce a dry cough, dyspnea, and pleuritic or anginal chest pain. In most cases, though, the cough produces blood-tinged sputum. Tachycardia and low-grade fever are also common; less common signs and symptoms include massive hemoptysis, chest splinting, leg edema and, with a large embolus, cyanosis, syncope, and distended jugular veins. The patient may also have a pleural friction rub, diffuse wheezing, dullness on percussion, and decreased breath sounds.

◆ ***Sarcoidosis.*** In this disorder, a nonproductive cough is accompanied by dyspnea, substernal pain, and malaise. The patient may also develop fatigue, arthralgia, myalgia, weight loss, tachypnea, crackles, lymphadenopathy, hepatosplenomegaly, skin lesions, vision impairment, difficulty swallowing, and arrhythmias.

◆ ***Severe acute respiratory syndrome (SARS).*** SARS is an acute infectious disease of unknown etiology; however, a novel coronavirus has been implicated as a possible cause. Although most cases have been reported in Asia (China, Vietnam, Singapore, Thailand), cases have cropped up in Europe and North America. The incubation period is 2 to 7 days, and the illness generally begins with a fever (usually greater than 100.4° F [38° C]). Other symptoms include headache, malaise, a nonproductive cough, and dyspnea. The severity of the illness is highly variable, ranging from mild illness to pneumonia and, in some cases, progressing to respiratory failure and death.

◆ ***Sinusitis (chronic).*** This disorder can cause a chronic nonproductive cough due to postnasal drip. The patient's nasal mucosa may appear inflamed, and he may have nasal congestion and profuse drainage. Usually, his breath smells musty.

◆ ***Tracheobronchitis (acute).*** Initially, this disorder produces a dry cough that later becomes productive as secretions increase. Chills, sore throat, slight fever, muscle and back pain, and substernal tightness generally precede the cough's onset. Rhonchi and wheezing are usually heard. Severe illness causes a fever of 101° to 102° F (38.3° to 38.9° C) and possibly bronchospasm, severe wheezing, and increased coughing.

◆ ***Tularemia.*** Also known as "rabbit fever," this infectious disease is caused by the gram-negative, non–spore-forming bacterium *Francisella tularensis*. This organism is found in wild animals, water, and moist soil, typically in rural areas. It's transmitted to humans through the bite of an infected insect or tick, the handling of infected animal carcasses, the drinking of contaminated water, or the inhalation of the bacterium. It's considered a possible airborne agent for biological warfare. Signs and symptoms following inhalation of the organism include the abrupt onset of fever, chills, headache, generalized myalgia, a nonproductive cough, dyspnea, pleuritic chest pain, and empyema.

OTHER CAUSES

◆ ***Diagnostic tests.*** Pulmonary function tests and bronchoscopy may stimulate cough receptors and trigger coughing.

◆ ***Drugs.*** Certain drugs, such as angiotensin-converting enzyme inhibitors, may also cause a nonproductive cough.

◆ ***Treatments.*** Irritation of the carina during suctioning or deep endotracheal or tracheal tube placement can trigger a paroxysmal or hacking cough. Intermittent positive-pressure breathing or spirometry can also cause a nonproductive cough. Some inhalants, such as pentamidine, may stimulate coughing.

SPECIAL CONSIDERATIONS

A nonproductive, paroxysmal cough may induce life-threatening bronchospasm. The patient may need a bronchodilator to relieve his bronchospasm and open his airways. Unless he has chronic obstructive pulmonary disease, you may have to administer an antitussive and a sedative to suppress the cough.

To relieve mucous membrane inflammation and dryness, humidify the air in the patient's room, or instruct him to use a humidifier at home. Tell him to avoid using aerosols, powders, and other respiratory irritants—especially cigarettes. Make sure that the patient receives adequate fluids and nutrition.

As indicated, prepare the patient for diagnostic tests, such as X-rays, a lung scan, bronchoscopy, and pulmonary function tests.

PEDIATRIC POINTERS

A nonproductive cough can be difficult to evaluate in infants and young children because it can't be voluntarily induced and must be observed.

A sudden onset of paroxysmal nonproductive coughing may indicate aspiration of a foreign body—a common danger in children, especially those between ages 6 months and 4 years. Nonproductive coughing can also result from several disorders that commonly affect infants and children. In asthma, a characteristic nonproductive "tight" cough can arise suddenly or insidiously as an attack begins. The cough usually becomes productive toward the end of the attack. In bacterial pneumonia, a nonproductive, hacking cough arises suddenly and becomes productive in 2 to 3 days. Acute bronchiolitis, which has a peak incidence at age 6, produces paroxysms of nonproductive coughing that become more frequent as the disease progresses. Acute otitis media, which is common in infants and young children because of their short eustachian tubes, also produces nonproductive coughing.

A child with measles typically has a slight nonproductive, hacking cough that increases in severity. The earliest sign of cystic fibrosis may be a nonproductive, paroxysmal cough from retained secretions. Life-threatening pertussis produces a cough that becomes paroxysmal with an inspiratory "whoop" or crowing sound. Airway hyperactivity causes a chronic nonproductive cough that increases with exercise or exposure to cold air. Psychogenic coughing may occur when a child is under stress, emotionally stimulated, or seeking attention.

Geriatric pointers

Always ask elderly patients about a nonproductive cough because it may be an indication of a serious acute or chronic illness.

Patient counseling

Explain to the patient why nonproductive coughs should be suppressed and productive coughs encouraged. Encourage the patient to use a respirator in the presence of airway irritants such as paint fumes and dust.

Cough, productive

Productive coughing is the body's mechanism for clearing airway passages of accumulated secretions that normal mucociliary action doesn't remove. It's a sudden, forceful, noisy expulsion of air (from the lungs) that contains sputum or blood (or both). The sputum's color, consistency, and odor provide important clues about the patient's condition. A productive cough can occur as a single cough or as paroxysmal coughing, and it can be voluntarily induced but is usually a reflexive response to stimulation of the airway mucosa.

Usually due to a cardiovascular or respiratory disorder, a productive cough commonly results from an acute or chronic infection that causes inflammation, edema, and increased mucus production in the airways. However, this sign can also result from acquired immunodeficiency syndrome. Inhalation of antigenic or irritating substances or foreign bodies also can cause a productive cough. In fact, the most common cause of chronic productive coughing is cigarette smoking, which produces mucoid sputum ranging in color from clear to yellow to brown.

Many patients minimize or overlook a chronic productive cough or accept it as normal. Such patients may not seek medical attention until an associated problem—such as dyspnea, hemoptysis, chest pain, weight loss, or recurrent respiratory tract infections—develops. The delay can have serious consequences because productive coughing is associated with several life-threatening disorders and can also herald airway occlusion from excessive secretions.

EMERGENCY INTERVENTIONS *A patient with a productive cough can develop acute respiratory distress from thick or excessive secretions, bronchospasm, or fatigue, so examine him before you take his history. Take vital signs and check the rate, depth, and rhythm of respirations. Keep his airway patent, and be prepared to provide supplemental oxygen if he becomes restless or confused, or if his respirations become shallow, irregular, rapid, or slow. Look for stridor, wheezing, choking, or gurgling. Be alert for nasal flaring and cyanosis.*

A productive cough may signal a life-threatening disorder. For example, coughing due to pulmonary edema produces thin, frothy, pink sputum, and coughing due to an asthma attack produces thick, mucoid sputum.

History and physical examination

When the patient's condition permits, ask when the cough began and how much sputum he's coughing up each day. (The normal tracheobronchial tree can produce up to 3 oz [89 ml] of sputum per day.) At what time of day does he cough up the most sputum? Is his sputum production affected by what or when he eats, his activities, or his environment? Ask him if he has noticed an increase in sputum production since his coughing began. This may result from external stimuli or from such internal causes as chronic bronchial infection or a lung abscess. Also ask about the color, odor, and consistency of the sputum. Blood-tinged or rust-colored sputum may result from trauma due to coughing or from an underlying condition, such as a pulmonary infection or a tumor. Foul-smelling sputum may result from an anaerobic infection, such as bronchitis or a lung abscess.

How does the cough sound? A hacking cough results from laryngeal involvement, whereas a "brassy" cough indicates major airway involvement. Does the patient feel any pain associated with his productive cough? If so, ask about its location and severity and whether it radiates to other areas. Does coughing, changing body position, or inspiration increase or help relieve his pain?

Next, ask the patient about his cigarette, drug, and alcohol use and whether his weight or appetite has changed. Find out if he has a history of asthma, allergies, or respiratory disorders, and ask about recent illnesses, surgery, or trauma. What medications is he taking? Does he work around chemicals or respiratory irritants such as silicone?

Examine the patient's mouth and nose for congestion, drainage, or inflammation. Note his breath odor: Halitosis can be a sign of pulmonary infection. Inspect his neck for distended veins, and palpate it for tenderness, masses, and enlarged lymph nodes. Observe his chest for accessory muscle use, retractions, and uneven chest expansion, and percuss it for dullness, tympany, or flatness. Finally, auscultate for pleural friction rub and abnormal breath sounds, including rhonchi, crackles, or wheezing. (See *Productive cough: Causes and associated findings,* pages 182 and 183.)

MEDICAL CAUSES

◆ ***Actinomycosis.*** This disorder begins with a cough that produces purulent sputum. Fever, weight loss, fatigue, weakness, dyspnea, night sweats, pleuritic chest pain, and hemoptysis may also occur.

◆ ***Aspiration pneumonitis.*** This disorder causes coughing that produces pink, frothy, possibly purulent sputum. The patient also has marked dyspnea, fever, tachypnea, tachycardia, wheezing, and cyanosis.

◆ ***Asthma (acute).*** A severe asthma attack, which can be life-threatening, may produce tenacious mucoid sputum and mucus plugs. Such an attack typically starts with a dry cough and mild wheezing, then progresses to severe dyspnea, audible wheezing, chest tightness, and a productive cough. Other findings include apprehension, prolonged expiration, intercostal and supraclavicular retraction on inspiration, accessory muscle use, rhonchi, crackles, flaring nostrils, tachypnea, tachycardia, diaphoresis, and flushing or cyanosis. Attacks commonly occur at night or during sleep.

◆ ***Bronchiectasis.*** The chronic cough of this disorder produces copious mucopurulent sputum that has characteristic layering (top, frothy; middle, clear; bottom, dense with purulent particles). The patient has halitosis: His sputum may smell foul or sickeningly sweet. Other characteristic findings include hemoptysis, persistent coarse crackles over the affected lung area, occasional wheezing, rhonchi, exertional dyspnea, weight loss, fatigue, malaise, weakness, recurrent fever, and late-stage finger clubbing.

◆ ***Bronchitis (chronic).*** The cough associated with chronic bronchitis may be nonproductive initially; eventually, however, it produces mucoid sputum that becomes purulent. Secondary infection can also cause mucopurulent sputum, which may become blood tinged and foul smelling. The cough, which may be paroxysmal during exercise, usually occurs when the patient is recumbent or rises from sleep.

The patient also exhibits prolonged expiration, accessory muscle use, barrel chest, tachypnea, cyanosis, wheezing, exertional dyspnea, scattered rhonchi, coarse crackles (which can be precipitated by coughing), and late-stage clubbing.

◆ ***Chemical pneumonitis.*** This disorder causes a cough with purulent sputum. It may also cause dyspnea, wheezing, orthopnea, fever, malaise, crackles, laryngitis, rhinitis, and mucous membrane irritation of the conjunctivae, throat, and nose. Signs and symptoms may increase for 24 to 48 hours after exposure, then resolve; in severe pneumonitis, however, they may recur 2 to 5 weeks later.

◆ ***Common cold.*** The common cold may cause a productive cough with mucoid or mucopurulent sputum, but it usually starts with a dry, hacking cough, sore throat, sneezing, rhinorrhea, and nasal congestion. Headache, malaise, fatigue, myalgia, and arthralgia may also occur.

◆ ***Emphysema.*** This disorder causes a chronic productive cough with scant mucoid, translucent,

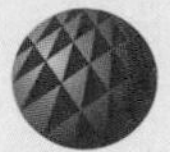

SIGNS & SYMPTOMS

Productive cough: Causes and associated findings

Common causes	Chest pain	Crackles	Cyanosis	Decreased breath sounds	Dyspnea	Fatigue	Fever	Rhonchi	Sore throat	Tachycardia	Tachypnea	Weight loss	Wheezing
	Major associated signs and symptoms												
Actinomycosis	●				●	●	●					●	
Aspiration pneumonitis		●	●		●	●	●	●		●	●		●
Asthma (acute)	●	●	●		●			●		●	●		●
Bronchiectasis		●			●	●	●	●				●	●
Bronchitis (chronic)		●	●		●			●			●		●
Chemical pneumonitis		●			●		●	●			●		●
Common cold						●	●		●				
Legionnaires' disease	●	●			●	●	●			●	●		
Lung abscess (ruptured)	●	●			●	●	●					●	
Lung cancer	●				●	●	●					●	●
Nocardiosis	●			●		●	●					●	
North American blastomycosis	●					●	●					●	
Plague	●				●		●				●		
Pneumonia (bacterial)	●	●	●		●	●	●	●		●	●		
Pneumonia (mycoplasmal)	●	●				●	●		●				
Psittacosis	●	●					●				●		
Pulmonary coccidioidomycosis	●						●	●	●				●
Pulmonary edema		●	●		●	●	●			●	●		

Productive cough: Causes and associated findings *(continued)*

Major associated signs and symptoms

Common causes	Chest pain	Crackles	Cyanosis	Decreased breath sounds	Dyspnea	Fatigue	Fever	Rhonchi	Sore throat	Tachycardia	Tachypnea	Weight loss	Wheezing
Pulmonary emphysema				●	●			●			●	●	
Pulmonary embolism	●	●	●		●		●			●	●		●
Pulmonary tuberculosis	●	●			●	●	●	●				●	
Silicosis		●			●	●					●	●	
Tracheobronchitis	●	●					●	●	●				●

grayish white sputum that can become mucopurulent. Patients with emphysema are typically thin and have the characteristic pink or red complexion ("pink puffer" appearance). They may also exhibit increased accessory muscle use, tachypnea, grunting expirations through pursed lips, diminished breath sounds, exertional dyspnea, rhonchi, barrel chest, anorexia, and weight loss. Clubbing is a late sign.

◆ ***Legionnaires' disease.*** This disorder causes a cough that produces scant mucoid, nonpurulent and, possibly, blood-streaked sputum. Prodromal signs and symptoms typically include malaise, fatigue, weakness, anorexia, diffuse myalgia, and possibly diarrhea. Within 12 to 48 hours, the patient develops a dry cough and a sudden high fever with chills. Many patients also have pleuritic chest pain, headache, tachypnea, tachycardia, nausea, vomiting, dyspnea, crackles, mild temporary amnesia, disorientation, confusion, flushing, mild diaphoresis, and prostration.

◆ ***Lung abscess (ruptured).*** The cardinal sign of a ruptured lung abscess is a cough that produces copious amounts of purulent, foul-smelling and, possibly, blood-tinged sputum. A ruptured abscess can also cause diaphoresis, anorexia, clubbing, weight loss, weakness, fatigue, fever with chills, dyspnea, headache, malaise, pleuritic chest pain, halitosis, inspiratory crackles, and tubular or amphoric breath sounds. The patient's chest is dull on percussion on the affected side.

◆ ***Lung cancer.*** One of the earliest signs of bronchogenic carcinoma is a chronic cough that produces small amounts of purulent (or mucopurulent), blood-streaked sputum. In a patient with bronchoalveolar cancer, however, coughing produces large amounts of frothy sputum. Other signs and symptoms of lung cancer include dyspnea, anorexia, fatigue, weight loss, chest pain, fever, diaphoresis, wheezing, and clubbing.

◆ ***Nocardiosis.*** This disorder causes a productive cough (with purulent, thick, tenacious, and possibly blood-tinged sputum) and fever that may last several months. Other findings include night sweats, pleuritic pain, anorexia, weight loss, malaise, fatigue, and diminished or absent breath sounds. The patient's chest is dull on percussion.

◆ ***North American blastomycosis.*** This chronic disorder may produce a dry hacking cough or a productive cough with bloody or purulent sputum. Other findings include pleuritic chest pain, fever, chills, anorexia, weight loss, malaise, fatigue, night sweats, cutaneous lesions (small, painless, nonpruritic macules or papules), and prostration.

◆ ***Plague.*** Caused by *Yersinia pestis,* plague is one of the most virulent and, if untreated, most lethal bacterial infections known. Most cases are sporadic, but the potential for epidemic spread still exists. Clinical forms include bubonic (the most common), septicemic, and pneumonic plagues. The bubonic form is transmitted to man from the bite of infected fleas. Signs and symptoms include fever, chills, and swollen, inflamed, and tender lymph nodes near the site of the fleabite. Septicemic plague may develop as a complication of untreated bubonic or pneumonic plague and occurs when plague bacteria enter the bloodstream and multiply. The pneumonic form can be contracted by inhaling respiratory droplets from an infected person or inhaling the organism that has been dispersed in the air through biological warfare. The onset is usually sudden with chills, fever, headache, and myalgia. Pulmonary signs and symptoms include a productive cough, chest pain, tachypnea, dyspnea, hemoptysis, increasing respiratory distress, and cardiopulmonary insufficiency.

◆ ***Pneumonia.*** Bacterial pneumonia initially produces a dry cough that becomes productive. Associated signs and symptoms develop suddenly and include shaking chills, high fever, myalgia, headache, pleuritic chest pain that increases with chest movement, tachypnea, tachycardia, dyspnea, cyanosis, diaphoresis, decreased breath sounds, fine crackles, and rhonchi.

Mycoplasmal pneumonia may cause a cough that produces scant blood-flecked sputum. In most cases, however, a nonproductive cough starts 2 to 3 days after the onset of malaise, headache, fever, and sore throat. Paroxysmal coughing causes substernal chest pain. Patients may develop crackles but generally don't appear seriously ill.

◆ ***Psittacosis.*** As this disorder progresses, the characteristic hacking cough, nonproductive at first, may later produce a small amount of mucoid, blood-streaked sputum. The infection may begin abruptly with chills, fever, headache, myalgia, and prostration. Other signs and symptoms include tachypnea, fine crackles, chest pain (rare), epistaxis, photophobia, abdominal distention and tenderness, nausea, vomiting, and a faint macular rash. Severe psittacosis may produce stupor, delirium, and coma.

◆ ***Pulmonary coccidioidomycosis.*** This disorder causes a nonproductive or slightly productive cough with fever, occasional chills, pleuritic chest pain, sore throat, headache, backache, malaise, marked weakness, anorexia, hemoptysis, and an itchy macular rash. Rhonchi and wheezing may be heard. The disease may spread to other areas, causing arthralgia, swelling of the knees and ankles, and erythema nodosum or erythema multiforme.

◆ ***Pulmonary edema.*** When severe, this life-threatening disorder causes a cough that produces frothy, blood-tinged sputum. Early signs and symptoms include exertional dyspnea, paroxysmal nocturnal dyspnea followed by orthopnea, and a cough that may be nonproductive initially. Fever, fatigue, tachycardia, tachypnea, dependent crackles, and ventricular gallop may also occur. As the patient's respirations become increasingly rapid and labored, he develops more diffuse crackles and the productive cough, worsening tachycardia, and possibly arrhythmias. His skin becomes cold, clammy, and cyanotic; his blood pressure falls; and his pulse becomes thready.

◆ ***Pulmonary embolism.*** This life-threatening disorder causes a cough that may be nonproductive or may produce blood-tinged sputum. Usually, the first symptom of a pulmonary embolism is severe dyspnea, which may be accompanied by angina or pleuritic chest pain. The patient experiences marked anxiety, a low-grade fever, tachycardia, tachypnea, and diaphoresis. Less common signs include massive hemoptysis, chest splinting, leg edema and, in a large embolus, cyanosis, syncope, and distended jugular veins. The patient may also have a pleural friction rub, diffuse wheezing, crackles, chest dullness on percussion, decreased breath sounds, and signs of circulatory collapse.

◆ ***Pulmonary tuberculosis.*** This disorder causes a mild to severe productive cough along with some combination of hemoptysis, malaise, dyspnea, and pleuritic chest pain. Sputum may be scant and mucoid or copious and purulent. Typically, the patient experiences night sweats, easy fatigability, and weight loss. His breath sounds are amphoric. He may exhibit chest dullness on percussion and, after coughing, increased tactile fremitus with crackles.

◆ ***Silicosis.*** A productive cough with mucopurulent sputum is the earliest sign of this disorder. The patient also has exertional dyspnea, tachypnea, weight loss, fatigue, general weakness, and recurrent respiratory infections.

Auscultation reveals end-inspiratory, fine crackles at the lung bases.

◆ ***Tracheobronchitis.*** Inflammation initially causes a nonproductive cough followed by chills, sore throat, slight fever, muscle and back pain, and substernal tightness. As secretions increase, the cough produces mucoid, mucopurulent, or purulent sputum. The patient typically has rhonchi and wheezing; he may also develop crackles. Severe tracheobronchitis may cause a fever of 101° to 102° F (38.3° to 38.9° C) and bronchospasm.

Other causes

◆ ***Diagnostic tests.*** Bronchoscopy and pulmonary function tests may increase productive coughing.

◆ ***Drugs.*** Expectorants, such as ammonium chloride, guaifenesin, potassium iodide, and terpin hydrate, increase productive coughing.

◆ ***Respiratory therapy.*** Intermittent positive-pressure breathing, nebulizer therapy, and incentive spirometry can help loosen secretions and cause or increase productive coughing.

Special considerations

Avoid taking measures to suppress a productive cough because retention of sputum may interfere with alveolar aeration or impair pulmonary resistance to infection. Expect to give a mucolytic and an expectorant, and increase the patient's intake of oral fluids to thin his secretions and increase their flow. In addition, you may give a bronchodilator to relieve bronchospasms and open airways. An antibiotic may be ordered to treat underlying infection.

Humidify the air around the patient; this will relieve mucous membrane inflammation and help loosen dried secretions. Provide pulmonary physiotherapy, such as postural drainage with vibration and percussion, to loosen secretions. Aerosol therapy may be necessary.

Provide the patient with uninterrupted rest periods. Keep him from using respiratory irritants. If he's confined to bed rest, change his position often to promote the drainage of secretions.

Prepare the patient for diagnostic tests, such as chest X-rays, bronchoscopy, a lung scan, and pulmonary function tests. Collect sputum specimens for culture and sensitivity testing.

Pediatric pointers

Because his airway is narrow, a child with a productive cough can quickly develop airway occlusion and respiratory distress from thick or excessive secretions. Causes of a productive cough in children include asthma, bronchiectasis, bronchitis, acute bronchiolitis, cystic fibrosis, and pertussis.

When caring for a child with a productive cough, expect to administer an expectorant, but not a cough suppressant. To soothe inflamed mucous membranes and prevent drying of secretions, provide humidified air or oxygen. Remember, high humidity can induce bronchospasm in a hyperactive child or produce overhydration in an infant.

Geriatric pointers

Always ask elderly patients about a productive cough because this sign may indicate a serious acute or chronic illness.

Patient counseling

Encourage the patient not to smoke because doing so can aggravate his condition. Explain that quitting even after decades of smoking is helpful. Teach him how to breathe deeply, to cough effectively and, if appropriate, to splint his incision when he coughs. Tell him to sit or stand upright when coughing, if possible, to maximize chest expansion. Teach the patient and his family how to use chest percussion to loosen secretions.

Tell the patient to cover his mouth and nose with a tissue when he coughs and to dispose of contaminated tissues properly, to protect himself and others from the cough and secretions. Be sure to provide a container for tissues and sputum.

Crackles

[Rales, crepitations]

A common finding in patients with certain cardiovascular and pulmonary disorders, crackles are nonmusical clicking or rattling noises heard during auscultation of breath sounds. They usually occur during inspiration and recur constantly from one respiratory cycle to the next. They can be unilateral or bilateral and moist or dry. They're characterized by their pitch, loudness, location, persistence, and occurrence during the respiratory cycle.

Crackles indicate abnormal movement of air through fluid-filled airways. They can be irregularly dispersed, as in pneumonia, or localized, as in bronchiectasis. (A few basilar crackles can be heard in normal lungs after prolonged shallow breathing. These normal crackles clear with a few deep breaths.) Crackles usually indicate the degree of an underlying illness. When crackles result from a generalized disorder, they usually occur in the less distended and more dependent areas of the lungs, such as the lung bases, when the patient is standing. Crackles caused by air passing through inflammatory exudate may not be audible if the involved portion of the lung isn't being ventilated because of shallow respirations. (See *How crackles occur*.)

EMERGENCY INTERVENTIONS *Quickly take the patient's vital signs, and examine him for signs of respiratory distress or airway obstruction. Check the depth and rhythm of respirations. Is he struggling to breathe? Check for increased accessory muscle use and chest wall motion, retractions, stridor, or nasal flaring. Provide supplemental oxygen. Endotracheal intubation may be necessary.*

HISTORY AND PHYSICAL EXAMINATION

If the patient also has a cough, ask when it began and if it's constant or intermittent. Find out what the cough sounds like and whether he's coughing up sputum or blood. If the cough is productive, determine the sputum's consistency, amount, odor, and color.

Ask the patient if he has any pain. If so, where is it located? When did he first notice it? Does it radiate to other areas? Also, ask the patient if movement, coughing, or breathing worsens or helps relieve his pain. Note the patient's position: Is he lying still or moving about restlessly?

Obtain a brief medical history. Does the patient have cancer or any known respiratory or cardiovascular problems? Ask about recent surgery, trauma, or illness. Does he smoke or drink alcohol? Is he experiencing hoarseness or difficulty swallowing? Find out which medications he's taking. Also, ask about recent weight loss, anorexia, nausea, vomiting, fatigue, weakness, vertigo, and syncope. Has the patient been exposed to irritants, such as vapors, fumes, or smoke?

Next, perform a physical examination. Examine the patient's nose and mouth for signs of infection, such as inflammation or increased secretions. Note his breath odor: Halitosis could indicate pulmonary infection. Check his neck for masses, tenderness, swelling, lymphadenopathy, or venous distention.

Inspect the patient's chest for abnormal configuration or uneven expansion. Percuss for dullness, tympany, or flatness. Auscultate his lungs for abnormal, diminished, or absent breath sounds. Listen to his heart for abnormal sounds, and check his hands and feet for edema or clubbing. (See *Crackles: Causes and associated findings*, page 188.)

MEDICAL CAUSES

◆ ***Acute respiratory distress syndrome.*** This life-threatening disorder causes diffuse fine to coarse crackles that are usually heard in the dependent portions of the lungs. It also produces cyanosis, nasal flaring, tachypnea, tachycardia, grunting respirations, rhonchi, dyspnea, anxiety, and decreased level of consciousness.

◆ ***Asthma (acute).*** A severe attack usually occurs at night or during sleep, causing dry, whistling crackles. An attack typically starts with a dry cough and mild wheezing and progresses to severe dyspnea, audible wheezing, chest tightness, and a productive cough. Other findings include apprehension, prolonged expirations, rhonchi, intercostal and supraclavicular retractions on inspiration, accessory muscle use, flaring nostrils, tachypnea, tachycardia, diaphoresis, and flushing or cyanosis.

◆ ***Bronchiectasis.*** In this disorder, persistent coarse crackles are heard over the affected area of the lung. They're accompanied by a chronic cough that produces copious amounts of mucopurulent sputum. Other characteristics include halitosis, occasional wheezing, exertional dyspnea, rhonchi, weight loss, fatigue, malaise, weakness, recurrent fever, and late-stage clubbing.

◆ ***Bronchitis (chronic).*** This disorder causes coarse crackles that are usually heard at the lung bases as well as prolonged expirations, wheezing, rhonchi, exertional dyspnea, tachypnea, and a persistent productive cough from increased bronchial secretions. Clubbing and cyanosis may also occur.

◆ ***Chemical pneumonitis.*** In acute chemical pneumonitis, diffuse fine to coarse, moist crackles accompany a productive cough with purulent sputum, dyspnea, wheezing, orthopnea, fever, malaise, and mucous membrane irritation. Signs and symptoms may worsen for 24 to 48 hours after exposure, then resolve; if severe, however, they may recur 2 to 5 weeks later.

◆ ***Interstitial fibrosis of the lungs.*** Cellophane-like crackles can be heard over all lobes in this disorder. As the disease progresses, a

How crackles occur

Crackles occur when air passes through fluid-filled airways, causing collapsed alveoli to pop open as the airway pressure equalizes. They can also occur when membranes lining the chest cavity and the lungs become inflamed. The illustrations below show a normal alveolus and two pathologic alveolar changes that cause crackles.

NORMAL ALVEOLUS

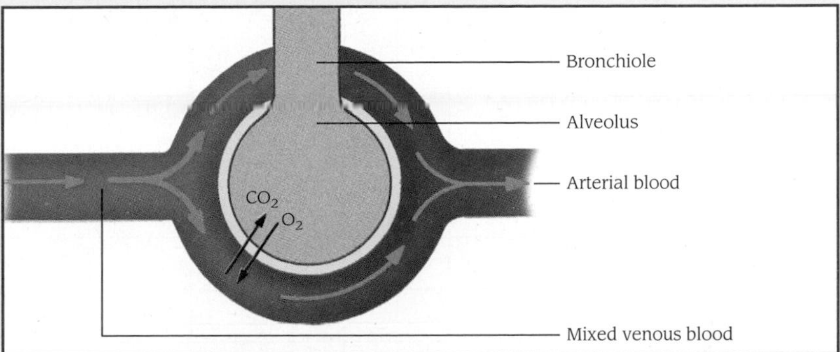

ALVEOLUS IN PULMONARY EDEMA

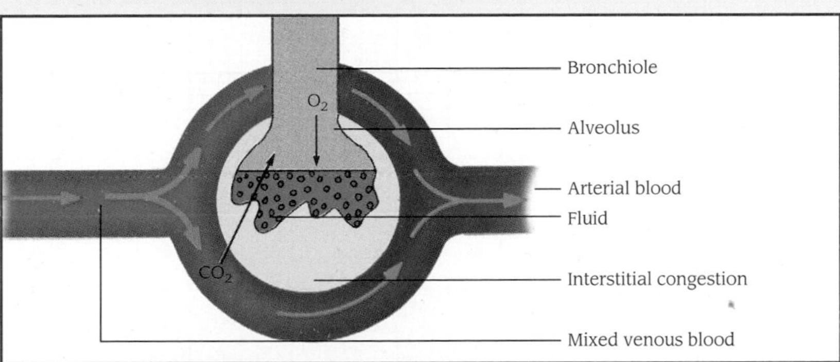

ALVEOLUS IN INFLAMMATION

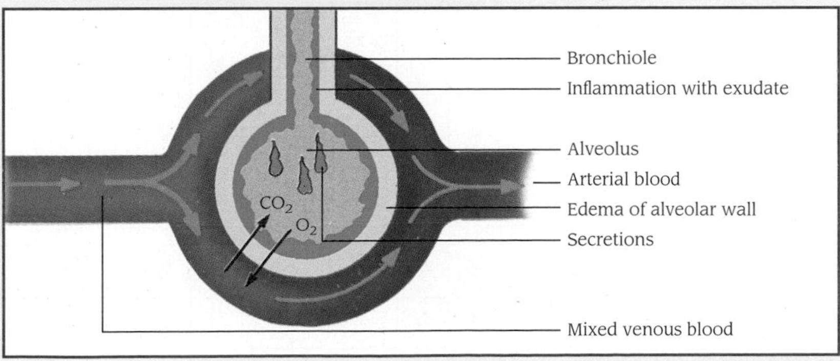

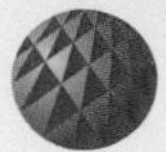

SIGNS & SYMPTOMS

Crackles: Causes and associated findings

Major associated signs and symptoms

Common causes	Chest pain	Cough	Cyanosis	Dyspnea	Fatigue	Fever	Hemoptysis	Rhonchi	Tachycardia	Tachypnea	Vomiting	Weakness	Weight loss
Acute respiratory distress syndrome			●	●				●	●	●			
Asthma (acute)	●	●	●	●				●	●	●			
Bronchiectasis		●		●	●	●		●				●	●
Bronchitis (chronic)		●	●	●			●	●		●			
Chemical pneumonitis		●		●		●		●		●			
Interstitial fibrosis of the lungs	●	●	●	●	●					●			●
Legionnaires' disease	●	●		●	●	●	●		●	●	●	●	
Lung abscess	●	●		●	●	●	●					●	●
Pneumonia (bacterial)	●	●	●	●	●	●		●	●	●			
Pneumonia (mycoplasmal)		●				●	●			●			
Pneumonia (viral)		●				●				●			
Psittacosis	●	●				●				●	●		
Pulmonary edema		●	●	●			●		●	●			
Pulmonary embolism	●	●	●	●		●	●		●	●			
Pulmonary tuberculosis	●	●		●	●	●	●					●	●
Sarcoidosis		●		●	●					●		●	●
Silicosis		●		●	●					●		●	●
Tracheobronchitis	●	●				●		●					

nonproductive cough, dyspnea, fatigue, weight loss, cyanosis, and pleuritic chest pain develop.

◆ ***Legionnaires' disease.*** This disorder causes diffuse moist crackles and a cough producing scant mucoid, nonpurulent and, possibly, blood-streaked sputum. Prodromal signs and symptoms usually include malaise, fatigue, weakness, anorexia, diffuse myalgia and, possibly, diarrhea. Within 12 to 48 hours, the patient develops a dry cough and a sudden high fever with chills. He may also have pleuritic chest pain, headache, dyspnea, tachypnea, tachycardia, nausea, vomiting, mild temporary amnesia, confusion, flushing, mild diaphoresis, and prostration.

◆ ***Lung abscess.*** This disorder produces fine to medium, moist inspiratory crackles. The onset is insidious; signs and symptoms include sweats, anorexia, weight loss, fever, fatigue, weakness, dyspnea, clubbing, pleuritic chest pain, pleural friction rub, and a cough producing copious amounts of foul-smelling, purulent and, possibly, blood-tinged sputum. The patient's breath sounds are hollow and tubular or amphoric; the affected side of his chest is dull on percussion.

◆ ***Pneumonia.*** Bacterial pneumonia produces diffuse fine crackles, sudden shaking chills, high fever, tachypnea, pleuritic chest pain, cyanosis, grunting respirations, nasal flaring, decreased breath sounds, myalgia, headache, tachycardia, dyspnea, cyanosis, diaphoresis, and rhonchi. The patient also has a dry cough that later becomes productive.

Mycoplasmal pneumonia produces medium to fine crackles with a nonproductive cough, malaise, sore throat, headache, and fever. The patient may have blood-flecked sputum. In viral pneumonia, diffuse crackles develop gradually and may be accompanied by a nonproductive cough, malaise, headache, anorexia, low-grade fever, and decreased breath sounds.

◆ ***Psittacosis.*** Diffuse fine crackles may be heard as this disorder progresses. Accompanying findings include a characteristic hacking, productive cough, chills, fever, headache, myalgia, and prostration. Other features include tachypnea, chest pain (rare), epistaxis, photophobia, abdominal distention and tenderness, nausea, vomiting, and a faint macular rash.

◆ ***Pulmonary edema.*** Moist, bubbling crackles on inspiration are one of the first signs of life-threatening pulmonary edema. Other early findings include exertional dyspnea; paroxysmal nocturnal dyspnea, then orthopnea; and coughing, which may be initially nonproductive but later produces frothy, bloody sputum. Related clinical effects include tachycardia, tachypnea, and a ventricular gallop (a third heart sound [S_3]). As the patient's respirations become increasingly rapid and labored, he develops more diffuse crackles, worsening tachycardia, hypotension, a rapid and thready pulse, cyanosis, and cold, clammy skin.

◆ ***Pulmonary embolism.*** This life-threatening disorder can cause fine to coarse crackles and a cough that may be dry or may produce blood-tinged sputum. Usually, the first sign of pulmonary embolism is severe dyspnea, which may be accompanied by angina or pleuritic chest pain. The patient has marked anxiety, a low-grade fever, tachycardia, tachypnea, and diaphoresis. Less-common signs include massive hemoptysis, chest splinting, leg edema and, with a large embolus, cyanosis, syncope, and distended jugular veins. The patient may also have a pleural friction rub, diffuse wheezing, chest dullness on percussion, decreased breath sounds, and signs of circulatory collapse.

◆ ***Pulmonary tuberculosis.*** In this disorder, fine crackles occur after coughing along with some combination of hemoptysis, malaise, dyspnea, and pleuritic chest pain. Sputum may be scant and mucoid or copious and purulent. Typically, the patient is easily fatigued and experiences night sweats, weakness, and weight loss. His breath sounds are amphoric.

◆ ***Sarcoidosis.*** This disorder produces fine, bibasilar, end-inspiratory crackles and, rarely, wheezing. The patient doesn't have a fever but does have malaise, fatigue, weakness, weight loss, a cough, dyspnea, and tachypnea.

◆ ***Silicosis.*** This disorder produces fine end-inspiratory crackles heard at the lung bases. The earliest sign of silicosis is a productive cough with mucopurulent sputum. The patient also exhibits exertional dyspnea, tachypnea, weight loss, fatigue, general weakness, and recurrent respiratory tract infections.

◆ ***Tracheobronchitis.*** In its acute form, this disorder produces moist or coarse crackles along with a productive cough, rhonchi, wheezing, chills, sore throat, a slight fever, muscle and back pain, and substernal tightness. Severe tracheobronchitis may cause a moderate fever and bronchospasm.

Special considerations

To keep the patient's airway patent and facilitate his breathing, elevate the head of his bed.

To liquefy thick secretions and relieve mucous membrane inflammation, administer fluids, humidified air, or oxygen. Diuretics may be needed if crackles result from cardiogenic pulmonary edema. Turn the patient every 1 to 2 hours, and encourage him to breathe deeply.

Plan daily uninterrupted rest periods to help the patient relax and sleep. Prepare the patient for diagnostic tests, such as chest X-rays, a lung scan, and sputum analysis.

Pediatric pointers

Crackles in an infant or a child may indicate a serious cardiovascular or respiratory disorder. Pneumonias produce sudden diffuse crackles in children. Esophageal atresia and tracheoesophageal fistula can cause bubbling, moist crackles due to aspiration of food or secretions into the lungs—especially in neonates. Pulmonary edema causes fine crackles at the base of the lungs, and bronchiectasis produces moist crackles. Cystic fibrosis produces widespread fine to coarse inspiratory crackles and wheezing in infants. Sickle cell anemia may produce crackles when it causes pulmonary infarction or infection.

Geriatric pointers

Crackles that clear after deep breathing may indicate mild basilar atelectasis. In elderly patients, auscultate lung bases before and after auscultating apices.

Patient counseling

Teach the patient how to cough effectively and splint incision areas if appropriate. Encourage him to avoid smoking and using aerosols, powders, or other products that might irritate his airways.

Crepitation, bony

[Bony crepitus]

Bony crepitation is a palpable vibration or an audible crunching sound that results when one bone grates against another. This sign commonly results from a fracture, but it can also occur when bones that have been stripped of their protective articular cartilage grind against each other as they articulate—for example, in patients with advanced arthritic or degenerative joint disorders.

Eliciting bony crepitation can help confirm the diagnosis of a fracture, but it can also cause further soft tissue, nerve, or vessel injury. Always evaluate distal pulses and perform neurologic checks distal to the suspected fracture site before manipulating an extremity. In addition, rubbing fractured bone ends together can convert a closed fracture into an open one if a bone end penetrates the skin. Therefore, after the initial detection of crepitation in a patient with a fracture, avoid subsequent elicitation of this sign.

History and physical examination

If you detect bony crepitation in a patient with a suspected fracture, ask him if he feels any pain and if he can point to the painful area. To prevent lacerating nerves, blood vessels, or other structures, immobilize the affected area by applying a splint that includes the joints above and below the affected area. Elevate the affected area, if possible, and apply cold packs. Inspect for abrasions or lacerations. Find out how and when the injury occurred. Palpate pulses distal to the injury site, and check the skin for pallor or coolness. Test motor and sensory function distal to the injury site.

If the patient doesn't have a suspected fracture, ask about a history of osteoarthritis or rheumatoid arthritis. Do any medications help ease arthritic discomfort? Take the patient's vital signs and test joint range of motion.

Medical causes

- ***Fracture.*** In addition to bony crepitation, a fracture causes acute local pain, hematoma, edema, and decreased range of motion. Other findings may include deformity, point tenderness, discoloration of the limb, and loss of limb function. Neurovascular damage may cause increased capillary refill time, diminished or absent pulses, mottled cyanosis, paresthesia, and decreased sensation (all distal to the fracture site). An open fracture produces an obvious skin wound.
- ***Osteoarthritis.*** Joint crepitation may be elicited during range-of-motion testing in advanced osteoarthritis. Soft fine crepitus on palpation may indicate roughening of the articular cartilage; coarse grating may indicate badly damaged cartilage. The cardinal symptom of osteoarthritis is joint pain, especially during motion and weight bearing. Other findings include joint stiffness that typically occurs after resting and subsides within a few minutes after the patient begins moving.

◆ ***Rheumatoid arthritis.*** In advanced rheumatoid arthritis, bony crepitation is heard when the affected joint is rotated. However, this disorder usually develops insidiously, producing nonspecific signs and symptoms, such as fatigue, malaise, anorexia, a persistent low-grade fever, weight loss, lymphadenopathy, and vague arthralgias and myalgia. Later, more specific and localized articular signs develop, commonly at the proximal finger joints. These signs usually occur bilaterally and symmetrically and may extend to the wrists, knees, elbows, and ankles. The affected joints stiffen after inactivity. The patient also has increased warmth, swelling, and tenderness of affected joints as well as limited range of motion.

Special considerations

If a fracture is suspected, prepare the patient for X-rays of the affected area, and reexamine his neurovascular status frequently. Keep the affected part immobilized and elevated until treatment begins. Give an analgesic to relieve pain.

Pediatric pointers

Bony crepitation in a child usually occurs after a fracture. Obtain an accurate history of the injury, and be alert for the possibility of child abuse. In a teenager, bony crepitation and pain in the patellofemoral joint help diagnose chondromalacia of the patella.

Geriatric pointers

Degenerative joint changes, which have usually begun by age 20 or 30, progress more rapidly after age 40 and occur primarily in weight-bearing joints, such as the lumbar spine, hips, knees, and ankles.

Crepitation, subcutaneous

[Subcutaneous crepitus, subcutaneous emphysema]

When bubbles of air or other gases (such as carbon dioxide) are trapped in subcutaneous tissue, palpation or stroking of the skin produces a crackling sound called *subcutaneous crepitation* or *subcutaneous emphysema.* The bubbles feel like small, unstable nodules and aren't painful, even though subcutaneous crepitation is commonly associated with painful disorders. Usually, the affected tissue is visibly edematous; this can lead to life-threatening airway occlusion if the edema affects the neck or upper chest.

The air or gas bubbles enter the tissues through open wounds from the action of anaerobic microorganisms or from traumatic or spontaneous rupture or perforation of pulmonary or GI organs.

History and physical examination

Because subcutaneous crepitation can indicate a life-threatening disorder, you'll need to perform a rapid initial evaluation and intervene if necessary. (See *Managing subcutaneous crepitation,* page 192.)

When the patient's condition permits, palpate the affected skin to evaluate the location and extent of subcutaneous crepitation and to obtain baseline information. Repalpate frequently to determine if the crepitation is increasing. Ask the patient if he's experiencing any pain or having difficulty breathing. If he's in pain, find out where the pain is located, how severe it is, and when it began. Ask about recent thoracic surgery, diagnostic tests, and respiratory therapy or a history of trauma or chronic pulmonary disease.

Medical causes

◆ ***Gas gangrene.*** Subcutaneous crepitation is the hallmark of this rare, but commonly fatal, infection that's caused by anaerobic microorganisms. It's accompanied by local pain, swelling, and discoloration as well as bullae and necrosis. The skin over the wound may rupture, revealing dark red or black necrotic muscle and a foul-smelling, watery or frothy discharge. Related findings include tachycardia, tachypnea, a moderate fever, cyanosis, and lassitude.

◆ ***Orbital fracture.*** This fracture allows air from the nasal sinuses to escape into subcutaneous tissue, causing subcutaneous crepitation of the eyelid and orbit. The most common sign of an orbital fracture is periorbital ecchymosis. Visual acuity is usually normal, although a swollen eyelid may prevent accurate testing. The patient has facial edema, diplopia, a hyphema and, occasionally, a dilated or unreactive pupil on the affected side. Extraocular movements may also be affected.

◆ ***Pneumothorax.*** Severe pneumothorax produces subcutaneous crepitation in the upper chest and neck. In many cases, the patient has chest pain that's unilateral, rarely localized initially, and increased on inspiration. Dyspnea, anxiety, restlessness, tachypnea, cyanosis,

EMERGENCY INTERVENTION

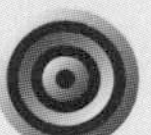

Managing subcutaneous crepitation

Subcutaneous crepitation occurs when air or gas bubbles escape into tissues. It may signal a life-threatening rupture of an air-filled or gas-producing organ or a fulminating anaerobic infection.

Organ rupture

If the patient shows signs of respiratory distress—such as severe dyspnea, tachypnea, accessory muscle use, nasal flaring, air hunger, or tachycardia—quickly test for Hamman's sign to detect trapped air bubbles in the mediastinum.

To test for Hamman's sign, help the patient assume a left-lateral recumbent position. Then place your stethoscope over the precordium. If you hear a loud crunching sound that synchronizes with his heartbeat, the patient has a positive Hamman's sign.

Depending on which organ is ruptured, be prepared for endotracheal intubation, an emergency tracheotomy, or chest tube insertion. Start administering supplemental oxygen immediately. Start an I.V. catheter to administer fluids and medication, and connect the patient to a cardiac monitor.

Anaerobic infection

If the patient has an open wound with a foul odor and local swelling and discoloration, you must act quickly. Take the patient's vital signs, checking especially for fever, tachycardia, hypotension, and tachypnea. Next, start an I.V. catheter to administer fluids and medication, and provide supplemental oxygen.

In addition, be prepared for emergency surgery to drain and debride the wound. If the patient's condition is life-threatening, you may need to prepare him for transfer to a facility with a hyperbaric chamber.

---

tachycardia, accessory muscle use, asymmetrical chest expansion, and a nonproductive cough can also occur. On the affected side, breath sounds are absent or decreased, hyperresonance or tympany may be heard, and decreased vocal fremitus may be present.

◆ ***Rupture of the esophagus.*** A ruptured esophagus usually produces subcutaneous crepitation in the neck, chest wall, or supraclavicular fossa, although this sign doesn't always occur. In a rupture of the cervical esophagus, the patient has excruciating pain in the neck or supraclavicular area, his neck is resistant to passive motion, and he has local tenderness, soft-tissue swelling, dysphagia, odynophagia, and orthostatic vertigo.

Life-threatening rupture of the intrathoracic esophagus can produce mediastinal emphysema confirmed by a positive Hamman's sign. The patient has severe retrosternal, epigastric, neck, or scapular pain and edema of the chest wall and neck. He may also display dyspnea, tachypnea, asymmetrical chest expansion, nasal flaring, cyanosis, diaphoresis, tachycardia, hypotension, dysphagia, and fever.

◆ ***Rupture of the trachea or major bronchus.*** This life-threatening injury produces abrupt subcutaneous crepitation of the neck and anterior chest wall. The patient has severe dyspnea with nasal flaring, tachycardia, accessory muscle use, hypotension, cyanosis, extreme anxiety and, possibly, hemoptysis and mediastinal emphysema confirmed by a positive Hamman's sign.

Other causes

◆ ***Diagnostic tests.*** Endoscopic tests, such as bronchoscopy and upper GI tract endoscopy, can cause rupture or perforation of respiratory or GI organs, producing subcutaneous crepitation.

◆ ***Respiratory treatments.*** Mechanical ventilation and intermittent positive-pressure breathing can rupture alveoli, producing subcutaneous crepitation.

◆ ***Thoracic surgery.*** Subcutaneous crepitation can occur if air escapes into the tissue in the area of the incision.

Special considerations

Monitor the patient's vital signs, especially respirations, frequently. Because excessive edema from subcutaneous crepitation in the neck and upper chest can cause airway obstruction, be alert for signs of respiratory distress such as dyspnea. Tell the patient that the affected tissues will eventually absorb the air or gas bubbles, decreasing the subcutaneous crepitation.

Pediatric pointers

Children may develop subcutaneous crepitation in the neck from ingestion of corrosive substances that perforate the esophagus.

PATIENT COUNSELING

Warn patients with asthma or chronic bronchitis to be alert for subcutaneous crepitation, which can signal pneumothorax, a dangerous complication.

Cry, high-pitched

[Cerebral cry]

A high-pitched cry is a brief, sharp, piercing vocal sound produced by a neonate or an infant. Whether acute or chronic, this cry is a late sign of increased intracranial pressure (ICP). The acute onset of a high-pitched cry demands emergency treatment to prevent permanent brain damage or death.

Any change in the volume of one of the brain's components—brain tissue, cerebrospinal fluid, or blood—may cause increased ICP. In neonates, increased ICP may result from intracranial bleeding associated with birth trauma or from congenital malformations, such as craniostenosis and Arnold-Chiari syndrome. In fact, a high-pitched cry may be an early sign of a congenital malformation. In infants, increased ICP may result from meningitis, head trauma, or child abuse.

HISTORY AND PHYSICAL EXAMINATION

Take the infant's vital signs, and then obtain a brief history. Did the infant fall recently or experience even minor head trauma? Be sure to ask the mother about any changes in the infant's behavior during the past 24 hours: Has he been vomiting? Has he seemed restless or unlike himself? Has his sucking reflex diminished? Does he cry when moved? Suspect child abuse if the infant's history is inconsistent with physical findings.

Next, perform a neurologic examination. Remember that neurologic responses in neonates and young infants are primarily reflex responses. Determine the infant's level of consciousness (LOC). Is he awake, irritable, or lethargic? Does he reach for an attractive object or turn toward the sound of a rattle? Observe his posture. Is he in the normal flexed position or in extension or opisthotonos? Examine muscle tone and observe the infant for signs of a seizure, such as a tremor and twitching.

Examine the size and shape of the infant's head. Is the anterior fontanel bulging? Measure the infant's head circumference, and check pupillary size and response to light. Unilateral or bilateral dilation and a sluggish response to light may accompany increased ICP. Finally, test the infant's reflexes; expect Moro's reflex to be diminished.

After completing your examination, elevate the infant's head to promote cerebral venous drainage and decrease ICP. Start an I.V. catheter, and give a diuretic and a corticosteroid to decrease ICP. Be sure to keep endotracheal (ET) intubation equipment close by to secure an airway.

MEDICAL CAUSES

◆ ***Increased ICP.*** A high-pitched cry is a late sign of increased ICP. Typically, the infant also displays bulging fontanels, increased head circumference, and widened sutures. Earlier signs and symptoms of increasing ICP include seizures, bradycardia, dilated pupils, decreased LOC, increased systolic blood pressure, widened pulse pressure, altered respiratory pattern and, possibly, vomiting.

SPECIAL CONSIDERATIONS

An infant with increased ICP requires specialized care and monitoring in the intensive care unit. For example, you'll need to monitor his vital signs and neurologic status to detect subtle changes in his condition. Also, monitor intake and output and ICP. Restrict fluids and administer a diuretic. Increase the head of the bed 30 degrees, if the infant's condition permits, and keep the head midline. Perform nursing care judiciously because procedures may further increase ICP. For an infant with severely increased ICP, ET intubation and mechanical hyperventilation may be needed to decrease serum carbon dioxide levels and constrict cerebral blood vessels. Hyperventilation is used for acute increases in ICP after carefully weighing the risks and benefits. Alternatively, a barbiturate coma or hypothermia therapy may be needed to decrease the infant's metabolic rate.

Remember to avoid jostling the infant, which may aggravate increased ICP. Comfort him and maintain a calm, quiet environment because the infant's crying or exposure to environmental stimuli may also worsen increased ICP.

Cyanosis

A bluish or bluish black discoloration of the skin and mucous membranes, cyanosis results from excessive concentration of unoxygenated hemoglobin in the blood. This common sign may develop abruptly or gradually. It can be classified as central or peripheral, although the two types may coexist.

Central cyanosis reflects inadequate oxygenation of systemic arterial blood caused by right-to-left cardiac shunting, pulmonary disease, or hematologic disorders. It may occur anywhere on the skin and also on the mucous membranes of the mouth, lips, and conjunctivae.

Peripheral cyanosis reflects sluggish peripheral circulation caused by vasoconstriction, reduced cardiac output, or vascular occlusion. It may be widespread or may affect only one extremity; however, it doesn't affect mucous membranes. Typically, peripheral cyanosis appears on exposed areas, such as the fingers, nail beds, feet, nose, and ears.

Although cyanosis is an important sign of cardiovascular and pulmonary disorders, it isn't always an accurate gauge of oxygenation. Several factors contribute to its development: hemoglobin concentration and oxygen saturation, cardiac output, and partial pressure of arterial oxygen (Pao_2). Cyanosis is usually undetectable until the oxygen saturation of hemoglobin falls below 80%. Severe cyanosis is quite obvious, whereas mild cyanosis is more difficult to detect, even in natural bright light. In dark-skinned patients, cyanosis is most apparent in the mucous membranes and nail beds.

Transient, nonpathologic cyanosis may result from environmental factors. For example, peripheral cyanosis may result from cutaneous vasoconstriction after brief exposure to cold air or water, and central cyanosis may result from reduced Pao_2 at high altitudes.

EMERGENCY INTERVENTIONS *If the patient displays sudden, localized cyanosis and other signs of arterial occlusion, protect the affected limb from injury, but don't massage it. If you see central cyanosis stemming from a pulmonary disorder or shock, perform a rapid evaluation. Take immediate steps to maintain an airway, assist breathing, and monitor circulation.*

History and physical examination

If cyanosis accompanies less acute conditions, perform a thorough examination. Begin with a history, focusing on cardiac, pulmonary, and hematologic disorders. Ask about previous surgery. Then begin the physical examination by taking vital signs. Inspect the skin and mucous membranes to determine the extent of cyanosis. Ask the patient when he first noticed the cyanosis. Does it subside and recur? Is it aggravated by cold, smoking, or stress? Is it alleviated by massage or rewarming? Check the skin for coolness, pallor, redness, pain, and ulceration. Also note clubbing.

Next, evaluate the patient's level of consciousness. Ask about headaches, dizziness, or blurred vision. Then test his motor strength. Ask about pain in the arms and legs (especially with walking) and about abnormal sensations, such as numbness, tingling, and coldness.

Ask about chest pain and its severity. Can the patient identify any aggravating or alleviating factors? Palpate peripheral pulses, and test capillary refill time. Also, check for edema. Auscultate heart rate and rhythm, especially noting gallops and murmurs. Also auscultate the abdominal aorta and femoral arteries to detect any bruits.

Does the patient have a cough? Is it productive? If so, have the patient describe the sputum. Evaluate respiratory rate and rhythm. Check for nasal flaring and use of accessory muscles. Ask about sleep apnea. Does the patient sleep with his head propped up on pillows? Inspect the patient for asymmetrical chest expansion or barrel chest. Percuss the lungs for dullness or hyperresonance, and auscultate for decreased or adventitious breath sounds.

Inspect the abdomen for ascites, and test for shifting dullness or a fluid wave. Percuss and palpate the abdomen for liver enlargement and tenderness. Also, ask about nausea, anorexia, and weight loss.

Medical causes

◆ ***Arteriosclerotic occlusive disease (chronic).*** In this disorder, peripheral cyanosis occurs in the legs whenever they're in a dependent position. Associated signs and symptoms include intermittent claudication and burning pain at rest, paresthesia, pallor, muscle atrophy, weak leg pulses, and impotence. Leg ulcers and gangrene are late signs.

◆ ***Blast lung injury.*** Cyanosis is a serious sign of blast lung injury. The impact of this condition on the lungs of affected individuals varies and may include tearing, contusion, edema, and hemorrhage. Other signs and symptoms may include chest pain, wheezing, hemoptysis, and dyspnea. Treatment for patients with blast lung injury typically involves high-flow oxygen, careful fluid management, possible intubation, and close observation in an intensive care setting.

◆ ***Bronchiectasis.*** This disorder produces chronic central cyanosis. Its classic sign, though, is a chronic productive cough with copious, foul-smelling, mucopurulent sputum or hemoptysis. Auscultation reveals rhonchi and coarse crackles during inspiration. Other signs and symptoms include dyspnea, recurrent fever and chills, weight loss, malaise, clubbing, and signs of anemia.

◆ ***Buerger's disease.*** In this disorder, exposure to cold initially causes the feet to become cold, cyanotic, and numb; later, they become red, hot, and tingly. Intermittent claudication of the instep, a characteristic sign, is aggravated by exercise and smoking and relieved by rest. Associated signs and symptoms include weak peripheral pulses and, in later stages, ulceration, muscle atrophy, and gangrene.

◆ ***Chronic obstructive pulmonary disease (COPD).*** Chronic central cyanosis occurs in advanced COPD and may be aggravated by exertion. Associated signs and symptoms include exertional dyspnea, a productive cough with thick sputum, anorexia, weight loss, purse-lip breathing, tachypnea, and accessory muscle use. Examination reveals wheezing and hyperresonant lung fields. Barrel chest and clubbing are late signs. Tachycardia, diaphoresis, and flushing may also accompany COPD.

◆ ***Deep vein thrombosis.*** In this disorder, acute peripheral cyanosis in the affected extremity is associated with tenderness, painful movement, edema, warmth, and prominent superficial veins. Homans' sign can also be elicited.

◆ ***Heart failure.*** Acute or chronic cyanosis may occur in patients with heart failure. It may be central, peripheral, or both and is typically a late sign. In left-sided heart failure, central cyanosis occurs with tachycardia, fatigue, dyspnea, cold intolerance, orthopnea, a cough, ventricular or atrial gallop, bibasilar crackles, and diffuse apical impulse. In right-sided heart failure, peripheral cyanosis occurs with fatigue, peripheral edema, ascites, jugular vein distention, and hepatomegaly.

◆ ***Lung cancer.*** This disease causes chronic central cyanosis accompanied by fever, weakness, anorexia, weight loss, dyspnea, chest pain, hemoptysis, and wheezing. Atelectasis causes mediastinal shift, decreased diaphragmatic excursion, asymmetrical chest expansion, a dull percussion note, and diminished breath sounds.

◆ ***Peripheral arterial occlusion (acute).*** This disorder produces acute cyanosis of one arm or leg or, occasionally, of both legs. The cyanosis is accompanied by sharp or aching pain that worsens when the patient moves. The affected extremity also exhibits paresthesia, weakness, and pale, cool skin. Examination reveals decreased or absent pulse and increased capillary refill time.

◆ ***Pneumonia.*** In pneumonia, acute central cyanosis is usually preceded by fever, shaking chills, a cough with purulent sputum, crackles, rhonchi, and pleuritic chest pain that's exacerbated by deep inspiration. Associated signs and symptoms include tachycardia, dyspnea, tachypnea, diminished breath sounds, diaphoresis, myalgia, fatigue, headache, and anorexia.

◆ ***Pneumothorax.*** A cardinal sign of pneumothorax, acute central cyanosis is accompanied by dyspnea; sharp chest pain that's exacerbated by movement, deep breathing, and coughing; and asymmetrical chest wall expansion. The patient may also exhibit rapid, shallow respirations; a weak, rapid pulse; pallor; jugular vein distention; anxiety; and absence of breath sounds over the affected lobe.

◆ ***Polycythemia vera.*** A ruddy complexion that can appear cyanotic is characteristic in this chronic myeloproliferative disorder. Other findings include hepatosplenomegaly, headache, dizziness, fatigue, aquagenic pruritus, blurred vision, chest pain, intermittent claudication, and coagulation defects.

◆ ***Pulmonary edema.*** In this disorder, acute central cyanosis occurs with dyspnea; orthopnea; frothy, blood-tinged sputum; tachycardia; tachypnea; dependent crackles; ventricular gallop; cold, clammy skin; weak, thready pulse; hypotension; and confusion.

◆ ***Pulmonary embolism.*** Acute central cyanosis occurs when a large embolus causes significant obstruction of the pulmonary circulation. Syncope and jugular vein distention may also occur. Other common signs and symptoms include dyspnea, chest pain, tachycardia, paradoxical pulse, a dry cough or a productive cough with blood-tinged sputum, low-grade fever, restlessness, and diaphoresis.

◆ ***Raynaud's disease.*** In Raynaud's disease, exposure to cold or stress initially causes the fingers or hands to blanch and turn cold, then to become cyanotic, and finally to redden with return of normal temperature. Numbness and tingling may also occur. Raynaud's phenomenon describes the same presentation when associated with other disorders, such as rheumatoid arthritis, scleroderma, or lupus erythematosus.

◆ ***Shock.*** In shock, acute peripheral cyanosis develops in the hands and feet, which may also be cold, clammy, and pale. Other characteristic signs and symptoms include lethargy, confusion, increased capillary refill time, and a rapid, weak pulse. Tachypnea, hyperpnea, and hypotension may also be present.

◆ ***Sleep apnea.*** Chronic and severe sleep apnea causes pulmonary hypertension and cor pulmonale (right-sided heart failure), which can produce chronic cyanosis.

Special considerations

Provide supplemental oxygen to relieve dyspnea, improve oxygenation, and decrease cyanosis. Be sure to deliver small doses (2 L/minute) to patients with COPD, who may retain carbon dioxide. Use a low-flow oxygen rate for mild COPD exacerbations. However, for acute situations, a high-flow oxygen rate may be needed initially. Remember to pay attention to the patient's respiratory drive and adjust the amount of oxygen accordingly. Position the patient comfortably to ease breathing. Administer a diuretic, a bronchodilator, an antibiotic or a cardiac drug as needed. Make sure that the patient gets sufficient rest between activities to prevent dyspnea.

Prepare the patient for such tests as arterial blood gas analysis and a complete blood count to determine the cause of cyanosis.

Pediatric pointers

Many pulmonary disorders responsible for cyanosis in adults also cause cyanosis in children. In addition, central cyanosis may result from cystic fibrosis, asthma, airway obstruction by a foreign body, acute laryngotracheobronchitis, or epiglottiditis. It may also result from a congenital heart defect, such as transposition of the great vessels, that causes right-to-left intracardiac shunting.

In children, circumoral cyanosis may precede generalized cyanosis. Acrocyanosis (also called "glove and bootee" cyanosis) may occur in infants from excessive crying or exposure to cold. Exercise and agitation enhance cyanosis, so provide regular rest periods and make the child comfortable. Also, administer supplemental oxygen during cyanotic episodes.

Geriatric pointers

Because elderly patients have reduced tissue perfusion, peripheral cyanosis can occur even with a slight decrease in cardiac output or systemic blood pressure.

Patient counseling

Teach patients with chronic cardiopulmonary diseases, such as heart failure, asthma, or COPD, to recognize cyanosis as a sign of severe disease and to get immediate medical attention when it occurs.

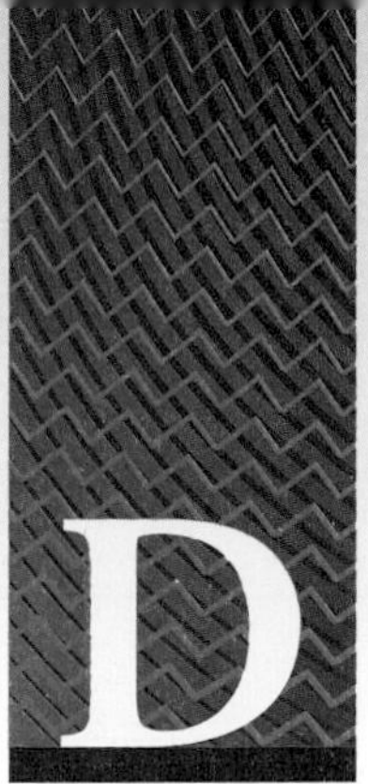

Decerebrate posture

[Decerebrate rigidity, abnormal extensor reflex]

Decerebrate posture is characterized by adduction (internal rotation) and extension of the arms, with the wrists pronated and the fingers flexed. The legs are stiffly extended, with forced plantar flexion of the feet. In severe cases, the back is acutely arched (opisthotonos). This sign indicates upper brain stem damage, which may result from primary lesions, such as infarction, hemorrhage, or tumor; metabolic encephalopathy; head injury; or brain stem compression associated with increased intracranial pressure (ICP).

Decerebrate posture may be elicited by noxious stimuli or may occur spontaneously. It may be unilateral or bilateral. With concurrent brain stem and cerebral damage, decerebrate posture may affect only the arms, with the legs remaining flaccid. Or, decerebrate posture may affect one side of the body and decorticate posture the other. The two postures may also alternate as the patient's neurologic status fluctuates. Generally, the duration of each posturing episode correlates with the severity of brain stem damage. (See *Comparing decerebrate and decorticate postures,* page 198.)

EMERGENCY INTERVENTIONS *Your first priority is to ensure a patent airway. Insert an artificial airway and institute measures to prevent aspiration. (Don't disrupt spinal alignment if you suspect spinal cord injury.) Suction the patient as necessary.*

Next, examine spontaneous respirations. Give supplemental oxygen, and ventilate the patient with a handheld resuscitation bag if necessary. Intubation and mechanical ventilation may be indicated. Keep emergency resuscitation equipment handy, but be sure to check the patient's chart for a do-not-resuscitate order.

History and physical examination

After taking vital signs, determine the patient's level of consciousness (LOC). Use the Glasgow Coma Scale (GCS) as a reference. Decerebrate posturing indicates the second-lowest measure of motor response, according to the GCS. Patients exhibiting this abnormal posturing have a decreased LOC and may be in a comatose state. Evaluate the pupils for size, equality, and response to light. Test deep tendon reflexes (DTRs) and cranial nerve reflexes, and check for doll's eye sign.

Next, explore the history of the patient's coma. If you're unable to obtain this information, look for clues to the causative disorder, such as hepatomegaly, cyanosis, diabetic skin changes, needle tracks, or obvious trauma. If a family member is available, find out when the patient's LOC began deteriorating. Did it occur abruptly? What did the patient complain of before he lost consciousness? Does he have a history of diabetes, liver disease, cancer, blood clots, or aneurysm? Ask about any accident or traumatic injury responsible for the coma.

Comparing decerebrate and decorticate postures

Decerebrate posture results from damage to the upper brain stem. In this posture, the arms are adducted and extended, with the wrists pronated and the fingers flexed. The legs are stiffly extended, with plantar flexion of the feet.

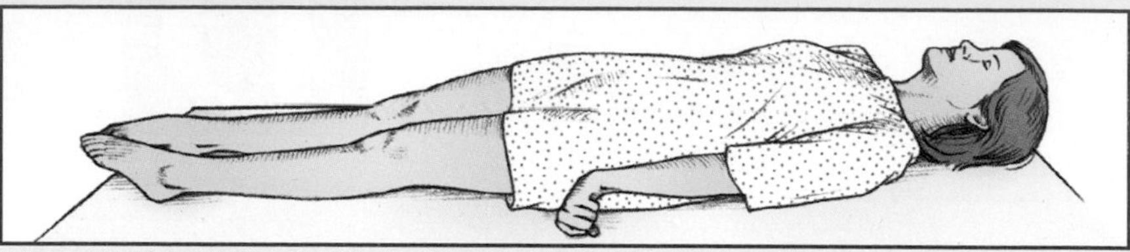

Decorticate posture results from damage to one or both corticospinal tracts. In this posture, the arms are adducted and the elbows are flexed, with the wrists and fingers flexed on the chest. The legs are stiffly extended and internally rotated, with plantar flexion of the feet.

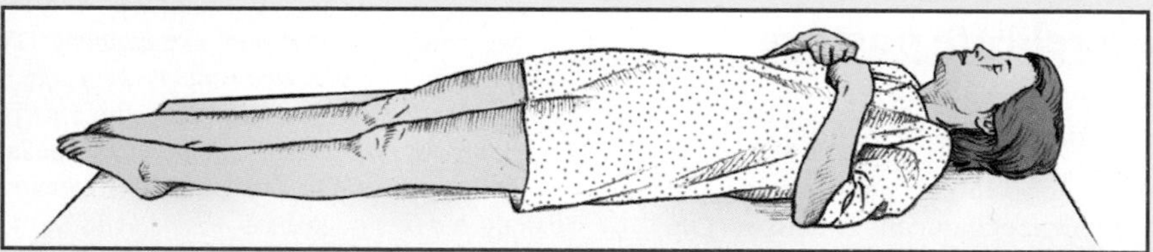

MEDICAL CAUSES

◆ ***Brain stem infarction.*** Decerebrate posture may be elicited when this primary lesion produces a coma. Associated signs and symptoms vary with the severity of the infarct and may include cranial nerve palsies, bilateral cerebellar ataxia, and sensory loss. In a deep coma, all normal reflexes are usually lost, resulting in absence of doll's eye sign, a positive Babinski's reflex, and flaccidity.

◆ ***Brain stem tumor.*** In a brain stem tumor, decerebrate posture is a late sign that accompanies a coma. Early findings commonly include hemiparesis or quadriparesis, cranial nerve palsies, vertigo, dizziness, ataxia, and vomiting.

◆ ***Cerebral lesion.*** Whether the cause is trauma, tumor, abscess, or infarction, any cerebral lesion that increases ICP may also produce decerebrate posture, which is typically a late sign. Associated findings vary with the lesion's site and extent but commonly include a coma, abnormal pupil size and response to light, and the classic triad of increased ICP—bradycardia, increasing systolic blood pressure, and widening pulse pressure.

◆ ***Hepatic encephalopathy.*** A late sign in this disorder, decerebrate posture occurs with a coma resulting from increased ICP and ammonia toxicity. Associated signs include fetor hepaticus (foul-smelling breath), a positive Babinski's reflex, and hyperactive DTRs.

◆ ***Hypoglycemic encephalopathy.*** Characterized by extremely low blood glucose levels, this disorder may produce decerebrate posture and a coma. It also causes dilated pupils, bradypnea, and bradycardia. Muscle spasms, twitching, and seizures eventually progress to flaccidity.

◆ ***Hypoxic encephalopathy.*** Severe hypoxia may produce decerebrate posture—the result of brain stem compression associated with anaerobic metabolism and increased ICP. Other findings include a coma, a positive Babinski's reflex, absence of doll's eye sign, hypoactive DTRs, and possibly fixed pupils and respiratory arrest.

◆ ***Pontine hemorrhage.*** Typically, this life-threatening disorder rapidly leads to decerebrate posture with a coma. Accompanying signs include total paralysis, absence of doll's eye sign, a positive Babinski's reflex, and small, reactive pupils.

◆ ***Posterior fossa hemorrhage.*** This subtentorial lesion causes decerebrate posture. Its early signs and symptoms include vomiting, headache, vertigo, ataxia, stiff neck, drowsiness, papilledema, and cranial nerve palsies. The patient eventually slips into a coma and may experience respiratory arrest.

OTHER CAUSES

◆ ***Diagnostic tests.*** Removal of spinal fluid during a lumbar puncture to relieve high ICP may precipitate cerebral compression of the brain stem and cause decerebrate posture and a coma.

SPECIAL CONSIDERATIONS

Help prepare the patient for diagnostic tests that will determine the cause of his decerebrate posture. These include skull X-rays, computed tomography scan, magnetic resonance imaging, cerebral angiography, digital subtraction angiography, EEG, brain scan, and ICP monitoring.

Monitor the patient's neurologic status and vital signs every 30 minutes or as indicated. Also, be alert for signs of increased ICP (bradycardia, increasing systolic blood pressure, and widening pulse pressure) and neurologic deterioration (altered respiratory pattern and abnormal temperature).

Inform the patient's family that decerebrate posture is a reflex response—not a voluntary response to pain or a sign of recovery. Offer emotional support.

PEDIATRIC POINTERS

Children younger than age 2 may not display decerebrate posture because the nervous system is still immature. However, if this posture occurs, it's usually the more severe opisthotonos. In fact, opisthotonos is more common in infants and young children than in adults and is usually a terminal sign. In children, the most common cause of decerebrate posture is head injury. It also occurs in Reye's syndrome—the result of increased ICP causing brain stem compression.

Decorticate posture

[Decorticate rigidity, abnormal flexor response]

A sign of corticospinal damage, decorticate posture is characterized by adduction of the arms and flexion of the elbows, with wrists and fingers flexed on the chest. The legs are extended and internally rotated, with plantar flexion of the feet. This posture may occur unilaterally or bilaterally. It usually results from a stroke or head injury. It may be elicited by noxious stimuli or may occur spontaneously. The intensity of the required stimulus, the duration of the posture, and the frequency of spontaneous episodes vary with the severity and location of the cerebral injury.

Although a serious sign, decorticate posture carries a more favorable prognosis than decerebrate posture. However, decorticate posture may progress to decerebrate posture if the causative disorder extends lower in the brain stem. (See *Comparing decerebrate and decorticate postures.*)

EMERGENCY INTERVENTIONS *Obtain vital signs and evaluate the patient's level of consciousness (LOC). If his consciousness is impaired, insert an oropharyngeal airway, and take measures to prevent aspiration (unless spinal cord injury is suspected). Evaluate the patient's respiratory rate, rhythm, and depth. Prepare to assist respirations with a handheld resuscitation bag or with intubation and mechanical ventilation if necessary. Also, institute seizure precautions.*

HISTORY AND PHYSICAL EXAMINATION

Test the patient's motor and sensory function. Evaluate pupil size, equality, and response to light. Then test cranial nerve function and deep tendon reflexes. Ask family members if the patient experienced headache, dizziness, nausea, changes in vision, numbness, or tingling. When did the patient first notice these symptoms? Is his family aware of any behavioral changes? Also, ask about a history of cerebrovascular disease, cancer, meningitis, encephalitis, upper respiratory tract infection, bleeding or clotting disorders, or recent trauma.

MEDICAL CAUSES

◆ ***Brain abscess.*** Decorticate posture may occur in a brain abscess. Accompanying findings vary depending on the size and location of the abscess but may include aphasia, hemiparesis, headache, dizziness, seizures, nausea, and vomiting. The patient may also experience behavioral changes, altered vital signs, and decreased LOC.

◆ ***Brain tumor.*** A brain tumor may produce decorticate posture that's usually bilateral—the result of increased intracranial pressure (ICP) associated with tumor growth. Related signs and symptoms include headache, behavioral changes, memory loss, diplopia, blurred vision or vision loss, seizures, ataxia, dizziness, apraxia, aphasia, paresis, sensory loss, paresthesia, vomiting, papilledema, and signs of hormonal imbalance.

◆ ***Head injury.*** Decorticate posture may result from a head injury, depending on the site and severity of the injury. Associated signs and symptoms include headache, nausea and vomiting, dizziness, irritability, decreased LOC, aphasia, hemiparesis, unilateral numbness, seizures, and pupillary dilation.

◆ ***Stroke.*** Typically, a stroke involving the cerebral cortex produces unilateral decorticate posture, also called spastic hemiplegia. Other signs and symptoms include hemiplegia (contralateral to the lesion), dysarthria, dysphagia, unilateral sensory loss, apraxia, agnosia, aphasia, memory loss, decreased LOC, urine retention, urinary incontinence, and constipation. Ocular effects include homonymous hemianopsia, diplopia, and blurred vision.

Special considerations
Monitor the patient's neurologic status and vital signs every 30 minutes to 2 hours. Be alert for signs of increased ICP, including bradycardia, increasing systolic blood pressure, and widening pulse pressure and subtle signs of neurologic deterioration.

Pediatric pointers
Decorticate posture is an unreliable sign before age 2 because of nervous system immaturity. In children, this posture usually results from head injury, but it may also occur in Reye's syndrome.

Deep tendon reflexes, hyperactive

A hyperactive deep tendon reflex (DTR) is an abnormally brisk muscle contraction that occurs in response to a sudden stretch induced by sharply tapping the muscle's tendon of insertion. This elicited sign may be graded as brisk or pathologically hyperactive. Hyperactive DTRs are commonly accompanied by clonus.

The corticospinal tract and other descending tracts govern the reflex arc—the relay cycle that produces any reflex response. A corticospinal lesion above the level of the reflex arc being tested may result in hyperactive DTRs. Abnormal neuromuscular transmission at the end of the reflex arc may also cause hyperactive DTRs. For example, a deficiency of calcium or magnesium may cause hyperactive DTRs because these electrolytes regulate neuromuscular excitability. (See *The reflex arc,* pages 202 and 203.)

Although hyperactive DTRs typically accompany other neurologic findings, they usually lack specific diagnostic value.

History and physical examination
After eliciting hyperactive DTRs, take the patient's history. Ask about spinal cord injury or other trauma and about prolonged exposure to cold, wind, or water. Could the patient be pregnant? A positive response to any of these questions requires prompt evaluation to rule out life-threatening autonomic hyperreflexia, tetanus, preeclampsia, or hypothermia. Ask about the onset and progression of associated signs and symptoms. Next, perform a neurologic examination. Evaluate level of consciousness, and test motor and sensory function in the limbs. Ask about paresthesia. Check for ataxia or tremors and for speech and visual deficits. Test for Chvostek's sign (an abnormal spasm of the facial muscles elicited by light taps on the facial nerve in patients who have hypocalcemia) and Trousseau's sign (a carpal spasm induced by inflating a sphygmomanometer cuff on the upper arm to a pressure exceeding systolic blood pressure for 3 minutes in patients who have hypocalcemia or hypomagnesemia) and for carpopedal spasm. Ask about vomiting or altered urination habits. Be sure to take vital signs.

Medical causes
◆ ***Amyotrophic lateral sclerosis.*** This disorder produces generalized hyperactive DTRs accompanied by weakness of the hands and forearms and spasticity of the legs. Eventually, the patient develops atrophy of the neck and tongue muscles, fasciculations, weakness of the legs and, possibly, bulbar signs (dysphagia, dysphonia, facial weakness, and dyspnea).

◆ ***Brain tumor.*** A cerebral tumor causes hyperactive DTRs on the side opposite the lesion. Associated signs and symptoms develop slowly and may include unilateral paresis or paralysis, anesthesia, visual field deficits, spasticity, and a positive Babinski's reflex.

◆ ***Hepatic encephalopathy.*** Generalized hyperactive DTRs occur late and are accompanied by a positive Babinski's reflex, fetor hepaticus, and a coma.

◆ ***Hypocalcemia.*** This disorder may produce sudden or gradual onset of generalized hyperactive DTRs with paresthesia, muscle twitching and cramping, positive Chvostek's and Trousseau's signs, carpopedal spasm, and tetany.

◆ ***Hypomagnesemia.*** This disorder results in gradual onset of generalized hyperactive DTRs accompanied by muscle cramps, hypotension, tachycardia, paresthesia, ataxia, tetany and, possibly, seizures.

◆ ***Hypothermia.*** Mild hypothermia (90° to 94° F [32.2° to 34.4° C]) produces generalized hyperactive DTRs. Other signs and symptoms include shivering, fatigue, weakness, lethargy, slurred speech, ataxia, muscle stiffness, tachycardia, diuresis, bradypnea, hypotension, and cold, pale skin.

◆ ***Multiple sclerosis.*** Typically, hyperactive DTRs are preceded by weakness and paresthesia in one or both arms or legs. Associated signs include clonus and a positive Babinski's reflex. Passive flexion of the patient's neck may cause a tingling sensation down his back. Later, ataxia, diplopia, vertigo, vomiting, urine retention, or urinary incontinence may occur.

◆ ***Preeclampsia.*** Occurring in pregnancy of at least 20 weeks' duration, preeclampsia may cause gradual onset of generalized hyperactive DTRs. Accompanying signs and symptoms include increased blood pressure; abnormal weight gain; edema of the face, fingers, and abdomen after bed rest; albuminuria; oliguria; severe headache; blurred or double vision; epigastric pain; nausea and vomiting; irritability; cyanosis; dyspnea; and crackles. If preeclampsia progresses to eclampsia, the patient develops seizures.

◆ ***Spinal cord lesion.*** Incomplete spinal cord lesions cause hyperactive DTRs below the level of the lesion. In a traumatic lesion, hyperactive DTRs follow resolution of spinal shock. In a neoplastic lesion, hyperactive DTRs gradually replace normal DTRs. Other signs and symptoms are paralysis and sensory loss below the level of the lesion, urine retention and overflow incontinence, and alternating constipation and diarrhea. A lesion above T6 may also produce autonomic hyperreflexia with diaphoresis and flushing above the level of the lesion, headache, nasal congestion, nausea, increased blood pressure, and bradycardia.

◆ ***Stroke.*** Any stroke that affects the origin of the corticospinal tracts causes sudden onset of hyperactive DTRs on the side opposite the lesion. The patient may also have unilateral paresis or paralysis, anesthesia, visual field deficits, spasticity, and a positive Babinski's reflex.

◆ ***Tetanus.*** In this disorder, sudden onset of generalized hyperactive DTRs accompanies tachycardia, diaphoresis, low-grade fever, painful and involuntary muscle contractions, trismus (lockjaw), and risus sardonicus (a masklike grin).

SPECIAL CONSIDERATIONS

Prepare the patient for diagnostic tests to evaluate hyperactive DTRs. These may include laboratory tests for serum calcium magnesium and ammonia levels, magnetic resonance imaging, computed tomography scan, lumbar puncture, spinal X-rays, and myelography.

If motor weakness accompanies hyperactive DTRs, perform or encourage range-of-motion exercises to preserve muscle integrity and prevent deep vein thrombosis. Also, reposition the patient frequently, provide a special mattress, and massage his back and ensure adequate nutrition to prevent skin breakdown. Administer a muscle relaxant and a sedative to relieve severe muscle contractions. Keep emergency resuscitation equipment on hand. Provide a quiet, calm atmosphere to decrease neuromuscular excitability. Assist with activities of daily living, and provide emotional support.

PEDIATRIC POINTERS

Hyperreflexia may be a normal sign in neonates. After age 6, reflex responses are similar to those of adults. When testing DTRs in small children, use distraction techniques to promote reliable results.

Cerebral palsy commonly causes hyperactive DTRs in children. Reye's syndrome causes generalized hyperactive DTRs in stage II and absent DTRs in stage V. Adult causes of hyperactive DTRs may also appear in children.

Deep tendon reflexes, hypoactive

A hypoactive deep tendon reflex (DTR) is an abnormally diminished muscle contraction that occurs in response to a sudden stretch induced by sharply tapping the muscle's tendon of

(Text continues on page 204.)

The reflex arc

The reflex arc is the transmission of sensory impulses to a motor neuron via the dorsal root. The motor neuron delivers the impulse to a muscle or gland, producing an immediate response.

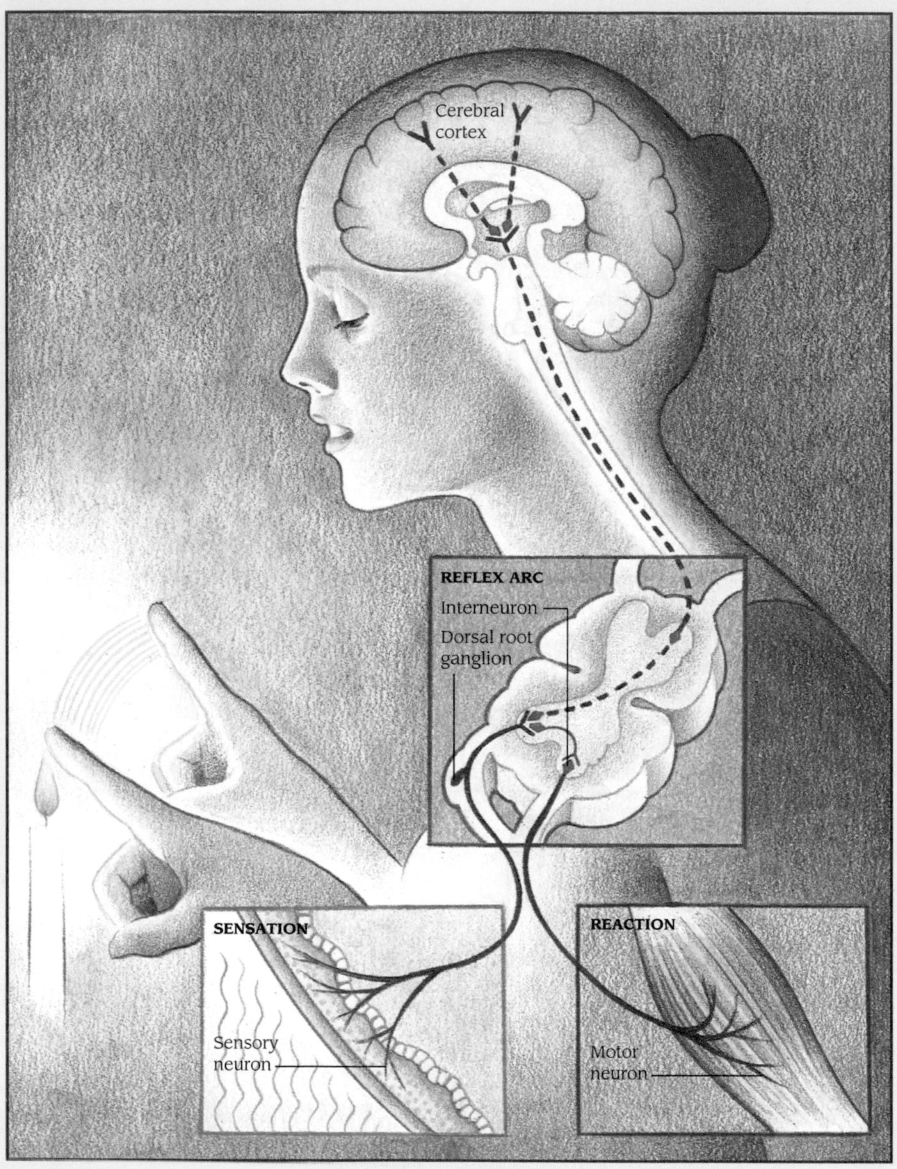

BICEPS REFLEX
(C 5–6 INNERVATION)

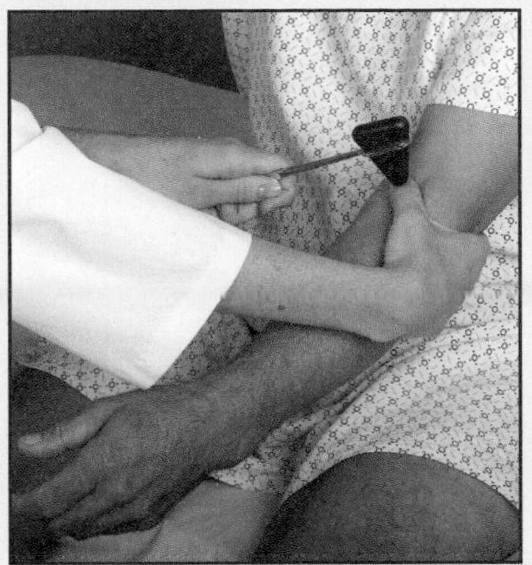

TRICEPS REFLEX
(C 7–8 INNERVATION)

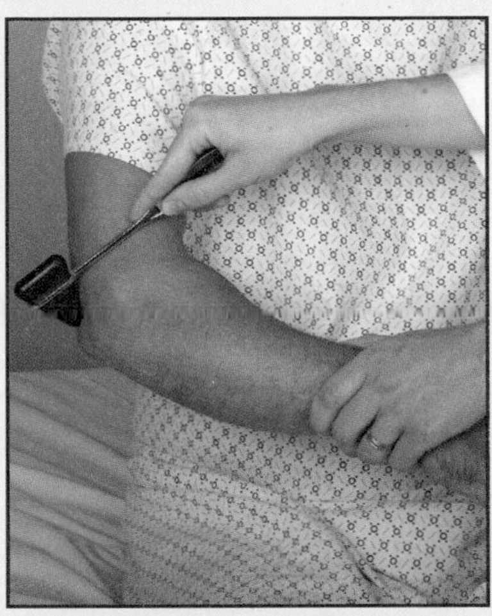

PATELLAR REFLEXES
(L 2–4 INNERVATION)

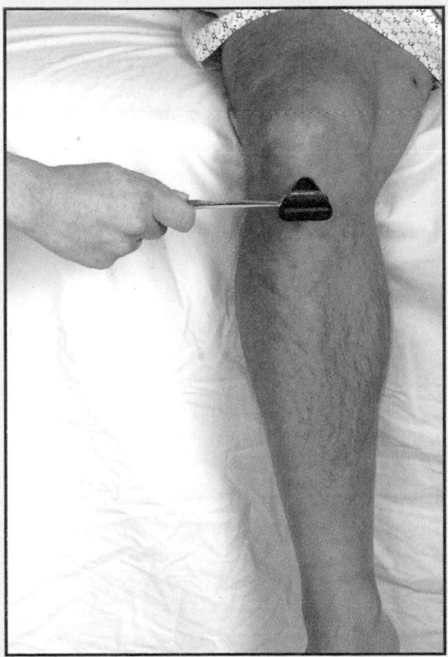

BRACHIORADIALIS REFLEX
(C 5–6 INNERVATION)

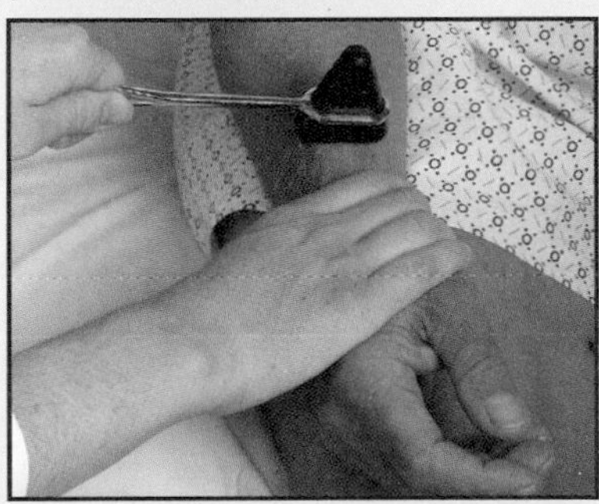

ACHILLES TENDON REFLEX
(S 1–2 INNERVATION)

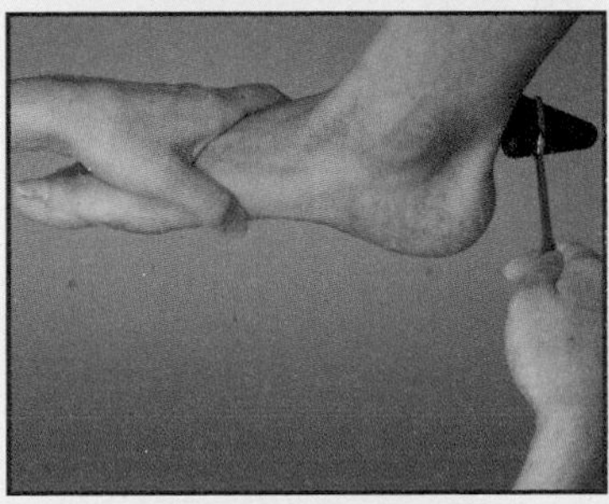

Documenting deep tendon reflexes

Record the patient's deep tendon reflex scores by drawing a stick figure and entering the grades on this scale at the proper location. The figure shown here indicates hypoactive deep tendon reflexes in the legs; other reflexes are normal.

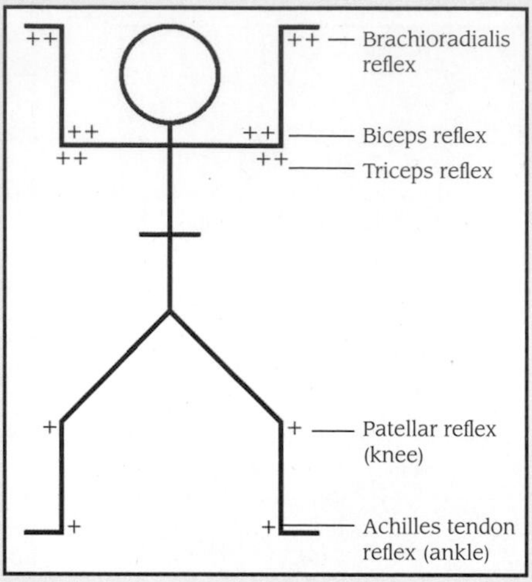

KEY:

0 = absent

\+ = hypoactive (diminished)

++ = normal

+++ = brisk (increased)

++++ = hyperactive (clonus may be present)

insertion. It may be graded as minimal (+) or absent (0). Symmetrically reduced (+) reflexes may be normal.

Normally, a DTR depends on an intact receptor, intact sensory-motor nerve fiber, an intact neuromuscular-glandular junction, and a functional synapse in the spinal cord. Hypoactive DTRs may result from damage to the reflex arc involving the specific muscle, the peripheral nerve, the nerve roots, or the spinal cord at that level. Hypoactive DTRs are an important sign of many disorders, especially when they appear with other neurologic signs and symptoms. (See *Documenting deep tendon reflexes*.)

History and physical examination

After eliciting hypoactive DTRs, obtain a thorough history from the patient or a family member. Have him describe current signs and symptoms in detail. Then take a family and drug history.

Next, evaluate the patient's level of consciousness. Test motor function in his limbs, and palpate for muscle atrophy or increased mass. Test sensory function, including pain, touch, temperature, and vibration sensation. Ask about paresthesia. To observe gait and coordination, have the patient take several steps. To check for Romberg's sign, ask him to stand with his feet together and his eyes closed. During conversation, evaluate his speech. Check for signs of vision or hearing loss. Abrupt onset of hypoactive DTRs accompanied by muscle weakness may occur in life-threatening Guillain-Barré syndrome, botulism, or spinal cord lesions with spinal shock.

Look for autonomic nervous system effects by taking vital signs and monitoring for increased heart rate and blood pressure. Also, inspect the skin for pallor, dryness, flushing, or diaphoresis. Auscultate for hypoactive bowel sounds, and palpate for bladder distention. Ask about nausea, vomiting, constipation, and incontinence.

Medical causes

◆ ***Botulism.*** In this disorder, generalized hypoactive DTRs accompany progressive descending muscle weakness. Initially, the patient usually complains of blurred and double vision and, occasionally, anorexia, nausea, and vomiting. Other early bulbar findings include vertigo, hearing loss, dysarthria, and dysphagia. The patient may have signs of respiratory distress and severe constipation marked by hypoactive bowel sounds.

◆ ***Cerebellar dysfunction.*** This disorder may produce hypoactive DTRs by increasing the level of inhibition through long tracts upon spinal motor neurons. Associated clinical findings vary depending on the cause and location of the dysfunction.

◆ ***Eaton-Lambert syndrome.*** This disorder produces generalized hypoactive DTRs. Early signs include difficulty rising from a chair, climbing stairs, and walking. The patient may complain of achiness, paresthesia, and muscle weakness that's most severe in the morning. Weakness improves with mild exercise and worsens with strenuous exercise.

◆ ***Guillain-Barré syndrome.*** This disorder causes bilateral hypoactive DTRs that progress from hypotonia to areflexia in several days. Guillain-Barré syndrome typically causes muscle weakness that begins in the legs and then extends to the arms and, possibly, to the trunk and neck muscles. Occasionally, weakness may progress to total paralysis. Other signs and symptoms include cranial nerve palsies, pain, paresthesia, and signs of brief autonomic dysfunction, such as sinus tachycardia or bradycardia, flushing, fluctuating blood pressure, and anhidrosis or episodic diaphoresis.

Usually, muscle weakness and hypoactive DTRs peak in severity within 10 to 14 days; then symptoms begin to clear. However, in severe cases, residual hypoactive DTRs and motor weakness may persist.

◆ ***Peripheral neuropathy.*** Characteristic of end-stage diabetes mellitus, renal failure, and alcoholism, and as an adverse effect of various medications, peripheral neuropathy results in progressive hypoactive DTRs. Other effects include motor weakness, sensory loss, paresthesia, tremors and, possibly, signs of autonomic dysfunction, such as orthostatic hypotension and incontinence.

◆ ***Polymyositis.*** In this disorder, hypoactive DTRs accompany muscle weakness, pain, stiffness, spasms and, possibly, increased size or atrophy. These effects are usually temporary; their location varies with the affected muscles.

◆ ***Spinal cord lesions.*** Spinal cord injury or complete transection produces spinal shock, resulting in hypoactive DTRs (areflexia) below the level of the lesion. Associated signs and symptoms include quadriplegia or paraplegia, flaccidity, loss of sensation below the level of the lesion, and dry, pale skin. Also characteristic are urine retention with overflow incontinence, hypoactive bowel sounds, constipation, and genital reflex loss. Hypoactive DTRs and flaccidity are usually transient; reflex activity may return within several weeks.

◆ ***Syringomyelia.*** Permanent bilateral hypoactive DTRs occur early in this slowly progressive disorder. Other signs and symptoms are muscle weakness and atrophy; loss of sensation usually extending in a capelike fashion over the arms, shoulders, neck, back, and occasionally the legs; deep, boring pain (despite analgesia) in the limbs; and signs of brain stem involvement (nystagmus, facial numbness, unilateral vocal cord paralysis or weakness, and unilateral tongue atrophy). Syringomyelia is more common in males than in females.

◆ ***Tabes dorsalis.*** This progressive disorder results in bilateral hypoactive DTRs in the legs and occasionally the arms. Associated signs and symptoms include sharp pain and paresthesia of the legs, face, or trunk; visceral pain with retching and vomiting; sensory loss in the legs; ataxic gait with a positive Romberg's sign; urine retention and urinary incontinence; and arthropathies.

Other causes

◆ ***Drugs.*** Barbiturates and paralyzing drugs, such as pancuronium, may cause hypoactive DTRs.

Special considerations

Help the patient perform his daily activities. Try to strike a balance between promoting independence and ensuring his safety. Encourage him to walk with assistance. Make sure personal care articles are within easy reach, and provide an obstacle-free course from his bed to the bathroom.

If the patient has sensory deficits, protect him from injury from heat, cold, or pressure. Test his bath water, and reposition him frequently, ensuring a soft, smooth bed surface. Keep his skin clean and dry to prevent breakdown. Perform or encourage range-of-motion exercises. Also encourage a balanced diet with plenty of protein and adequate hydration.

Pediatric pointers

Hypoactive DTRs commonly occur in children with muscular dystrophy, Friedreich's ataxia, syringomyelia, or a spinal cord injury. They also accompany progressive muscular atrophy, which affects preschoolers and adolescents.

Use distraction techniques to test DTRs; assess motor function by watching the infant or child at play.

Depression

Depression is a mood disturbance characterized by feelings of sadness, despair, and loss of interest or pleasure in activities. These feelings may be accompanied by somatic complaints, such as changes in appetite, sleep disturbances, restlessness or lethargy, and decreased concentration. The patient also may have thoughts of death, suicide, or injuring herself.

Clinical depression must be distinguished from "the blues," periodic bouts of dysphoria that are less persistent and severe than the clinical disorder. The criterion for major depression is one or more episodes of depressed mood, or decreased interest or ability to take pleasure in all or most activities, lasting at least 2 weeks.

Major depression strikes 10% to 15% of adults, affecting all racial, ethnic, age, and socioeconomic groups. It's twice as common in women as in men and is especially prevalent among adolescents. Depression has numerous causes, including genetic and family history, medical and psychiatric disorders, and the use of certain drugs. It can also occur in the postpartum period. A complete psychiatric and physical examination should be conducted to exclude possible medical causes.

HISTORY AND PHYSICAL EXAMINATION

During the examination, determine how the patient feels about herself, her family, and her environment. Your goal is to explore the nature of her depression, the extent to which other factors affect it, and her coping mechanisms and their effectiveness. Begin by asking what's bothering her. How does her current mood differ from her usual mood? Then ask her to describe the way she feels about herself. What are her plans and dreams? How realistic are they? Is she generally satisfied with what she has accomplished in her work, relationships, and other interests? Ask about changes in her social interactions, sleep patterns, appetite, normal activities, or ability to make decisions and concentrate. Determine patterns of drug and alcohol use. Listen for clues that she may be suicidal. (See *Suicide: Caring for the high-risk patient.*)

Ask the patient about her family—its patterns of interaction and characteristic responses to success and failure. What part does she feel she plays in her family life? Find out if other family members have been depressed and whether anyone important to her has been sick or has died in the past year. Finally, ask the patient about her environment. Has her lifestyle changed in the past month? Six months? Year? When she's feeling blue, where does she go and what does she do to feel better? Find out how she feels about her role in the community and the resources that are available to her. Try to determine if she has an adequate support network to help her cope with her depression.

CULTURAL CUE *Patients who don't speak English fluently may have difficulty communicating their feelings and thoughts. Consider using someone outside the family as an interpreter to allow the patient to express her feelings more freely.*

MEDICAL CAUSES

◆ ***Organic disorders.*** Various organic disorders and chronic illnesses produce mild, moderate, or severe depression. Among these are metabolic and endocrine disorders, such as hypothyroidism, hyperthyroidism, and diabetes; infectious diseases, such as influenza, hepatitis, and encephalitis; degenerative diseases, such as Alzheimer's disease, multiple sclerosis, and multi-infarct dementia; and neoplastic disorders such as cancer.

◆ ***Psychiatric disorders.*** Affective disorders are typically characterized by abrupt mood swings from depression to elation (mania) or by prolonged episodes of either mood. In fact, severe depression may last for weeks. More moderate depression occurs in cyclothymic disorders and usually alternates with moderate mania. Moderate depression that's more or less constant over a 2-year period typically results from dysthymic disorders. Also, chronic anxiety disorders, such as panic and obsessive-compulsive disorder, may be accompanied by depression.

OTHER CAUSES

◆ ***Alcohol abuse.*** Long-term alcohol use, intoxication, or withdrawal commonly produces depression.

◆ ***Drugs.*** Various drugs cause depression as an adverse effect. Among the more common are barbiturates, chemotherapeutic drugs such as asparaginase, anticonvulsants such as diazepam, and antiarrhythmics such as disopyramide. Other depression-inducing drugs include centrally acting antihypertensives, such as reserpine (common with high doses), methyldopa,

Suicide: Caring for the high-risk patient

One of the most common factors contributing to suicide is hopelessness, an emotion that many depressed patients experience. As a result, you'll need to regularly assess a depressed patient for suicidal tendencies.

The patient may provide specific clues about her intentions. For example, you may notice her talking frequently about death or the futility of life, concealing potentially harmful items (such as knives and belts), hoarding medications, giving away personal belongings, or getting her legal and financial affairs in order. If you suspect that a patient is suicidal, follow these guidelines:

◆ First, try to determine the patient's suicide potential. Find out how upset she is. Does she have a simple, straightforward suicide plan that's likely to succeed? Does she have a strong support system (family, friends, a therapist)? A patient with low to moderate suicide potential is noticeably depressed but has a support system. She may have thoughts of suicide, but no specific plan. A patient with high suicide potential feels profoundly hopeless and has a minimal or no support system. She thinks about suicide frequently and has a plan that's likely to succeed.

◆ Next, observe precautions. Ensure the patient's safety by removing any objects she could use to harm herself, such as knives, scissors, razors, belts, electric cords, shoelaces, and drugs. Know her whereabouts and what she's doing at all times; this may require one-on-one surveillance and placing the patient in a room that's close to your station. Always have someone accompany her when she leaves the unit.

◆ Be alert for in-hospital suicide attempts, which typically occur when there's a low staff-to-patient ratio—for example, between shifts, during evening and night shifts, or when a critical event such as a code draws attention away from the patient.

◆ Finally, arrange for follow-up counseling. Recognize suicidal ideation and behavior as a desperate cry for help. Contact a mental health professional for a referral.

and clonidine; beta-adrenergic blockers such as propranolol; indomethacin; cycloserine; corticosteroids; and hormonal contraceptives.

◆ ***Postpartum period.*** Although its cause hasn't been determined, postpartum depression occurs in about 10% to 20% of women who have given birth. Symptoms range from mild postpartum blues to an intense, suicidal, depressive psychosis.

SPECIAL CONSIDERATIONS

Caring for a depressed patient takes time, tact, and energy. It also requires an awareness of your own vulnerability to feelings of despair that can stem from interacting with a depressed patient. Help the patient set realistic goals; encourage her to promote feelings of self-worth by expressing her opinions and making decisions. Try to determine her suicide potential, and take steps to help ensure her safety. The patient may require close surveillance to prevent a suicide attempt.

Make sure the patient receives adequate nourishment and rest, and keep her environment free from stress and excessive stimulation. Arrange for ordered diagnostic tests to determine if her depression has an organic cause, and administer prescribed drugs. Also arrange for follow-up counseling, or contact a mental health professional for a referral.

PEDIATRIC POINTERS

Because emotional lability is normal in adolescence, depression can be difficult to assess and diagnose in teenagers. Clues to underlying depression may include somatic complaints, sexual promiscuity, poor grades, and abuse of alcohol or drugs.

Use of a family systems model usually helps determine the cause of depression in adolescents. Once family roles are determined, family therapy or group therapy with peers may help the patient overcome her depression. In severe cases, an antidepressant may be required.

GERIATRIC POINTERS

Many elderly patients have physical complaints, somatic complaints, agitation, or changes in intellectual functioning (memory impairment), making the diagnosis of depression difficult in these patients. Depressed older adults who are age 85 and older, have low self-esteem, and need to be in control have the highest risk of suicide. Even a frail nursing home resident with these characteristics may have the strength to kill herself.

Understanding diaphoresis

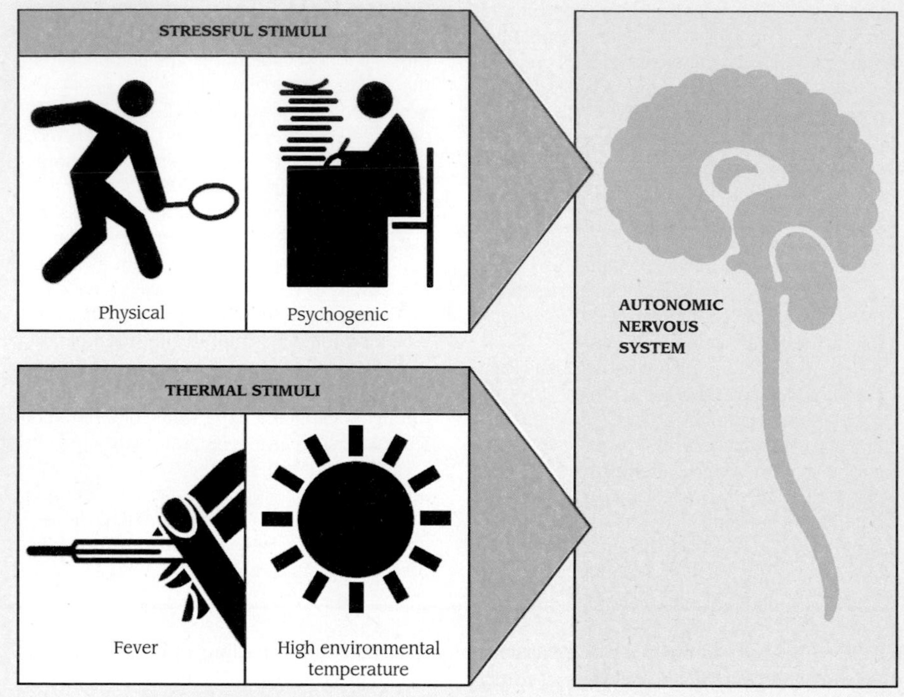

Diaphoresis

Diaphoresis is profuse sweating, sometimes amounting to more than 1 L of sweat per hour. This sign represents an autonomic nervous system response to physical or psychogenic stress, fever, or high environmental temperature. When caused by stress, diaphoresis may be generalized or limited to the palms, soles, and forehead. When caused by fever or high environmental temperature, it's usually generalized.

Diaphoresis usually begins abruptly and may be accompanied by other autonomic system signs, such as tachycardia and increased blood pressure. However, this sign also varies with age because sweat glands function immaturely in infants and are less active in elderly people. As a result, patients in these age-groups may fail to display diaphoresis associated with its common causes. Intermittent diaphoresis may accompany chronic disorders characterized by recurrent fever; isolated diaphoresis may mark an episode of acute pain or fever. Night sweats may characterize intermittent fever because body temperature tends to return to normal between 2 A.M. and 4 A.M. before rising again. (Temperature is usually lowest around 6 A.M.)

Diaphoresis is a normal response to high external temperature. Acclimatization usually requires several days of exposure to high temperatures; during this process, diaphoresis helps maintain normal body temperature. Diaphoresis also commonly occurs during menopause, preceded by a sensation of intense heat (a hot flash). Other causes include exercise or exertion that accelerates metabolism, creating internal heat, and mild to moderate anxiety that helps initiate the fight-or-flight response. (See *Understanding diaphoresis*.)

History and Physical Examination

If the patient is diaphoretic, quickly rule out the possibility of a life-threatening cause. (See *When diaphoresis spells crisis,* page 210.) Begin

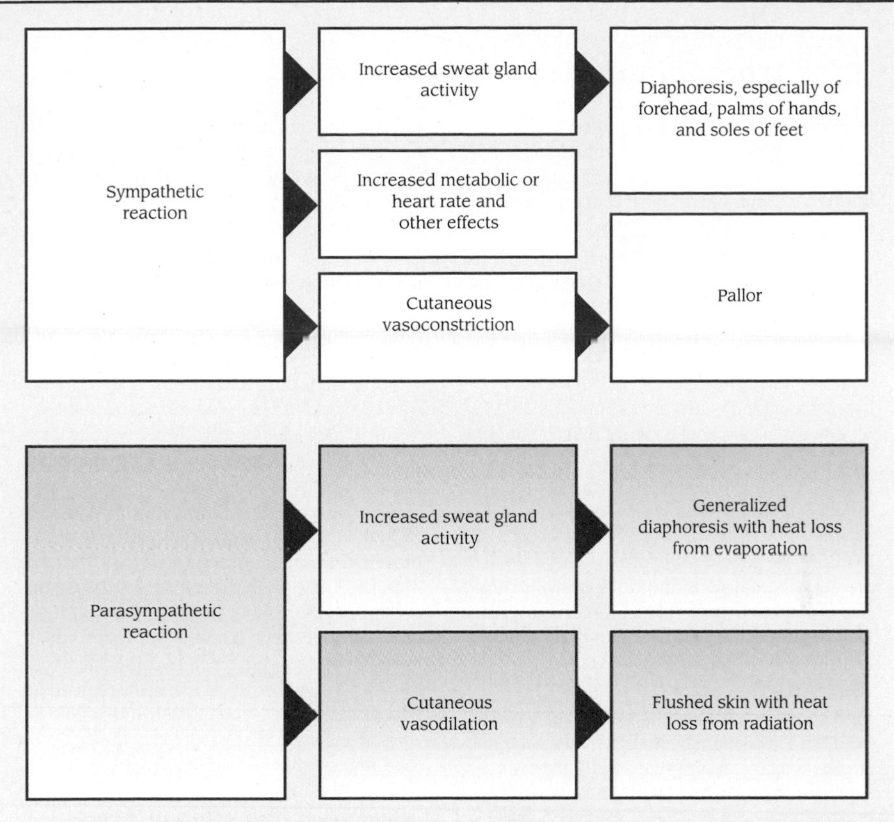

the history by having the patient describe his chief complaint. Then explore associated signs and symptoms. Note general fatigue and weakness. Does the patient have insomnia, headache, and changes in vision or hearing? Is he often dizzy? Does he have palpitations? Ask about pleuritic pain, cough, sputum, difficulty breathing, nausea, vomiting, abdominal pain, and altered elimination habits. Ask the female patient about amenorrhea and any changes in her menstrual cycle. Is she menopausal? Ask about paresthesia, muscle cramps or stiffness, and joint pain. Has she noticed any changes in elimination habits? Note weight loss or gain. Has she had to change her glove or shoe size lately?

Complete the history by asking about travel to tropical countries. Note recent exposure to high environmental temperatures or to pesticides. Did the patient recently experience an insect bite? Check for a history of partial gastrectomy or of drug or alcohol abuse. Finally, obtain a thorough drug history.

Next, perform a physical examination. First, determine the extent of diaphoresis by inspecting the trunk and extremities as well as the palms, soles, and forehead. Also, check the patient's clothing and bedding for dampness. Note whether diaphoresis occurs during the day or at night. Observe the patient for flushing, abnormal skin texture or lesions, and an increased amount of coarse body hair. Note poor skin turgor and dry mucous membranes. Check for splinter hemorrhages and Plummer's nails (separation of the fingernail ends from the nail beds).

Then evaluate the patient's mental status and take his vital signs. Observe the patient for fasciculations and flaccid paralysis. Be alert for seizures. Note the patient's facial expression, and examine the eyes for pupillary dilation or constriction, exophthalmos, and excessive tearing. Test visual fields. Also, check for hearing loss and for tooth or gum disease. Percuss the lungs for dullness, and auscultate for crackles, diminished or

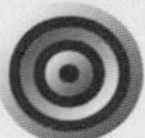

EMERGENCY INTERVENTION

When diaphoresis spells crisis

Diaphoresis is an early sign of certain life-threatening disorders. These guidelines will help you promptly detect such disorders and intervene to minimize harm to the patient.

Hypoglycemia

If you observe diaphoresis in a patient who complains of blurred vision, ask him about increased irritability and anxiety. Has the patient been unusually hungry lately? Does he have tremors? Take the patient's vital signs, noting hypotension and tachycardia. Then ask about a history of type 2 diabetes or antidiabetic therapy. If you suspect hypoglycemia, evaluate the patient's blood glucose level using a glucose reagent strip, or send a serum sample to the laboratory. Administer I.V. glucose 50% as ordered to return the patient's glucose level to normal. Monitor his vital signs and cardiac rhythm. Ensure a patent airway, and be prepared to assist with breathing and circulation, if necessary.

Heatstroke

If you observe profuse diaphoresis in a weak, tired, and apprehensive patient, suspect heatstroke, which can progress to circulatory collapse. Take vital signs, noting a normal or subnormal temperature. Check for ashen gray skin and dilated pupils. Was the patient recently exposed to high temperatures and humidity? Was he wearing heavy clothing or performing strenuous physical activity at the time? Also, ask if he takes a diuretic, which interferes with normal sweating.

Then take the patient to a cool room, remove his clothing, and use a fan to direct cool air over his body. Insert an I.V. catheter, and prepare for electrolyte and fluid replacement. Monitor the patient for signs of shock. Check his urine output carefully along with other sources of output (such as tubes, drains, and ostomies).

Autonomic hyperreflexia

If you observe diaphoresis in a patient with a spinal cord injury above T6 or T7, ask if he has a pounding headache, restlessness, blurred vision, or nasal congestion. Take the patient's vital signs, noting bradycardia or extremely elevated blood pressure. If you suspect autonomic hyperreflexia, quickly rule out its common complications. Examine the patient for eye pain associated with intraocular hemorrhage and for facial paralysis, slurred speech, or limb weakness associated with intracerebral hemorrhage.

Quickly reposition the patient to remove any pressure stimuli. Also, check for a distended bladder or fecal impaction. Remove any kinks from the urinary catheter if necessary, and administer a suppository or manually remove impacted feces. If you can't locate and relieve the causative stimulus, start an I.V. catheter. Prepare to administer hydralazine for hypertension.

Myocardial infarction or heart failure

If the diaphoretic patient complains of chest pain and dyspnea, or has arrhythmias or electrocardiogram changes, suspect a myocardial infarction or heart failure. Connect the patient to a cardiac monitor, ensure a patent airway, and administer supplemental oxygen. Start an I.V. catheter, and administer morphine. Be prepared to begin emergency resuscitation if cardiac or respiratory arrest occurs.

bronchial breath sounds, and increased vocal fremitus. Look for decreased respiratory excursion. Palpate for lymphadenopathy and hepatosplenomegaly.

MEDICAL CAUSES

◆ ***Acquired immunodeficiency syndrome.*** Night sweats may be an early feature, occurring either as a manifestation of the disease itself or secondary to an opportunistic infection. The patient also displays fever, fatigue, lymphadenopathy, anorexia, dramatic and unexplained weight loss, diarrhea, and a persistent cough.

◆ ***Acromegaly.*** In this slowly progressive disorder, diaphoresis is a sensitive gauge of disease activity, which involves hypersecretion of growth hormone and increased metabolic rate. The patient has a hulking appearance with an enlarged supraorbital ridge and thickened ears and nose. Other signs and symptoms include warm, oily, thickened skin; enlarged hands, feet, and jaw; joint pain; weight gain; hoarseness; and increased coarse body hair. Increased blood pressure, severe headache, and visual field deficits or blindness may also occur.

◆ ***Anxiety disorders.*** Acute anxiety characterizes panic, whereas chronic anxiety characterizes phobias, conversion disorders, obsessions, and compulsions. Whether acute or chronic, anxiety may cause sympathetic stimulation, resulting in diaphoresis. The diaphoresis is most dramatic on the palms, soles, and forehead and is accompanied by palpitations, tachycardia, tachypnea, tremors, and GI distress. Psychological signs and symptoms—fear, difficulty concentrating, and behavior changes—also occur.

◆ ***Autonomic hyperreflexia.*** Occurring after resolution of spinal shock in a spinal cord injury above T6, hyperreflexia causes profuse diaphoresis, pounding headache, blurred vision, and dramatically elevated blood pressure. Diaphoresis occurs above the level of the injury, especially on the forehead, and is accompanied by flushing. Other findings include restlessness, nausea, nasal congestion, and bradycardia.

◆ ***Drug and alcohol withdrawal syndromes.*** Withdrawal from alcohol or an opioid analgesic may cause generalized diaphoresis, dilated pupils, tachycardia, tremors, and altered mental status (confusion, delusions, hallucinations, agitation). Associated signs and symptoms include severe muscle cramps, generalized paresthesia, tachypnea, increased or decreased blood pressure and, possibly, seizures. Nausea and vomiting are common.

◆ ***Empyema.*** Pus accumulation in the pleural space leads to drenching night sweats and fever. The patient also complains of chest pain, cough, and weight loss. Examination reveals decreased respiratory excursion on the affected side and absent or distant breath sounds.

◆ ***Heart failure.*** Typically, diaphoresis follows fatigue, dyspnea, orthopnea, and tachycardia in patients with left-sided heart failure, and jugular vein distention and dry cough in patients with right-sided heart failure. Other features include tachypnea, cyanosis, dependent edema, crackles, ventricular gallop, and anxiety.

◆ ***Heat exhaustion.*** Although this condition is marked by failure of heat to dissipate, it initially may cause profuse diaphoresis, fatigue, weakness, and anxiety. These signs and symptoms may progress to circulatory collapse and shock (marked by confusion, thready pulse, hypotension, tachycardia, and cold, clammy skin). Other features include an ashen gray appearance, dilated pupils, and normal or subnormal temperature.

◆ ***Hodgkin's disease.*** Especially in elderly patients, early features of Hodgkin's disease may include night sweats, fever, fatigue, pruritus, and weight loss. Usually, however, this disease initially causes painless swelling of a cervical lymph node. Occasionally, a Pel-Ebstein fever pattern is present—several days or weeks of fever and chills alternating with afebrile periods with no chills. Systemic signs and symptoms—such as weight loss, fever, and night sweats—indicate a poor prognosis Progressive lymphadenopathy eventually causes widespread effects, such as hepatomegaly and dyspnea.

◆ ***Hypoglycemia.*** Rapidly induced hypoglycemia may cause diaphoresis accompanied by irritability, tremors, hypotension, blurred vision, tachycardia, hunger, and loss of consciousness.

◆ ***Immunoblastic lymphadenopathy.*** Resembling Hodgkin's disease but rarer, this disorder causes episodic diaphoresis along with fever, weight loss, weakness, generalized lymphadenopathy, rash, and hepatosplenomegaly.

◆ ***Infective endocarditis (subacute).*** Generalized night sweats occur early in this disorder and are accompanyied by intermittent low-grade fever, weakness, fatigue, anorexia, weight loss, and arthralgia. A sudden change in a murmur or the discovery of a new murmur is a classic sign. Petechiae and splinter hemorrhages are also common.

◆ ***Liver abscess.*** Signs and symptoms vary, depending on the extent of the abscess, but commonly include diaphoresis, right-upper-quadrant pain, weight loss, fever, chills, nausea, vomiting, and signs of anemia.

◆ ***Lung abscess.*** Drenching night sweats are common in this disorder. Its chief sign, however, is a cough that produces copious amounts of purulent, foul-smelling, and typically blood-tinged sputum. Associated findings include fever with chills, pleuritic chest pain, dyspnea, weakness, anorexia, weight loss, headache, malaise, clubbing, tubular or amphoric breath sounds, and dullness on percussion.

◆ ***Malaria.*** Profuse diaphoresis marks the third stage of paroxysmal malaria, preceded by chills (first stage) and high fever (second stage). Headache, arthralgia, and hepatosplenomegaly may also occur. In the benign form of malaria, these paroxysms alternate with periods of well-being. The severe form may progress to delirium, seizures, and coma.

◆ ***Ménière's disease.*** Characterized by severe vertigo, tinnitus, and hearing loss, this disorder may also cause diaphoresis, nausea, vomiting, and nystagmus. Hearing loss may be progressive and tinnitus may persist between attacks.

◆ ***Myocardial infarction.*** Diaphoresis usually accompanies acute, substernal, radiating chest pain in this life-threatening disorder. Associated signs and symptoms include anxiety, dyspnea, nausea, vomiting, tachycardia, irregular pulse, blood pressure change, fine crackles, pallor, and clammy skin.

◆ ***Pheochromocytoma.*** This disorder commonly produces diaphoresis, but its cardinal sign is persistent or paroxysmal hypertension. Other effects include headache, palpitations, tachycardia, anxiety, tremors, pallor, flushing, paresthesia, abdominal pain, tachypnea, nausea, vomiting, and orthostatic hypotension.

◆ ***Pneumonia.*** In patients with pneumonia, intermittent, generalized diaphoresis accompanies fever, chills, and pleuritic chest pain that increases with deep inspiration. Other features are tachypnea, dyspnea, a productive cough (with scant and mucoid or copious and purulent sputum), headache, fatigue, myalgia, abdominal pain, anorexia, and cyanosis. Auscultation reveals bronchial breath sounds.

◆ ***Relapsing fever.*** Profuse diaphoresis marks resolution of the crisis stage of this disorder, which typically produces attacks of high fever accompanied by severe myalgia, headache, arthralgia, diarrhea, vomiting, coughing, and eye or chest pain. Splenomegaly is common, but hepatomegaly and lymphadenopathy may also occur. The patient may develop a transient macular rash. Between 3 and 10 days after onset, the febrile attack abruptly terminates in chills with increased pulse and respiratory rates. Diaphoresis, flushing, and hypotension may then lead to circulatory collapse and death. Relapse invariably occurs if the patient survives the initial attack.

◆ ***Tetanus.*** This disorder commonly causes profuse sweating accompanied by low-grade fever, tachycardia, and hyperactive deep tendon reflexes. Early restlessness and pain and stiffness in the jaw, abdomen, and back progress to spasms associated with lockjaw, risus sardonicus, dysphagia, and opisthotonos. Laryngospasm may result in cyanosis or sudden death by asphyxiation.

◆ ***Thyrotoxicosis.*** This disorder commonly produces diaphoresis accompanied by heat intolerance, weight loss despite increased appetite, tachycardia, palpitations, an enlarged thyroid, dyspnea, nervousness, diarrhea, tremors, Plummer's nails and, possibly, exophthalmos. Gallops may also occur.

◆ ***Tuberculosis (TB).*** Although many patients with primary infection are asymptomatic, TB may cause night sweats, low-grade fever, fatigue, weakness, anorexia, and weight loss. In reactivation, a productive cough with mucopurulent sputum, occasional hemoptysis, and chest pain may be present.

OTHER CAUSES

◆ ***Drugs.*** Sympathomimetics, certain antipsychotics, thyroid hormone, corticosteroids, and antipyretics may cause diaphoresis. Aspirin and acetaminophen poisoning also cause this sign.

◆ ***Dumping syndrome.*** The result of rapid emptying of gastric contents into the small intestine after partial gastrectomy, dumping syndrome causes diaphoresis, palpitations, profound weakness, epigastric distress, nausea, and explosive diarrhea soon after eating.

◆ ***Envenomation.*** Depending on the type of bite, neurotoxic effects may include diaphoresis, chills (with or without fever), weakness, dizziness, blurred vision, increased salivation, nausea and vomiting and, possibly, paresthesia and muscle fasciculations. Local features may include ecchymosis and progressively severe pain and edema. Palpation reveals tender regional lymph nodes.

◆ ***Pesticide poisoning.*** Among the toxic effects of pesticides are diaphoresis, nausea, vomiting, diarrhea, blurred vision, miosis, and excessive lacrimation and salivation. The patient may also display fasciculations, muscle weakness, and flaccid paralysis. Signs of respiratory depression and coma may also occur.

SPECIAL CONSIDERATIONS

After an episode of diaphoresis, sponge the patient's face and body and change wet clothes and sheets. To prevent skin irritation, dust skin folds in the groin and axillae and under pendulous breasts with cornstarch, or tuck gauze or cloth into the folds. Encourage regular bathing.

Replace fluids and electrolytes. Regulate infusions of I.V. saline or Ringer's lactate solution, and monitor urine output. Encourage intake of oral fluids high in electrolytes (such as Gatorade). Enforce bed rest and maintain a quiet environment. Keep the patient's room temperature moderate to prevent additional diaphoresis.

Prepare the patient for diagnostic tests, such as blood tests, cultures, chest X-rays, immunologic studies, biopsy, computed tomography scan, and audiometry. Monitor the patient's vital signs, including temperature.

Pediatric pointers

Diaphoresis in children commonly results from environmental heat or overdressing the child; it's usually most apparent around the head. Other causes include drug withdrawal associated with maternal addiction, heart failure, thyrotoxicosis, and the effects of such drugs as antihistamines, ephedrine, haloperidol, and thyroid hormone.

Assess fluid status carefully. Some fluid loss through diaphoresis may precipitate hypovolemia more rapidly in a child than an adult. Monitor input and output, weigh the child daily, and note the duration of each episode of diaphoresis.

Geriatric pointers

Elderly patients with TB may exhibit a change in activity or weight rather than the hallmark symptoms of fever and night sweats. Also, keep in mind that older patients may not exhibit diaphoresis because of a decreased sweating mechanism. For this reason, they're at increased risk for developing heatstroke in high temperatures.

Diarrhea

Usually a chief sign of an intestinal disorder, diarrhea is an increase in the volume of stools compared with the patient's normal bowel elimination habits. It varies in severity and may be acute or chronic. Acute diarrhea may result from acute infection, stress, fecal impaction, or the effect of a drug. Chronic diarrhea may result from chronic infection, obstructive and inflammatory bowel disease, malabsorption syndrome, an endocrine disorder, or GI surgery. Periodic diarrhea may result from food intolerance or from ingestion of spicy or high-fiber foods or caffeine.

One or more pathophysiologic mechanisms may contribute to diarrhea. (See *What causes diarrhea,* page 214.) The fluid and electrolyte imbalances it produces may precipitate life-threatening arrhythmias or hypovolemic shock.

EMERGENCY INTERVENTIONS *If the patient's diarrhea is profuse, check for signs of shock—tachycardia, hypotension, and cool, pale, clammy skin. If you detect these signs, place the patient in the supine position and elevate his legs 20 degrees. Insert an I.V. catheter for fluid replacement. Monitor the patient for electrolyte imbalances, and look for an irregular pulse, muscle weakness, anorexia, and nausea and vomiting. Keep emergency resuscitation equipment handy.*

History and physical examination

If the patient isn't in shock, proceed with a brief physical examination. Evaluate hydration, check skin turgor and mucous membranes, and take blood pressure with the patient lying, sitting, and standing. Inspect the abdomen for distention, and palpate for tenderness. Auscultate bowel sounds. Check for tympany over the abdomen. Take the patient's temperature, and note any chills. Also, look for a rash. Conduct a rectal examination and a pelvic examination if indicated.

Explore signs and symptoms associated with diarrhea. Does the patient have abdominal pain and cramps? Difficulty breathing? Is he weak or fatigued? Find out his drug history. Has he had GI surgery or radiation therapy recently? Ask the patient to briefly describe his diet. Does he have any known food allergies? Lastly, find out if he's under unusual stress.

Medical causes

◆ ***Anthrax, GI.*** This disease follows ingestion of contaminated meat from an animal infected with *Bacillus anthracis*. Early signs and symptoms include decreased appetite, nausea, vomiting, and fever. Later signs and symptoms include severe bloody diarrhea, abdominal pain, and hematemesis.

◆ ***Carcinoid syndrome.*** In this disorder, severe diarrhea occurs with flushing—usually of the head and neck—that's commonly caused by emotional stimuli or the ingestion of food, hot water, or alcohol. Associated signs and symptoms include abdominal cramps, dyspnea, anorexia, weight loss, weakness, palpitations, valvular heart disease, and depression.

◆ ***Cholera.*** After ingesting water or food contaminated by the bacterium *Vibrio cholerae,* the patient experiences abrupt watery diarrhea and vomiting. Other signs and symptoms include thirst (due to severe water and electrolyte loss), weakness, muscle cramps, decreased skin turgor, oliguria, tachycardia, and hypotension.

What causes diarrhea

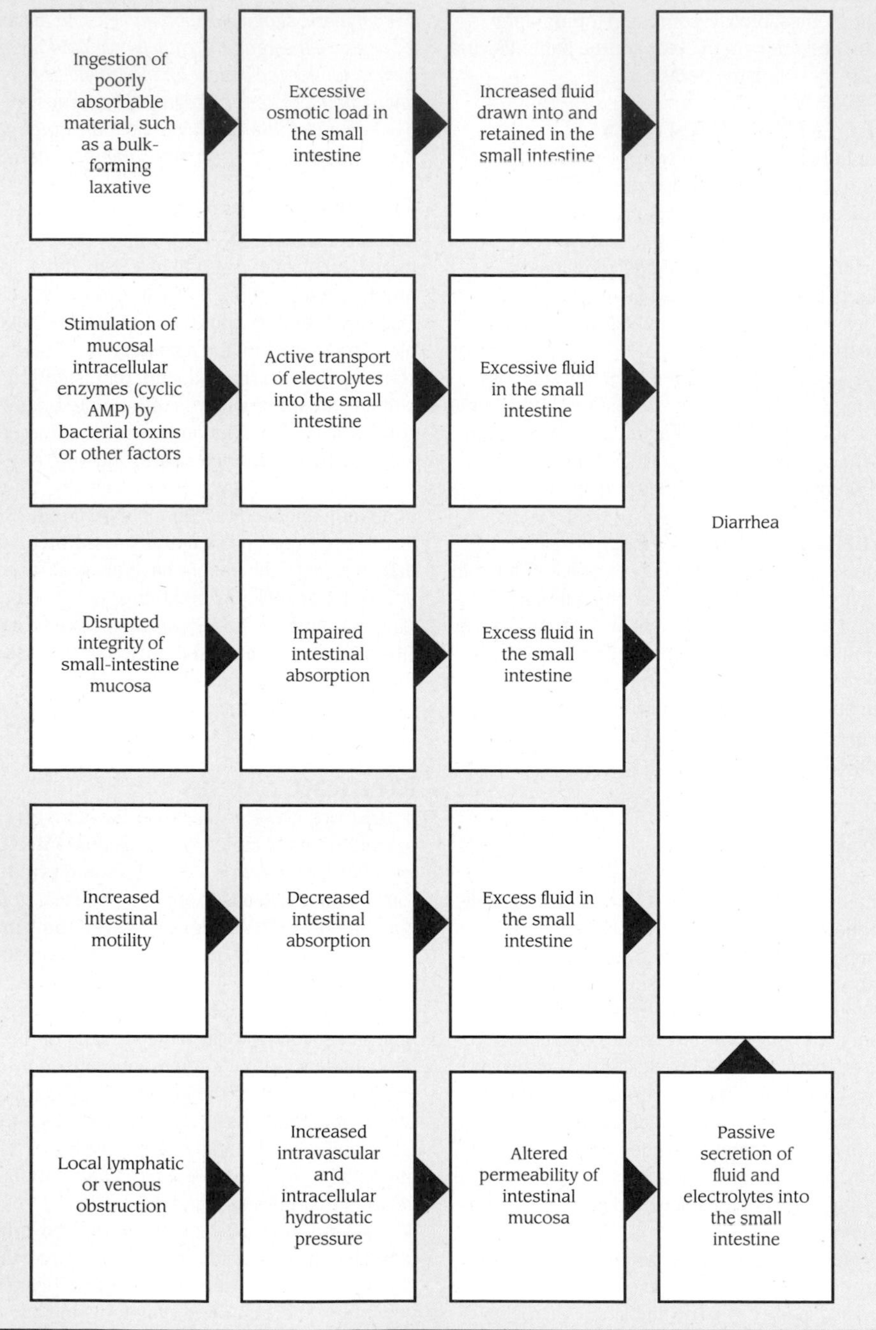

Without treatment, death can occur within hours.

◆ **Clostridium difficile *infection.*** The patient may be asymptomatic or may have soft, unformed stools or watery diarrhea that may be foul smelling or grossly bloody; abdominal pain, cramping, and tenderness; fever; and a white blood cell count as high as 20,000/µl. In severe cases, the patient may develop toxic megacolon, colonic perforation, or peritonitis.

◆ ***Crohn's disease.*** This recurring inflammatory disorder produces diarrhea, abdominal pain with guarding and tenderness, and nausea. The patient may also display fever, chills, weakness, anorexia, and weight loss.

◆ **Escherichia coli *O157:H7.*** Watery or bloody diarrhea, nausea, vomiting, fever, and abdominal cramps occur after the patient eats undercooked beef or other foods contaminated with this particular strain of bacteria. Hemolytic uremic syndrome, which causes red blood cell destruction and eventually acute renal failure, is a complication of *E. coli* O157:H7 in children age 5 and younger and elderly people.

◆ ***Infections.*** Acute viral, bacterial, and protozoal infections (such as cryptosporidiosis) cause the sudden onset of watery diarrhea as well as abdominal pain or cramps, nausea, vomiting, and fever. Significant fluid and electrolyte loss may cause signs of dehydration and shock. Chronic tuberculosis and fungal and parasitic infections may produce a less severe but more persistent diarrhea, accompanied by epigastric distress, vomiting, weight loss and, possibly, passage of blood and mucus.

◆ ***Intestinal obstruction.*** Partial intestinal obstruction increases intestinal motility, resulting in diarrhea, abdominal pain with tenderness and guarding, nausea and, possibly, distention.

◆ ***Irritable bowel syndrome.*** Diarrhea alternates with constipation or normal bowel function. Related findings include abdominal pain, tenderness, and distention; dyspepsia; and nausea.

◆ ***Ischemic bowel disease.*** This life-threatening disorder causes bloody diarrhea with abdominal pain. If severe, shock may occur, requiring surgery.

◆ ***Lactose intolerance.*** Diarrhea occurs within several hours of ingesting milk or milk products in patients with this disorder. It's accompanied by cramps, abdominal pain, borborygmi, bloating, nausea, and flatus.

◆ ***Large-bowel cancer.*** In this disorder, bloody diarrhea is seen with a partial obstruction. Other signs and symptoms include abdominal pain, anorexia, weight loss, weakness, fatigue, exertional dyspnea, and depression.

◆ ***Listeriosis.*** This infection, caused by ingestion of food contaminated with the bacterium *Listeria monocytogenes,* primarily affects pregnant women, neonates, and those with weakened immune systems. Characteristic findings include diarrhea, fever, myalgia, abdominal pain, nausea, and vomiting. Fever, headache, nuchal rigidity, and altered level of consciousness may occur if the infection spreads to the nervous system and causes meningitis.

GENDER CUE *Listeriosis during pregnancy may lead to premature delivery, infection of the neonate, or stillbirth.*

◆ ***Malabsorption syndrome.*** Occurring after meals, diarrhea is accompanied by steatorrhea, abdominal distention, and muscle cramps. The patient also displays anorexia, weight loss, bone pain, anemia, weakness, and fatigue. He may bruise easily and have night blindness.

◆ ***Pseudomembranous enterocolitis.*** This potentially life-threatening disorder commonly follows antibiotic administration. It produces copious watery, green, foul-smelling, bloody diarrhea that rapidly precipitates signs of shock. Other signs and symptoms include colicky abdominal pain, distention, fever, and dehydration.

◆ ***Q fever.*** This infection is caused by the bacterium *Coxiella burnetii* and causes diarrhea along with fever, chills, severe headache, malaise, chest pain, and vomiting. In severe cases, hepatitis or pneumonia may follow.

◆ ***Rotavirus gastroenteritis.*** This disorder commonly starts with a fever, nausea, and vomiting, followed by diarrhea. The illness can be mild to severe and last from 3 to 9 days. Diarrhea and vomiting may result in dehydration.

◆ ***Thyrotoxicosis.*** In this disorder, diarrhea is accompanied by nervousness, tremors, diaphoresis, weight loss despite increased appetite, dyspnea, palpitations, tachycardia, enlarged thyroid, heat intolerance and, possibly, exophthalmos.

◆ ***Ulcerative colitis.*** The hallmark of this disorder is recurrent bloody diarrhea with pus or mucus. Other signs and symptoms include tenesmus, hyperactive bowel sounds, cramping lower abdominal pain, low-grade fever, anorexia and, possibly, nausea and vomiting. Weight loss, anemia, and weakness are late findings.

◆ ***Vancomycin-resistant enterococci (VRE) infection.*** Enterococci are bacteria naturally present in the intestinal tract of all people; however, some strains of enterococci have become resistant to vancomycin. Serious VRE infections may occur in hospitalized patients with such comorbidities as cancer, kidney disease, or immune deficiencies. Elderly patients and those hospitalized for long periods are also at risk for developing VRE infections. Symptoms of VRE infection depend on where the infection is; patients with VRE infections may have diarrhea, fever, and fatigue.

OTHER CAUSES

◆ ***Drugs.*** Many antibiotics—such as ampicillin, cephalosporins, tetracyclines, and clindamycin—cause diarrhea. Other drugs that may cause diarrhea include magnesium-containing antacids, lactulose, dantrolene, ethacrynic acid, mefenamic acid, methotrexate, metyrosine and, with high doses, cardiac glycosides and quinidine. Laxative abuse can cause acute or chronic diarrhea.

◆ ***Foods.*** Foods that contain certain oils may inhibit the food's absorption, causing acute uncontrollable diarrhea and rectal leakage.

HERB ALERT *Herbal remedies, such as ginkgo biloba, ginseng, and licorice, may cause diarrhea.*

◆ ***Lead poisoning.*** Alternating diarrhea and constipation may be accompanied by abdominal pain, anorexia, nausea, and vomiting. The patient complains of a metallic taste, headache, and dizziness and displays a bluish gingival lead line.

◆ ***Treatments.*** Gastrectomy, gastroenterostomy, and pyloroplasty may produce diarrhea. High-dose radiation therapy may produce enteritis associated with diarrhea.

SPECIAL CONSIDERATIONS

When appropriate, administer an analgesic for pain and an opiate as ordered to decrease intestinal motility, unless the patient may have a stool infection. Ensure the patient's privacy during defecation, and empty bedpans promptly. Clean the perineum thoroughly, and apply ointment to prevent skin breakdown. Quantify the amount of liquid stool and carefully observe intake and output.

Stress the need for medical follow-up to patients with inflammatory bowel disease (particularly ulcerative colitis), who have an increased risk of developing colon cancer.

PEDIATRIC POINTERS

Diarrhea in children commonly results from infection, although chronic diarrhea may result from malabsorption syndrome, an anatomic defect, or allergies. Because dehydration and electrolyte imbalance occur rapidly in children, diarrhea can be life-threatening. Diligently monitor all episodes of diarrhea, and replace lost fluids immediately.

GERIATRIC POINTERS

In the elderly patient with new-onset segmental colitis, always consider ischemia before labeling the patient as having Crohn's disease.

PATIENT COUNSELING

Explain the purpose of diagnostic tests to the patient. These tests may include blood studies, stool cultures, X-rays, and endoscopy.

Administer I.V. fluid replacements to help the patient maintain adequate hydration. Measure liquid stools and weigh the patient daily. Monitor electrolyte levels and hematocrit.

Advise the patient to avoid spicy or high-fiber foods (such as fruits), caffeine, high-fat foods, and milk. Suggest smaller, more frequent meals if he has had GI surgery or disease. If appropriate, teach the patient stress-reducing measures, such as guided imagery and deep-breathing techniques, or recommend counseling.

Diplopia

Diplopia is double vision—seeing one object as two. This symptom results when extraocular muscles fail to work together, causing images to fall on noncorresponding parts of the retinas. What causes this muscle incoordination? Orbital lesions, the effects of surgery, or impaired function of the cranial nerves (CNs) that supply extraocular muscles—oculomotor (CN III), trochlear (CN IV), and abducens (CN VI)—may be responsible. (See *Testing extraocular muscles.*)

Diplopia usually begins intermittently and affects near or far vision exclusively. It can be classified as monocular or binocular. More common binocular diplopia may result from ocular deviation or displacement, extraocular muscle palsies, or psychoneurosis, or it may occur after retinal surgery. Monocular diplopia

Testing extraocular muscles

The coordinated action of six muscles controls eyeball movements. To test the function of each muscle and the cranial nerve that innervates it, ask the patient to look in the direction controlled by that muscle. The six directions you can test make up the *cardinal fields of gaze.* The patient's inability to turn the eye in the designated direction indicates muscle weakness or paralysis.

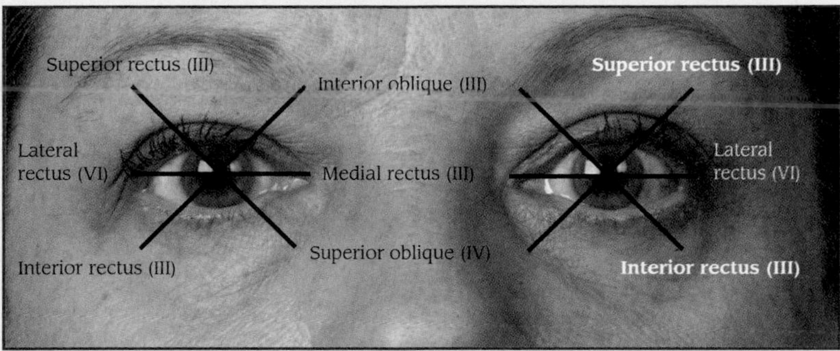

may result from an early cataract, retinal edema or scarring, iridodialysis, a subluxated lens, a poorly fitting contact lens, or an uncorrected refractive error such as astigmatism. Diplopia may also occur in hysteria or malingering.

History and physical examination

If the patient complains of double vision, first check his neurologic status. Evaluate his level of consciousness (LOC); pupil size, equality, and response to light; and motor and sensory function. Then take his vital signs. Briefly ask about associated symptoms. First find out about associated neurologic symptoms, especially a severe headache, because diplopia can accompany serious disorders.

Next, continue with a more detailed examination. Find out when the patient first noticed diplopia. Are the images side by side (horizontal), one above the other (vertical), or a combination? Does diplopia affect near or far vision? Does it affect certain directions of gaze? Ask if diplopia has worsened, remained the same, or subsided. Does its severity change throughout the day? Diplopia that worsens or appears in the evening may indicate myasthenia gravis. Find out if the patient can correct diplopia by tilting his head. If so, ask him to show you. (If the patient has a fourth cranial nerve lesion, tilting the head toward the opposite shoulder causes compensatory tilting of the unaffected eye. If he has incomplete sixth cranial nerve palsy, tilting the head toward the side of the paralyzed muscle may relax the affected lateral rectus muscle.)

Explore associated symptoms such as eye pain. Ask about hypertension, diabetes mellitus, allergies, and thyroid, neurologic, or muscular disorders. Also, note a history of extraocular muscle disorders, trauma, or eye surgery.

Observe the patient for ocular deviation, ptosis, exophthalmos, eyelid edema, and conjunctival injection. Distinguish monocular from binocular diplopia by asking the patient to occlude one eye at a time. If he still sees double out of one eye, he has monocular diplopia. Test visual acuity and extraocular muscles. Also, check vital signs.

Medical causes

- ***Alcohol intoxication.*** Diplopia, a common symptom of this disorder, may be accompanied by confusion, slurred speech, halitosis, staggering gait, behavior changes, nausea, vomiting and, possibly, conjunctival injection.
- ***Botulism.*** The hallmark signs of botulism are diplopia, dysarthria, dysphagia, and ptosis. Early findings include dry mouth, sore throat, vomiting, and diarrhea. Later, descending weakness or paralysis of extremity and trunk muscles causes hyporeflexia and dyspnea.

◆ ***Brain tumor.*** Diplopia may be an early symptom of a brain tumor. Associated signs and symptoms vary with the tumor's size and location but may include eye deviation, emotional lability, decreased LOC, headache, vomiting, absence or generalized tonic-clonic seizures, hearing loss, visual field deficits, abnormal pupillary responses, nystagmus, motor weakness, and paralysis.

◆ ***Cavernous sinus thrombosis.*** This disorder may produce diplopia and limited eye movement. Associated signs and symptoms include exophthalmos, orbital and eyelid edema, diminished or absent pupillary responses, impaired visual acuity, papilledema, and fever.

◆ ***Diabetes mellitus.*** Among the long-term effects of this disorder may be diplopia due to isolated third cranial nerve palsy. Diplopia typically begins suddenly and may be accompanied by pain.

◆ ***Encephalitis.*** Initially, this disorder may cause a brief episode of diplopia and eye deviation. However, it usually begins with sudden onset of high fever, severe headache, and vomiting. As the inflammation progresses, the patient may display signs of meningeal irritation, decreased LOC, seizures, ataxia, and paralysis.

◆ ***Head injury.*** Potentially life-threatening head injuries may cause diplopia, depending on the site and extent of the injury. Associated signs and symptoms include eye deviation, pupillary changes, headache, decreased LOC, altered vital signs, nausea, vomiting, and motor weakness or paralysis.

◆ ***Intracranial aneurysm.*** This life-threatening disorder initially produces diplopia and eye deviation, perhaps accompanied by ptosis and a dilated pupil on the affected side. The patient complains of a recurrent, severe, unilateral, frontal headache. After the aneurysm ruptures, the headache becomes violent. Associated signs and symptoms include neck and spinal pain and rigidity, decreased LOC, tinnitus, dizziness, nausea, vomiting, and unilateral muscle weakness or paralysis.

◆ ***Multiple sclerosis (MS).*** Diplopia, a common early symptom of MS, is usually accompanied by blurred vision and paresthesia. As MS progresses, signs and symptoms may include nystagmus, constipation, muscle weakness, paralysis, spasticity, hyperreflexia, intention tremor, gait ataxia, dysphagia, dysarthria, impotence, emotional lability, and urinary frequency, urgency, and incontinence.

◆ ***Myasthenia gravis.*** This disorder initially produces diplopia and ptosis, which worsen throughout the day. It then progressively involves other muscles, resulting in blank facial expression; nasal voice; difficulty chewing, swallowing, and making fine hand movements and, possibly, signs of life-threatening respiratory muscle weakness.

◆ ***Ophthalmologic migraine.*** Most common in young adults, this disorder results in diplopia that persists for days after the headache resolves. Accompanying signs and symptoms include severe unilateral pain, ptosis, and extraocular muscle palsies. Irritability, depression, or slight confusion may also occur.

◆ ***Orbital blowout fracture.*** This fracture usually causes monocular diplopia affecting the upward gaze. However, with marked periorbital edema, diplopia may affect other directions of gaze. This fracture commonly causes periorbital ecchymosis but doesn't affect visual acuity, although eyelid edema may prevent accurate testing. Subcutaneous crepitation of the eyelid and orbit is typical. Occasionally, the patient's pupil is dilated and unreactive, and he may have a hyphema.

◆ ***Orbital cellulitis.*** Inflammation of the orbital tissues and eyelids causes sudden diplopia as well as eye deviation and pain, purulent drainage, eyelid edema, chemosis and redness, exophthalmos, nausea, and fever.

◆ ***Orbital tumor.*** An enlarging tumor can cause diplopia, exophthalmos and, possibly, blurred vision.

◆ ***Stroke.*** Diplopia characterizes this life-threatening disorder when it affects the vertebrobasilar artery. Other signs and symptoms include unilateral motor weakness or paralysis, ataxia, decreased LOC, dizziness, aphasia, visual field deficits, circumoral numbness, slurred speech, dysphagia, and amnesia.

◆ ***Thyrotoxicosis.*** Diplopia occurs when exophthalmos characterizes the disorder. It usually begins in the upper field of gaze because of infiltrative myopathy involving the inferior rectus muscle. It's accompanied by impaired eye movement, excessive tearing, eyelid edema and, possibly, inability to close the eyelids. Other cardinal findings include tachycardia, palpitations, weight loss, diarrhea, tremors, an enlarged thyroid, dyspnea, nervousness, diaphoresis, and heat intolerance.

◆ ***Transient ischemic attack (TIA).*** A TIA, which may be a warning sign of a future stroke, is generally accompanied by diplopia, dizziness, tinnitus, hearing loss, and numbness. It can last for a few seconds or up to 24 hours.

Other causes

◆ ***Eye surgery.*** Fibrosis associated with eye surgery may restrict eye movement, resulting in diplopia.

Special considerations

Continue to monitor vital signs and neurologic status if you suspect an acute neurologic disorder. Prepare the patient for neurologic tests such as a computed tomography scan. Provide a safe environment. If the patient has severe diplopia, remove sharp obstacles and assist him with ambulation. Also, institute seizure precautions if indicated.

Pediatric pointers

Strabismus, which can be congenital or acquired at an early age, produces diplopia; however, diplopia is a rare complaint in young children because the brain rapidly compensates for double vision by suppressing one image. School-age children who complain of double vision require a careful examination to rule out serious disorders such as a brain tumor.

Dizziness

A common symptom, dizziness is a sensation of imbalance or faintness, sometimes associated with giddiness, weakness, confusion, and blurred or double vision. Episodes of dizziness are usually brief; they may be mild or severe with an abrupt or gradual onset. Dizziness may be aggravated by standing up quickly and alleviated by lying down and by rest.

Dizziness typically results from inadequate blood flow and oxygen supply to the cerebrum and spinal cord. It's a key symptom in certain serious disorders, such as hypertension and vertebrobasilar artery insufficiency, and it may also occur in anxiety, respiratory and cardiovascular disorders, and postconcussion syndrome.

Dizziness is commonly confused with vertigo—a sensation of revolving in space or of surroundings revolving around oneself. However, unlike dizziness, vertigo is commonly accompanied by nausea, vomiting, nystagmus, staggering gait, and tinnitus or hearing loss. Dizziness and vertigo may occur together, as in postconcussion syndrome.

EMERGENCY INTERVENTIONS *If the patient complains of dizziness, first ensure his safety by preventing falls, and then determine the severity and onset of the dizziness. Ask the patient to describe it. Is it associated with headache or blurred vision? Next, take the patient's blood pressure while he's lying, sitting, and standing to check for orthostatic hypotension. Ask about a history of high blood pressure. Determine if the patient is at risk for hypoglycemia. Tell the patient to lie down, and recheck his vital signs every 15 minutes. Insert an I.V. catheter, and prepare to administer medications as ordered.*

History and physical examination

Ask about a history of diabetes and cardiovascular disease. Is the patient taking drugs prescribed for high blood pressure? If so, when did he take his last dose?

If the patient's blood pressure is normal, obtain a more complete history. Ask if he's had a myocardial infarction, heart failure, kidney disease, or atherosclerosis, which may predispose him to cardiac arrhythmias, hypertension, and a transient ischemic attack. Does he have a history of anemia, chronic obstructive pulmonary disease, anxiety disorders, or head injury? Obtain a complete drug history.

Next, explore the patient's dizziness. How often does it occur? How long does each episode last? Does the dizziness abate spontaneously? Does it lead to loss of consciousness? Find out if dizziness is triggered by sitting or standing up suddenly or by stooping over. Does being in a crowd make the patient feel dizzy? Ask about emotional stress. Has the patient been irritable or anxious lately? Does he have insomnia or difficulty concentrating? Look for fidgeting and eyelid twitching. Does the patient startle easily? Also, ask about palpitations, chest pain, diaphoresis, shortness of breath, and chronic cough.

Next, perform a physical examination. Begin with a quick neurocheck, assessing the patient's level of consciousness (LOC), motor and sensory function, and reflexes. Then inspect for poor skin turgor and dry mucous membranes, signs of dehydration. Auscultate heart rate and rhythm. Inspect for barrel chest, clubbing, cyanosis, and use of accessory muscles. Also auscultate breath sounds. Take the patient's blood pressure while he's lying, sitting, and standing to check for orthostatic hypotension. Test capillary refill time in the extremities, and palpate for edema.

Medical causes

◆ ***Anemia.*** Anemia typically causes dizziness that's aggravated by postural changes or exertion. Other signs and symptoms include pallor, dyspnea, fatigue, tachycardia, bounding pulse, and increased capillary refill time.

◆ ***Cardiac arrhythmias.*** Dizziness lasts for several seconds or longer and may precede fainting in arrhythmias. The patient may experience palpitations; irregular, rapid, or thready pulse and, possibly, hypotension. He may also experience weakness, blurred vision, paresthesia, and confusion.

◆ ***Carotid sinus hypersensitivity.*** This disorder is characterized by brief episodes of dizziness that usually terminate in fainting. These episodes are precipitated by stimulation of one or both carotid arteries by seemingly minor sensations or actions, such as wearing a tight collar or moving the head. Associated signs and symptoms include sweating, nausea, and pallor.

◆ ***Emphysema.*** Dizziness may follow exertion or the chronic productive cough that's characteristic of this disorder. Associated signs and symptoms include dyspnea, anorexia, weight loss, malaise, use of accessory muscles, pursed-lip breathing, tachypnea, peripheral cyanosis, and diminished breath sounds. Barrel chest and clubbing may occur.

◆ ***Generalized anxiety disorder.*** This disorder produces persistent anxiety (for at least 1 month), insomnia, difficulty concentrating, irritability and, possibly, continuous dizziness that may intensify as the anxiety worsens. The patient may show signs of motor tension—for example, twitching or fidgeting, muscle aches, a furrowed brow, and a tendency to be startled. He may also display signs of autonomic hyperactivity, such as diaphoresis, palpitations, cold and clammy hands, dry mouth, paresthesia, indigestion, hot or cold flashes, frequent urination, diarrhea, a lump in the throat, pallor, and increased pulse and respiratory rates.

◆ ***Hypertension.*** In patients with hypertension, dizziness may precede fainting, but it may also be relieved by rest. Other common signs and symptoms include headache and blurred vision. Retinal changes include hemorrhage, sclerosis of retinal blood vessels, exudate, and papilledema.

◆ ***Hyperventilation syndrome.*** Episodes of hyperventilation cause dizziness that usually lasts a few minutes; however, if these episodes occur frequently, dizziness may persist between them. Other effects include apprehension, diaphoresis, pallor, dyspnea, chest tightness, palpitations, trembling, fatigue, and peripheral and circumoral paresthesia.

◆ ***Hypoglycemia.*** Dizziness is a central nervous system (CNS) disturbance that can result from fasting hypoglycemia. It's generally accompanied by headache, clouding of vision, restlessness, and mental status changes.

◆ ***Hypovolemia.*** Dizziness may be accompanied by other signs of fluid volume deficit, such as dry mucous membranes, decreased blood pressure, and increased heart rate.

◆ ***Orthostatic hypotension.*** This condition produces dizziness that may terminate in fainting or disappear with rest. Related findings include dim vision, spots before the eyes, pallor, diaphoresis, hypotension, tachycardia and, possibly, signs of dehydration.

◆ ***Panic disorder.*** Dizziness may accompany acute attacks of panic in patients with this disorder. Other findings include anxiety, dyspnea, palpitations, chest pain, a choking or smothering sensation, vertigo, paresthesia, hot and cold flashes, diaphoresis, and trembling or shaking. The patient may feel like he's dying or losing his mind.

◆ ***Postconcussion syndrome.*** Occurring 1 to 3 weeks after a head injury, this syndrome is marked by dizziness, headache (throbbing, aching, bandlike, or stabbing), emotional lability, alcohol intolerance, fatigue, anxiety and, possibly, vertigo. Dizziness and other symptoms are intensified by mental or physical stress. The syndrome may persist for years, but symptoms eventually abate.

◆ ***Rift Valley fever.*** Typical signs and symptoms of this disorder include dizziness, fever, myalgia, weakness, and back pain. A small percentage of patients may develop encephalitis or may progress to hemorrhagic fever, which can lead to shock and hemorrhage. Inflammation of the retina may result in some permanent vision loss.

◆ ***Transient ischemic attack (TIA).*** Lasting from a few seconds to 24 hours, a TIA commonly signals an impending stroke and may be triggered by turning the head to the side. Besides dizziness of varying severity, TIAs are marked by unilateral or bilateral diplopia, blindness or visual field deficits, ptosis, tinnitus, hearing loss, paresis, and numbness. Other findings may include dysarthria, dysphagia, vomiting, hiccups, confusion, decreased LOC, and pallor.

Other causes

◆ ***Drugs.*** Anxiolytics, CNS depressants, opioids, decongestants, antihistamines, antihypertensives, and vasodilators commonly cause dizziness.

HERB ALERT *Herbal remedies, such as St. John's wort, can produce dizziness.*

Special considerations

Prepare the patient for diagnostic tests, such as blood studies, arteriography, computed tomography scan, EEG, magnetic resonance imaging, and tilt-table studies.

Pediatric pointers

Dizziness is less common in children than in adults. Many children have difficulty describing this symptom and instead complain of tiredness, stomachache, or feeling sick. If you suspect dizziness, also assess the patient for vertigo, a more common symptom in children that may result from a vision disorder, an ear infection, or antibiotic therapy.

Patient counseling

Teach the patient ways to control dizziness. If he's hyperventilating, have him breathe and rebreathe into his cupped hands or a paper bag. If he experiences dizziness in an upright position, tell him to lie down and rest and then to rise slowly. Advise the patient with carotid sinus hypersensitivity to avoid wearing garments that constrict the neck. Instruct the patient who risks a TIA from vertebrobasilar insufficiency to turn his body instead of sharply turning his head to one side.

Doll's eye sign, absent

[Negative oculocephalic reflex]

An indicator of brain stem dysfunction, the absence of the doll's eye sign is detected by rapid, gentle turning of the patient's head from side to side. The eyes remain fixed in midposition, instead of the normal response of moving laterally toward side opposite the direction the head is turned. (See *Testing for absent doll's eye sign*.)

The absence of doll's eye sign indicates injury to the midbrain or pons, involving cranial nerves III and VI. It typically accompanies a coma caused by lesions of the cerebellum and brain stem. This sign usually can't be relied upon in a conscious patient because he can control eye movements voluntarily. Absent

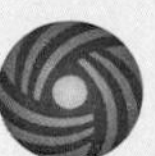

EXAMINATION TIP

Testing for absent doll's eye sign

To evaluate the patient's oculocephalic reflex, hold her upper eyelids open and quickly (but gently) turn her head from side to side, noting eye movements with each head turn.

In absent doll's eye sign, the eyes remain fixed in midposition.

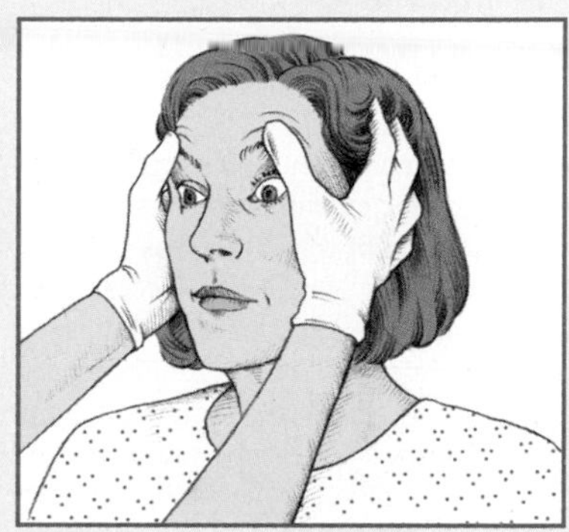

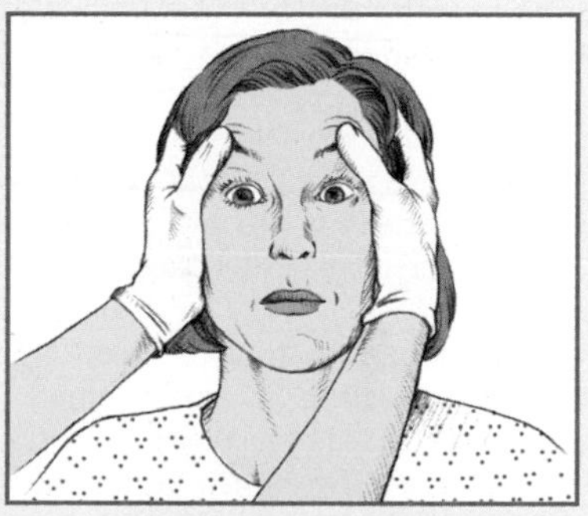

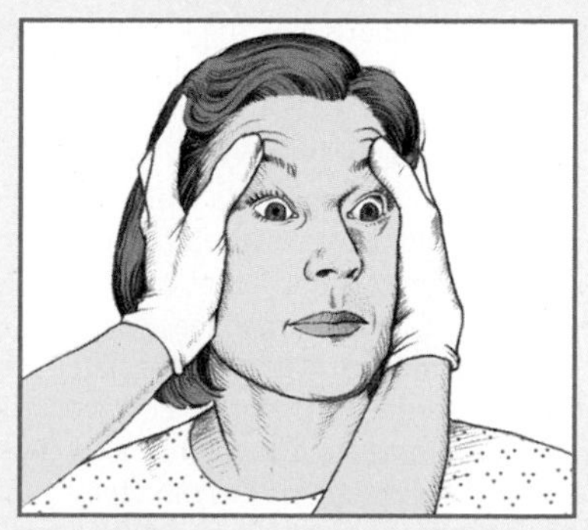

doll's eye sign is necessary for a diagnosis of brain death.

A variant of absent doll's eye sign that develops gradually is known as *abnormal doll's eye sign.* Because conjugate eye movement is lost, one eye may move laterally while the other remains fixed or moves in the opposite direction. An abnormal doll's eye sign usually accompanies metabolic coma or increased intracranial pressure (ICP). Associated brain stem dysfunction may be reversible or may progress to deeper coma in patients with this sign.

History and physical examination

After detecting an absent doll's eye sign, perform a neurologic examination. First, evaluate the patient's level of consciousness (LOC), using the Glasgow Coma Scale. Note decerebrate or decorticate posture. Examine the pupils for size, equality, and response to light. Check for signs of increased ICP—increased systolic blood pressure, widening pulse pressure, and bradycardia.

Medical causes

◆ ***Brain stem infarction.*** This infarction causes absent doll's eye sign with a coma. It also causes limb paralysis, cranial nerve palsies (facial weakness, diplopia, blindness or visual field deficits, and nystagmus), bilateral cerebellar ataxia, variable sensory loss, a positive Babinski's reflex, decerebrate posture, and muscle flaccidity.

◆ ***Brain stem tumor.*** Absent doll's eye sign accompanies a coma in this type of tumor. This sign may be preceded by hemiparesis, nystagmus, extraocular nerve palsies, facial pain or sensory loss, facial paralysis, diminished corneal reflex, tinnitus, hearing loss, dysphagia, drooling, vertigo, dizziness, ataxia, and vomiting.

◆ ***Central midbrain infarction.*** Accompanying absent doll's eye sign are a coma, Weber's syndrome (oculomotor palsy with contralateral hemiplegia), contralateral ataxic tremor, nystagmus, and pupillary abnormalities.

◆ ***Cerebellar lesion.*** Whether associated with abscess, hemorrhage, or tumor, a cerebellar lesion that progresses to a coma may also cause an absent doll's eye sign. The coma may be preceded by headache, nystagmus, ocular deviation to the side of the lesion, unequal pupils, dysarthria, dysphagia, ipsilateral facial paresis, and cerebellar ataxia. Characteristic signs of increased ICP may also occur, including decreased LOC, abnormal pupillary responses, increased systolic blood pressure, widening pulse pressure, bradycardia, altered respiratory pattern, papilledema, and vomiting.

◆ ***Pontine hemorrhage.*** Absent doll's eye sign and a coma develop within minutes in this life-threatening disorder. Other ominous signs—such as complete paralysis, decerebrate posture, a positive Babinski's reflex, and small, reactive pupils—may rapidly progress to death.

◆ ***Posterior fossa hematoma.*** A subdural hematoma at this location typically causes absent doll's eye sign and a coma. These signs may be preceded by characteristic signs and symptoms, such as headache, vomiting, drowsiness, confusion, unequal pupils, dysphagia, cranial nerve palsies, stiff neck, and cerebellar ataxia.

Other causes

◆ ***Drugs.*** Barbiturates may produce severe central nervous system depression, resulting in a coma and absent doll's eye sign.

Special considerations

Don't attempt to elicit doll's eye sign in a comatose patient with a suspected cervical spine injury; doing so risks spinal cord damage. Instead, evaluate the oculovestibular reflex with the cold caloric test. Normally, instilling cold water in the ear causes the eyes to move slowly toward the irrigated ear. Cold caloric testing may also be done to confirm an absent doll's eye sign.

Continue to monitor vital signs and neurologic status in the patient with an absent doll's eye sign.

Pediatric pointers

Normally, doll's eye sign isn't present for the first 10 days after birth, and it may be irregular until age 2. After that, this sign reliably indicates brain stem dysfunction. An absent doll's eye sign in children may accompany a coma associated with head injury, near drowning, suffocation, or brain stem astrocytoma.

Drooling

Drooling—the flow of saliva from the mouth—results from a failure to swallow or retain saliva or from excess salivation. It may stem from facial muscle paralysis or weakness that prevents mouth closure, from neuromuscular disorders or local pain that causes dysphagia or, less commonly, from the effects of drugs or toxins that induce salivation. Drooling may be scant or copious (up to 1 L daily) and may cause circumoral irritation. Because it signals an inability to handle secretions, drooling warns of potential aspiration.

History and physical examination

If you observe the patient drooling, first determine the amount. Is it scant or copious? When did it begin? Ask the patient if his pillow is wet in the morning. Also, inspect for circumoral irritation.

Then explore associated signs and symptoms. Ask about sore throat and difficulty swallowing, chewing, speaking, or breathing. Have the patient describe any pain or stiffness in the face and neck and any muscle weakness in the face and extremities. Has he noticed any mental status changes, such as drowsiness or agitation? Ask about changes in vision, hearing, and sense of taste. Also ask about anorexia, weight loss, fatigue, nausea, vomiting, and altered elimination habits. Has the patient recently had a cold or other infection? Was he recently bitten by an animal or exposed to pesticides? Finally, obtain a complete drug history.

Next, perform a physical examination, starting with vital signs. Inspect the face for signs of paralysis or an abnormal expression. Examine the mouth and neck for swelling, the throat for edema and redness, and the tonsils for exudate. Note halitosis. Examine the tongue for bilateral furrowing (trident tongue). Look for pallor, skin lesions, and frontal baldness. Carefully assess any bite or puncture marks.

Assess cranial nerves II through XII. Then check pupillary size and response to light. Assess the patient's speech. Evaluate muscle strength and palpate for tenderness or atrophy. Also palpate for lymphadenopathy, especially in the cervical area. Observe the patient's ability to swallow. Test for poor balance, hyperreflexia, and a positive Babinski's reflex. Also, assess sensory function for paresthesia.

Medical causes

◆ ***Achalasia.*** Progressively severe dysphagia may cause copious drooling late in this disorder. When the patient lies down, food and saliva in the dilated esophagus flow back to the pharynx and mouth, resulting in drooling. Coughing or choking and aspiration may follow regurgitation. Other findings include weight loss and, possibly, spasms or substernal pain after eating.

◆ ***Acoustic neuroma.*** When this malignant tumor involves the facial nerve, it produces facial weakness or paralysis with scant to copious drooling. The drooling is followed by tinnitus, unilateral hearing loss, and vertigo. Other symptoms include dysphagia, poor balance, and ear or eye pain.

◆ ***Amyotrophic lateral sclerosis.*** Brain stem involvement in this degenerative disorder weakens muscles of the face and tongue, resulting in constant scant to copious drooling. The drooling is accompanied by dysarthria and difficulty chewing, swallowing, and breathing. Fasciculations are common along with muscle atrophy and weakness, especially in the forearms and hands, and hyperreflexia and spasticity in the legs.

◆ ***Bell's palsy.*** Drooling accompanies the gradual onset of facial hemiplegia in Bell's palsy. The affected side of the face sags and is expressionless, the nasolabial fold flattens, and the palpebral fissure (distance between upper and lower eyelids) widens. The patient usually complains of pain in or behind the ear. Other cardinal signs and symptoms include a unilateral diminished or absent corneal reflex, decreased lacrimation, Bell's phenomenon (upward deviation of the eye with attempt at eyelid closure), and partial loss of taste or abnormal taste sensation.

◆ ***Diphtheria.*** In this infection, moderate drooling results from dysphagia associated with sore throat. The hallmark of diphtheria, however, is a bluish white, gray, or black membrane over the mucous membranes of the tonsils, pharynx, larynx, soft palate, and nose. This membrane causes pooling of saliva, which aggravates drooling. Other signs and symptoms include fever, pallor, tachycardia, halitosis, noisy respirations, cervical lymphadenopathy, purpuric skin lesions, drowsiness, and delirium.

◆ ***Esophageal tumor.*** In this type of tumor, copious and persistent drooling is typically preceded by weight loss and progressively severe dysphagia. Other signs and symptoms include substernal, back, or neck pain and blood-flecked regurgitation.

◆ ***Glossopharyngeal neuralgia.*** Drooling may accompany the sharp paroxysms of pain that characterize this rare disorder. The pain may be precipitated by swallowing, talking, chewing, or coughing or by external pressure on the ear; it may affect the posterior pharynx, the ear, or the base of the tongue or jaw. Associated findings include hoarseness, soft palate deviation to the unaffected side, absent gag reflex, partial loss of taste, and trapezius and sternocleidomastoid muscle weakness.

◆ ***Guillain-Barré syndrome.*** The hallmark of this polyneuritis is ascending muscle weakness that typically starts in the legs and extends to the arms and face within 24 to 72 hours. Facial diplegia and dysphagia set the stage for scant to copious drooling, which is accompanied by dysarthria, nasal voice tone, and a diminished or absent corneal reflex. Other signs and symptoms include paresthesia, signs of respiratory distress, and signs of sympathetic dysfunction, such as orthostatic hypotension, loss of bowel and bladder control, diaphoresis, and tachycardia.

◆ ***Hypocalcemia.*** The chief feature of hypocalcemia is tetany, characterized by muscle twitching, cramps, and seizures; carpopedal spasm; and positive Chvostek's and Trousseau's signs. Moderate to copious drooling may accompany the resultant dysphagia. In severe hypocalcemia, the patient may have laryngeal spasm with stridor, cyanosis, and generalized tonic-clonic seizures.

◆ ***Ludwig's angina.*** In this disorder, moderate to copious drooling stems from dysphagia and local swelling of the floor of the mouth, causing tongue displacement. Submandibular swelling of the neck and signs of respiratory distress may also occur.

◆ ***Myasthenia gravis.*** Facial and pharyngeal muscle weakness causes scant to copious drooling that's accompanied by difficulty swallowing, chewing, and speaking. Typically, drooling is preceded by diplopia and ptosis. The patient displays a masklike face and myasthenia snarl (smile with lips elevated but not retracted). Other features include a weak tongue with bilateral furrowing (trident tongue) and a sagging jaw if masseter muscles are affected. Skeletal muscle weakness is characteristic; muscles typically weaken throughout the day, especially after exercise.

◆ ***Myotonic dystrophy.*** Facial weakness and a sagging jaw account for constant drooling in this disorder. Other characteristic findings include myotonia (inability to relax a muscle after its contraction), muscle wasting, cataracts, testicular atrophy, frontal baldness, ptosis, and a nasal, monotone voice.

◆ ***Paralytic poliomyelitis.*** When this infection involves the brain stem, it may produce facial paralysis and dysphagia, resulting in scant to copious drooling. Typically, the drooling is preceded by fever, headache, nuchal rigidity, and intense muscle aches. The patient then develops fasciculations and usually asymmetrical paralysis in the lower legs and trunk that's associated with transient urine retention.

◆ ***Parkinson's disease.*** In this degenerative disorder, the neck is flexed forward, so saliva isn't directed to the back of the mouth; the result is drooling. Other cardinal features include a pill-rolling tremor, rigidity, bradykinesia, a shuffling gait, stooped posture, masklike facies, dysarthria, and a high-pitched, monotone voice.

◆ ***Peritonsillar abscess.*** A severe sore throat causes dysphagia with moderate to copious drooling in this type of abscess. Accompanying signs and symptoms are high fever, rancid breath, and enlarged, reddened, edematous tonsils that may be covered by a soft gray exudate. Palpation may reveal cervical lymphadenopathy.

◆ ***Rabies.*** When this acute central nervous system infection advances to the brain stem, it produces drooling (commonly referred to as "foaming at the mouth") from excessive salivation, facial palsy, or extremely painful pharyngeal spasms that prohibit swallowing. It's accompanied by hydrophobia in about 50% of patients. Seizures and hyperactive deep tendon reflexes (DTRs) may also occur before the patient develops generalized flaccid paralysis and a coma.

◆ ***Retropharyngeal abscess.*** This disorder causes painful swallowing, resulting in moderate to copious drooling. The patient complains of a lump in his throat that he can't swallow and of dyspnea in the sitting position that disappears when he lies down. Other cardinal signs and symptoms include coughing, snoring, choking, noisy breathing, and a "cry of a duck" voice tone. Cervical lymphadenopathy, pharyngeal edema and redness, and a high fever may also occur.

◆ ***Seizures (generalized).*** This tonic-clonic muscular reaction causes excessive salivation and frothing at the mouth accompanied by loss of consciousness and cyanosis. In the unresponsive postictal state, the patient may also drool.

◆ ***Stroke.*** Facial paralysis associated with stroke results in scant to copious drooling. Other signs and symptoms include diplopia, visual field deficits, dysarthria, hearing loss, paresthesia, paralysis, ataxia, headache, dizziness, confusion, nausea, vomiting, unilateral or bilateral hyperactive DTRs, and a positive Babinski's reflex.

◆ ***Tetanus.*** This acute infection may produce scant to copious drooling associated with dysphagia. Typically, drooling is preceded by restlessness and pain and stiffness in the jaw, abdomen, and back that progress to tonic spasms. A locked jaw and a grotesque grinning expression (risus sardonicus) are characteristic signs. Profuse sweating, low-grade fever, and tachycardia are also common.

OTHER CAUSES

- ***Drugs.*** Such drugs as clonazepam, ethionamide, and haloperidol can all cause excessive salivation, which may result in drooling.
- ***Envenomation.*** Some snakebites trigger excess salivation, resulting in drooling. The drooling is accompanied by other neurotoxic effects, such as diaphoresis, chills, weakness, dizziness, nausea, vomiting, paresthesia, fasciculations, and tender lymphadenopathy. Local swelling, pain, and ecchymoses may occur.
- ***Pesticide poisoning.*** Toxic effects of pesticides may include excess salivation with drooling, diaphoresis, nausea and vomiting, involuntary urination and defecation, blurred vision, miosis, increased lacrimation, fasciculations, weakness, flaccid paralysis, signs of respiratory distress, and coma.

SPECIAL CONSIDERATIONS

Be alert for aspiration in the drooling patient. Position him upright or on his side. Provide frequent mouth care, and suction as necessary to control drooling. Be prepared to perform a tracheostomy and intubation, to administer oxygen, or to execute an abdominal thrust.

Help the patient cope with drooling by providing a covered, opaque collecting jar to decrease odor and prevent transmission of infection. Keep tissues handy and drape a towel across the patient's chest at mealtime. Encourage oral hygiene. Also, teach the patient exercises to help strengthen facial muscles, if appropriate. Assist the patient with meticulous skin care, especially around the mouth and in the neck area, to prevent skin breakdown. Cornstarch may be placed on the neck to reduce the risk of maceration.

PEDIATRIC POINTERS

Normally, an infant can't control saliva flow until about age 1, when muscular reflexes that initiate swallowing and lip closure mature. Salivation and drooling typically increase with teething, which begins at about the fifth month and continues until about age 2. Excessive salivation and drooling may also occur in response to hunger or anticipation of feeding, and in association with nausea.

Common causes of drooling in children include epiglottiditis, retropharyngeal abscess, severe tonsillitis, stomatitis, herpetic lesions, esophageal atresia, cerebral palsy, mental deficiency, and drug withdrawal in neonates of addicted mothers. It may also result from a foreign body in the esophagus, causing dysphagia.

Dysarthria

Dysarthria, poorly articulated speech, is characterized by slurring and a labored, irregular rhythm. It may be accompanied by a nasal voice tone caused by palate weakness. Whether it occurs abruptly or gradually, dysarthria is usually evident in ordinary conversation. It's confirmed by asking the patient to produce a few simple sounds and words, such as "ba," "sh," and "cat." However, dysarthria is occasionally confused with aphasia, loss of the ability to produce or comprehend speech.

Dysarthria results from brain stem damage that affects cranial nerves IX, X, or XII. Degenerative neurologic disorders and cerebellar disorders commonly cause dysarthria. In fact, dysarthria is a cardinal sign of olivopontocerebellar degeneration. It may also result from ill-fitting dentures. (See *Dysarthria: Causes and associated findings,* pages 226 and 227.)

EMERGENCY INTERVENTIONS *If the patient displays dysarthria, ask him about associated difficulty swallowing. Then determine respiratory rate and depth. Measure vital capacity with a Wright respirometer if available. Assess blood pressure and heart rate. Tachycardia, slightly increased blood pressure, and shortness of breath are usually early signs of respiratory muscle weakness.*

Ensure a patent airway. Place the patient in Fowler's position and suction him if necessary. Administer oxygen and keep emergency resuscitation equipment nearby. Anticipate intubation and mechanical ventilation in progressive respiratory muscle weakness. Withhold oral fluids in the patient with associated dysphagia.

If dysarthria isn't accompanied by respiratory muscle weakness and dysphagia, continue to assess for other neurologic deficits. Compare muscle strength and tone in the limbs, and evaluate tactile sensation. Ask the patient about numbness or tingling. Test deep tendon reflexes (DTRs), and note gait ataxia. Assess cerebellar function by observing

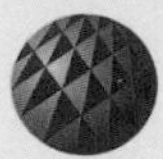

SIGNS & SYMPTOMS

Dysarthria: Causes and associated findings

Common causes	Major associated signs and symptoms: Aphasia	Ataxia	Bradykinesia	Diplopia	Drooling	Dysphagia	Dyspnea	Fasciculations	Gait, propulsive	Hyperreflexia	Hypotension	Level of consciousness, decreased	Masklike facies
Alcoholic cerebellar degeneration		●		●							●	●	
Amyotrophic lateral sclerosis					●	●	●	●		●			
Basilar artery insufficiency		●		●									
Botulism				●		●	●						
Manganese poisoning					●				●			●	
Mercury poisoning		●										●	
Multiple sclerosis		●		●		●				●			
Myasthenia gravis				●	●	●	●						
Olivopontocerebellar degeneration		●											
Parkinson's disease			●		●	●			●				●
Shy-Drager syndrome		●	●								●		●
Stroke (brain stem)				●	●	●	●					●	
Stroke (cerebral)	●				●	●				●			

rapid alternating movement, which should be smooth and coordinated. Next, test visual fields and ask about double vision. Check for signs of facial weakness such as ptosis. Finally, determine level of consciousness (LOC) and mental status.

History and physical examination

Explore dysarthria completely. When did it begin? Has it gotten better? Speech improves with resolution of a transient ischemic attack, but not in a completed stroke. Ask if dysarthria worsens during the day. Then obtain a drug and alcohol history. Also, ask about a history of seizures. Observe dentures for a proper fit.

Medical causes

◆ ***Alcoholic cerebellar degeneration.*** This disorder commonly causes chronic, progressive dysarthria along with ataxia, diplopia,

	Muscle atrophy	Muscle weakness	Ptosis	Spasticity	Tremor	Vertigo	Visual field deficits
	●	●		●			
		●				●	●
		●	●				
		●		●	●		
		●			●		
		●		●	●		
		●	●				
				●			
		●			●		
		●		●			
		●		●			

ophthalmoplegia, hypotension, and altered mental status.

◆ ***Amyotrophic lateral sclerosis.*** Dysarthria occurs when this disorder affects the bulbar nuclei; it may worsen as the disease progresses. Other signs and symptoms include dysphagia; difficulty breathing; muscle atrophy and weakness, especially of the hands and feet; fasciculations; spasticity; hyperactive DTRs in the legs; and occasionally excessive drooling. Progressive bulbar palsy may cause crying spells or inappropriate laughter.

◆ ***Basilar artery insufficiency.*** This disorder causes random, brief episodes of bilateral brain stem dysfunction, resulting in dysarthria. Accompanying it are diplopia, vertigo, facial numbness, ataxia, paresis, and visual field loss, all of which can last from minutes to hours.

◆ ***Botulism.*** The hallmark of this disorder is acute cranial nerve dysfunction that causes dysarthria, dysphagia, diplopia, and ptosis. Early findings include dry mouth, sore throat, weakness, vomiting, and diarrhea. Later, descending weakness or paralysis of muscles in the extremities and trunk causes hyporeflexia and dyspnea.

◆ ***Multiple sclerosis.*** When demyelination affects the brain stem and cerebellum, the patient displays dysarthria accompanied by nystagmus, blurred or double vision, dysphagia, ataxia, and intention tremor. Exacerbations and remissions of these signs and symptoms are common. Other findings include paresthesia, spasticity, intention tremor, hyperreflexia, muscle weakness or paralysis, constipation, emotional lability, and urinary frequency, urgency, and incontinence.

◆ ***Myasthenia gravis.*** This neuromuscular disorder causes dysarthria associated with a nasal voice tone. Typically, the dysarthria worsens during the day and may temporarily improve with short rest periods. Other findings include dysphagia, drooling, facial weakness, diplopia, ptosis, dyspnea, and muscle weakness.

◆ ***Olivopontocerebellar degeneration.*** Dysarthria, a cardinal sign of this disorder, accompanies cerebellar ataxia and spasticity.

◆ ***Parkinson's disease.*** This disorder produces dysarthria and a monotone voice. It also produces muscle rigidity, bradykinesia, an involuntary tremor that usually begins in the fingers, difficulty walking, muscle weakness, and stooped posture. Other findings include masklike facies, dysphagia and, occasionally, drooling.

◆ ***Shy-Drager syndrome.*** Marked by chronic orthostatic hypotension, this syndrome eventually causes dysarthria as well as cerebellar ataxia, bradykinesia, masklike facies, dementia, impotence and, possibly, stooped posture and incontinence.

◆ ***Stroke (brain stem).*** This type of stroke is characterized by bulbar palsy, resulting in the triad of dysarthria, dysphonia, and dysphagia. The dysarthria is most severe at the onset of the stroke; it may lessen or disappear with rehabilitation and training. Other findings include facial weakness, diplopia, hemiparesis, spasticity, drooling, dyspnea, and decreased LOC.

◆ ***Stroke (cerebral).*** A massive bilateral stroke causes pseudobulbar palsy. Bilateral weakness produces dysarthria that's most severe at the stroke's onset. This sign is accompanied by dysphagia, drooling, dysphonia, bilateral hemianopsia, and aphasia. Sensory loss, spasticity, and hyperreflexia may also occur.

Other causes

◆ ***Drugs.*** Dysarthria can occur when anticonvulsant dosage is too high. Ingestion of large doses of barbiturates may also cause dysarthria.

◆ ***Manganese poisoning.*** Chronic manganese poisoning causes progressive dysarthria accompanied by weakness, fatigue, confusion, hallucinations, drooling, hand tremors, limb stiffness, spasticity, gross rhythmic movements of the trunk and head, and a propulsive gait.

◆ ***Mercury poisoning.*** Chronic mercury poisoning causes progressive dysarthria accompanied by weakness, fatigue, depression, lethargy, irritability, confusion, ataxia, and tremors.

Special considerations

Encourage the patient with dysarthria to speak slowly so that he can be understood. Give him time to express himself, and encourage him to use gestures. Dysarthria usually requires consultation with a speech pathologist.

Pediatric pointers

Dysarthria in children usually results from brain stem glioma, a slow-growing tumor that primarily affects children. It may also result from cerebral palsy.

Dysarthria may be difficult to detect, especially in an infant or a young child who hasn't perfected speech. Be sure to look for other neurologic deficits, too. Encourage a child with dysarthria to speak; a child's potential for rehabilitation is typically greater than an adult's.

Dysmenorrhea

Dysmenorrhea—painful menstruation—affects more than 50% of menstruating women; in fact, it's the leading cause of lost time from school and work among women of childbearing age. Dysmenorrhea may involve sharp, intermittent pain or dull, aching pain. It's usually characterized by mild to severe cramping or colicky pain in the pelvis or lower abdomen that may radiate to the thighs and lower sacrum. This pain may precede menstruation by several days or may accompany it. The pain gradually subsides as bleeding tapers off.

Dysmenorrhea may be idiopathic, as in premenstrual syndrome (PMS) and primary dysmenorrhea. It commonly results from endometriosis and other pelvic disorders. It may also result from structural abnormalities such as an imperforate hymen. Stress and poor health may aggravate dysmenorrhea; rest and mild exercise may relieve it.

History and physical examination

If the patient complains of dysmenorrhea, have her describe it fully. Is it intermittent or continuous? Sharp, cramping, or aching? Ask where the pain is located and whether it's bilateral. How long has she been experiencing it? When does the pain begin and end, and when is it severe? Does it radiate to the back? Explore associated signs and symptoms, such as nausea and vomiting, altered elimination habits, bloating, water retention, pelvic or rectal pressure, and unusual fatigue, irritability, or depression.

Then obtain a menstrual and sexual history. Ask the patient if her menstrual flow is heavy or scant. Have her describe any vaginal discharge between menses. Does she experience pain during sexual intercourse? Does it occur with menses? Find out what relieves her cramps. Does she take pain medication? Is it effective? Note her method of contraception, and ask about a history of pelvic infection. Does she have any signs and symptoms of urinary system obstruction, such as pyuria, urine retention, or incontinence? Determine how she copes with stress. Determine her risk for sexually transmitted diseases.

Next, perform a focused physical examination. Take vital signs, noting fever and accompanying chills. Inspect the abdomen for distention, and palpate for tenderness and masses. Note costovertebral angle tenderness.

Medical causes

◆ ***Adenomyosis.*** In this disorder, endometrial tissue invades the myometrium, resulting in severe dysmenorrhea with pain radiating to the back or rectum, menorrhagia, and a symmetrically enlarged, globular uterus that's usually softer on palpation than a uterine myoma.

◆ ***Cervical stenosis.*** This structural disorder causes dysmenorrhea and scant or absent menstrual flow.
◆ ***Endometriosis.*** In this disorder, steady, aching pain typically begins before menses and peaks at the height of menstrual flow, but it may also occur between menstrual periods. The pain may arise at the endometrial deposit site or may radiate to the perineum or rectum. Associated signs and symptoms include premenstrual spotting, dyspareunia, infertility, nausea and vomiting, painful defecation, and rectal bleeding and hematuria during menses. A tender, fixed adnexal mass is usually palpable on bimanual examination.
◆ ***Pelvic inflammatory disease.*** Chronic infection produces dysmenorrhea accompanied by fever; malaise; a foul-smelling, purulent vaginal discharge; menorrhagia; dyspareunia; severe abdominal pain; nausea and vomiting; and diarrhea. A pelvic examination may reveal cervical motion tenderness and bilateral adnexal tenderness.
◆ ***PMS.*** The cramping pain of PMS usually begins with menstrual flow and persists for several hours or days, diminishing as flow decreases. Abdominal bloating, breast tenderness, palpitations, diaphoresis, flushing, depression, and irritability commonly precede menses by several days to 2 weeks. Other findings include nausea, vomiting, diarrhea, and headache. Because PMS usually follows an ovulatory cycle, it rarely occurs during the first 12 months of menses, which may be anovulatory.
◆ ***Primary (idiopathic) dysmenorrhea.*** Increased prostaglandin secretion intensifies uterine contractions, apparently causing mild to severe spasmodic cramping pain in the lower abdomen, which radiates to the sacrum and inner thighs. The cramping abdominal pain peaks a few hours before menses. Patients may also experience nausea and vomiting, fatigue, diarrhea, and headache.
◆ ***Uterine leiomyomas.*** If these tumors twist or degenerate after circulatory occlusion or infection or if the uterus contracts in an attempt to expel them, they may cause constant or intermittent lower abdominal pain that worsens with menses. Associated signs and symptoms include backache, constipation, menorrhagia, and urinary frequency or retention. Palpation may reveal the tumor mass and an enlarged uterus. The tumors are almost always nontender.

Relief for dysmenorrhea

To relieve cramping and other symptoms caused by primary dysmenorrhea or an intrauterine device, the patient may receive a prostaglandin inhibitor, such as aspirin, ibuprofen, indomethacin, or naproxen. These nonsteroidal anti-inflammatory drugs block prostaglandin synthesis early in the inflammatory reaction, thereby inhibiting prostaglandin action at receptor sites. They also have analgesic and antipyretic effects.

Make sure you and your patient are informed about the adverse effects and cautions associated with these drugs.

Adverse effects

Alert the patient to the possible adverse effects of prostaglandin inhibitors. Central nervous system effects include dizziness, headache, and vision disturbances. GI effects include nausea, vomiting, heartburn, and diarrhea. Advise the patient to take the drug with milk or after meals to reduce gastric irritation.

Contraindications

Because prostaglandin inhibitors are potentially teratogenic, be sure to rule out the possibility of pregnancy before starting the patient on this therapy. Advise any patient who suspects she's pregnant to delay therapy until menses begins.

Other cautions

If the patient has cardiac decompensation, hypertension, renal dysfunction, an ulcer, or a coagulation defect (and is receiving ongoing anticoagulant therapy), use caution when administering a prostaglandin inhibitor. Because a patient who is hypersensitive to aspirin may also be hypersensitive to other prostaglandin inhibitors, watch for signs of gastric ulceration and bleeding.

Other causes

◆ ***Intrauterine devices.*** These devices may cause severe cramping and heavy menstrual flow.

Special considerations

In the past, women with dysmenorrhea were considered neurotic. Although current research suggests that prostaglandins contribute to this symptom, old attitudes persist. Encourage the patient to view dysmenorrhea as a medical problem, not as a sign of maladjustment.

Pediatric pointers

Dysmenorrhea is rare during the first year of menstruation, before the menstrual cycle becomes ovulatory. However, the incidence of dysmenorrhea is generally higher among adolescents than older women. Teach the adolescent about dysmenorrhea. Dispel myths about it, and inform her that it's a common medical problem. Encourage good hygiene, nutrition, and exercise.

Patient counseling

If dysmenorrhea is idiopathic, advise the patient to place a heating pad on her abdomen to relieve the pain. This therapy reduces abdominal muscle tension and increases blood flow.

Effleurage, a light circular massage with the fingertips, may also provide relief. Other comfort measures include drinking warm beverages, taking a warm shower, performing waist-bending and pelvic-rocking exercises, and walking. Inform the patient that increasing aerobic exercise and dietary intake of vitamin B_1 and fish oil capsules have also proved effective in relieving dysmenorrhea.

Inform the patient that taking a nonsteroidal anti-inflammatory drug (NSAID) 1 to 2 days before the onset of menses is usually helpful. If she isn't trying to get pregnant, taking monophasic birth control pills is also beneficial. Warn the patient that both of these treatments may reduce menstrual flow and duration. Be sure to rule out the possibility of pregnancy before starting contraceptive or NSAID therapy. Explain the actions and adverse effects of these drugs. (See *Relief for dysmenorrhea,* page 229.)

Dyspareunia

A major obstacle to sexual enjoyment, dyspareunia is painful or difficult coitus. Although most sexually active women occasionally experience mild dyspareunia, persistent or severe dyspareunia is cause for concern. Dyspareunia may occur with attempted penetration or during or after coitus. It may stem from friction of the penis against perineal tissue or from jarring of deeper adnexal structures. The location of pain helps determine its cause.

Dyspareunia commonly accompanies pelvic disorders. However, it may also result from diminished vaginal lubrication associated with aging, the effects of drugs, and psychological factors—most notably, fear of pain or injury. A cycle of fear, pain, and tension may become established, in which repeated episodes of painful coitus condition the patient to anticipate pain, causing fear, which prevents sexual arousal and adequate vaginal lubrication. Contraction of the pubococcygeal muscle also occurs, making penetration still more difficult and traumatic.

Psychological factors include guilty feelings about sex, fear of pregnancy or of injury to the fetus during pregnancy, and anxiety caused by a disrupted sexual relationship or by a new sexual partner. Inadequate vaginal lubrication associated with insufficient foreplay and mental or physical fatigue may also cause dyspareunia.

History and physical examination

Begin by asking the patient to describe the pain. Does it occur with attempted penetration or deep thrusting? How long does it last? Is the pain intermittent or does it always accompany intercourse? Ask whether changing coital position or using a vaginal lubricant relieves the pain.

Next, ask about a history of pelvic, vaginal, or urinary tract infection. Does the patient have signs and symptoms of a current infection? Have her describe any discharge. Also, ask about malaise, headache, fatigue, abdominal or back pain, nausea and vomiting, and diarrhea or constipation.

Obtain a sexual and menstrual history. Determine whether dyspareunia is related to the patient's menstrual cycle. Are her cycles regular? Ask about dysmenorrhea and metrorrhagia. Has the patient had a baby? If so, did she have an episiotomy? Note whether she's breast-feeding. Ask about previous abortion, sexual abuse, or pelvic surgery. Also, find out what contraceptive method the patient uses. Does her partner use condoms? Does he or could he have a latex allergy? Then try to determine her attitude toward sexual intimacy. Does she feel tense during coitus? Is she satisfied with the length of foreplay? Does she usually achieve orgasm? Ask about a history of rape, incest, or sexual abuse as a child.

Next, perform a physical examination, starting with vital signs. Palpate the abdomen for tenderness, pain, or masses and for inguinal lymphadenopathy. Finally, inspect the genitalia for lesions and vaginal discharge.

MEDICAL CAUSES

◆ ***Allergies.*** Allergic reactions to diaphragms or condoms may result in dyspareunia.

◆ ***Atrophic vaginitis.*** In postmenopausal and breast-feeding women, decreased estrogen secretion may lead to inadequate vaginal lubrication and dyspareunia, which intensifies as intercourse continues. Accompanying signs and symptoms include pruritus, burning, bleeding, and vaginal tenderness. Patients may complain of a watery discharge at the same time that they're feeling "dry."

◆ ***Bartholinitis.*** This inflammatory disorder may produce throbbing pain accompanied by vulvar tenderness during intercourse. The patient may also complain of pain with walking or sitting. Chronic inflammation causes a purulent discharge from the infected cyst.

◆ ***Cervicitis.*** This inflammatory disorder causes pain with deep penetration. It may also cause dull lower abdominal pain, a purulent vaginal discharge, backache, and metrorrhagia.

◆ ***Condylomata acuminata.*** These papular, mosaic, warty growths occur on the vulva, vaginal and cervical walls, and perianal area. They may bleed, itch, cause burning or paresthesia in the vaginal introitus, and become tender during and after intercourse. A profuse, odorless vaginal discharge may also occur.

◆ ***Cystitis.*** Dyspareunia may occur if the patient has inflammation or infection of the bladder. Associated findings include dysuria; urinary urgency, frequency, or incontinence; pyuria; and, after coitus, hematuria.

◆ ***Endometriosis.*** This disorder causes intense pain during deep coital penetration. In addition, aching pain may occur during gentle thrusting or during a pelvic examination. The pain is usually in the lower abdomen or behind the uterus and may be worse on one side. It may be relieved by changing coital positions. Other signs and symptoms include dysmenorrhea, irregular menses, infertility, painful urination or defecation, and rectal bleeding and hematuria during menses. Typically, a tender, fixed adnexal mass is palpable on bimanual examination.

◆ ***Herpes genitalis.*** During intercourse, friction against lesions on the labia, vulva, vagina, or perianal skin causes pain and itching. The lesions are fluid-filled and usually painless at first, but may rupture and form shallow, painful ulcers with erythema and edema. Related findings include leukorrhea, fever, malaise, headache, inguinal lymphadenopathy, myalgia, and dysuria.

◆ ***Occlusive or rigid hymen.*** Dyspareunia may prevent penetration in this condition.

◆ ***Ovarian cyst or tumor.*** In this disorder, lower abdominal pain accompanies deep penetration during intercourse. Other signs and symptoms include chronic lower back pain; a tender, palpable abdominal mass; constipation; urinary frequency; menstrual irregularities; and hirsutism.

◆ ***Pelvic inflammatory disease.*** Deep penetration causes severe pain that's unrelieved by changing coital positions. Uterine tenderness may also occur with gentle thrusting or during a pelvic examination. This disorder also causes fever; malaise; a foul-smelling, purulent vaginal discharge; menorrhagia; dysmenorrhea; a soft, enlarged uterus; severe abdominal pain; nausea and vomiting; cervical motion tenderness; and diarrhea.

◆ ***Uterine prolapse.*** Sharp or aching pain occurs when the penis strikes the descended cervix of a patient with uterine prolapse. Other effects are dysmenorrhea, pelvic pressure, leukorrhea, urine retention and urinary incontinence, and chronic lower back pain.

◆ ***Vaginitis.*** This infection produces dyspareunia along with vulvar pain, burning, and itching during and for several hours after coitus. These symptoms may be aggravated by sexual arousal aside from intercourse. Vaginal discharge is typical; the type varies with the causative organism. *Candida albicans* produces a curdlike, odorless to musty-smelling discharge; *Trichomonas vaginalis* produces a yellow-green, frothy, fish-smelling discharge; bacterial vaginosis and *Neisseria gonorrhoeae* produce a profuse whitish yellow, foul-smelling discharge. Pruritus and dysuria may also occur.

OTHER CAUSES

◆ ***Contraceptive and hygienic products.*** Some spermicidal jellies, douches, and vaginal creams and deodorants cause irritation and edema, resulting in dyspareunia.

◆ ***Diaphragms and intrauterine devices.*** An ill-fitting diaphragm may produce cramps with intercourse. An incorrectly placed intrauterine device may cause dyspareunia during orgasm.

◆ ***Drugs.*** Antihistamines, decongestants, and nonsteroidal anti-inflammatory drugs decrease lubrication, resulting in dyspareunia.

◆ ***Episiotomy.*** If the episiotomy scar constricts the vaginal introitus or narrows the vaginal barrel, the patient may experience perineal pain with coitus.

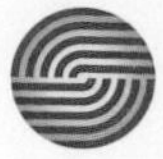

PATIENT-TEACHING AID

How to do Kegel exercises

Dear Patient:
Repeated painful intercourse may cause involuntary contraction of the pubococcygeal (PC) muscle, which encircles your urinary opening and vagina. When this happens, intercourse becomes even more difficult. Below are some isometric exercises—called Kegel exercises—that can strengthen the PC muscle and help you gain voluntary control of it.

◆ Begin by sitting on the toilet with your legs spread. Then, without moving your legs, start and stop the flow of urine. The PC muscle is the one that contracts to help control urine flow.

◆ Now that you've identified the PC muscle, you can exercise it regularly. Like most isometric exercises, Kegel exercises can be performed almost anywhere—while sitting at your desk, lying in bed, standing in line, and especially while urinating. As you perform these exercises, remember to breathe naturally—don't hold your breath.

Now, periodically contract the PC muscle as you did to stop the urine flow. Count slowly to three and then relax the muscle.

◆ Next, contract and relax the PC muscle as quickly as possible, without using your stomach or buttock muscles.

◆ Finally, slowly contract the entire vaginal area. Then bear down, using your abdominal muscles and your PC muscle.

For the first week, repeat each exercise 10 times (1 set) for 5 sets daily. Then each week, add 5 repetitions of each exercise (15, 20, and so forth). Keep doing 5 sets daily.

After about 2 weeks of practice, you'll notice improvement.

◆ ***Pelvic irradiation.*** Radiation therapy for pelvic cancer may cause pelvic and vaginal scarring, resulting in dyspareunia.

Special considerations

Prepare the patient for a pelvic examination. Explain that it involves inspection of the vagina and cervix and bimanual palpation of the uterus, fallopian tubes, and ovaries. Remind her to breathe deeply and evenly during the examination. If an antimicrobial or anti-inflammatory drug is prescribed, teach her how to apply the cream or insert the vaginal suppository.

Pediatric pointers

Dyspareunia can also be an adolescent problem. Although about 40% of adolescents are sexually active by age 19, most are reluctant to initiate a frank sexual discussion. Obtain a thorough sexual history by asking the patient direct but nonjudgmental questions.

Geriatric pointers

In postmenopausal women, the absence of estrogen reduces vaginal diameter and elasticity, which causes tearing of the vaginal mucosa during intercourse. These tears as well as inflammatory reactions to bacterial invasion cause fibrous adhesions that occlude the vagina. Dyspareunia can result from any of these conditions.

Patient counseling

Encourage the patient to discuss dyspareunia openly. A woman may hesitate to report dyspareunia because of embarrassment and modesty.

To minimize dyspareunia, advise the patient to apply a vaginal lubricant before intercourse, to attempt different coital positions, and to increase foreplay time. Teach her Kegel exercises to reduce muscle tension. (See *How to do Kegel exercises*.)

Dyspepsia

Dyspepsia refers to an uncomfortable fullness after meals that's associated with nausea, belching, heartburn and, possibly, cramping and abdominal distention. Frequently aggravated by spicy, fatty, or high-fiber foods and by excessive caffeine intake, dyspepsia without other pathology indicates impaired digestive function.

Dyspepsia is primarily caused by GI disorders and, to a lesser extent, by cardiac, pulmonary, and renal disorders and by the effects of drugs. It apparently results when altered gastric secretions lead to excessive stomach acidity. This symptom may also result from emotional upset and overly rapid eating or improper chewing. It usually occurs a few hours after eating and lasts for a variable period of time. Its severity depends on the amount and type of food eaten and on GI motility. Additional food or an antacid may relieve the discomfort. (See *Dyspepsia: Causes and associated findings,* page 234.)

History and physical examination

If the patient complains of dyspepsia, begin by asking him to describe it in detail. How often and when does it occur, specifically in relation to meals? Do any drugs or activities relieve or aggravate it? Has the patient had nausea, vomiting, melena, hematemesis, cough, or chest pain? Ask if he's taking any prescription drugs and if he has recently had surgery. Does he have a history of renal, cardiovascular, or pulmonary disease? Has he noticed any change in the amount or color of his urine?

Ask the patient if he's experiencing an unusual or overwhelming amount of emotional stress. Determine the patient's coping mechanisms and their effectiveness.

Focus the physical examination on the abdomen. Inspect it for distention, ascites, scars, obvious hernias, jaundice, uremic frost, and bruising. Then auscultate it for bowel sounds and characterize their motility. Palpate and percuss the abdomen, noting any tenderness, pain, organ enlargement, or tympany.

Finally, examine other body systems. Ask about behavior changes, and evaluate level of consciousness. Auscultate for gallops and crackles. Percuss the lungs to detect consolidation. Note peripheral edema and any swelling of lymph nodes.

Medical causes

◆ ***Cholelithiasis.*** Dyspepsia may occur with gallstones, commonly after intake of fatty foods. Biliary colic, a more common symptom of gallstones, causes acute pain that may radiate to the back, shoulders, and chest. The patient may also have diaphoresis, tachycardia, chills, low-grade fever, petechiae, bleeding tendencies, jaundice with pruritus, dark urine, and clay-colored stools.

◆ ***Cirrhosis.*** In this chronic disorder, dyspepsia varies in intensity and duration and is relieved by ingestion of an antacid. Other GI effects are anorexia, nausea, vomiting, flatulence, diarrhea, constipation, abdominal distention, and epigastric or right-upper-quadrant pain. Weight loss, jaundice, hepatomegaly, ascites, dependent edema, fever, bleeding tendencies, and muscle weakness are also common. Skin changes include severe pruritus, extreme dryness, easy bruising, and lesions, such as telangiectasis and palmar erythema. Gynecomastia or testicular atrophy may also occur.

◆ ***Duodenal ulcer.*** A primary symptom of duodenal ulcer, dyspepsia ranges from a vague feeling of fullness or pressure to a boring or aching sensation in the middle or right epigastrium. It usually occurs 1½ to 3 hours after eating and is relieved by food or an antacid. The pain may awaken the patient at night with heartburn and fluid regurgitation. Abdominal tenderness and weight gain may occur; vomiting and anorexia are rare.

◆ ***Gastric dilation (acute).*** Epigastric fullness is an early symptom of this life-threatening disorder. Accompanying dyspepsia are nausea and vomiting, upper abdominal distention, a succussion splash, and apathy. The patient may display signs and symptoms of dehydration, such as poor skin turgor and dry mucous membranes, and of electrolyte imbalance, such as irregular pulse and muscle weakness. Gastric bleeding may produce hematemesis and melena.

◆ ***Gastric ulcer.*** Dyspepsia and heartburn after eating may occur in the early stages of a gastric ulcer. The cardinal symptom, however, is epigastric pain that may occur with vomiting, fullness, and abdominal distention and may not be relieved by food. Weight loss and GI bleeding are also characteristic.

◆ ***Gastritis (chronic).*** In this disorder, dyspepsia is relieved by antacids; lessened by smaller, more frequent meals; and aggravated by spicy foods or excessive caffeine. It occurs with anorexia, a feeling of fullness, vague epigastric pain, belching, nausea, and vomiting.

◆ ***GI cancer.*** This type of cancer usually produces chronic dyspepsia. Other features include anorexia, fatigue, jaundice, melena, hematemesis, constipation, and abdominal pain.

◆ ***Heart failure.*** Common in right-sided heart failure, transient dyspepsia may occur with chest tightness and a constant ache or sharp pain in the right upper quadrant. Heart failure also typically causes hepatomegaly, anorexia, nausea, vomiting, bloating, ascites, tachycardia, jugular vein distention, tachypnea, dyspnea, and orthopnea. Other findings include dependent edema, anxiety, fatigue, diaphoresis, hypotension, cough, crackles, ventricular and atrial gallops, nocturia, elevated diastolic blood pressure, and cool, pale skin.

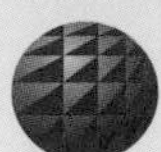

SIGNS & SYMPTOMS

Dyspepsia: Causes and associated findings

Major associated signs and symptoms

Common causes	Abdominal distention	Abdominal pain	Anorexia	Bruising, easy	Chest pain	Cough	Edema	Hepatomegaly	Jaundice	Nausea/vomiting	Oliguria	Tachycardia	Weight loss
Cholelithiasis		●							●	●		●	
Cirrhosis	●	●	●	●			●	●	●	●			●
Duodenal ulcer		●								●			
Gastric dilation (acute)	●									●			
Gastric ulcer	●	●								●			●
Gastritis (chronic)		●	●							●			
GI cancer		●	●						●				
Heart failure		●	●		●	●	●	●		●		●	
Hepatitis			●					●	●	●			
Hiatal hernia		●			●					●			
Pancreatitis (chronic)		●	●						●	●			●
Pulmonary embolism					●	●						●	
Pulmonary tuberculosis			●			●							●
Uremia		●	●				●			●	●		

◆ ***Hepatitis.*** Dyspepsia occurs in two of the three stages of hepatitis. The preicteric phase produces moderate to severe dyspepsia, fever, malaise, arthralgia, coryza, myalgia, nausea, vomiting, an altered sense of taste or smell, and hepatomegaly. Jaundice marks the onset of the icteric phase, which also includes continued dyspepsia, anorexia, irritability, and severe pruritus. As jaundice clears, dyspepsia and other GI effects also diminish. In the recovery phase, only fatigue remains.

◆ ***Hiatal hernia.*** In this disorder, dyspepsia results when the lower portion of the esophagus and the upper portion of the stomach rise into the chest as abdominal pressure increases.

◆ ***Pancreatitis (chronic).*** Dyspepsia is usually accompanied by severe continuous or intermittent epigastric pain that radiates to the back or through the abdomen. Anorexia, nausea, vomiting, jaundice, dramatic weight loss, hyperglycemia, and steatorrhea may also occur. The patient may have Turner's or Cullen's sign.

◆ ***Pulmonary embolism.*** Sudden dyspnea characterizes this potentially fatal disorder; however, dyspepsia may occur as an oppressive, severe, substernal discomfort. Other findings include anxiety, tachycardia, tachypnea, cough, pleuritic chest pain, hemoptysis, syncope, cyanosis, jugular vein distention, and hypotension.

◆ ***Pulmonary tuberculosis.*** Vague dyspepsia may occur along with anorexia, malaise, and weight loss. Common associated findings include high fever, night sweats, palpitations on mild exertion, a productive cough, dyspnea, adenopathy, and occasional hemoptysis.

◆ ***Uremia.*** Of the many GI complaints associated with uremia, dyspepsia may be the earliest and most important. Others include anorexia, nausea, vomiting, bloating, diarrhea, abdominal cramps, epigastric pain, and weight gain. As the renal system deteriorates, the patient may experience edema, pruritus, pallor, hyperpigmentation, uremic frost, ecchymoses, sexual dysfunction, poor memory, irritability, headache, drowsiness, muscle twitching, seizures, and oliguria.

Other causes

◆ ***Drugs.*** Nonsteroidal anti-inflammatory drugs, especially aspirin, commonly cause dyspepsia. Diuretics, antibiotics, antihypertensives, corticosteroids, and many other drugs can also cause dyspepsia, depending on the patient's tolerance of the dosage.

◆ ***Surgery.*** After GI or other surgery, postoperative gastritis can cause dyspepsia, which usually disappears in a few weeks.

Special considerations

Changing the patient's position usually doesn't relieve dyspepsia, but providing food or an antacid may, so have food available at all times, and give an antacid 30 minutes before or 1 hour after a meal. Because various drugs can cause dyspepsia, give these after meals, if possible.

Provide a calm environment to reduce stress, and make sure the patient gets plenty of rest. Discuss other ways to deal with stress, such as deep breathing and guided imagery. In addition, prepare the patient for endoscopy to determine the cause of dyspepsia.

Pediatric pointers

Dyspepsia may occur in adolescents with peptic ulcer disease, but it isn't relieved by food. It may also occur in congenital pyloric stenosis, but projectile vomiting after meals is a more characteristic sign. It may also result from lactose intolerance.

Geriatric pointers

Most older patients with chronic pancreatitis experience less severe pain than younger adults; some have no pain at all.

Patient counseling

Advise the patient to eat frequent small meals and to avoid foods known to cause symptoms as well as coffee, tea, chocolate, alcohol, and tobacco.

Dysphagia

Dysphagia—difficulty swallowing—is a common symptom that's usually easy to localize. It may be constant or intermittent and is classified by the phase of swallowing it affects. (See *Classifying dysphagia,* page 236.) Among the factors that interfere with swallowing are severe pain, obstruction, abnormal peristalsis, impaired gag reflex, and excessive, scanty, or thick oral secretions.

Dysphagia is the most common—and sometimes the only—symptom of esophageal disorders. However, it may also result from oropharyngeal, respiratory, neurologic, and collagen disorders or from the effects of toxins and treatments. Dysphagia increases the risk of choking and aspiration and may lead to malnutrition and dehydration.

EMERGENCY INTERVENTIONS *If the patient suddenly complains of dysphagia and displays signs of respiratory distress, such as dyspnea and stridor, suspect an airway obstruction and quickly perform abdominal thrusts. Prepare to administer oxygen by mask or nasal cannula or to assist with endotracheal intubation.*

History and physical examination

If the patient's dysphagia doesn't suggest an airway obstruction, begin a health history. Ask the patient if swallowing is painful. If so, is the pain constant or intermittent? Have the patient point to where dysphagia feels most intense. Does eating alleviate or aggravate the symptom? Are solids or liquids more difficult to swallow? If the answer is liquids, ask if hot, cold, and lukewarm

Classifying dysphagia

Because swallowing occurs in three distinct phases, dysphagia can be classified by the phase that it affects. Each phase suggests a specific pathology for dysphagia.

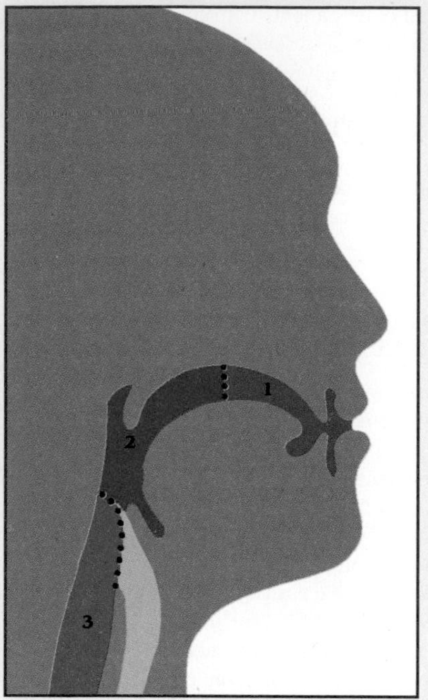

Phase 1
Swallowing begins in the *transfer phase* with chewing and moistening of food with saliva. The tongue presses against the hard palate to transfer the chewed food to the back of the throat; cranial nerve V then stimulates the swallowing reflex. Phase 1 dysphagia typically results from a neuromuscular disorder.

Phase 2
In the *transport phase,* the soft palate closes against the pharyngeal wall to prevent nasal regurgitation. At the same time, the larynx rises and the vocal cords close to keep food out of the lungs; breathing stops momentarily as the throat muscles constrict to move food into the esophagus. Phase 2 dysphagia usually indicates spasm or cancer.

Phase 3
Peristalsis and gravity work together in the *entrance phase* to move food through the esophageal sphincter and into the stomach. Phase 3 dysphagia results from lower esophageal narrowing by diverticula, esophagitis, and other disorders.

fluids affect him differently. Does the symptom disappear after he tries to swallow a few times? Is swallowing easier if he changes position? Ask if he has recently experienced vomiting, regurgitation, weight loss, anorexia, hoarseness, dyspnea, or a cough.

To evaluate the patient's swallowing reflex, place your finger along his thyroid notch and instruct him to swallow. If you feel his larynx rise, the reflex is intact. Next, have him cough to assess his cough reflex. Check his gag reflex if you're sure he has a good swallow or cough reflex. Listen closely to his speech for signs of muscle weakness. Does he have aphasia or dysarthria? Is his voice nasal, hoarse, or breathy? Assess the patient's mouth carefully. Check for dry mucous membranes and thick, sticky secretions. Observe for tongue and facial weakness and obvious obstructions (for example, enlarged tonsils). Assess the patient for disorientation, which may make him neglect to swallow.

Medical causes

◆ ***Achalasia.*** Most common in patients ages 20 to 40, this disorder produces phase 3 dysphagia for solids and liquids. The dysphagia develops gradually and may be precipitated or exacerbated by stress. Occasionally, it's preceded by esophageal colic. Regurgitation of undigested food, especially at night, may cause wheezing, coughing, or choking as well as halitosis. Weight loss, cachexia, hematemesis and, possibly, heartburn are late findings.

◆ ***Airway obstruction.*** Life-threatening upper airway obstruction is marked by signs of respiratory distress, such as crowing and stridor. Phase 2 dysphagia occurs with gagging and dysphonia. When hemorrhage obstructs the trachea, dysphagia is usually painless and rapid in onset. When inflammation causes the obstruction, dysphagia may be painful and develop slowly.

◆ ***Amyotrophic lateral sclerosis.*** Besides dysphagia, this disorder causes muscle weakness and atrophy, fasciculations, dysarthria, dyspnea, shallow respirations, tachypnea, slurred speech, hyperactive deep tendon reflexes, and emotional lability.

◆ ***Botulism.*** This type of food poisoning causes phase 1 dysphagia and dysuria, usually within 36 hours of toxin ingestion. Other early findings include blurred or double vision, dry mouth, sore throat, nausea, vomiting, and diarrhea. Symmetrical descending weakness or paralysis occurs gradually.

◆ ***Bulbar paralysis.*** Phase 1 dysphagia occurs along with drooling, difficulty chewing, dysarthria, and nasal regurgitation in this disorder. Dysphagia for both solids and liquids is painful and progressive. Accompanying features may include arm and leg spasticity, hyperreflexia, and emotional lability.

◆ ***Dysphagia lusoria.*** This disorder is caused by compression of the esophagus by a congenital vascular abnormality (usually an aberrant right subclavian artery arising from the left side of the aortic arch). Phase 3 dysphagia symptoms may start in childhood or may develop later from changes in the aberrant vessel such as arteriosclerosis.

◆ ***Esophageal cancer.*** Phase 2 or 3 dysphagia is the earliest and most common symptom of esophageal cancer. Typically, this painless, progressive symptom is accompanied by rapid weight loss. As the cancer advances, dysphagia becomes painful and constant. In addition, the patient complains of steady chest pain, cough with hemoptysis, hoarseness, and sore throat. He may also develop nausea and vomiting, fever, hiccups, hematemesis, melena, and halitosis.

◆ ***Esophageal compression (external).*** Usually caused by a dilated carotid or aortic aneurysm, this rare condition causes phase 3 dysphagia as the primary symptom. Other features depend on the cause of the compression.

◆ ***Esophageal diverticulum.*** This disorder causes phase 3 dysphagia when the enlarged diverticulum obstructs the esophagus. Associated signs and symptoms include food regurgitation, chronic cough, hoarseness, chest pain, and halitosis.

◆ ***Esophageal leiomyoma.*** A relatively rare benign tumor, esophageal leiomyoma may cause phase 3 dysphagia along with retrosternal pain or discomfort. In addition, the patient experiences weight loss and a feeling of fullness.

◆ ***Esophageal obstruction by foreign body.*** Sudden onset of phase 2 or 3 dysphagia, gagging, coughing, and esophageal pain characterize this potentially life-threatening condition. Dyspnea may occur if the obstruction compresses the trachea.

◆ ***Esophageal spasm.*** The most striking symptoms of this disorder are phase 2 dysphagia for solids and liquids and dull or squeezing substernal chest pain. The pain may last up to an hour and may radiate to the neck, arm, back, or jaw; however, it may be relieved by drinking a glass of water. Bradycardia may also occur.

◆ ***Esophageal stricture.*** Usually caused by scar tissue or ingestion of a chemical, this condition causes phase 3 dysphagia. Drooling, tachypnea, and gagging may also be evident.

◆ ***Esophagitis.*** Corrosive esophagitis, resulting from ingestion of alkalies or acids, causes severe phase 3 dysphagia. Accompanying it are marked salivation, hematemesis, tachypnea, fever, and intense pain in the mouth and anterior chest that's aggravated by swallowing. Signs of shock, such as hypotension and tachycardia, may also occur.

Candidal esophagitis causes phase 2 dysphagia, sore throat and, possibly, retrosternal pain on swallowing. In reflux esophagitis, phase 3 dysphagia is a late symptom that usually accompanies stricture development. The patient complains of heartburn, which is aggravated by strenuous exercise, bending over, or lying down and is relieved by sitting up or taking an antacid.

Other features include regurgitation; frequent, effortless vomiting; a dry, nocturnal cough; and substernal chest pain that may mimic angina pectoris. If the esophagus ulcerates, signs of bleeding, such as melena and hematemesis, may occur along with weakness and fatigue.

◆ ***Gastric carcinoma.*** Infiltration of the cardia or esophagus by gastric carcinoma causes phase 3 dysphagia along with nausea, vomiting, and pain that may radiate to the neck, back, or retrosternum. In addition, perforation causes massive bleeding with coffee-ground vomitus or melena.

◆ ***Hypocalcemia.*** Although tetany is its primary sign, severe hypocalcemia may cause neuromuscular irritability, producing phase 1 dysphagia associated with numbness and tingling in the nose, ears, fingertips, and toes and around the mouth. Carpopedal spasms, muscle twitching, and laryngeal spasms may also occur.

◆ ***Laryngeal cancer (extrinsic).*** Phase 2 dysphagia and dyspnea develop late in this disorder. Accompanying features include muffled voice, stridor, pain, halitosis, weight loss, ipsilateral otalgia, chronic cough, and cachexia. Palpation reveals enlarged cervical nodes.

◆ ***Laryngeal nerve damage.*** Commonly the result of radical neck surgery, superior laryngeal nerve damage may produce painless phase 2 dysphagia.

◆ ***Lower esophageal ring.*** Narrowing of the lower esophagus can cause an attack of phase 3 dysphagia that may recur several weeks or months later. During the attack, the patient complains of a foreign body sensation in the lower esophagus, which may be relieved by drinking water or vomiting. Esophageal rupture produces severe lower chest pain followed by a feeling of something giving way.

◆ ***Mediastinitis.*** Varying with the extent of esophageal perforation, mediastinitis can cause insidious or rapid onset of phase 3 dysphagia. The patient displays chills, fever, and severe retrosternal chest pain that may radiate to the epigastrium, back, or shoulder. The pain may be aggravated by breathing, coughing, or sneezing. Other findings include tachycardia, subcutaneous crepitation in the suprasternal notch, and falling blood pressure.

◆ ***Myasthenia gravis.*** Fatigue and progressive muscle weakness characterize this disorder and account for painless phase 1 dysphagia and possibly choking. Typically, dysphagia follows ptosis and diplopia. Other features include masklike facies, nasal voice, frequent nasal regurgitation, and head bobbing. Shallow respirations and dyspnea may occur with respiratory muscle weakness. Signs and symptoms worsen during menses and with exposure to stress, cold, or infection.

◆ ***Oral cavity tumor.*** Painful phase 1 dysphagia is accompanied by hoarseness and ulcerating lesions in patients with this type of tumor.

◆ ***Parkinson's disease.*** Usually a late symptom, phase 1 dysphagia is painless but progressive and may cause choking. Other signs and symptoms include bradykinesia, tremors, muscle rigidity, dysarthria, masklike facies, muffled voice, increased salivation and lacrimation, constipation, stooped posture, a propulsive gait, incontinence, and sexual dysfunction.

◆ ***Pharyngitis (chronic).*** This condition causes painful phase 2 dysphagia for solids and liquids. Rarely serious, it's accompanied by a dry, sore throat; a cough; and thick mucus in the throat.

◆ ***Plummer-Vinson syndrome.*** This syndrome causes phase 3 dysphagia for solids in some women with severe iron deficiency anemia. Related features include upper esophageal pain; atrophy of the oral or pharyngeal mucous membranes; tooth loss; a smooth, red, sore tongue; dry mouth; chills; inflamed lips; spoon-shaped nails; pallor; and splenomegaly.

◆ ***Rabies.*** Severe phase 2 dysphagia for liquids results from painful pharyngeal muscle spasms occurring late in this rare, life-threatening disorder. In fact, the patient may become dehydrated and possibly apneic. Dysphagia also causes drooling and, in 50% of patients, hydrophobia. Eventually, rabies causes progressive flaccid paralysis that leads to peripheral vascular collapse, coma, and death.

◆ ***Scleroderma (progressive systemic sclerosis).*** Typically, dysphagia is preceded by Raynaud's phenomenon in patients with this disorder. The dysphagia may be mild at first and described as a feeling of food sticking behind the breastbone. The patient also complains of heartburn after meals that's aggravated by lying down. As the disease progresses, dysphagia worsens until only liquids can be swallowed. It may be accompanied by other GI effects, including weight loss, abdominal distention, diarrhea, and malodorous, floating stools. Other characteristic late features include joint pain and stiffness, masklike facies, and thick, taut, shiny skin.

◆ ***Syphilis.*** Rarely, tertiary-stage syphilis causes ulceration and stricture of the upper esophagus, resulting in phase 3 dysphagia. The dysphagia may be accompanied by regurgitation after meals and heartburn that's aggravated by lying down or bending over.

◆ ***Systemic lupus erythematosus.*** This disorder may cause progressive phase 2 dysphagia. However, its primary signs and symptoms include nondeforming arthritis, a characteristic butterfly rash, and photosensitivity.

◆ ***Tetanus.*** Phase 1 dysphagia usually develops about 1 week after the patient receives a puncture wound. Other characteristics include marked muscle hypertonicity, hyperactive deep tendon reflexes, tachycardia, diaphoresis, drooling, and low-grade fever. Painful, involuntary muscle spasms account for lockjaw (trismus), risus sardonicus, opisthotonos, boardlike abdominal rigidity, and intermittent tonic seizures.

OTHER CAUSES

◆ ***Lead poisoning.*** Painless, progressive dysphagia may result from lead poisoning. Related findings include a lead line on the gums, metallic taste, papilledema, ocular palsy, footdrop or wristdrop, and signs of hemolytic anemia, such as abdominal pain and fever. The patient may be depressed and display severe mental impairment and seizures.

◆ ***Procedures.*** A recent tracheostomy or repeated or prolonged intubation may cause temporary dysphagia.

◆ ***Radiation therapy.*** When usd to treat oral cancer, radiation therapy may cause scant salivation and temporary dysphagia.

SPECIAL CONSIDERATIONS

Stimulate salivation by talking with the patient about food, adding a lemon slice or dill pickle to his tray, and providing mouth care before and after meals. Moisten his food with a little liquid if he has decreased salivation. Administer an anticholinergic or antiemetic to control excess salivation. If he has a weak or absent cough reflex, begin tube feedings or esophageal drips of special formulas.

Consult with the dietitian to select foods with distinct temperatures and textures. The patient should avoid sticky foods, such as bananas and peanut butter. If the patient produces mucus, avoid uncooked milk products. Arrange for a therapist to assess the patient for his aspiration risk and to teach him swallowing exercises that may help decrease his risk. At mealtimes, take measures to minimize the patient's risk of choking and aspiration. Place the patient in an upright position, and have him flex his neck forward slightly and keep his chin at midline. Instruct the patient to swallow multiple times before taking the next bite or sip. Separate solids from liquids; it depends on the individual whether solids or liquids are harder to swallow.

Prepare the patient for diagnostic tests, including endoscopy, esophageal manometry, esophagography, and the esophageal acidity test, to pinpoint the cause of dysphagia.

PEDIATRIC POINTERS

In looking for dysphagia in an infant or a small child, pay close attention to his sucking and swallowing ability. Coughing, choking, or regurgitation during feeding suggests dysphagia.

Corrosive esophagitis and esophageal obstruction by a foreign body are more common causes of dysphagia in children than in adults. However, dysphagia may also result from congenital anomalies, such as annular stenosis, dysphagia lusoria, and esophageal atresia.

GERIATRIC POINTERS

Dysphagia is commonly the presenting complaint of patients older than age 50 with head or neck cancer. The incidence of these cancers increases markedly in this age-group.

PATIENT COUNSELING

Advise the patient to prepare foods that are easy to swallow.

Dyspnea

Typically a symptom of cardiopulmonary dysfunction, dyspnea is the sensation of difficult or uncomfortable breathing. It's usually described as shortness of breath. Its severity varies greatly and is usually unrelated to the severity of the underlying cause. Dyspnea may arise suddenly or slowly and may subside rapidly or persist for years.

Most people normally experience dyspnea when they exert themselves, and its severity depends on their physical condition. In a healthy person, dyspnea is quickly relieved by rest. Pathologic causes of dyspnea include pulmonary, cardiac, neuromuscular, and allergic disorders. It may also be caused by anxiety. (See *Dyspnea: Causes and associated findings,* pages 240 to 243.).

EMERGENCY INTERVENTIONS *If a patient complains of shortness of breath, quickly look for signs of respiratory distress, such as tachypnea, cyanosis, restlessness, and accessory muscle use. Prepare to administer oxygen by nasal cannula, mask, or endotracheal tube. Ensure patent I.V. access, and begin cardiac monitoring and oxygen saturation monitoring to detect arrhythmias and low oxygen saturation, respectively. Expect to insert a chest tube for severe pneumothorax and to administer continuous positive airway pressure.*

HISTORY AND PHYSICAL EXAMINATION

If the patient can answer questions without increasing his distress, take a complete history. (See *Differential diagnosis: Dyspnea,* pages 244 and 245.) Ask if the shortness of breath began suddenly or gradually. Is it constant or intermittent? Does it occur during activity or while at rest? If the patient has had dyspneic attacks before, ask if they're increasing in severity. Can he identify what aggravates or alleviates these attacks? Does he have a productive or

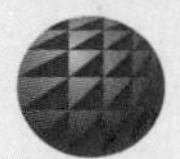

SIGNS & SYMPTOMS

Dyspnea: Causes and associated findings

Major associated signs and symptoms

Common causes	Accessory muscle use	Blood pressure, decreased	Breath sounds, decreased	Chest pain	Cough, nonproductive	Cough, productive	Crackles	Cyanosis	Diaphoresis	Edema	Fasciculations	Fever
Acute respiratory distress syndrome	●	●					●	●				●
Amyotrophic lateral sclerosis											●	
Anemia												
Anthrax (inhalation)				●								●
Aspiration of a foreign body	●	●	●		●			●	●			
Asthma	●				●			●	●			
Avian influenza					●							●
Blast lung injury				●				●				
Cardiac arrhythmia				●					●			
Cor pulmonale	●					●		●		●		
Emphysema	●		●		●							
Flail chest	●	●	●	●				●				
Guillain-Barré syndrome												
Heart failure	●	●			●					●		
Inhalation injury						●	●					
Interstitial fibrosis				●	●				●			
Lung cancer				●		●						●
Monkeypox												●
Myasthenia gravis												

	Muscle weakness	Nausea	Jugular vein distention	Orthopnea	Stridor	Tachycardia	Tachypnea	Weight loss
						●	●	
	●						●	
	●					●	●	
					●			
					●		●	
						●	●	
						●		
			●				●	
							●	●
						●	●	
	●							
			●	●		●	●	
				●			●	
								●
								●
	●						●	

(continued)

nonproductive cough or chest pain? Ask about recent trauma, and note a history of upper respiratory tract infection, deep vein phlebitis, or other disorders. Ask the patient if he smokes or is exposed to toxic fumes or irritants on the job. Find out if he also has orthopnea, paroxysmal nocturnal dyspnea, or progressive fatigue.

CULTURAL CUE *Because dyspnea is subjective and is exacerbated by anxiety, patients from cultures that are highly emotional may complain of shortness of breath sooner than those who are more stoic about symptoms of illness.*

During the physical examination, look for signs of chronic dyspnea such as accessory muscle hypertrophy (especially in the shoulders and neck). Also look for pursed-lip exhalation, clubbing, peripheral edema, barrel chest, diaphoresis, and jugular vein distention.

Check blood pressure and auscultate the lungs for crackles, abnormal heart sounds or rhythms, egophony, bronchophony, and whispered pectoriloquy. Finally, palpate the abdomen for hepatomegaly, and assess the patient for edema.

MEDICAL CAUSES

◆ ***Acute respiratory distress syndrome (ARDS).*** This life-threatening form of noncardiogenic pulmonary edema usually produces acute dyspnea as the first complaint. As respiratory distress progresses, the patient develops restlessness, anxiety, decreased mental acuity, tachycardia, and crackles and rhonchi in both lung fields. Other findings include cyanosis, tachypnea, motor dysfunction, and intercostal and suprasternal retractions. Severe ARDS can produce signs of shock, such as hypotension and cool, clammy skin.

◆ ***Amyotrophic lateral sclerosis.*** Also known as *Lou Gehrig's disease,* this disorder causes slow onset of dyspnea that worsens with time. Other features include dysphagia, dysarthria, muscle weakness and atrophy, fasciculations, shallow respirations, tachypnea, and emotional lability.

◆ ***Anemia.*** Dyspnea usually develops gradually in anemia, which commonly causes fatigue, weakness, and syncope; severe anemia may also cause tachycardia, tachypnea, restlessness, anxiety, and thirst.

◆ ***Anthrax, inhalation.*** Anthrax is an acute infectious disease that's caused by the gram-positive, spore-forming bacterium *Bacillus anthracis.*

Dyspnea: Causes and associated findings *(continued)*

Common causes	Accessory muscle use	Blood pressure, decreased	Breath sounds, decreased	Chest pain	Cough, nonproductive	Cough, productive	Crackles	Cyanosis	Diaphoresis	Edema	Fasciculations	Fever
Myocardial infarction		●		●					●			
Plague				●		●						●
Pleural effusion			●		●							●
Pneumonia			●	●		●	●	●	●			●
Pneumothorax	●	●	●	●	●			●				
Poliomyelitis (bulbar)												●
Popcorn lung disease					●							●
Pulmonary edema	●	●			●	●	●	●	●			
Pulmonary embolism		●	●	●	●	●	●	●	●	●		●
Sepsis												●
Severe acute respiratory syndrome					●							●
Shock		●										
Tuberculosis				●			●		●			●
Tularemia				●	●							●

Although the disease most commonly occurs in wild and domestic grazing animals, such as cattle, sheep, and goats, the spores can live in the soil for many years. The disease can occur in humans exposed to infected animals, tissue from infected animals, or biological agents. Most natural cases occur in agricultural regions worldwide. Anthrax may occur in cutaneous, inhalation, or GI forms.

Inhalation anthrax is caused by inhalation of aerosolized spores. The disease generally occurs in two stages with a period of recovery after the initial signs and symptoms. Dyspnea is a symptom of the second stage of this disorder along with fever, stridor and hypotension; the patient usually dies within 24 hours. Initial signs and symptoms are flulike and include fever, chills, weakness, cough, and chest pain.

	Muscle weakness	Nausea	Jugular vein distention	Orthopnea	Stridor	Tachycardia	Tachypnea	Weight loss
		●				●		
							●	
						●	●	
						●	●	
						●	●	
								●
			●	●		●	●	
						●	●	
						●	●	
						●	●	
								●

◆ ***Aspiration of a foreign body.*** Acute dyspnea marks this life-threatening condition, along with paroxysmal intercostal, suprasternal, and substernal retractions. The patient may also display accessory muscle use, inspiratory stridor, tachypnea, decreased or absent breath sounds, asymmetrical chest expansion, anxiety, cyanosis, diaphoresis, and hypotension.

◆ ***Asthma.*** Acute dyspneic attacks occur in this chronic disorder along with audible wheezing, a dry cough, accessory muscle use, nasal flaring, intercostal and supraclavicular retractions, tachypnea, tachycardia, diaphoresis, prolonged expiration, flushing or cyanosis, and apprehension. Medications that block beta receptors can exacerbate asthma attacks.

◆ ***Avian influenza.*** These potentially life-threatening viruses are spread to humans through contact with infected poultry or surfaces contaminated with infected bird excretions. Within 1 to 5 days of exposure to avian influenza, the patient typically develops flulike symptoms, such as fever, sore throat, cough, and muscle aches. Those with severe forms of the virus may develop dyspnea caused by acute respiratory distress or pneumonia. To date, the most virulent strain of this virus has not yet surfaced in humans in the United States, but a recent outbreak in Asian countries has had a mortality rate of about 50% among infected humans.

◆ ***Blast lung injury.*** The result of a forceful percussive wave following an explosive detonation, blast lung injury is commonly characterized by dyspnea and hypoxia. Worldwide terrorist activity has recently increased the incidence of this condition, which may also cause cyanosis, chest pain, wheezing, and hemopytsis. Chest X-ray, the primary diagnostic tool, reveals a characteristic "butterfly" pattern. Many of these patients suffer concomitant injuries and require complex management, usually in an intensive care setting.

◆ ***Cardiac arrhythmias.*** Acute or gradual dyspnea can result from decreased cardiac output in a patient with arrhythmias. The pulse rate may be rapid, slow, or irregular, with frequent premature or escape beats. Alternating pulse may be present. Other symptoms include palpitations, chest pain, diaphoresis, light-headedness, weakness, and vertigo.

◆ ***Cor pulmonale.*** Chronic dyspnea begins gradually with exertion and progressively worsens until it occurs even at rest. Most patients with cor pulmonale have an underlying cardiac or pulmonary disease. Other findings may include a chronic productive cough, wheezing, tachypnea, jugular vein distention, dependent edema, hepatomegaly, increasing fatigue, weakness, and light-headedness.

◆ ***Emphysema.*** This chronic disorder gradually causes progressive exertional dyspnea as well

(Text continues on page 246.)

Differential diagnosis: Dyspnea

History of present illness

Focused physical examination: Abdomen; respiratory, cardiovascular, and neurologic systems

Asthma, acute

Signs and symptoms
- ◆ Acute dyspneic attacks
- ◆ Audible or auscultated wheezing
- ◆ Dry cough
- ◆ Hyperpnea
- ◆ Chest tightness
- ◆ Accessory muscle use
- ◆ Nasal flaring
- ◆ Intercostal and supraclavicular retractions
- ◆ Tachypnea
- ◆ Tachycardia
- ◆ Diaphoresis
- ◆ Prolonged expiration
- ◆ Flushing or cyanosis
- ◆ Apprehension

Diagnosis: Laboratory tests (complete blood count [CBC], arterial blood gas [ABG] analysis, allergy skin testing), pulmonary function tests, chest X-ray, peak flow meter

Treatment: Avoidance of allergens and tobacco, medication (beta-adrenergic blockers, inhaled $beta_2$-agonists, inhaled corticosteroid [cromolyn if age younger than 12], leukotriene receptor agonist, systemic corticosteroids during infections and exacerbations, mast cell stabilizer), peak expiratory flow monitoring

Follow-up: For acute exacerbation, return visit within 24 hours, then every 3 to 5 days, then every 1 to 3 months; referral to pulmonologist, if the treatment is ineffective

Pulmonary embolism

Signs and symptoms
- ◆ Acute dyspnea
- ◆ Sudden pleuritic chest pain
- ◆ Tachycardia
- ◆ Low-grade fever
- ◆ Tachypnea
- ◆ Nonproductive or productive cough with blood-tinged sputum
- ◆ Pleural friction rub
- ◆ Crackles
- ◆ Possible hemoptysis
- ◆ Diffuse wheezing
- ◆ Dullness on percussion
- ◆ Decreased breath sounds
- ◆ Diaphoresis
- ◆ Restlessness
- ◆ Acute anxiety
- ◆ Signs of shock (possibly)

Diagnosis: Imaging studies (chest X-ray, pulmonary $\dot{V}/\dot{Q}$ scan or pulmonary angiography, spiral chest computed tomography scan), electrocardiography (ECG)

Treatment: Oxygen therapy, medication (anticoagulants, thrombolytic therapy)

Follow-up: Reevaluation within the first week after hospitalization

Common signs and symptoms
- Gradually developing dyspnea
- Chronic paroxysmal nocturnal dyspnea
- Ortopnea
- Tachypnea
- Tachycardia
- Palpitations
- S_3
- Fatigue
- Dependent peripheral edema
- Hepatomegaly
- Dry cough
- Anorexia
- Weight gain
- Loss of mental acuity
- Hemoptysis

Common signs and symptoms
- Acute dyspnea
- Sudden, stabbing chest pain that may radiate to the arms, face, back, or abdomen
- Anxiety
- Restlessness
- Dry cough
- Cyanosis
- Decreased vocal fremitus
- Tachypnea
- Tympany
- Decreased or absent breath sounds on the affected side
- Asymmetrical chest expansion
- Splinting
- Accessory muscle use

Heart failure

Acute onset heart failure

Additional signs and symptoms
- Jugular vein distention (JVD)
- Bibasilar crackles
- Oliguria
- Hypotension

Diagnosis: Physical examination, laboratory tests (CBC, cardiac enzymes), imaging studies (chest X-ray, echocardiogram), ECG
Treatment: Medication (angiotensin-converting enzyme inhibitor, diuretics, carvedilol [possibly], digoxin [possibly]), inotropic agents
Follow-up: Return visit within 1 week after discharge, at 4 weeks, and then every 3 months; referral to cardiologist if chronic

Pneumothorax

Diagnosis: ABG, chest X-ray
Treatment: Chest tube insertion, oxygen therapy
Follow-up: Return visit in 1 to 2 weeks after hospitalization

Tension pneumothorax

Additional signs and symptoms
- Tracheal deviation
- Decreased blood pressure
- Tachycardia
- JVD

Diagnosis: ABG, chest X-ray
Treatment: Immediate needle decompression followed by chest tube insertion, oxygen therapy
Follow-up: Return visit in 1 to 2 weeks after hospitalization

Additional differential diagnoses: acute respiratory distress syndrome ◆ anemia ◆ aspiration of a foreign body ◆ cardiac arrhythmias ◆ chronic obstructive pulmonary disease ◆ cor pulmonale ◆ emphysema ◆ flail chest ◆ inhalation injury ◆ interstitial fibrosis ◆ lung cancer ◆ myocardial infarction ◆ pleural effusion ◆ pneumonia ◆ pulmonary edema

as barrel chest, accessory muscle hypertrophy, diminished breath sounds, anorexia, weight loss, malaise, peripheral cyanosis, tachypnea, pursed-lip breathing, prolonged expiration and, possibly, a chronic productive cough. Clubbing is a late sign. The patient may have a history of smoking, an alpha$_1$-antitrypsin deficiency, or exposure to an occupational irritant.

◆ ***Flail chest.*** In this condition, dyspnea results suddenly from multiple rib fractures and is accompanied by paradoxical chest movement, severe chest pain, hypotension, tachypnea, tachycardia, and cyanosis. Bruising and decreased or absent breath sounds occur over the affected side.

◆ ***Guillain-Barré syndrome.*** This syndrome, which usually follows a fever and upper respiratory tract infection, causes slowly worsening dyspnea along with fatigue, ascending muscle weakness and, eventually, paralysis.

◆ ***Heart failure.*** Dyspnea usually develops gradually in patients with heart failure. Chronic paroxysmal nocturnal dyspnea, orthopnea, tachypnea, tachycardia, palpitations, ventricular gallop, fatigue, dependent peripheral edema, hepatomegaly, dry cough, weight gain, and loss of mental acuity may occur. With acute onset, heart failure may produce jugular vein distention, bibasilar crackles, oliguria, and hypotension.

◆ ***Interstitial fibrosis.*** Besides dyspnea, this disorder causes chest pain, a dry cough, crackles, weight loss and, possibly, cyanosis and pleural friction rub.

◆ ***Lung cancer.*** Dyspnea develops slowly and worsens progressively in late-stage lung cancer. Other findings include fever, hemoptysis, a productive cough, wheezing, clubbing, chest pain, and pleural friction rub.

◆ ***Monkeypox.*** Dyspnea is one of the less common symptoms of this rare viral disease. Infected individuals may also experience fever, muscle aches, sore throat, chills, and lymphadenopathy. A papular rash appears 1 to 3 days after the fever begins. The virus is similar to smallpox; however, the symptoms are milder and the disease is rarely fatal in developed countries.

◆ ***Myasthenia gravis.*** This neuromuscular disorder causes bouts of dyspnea as the respiratory muscles weaken. In myasthenic crisis, acute respiratory distress may occur, with shallow respirations and tachypnea.

◆ ***Myocardial infarction.*** Sudden dyspnea occurs with crushing substernal chest pain that may radiate to the back, neck, jaw, and arms. Other signs and symptoms include nausea, vomiting, diaphoresis, vertigo, hypertension or hypotension, tachycardia, anxiety, and pale, cool, clammy skin.

◆ ***Plague.*** Caused by *Yersinia pestis,* plague is one of the most virulent and, if untreated, most lethal bacterial infections known. Clinical forms include bubonic (the most common), septicemic, and pneumonic plagues. The pneumonic form can be contracted by inhaling respiratory droplets from an infected person or inhaling the organism that has been dispersed in the air through biological warfare. Among the symptoms of the pneumonic form are dyspnea, a productive cough, chest pain, tachypnea, hemoptysis, increasing respiratory distress, and cardiopulmonary insufficiency.

◆ ***Pleural effusion.*** Dyspnea develops slowly and worsens progressively in this disorder. Initial findings include a pleural friction rub accompanied by pleuritic pain that worsens with coughing or deep breathing. Other findings include a dry cough; dullness on percussion; egophony, bronchophony, and whispered pectoriloquy; tachycardia; tachypnea; weight loss; and decreased breath sounds, chest motion, and tactile fremitus. Fever may occur if infection is present.

◆ ***Pneumonia.*** Dyspnea occurs suddenly in pneumonia and is usually accompanied by fever, shaking chills, pleuritic chest pain that worsens with deep inspiration, and a productive cough. Fatigue, headache, myalgia, anorexia, abdominal pain, crackles, rhonchi, tachycardia, tachypnea, cyanosis, decreased breath sounds, and diaphoresis may also occur.

◆ ***Pneumothorax.*** This life-threatening disorder causes acute dyspnea unrelated to the severity of pain. Sudden, stabbing chest pain may radiate to the arms, face, back, or abdomen. Other signs and symptoms include anxiety, restlessness, dry cough, cyanosis, decreased vocal fremitus, tachypnea, tympany, decreased or absent breath sounds on the affected side, asymmetrical chest expansion, splinting, and accessory muscle use. In patients with tension pneumothorax, tracheal deviation occurs in addition to these typical findings. Decreased blood pressure and tachycardia may also occur.

◆ ***Poliomyelitis (bulbar).*** Dyspnea develops gradually in this disorder and worsens progressively. Additional signs and symptoms include fever, facial weakness, dysphasia, hypoactive deep tendon reflexes, decreased mental acuity, dysphagia, nasal regurgitation, and hypopnea.
◆ ***Popcorn lung disease.*** Popcorn lung disease occurs in factory workers who experience respiratory symptoms after inhaling butter flavoring chemicals such as diacetyl, used in the manufacture of microwave popcorn. The patient typically complains of gradual onset of a nonproductive cough that worsens over time, progressive shortness of breath, and unusual fatigue. Clinical findings include wheezing, chest pain, fever, night sweats, and weight loss. Bronchiolitis fibrosa obliterans, an irreversible fixed airway obstructive lung disorder, is the most severe condition reported.
◆ ***Pulmonary edema.*** Commonly preceded by signs of heart failure, such as jugular vein distention and orthopnea, this life-threatening disorder causes acute dyspnea. Other features include tachycardia, tachypnea, crackles in both lung fields, a ventricular gallop (third heart sound [S_3]), oliguria, thready pulse, hypotension, diaphoresis, cyanosis, and marked anxiety. The patient's cough may be dry or may produce copious amounts of pink, frothy sputum.
◆ ***Pulmonary embolism.*** This life-threatening disorder is characterized by acute dyspnea that's usually accompanied by sudden pleuritic chest pain. Related findings include tachycardia, low-grade fever, tachypnea, a nonproductive cough or a productive cough with blood-tinged sputum, pleural friction rub, crackles, diffuse wheezing, dullness on percussion, decreased breath sounds, diaphoresis, restlessness, and acute anxiety. A massive embolism may cause signs of shock, such as hypotension and cool, clammy skin.
◆ ***Sepsis.*** This potentially fatal disorder gradually causes dyspnea along with chills and sudden fever. As dyspnea worsens, it may be accompanied by tachycardia, tachypnea, restlessness, anxiety, decreased mental acuity, and warm, flushed, dry skin. Late findings include hypotension; oliguria; cool, clammy skin; and rapid, thready pulse.
◆ ***Severe acute respiratory syndrome (SARS).*** SARS is an acute infectious disease of unknown etiology; however, a novel coronavirus has been implicated as a possible cause. Although most cases have been reported in Asia (China, Vietnam, Singapore, Thailand), cases have cropped up in Europe and North America. After an incubation period of 2 to 7 days, the illness generally begins with a fever (usually greater than 100.4° F [38° C]). Other symptoms include headache, malaise, a nonproductive cough, and dyspnea. The severity of the illness is highly variable, ranging from mild illness to pneumonia and, in some cases, progressing to respiratory failure and death.
◆ ***Shock.*** Dyspnea arises suddenly and worsens progressively in this life-threatening disorder. Related findings include severe hypotension, tachypnea, tachycardia, decreased peripheral pulses, decreased mental acuity, restlessness, anxiety, and cool, clammy skin.
◆ ***Tuberculosis.*** Dyspnea commonly occurs with chest pain, crackles, and a productive cough. Other findings are night sweats, fever, anorexia and weight loss, vague dyspepsia, palpitations on mild exertion, and dullness on percussion.
◆ ***Tularemia.*** Also known as "rabbit fever," this infectious disease causes dyspnea along with fever, chills, headache, generalized myalgia, a nonproductive cough, pleuritic chest pain, and empyema.

Other causes

◆ ***Inhalation injury.*** Dyspnea may develop suddenly or over several hours after inhalation of chemicals or hot gases. Increasing hoarseness, a persistent cough, sooty or bloody sputum, and oropharyngeal edema may also be present. The patient may also exhibit thermal burns, singed nasal hairs, and orofacial burns as well as crackles, rhonchi, wheezing, and signs of respiratory distress.

Special considerations

Monitor the dyspneic patient closely. Be as calm and reassuring as possible to reduce his anxiety, and help him into a comfortable position—usually high Fowler's or a forward-leaning position. Support him with pillows, loosen his clothing, and administer oxygen if appropriate.

Prepare the patient for diagnostic studies, such as arterial blood gas analysis, chest X-rays, and pulmonary function tests. Administer a bronchodilator, an antiarrhythmic, a diuretic, and an analgesic, as needed, to dilate bronchioles, correct cardiac arrhythmias, promote fluid excretion, and relieve pain, respectively.

Pediatric pointers

Normally, a child's respirations are abdominal in infancy and gradually change to costal by age 7. Suspect dyspnea in an infant who breathes costally, in an older child who breathes abdominally, or in any child who uses his neck or shoulder muscles to help him breathe.

Both acute epiglottiditis and laryngotracheobronchitis (croup) can cause severe dyspnea in a child and may even lead to respiratory or cardiovascular collapse. Expect to administer oxygen, using a hood or cool mist tent.

Geriatric pointers

Older patients with dyspnea related to chronic illness may not be aware initially of a significant change in their breathing pattern.

Patient counseling

Tell the patient that oxygen therapy isn't necessarily indicated for dyspnea. Encourage a patient with chronic dyspnea to pace his daily activities.

Dystonia

Dystonia is marked by slow, involuntary movements of large-muscle groups in the limbs, trunk, and neck. This extrapyramidal sign may involve flexion of the foot, hyperextension of the legs, extension and pronation of the arms, arching of the back, and extension and rotation of the neck (spasmodic torticollis). It's typically aggravated by walking and emotional stress and relieved by sleep. Dystonia may be intermittent—lasting just a few minutes—or continuous and painful. Occasionally, it causes permanent contractures, resulting in a grotesque posture. Although dystonia may be hereditary or idiopathic, it usually results from extrapyramidal disorders or the use of certain drugs.

EXAMINATION TIP

Recognizing dystonia

Dystonia, chorea, and athetosis may occur simultaneously. To differentiate among these three, keep the following points in mind:

- *Dystonic movements* are slow and twisting and involve large-muscle groups in the head, neck (as shown below), trunk, and limbs. They may be intermittent or continuous.
- *Choreiform movements* are rapid, highly complex, and jerky.
- *Athetoid movements* are slow, sinuous, and writhing, but always continuous; they typically affect the hands and extremities.

DYSTONIA OF THE NECK (SPASMODIC TORTICOLLIS)

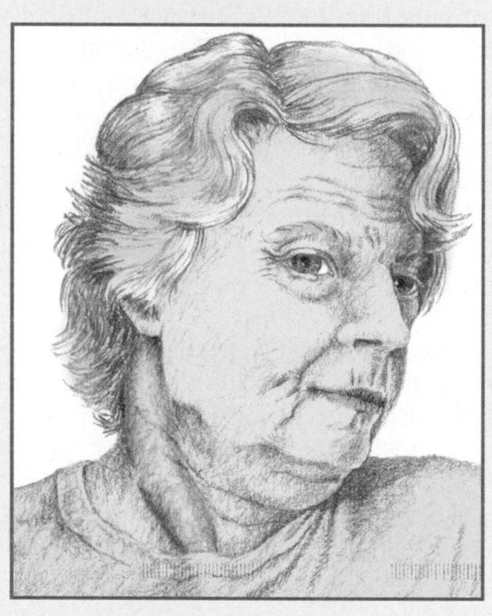

History and physical examination

If possible, include the patient's family in history taking; they may be more aware of behavior changes than the patient is. Begin by asking them when dystonia occurs. Is it aggravated by emotional upset? Does it disappear during sleep? Is there a family history of dystonia? Obtain a drug history, noting especially the use of a phenothiazine or an antipsychotic. Dystonia is a common adverse effect of these drugs, and the dosage may need to be adjusted to minimize this effect.

Next, examine the patient's coordination and voluntary muscle movement. Observe his gait as he walks across the room; then have him squeeze your fingers to assess muscle strength. (See *Recognizing dystonia*.) Check coordination by having him touch your fingertip and then his nose repeatedly. Follow this by testing gross motor movement of the leg: Have him place his heel on one knee, slide it down his shin to the top of his great toe, and then return it to his knee. Finally, assess fine-motor movement by asking him to touch each finger to his thumb in succession.

Medical causes

◆ ***Alzheimer's disease.*** Dystonia is a late sign of this disorder, which is marked by slowly progressive dementia. The patient typically displays decreased attention span, amnesia, agitation, an inability to carry out activities of daily living, dysarthria, and emotional lability.

◆ ***Dystonia musculorum deformans.*** Prolonged, generalized dystonia is the hallmark of this disorder, which usually develops in childhood and worsens with age. Initially, it causes foot inversion, which is followed by growth retardation and scoliosis. Late signs include twisted, bizarre postures, limb contractures, and dysarthria.

◆ ***Hallervorden-Spatz disease.*** This degenerative disease causes dystonic trunk movements accompanied by choreoathetosis, ataxia, myoclonus, and generalized rigidity. The patient also exhibits a progressive intellectual decline and dysarthria.

◆ ***Huntington's disease.*** Dystonic movements mark the preterminal stage of Huntington's disease. Characterized by progressive intellectual decline, this disorder leads to dementia and emotional lability. The patient displays choreoathetosis accompanied by dysarthria, dysphagia, facial grimacing, and a wide-based, prancing gait.

◆ ***Olivopontocerebellar atrophy.*** Ataxia, an early sign in this rare disorder, slowly progresses to dystonia. Other findings include dysarthria, action tremor, bradykinesia, and visual deterioration.

◆ ***Parkinson's disease.*** Dystonic spasms are common in this disease. Other classic features include uniform or jerky rigidity, pill-rolling tremor, bradykinesia, dysarthria, dysphagia, drooling, masklike facies, monotone voice, stooped posture, and a propulsive gait.

◆ ***Pick's disease.*** Dystonia appears as a late sign in this rare disorder, which resembles Alzheimer's disease.

◆ ***Supranuclear ophthalmoplegia.*** Also known as Steele-Richardson-Olszewski syndrome, this rare disorder affects mainly middle-aged people, causing intermittent dystonia with extreme neck flexion or extension. Other signs and symptoms include impaired extraocular movement, diminished voice volume, dysarthria, truncal rigidity, dementia, ataxia, masklike facies, and dysphagia.

◆ ***Wilson's disease.*** Progressive dystonia and chorea of the arms and legs mark this disorder. Other common signs and symptoms include hoarseness, bradykinesia, behavior changes, dysphagia, drooling, dysarthria, tremors, and Kayser-Fleischer rings (rusty-brown rings at the periphery of the cornea).

Other causes

◆ ***Drugs.*** Phenothiazines can cause dystonia. Aliphatics such as chlorpromazine cause it occasionally, and piperidines rarely cause it.

Haloperidol, loxapine, and other antipsychotics usually produce acute facial dystonia, as do risperidone, metyrosine, antiemetic doses of metoclopramide, and excessive doses of levodopa.

Special considerations

Encourage the patient to obtain adequate sleep and avoid emotional upset. Avoid range-of-motion exercises, which can aggravate dystonia. If dystonia is severe, protect the patient from injury by raising and padding his bed rails. Provide an uncluttered environment if he's ambulatory.

Pediatric pointers

Children don't exhibit dystonia until after they can walk. Even so, it rarely occurs until after age 10. Common causes include Fahr's syndrome, dystonia musculorum deformans, athetoid cerebral palsy, and the residual effects of anoxia at birth.

Dysuria

Dysuria—painful or difficult urination—is commonly accompanied by urinary frequency, urgency, or hesitancy. This symptom usually reflects lower urinary tract infection (UTI)—a common disorder, especially in women. (See *Preventing urinary tract infections,* page 250.)

Dysuria results from lower urinary tract irritation or inflammation, which stimulates nerve endings in the bladder and urethra. The onset

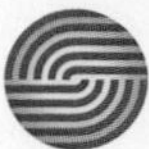

PATIENT-TEACHING AID

Preventing urinary tract infections

Dear Patient:
To prevent recurrent urinary tract infections, follow these guidelines:

- Drink at least 10 glasses of fluid, especially water, daily. This helps flush bacteria from the urinary tract.
- Empty your bladder completely every 2 to 3 hours or as soon as you feel the urge to urinate.
- Wipe your perineum from front to back after urinating or defecating to prevent contamination with fecal material.
- Wear cotton underpants, which allow better ventilation and absorption than synthetic ones.
- Take showers instead of baths. If you must bathe, don't use bubble bath salts, bath oil, perfume, or other chemical irritants in the water. Also, avoid using feminine deodorants, douches, and similar irritants. Avoid using menstrual pads, which may also act as irritants.
- Urinate before and after intercourse.
- Include meats, eggs, cheese, nuts, prunes, plums, whole grains, and especially cranberry juice in your daily intake. These foods acidify the urine, which helps decrease bacterial growth. Avoid foods containing baking soda or powder, such as most baked goods.
- Avoid coffee, citrus juices, and alcohol, which tend to irritate the bladder.
- Seek medical help for any unusual vaginal discharge, which suggests infection.

of pain provides clues to its cause. For example, pain just before voiding usually indicates bladder irritation or distention, whereas pain at the start of urination typically results from bladder outlet irritation. Pain at the end of voiding may signal bladder spasms; in women, it may indicate vaginal candidiasis. (See *Dysuria: Causes and associated findings*, pages 252 and 253.)

History and physical examination

If the patient complains of dysuria, have him describe its severity and location. When did he first notice it? Did anything precipitate it? Does anything aggravate or alleviate it?

Next, ask about previous urinary or genital tract infections. Has the patient recently undergone an invasive procedure, such as cystoscopy or urethral dilatation, or had a urinary catheter inserted? Also, ask if he has a history of intestinal disease. Ask the female patient about menstrual disorders and use of products that irritate the urinary tract, such as bubble bath salts, feminine deodorants, contraceptive gels, or perineal lotions. Also ask her about vaginal discharge or pruritus.

During the physical examination, inspect the urethral meatus for discharge, irritation, or other abnormalities. A pelvic or rectal examination may be necessary.

Medical causes

◆ ***Appendicitis.*** Occasionally, appendicitis causes dysuria that persists throughout voiding and is accompanied by bladder tenderness. Appendicitis is characterized by periumbilical abdominal pain that shifts to McBurney's point, anorexia, nausea, vomiting, constipation, slight fever, abdominal rigidity and rebound tenderness, and tachycardia.

◆ ***Bladder cancer.*** In this predominantly male disorder, dysuria throughout voiding is a late symptom associated with urinary frequency and urgency, nocturia, hematuria, and perineal, back, or flank pain.

CULTURAL CUE *Bladder cancer is twice as common in White males as in Blacks. It's relatively uncommon in Asians, Hispanics, and Native Americans.*

◆ ***Cystitis.*** Dysuria throughout voiding is common in all types of cystitis, as are urinary frequency, nocturia, straining to void, and hematuria. Bacterial cystitis, the most common cause of dysuria in women, may also produce urinary urgency, perineal and lower back pain, suprapubic discomfort, fatigue and, possibly, a low-grade fever. In chronic interstitial cystitis, dysuria is accentuated at the end of voiding. In tubercular cystitis, symptoms may also include urinary urgency, flank pain, fatigue, and anorexia. In viral cystitis, severe dysuria occurs with gross hematuria, urinary urgency, and fever.

GENDER CUE *Women are more prone to develop cystitis than men because they have a shorter urethra. For men, age is a factor: Older men have a 15% higher risk of developing cystitis.*

◆ ***Diverticulitis.*** Inflammation near the bladder may cause dysuria throughout voiding. Other effects include urinary frequency and urgency, nocturia, hematuria, fever, abdominal pain and tenderness, perineal pain, constipation or diarrhea and, possibly, an abdominal mass.

◆ ***Paraurethral gland inflammation.*** Dysuria throughout voiding is accompanied by urinary frequency and urgency, diminished urine stream, mild perineal pain and, occasionally, hematuria in this disorder.

◆ ***Prostatitis.*** Acute prostatitis commonly causes dysuria throughout or toward the end of voiding as well as a diminished urine stream, urinary frequency and urgency, hematuria, suprapubic fullness, fever, chills, fatigue, myalgia, nausea, vomiting, and constipation. In chronic prostatitis, urethral narrowing causes dysuria throughout voiding. Related effects are urinary frequency and urgency; diminished urine stream; perineal, back, and buttocks pain; urethral discharge; nocturia; and, at times, hematospermia and ejaculatory pain.

◆ ***Pyelonephritis (acute).*** More common in females than in males, this disorder causes dysuria throughout voiding. Other features include persistent high fever with chills, costovertebral angle tenderness, unilateral or bilateral flank pain, weakness, urinary urgency and frequency, nocturia, straining on urination, and hematuria. Nausea, vomiting, and anorexia may also occur.

◆ ***Reiter's syndrome.*** In this predominantly male disorder, dysuria occurs 1 to 2 weeks after sexual contact. Initially, the patient has a mucopurulent discharge, urinary urgency and frequency, meatal swelling and redness, suprapubic pain, anorexia, weight loss, and low-grade fever. Hematuria, conjunctivitis, arthritic symptoms, a papular rash, and oral and penile lesions may follow.

◆ ***Urethral syndrome.*** Occurring in sexually active women, this syndrome mimics urethritis. Dysuria throughout voiding may occur with urinary frequency, diminished urine stream, suprapubic aching and cramping, tenesmus, and low back and unilateral flank pain. In the absence of pyuria, symptoms will usually resolve without intervention.

◆ ***Urethritis.*** Primarily found in sexually active males, this infection causes dysuria throughout voiding. It's accompanied by a reddened meatus and a copious, yellow, purulent discharge (gonorrheal infection) or a white or clear mucoid discharge (nongonorrheal infection).

◆ ***Urinary obstruction.*** Outflow obstruction by urethral strictures or calculi produces dysuria throughout voiding. (In a complete obstruction, bladder distention develops and dysuria precedes voiding.) Other features are diminished urine stream, urinary frequency and urgency, and a sensation of fullness or bloating in the lower abdomen or groin.

◆ ***Vaginitis.*** Characteristically, dysuria occurs throughout voiding as urine touches inflamed or ulcerated labia. Other findings include urinary frequency and urgency, nocturia, hematuria, perineal pain, and vaginal discharge and odor.

OTHER CAUSES

◆ ***Chemical irritants.*** Dysuria may result from irritating substances, such as bubble bath salts and feminine deodorants; it's usually most intense at the end of voiding. Spermicides may cause dysuria in both sexes as well as urinary frequency and urgency, a diminished urine stream and, possibly, hematuria.

◆ ***Drugs.*** Monoamine oxidase inhibitors and metyrosine can cause dysuria.

SPECIAL CONSIDERATIONS

Monitor vital signs and intake and output. Administer prescribed drugs, and prepare the patient for such tests as urinalysis and cystoscopy.

GERIATRIC POINTERS

Be aware that elderly patients tend to underreport their symptoms, even though older men have an increased incidence of nonsexually related UTIs and postmenopausal women have an increased incidence of noninfectious dysuria.

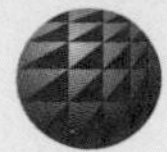

SIGNS & SYMPTOMS

Dysuria: Causes and associated findings

Major associated signs and symptoms

Common causes	Abdominal pain	Anorexia	Back pain	Constipation	Costovertebral angle tenderness	Erythema of meatus	Fatigue	Fever	Flank pain	Hematuria	Nausea	Nocturia	Perineal pain	Straining to void
Appendicitis	●	●		●				●			●			
Bladder cancer			●						●	●		●	●	
Cystitis (bacterial)			●				●	●		●		●	●	●
Cystitis (chronic interstitial)										●		●		●
Cystitis (tubercular)		●					●		●	●		●		●
Cystitis (viral)								●		●		●		●
Diverticulitis	●			●				●		●		●	●	
Paraurethral gland inflammation										●			●	
Prostatitis (acute)				●			●	●		●	●		●	
Prostatitis (chronic)			●										●	
Pyelonephritis (acute)		●			●			●	●	●	●	●		●
Reiter's syndrome		●				●		●		●				
Urethral syndrome			●						●					●
Urethritis						●								
Urinary obstruction														
Vaginitis										●		●	●	

	Suprapubic pain	Urethral discharge	Urinary frequency	Urine stream, diminished	Urinary urgency	Vaginal discharge	Vomiting	Weakness
							●	
			●		●			
	●		●		●			
			●					
			●		●			
			●		●			
			●		●			
			●	●	●			
			●	●	●		●	
		●	●	●	●			
			●		●		●	●
	●	●	●		●			
	●		●	●				
		●						
			●	●	●			
			●		●	●		

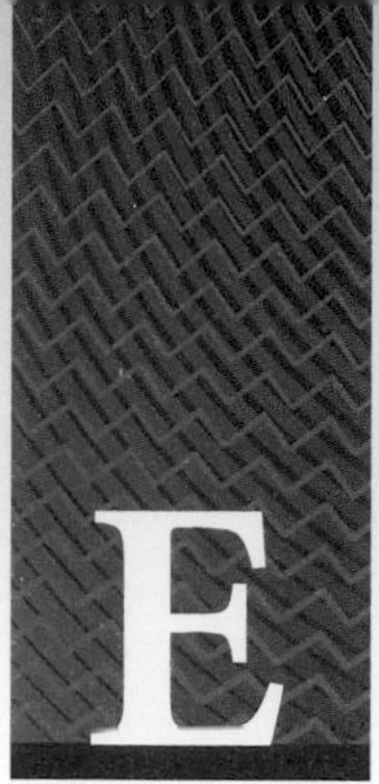

Earache

[Otalgia]

Earaches usually result from disorders of the external and middle ear associated with infection, obstruction, or trauma. Their severity ranges from a feeling of fullness or blockage to deep, boring pain. At times, it may be difficult to determine the precise location of the earache. Earaches can be intermittent or continuous and may develop suddenly or gradually.

History and physical examination

Ask the patient to characterize his earache. How long has he had it? Is it intermittent or continuous? Is it painful or slightly annoying? Can he localize the site of the pain? Does he have pain in any other areas, such as the jaw?

Ask about recent ear injury or other trauma. Does swimming or showering trigger ear discomfort? Is discomfort associated with itching? If so, find out where the itching is most intense and when it began. Ask about ear drainage and, if present, have the patient characterize it. Does he hear ringing, "swishing," or other noises in his ears? Ask about dizziness or vertigo. Does it worsen when the patient changes position? Does he have difficulty swallowing, hoarseness, neck pain, or pain when he opens his mouth?

Find out if the patient has recently had a head cold or problems with his eyes, mouth, teeth, jaws, sinuses, or throat. Disorders in these areas may refer pain to the ear along the cranial nerves.

Finally, find out if the patient has recently flown, been to a high-altitude location, or been scuba diving.

Begin your physical examination by inspecting the external ear for redness, drainage, swelling, or deformity. Then apply pressure to the mastoid process and tragus to elicit any tenderness. Using an otoscope, examine the external auditory canal for lesions, bleeding or discharge, impacted cerumen, foreign bodies, tenderness, or swelling. Examine the tympanic membrane: Is it intact? Is it pearly gray (normal)? Look for tympanic membrane landmarks: the cone of light, umbo, pars tensa, and the handle and short process of the malleus. (See *Using an otoscope correctly*.) Perform the watch tick, whispered voice, Rinne, and Weber's tests to assess for hearing loss.

Medical causes

◆ ***Abscess (extradural).*** Severe earache accompanied by a persistent ipsilateral headache, malaise, and recurrent mild fever characterizes this serious complication of middle ear infection.

◆ ***Barotrauma (acute).*** Earache associated with barotrauma ranges from mild pressure to severe pain. Tympanic membrane ecchymosis or bleeding into the tympanic cavity may occur, producing a blue drumhead; the eardrum usually isn't perforated.

◆ ***Cerumen impaction.*** Impacted cerumen (earwax) may cause a sensation of blockage or fullness in the ear. Additional features include

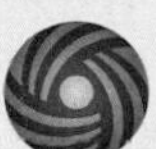

EXAMINATION TIP

Using an otoscope correctly

When the patient reports an earache, use an otoscope to inspect ear structures closely. Follow these techniques to obtain the best view and ensure patient safety.

Child younger than age 3

To inspect an infant's or a young child's ear, grasp the *lower part* of the auricle and pull it *down and back* to straighten the upward S curve of the external canal. Then gently insert the speculum no more than 1/2" (1.2 cm) into the canal.

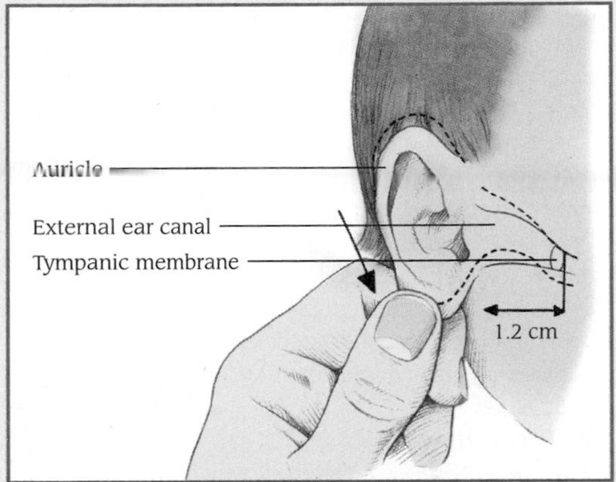

Adult

To inspect an adult's ear, grasp the *upper part* of the auricle and pull it *up and back* to straighten the external canal. Then insert the speculum about 1" (2.5 cm) into the canal. Also use this technique for children ages 3 and older.

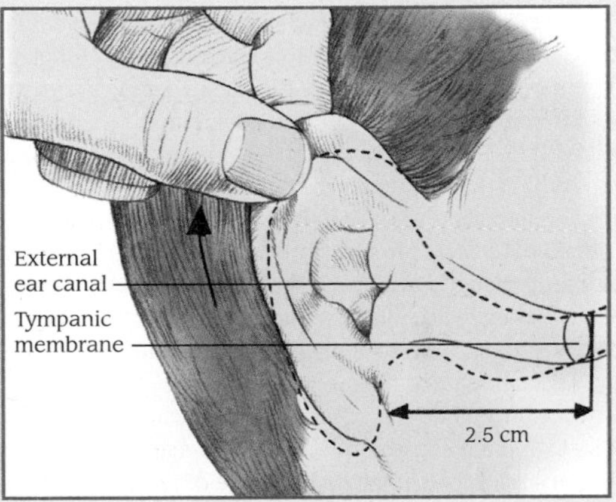

partial hearing loss, itching and, possibly, dizziness.

◆ ***Chondrodermatitis nodularis chronica.*** Chondrodermatitis nodularis chronica produces small, painful, indurated areas along the auricle's upper rim.

◆ ***Ear canal obstruction by an insect.*** An insect lodged in the ear canal may cause severe pain and distressing noise.

◆ ***Frostbite.*** Prolonged exposure to cold may cause burning or tingling pain in the ear, followed by numbness. The ear appears mottled and gray or white; it turns purplish blue as it's warmed.

◆ ***Furunculosis.*** Infected hair follicles in the outer ear canal may produce severe, localized ear pain associated with a pus-filled furuncle (boil). The pain is aggravated by jaw movement and relieved by rupture or incision of the furuncle. Pinna tenderness, swelling of the auditory meatus, partial hearing loss, and a feeling of fullness in the ear canal may also occur.

◆ ***Herpes zoster oticus (Ramsay Hunt syndrome).*** Herpes zoster oticus causes burning or stabbing ear pain that's commonly associated with ear vesicles. The patient also complains of hearing loss and vertigo. Associated signs and symptoms include transient ipsilateral facial paralysis, partial loss of taste, tongue vesicles, and nausea and vomiting.

◆ ***Keratosis obturans.*** Mild ear pain, otorrhea, and tinnitus are common in keratosis obturans. Inspection reveals a white glistening plug obstructing the external meatus.

◆ ***Mastoiditis (acute).*** Mastoiditis causes a dull ache behind the ear accompanied by low-grade fever (99° F to 100° F [37.2° C to 37.8° C]). The eardrum appears dull and edematous and may perforate, and soft tissue near the eardrum may sag. A purulent discharge is seen in the external canal.

◆ ***Ménière's disease.*** Ménière's disease is an inner ear disorder that can produce a sensation of fullness in the affected ear. Its classic effects, however, include severe vertigo, tinnitus, and sensorineural hearing loss. The patient may also experience nausea and vomiting, diaphoresis, and nystagmus.

◆ ***Middle ear tumor.*** Deep, boring ear pain and facial paralysis are late signs of a malignant tumor.

◆ ***Myringitis bullosa.*** Myringitis bullosa is a rare bacterial infection that causes sudden, severe ear pain that radiates over the mastoid and lasts for up to 48 hours. Small serous or blood-filled vesicles may dot the reddened tympanic membrane. Transient hearing loss and a serosanguineous discharge may also occur.

◆ ***Otitis externa.*** Earache characterizes both acute and malignant otitis externa. Acute otitis externa begins with mild to moderate ear pain that occurs with tragus manipulation. The pain may be accompanied by low-grade fever, sticky yellow or purulent ear discharge, partial hearing loss, and a feeling of blockage. Later, ear pain intensifies, causing the entire side of the head to ache and throb. Fever may reach 104° F (40° C). Examination reveals swelling of the tragus, external meatus, and external canal; eardrum erythema; and lymphadenopathy. The patient also complains of dizziness and malaise.

Malignant otitis externa causes sudden ear pain that's aggravated by moving the auricle or tragus. The pain is accompanied by intense itching, purulent ear discharge, fever, parotid gland swelling, and trismus. Examination reveals a swollen external canal with exposed cartilage and temporal bone. Cranial nerve palsy may occur.

◆ ***Otitis media (acute).*** Otitis media is a middle ear inflammation that can be serous or suppurative. *Acute serous otitis media* may cause a feeling of fullness in the ear, hearing loss, and a vague sensation of top-heaviness. The eardrum may be slightly retracted, amber colored, and marked by air bubbles and a meniscus, or it may be blue-black from hemorrhage.

Acute suppurative otitis media is characterized by severe deep, throbbing ear pain; hearing loss; and fever that may reach 102° F (38.9° C). The pain increases steadily over several hours or days and may be aggravated by pressure on the mastoid antrum. Perforation of the eardrum is possible. Before rupture, the eardrum appears bulging and fiery red. Rupture causes purulent drainage and relieves the pain.

Chronic otitis media usually isn't painful except during exacerbations. Persistent pain and discharge from the ear suggest cancer or osteomyelitis of the skull base.

◆ ***Perichondritis.*** Perichondritis can cause ear pain accompanied by warmth and tenderness in the outer ear and a reddened, doughlike auricle.

◆ ***Petrositis.*** The result of acute otitis media, this infection produces deep ear pain with headache and pain behind the eye. Other findings are diplopia, loss of lateral gaze, vomiting, sensorineural hearing loss, vertigo and, possibly, nuchal rigidity.

◆ ***Temporomandibular joint infection.*** Typically unilateral, temporomandibular joint infection produces ear pain that's referred from the jaw joint. The pain is aggravated by pressure on the joint with jaw movement; it commonly radiates to the temporal area or the entire side of the head.

Special considerations

Administer an analgesic, and apply heat to relieve discomfort. Instill eardrops if necessary. Teach the patient how to instill drops if they're prescribed for home use.

Pediatric pointers

Common causes of earache in children are acute otitis media and insertion of foreign bodies that become lodged or infected. Be alert for nonverbal clues to earache in a young child, such as crying or ear tugging.

To examine the child's ears, place him in a supine position with his arms extended and held securely by his parent. Then hold the otoscope with the handle pointing toward the top of the child's head, and brace it against him using one or two fingers. Because an ear examination may upset the child with an earache, save it for the end of your physical examination.

Edema, generalized

A common sign in severely ill patients, generalized edema is the excessive accumulation of interstitial fluid throughout the body. Its severity varies widely; slight edema may be difficult to detect, especially if the patient is obese, whereas massive edema is immediately apparent.

Generalized edema is typically chronic and progressive. It may result from cardiac, renal, endocrine, or hepatic disorders as well as from severe burns, malnutrition, or the effects of certain drugs and treatments.

Common factors responsible for edema are hypoalbuminemia and excess sodium ingestion or retention, both of which influence plasma osmotic pressure. (See *Understanding fluid balance,* page 258.) Cyclic edema associated with increased aldosterone secretion may occur in premenopausal women.

EMERGENCY INTERVENTIONS *Quickly determine the location and severity of edema, including the degree of pitting. (See* Edema: Pitting or nonpitting? *page 259.) If the patient has severe edema, promptly take his vital signs, and check for jugular vein distention and cyanotic lips. Auscultate the lungs and heart. Be alert for signs of heart failure or pulmonary congestion, such as crackles, muffled heart sounds, or ventricular gallop. Unless the patient is hypotensive, place him in Fowler's position to promote lung expansion. Prepare to administer oxygen and an I.V. diuretic. Have emergency resuscitation equipment nearby.*

History and physical examination

When the patient's condition permits, obtain a complete medical history. First, note when the edema began. Is the edema worse in the morning or at the end of the day? Is it accompanied by shortness of breath or pain in the arms or legs? Find out how much weight the patient has gained. Has his urine output changed in quantity or quality? Is the edema generalized or localized, dependent or nondependent?

Next, ask about previous burns or cardiac, renal, hepatic, endocrine, or GI disorders. Have the patient describe his diet so you can determine whether he suffers from protein malnutrition. Explore his drug history, and note recent I.V. therapy.

Begin the physical examination by comparing the patient's arms and legs for symmetrical edema. Also, note ecchymoses and cyanosis. Assess the back, sacrum, and hips of the bedridden patient for dependent edema. Palpate peripheral pulses, noting whether hands and feet feel cold. Finally, perform a complete cardiac and respiratory assessment.

Medical causes

◆ ***Angioneurotic edema or angioedema.*** Recurrent attacks of acute, painless, nonpitting edema involving the skin and mucous membranes—especially those of the respiratory tract, face, neck, lips, larynx, hands, feet, genitalia, or viscera—may be the result of a food or drug allergy or emotional stress, or they may be hereditary. Abdominal pain, nausea, vomiting, and diarrhea accompany visceral edema; dyspnea and stridor accompany life-threatening laryngeal edema.

◆ ***Burns.*** Edema and associated tissue damage vary with the severity of the burn. Severe generalized edema (4+) may occur within 2 days of a major burn; localized edema may occur with a less severe burn.

◆ ***Cirrhosis.*** A late sign of chronic cirrhosis, edema usually starts in the legs and thighs and may progress to anasarca. Accompanying signs and symptoms include abdominal pain, anorexia, nausea and vomiting, hepatomegaly, ascites, jaundice, pruritus, bleeding tendencies, musty breath, lethargy, mental changes, and asterixis.

◆ ***Heart failure.*** Severe, generalized pitting edema—occasionally anasarca—may follow leg edema late in heart failure. The edema may improve with exercise or elevation of the limbs and is typically worse at the end of the day. Among other classic late findings are hemoptysis, cyanosis, marked hepatomegaly, clubbing, crackles, and a ventricular gallop. Typically, the patient has tachypnea, palpitations, hypotension, weight gain despite anorexia, nausea, slowed mental response, diaphoresis, and pallor. Dyspnea, orthopnea, tachycardia, and fatigue typify left-sided heart failure; jugular vein distention, hepatomegaly, and peripheral edema typify right-sided heart failure.

◆ ***Malnutrition.*** Anasarca in this disorder may mask dramatic muscle wasting. Malnutrition also typically causes muscle weakness; lethargy; anorexia; diarrhea; apathy; dry, wrinkled skin; and signs of anemia, such as dizziness and pallor.

◆ ***Myxedema.*** In this severe form of hypothyroidism, generalized nonpitting edema is accompanied by dry, flaky, inelastic, waxy, pale skin; a puffy face; and an upper eyelid droop. Observation also reveals masklike facies, hair

Understanding fluid balance

Normally, fluid moves freely between the interstitial and intravascular spaces to maintain homeostasis. Four basic types of pressure control fluid shifts across the capillary membrane that separates these spaces:
- capillary hydrostatic pressure (the internal fluid pressure on the capillary membrane)
- interstitial fluid pressure (the external fluid pressure on the capillary membrane)
- osmotic pressure (the fluid-attracting pressure from protein concentration within the capillary)
- interstitial osmotic pressure (the fluid-attracting pressure from protein concentration outside the capillary).

Here's how these pressures maintain homeostasis. Normally, capillary hydrostatic pressure is greater than plasma osmotic pressure at the capillary's arterial end, forcing fluid out of the capillary. At the capillary's venous end, the reverse is true: The plasma osmotic pressure is greater than the capillary hydrostatic pressure, drawing fluid into the capillary. Normally, the lymphatic system transports excess interstitial fluid back to the intravascular space.

Edema results when this balance is upset by increased capillary permeability, lymphatic obstruction, persistently increased capillary hydrostatic pressure, decreased plasma osmotic or interstitial fluid pressure, or dilation of precapillary sphincters.

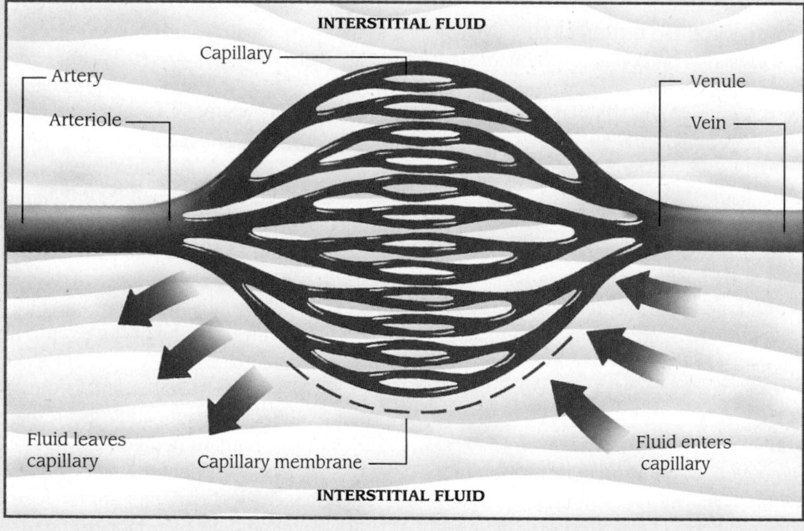

loss or coarsening, and psychomotor slowing. Associated findings include hoarseness, weight gain, fatigue, cold intolerance, bradycardia, hypoventilation, constipation, abdominal distention, menorrhagia, impotence, and infertility.

◆ ***Nephrotic syndrome.*** Although nephrotic syndrome is characterized by generalized pitting edema, the edema is initially localized around the eyes. Anasarca develops in severe cases, increasing body weight by up to 50%. Other common signs and symptoms are ascites, anorexia, fatigue, malaise, depression, and pallor.

◆ ***Pericardial effusion.*** In pericardial effusion, generalized pitting edema may be most prominent in the arms and legs. It may be accompanied by chest pain, dyspnea, orthopnea, a nonproductive cough, pericardial friction rub, jugular vein distention, dysphagia, and fever.

◆ ***Pericarditis (chronic constructive).*** Like right-sided heart failure, this disorder usually begins with pitting edema of the arms and legs that may progress to generalized edema. Other signs and symptoms include ascites, Kussmaul's sign, dyspnea, fatigue, weakness, abdominal distention, and hepatomegaly.

◆ ***Protein-losing enteropathy.*** Increased albumin levels lead to progressive generalized pitting edema in this disorder. The patient may

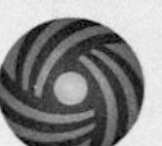

EXAMINATION TIP

Edema: Pitting or nonpitting?

To differentiate pitting from nonpitting edema, press your finger against a swollen area for 5 seconds, and then quickly remove it.

In pitting edema, pressure forces fluid into the underlying tissues, causing an indentation that fills slowly. To determine the severity of pitting edema, estimate the indentation's depth in centimeters: 1+ (1 cm), 2+ (2 cm), 3+ (3 cm), or 4+ (4 cm).

In nonpitting edema, pressure leaves no indentation because fluid has coagulated in the tissues. Typically, the skin feels unusually tight and firm.

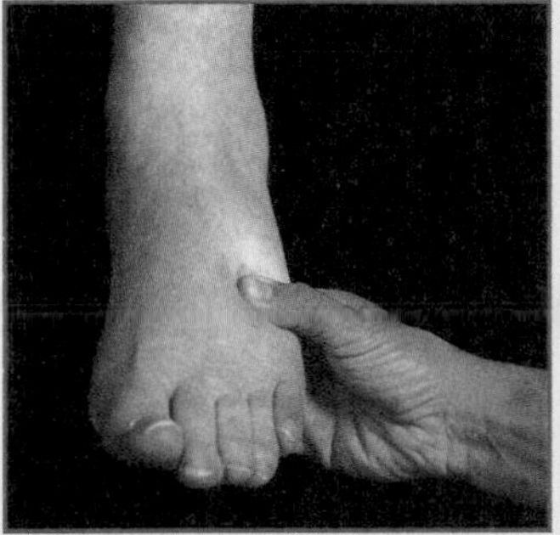

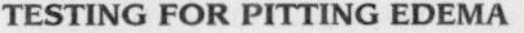

TESTING FOR PITTING EDEMA

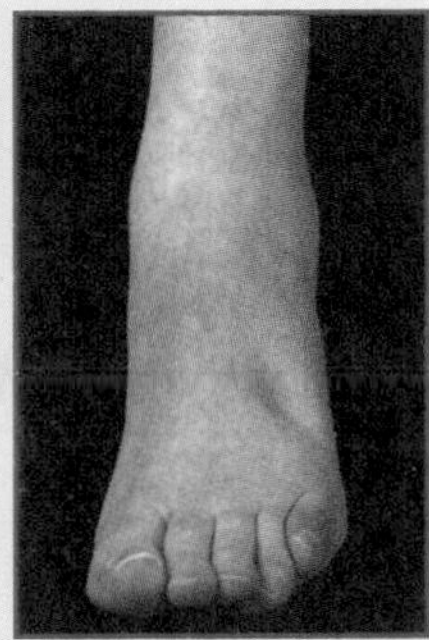

PITTING EDEMA

also have a mild fever and abdominal pain with bloody diarrhea and steatorrhea.

◆ ***Renal failure.*** Generalized pitting edema is a late sign of acute renal failure. In chronic failure, edema is less likely to become generalized; its severity depends on the degree of fluid overload. Both forms of renal failure cause oliguria, anorexia, nausea and vomiting, drowsiness, confusion, hypertension, dyspnea, crackles, dizziness, and pallor.

◆ ***Septic shock.*** A late sign of this life-threatening disorder, generalized edema typically develops rapidly. The edema is pitting and moderately severe. Accompanying it may be cool skin, hypotension, oliguria, tachycardia, cyanosis, thirst, anxiety, and signs of respiratory failure.

Other causes

◆ ***Drugs.*** Any drug that causes sodium retention may aggravate or cause generalized edema. Examples include antihypertensives, corticosteroids, androgenic and anabolic steroids, estrogens, and nonsteroidal anti-inflammatory drugs, such as ibuprofen and naproxen.

◆ ***Treatments.*** I.V. saline solution infusions and internal feedings may cause sodium and fluid overload, resulting in generalized edema, especially in patients with cardiac or renal disease.

Special considerations

Position the patient with his limbs above heart level to promote drainage. Periodically reposition him to avoid pressure ulcers. If the patient develops dyspnea, lower his limbs, elevate the head of the bed, and administer oxygen. Massage areas where dependent edema has formed (for example, the back, sacrum, hips, and buttocks). Prevent skin breakdown in these areas by placing a pressure mattress on the patient's bed. Restrict fluids and sodium, and administer a diuretic.

Monitor intake and output and daily weight. Also monitor serum electrolyte levels, especially sodium and albumin. Prepare the patient for blood and urine tests, X-rays, echocardiography, or an electrocardiogram.

Pediatric pointers

Renal failure in children commonly causes generalized edema. Monitor fluid balance closely. Remember that fever or diaphoresis can lead to fluid loss, so promote fluid intake.

Kwashiorkor (protein-deficiency malnutrition) is more common in children than in adults and causes anasarca.

Geriatric pointers

Elderly patients are more likely to develop edema for several reasons, including decreased cardiac and renal function and, in some cases, poor nutritional status. Use caution when giving older patients I.V. fluids or medications that can raise sodium levels and thereby increase fluid retention.

Patient counseling

Teach patients with known heart failure or renal failure to watch for edema; explain that it's an important sign of decompensation that indicates the need for immediate adjustment of therapy. Also teach patients to weigh themselves every day at the same time with the same clothes on to track if they have an increase in weight, which may correspond to increased fluid retention.

Edema of the arm

The result of excess interstitial fluid in the arm, this type of edema may be unilateral or bilateral and may develop gradually or abruptly. It may be aggravated by immobility and alleviated by arm elevation and exercise.

Arm edema signals a localized fluid imbalance between the vascular and interstitial spaces. (See *Understanding fluid balance,* page 258.) It commonly results from trauma, venous disorders, toxins, or certain treatments.

EMERGENCY INTERVENTIONS *Remove rings, bracelets, and watches from the patient's affected arm because they may act as a tourniquet. Make sure the patient's sleeves don't inhibit drainage of fluid or blood flow.*

History and physical examination

When taking the patient's history, one of the first questions to ask is "How long has your arm been swollen?" Then find out if the patient also has arm pain, numbness, or tingling. Does exercise or arm elevation decrease the edema? Ask about recent arm injury, such as burns or insect stings. Also, note recent I.V. therapy, surgery, or radiation therapy for breast cancer.

Determine the edema's severity by comparing the size and symmetry of both arms. Use a tape measure to determine the exact girth. Be sure to note whether the edema is unilateral or bilateral, and test for pitting. (See *Edema: Pitting or nonpitting?* page 259.) Next, examine and compare the color and temperature of both arms. Look for erythema and ecchymoses and for wounds that suggest injury. Palpate and compare the radial and brachial pulses. Finally, look for arm tenderness and decreased sensation or mobility. If you detect signs of neurovascular compromise, elevate the arm.

Medical causes

◆ ***Angioneurotic edema.*** Angioneurotic edema is a common reaction that's characterized by sudden onset of painless, nonpruritic edema in the hands, feet, eyelids, lips, face, neck, genitalia, or viscera. Although these swellings usually don't itch, they may burn and tingle. If edema spreads to the larynx, signs of respiratory distress may occur.

◆ ***Arm trauma.*** Shortly after a crush injury, severe edema may affect the entire arm. It may be accompanied by ecchymoses or superficial bleeding, pain or numbness, and paralysis.

◆ ***Burns.*** Mild to severe edema, pain, and tissue damage may occur up to 2 days after an arm burn.

◆ ***Superior vena cava syndrome.*** Bilateral arm edema usually progresses slowly in this disorder and is accompanied by facial and neck edema. Dilated veins mark these edematous areas. The patient also complains of headache, vertigo, and vision disturbances.

◆ ***Thrombophlebitis.*** Thrombophlebitis, which can result from peripherally inserted central catheters or arm portacaths, may cause arm edema, pain, and warmth. Deep vein thrombophlebitis can also produce cyanosis, fever, chills, and malaise; superficial thrombophlebitis also causes redness, tenderness, and induration along the vein.

Other causes

◆ ***Envenomation.*** Envenomation by snakes, aquatic animals, or insects initially may cause edema around the bite or sting that quickly spreads to the entire arm. Pain, erythema, and pruritus at the site are common; paresthesia occurs occasionally. Later, the patient may develop generalized signs and symptoms, such as nausea, vomiting, weakness, muscle cramps, fever, chills, hypotension, headache and, in severe cases, dyspnea, seizures, and paralysis.

◆ ***Treatments.*** Localized arm edema may result from infiltration of I.V. fluid into the interstitial tissue. A radical or modified radical mastectomy that disrupts lymphatic drainage may cause edema of the entire arm, as can axillary lymph node dissection. Also, radiation therapy for breast cancer may produce arm edema immediately after treatment or months later.

Special considerations

Treatment of the patient with arm edema varies according to the underlying cause. General care measures include elevation of the arm, frequent repositioning, and appropriate use of bandages and dressings to promote drainage and circulation. Provide meticulous skin care to prevent breakdown and formation of pressure ulcers.

Also, administer an analgesic and anticoagulant as needed.

Pediatric pointers

Arm edema rarely occurs in children, except as part of generalized edema, but it may result from arm trauma, such as burns and crush injuries.

Patient counseling

Warn the patient who has undergone a mastectomy or axillary lymph node dissection of the possibility of arm edema, and advise her not to have blood pressure measurements taken or phlebotomies performed on the affected arm. Teach the patient how to perform arm exercises after surgery to prevent lymphedema.

Edema of the face

Facial edema refers to either localized swelling—around the eyes, for example—or more generalized facial swelling that may extend to the neck and upper arms. Occasionally painful, this sign may develop gradually or abruptly. Sometimes it precedes onset of peripheral or generalized edema. Mild facial edema may be difficult to detect; the patient or someone who's familiar with his appearance may report it before it's noticed during assessment.

Facial edema results from disruption of the hydrostatic and osmotic pressures that govern fluid movement between the arteries, veins, and lymphatics. (See *Understanding fluid balance,* page 258.) It may result from venous, inflammatory, and certain systemic disorders; trauma; allergy; malnutrition; or the effects of certain drugs, tests, and treatments.

EMERGENCY INTERVENTIONS *If the patient has facial edema associated with burns or if he reports recent exposure to an allergen, quickly evaluate his respiratory status: Edema may also affect his upper airway, causing a life-threatening obstruction. If you detect audible wheezing, inspiratory stridor, or other signs of respiratory distress, administer epinephrine. For patients in severe distress—with absent breath sounds and cyanosis—tracheal intubation, cricothyroidotomy, or tracheotomy may be required. Always administer oxygen.*

History and physical examination

If the patient isn't in severe distress, take his health history. Ask if facial edema developed suddenly or gradually. Is it more prominent in early morning, or does it worsen throughout the day? Has the patient gained weight? If so, how much and over what length of time? Has he noticed a change in his urine color or output? In his appetite? Take a drug history and ask about recent facial trauma.

Begin the physical examination by characterizing the edema. Is it localized to one part of the face, or does it affect the entire face or other parts of the body? Determine if the edema is pitting or nonpitting, and grade its severity. (See *Edema: Pitting or nonpitting?* page 259.) Next, take vital signs and assess neurologic status. Examine the oral cavity to evaluate dental hygiene and look for signs of infection. Visualize the oropharynx and look for any soft-tissue swelling.

Medical causes

◆ ***Abscess, periodontal.*** This type of abscess, which usually results from poor oral hygiene, is commonly caused by anaerobic organisms. It can cause edema of the side of the face, pain, warmth, erythema, and a purulent discharge around the affected tooth.

◆ ***Abscess, peritonsillar.*** This complication of tonsillitis may cause unilateral facial edema. Other key signs and symptoms include severe throat pain, neck swelling, drooling, cervical adenopathy, fever, chills, and malaise.

◆ ***Allergic reaction.*** Facial edema may characterize both a local allergic reaction and anaphylaxis. A local reaction produces facial edema, erythema, and urticaria. In life-threatening anaphylaxis, angioneurotic facial edema may occur with urticaria and flushing. (See *Recognizing angioneurotic edema,* page 262.) Airway edema causes hoarseness, stridor, and bronchospasm with dyspnea and tachypnea. Signs of shock, such as hypotension and cool, clammy skin, may also occur.

◆ ***Cavernous sinus thrombosis.*** Cavernous sinus thrombosis is a rare but serious disorder that may begin with unilateral edema that quickly progresses to bilateral edema of the forehead, base of the nose, and eyelids. It may also produce chills, fever, headache, nausea, lethargy, exophthalmos, and eye pain.

◆ ***Chalazion.*** A chalazion causes localized swelling and tenderness of the affected eyelid, accompanied by a small red lump on the conjunctival surface.

◆ ***Conjunctivitis.*** Conjunctivitis is an inflammation that causes eyelid edema, excessive

Recognizing angioneurotic edema

Most dramatic in the lips, eyelids, and tongue, angioneurotic edema commonly results from an allergic reaction. It's characterized by rapid onset of painless, nonpitting, subcutaneous swelling that usually resolves in 1 to 2 days. This type of edema may also involve the hands, feet, genitalia, and viscera; laryngeal edema may cause life-threatening airway obstruction.

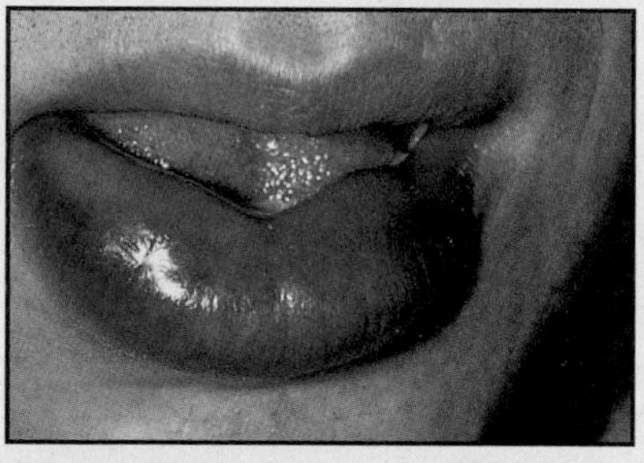

tearing, and itchy, burning eyes. Inspection reveals a thick purulent discharge, crusty eyelids, and conjunctival injection. Corneal involvement causes photophobia and pain.

◆ ***Corneal ulcers, fungal.*** Accompanying red, edematous eyelids in this disorder are conjunctival injection, intense pain, photophobia, and severely impaired visual acuity. Copious amounts of a purulent eye discharge make the eyelids sticky and crusted. The characteristic dense, central ulcer grows slowly, is whitish gray, and is surrounded by progressively clearer rings.

◆ ***Dacryoadenitis.*** Severe periorbital swelling characterizes dacryoadenitis, which may also cause conjunctival injection, a purulent discharge, and temporal pain.

◆ ***Dacryocystitis.*** Lacrimal sac inflammation causes prominent eyelid edema and constant tearing. In acute cases, pain and tenderness near the tear sac accompany a purulent discharge.

◆ ***Dermatomyositis.*** Periorbital edema and a heliotropic rash develop gradually in this rare disease. An itchy, lilac-colored rash appears on the bridge of the nose, cheeks, and forehead. Localized or diffuse erythema, eye pain, and fever may also occur.

◆ ***Facial burns.*** Burns may cause extensive edema that impairs respiration. Additional findings include singed nasal hairs, red mucosa, sooty sputum, and signs of respiratory distress such as inspiratory stridor.

◆ ***Facial trauma.*** The extent of edema varies with the type of injury. For example, a contusion may cause localized edema, whereas a nasal or maxillary fracture causes more generalized edema. Associated features also depend on the type of injury.

◆ ***Frontal sinus cancer.*** This rare form of cancer causes cheek edema on the affected side, reddened skin over the sinus, unilateral nasal bleeding or discharge, and exophthalmos. Pain over the forehead and unilateral hypoesthesia or anesthesia may occur later.

◆ ***Herpes zoster ophthalmicus (shingles).*** In herpes zoster ophthalmicus, edematous and red eyelids are usually accompanied by excessive tearing and a serous discharge. Severe unilateral facial pain may occur several days before vesicles erupt.

◆ ***Hordeolum (stye).*** Typically, a hordeolum produces localized eyelid edema, erythema, and pain.

◆ ***Malnutrition.*** Severe malnutrition causes facial edema followed by swelling of the feet and legs. Associated signs and symptoms include muscle atrophy and weakness; anorexia; diarrhea; lethargy; dry, wrinkled skin; sparse, brittle, easily plucked hair; and decreased pulse and respiratory rates.

◆ ***Melkersson's syndrome.*** Facial edema (especially of the lips), facial paralysis, and folds in the tongue are the three characteristic signs of this rare disorder.

◆ ***Myxedema.*** Myxedema eventually causes generalized facial edema, waxy dry skin, hair loss or coarsening, and other signs of hypothyroidism.

◆ ***Nephrotic syndrome.*** Commonly the first sign of nephrotic syndrome, periorbital edema precedes dependent and abdominal edema. Associated findings include weight gain, nausea, anorexia, lethargy, fatigue, and pallor.

◆ ***Orbital cellulitis.*** Sudden onset of periorbital edema marks this inflammatory disorder. It may be accompanied by a unilateral purulent discharge, hyperemia, exophthalmos, conjunctival injection, impaired extraocular movements, fever, and extreme orbital pain.

◆ ***Osteomyelitis.*** When osteomyelitis affects the frontal bone, it may cause forehead edema as well as fever, chills, headache, and cool, pallid skin.

◆ ***Preeclampsia.*** Edema of the face, hands, and ankles is an early sign of this disorder of pregnancy. Other characteristics include excessive weight gain, severe headache, blurred vision, hypertension, and midepigastric pain.

◆ ***Rhinitis, allergic.*** In allergic rhinitis, red and edematous eyelids are accompanied by paroxysmal sneezing, itchy nose and eyes, and profuse, watery rhinorrhea. The patient may also develop nasal congestion, excessive tearing, headache, sinus pain, and sometimes malaise and fever.

◆ ***Sinusitis.*** Frontal sinusitis causes edema of the forehead and eyelids. Maxillary sinusitis produces edema in the maxillary area as well as malaise, gingival swelling, and trismus. Both types are also accompanied by facial pain, fever, nasal congestion, a purulent nasal discharge, and red, swollen nasal mucosa.

◆ ***Superior vena cava syndrome.*** Superior vena cava syndrome gradually produces facial and neck edema accompanied by thoracic or jugular vein distention. It also causes central nervous system symptoms, such as headache, vision disturbances, and vertigo.

◆ ***Trachoma.*** In trachoma, edema affects the eyelid and conjunctiva and is accompanied by eye pain, excessive tearing, photophobia, and eye discharge. Examination reveals an inflamed preauricular node and visible conjunctival follicles.

◆ ***Trichinosis.*** This relatively rare infectious disorder causes sudden onset of eyelid edema with fever (102° F to 104° F [38.9° C to 40° C]), conjunctivitis, muscle pain, itching and burning skin, sweating, skin lesions, and delirium.

OTHER CAUSES

◆ ***Diagnostic tests.*** An allergic reaction to contrast media used in radiologic tests may produce facial edema.

◆ ***Drugs.*** Long-term use of glucocorticoids may produce facial edema. Any drug that causes an allergic reaction (aspirin, antipyretics, penicillin, and sulfa preparations, for example) may have the same effect.

HERB ALERT *Ingestion of the fruit pulp of ginkgo biloba can cause severe erythema and edema and the rapid formation of vesicles. Feverfew and chrysanthemum parthenium can cause swelling of the lips, irritation of the tongue, and mouth ulcers. Licorice may cause facial edema and water retention or bloating, especially if used before menses.*

◆ ***Surgery and transfusion.*** Facial edema may result from cranial, nasal, or jaw surgery or from a blood transfusion that causes an allergic reaction.

SPECIAL CONSIDERATIONS

Administer an analgesic for pain, and apply cream to reduce itching. Unless contraindicated, apply cold compresses to the patient's eyes to decrease edema. Elevate the head of the bed to help drain the accumulated fluid. Urine and blood tests are commonly ordered to help diagnose the cause of facial edema.

PEDIATRIC POINTERS

Normally, periorbital tissue pressure is lower in a child than in an adult. As a result, children are more likely to develop periorbital edema. In fact, periorbital edema is more common than peripheral edema in children with such disorders as heart failure and acute glomerulonephritis. Pertussis may also cause periorbital edema.

Edema of the leg

Leg edema is a common sign that results when excess interstitial fluid accumulates in one or both legs. It may affect just the foot and ankle or extend to the thigh, and may be slight or dramatic and pitting or nonpitting.

Leg edema may result from venous disorders, trauma, and certain bone and cardiac disorders that disturb normal fluid balance. (See *Understanding fluid balance,* page 258.) It may result from nephrotic syndrome, cirrhosis, acute or chronic thrombophlebitis, chronic venous insufficiency (most common), cellulitis, lymphedema, and the use of certain drugs. However, several nonpathologic mechanisms may also cause leg edema. For example, prolonged sitting, standing, or immobility may cause bilateral orthostatic edema. This pitting edema usually affects the foot and disappears with rest and leg elevation. Increased venous pressure late in pregnancy may cause ankle edema. Constricting garters or pantyhose may mechanically cause lower-extremity edema.

HISTORY AND PHYSICAL EXAMINATION

To evaluate the patient, first ask how long he has had the edema. Did it develop suddenly or gradually? Does it decrease if he elevates his legs? Is it painful when touched or when he walks? Is it worse in the morning, or does it get progressively worse during the day? Ask about a recent leg injury or any recent surgery or illness that may have immobilized the patient.

Does he have a history of cardiovascular disease? Finally, obtain a drug history.

Begin the physical examination by examining each leg for pitting edema. (See *Edema: Pitting or nonpitting?* page 259.) Because leg edema may compromise arterial blood flow, palpate or use a handheld Doppler device to auscultate peripheral pulses to detect any insufficiency. Observe leg color and look for unusual vein patterns. Then palpate for warmth, tenderness, and cords, and gently squeeze the calf muscle against the tibia to check for deep pain. If leg edema is unilateral, dorsiflex the foot to look for Homans' sign, which is indicated by calf pain. Finally, note skin thickening or ulceration in the edematous areas.

Medical causes

◆ ***Burns.*** Mild to severe edema, pain, and tissue damage may occur up to 2 days after a leg burn.

◆ ***Cellulitis.*** Caused by a streptococcal or staphylococcal infection that usually affects the legs, cellulitis produces pitting edema and orange peel skin along with erythema, warmth, and tenderness in the infected area.

◆ ***Cirrhosis.*** Cirrhosis commonly causes bilateral edema, which is associated with ascites, jaundice, and abdominal swelling.

◆ ***Heart failure.*** Bilateral leg edema is an early sign of right-sided heart failure. Other signs and symptoms include weight gain despite anorexia, nausea, chest tightness, hypotension, pallor, tachypnea, exertional dyspnea, orthopnea, paroxysmal nocturnal dyspnea, palpitations, a ventricular gallop, and inspiratory crackles. Pitting ankle edema, hepatomegaly, hemoptysis, and cyanosis signal more advanced heart failure.

◆ ***Hypoproteinemia.*** Malnourished patients may develop bilateral leg edema secondary to decreased protein and osmotic pressures.

◆ ***Leg trauma.*** Mild to severe localized edema may form around the trauma site.

◆ ***Nephrotic syndrome.*** Nephrotic syndrome is commonly seen in children and results in bilateral leg edema. It's associated with polyuria and eyelid swelling.

◆ ***Osteomyelitis.*** When this bone infection affects the lower leg, it usually produces localized, mild to moderate edema, which may spread to the adjacent joint. Edema typically follows fever, localized tenderness, and pain that increases with leg movement.

◆ ***Phlegmasia cerulea dolens.*** Severe unilateral leg edema and cyanosis may spread to the abdomen and flank in this rare form of venous thrombosis. Other signs and symptoms include pain, cold skin, absent pulse in the affected leg, and signs of shock, such as hypotension and tachycardia.

◆ ***Rupture of the gastrocnemius muscle.*** Ruptured gastrocnemius muscle can cause leg edema and often occurs in runners. Pain is usually sudden, and ecchymosis is evident on the ankles.

◆ ***Rupture of a popliteal (Baker's) cyst.*** A ruptured popliteal cyst can cause sudden onset of unilateral calf pain and edema, usually after walking or exercising. This type of cyst is common in patients with arthritis. It can compress vascular structures and cause severe edema and thrombophlebitis.

◆ ***Thrombophlebitis.*** Both deep and superficial vein thrombosis may cause unilateral mild to moderate edema. Deep vein thrombophlebitis may be asymptomatic or may cause mild to severe pain, warmth, and cyanosis in the affected leg as well as fever, chills, and malaise. Superficial vein thrombophlebitis typically causes pain, warmth, redness, tenderness, and induration along the affected vein.

◆ ***Venous insufficiency (chronic).*** Moderate to severe unilateral or bilateral leg edema occurs in patients with this disorder, which generally affects females. Initially soft and pitting, the edema later becomes hard as tissues thicken. Other signs include darkened skin and painless, easily infected stasis ulcers around the ankle.

Other causes

◆ ***Coronary artery bypass surgery.*** Unilateral venous insufficiency may follow saphenous vein retrieval. Edema often occurs in the affected leg or ankle and usually resolves after 6 to 8 weeks.

◆ ***Diagnostic tests.*** Venography is a rare cause of leg edema.

◆ ***Drugs.*** Estrogen, hormonal contraceptives, lithium, nonsteroidal anti-inflammatory drugs, vasodilators, and drugs that cause sodium retention can cause bilateral leg edema.

◆ ***Envenomation.*** Mild to severe localized edema may develop suddenly at the site of a bite or sting along with erythema, pain, urticaria, pruritus, and a burning sensation.

Special considerations

Provide an analgesic and an antibiotic as needed. Have the patient avoid prolonged sitting or standing, and elevate his legs as necessary. A compression boot (Unna's boot) may be used to help reduce edema. Monitor the patient's intake and output, and check his weight and leg circumference daily to detect any change in the edema. Prepare him for diagnostic tests, such as blood and urine studies and X-rays. Determine the need for dietary modifications, such as water and sodium restrictions. Monitor the affected extremity for skin breakdown.

Pediatric pointers

Uncommon in children, leg edema may result from osteomyelitis, leg trauma or, rarely, heart failure.

Patient counseling

Show the patient with leg edema how to apply antiembolism stockings or bandages to promote venous return. Encourage him to perform leg exercises.

Enophthalmos

Enophthalmos is the backward displacement of the eye into the orbit. This sign may develop suddenly or gradually and may be severe or mild. Enophthalmos usually results from trauma, but it may also be due to severe dehydration and eye disorders. In elderly people, senile atrophy of orbital fat may produce physiologic enophthalmos.

Because enophthalmos allows the upper lid to droop over the sunken eye, this sign is commonly mistaken for ptosis. However, exophthalmometry can differentiate these two signs. (See *Differentiating enophthalmos from ptosis,* page 266.)

History and physical examination

Begin by asking the patient how long he has had enophthalmos. Is it accompanied by headache or eye pain? If so, ask him to describe its severity and location. Next, ask about a history of trauma, cancer, or other eye disorders.

If you suspect an orbital fracture, *don't* open the patient's eye or place any pressure on the eyeball; this risks ocular laceration. Apply a metal or plastic eye shield until the ophthalmologist can perform a complete examination.

Otherwise, perform a visual acuity test, with and without correction. Then evaluate extraocular movements, and determine intraocular pressure with a Schiøtz tonometer. Using a direct ophthalmoscope, check for papilledema and other abnormalities. Check pupil response to light, and note eyelid drooping.

Assess the patient for signs and symptoms of dehydration, such as dry mucous membranes, poor skin turgor, and hypotension.

Medical causes

- ***Crouzon's disease (craniofacial dysostosis).*** Typically, enophthalmos occurs along with an abnormally wide distance between the pupils in this disorder. Other findings include mental deficiency, astigmatism, epicanthal folds, skull deformity and, occasionally, ocular deviation.
- ***Dehydration.*** Mild to severe enophthalmos may accompany severe dehydration. Typically, the patient also displays poor skin turgor, dry mucous membranes, extreme thirst, weight loss, fatigue, tachycardia, hypotension, nausea, vomiting, and diarrhea.
- ***Duane's syndrome.*** In this congenital syndrome, transient enophthalmos occurs when the patient looks to the side. Visual acuity is usually normal, but horizontal eye movement is impaired.
- ***Orbital fracture.*** In this type of fracture, enophthalmos may not be apparent until edema subsides. The affected eyeball is displaced downward and inward and is surrounded by ecchymosis. Other findings include diplopia in the affected eye, eye or head pain, subconjunctival hemorrhage, and a dilated or unreactive pupil.
- ***Pancoast's syndrome.*** This syndrome produces enophthalmos, ptosis, miosis, shoulder pain, and paresthesia of the hand and arm of the same side.
- ***Parinaud's syndrome.*** In patients with this disorder, enophthalmos occurs with nystagmus when the patient tries to look up. Ocular muscles show absent voluntary movement but normal conjugate movement. Other signs include lid retraction, ptosis, dilated pupils with poor or absent light response, and papilledema.
- ***Parry-Romberg syndrome.*** This syndrome produces enophthalmos and may cause irises of different color, facial hemiatrophy, miotic pupils with a sluggish response to dim light, nystagmus, ocular muscle paralysis, and ptosis.

Special considerations

Regularly monitor vital signs and evaluate pupillary response to light. Prepare the trauma patient for skull X-rays and an eye examination.

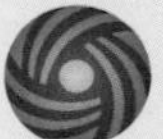

EXAMINATION TIP

Differentiating enophthalmos from ptosis

In patients with enophthalmos, the eye is displaced backward in its socket, causing the upper eyelid to droop. In those with ptosis, eyelid drooping is also characteristic, but it results from muscle weakness or cranial nerve paralysis.

To differentiate enophthalmos from ptosis, use an exophthalmometer to measure the distance between the orbital rim and the tip of the cornea. Have the patient stand against the wall and look into your eyes. Place the device on the patient's face like a pair of glasses, adjust it to fit snugly at the orbital rims, and note the bar reading. Then look into the 45-degree-angle mirrors, and measure the corneal apex by lining it up visually against the millimeter scale.

Normally, the corneal apex is 12 to 24 mm in front of the orbital rim, and the difference between the eyes is less than 2 mm. In patients with enophthalmos, the reading in one or both eyes may be less than 12 mm; in those with ptosis, the readings are within the normal range.

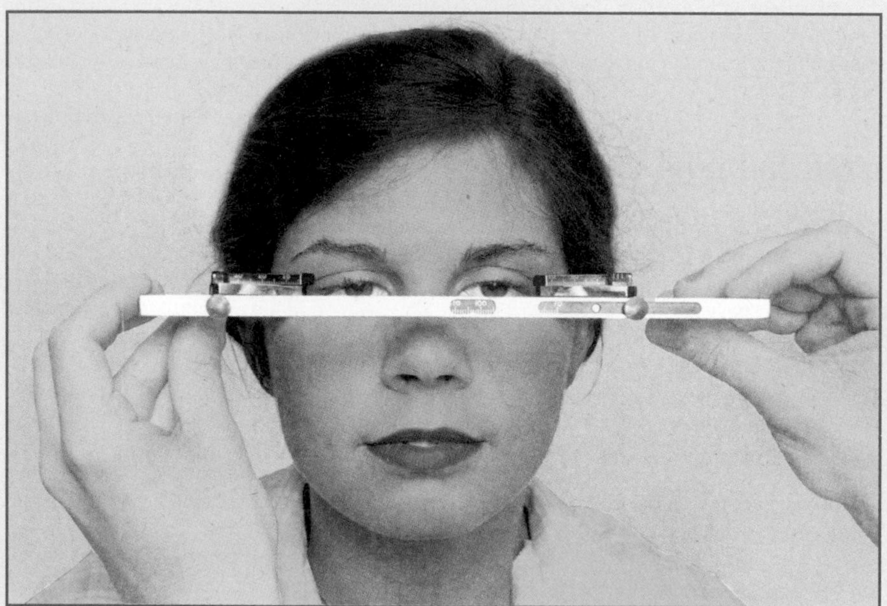

Pediatric pointers

In neonates, enophthalmos usually results from microphthalmos (abnormally small eyes). Later, its causes are the same as those for adults.

Enuresis

Enuresis usually refers to nighttime urinary incontinence in girls age 5 and older and boys age 6 and older. This sign rarely continues into adulthood but may occur in some adults with sleep apnea. It's most common in boys and may be classified as primary or secondary. In primary enuresis, a child has never achieved bladder control; in secondary enuresis, a child who achieved bladder control for at least 3 months has lost it.

Factors that may contribute to enuresis are delayed development of detrusor muscle control, unusually deep or sound sleep, organic disorders (such as a urinary tract infection [UTI] or obstruction), and psychological stress. Psychological stress, probably the most important factor, commonly results from the birth of a sibling, the death of a parent or loved one, divorce, or premature, rigorous

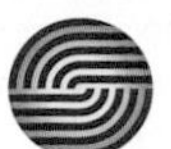

PATIENT-TEACHING AID

Helping your child have dry nights

Dear Parent:
Although no single treatment for bed-wetting is always effective, by following these recommendations you can help your child achieve bladder control:

- Restrict your child's intake of fluids—especially colas—after supper.
- Make sure your child urinates before bedtime. In addition, wake him once during the night to go to the bathroom.
- Reward your child after each dry night with praise and encouragement. Keep a progress chart, marking each dry night with a sticker.
- Reward your child with a book, a small toy, or a special activity for a certain number of consecutive dry nights.
- Always give your child emotional support. Never punish him if he wets the bed; instead reassure him that he'll learn to achieve bladder control. Remember that most children simply outgrow bed-wetting. However, wet and dry nights will alternate before your child develops a constant pattern of dryness.

toilet training. The child may be too embarrassed or ashamed to discuss his bed-wetting, which intensifies psychological stress and makes enuresis more likely—thus creating a vicious circle.

History and physical examination

When taking a history, include the parents as well as the child. First, determine the number of nights each week or month that the child wets the bed. Is there a family history of enuresis? Ask about the child's daily fluid intake. Does he drink much after supper? What are his typical sleep and voiding patterns? Find out if the child has ever had control of his bladder. If so, try to pinpoint what may have precipitated enuresis, such as an organic disorder or psychological stress. Does the bed-wetting occur both at home and away from home? Ask the parents how they have tried to manage the problem, and have them describe the child's toilet training. Observe the child's and parents' attitudes toward bed-wetting. Finally, ask the child if it hurts when he urinates.

Next, perform a physical examination to detect signs of neurologic or urinary tract disorders. Observe the child's gait to check for motor dysfunction, and test sensory function in the legs. Inspect the urethral meatus for erythema, and obtain a urine specimen. A rectal examination to evaluate sphincter control may be required.

Medical causes

- ***Detrusor muscle hyperactivity.*** Involuntary detrusor muscle contractions may cause primary or secondary enuresis associated with urinary urgency, frequency, and incontinence. Signs and symptoms of UTI are also common.
- ***Urinary tract obstruction.*** Although it usually causes daytime incontinence, this disorder may also produce primary or secondary enuresis as well as flank and lower back pain; upper abdominal distention; urinary frequency, urgency, hesitancy, and dribbling; dysuria; diminished urine stream; hematuria; and variable urine output.
- ***UTI.*** In children, most UTIs produce secondary enuresis. Associated features include urinary frequency and urgency, dysuria, straining to urinate, and hematuria. Low back pain, fatigue, and suprapubic discomfort may also occur.

Special considerations

Provide emotional support to the child and his family. Encourage the parents to accept and support the child. Tell them how to manage enuresis at home. (See *Helping your child have dry nights.*)

Bladder training may help control enuresis caused by detrusor muscle hyperactivity. An alarm device may be useful for children ages 8 and older. This moisture-sensitive device fits in his mattress and triggers an alarm when moistened, waking the child. The alarm conditions him to avoid bed-wetting and should be used only in cases in which enuresis is having adverse psychological effects on the child. Pharmacologic treatment with imipramine, desmopressin, or an anticholinergic may be helpful.

Epistaxis

A common sign, epistaxis (nosebleed) can be spontaneous or induced from the front or back of the nose. Most nosebleeds occur in the anterior-inferior nasal septum (Kiesselbach's plexus), but some occur at the point where the inferior turbinates meet the nasopharynx. Usually unilateral, they seem bilateral when blood runs from the bleeding side behind the nasal septum and out the opposite side. Epistaxis ranges from mild oozing to severe—possibly life-threatening—blood loss.

A rich supply of fragile blood vessels makes the nose particularly vulnerable to bleeding. Air moving through the nose can dry and irritate the mucous membranes, forming crusts that bleed when they're removed; dry mucous membranes are also more susceptible to infections, which can produce epistaxis as well. Trauma is another common cause of epistaxis. Additional causes include septal deviations; hematologic, coagulation, renal, and GI disorders; and certain drugs and treatments.

EMERGENCY INTERVENTIONS *If your patient has severe epistaxis, quickly take his vital signs. Be alert for tachypnea, hypotension, and other signs of hypovolemic shock. Insert a large-gauge I.V. catheter for rapid fluid and blood replacement, and attempt to control bleeding by pinching the nares closed. (However, if you suspect a nasal fracture,* don't *pinch the nares. Instead, place gauze under the patient's nose to absorb the blood.)*

Have a hypovolemic patient lie down and turn his head to the side to prevent blood from draining down the back of his throat, which could cause aspiration or vomiting of swallowed blood. If the patient isn't hypovolemic, have him sit upright and tilt his head forward. Constantly check airway patency. If the patient's condition is unstable, begin cardiac monitoring and give supplemental oxygen by mask.

History and physical examination

If your patient isn't in distress, take a history. Does he have a history of recent trauma? How often has he had nosebleeds in the past? Have the nosebleeds been long or unusually severe? Has the patient recently had surgery in the sinus area? Ask about a history of hypertension, bleeding or liver disorders, and other recent illnesses. Ask if the patient bruises easily. Find out what drugs he uses, especially anti-inflammatories such as aspirin and anticoagulants such as warfarin.

Begin the physical examination by inspecting the patient's skin for other signs of bleeding, such as ecchymoses and petechiae, and noting any jaundice, pallor, or other abnormalities. When examining a trauma patient, look for associated injuries, such as eye trauma or facial fractures.

Medical causes

◆ ***Angiofibroma (juvenile).*** This rare disorder usually occurs in males and is characterized by severe recurrent epistaxis and nasal obstruction.

◆ ***Aplastic anemia.*** This disorder develops insidiously, eventually producing nosebleeds as well as ecchymoses, retinal hemorrhages, menorrhagia, petechiae, bleeding from the mouth, and signs of GI bleeding. Fatigue, dyspnea, headache, tachycardia, and pallor may also occur.

◆ ***Barotrauma.*** Commonly seen in airline passengers and scuba divers, barotrauma may cause severe, painful epistaxis when the patient has an upper tract respiratory infection.

◆ ***Biliary obstruction.*** This disorder produces bleeding tendencies, including epistaxis. Typical features are colicky right-upper-quadrant pain after eating fatty food, nausea, vomiting, fever, flatulence and, possibly, jaundice.

◆ ***Cirrhosis.*** Epistaxis is a late sign that occurs along with other bleeding tendencies (bleeding gums, easy bruising, hematemesis, melena) in cirrhosis. Other typical late findings include ascites, abdominal pain, shallow respirations, hepatomegaly or splenomegaly, and fever of 101° F to 103° F (38.3° C to 39.4° C). The patient may also exhibit muscle atrophy, enlarged superficial abdominal veins, severe pruritus, extremely dry skin, poor tissue turgor, abnormal pigmentation, spider angiomas, palmar erythema and, possibly, jaundice and central nervous system disturbances.

◆ ***Coagulation disorders.*** Such disorders as hemophilia and thrombocytopenic purpura can cause epistaxis along with ecchymoses, petechiae, and bleeding from the gums, mouth, and I.V. puncture sites. Menorrhagia and signs of GI bleeding, such as melena and hematemesis, can also occur.

◆ ***Glomerulonephritis (chronic).*** This disorder produces epistaxis as well as hypertension, proteinuria, hematuria, headache, edema, oliguria, hemoptysis, nausea, vomiting, pruritus, dyspnea, malaise, and fatigue.

◆ ***Hepatitis.*** When hepatitis interferes with the clotting mechanism, epistaxis and other abnormal bleeding tendencies can result. Associated signs and symptoms typically include jaundice, clay-colored stools, pruritus, hepatomegaly, abdominal pain, fever, fatigue, weakness, dark amber urine, anorexia, nausea, and vomiting.

◆ ***Hereditary hemorrhagic telangiectasia (Rendu-Osler-Weber disease).*** This disease causes frequent, sometimes daily, epistaxis as well as hemoptysis and GI bleeding. It's characterized by telangiectases—pinpoint, purplish red spots or flat, spiderlike lesions—on the mucous membranes of the lips, mouth, tongue, nose, and GI tract and occasionally on the trunk and fingertips.

◆ ***Hypertension.*** Severe hypertension can produce severe epistaxis, usually in the posterior nose, with pulsation above the middle turbinate. It may be accompanied by dizziness, a throbbing headache, anxiety, peripheral edema, nocturia, nausea, vomiting, drowsiness, and mental impairment.

◆ ***Infectious mononucleosis.*** In patients with this infectious disorder, blood may ooze from the nose. Characteristic features include sore throat, cervical lymphadenopathy, and a fluctuating fever with an evening peak of 101° F to 102° F (38.3° C to 38.9° C).

◆ ***Influenza.*** When influenza affects the capillaries, a slow, oozing nosebleed results. Other signs and symptoms of influenza include a dry cough, chills, fever, malaise, myalgia, sore throat, hoarseness or loss of voice, conjunctivitis, facial flushing, headache, rhinitis, and rhinorrhea.

◆ ***Leukemia.*** In acute leukemia, sudden epistaxis is accompanied by a high fever and other types of abnormal bleeding, such as bleeding gums, ecchymoses, petechiae, easy bruising, and prolonged menses. These may follow less-noticeable signs and symptoms, such as weakness, lassitude, pallor, chills, recurrent infections, and a low-grade fever. Acute leukemia may also cause dyspnea, fatigue, malaise, tachycardia, palpitations, a systolic ejection murmur, and abdominal or bone pain.

In chronic leukemia, epistaxis is a late sign that may be accompanied by other types of abnormal bleeding, extreme fatigue, weight loss, hepatosplenomegaly, bone tenderness, edema, macular or nodular skin lesions, pallor, weakness, dyspnea, tachycardia, palpitations, and headache.

◆ ***Maxillofacial injury.*** A pumping arterial bleed usually causes severe epistaxis in a maxillofacial injury. Associated signs and symptoms include facial pain, numbness, swelling, and asymmetry; open-bite malocclusion or inability to open the mouth; diplopia; conjunctival hemorrhage; lip edema; and buccal, mucosal, and soft-palatal ecchymoses.

◆ ***Nasal fracture.*** A nasal fracture may cause unilateral or bilateral epistaxis with nasal swelling, pain, and deformity; crepitation of the nasal bones; and periorbital ecchymoses and edema.

◆ ***Nasal tumor.*** Blood may ooze from the nose when a tumor disrupts the nasal vasculature. Benign tumors usually bleed when touched, but malignant tumors produce spontaneous unilateral epistaxis along with a foul discharge, cheek swelling, and—in the late stage—pain.

◆ ***Orbital floor fracture.*** This type of trauma may damage the maxillary sinus mucosa and, on rare occasions, cause epistaxis. More typical features include periorbital edema and ecchymoses, diplopia, infraorbital numbness, enophthalmos, limited eye movement, and facial asymmetry.

◆ ***Polycythemia vera.*** A common sign of polycythemia vera, spontaneous epistaxis may be accompanied by bleeding gums; ecchymoses; ruddy cyanosis of the face, nose, ears, and lips; and congestion of the conjunctiva, retina, and oral mucous membranes. Other signs and symptoms vary according to the affected body system but may include headache, dizziness, tinnitus, vision disturbances, hypertension, chest pain, intermittent claudication, early satiety and fullness, marked splenomegaly, epigastric pain, pruritus, and dyspnea.

◆ ***Renal failure.*** Chronic renal failure is more likely than acute renal failure to cause epistaxis and a tendency to bruise easily. More common signs and symptoms are oliguria or anuria, anorexia, weight loss, abdominal pain, diarrhea, nausea, vomiting, tissue wasting, dry mucous membranes, uremic breath odor, Kussmaul's respirations, deteriorating mental status, and tachycardia.

Skin changes include pruritus, pallor, yellow-bronze pigmentation, purpura, excoriation, uremic frost, and brown arcs under the nail margins. Neurologic signs and symptoms may include muscle twitching, fasciculations, asterixis, paresthesia, and footdrop. Cardiovascular effects include hypertension, arrhythmias, signs of heart failure or pericarditis, and peripheral edema.

◆ ***Sarcoidosis.*** Oozing epistaxis may be accompanied by a nonproductive cough, substernal pain, malaise, and weight loss in this disorder. Related findings include tachycardia, arrhythmias, parotid gland enlargement, cervical lymphadenopathy, skin lesions, hepatosplenomegaly, and arthritis in the ankles, knees, and wrists.

◆ ***Scleroma.*** In this disorder, oozing epistaxis occurs with a watery nasal discharge that becomes foul-smelling and crusty. Progressive anosmia and turbinate atrophy may also occur.

◆ ***Sinusitis (acute).*** In this disorder, a bloody or blood-tinged nasal discharge may become purulent and copious after 24 to 48 hours. Associated signs and symptoms include nasal congestion, pain, and tenderness; malaise; headache; a low-grade fever; and red, edematous nasal mucosa.

◆ ***Skull fracture.*** Depending on the type of fracture, epistaxis can be direct (when blood flows directly down the nares) or indirect (when blood drains through the eustachian tube and into the nose). Abrasions, contusions, lacerations, or avulsions are common. A severe skull fracture may cause severe headache, decreased level of consciousness, hemiparesis, dizziness, seizures, projectile vomiting, and decreased pulse and respiratory rates.

A basilar fracture may also cause bleeding from the pharynx, ears, and conjunctivae as well as raccoon eyes and Battle's sign. Cerebrospinal fluid or even brain tissue may leak from the nose or ears. A sphenoid fracture may also cause blindness, whereas a temporal fracture may also cause unilateral deafness or facial paralysis.

◆ ***Syphilis.*** Epistaxis is most common in patients with tertiary syphilis, as posterior septum ulcerations produce a foul, bloody nasal discharge. It may be accompanied by a painful nasal obstruction and nasal deformity. Occasionally, primary syphilis causes painful nasal crusting and bleeding accompanied by the characteristic chancre sores.

◆ ***Systemic lupus erythematosus (SLE).*** Usually affecting women younger than age 50, SLE causes oozing epistaxis. More characteristic signs and symptoms include butterfly rash, lymphadenopathy, joint pain and stiffness, nausea, vomiting, myalgia, anorexia, and weight loss.

◆ ***Typhoid fever.*** Oozing epistaxis and dry cough are common signs of typhoid fever, which may also cause sudden chills and high fever, vomiting, abdominal distention, constipation or diarrhea, splenomegaly, hepatomegaly, "rose-spot" rash, jaundice, anorexia, weight loss, and profound fatigue.

Other causes

◆ ***Chemical irritants.*** Some chemicals—including phosphorus, sulfuric acid, ammonia, printer's ink, and chromates—irritate the nasal mucosa, producing epistaxis.

◆ ***Drugs.*** Anticoagulants, such as warfarin, and anti-inflammatories, such as aspirin, can cause epistaxis. Cocaine use, especially if frequent, can also cause epistaxis.

◆ ***Surgery and procedures.*** Epistaxis rarely results from facial or nasal surgery, including septoplasty, rhinoplasty, antrostomy, endoscopic sinus procedures, orbital decompression, and dental extraction.

◆ ***Vigorous nose blowing.*** This may rupture superficial blood vessels, especially in elderly people and young people, causing nosebleeds.

Special considerations

Until the bleeding is completely under control, continue to monitor the patient for signs of hypovolemic shock, such as tachycardia and clammy skin. If external pressure doesn't control the bleeding, insert cotton that has been impregnated with a vasoconstrictor and local anesthetic into the patient's nose.

If bleeding persists, expect to insert anterior or posterior nasal packing. (See *Controlling epistaxis with nasal packing.*) Administer humidified oxygen by face mask to a patient with posterior packing.

A complete blood count may be ordered to evaluate blood loss and detect anemia. Clotting studies, such as prothrombin time and activated partial thromboplastin time, may be required to test coagulation time. Prepare the patient for X rays if he has had a recent trauma.

Pediatric pointers

Children are more likely to experience anterior nosebleeds, usually the result of nose-picking or allergic rhinitis. Biliary atresia, cystic fibrosis, hereditary afibrinogenemia, and nasal

Controlling epistaxis with nasal packing

When direct pressure and cautery fail to control epistaxis, nasal packing may be required. Anterior packing may be used if the patient has severe bleeding in the anterior nose. This involves inserting horizontal layers of petroleum jelly gauze strips into the nostrils near the turbinates.

Posterior packing may be needed if the patient has severe bleeding in the posterior nose or if blood from anterior bleeding starts flowing backward. This type of packing consists of a gauze pack secured by three strong silk sutures. After the nose is anesthetized, sutures are pulled through the nostrils with a soft catheter and the pack is positioned behind the soft palate. Two of the sutures are tied to a gauze roll under the patient's nose, which keeps the pack in place. The third suture is taped to his cheek. Instead of a gauze pack, an indwelling urinary or nasal epistaxis catheter may be inserted through the nose into the area behind the soft palate and inflated with 10 ml of water to compress the bleeding point.

Precautions

If the patient has nasal packing, follow these guidelines:

- Watch for signs of respiratory distress such as dyspnea, which may occur if the packing slips and obstructs the airway.
- Keep emergency equipment (flashlights, scissors, and hemostat) at the patient's bedside. Expect to cut the cheek suture (or deflate the catheter) and remove the pack at the first sign of airway obstruction.
- Avoid tension on the cheek suture, which could cause the posterior pack to slip out of place.
- Keep the call bell within easy reach.
- Monitor vital signs frequently. Watch for signs of hypoxia, such as tachycardia and restlessness.
- Elevate the head of the patient's bed, and remind him to breathe through his mouth.
- Administer humidified oxygen as needed.
- Instruct the patient not to blow his nose for 48 hours after the packing is removed.

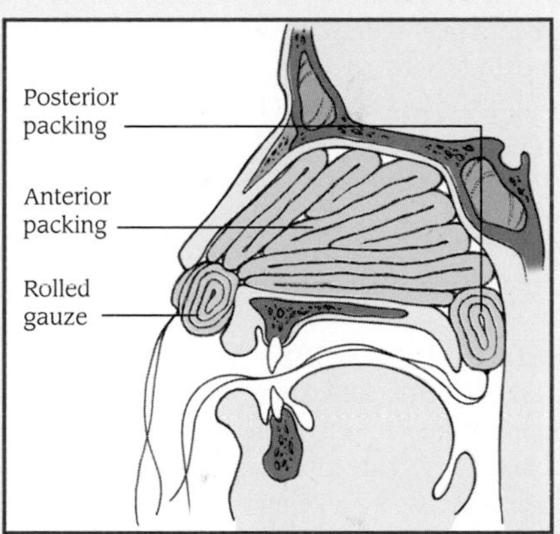

trauma due to a foreign body can also cause epistaxis. Rubeola may cause an oozing nosebleed along with the characteristic maculopapular rash. Two rare childhood diseases—pertussis and diphtheria—can also cause oozing epistaxis.

Suspect a bleeding disorder if you see excess umbilical cord bleeding at birth or profuse bleeding during circumcision. Epistaxis commonly begins at puberty in patients with hereditary hemorrhagic telangiectasia.

Geriatric pointers

Elderly patients are more likely to have posterior nosebleeds.

Patient counseling

Teach the patient proper pinching techniques for applying pressure to the nose. For prevention, tell him to apply liberal amounts of petroleum jelly to nostrils to prevent drying, cracking, and picking. Also recommend using of a humidifier at night and trimming fingernails.

Eructation

Eructation (belching) occurs when gas or acidic fluid rises from the stomach, producing a characteristic sound. Depending on the cause, eructation may vary in duration and intensity. Occasionally, this sign results from a GI disorder. More commonly, however, it results from aerophagia—the unconscious swallowing of air—or from ingestion of gas-producing food. Eructation may relieve associated symptoms, most notably nausea, heartburn, dyspepsia, and bloating.

History and physical examination

Focus your history on trying to decipher the cause of eructation. Ask the patient if belching occurs after drinking carbonated beverages. Does it occur immediately after eating or several hours later? Is it relieved by vomiting or an antacid? By changing position?

Determine whether the patient has associated abdominal pain or heartburn. If so, ask him to describe its location, duration, and intensity. Also ask him about recent weight loss, lack of appetite, heartburn, nausea, or vomiting. Has he noticed a change in bowel habits? Does he have difficulty breathing while he's lying down?

Begin the physical examination by taking the patient's vital signs. As you do so, note the patient's facial expression and posture. Does he appear to guard his abdomen? Is he sitting still or moving about?

Check for foul-smelling breath. Next, inspect the patient's abdomen for distention or visible peristalsis. Auscultate for bowel sounds and characterize their motility. Then palpate or percuss the abdomen for masses, tenderness, rigidity, and distention.

Medical causes

◆ ***Gastric outlet obstruction.*** This common complication of duodenal ulcer disease causes eructation, epigastric fullness and discomfort, anorexia, nausea, and vomiting.

◆ ***Hiatal hernia.*** In this disorder, eructation occurs after eating and is accompanied by heartburn, regurgitation of sour-tasting fluid, and abdominal distention. The patient complains of dull substernal or epigastric pain that may radiate to the shoulder. Other features include dysphagia, nausea, weight loss, dyspnea, tachypnea, a cough, and halitosis.

◆ ***Peptic ulcer.*** This common disorder may cause eructation, but its cardinal symptoms are heartburn and gnawing or burning stomach pain that's relieved by food, antacids, or antisecretories. Associated signs and symptoms include nausea, vomiting, melena, abdominal distention, early satiety, and epigastric tenderness.

◆ ***Superior mesenteric artery syndrome (acute).*** Eructation and halitosis are late signs of this uncommon syndrome. Typically, the eructation occurs after eating and is accompanied by regurgitation.

Special considerations

Place the patient in a side-lying or knee-chest position to help relieve eructation. If the patient is sensitive to gas-producing food, such as onions and cucumbers, adjust his diet as necessary. He may also need to be placed on a lactose-restricted diet.

Pediatric pointers

Aerophagia is a common cause of eructation in children, who commonly swallow air while eating or crying. Organic causes are rare and usually result from a congenital anomaly such as aganglionic megaduodenum.

Geriatric pointers

Older patients who have missing teeth or other dental problems and decreased salivary gland function tend to chew less, thereby swallowing larger pieces of food and more air. These factors combined with decreased gastric acid output and decreased motility cause increased eructation.

Patient counseling

To prevent aerophagia, advise patients to avoid chewing gum and smoking, to chew small pieces of food slowly and thoroughly, and to talk as little as possible while eating.

Erythema

[Erythroderma]

Dilated or congested blood vessels produce red skin, or erythema, the most common sign of skin inflammation or irritation. Erythema may be localized or generalized and may occur suddenly or gradually. Skin color can range from bright red in patients with acute conditions to pale violet or brown in those whose conditions are chronic. Erythema must be differentiated from purpura, which causes redness from bleeding into the skin. When pressure is applied directly to the skin, erythema blanches momentarily, but purpura doesn't.

Erythema usually results from changes in the arteries, veins, and small vessels that lead to increased small-vessel perfusion. Drugs and neurogenic mechanisms can allow extra blood to enter the small vessels. Erythema can also result from trauma and tissue damage; changes in supporting tissues, which increase vessel visibility; and a number of rare disorders. (See *Rare causes of erythema.*)

EMERGENCY INTERVENTIONS *If your patient suddenly develops progressive erythema with a rapid pulse, dyspnea, hoarseness, and agitation, quickly take his vital signs. These may be indications of anaphylactic shock. Provide emergency respiratory support and give epinephrine.*

HISTORY AND PHYSICAL EXAMINATION

If erythema isn't associated with anaphylaxis, obtain a detailed health history. (See *Differential diagnosis: Erythema*, pages 274 and 275.) Find out how long the patient has had the erythema and where it first began. Has he had any associated pain or itching? Has he recently had a fever, an upper respiratory tract infection, or joint pain? Does he have a history of skin disease or other illness? Does he or anyone in his family have allergies, asthma, or eczema? Find out if he has been exposed to someone who has had a similar rash or who is now ill. Did he have a recent fall or injury in the erythematous area?

Obtain a complete drug history, including recent immunizations. Ask about food intake and exposure to chemicals.

Begin the physical examination by assessing the extent, distribution, and intensity of erythema. Look for edema and other skin lesions, such as urticaria, scales, papules, and purpura. Examine the affected area for warmth, and gently palpate it to check for tenderness or crepitus.

CULTURAL CUE *Dark-skinned patients may have difficulty recognizing erythema; as a result, they may present with associated diseases in a more advanced state.*

Rare causes of erythema

In exceptional cases, your patient's erythema may be caused by one of these rare disorders:

- *acute febrile neutrophilic dermatosis,* which produces erythematous lesions on the face, neck, and extremities after a high fever
- *erythema abigne,* which produces lacy erythema and telangiectases after exposure to radiant heat
- *erythema chronicum migrans,* which produces erythematous macules and papules on the trunk, upper arms, or thighs after a tick bite
- *erythema gyratum repens,* which produces wavy bands of erythema and is commonly associated with internal malignancy
- *toxic epidermal necrolysis,* which causes severe, widespread erythema, tenderness, bullae formation, and exfoliation; this disorder is usually caused by medications and may be fatal because of epidermal destruction and its consequences.

MEDICAL CAUSES

◆ ***Allergic reactions.*** Foods, drugs, chemicals, and other allergens can cause an allergic reaction and erythema. A localized allergic reaction also produces hivelike eruptions and edema.

Anaphylaxis, a life-threatening reaction, produces relatively sudden erythema in the form of urticaria. It also produces flushing; facial edema; diaphoresis; weakness; sneezing; bronchospasm with dyspnea and tachypnea; shock with hypotension and cool, clammy skin; and possibly airway edema with hoarseness and stridor.

◆ ***Burns.*** In thermal burns, erythema and swelling appear first, possibly followed by deep or superficial blisters and other signs of damage that vary with the severity of the burn. Burns from ultraviolet rays, such as sunburn, cause delayed erythema and tenderness on exposed areas of the skin.

◆ ***Candidiasis.*** When this fungal infection affects the skin, it produces erythema and a scaly, papular rash under the breasts and at the axillae, neck, umbilicus, and groin (intertrigo). Small pustules commonly occur at the periphery of the rash (satellite pustulosis).

◆ ***Cellulitis.*** This bacterial infection of the skin and subcutaneous tissue causes erythema, tenderness, and edema.

◆ ***Dermatitis.*** Erythema commonly occurs in this family of inflammatory disorders. In *atopic dermatitis,* erythema and intense pruritus precede the development of small papules that may redden, weep, scale, and lichenify. These occur most commonly at skin folds of the extremities, neck, and eyelids.

Contact dermatitis occurs after exposure to an irritant. It quickly produces erythema and vesicles, blisters, or ulcerations on exposed skin.

Differential diagnosis: Erythema

History of present illness
Focused physical examination: Skin

Burns

Signs and symptoms
First degree
- Pressure that causes blanching of skin
- Tenderness at the site
- Involvement of superficial layers of the epidermis

Second-degree superficial partial-thickness
- Thin, fluid-filled blisters
- Pain at site
- Involvement of epidermis and some dermis

Second-degree deep partial-thickness
- Tenderness around site
- Development of blisters and edema
- Involvement of epidermis and dermis

Third degree
- Tough and leathery affected area
- Nontender
- Destruction of all skin elements

Diagnosis: History of exposure to heat, chemicals, or electricity; physical examination; chest X-ray for smoke inhalation

Treatment: Removal of cause of injury, rule of nines to estimate extent of injury and guide treatment, I.V. hydration, medication (analgesics, nonsteroidal anti-inflammatory drugs, topical antibacterial)

Follow-up: As needed (depending on severity of burn), referral to burn center if injury is severe

In *seborrheic dermatitis,* erythema appears with dull red or yellow lesions. Sharply marginated, these lesions are sometimes ring shaped and covered with greasy scales. They usually occur on the scalp, eyebrows, ears, and nasolabial folds, but they may form a butterfly rash on the face or move to the chest or to skin folds on the trunk. This disorder is common in patients infected with the human immunodeficiency virus and in infants (cradle cap).

◆ ***Dermatomyositis.*** This disorder, most common in women older than age 50, produces a dusky lilac rash on the face, neck, upper torso, and nail beds. Gottron's papules (violet, flat-topped lesions) may appear on finger joints.

◆ ***Erysipelas.*** This skin infection caused by group A beta-hemolytic streptococci is characterized by an abrupt onset of reddish, well-demarcated, tender, warm, sometimes elevated lesions, mainly on the face and neck but sometimes also on the extremities. Flaccid, pus-filled bullae may develop after 2 to 3 days. Extension into deeper tissues is rare. Other signs and symptoms include fever, chills, cervical lym-

Erythema multiforme	Seborrheic dermatitis	Atopic dermatitis	Contact dermatitis
Signs and symptoms ◆ Hivelike erythema with blisters ◆ Pathognomonic petechial or "iris" lesions ◆ Symmetrical lesions (less than 3 cm) on the face, hands, and feet ◆ Involvement of less than 20% of body surface area **Diagnosis:** Physical examination, skin biopsy **Treatment:** Treatment of underlying cause, medication (analgesics, antipruritics) **Follow-up:** None unless complications develop	**Signs and symptoms** ◆ Dull red or yellow lesions on the scalp, eyebrows, ears, and nasolabial folds ◆ Butterfly rash on the face, chest, or trunk **Diagnosis:** Physical examination, skin biopsy, allergy patch test **Treatment:** Medication (antiseborrheic shampoo, selenium or zinc lotion, steroid cream) **Follow-up:** Reevaluation every 2 to 12 weeks as necessary	**Signs and symptoms** ◆ Intense pruritus ◆ Small papules that redden, weep, scale, and lichenify, commonly occurring in skin folds of the extremities, neck, and eyelids **Diagnosis:** Physical examination, skin biopsy, allergy patch test **Treatment:** Topical corticosteroids **Follow-up:** Reevaluation every 2 to 12 weeks as necessary	**Signs and symptoms** ◆ History of exposure to irritant ◆ Vesicles, blisters, ulcerations that appear on exposed skin **Diagnosis:** Physical examination, skin biopsy, allergy patch test **Treatment:** Cool compresses with astringent, soaks with oatmeal, medication (topical and systemic corticosteroids, antihistamines, antibiotics) **Follow-up:** Reevaluation every 2 to 12 weeks as necessary

Additional differential diagnoses: allergic reaction ◆ candidiasis ◆ chronic liver disease ◆ dermatomyositis ◆ erysipelas ◆ erythema annulare centrifugum ◆ erythema marginatum rheumaticum ◆ erythema nodosum ◆ frostbite ◆ intertrigo ◆ necrotizing fasciitis ◆ polymorphous light eruption ◆ psoirasis ◆ Raynaud's disease ◆ rheumatoid arthritis ◆ rosacea ◆ rubella ◆ systemic lupus erythematosus ◆ thrombophlebitis ◆ toxic shock syndrome

phadenopathy, vomiting, headache, sore throat, warmth and tenderness in the affected area and, possibly, alopecia.

◆ ***Erythema annulare centrifugum.*** Small, pink infiltrated papules appear on the trunk, buttocks, and inner thighs, slowly spreading at the margins and clearing in the center. Itching, scaling, and tissue hardening may occur.

◆ ***Erythema marginatum rheumaticum.*** Associated with rheumatic fever, this disorder causes erythematous lesions that are superficial, flat, and slightly hardened. They shift, spread rapidly, and may last for hours or days, recurring after a time.

◆ ***Erythema multiforme.*** This acute inflammatory skin disease develops as a result of drug sensitivity after an infection (most commonly herpes simplex or a mycoplasmal infection), allergies, or pregnancy. One-half of the cases are of idiopathic origin.

Erythema multiforme minor produces reddish pink iris-shaped, urticarial, localized lesions with little or no mucous membrane involvement. Most lesions occur on flexor surfaces of the extremities. Burning or itching may occur before or in conjunction with lesion development. Lesions appear in crops and last 2 to 3 weeks. After 1 week, they become flat or hyperpigmented. Early signs and symptoms may include a mild fever, cough, and sore throat.

Erythema multiforme major usually occurs as a drug reaction; causes widespread symmetrical, bullous lesions that may become confluent; and includes erosions of the mucous membranes. Erythema is characteristically preceded by blisters on the lips, tongue, and buccal mucosa and a sore throat. Additional early signs and symptoms include cough, vomiting, diarrhea, coryza, and epistaxis. Later signs and symptoms include fever, prostration, difficulty with oral intake because of mouth and lip lesions, conjunctivitis due to ulceration, vulvitis, and balanitis. The most severe form of this disorder is known as Stevens-Johnson syndrome, a multisystem disorder that can occasionally be fatal. In addition to all signs and symptoms mentioned above, patients develop exfoliation of the skin from disruptions of bullae, although less than 10% of the body surface area is affected. These areas resemble second-degree thermal burns and should be cared for as such. Fever may rise to 102° F to 104° F (38.9° C to 40° C). The patient may also experience tachypnea; a weak, rapid pulse; chest pain; malaise; and muscle or joint pain.

◆ ***Erythema nodosum.*** Sudden bilateral eruption of tender erythematous nodules characterizes this disorder. These firm, round, protruding lesions usually appear in crops on the shins, knees, and ankles but may occur on the buttocks, arms, calves, and trunk as well. Other effects include mild fever, chills, malaise, muscle and joint pain and, possibly, swollen feet and ankles. Erythema nodosum is associated with various diseases, most notably inflammatory bowel disease, sarcoidosis, tuberculosis, and streptococcal and fungal infections.

◆ ***Frostbite.*** First-degree frostbite turns the affected body part a lifeless gray color, followed by an intense bluish red flush on rewarming. Blisters, lack of feeling, and tissue necrosis may follow.

◆ ***Gout.*** This disease, which generally affects men ages 40 to 60, is characterized by tight and erythematous skin over an inflamed, edematous joint.

◆ ***Intertrigo.*** In this superficial fungal infection, skin friction usually causes symmetrical erythema that may be accompanied by soreness and itching. Typically, erythema occurs in skin folds, such as in the groin; in severe cases, the skin may become bright red with erosion and maceration.

◆ ***Kawasaki syndrome.*** This acute illness of unknown cause, which primarily affects children younger than age 5, commonly produces a rash or erythema. No test is available for Kawasaki syndrome, which can cause serious heart damage and death if not detected and treated immediately. Additional characteristic signs include fever, conjunctival injection, and lymphadenopathy. Patients are treated with I.V. gamma globulin and aspirin.

◆ ***Liver disease (chronic).*** Any chronic liver disease, such as cirrhosis, can cause local vasodilation and palmar erythema along with jaundice, pruritus, spider angiomas, xanthomas, and characteristic systemic signs.

◆ ***Lupus erythematosus.*** Both discoid and systemic lupus erythematosus (SLE) can produce a characteristic butterfly rash. This erythematous eruption may range from a blush with swelling to a scaly, sharply demarcated, macular rash with plaques that may spread to the forehead, chin, ears, chest, and other sun-exposed parts of the body.

In discoid lupus erythematosus, other signs and symptoms may include telangiectasia, hyperpigmentation, ear and nose deformity, and mouth, tongue, and eyelid lesions.

In SLE, acute onset of erythema may be accompanied by photosensitivity and mucous membrane ulcers, especially in the nose and mouth. Mottled erythema may occur on the hands, with edema around the nails and macular reddish purple lesions on the fingers. Telangiectasia occurs at the base of the nails or eyelids along with purpura, petechiae, ecchymoses, and urticaria. Other findings vary according to the body systems affected but typically include low-grade fever, malaise, weakness, headache, arthralgia, arthritis, depression, lymphadenopathy, fatigue, anorexia, weight loss, nausea, vomiting, diarrhea, and constipation.

◆ ***Necrotizing fasciitis.*** This streptococcal infection usually begins with an area of mild erythema at the site of insult, which soon changes from red to purple and then blue. The appearance of fluid-filled blisters and bullae indicates the rapid progression of the necrotizing process. By days 7 to 10, dead skin begins to separate at the margins of the erythema, revealing extensive necrosis of the subcutaneous tissue. Other findings include fever, hypovolemia and, in later stages, hypotension and respiratory insufficiency—signs of overwhelming sepsis that require supportive care.

◆ ***Polymorphous light eruption.*** This condition produces erythema, vesicles, plaques, and multiple small papules on sun-exposed areas, which may later eczematize, lichenify, and excoriate. Pruritus may also occur.

◆ ***Psoriasis.*** Silvery white scales over a thickened erythematous base usually affect the elbows, knees, chest, scalp, and intergluteal folds. The fingernails may become thick and pitted.

◆ ***Raynaud's disease.*** In this disorder, the skin on the hands and feet typically blanches and cools after exposure to cold and stress and later becomes warm and purplish red.

◆ ***Rheumatoid arthritis.*** In a flare-up of this disorder, erythema occurs over the affected joints along with heat, swelling, pain, and stiffness. Earlier symptoms include malaise, fatigue, myalgia, prolonged morning stiffness, and clumsiness. As the disease progresses, muscle atrophy, palmar erythema, generalized edema, mottled skin, and structural deformities occur.

◆ ***Rosacea.*** Scattered erythema initially develops across the center of the face, followed by superficial telangiectases, papules, pustules, and nodules. Rhinophyma may occur on the lower half of the nose.

◆ ***Rubella.*** Typically, flat solitary lesions join to form a blotchy pink erythematous rash that spreads rapidly to the trunk and extremities in this disorder. Occasionally, small red lesions (Forschheimer spots) occur on the soft palate. Lesions clear in 4 to 5 days. The rash usually follows a fever (up to 102° F [38.9° C]), headache, malaise, sore throat, a gritty eye sensation, lymphadenopathy, pain in the joints, and coryza.

◆ ***Staphylococcal scalded skin syndrome.*** This endotoxin-mediated epidermolytic disease is caused by a clinically unapparent *Staphylococcus aureus* infection and primarily affects infants (Ritter's disease) and small children. It's characterized by erythema and widespread exfoliation of superficial epidermal layers, resembling scalded skin. Associated signs and symptoms include low-grade fever and irritability. Care must be taken to maintain hydration and prevent secondary infections of denuded areas; hospitalization is commonly required. Death may occur, especially in infants with extensive disease.

◆ ***Thrombophlebitis.*** Although this disorder is sometimes asymptomatic, it can produce erythema over the inflamed vein. Fever, chills, and malaise may accompany severe localized pain, warmth, and induration; distal edema; and a positive Homans' sign.

◆ ***Toxic shock syndrome.*** This infectious disorder, which is caused by a toxin-producing *S. aureus* infection, causes sudden, diffuse erythema in the form of a macular rash. It's accompanied by a sudden high fever, myalgia, vomiting, severe diarrhea, and sudden hypotension that may lead to shock. Desquamation occurs after 1 to 2 weeks, especially on the palms and soles. This syndrome usually affects young women and has been associated with the use of tampons during menses.

Other causes

◆ ***Drugs.*** Many drugs commonly cause erythema. (See *Drugs associated with erythema,* page 278.)

HERB ALERT *Ingestion of the fruit pulp of ginkgo biloba can cause severe erythema and edema of the mouth and rapid formation of vesicles. St. John's wort can cause heightened photosensitivity, resulting in erythema or "sunburn."*

◆ ***Radiation and other treatments.*** Radiation therapy may produce dull erythema and edema within 24 hours. As the erythema fades, the skin becomes light brown and mildly scaly. Any treatment that causes an allergic reaction can also cause erythema.

Special considerations

Because erythema can cause fluid loss, closely monitor and replace fluids and electrolytes, especially in patients with burns or widespread erythema. Be sure to withhold all medications until the cause of the erythema has been identified. Then expect to administer an antibiotic and a topical or systemic corticosteroid.

For a patient with itching skin, expect to give soothing baths or apply open wet dressings containing starch, bran, or sodium bicarbonate; also administer an antihistamine and an analgesic as needed. Advise a patient with leg erythema to keep his legs elevated above heart level. For a burn patient with erythema, immerse the affected area in cold water, or apply a sheet soaked in cold water to reduce pain, edema, and erythema.

Prepare the patient for diagnostic tests, such as skin biopsy to detect cancerous lesions, cultures to identify infectious organisms, and sensitivity studies to confirm allergies.

Drugs associated with erythema

Suspect drug-induced erythema in any patient who develops this sign within 1 week of starting a drug. Erythematous lesions can vary in size, shape, type, and amount, but they almost always appear suddenly and symmetrically on the trunk and inner arms. The following drugs can produce erythematous lesions:

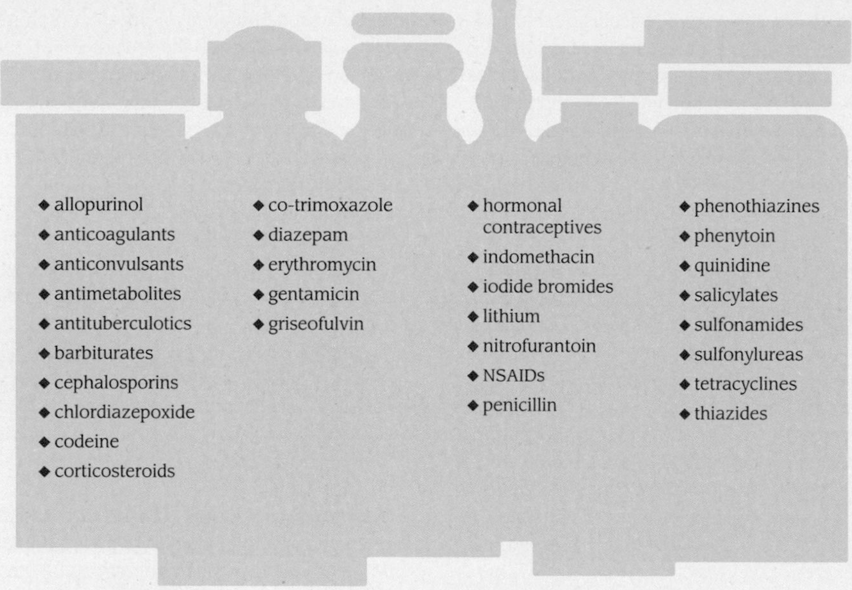

- allopurinol
- anticoagulants
- anticonvulsants
- antimetabolites
- antituberculotics
- barbiturates
- cephalosporins
- chlordiazepoxide
- codeine
- corticosteroids
- co-trimoxazole
- diazepam
- erythromycin
- gentamicin
- griseofulvin
- hormonal contraceptives
- indomethacin
- iodide bromides
- lithium
- nitrofurantoin
- NSAIDs
- penicillin
- phenothiazines
- phenytoin
- quinidine
- salicylates
- sulfonamides
- sulfonylureas
- tetracyclines
- thiazides

Some drugs—particularly barbiturates, hormonal contraceptives, salicylates, sulfonamides, and tetracycline—can cause a "fixed" drug eruption. In this type of reaction, lesions can appear in any body part and flake off after a few days, leaving a brownish purple pigmentation. Repeated drug administration causes the original lesions to recur and new ones to develop.

Pediatric pointers

Many newborns develop a pink papular rash (erythema toxicum neonatorum) that starts within the first 4 days after birth and spontaneously disappears by the 10th day. Neonates and infants can also develop erythema from infections and other disorders. For instance, candidiasis can produce thick white lesions over an erythematous base on the oral mucosa as well as diaper rash with beefy red erythema.

Roseola, rubeola, scarlet fever, granuloma annulare, and cutis marmorata also cause erythema in children.

Geriatric pointers

Many elderly patients have well-demarcated purple macules or patches, usually on the back of the hands and on the forearms. Known as actinic purpura, this condition results from blood leaking through fragile capillaries. The lesions disappear spontaneously.

Patient counseling

Teach patients with a chronic disease, such as SLE or psoriasis, about the character of their typical rashes so they can be alert to any flare-ups of their disease. Also, advise such patients to avoid sun exposure and to use sunblock when appropriate.

Exophthalmos

[Proptosis]

Exophthalmos—the abnormal protrusion of one or both eyeballs—may result from hemorrhage, edema, or inflammation behind the eye; extraocular muscle relaxation; or space-occupying intraorbital lesions and metastatic tumors. This sign may occur suddenly or gradually, causing mild to dramatic protrusion. Occasionally, the affected eye also pulsates. The most common cause of exophthalmos in adults is dysthyroid eye disease.

Exophthalmos is usually easily observed. However, lid retraction may mimic exophthalmos even when protrusion is absent. Similarly, ptosis in one eye may make the other eye appear exophthalmic by comparison. An exophthalmometer can differentiate these signs by measuring ocular protrusion.

History and physical examination

Begin by asking when the patient first noticed exophthalmos. Is it associated with pain in or around the eye? If so, ask him how severe it is and how long he has had it. Then ask about recent sinus infection or vision problems. Take the patient's vital signs, noting fever, which may accompany an eye infection. Next, evaluate the severity of exophthalmos with an exophthalmometer. (See *Detecting unilateral exophthalmos.*) If the eyes bulge severely, look for cloudiness on the cornea, which may indicate ulcer formation. Describe any eye discharge and observe for ptosis. Then check visual acuity, with and without correction, and evaluate extraocular movements. Palpate the patient's thyroid for enlargement or goiter.

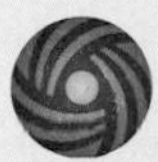

EXAMINATION TIP

Detecting unilateral exophthalmos

If one of the patient's eyes seems more prominent than the other, examine both eyes from above the patient's head. Look down across his face, gently draw his lids up, and compare the relationship of the corneas to the lower lids. Abnormal protrusion of one eye suggests unilateral exophthalmos.

Remember: Don't perform this test if you suspect eye trauma.

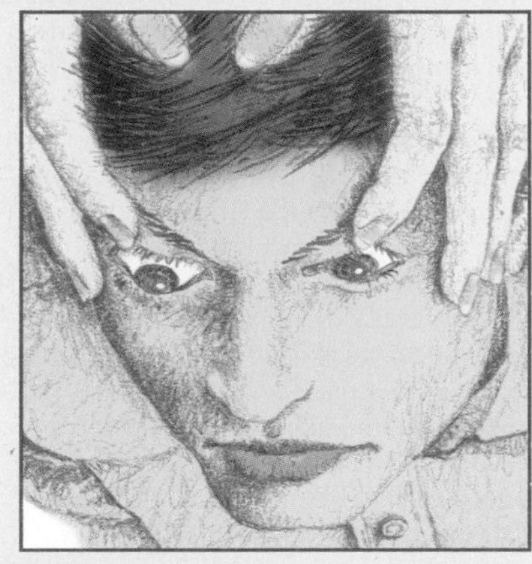

Medical causes

◆ ***Cavernous sinus thrombosis.*** This disorder usually causes sudden onset of pulsating unilateral exophthalmos. Accompanying it may be eyelid edema, decreased or absent pupillary reflexes, limited extraocular movement, and impaired visual acuity. Other features include high fever with chills, papilledema, headache, nausea, vomiting, somnolence and, rarely, seizures.

◆ ***Dacryoadenitis.*** Unilateral, slowly progressive exophthalmos is the most common sign of dacryoadenitis. Assessment may also reveal limited extraocular movement (especially on elevation and abduction), ptosis, eyelid edema and erythema, conjunctival injection, eye pain, and diplopia.

◆ ***Foreign body in the eye.*** When a foreign body enters the eye, exophthalmos may accompany other signs and symptoms of ocular trauma, such as eye pain, redness, and tearing.

◆ ***Hemangioma.*** Most common in young adults, this orbital tumor produces progressive exophthalmos, which may be mild or severe and unilateral or bilateral. Other signs and symptoms include ptosis, limited extraocular movement, and blurred vision.

◆ ***Hodgkin's disease.*** In this disorder, unilateral exophthalmos may develop gradually along with eyelid edema, diplopia, and a palpable eyelid mass. More characteristic findings include painless swelling of one or more lymph nodes, intermittent fever, weight loss, fatigue, malaise, night sweats, hepatosplenomegaly, and pruritus.

◆ ***Lacrimal gland tumor.*** Exophthalmos usually develops slowly in one eye, causing its downward displacement toward the nose. The patient may also have ptosis and eye deviation and pain.

◆ ***Leiomyosarcoma.*** Most common in people ages 45 and older, this tumor is characterized by slowly developing unilateral exophthalmos. Other effects include diplopia, impaired vision, and intermittent eye pain.

◆ ***Leukemia.*** When leukemia causes intraorbital hemorrhage, mild to moderate bilateral exophthalmos and lacrimal gland enlargement also result. Associated signs and symptoms include bleeding tendency, fever, arthralgia, pallor, weakness, hepatosplenomegaly and, possibly, lymphadenopathy.

◆ ***Lymphangioma.*** Hemorrhage of this congenital tumor causes unilateral or bilateral exophthalmos, among other signs.

◆ ***Neuroblastoma.*** This highly malignant tumor, the most common extracranial solid tumor of childhood, may produce exophthalmos.

◆ ***Ocular tuberculosis.*** Occasionally, this rare disease causes progressive exophthalmos accompanied by ptosis, painless eyelid edema and erythema, and enlarged lacrimal glands. Examination may reveal yellow or white fat deposits on the cornea and small white nodules in the iris.

◆ ***Optic nerve meningioma.*** This tumor usually produces unilateral exophthalmos and a swollen temple. Impaired visual acuity, visual field deficits, and headache may occur.

◆ ***Orbital cellulitis.*** Commonly the result of sinusitis, this ocular emergency causes sudden onset of unilateral exophthalmos, which may be mild or severe. Orbital cellulitis may also produce eye pain, conjunctival injection, tearing, eyelid edema and erythema, a purulent discharge, and limited extraocular movement as well as fever, headache, and malaise.

◆ ***Orbital choristoma.*** A common sign of this benign tumor, progressive exophthalmos may be associated with diplopia and blurred vision.

◆ ***Orbital emphysema.*** Air leaking from the sinus into the orbit usually causes unilateral exophthalmos. Palpation of the globe elicits crepitation.

◆ ***Orbital pseudotumor.*** Progressive unilateral exophthalmos characterizes this uncommon disorder. Limited extraocular movement, eyelid edema, eye pain, and diplopia may also occur.

◆ ***Parasite infestation.*** Usually, this disorder causes painless progressive exophthalmos in one eye that may spread to the other eye. Associated findings include limited extraocular movement, diplopia, eye pain, and impaired visual acuity.

◆ ***Scleritis (posterior).*** Gradual onset of mild to severe unilateral exophthalmos is common in scleritis. Other signs and symptoms include severe eye pain, diplopia, papilledema, limited extraocular movement, and impaired visual acuity.

◆ ***Thyrotoxicosis.*** Although a classic sign of this disorder, exophthalmos is absent in many patients. It's usually bilateral, progressive, and severe. Associated ocular features include ptosis, increased tearing, lid lag and edema, photophobia, conjunctival injection, diplopia, and decreased visual acuity. Other findings include an enlarged thyroid, nervousness, heat intolerance, weight loss despite increased appetite, sweating, diarrhea, tremors, palpitations, and tachycardia.

Special considerations

Exophthalmos usually makes the patient self-conscious, so provide privacy and emotional support. Protect the affected eye from trauma, especially drying of the cornea. However, *never* place a gauze eye pad or other object over the affected eye; removal could damage the corneal epithelium. If a slit-lamp examination is indicated, explain the procedure to the patient. If necessary, refer him to an ophthalmologist for a complete examination. The cause of exophthalmos determines the therapy. Prepare the patient for blood tests, such as a thyroid panel and a white blood cell count.

Pediatric pointers

In children around age 5, a rare tumor—optic nerve glioma—may cause exophthalmos. Rhabdomyosarcoma, a more common tumor, usually affects children between ages 4 and 12 and produces rapid onset of exophthalmos. In Hand-Schüller-Christian syndrome, exophthalmos typically accompanies signs of diabetes insipidus and bone destruction.

Eye discharge

Usually associated with conjunctivitis, an eye discharge is the excretion of any substance other than tears. This common sign may occur in one or both eyes, producing scant to copious discharge. The discharge may be purulent, frothy, mucoid, cheesy, serous, clear, or white and stringy. Sometimes, the discharge can be expressed by applying pressure to the tear sac, punctum, meibomian glands, or canaliculi.

An eye discharge commonly results from inflammatory and infectious eye disorders but may also occur in certain systemic disorders. (See *Sources of eye discharge*.) Because this sign may accompany a disorder that threatens vision, it must be assessed and treated immediately.

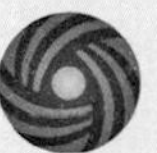

EXAMINATION TIP

Sources of eye discharge

An eye discharge can come from the tear sac, punctum, meibomian glands, or canaliculi. If the patient reports a discharge that isn't immediately apparent, you can express a sample by pressing your fingertip lightly over these structures. Then characterize the discharge, and note its source.

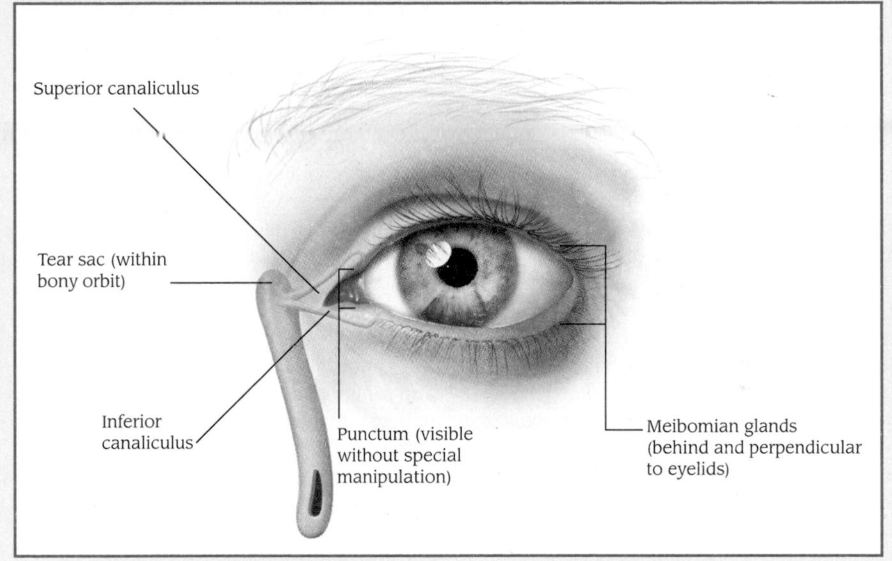

History and physical examination

Begin your evaluation by finding out when the discharge began. Does it occur at certain times of day or in connection with certain activities? If the patient complains of pain, ask him to show you its exact location and to describe its character. Is the pain dull, continuous, sharp, or stabbing? Do his eyes itch or burn? Do they tear excessively? Are they sensitive to light? Does he feel like something is in them?

After taking vital signs, carefully inspect the eye discharge. Note its amount, color, and consistency. Then test visual acuity, with and without correction. Examine external eye structures, beginning with the unaffected eye to prevent cross-contamination. Observe for eyelid edema, entropion, crusts, lesions, and trichiasis. Next, ask the patient to blink as you watch for impaired eyelid movement. If the eyes seem to bulge, measure them with an exophthalmometer. Test the six cardinal fields of gaze. Examine the eye for conjunctival injection and follicles and for corneal cloudiness or white lesions.

Medical causes

◆ ***Canaliculitis.*** This uncommon chronic disorder causes a scant purulent discharge, usually from the lower canaliculus of one eye. The eye is red and irritated, and its punctum bulges a bit.

◆ ***Conjunctivitis.*** Five types of conjunctivitis may cause an eye discharge with redness, hyperemia, foreign-body sensation, periocular edema, and tearing.

In *allergic conjunctivitis,* a bilateral ropey discharge is accompanied by itching and tearing.

Bacterial conjunctivitis causes a moderate purulent or mucopurulent discharge that may form sticky crusts on the eyelids during sleep. The discharge is commonly greenish white and usually occurs in one eye. The patient may also experience itching, burning, excessive tearing, and the sensation of a foreign body in the eye. Eye pain indicates corneal involvement. Preauricular adenopathy is uncommon.

Viral conjunctivitis, which is more common than the bacterial form, usually produces a serous, clear discharge and preauricular adenopathy. The history includes a runny nose, an upper respiratory tract infection, or recent contact with a person who had these signs. Onset is usually unilateral.

Fungal conjunctivitis produces a copious, thick, purulent discharge that makes the eyelids crusty and sticky. Also characteristic are eyelid edema, itching, burning, and tearing. Pain and photophobia occur only with corneal involvement.

Inclusion conjunctivitis causes a scant mucoid discharge—especially in the morning—in both eyes, accompanied by pseudoptosis and conjunctival follicles.

◆ ***Corneal ulcers.*** Both bacterial and fungal ulcers produce a copious, purulent unilateral eye discharge and crusty, sticky eyelids. Severe pain, photophobia, and impaired visual acuity may also occur.

Bacterial corneal ulcers are also characterized by an irregular gray-white area on the cornea, blurred vision, unilateral pupil constriction, and conjunctival injection.

Fungal corneal ulcers are also characterized by conjunctival injection and eyelid edema and erythema. A painless, dense, whitish gray central ulcer develops slowly and may be surrounded by progressively clearer rings.

◆ ***Dacryoadenitis.*** This disorder may cause a moderate purulent discharge associated with temporal eye pain, conjunctival injection, and severe eyelid edema and erythema. However, its most characteristic sign is unilateral exophthalmos.

◆ ***Dacryocystitis.*** A lacrimal sac infection may produce a scant but continuous purulent discharge that's easily expressed from the tear sac. Additional signs and symptoms include excessive tearing, pain, and tenderness near the tear sac. Eyelid inflammation and edema are most noticeable around the lacrimal punctum.

◆ ***Erythema multiforme major (Stevens-Johnson syndrome).*** Ocular effects of this disorder include a purulent discharge, severe eye pain, entropion, trichiasis, photophobia, and decreased tear formation. Also typical are erythematous, urticarial, bullous lesions that suddenly erupt over the skin.

◆ ***Herpes zoster ophthalmicus.*** This disorder yields a moderate to copious serous eye discharge accompanied by excessive tearing. Examination reveals eyelid edema and erythema, conjunctival injection, and a white, cloudy cornea. The patient also complains of eye pain and severe unilateral facial pain that occurs several days before vesicles erupt.

◆ ***Keratoconjunctivitis sicca.*** Better known as dry eye syndrome, this disorder typically causes a copious and continuous mucoid discharge and insufficient tearing. Accompanying signs and symptoms include eye pain, itching, burning, a foreign-body sensation, and dramatic conjunctival injection. The patient may also have difficulty closing his eyes.

◆ ***Meibomianitis.*** In this disorder, applying pressure on the meibomian glands may produce a continuous frothy, soft, foul-smelling, cheesy yellow eye discharge. The eyes also appear chronically red, with inflamed lid margins.

◆ ***Orbital cellulitis.*** Although exophthalmos is the most obvious sign of this disorder, a unilateral purulent eye discharge may also be present. Related findings include eyelid edema, conjunctival injection, orbital pain, impaired visual acuity, limited extraocular movement, headache, and fever.

◆ ***Pemphigus.*** This rare disorder may cause a thick, mucuslike discharge; eye pain, burning, and irritation; and blurred vision. Initially, the patient may develop unilateral or bilateral conjunctivitis that's unrelieved by treatment; later, entropion and, occasionally, corneal ulceration may occur.

◆ ***Psoriasis vulgaris.*** Usually, psoriasis vulgaris causes a substantial mucoid discharge in both eyes, accompanied by redness. The characteristic lesions it produces on the eyelids may extend into the conjunctivae, causing irritation, excessive tearing, and a foreign-body sensation.

◆ ***Trachoma.*** A bilateral eye discharge occurs in this disorder along with severe pain, excessive tearing, photophobia, eyelid edema, redness, and visible conjunctival follicles.

Special considerations

Apply warm soaks to soften crusts on the eyelids and lashes. Then gently wipe the eyes with a soft gauze pad. Carefully dispose of all used dressings, tissues, and cotton swabs to prevent the spread of infection. Also, be sure to sterilize ophthalmic equipment after use. Teach the patient how to avoid contaminating the unaffected eye.

Explain any ordered diagnostic tests, including culture and sensitivity studies to identify the infectious organism.

Pediatric pointers

The prophylactic eye medication (silver nitrate), no longer commonly used with neonates, causes eye irritation and discharge. In children, discharges usually result from eye trauma, eye infection, or upper respiratory tract infection.

PATIENT COUNSELING

Inform patients with bacterial or viral conjunctivitis that these disorders are contagious. Tell those with bacterial conjunctivitis to avoid contact with other people for 24 hours after receiving antibiotic treatment; not to share towels, pillows, or cosmetic eye products; and not to wear contact lenses until the conjunctivitis resolves. Tell patients with allergic conjunctivitis that this type of inflammation isn't contagious.

Eye pain

[Ophthalmalgia]

Eye pain may be described as a burning, throbbing, aching, or stabbing sensation in or around the eye. It may also be characterized as a foreign-body sensation. This sign varies from mild to severe; its duration and exact location provide clues to the causative disorder.

Eye pain usually results from corneal abrasion, but it may also be due to glaucoma or other eye disorders, trauma, and neurologic or systemic disorders. Any of these may stimulate nerve endings in the cornea or external eye, producing pain.

EMERGENCY INTERVENTIONS *If the patient's eye pain results from a chemical burn, remove contact lenses (if present) and irrigate the eye with at least 1 L of normal saline solution over 10 minutes. Evert the lids and wipe the fornices with a cotton-tipped applicator to remove any particles or chemicals. Eye pain from acute angle-closure glaucoma is an ocular emergency requiring immediate intervention to decrease intraocular pressure (IOP). If drug treatment doesn't reduce IOP, the patient will need laser iridotomy or surgical peripheral iridectomy to save his vision.*

HISTORY AND PHYSICAL EXAMINATION

If the patient's eye pain doesn't result from a chemical burn or from acute angle-closure glaucoma, take a complete history. Have the patient describe the pain fully. Is it an ache or a sharp pain? How long does it last? Is it accompanied by burning, itching, or a discharge? Find out when it began. Is it worse in the morning or late in the evening? Ask about recent trauma or surgery, especially if the patient complains of severe pain that developed suddenly. Does he have headaches? If so, find out how often and at what time of day they occur.

During the physical examination, *don't* manipulate the eye if you suspect trauma. Carefully assess the eyelids and conjunctivae for redness, inflammation, and swelling. Then examine the eyes for ptosis or exophthalmos. Finally, test visual acuity with and without correction, and assess extraocular movements. Characterize any discharge. (See *Examining the external eye*, page 284.)

MEDICAL CAUSES

◆ ***Acute angle-closure glaucoma.*** Blurred vision and sudden excruciating pain in and around the eye characterize this disorder; the pain may be so severe that it causes nausea, vomiting, and abdominal pain. Other findings are halo vision, rapidly decreasing visual acuity, and a fixed, nonreactive, moderately dilated pupil.

◆ ***Astigmatism.*** Uncorrected astigmatism commonly causes headaches and eye fatigue, aching, and redness. This disorder occurs in both older and younger people.

◆ ***Blepharitis.*** Burning pain in both eyelids is accompanied by conjunctival injection and an itching, sticky discharge. Related findings include a foreign-body sensation, eyelid ulcerations, and loss of eyelashes.

◆ ***Burns.*** In chemical burns, sudden severe eye pain may occur with erythema and blistering of the face and eyelids, photophobia, miosis, conjunctival injection, blurring, and inability to keep the eyelids open. In ultraviolet radiation burns, moderate to severe pain occurs about 12 hours after exposure along with photophobia and vision changes.

◆ ***Chalazion.*** A chalazion causes localized tenderness and swelling on the upper or lower eyelid. Eversion of the lid reveals conjunctival injection and a small red lump.

◆ ***Conjunctivitis.*** Some degree of eye pain and excessive tearing occur in four types of conjunctivitis. *Allergic conjunctivitis* causes mild, burning, bilateral pain accompanied by itching, conjunctival injection, and a characteristic ropey discharge.

Bacterial conjunctivitis causes pain only when it affects the cornea. Otherwise, it typically produces burning, a foreign-body sensation, a purulent discharge, and conjunctival injection.

If the cornea is affected, *fungal conjunctivitis* may cause pain and photophobia. Without

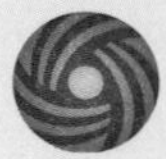

EXAMINATION TIP

Examining the external eye

For patients with eye pain or other ocular symptoms, examination of the external eye forms an important part of the ocular assessment. Here's how to examine the external eye.

First, inspect the eyelids for ptosis and incomplete closure. Also, observe the lids for edema, erythema, cyanosis, hematoma, and masses. Evaluate skin lesions, growths, swelling, and tenderness by gross palpation. Are the lids everted or inverted? Do the eyelashes turn inward? Have some of them been lost? Do the lashes adhere to one another or contain a discharge? Next, examine the lid margins, noting especially any debris, scaling, lesions, or unusual secretions. Also, watch for eyelid spasms.

Now gently retract the eyelid with your thumb and forefinger, and assess the conjunctiva for redness, cloudiness, follicles, and blisters or other lesions. Check for chemosis by pressing the lower lid against the eyeball and noting any bulging above this compression point. Observe the sclera, noting any change from its normal white color.

Next, shine a light across the cornea to detect scars, abrasions, or ulcers. Note any color changes, dots, or opaque or cloudy areas. Also, assess the anterior eye chamber, which should be clean, deep, shadow-free, and filled with clear aqueous humor.

Inspect the color, shape, texture, and pattern of the iris. Then assess the pupils' size, shape, and equality. Finally, evaluate their response to light. Are they sluggish, fixed, or unresponsive? Does pupil dilation or constriction occur only on one side?

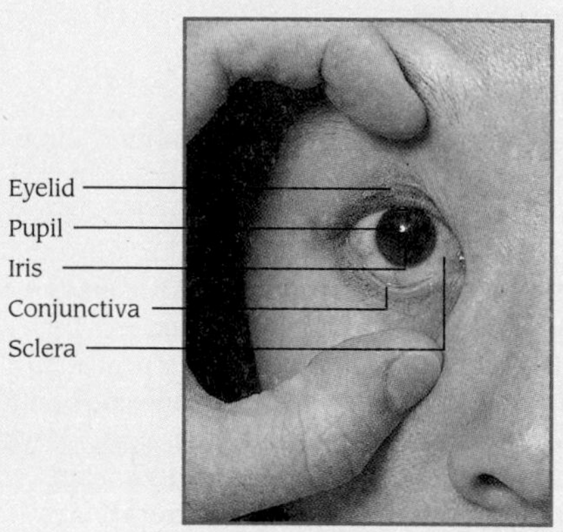

corneal involvement, it produces itching, burning eyes; a thick, purulent discharge; and conjunctival injection.

Viral conjunctivitis produces itching, red eyes; a foreign-body sensation; visible conjunctival follicles; and eyelid edema.

◆ ***Corneal abrasions.*** This type of injury typically produces a foreign-body sensation, excessive tearing, photophobia, and conjunctival injection.

◆ ***Corneal erosion (recurrent).*** In this disorder, severe pain occurs on waking and continues throughout the day. Accompanying the pain are conjunctival injection and photophobia.

◆ ***Corneal ulcers.*** Both bacterial and fungal corneal ulcers cause severe eye pain. They may also cause a purulent eye discharge, sticky eyelids, photophobia, and impaired visual acuity. In addition, bacterial corneal ulcers produce a grayish white, irregularly shaped ulcer on the cornea; unilateral pupil constriction; and conjunctival injection. Fungal corneal ulcers produce conjunctival injection, eyelid edema and erythema, and a dense, cloudy, central ulcer surrounded by progressively clearer rings.

◆ ***Dacryoadenitis.*** Temporal pain may affect both eyes in this disorder. Associated findings include exophthalmos, conjunctival injection, severe eyelid erythema and edema, and a purulent eye discharge.

◆ ***Dacryocystitis.*** Pain and tenderness near the tear sac characterize acute dacryocystitis. Additional signs include excessive tearing, a purulent discharge, eyelid erythema, and swelling around the lacrimal punctum.

◆ ***Episcleritis.*** Deep eye pain occurs as tissues over the sclera become inflamed. Related effects include photophobia, excessive tearing, conjunctival edema, and a red or purplish sclera.

◆ ***Erythema multiforme major.*** This disorder commonly produces severe eye pain, entropion, trichiasis, purulent conjunctivitis, photophobia, and decreased tear formation.

◆ ***Foreign bodies in the cornea and conjunctiva.*** Sudden severe pain is common in this condition, but vision usually remains intact.

Other findings include excessive tearing, photophobia, miosis, a foreign-body sensation, a dark speck on the cornea, and dramatic conjunctival injection.

◆ ***Glaucoma.*** Open-angle glaucoma may cause mild aching in the eyes as well as loss of peripheral vision, halo vision, and reduced visual acuity that isn't corrected by glasses. Acute angle-closure glaucoma may cause severe pain and pressure over the eye, blurred vision, halo vision, decreased visual acuity, and nausea and vomiting.

◆ ***Herpes zoster ophthalmicus.*** Eye pain occurs with severe unilateral facial pain, usually several days before vesicles erupt. Other signs include red, swollen eyelids; excessive tearing; a serous eye discharge; conjunctival injection; and a white, cloudy cornea.

◆ ***Hordeolum (stye).*** This lesion usually produces localized eye pain that increases as the stye grows. Eyelid erythema and edema are also common.

◆ ***Hyphema.*** Occurring after eye injury or surgery, hyphema accompanies sudden pain in and around the eye. Orbital and eyelid edema, conjunctival injection, and visual impairment may also occur.

◆ ***Interstitial keratitis.*** Associated with congenital syphilis, this corneal inflammation produces eye pain with photophobia, blurred vision, prominent conjunctival injection, and grayish pink corneas.

◆ ***Iritis (acute).*** Moderate to severe eye pain occurs with severe photophobia, dramatic conjunctival injection, and blurred vision. The constricted pupil may respond poorly to light.

◆ ***Keratoconjunctivitis sicca.*** This condition—known as dry eye syndrome—causes chronic burning pain in both eyes, itching, a foreign-body sensation, photophobia, dramatic conjunctival injection, and difficulty moving the eyelids. A copious mucoid discharge and inadequate tearing are typical.

◆ ***Lacrimal gland tumor.*** This neoplastic lesion usually produces unilateral eye pain, impaired visual acuity, and some degree of exophthalmos.

◆ ***Migraine headache.*** Migraines can produce head pain so severe that the eyes also ache. Nausea, vomiting, blurred vision, and light and noise sensitivity may also occur.

◆ ***Ocular laceration and intraocular foreign bodies.*** Penetrating eye injuries usually cause mild to severe unilateral eye pain and impaired visual acuity. Eyelid edema, conjunctival injection, and an abnormal pupillary response may also occur.

◆ ***Optic cellulitis.*** This disorder causes dull, aching pain in the affected eye, some degree of exophthalmos, eyelid edema and erythema, a purulent discharge, impaired extraocular movement and, occasionally, decreased visual acuity and fever.

◆ ***Optic neuritis.*** In this disorder, pain in and around the eye occurs with eye movement. Severe vision loss and tunnel vision develop but improve in 2 to 3 weeks. Pupils respond sluggishly to direct light but normally to consensual light.

◆ ***Orbital floor fracture.*** Sometimes called a blowout fracture, this injury causes eye pain, dramatic eyelid edema and, possibly, enophthalmos and diplopia.

◆ ***Orbital pseudotumor.*** This disorder causes deep, boring eye pain and diplopia in about 50% of patients. However, prominent exophthalmos and lateral ocular deviation are more characteristic. Eyelid edema and limited extraocular movement may also occur.

◆ ***Pemphigus.*** In this disorder, bilateral eye pain and irritation may be accompanied by blurred vision and a thick discharge. Blisters may develop on the conjunctiva alone or may extend to the nasal, oral, and vulvar mucous membranes as well as the skin.

◆ ***Scleritis.*** This inflammation produces severe eye pain and tenderness, conjunctival injection, bluish purple sclera and, possibly, photophobia and excessive tearing.

◆ ***Sclerokeratitis.*** Inflammation of the sclera and cornea causes pain, burning, irritation, and photophobia.

◆ ***Subdural hematoma.*** Following head trauma, a subdural hematoma commonly causes severe eye ache and headache. Related neurologic signs depend on the hematoma's location and size.

◆ ***Trachoma.*** Along with pain in the affected eye, trachoma causes excessive tearing, photophobia, an eye discharge, eyelid edema and erythema, and visible conjunctival follicles.

◆ ***Uveitis.*** Anterior uveitis causes sudden severe pain, dramatic conjunctival injection, photophobia, and a small, nonreactive pupil.

Posterior uveitis causes insidious onset of similar features, plus gradual blurring of vision and distorted pupil shape.

Lens-induced uveitis causes moderate eye pain, conjunctival injection, pupil constriction, and severely impaired visual acuity. In fact, the patient usually can perceive only light.

Other causes

◆ ***Treatments.*** Contact lenses may cause eye pain and a foreign-body sensation. Ocular surgery may also produce eye pain, ranging from a mild ache to a severe pounding or stabbing sensation.

Special considerations

To help ease eye pain, have the patient lie down in a darkened, quiet environment and close his eyes. Prepare him for diagnostic studies, including tonometry and orbital X-rays.

Pediatric pointers

Trauma and infection are the most common causes of eye pain in children. Be alert for nonverbal clues to pain, such as tightly shutting or frequently rubbing the eyes.

Geriatric pointers

Glaucoma, which can cause eye pain, usually affects older patients, becoming clinically significant after age 40. It usually occurs bilaterally and leads to slowly progressive vision loss, especially in peripheral visual fields.

Patient counseling

Tell the patient to seek medical help for eye pain, and stress the importance of meticulous compliance with drug therapy to prevent an increase in IOP.

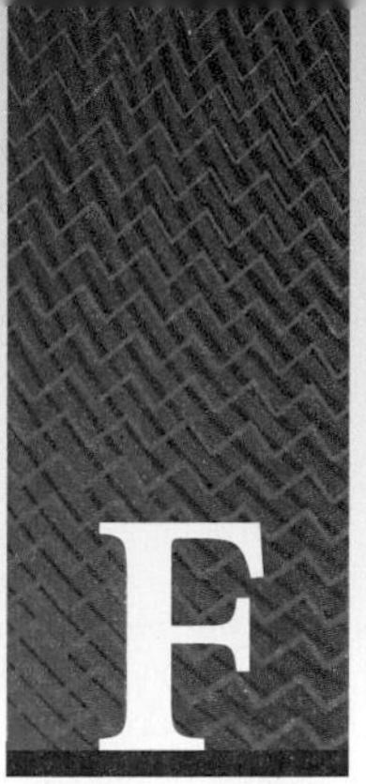

Facial pain

Facial pain may result from various neurologic, vascular, or infectious disorders. The most common cause of facial pain is trigeminal neuralgia (tic douloureux). In this disorder, intense, paroxysmal facial pain may occur along the pathway of a specific facial nerve or nerve branch, usually cranial nerve V (trigeminal nerve) or cranial nerve VII (facial nerve). Pain can also be referred to the face in disorders of the ear, nose, paranasal sinuses, teeth, neck, and jaw.

Atypical facial pain is a constant burning pain with limited distribution at onset; it typically spreads to the rest of the face and may involve the neck or back of the head as well. This type of facial pain is common in middle-aged women, especially those who are clinically depressed.

History and physical examination

Begin by characterizing the patient's facial pain. Is it stabbing, throbbing, or dull? When did it begin? How long has it lasted? What relieves or worsens it? Ask the patient to point to the painful area. If facial pain is recurrent, have him describe a typical episode. Review his medical and dental history, noting especially previous head trauma, dental disease, and infection.

Carefully examine the face and head. Inspect the ear for vesicles and changes in the tympanic membrane to rule out referred ear pain. Inspect the nose for deformity or asymmetry. Evaluate the condition of the mucous membranes and septum as well as the size and shape of the turbinates. Characterize any secretions. Palpate the frontal, ethmoid, and maxillary sinuses for tenderness and swelling.

Evaluate oral hygiene by inspecting the teeth for caries, percussing any diseased teeth for pain, and asking the patient about any sensitivity to hot, cold, or sweet liquids or foods. Have him open and close his mouth as you palpate the temporomandibular joint for tenderness, spasm, locking, and crepitus.

Examine the function of cranial nerves V and VII. To evaluate cranial nerve V, instruct the patient to clench his teeth. Then palpate the temporal and masseter muscles and evaluate muscle contraction. Test pain and sensation on his forehead, cheeks, and jaw. Next, test the corneal reflex by lightly touching the cornea with a piece of cotton.

To evaluate cranial nerve VII, inspect the face for symmetry and then have the patient perform facial movements that demonstrate facial muscle strength—raising his eyebrows, frowning, showing his teeth, closing his eyes tightly, and wrinkling his nose. (See *Major nerve pathways of the face,* page 288.)

Medical causes

◆ ***Angina pectoris.*** Occasionally, jaw pain may indicate angina pectoris. A more comprehensive history and evaluation is needed to determine cardiac origin.

◆ ***Dental caries.*** Caries in the mandibular molars can produce ear, preauricular, and temporal pain; caries in the maxillary teeth can produce

Major nerve pathways of the face

Cranial nerve V has three branches. The *ophthalmic branch* supplies sensation to the anterior scalp, forehead, upper nose, and cornea. The *maxillary branch* supplies sensation to the midportion of the face, lower nose, upper lip, and mucous membrane of the anterior palate. The *mandibular branch* supplies sensation to the lower face, lower jaw, mucous membrane of the cheek, and base of the tongue.

CRANIAL NERVE V

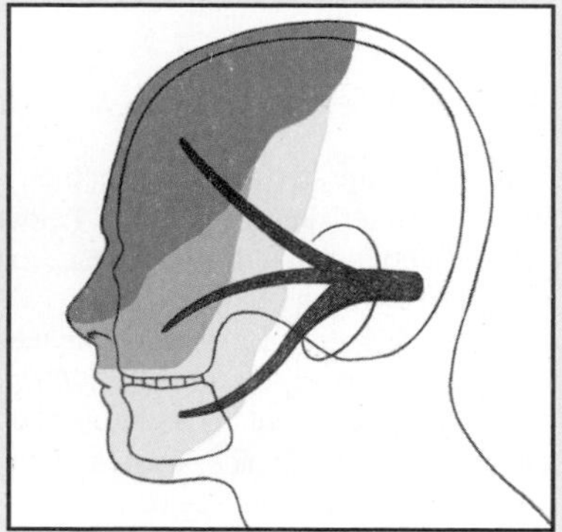

Cranial nerve VII innervates the facial muscles. Its motor branch controls the muscles of the forehead, eye orbit, and mouth.

CRANIAL NERVE VII

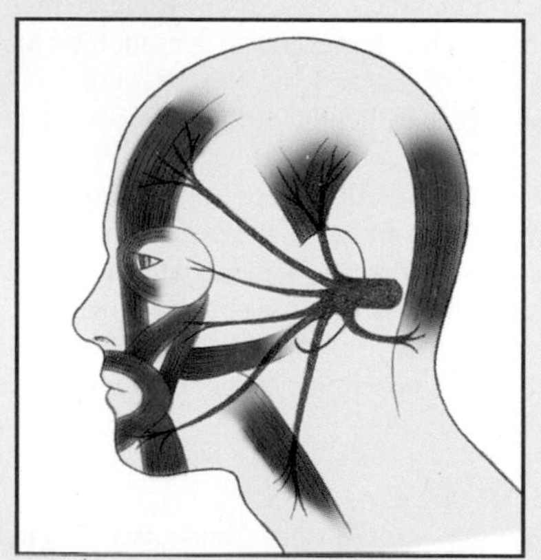

maxillary, orbital, retro-orbital, and parietal pain. Other dental causes of facial pain are an abnormal bite and faulty dentures. Facial pain related to chewing or temperature changes may suggest dental problems.

◆ ***Glaucoma.*** In glaucoma, an important cause of facial pain, the pain is usually located in the periorbital region.

◆ ***Glossopharyngeal neuralgia.*** The pain in this uncommon disorder is similar to that of trigeminal neuralgia. It typically occurs in the throat near the tonsillar fossa and may radiate to the ear and posterior aspect of the tongue. It may be aggravated by swallowing, chewing, talking, or yawning. No underlying structural abnormality is usually present.

◆ ***Herpes zoster oticus (Ramsay Hunt syndrome).*** This disorder causes severe pain around the ear, followed by vesicles in the ear and occasionally on the oral mucosa, tonsils, and posterior tongue. Other findings may include hearing loss, vertigo, and transient ipsilateral facial paralysis.

◆ ***Multiple sclerosis (MS).*** Facial pain in MS may resemble that of trigeminal neuralgia and is accompanied by jaw and facial weakness. Other common findings include visual blurring, diplopia, and nystagmus; sensory impairment such as paresthesia; generalized muscle weakness and gait abnormalities; urinary disturbances; and emotional lability.

◆ ***Postherpetic neuralgia.*** Burning, itching, prickly pain persists along any of the three trigeminal nerve divisions and worsens with contact or movement. Mild hypoesthesia or paresthesia and vesicles affect the area before the onset of pain.

◆ ***Sinus cancer.*** In ethmoid sinus cancer, facial pain is a late symptom, preceded by exophthalmos. In maxillary sinus cancer, persistent pain along the second division of cranial nerve V is a late symptom.

◆ ***Sinusitis (acute).*** *Acute maxillary sinusitis* produces unilateral or bilateral pressure, fullness, or burning pain over the cheekbone and upper teeth and around the eyes. Bending over increases the pain. Other findings include nasal congestion and purulent discharge; red, swollen nasal mucosa; tenderness and swelling over the cheekbone; fever; and malaise.

Acute frontal sinusitis commonly produces severe pain above or around the eyes, which worsens when the patient is in a supine position. It also causes nasal obstruction, inflamed nasal mucosa, fever, and tenderness and swelling above the eyes.

Acute ethmoid sinusitis produces pain at or around the inner corner of the eye and sometimes temporal headaches. Other findings include nasal congestion, purulent rhinorrhea, fever, and tenderness at the medial edge of the eye.

In *acute sphenoid sinusitis,* a deep-seated pain persists behind the eyes or nose or on the top of the head. The pain increases on bending forward and may be accompanied by fever.

◆ ***Sinusitis (chronic).*** *Chronic maxillary sinusitis* produces a feeling of pressure below the eyes or a chronic toothache. Discomfort typically worsens throughout the day. Nasal congestion and tenderness over the cheekbone are usually mild.

Chronic frontal sinusitis produces a persistent low-grade pain above the eyes. The patient usually has a history of trauma or long-standing inflammation.

Chronic ethmoid sinusitis is characterized by nasal congestion, an intermittent purulent nasal discharge, and low-grade discomfort at the medial corners of the eyes. Also common are recurrent sore throat, halitosis, ear fullness, and involvement of the other sinuses.

A low-grade, diffuse headache or retro-orbital discomfort is common in *chronic sphenoid sinusitis.*

◆ ***Sphenopalatine neuralgia.*** In this type of neuralgia, unilateral deep, boring pain occurs below the ear and may radiate to the eye, ear, cheek, nose, palate, maxillary teeth, temple, back of the head, neck, or shoulder. Attacks also cause increased tearing and salivation, rhinorrhea, a sensation of fullness in the ear, tinnitus, vertigo, taste disturbances, pruritus, and shoulder stiffness or weakness.

◆ ***Temporal arteritis.*** Unilateral pain occurs behind the eye or in the scalp, jaw, tongue, or neck. A typical episode consists of a severe throbbing or boring temporal headache with redness, swelling, and nodulation of the temporal artery.

◆ ***Temporomandibular joint syndrome.*** In this syndrome, intermittent pain, usually unilateral, is described as a severe, dull ache or an intense spasm that radiates to the cheek, temple, lower jaw, ear, or mastoid area. Associated findings include trismus, malocclusion, and clicking, crepitus, and tenderness in the temporomandibular joint.

◆ ***Trigeminal neuralgia.*** Paroxysms of intense pain, lasting up to 15 minutes, shoot along any or all of the three branches of the trigeminal nerve. The pain can be triggered by touching the nose, cheek, or mouth; by being exposed to hot or cold weather; by consuming hot or cold foods or beverages; or even by smiling or talking. Between attacks, the pain may diminish to a dull ache or may disappear. This disorder is most common in middle and later life, affecting more women than men.

SPECIAL CONSIDERATIONS

Prepare the patient for diagnostic tests, such as sinus, skull, or dental X-rays; sinus transillumination; and intracranial or sinus computed tomography scans. Give pain medications, and apply direct heat or administer a muscle relaxant to ease muscle spasms. Provide a humidifier, vaporizer, or decongestant to relieve nasal or sinus congestion.

PEDIATRIC POINTERS

Facial pain may be difficult to assess in a young child if his language skills aren't sufficiently developed for him to describe the pain. Be alert for subtle signs of pain, such as facial rubbing, irritability, or poor eating habits.

PATIENT COUNSELING

If appropriate, instruct the patient with trigeminal neuralgia to avoid stressful situations, hot and cold foods, and sudden jarring movements, which can trigger painful attacks.

Fasciculations

Fasciculations are local muscle contractions representing the spontaneous discharge of a muscle fiber bundle innervated by a single motor nerve filament. These contractions cause visible dimpling or wavelike twitching of the skin, but they aren't strong enough to cause a joint to move. Their frequency ranges from once every several seconds to two or three times per second; occasionally, myokymia—continuous, rapid fasciculations that cause a rippling effect—may occur. Because fasciculations are brief and painless, they commonly go undetected or are ignored.

Benign, nonpathologic fasciculations are common and normal. They often occur in tense, anxious, or overtired people and typically affect the eyelid, thumb, or calf. However, fasciculations may also indicate a severe neurologic disorder, most notably a diffuse motor neuron disorder that causes loss of control over muscle fiber discharge. They're also an early sign of pesticide poisoning.

EMERGENCY INTERVENTIONS *Begin by asking the patient about the nature, onset, and duration of the fasciculations. If the onset was sudden, ask about any precipitating events, such as exposure to pesticides. Pesticide poisoning, although uncommon, is a medical emergency requiring prompt and vigorous intervention. You may need to maintain airway patency, monitor vital signs, give oxygen, and perform gastric lavage or induce vomiting.*

HISTORY AND PHYSICAL EXAMINATION

If the patient isn't in severe distress, find out if he has experienced any sensory changes, such as paresthesia, or any difficulty speaking, swallowing, breathing, or controlling bowel or bladder function. Ask him if he's in pain.

Explore the patient's medical history for neurologic disorders, cancer, and recent infections. Also, ask him about his lifestyle, especially stress at home, on the job, or at school.

Ask the patient about his dietary habits and for a recall of his food and fluid intake in the recent past because electrolyte imbalances may also cause muscle twitching.

Perform a physical examination, looking for fasciculations while the affected muscle is at rest. Observe and test for motor and sensory abnormalities, particularly muscle atrophy and weakness, and decreased deep tendon reflexes. If you note these signs and symptoms, suspect motor neuron disease, and perform a comprehensive neurologic examination.

MEDICAL CAUSES

◆ ***Amyotrophic lateral sclerosis.*** In this progressive motor neuron disease, coarse fasciculations usually begin in the small muscles of the hands and feet, and then spread to the forearms and legs. Widespread, symmetrical muscle atrophy and weakness may result in dysarthria; difficulty chewing, swallowing, and breathing; and, occasionally, choking and drooling.

◆ ***Bulbar palsy.*** Fasciculations of the face and tongue commonly appear early in bulbar palsy. Progressive signs and symptoms include dysarthria, dysphagia, hoarseness, and drooling. Eventually, weakness spreads to the respiratory muscles.

◆ ***Guillain-Barré syndrome.*** Fasciculations may occur in Guillain-Barré syndrome, but the cardinal neurologic symptom is muscle weakness, which typically begins in the legs and spreads quickly to the arms and face. Other findings include paresthesia, incontinence, footdrop, tachycardia, dysphagia, and respiratory insufficiency.

◆ ***Herniated disk.*** Fasciculations of the muscles innervated by compressed nerve roots may be widespread and profound, but the hallmark of a herniated disk is severe low back pain that may radiate unilaterally to the leg. Coughing, sneezing, bending, and straining exacerbate the pain. Related effects include muscle weakness, atrophy, and spasms; paresthesia; footdrop; steppage gait; and hypoactive deep tendon reflexes in the leg.

◆ ***Poliomyelitis (spinal paralytic).*** Coarse fasciculations, usually transient but occasionally persistent, accompany progressive muscle weakness, spasms, and atrophy in this disorder. The patient may also exhibit decreased reflexes, paresthesia, coldness and cyanosis in the affected limbs, bladder paralysis, dyspnea, elevated blood pressure, and tachycardia.

◆ ***Spinal cord tumor.*** Fasciculations, muscle atrophy, and cramps may develop asymmetrically at first and then bilaterally as cord compression progresses. Motor and sensory changes distal to the tumor include weakness or paralysis, areflexia, paresthesia, and a tightening band of pain. Bowel and bladder control may be lost.

◆ ***Syringomyelia.*** In this disorder, fasciculations may occur along with Charcot's joints, areflexia, muscle atrophy, and deep, aching pain. Additional findings include thoracic scoliosis and loss of pain and temperature sensation over the neck, shoulders, and arms.

OTHER CAUSES

◆ ***Pesticide poisoning.*** Ingestion of organophosphate or carbamate pesticides commonly produces acute onset of long, wavelike fasciculations and muscle weakness that rapidly progresses to flaccid paralysis. Other common effects include nausea, vomiting, diarrhea, loss of bowel and bladder control, hyperactive bowel sounds, and abdominal cramping. Cardiopulmonary findings include bradycardia, dyspnea or bradypnea, and pallor or cyanosis. Seizures, vision disturbances (pupillary constriction or blurred vision), and increased secretions (tearing, salivation, pulmonary secretions, or diaphoresis) may also occur.

SPECIAL CONSIDERATIONS

Prepare the patient for diagnostic studies, such as spinal X-rays, myelography, computed tomography scan, magnetic resonance imaging, and electromyography with nerve conduction velocity tests. Prepare the patient for laboratory tests such as serum electrolyte levels. Help the patient with progressive neuromuscular degeneration perform activities of daily living, and provide appropriate assistive devices.

PEDIATRIC POINTERS

Fasciculations, particularly of the tongue, are an important early sign of Werdnig-Hoffmann disease.

PATIENT COUNSELING

Teach effective stress management techniques to the patient with stress-induced fasciculations.

Fatigue

Fatigue is a feeling of excessive tiredness, lack of energy, or exhaustion accompanied by a strong desire to rest or sleep. This common symptom is distinct from weakness, which involves the muscles, but may accompany it.

Fatigue is a normal and important response to physical overexertion, prolonged emotional stress, and sleep deprivation. However, it can also be a nonspecific symptom of a psychological or physiologic disorder, especially viral or bacterial infection and endocrine, cardiovascular, or neurologic disease.

Fatigue reflects both hypermetabolic and hypometabolic states in which nutrients needed for cellular energy and growth are lacking because of overly rapid depletion, impaired replacement mechanisms, insufficient hormone production, or inadequate nutrient intake or metabolism.

HISTORY AND PHYSICAL EXAMINATION

Obtain a careful history to identify the patient's fatigue pattern. Fatigue that worsens with activity and improves with rest generally indicates a physical disorder; the opposite pattern, a psychological disorder. Fatigue lasting longer than 4 months, constant fatigue that's unrelieved by rest, and transient exhaustion that quickly gives way to bursts of energy are findings associated with psychological disorders.

Ask about related symptoms and any recent viral or bacterial illness or stressful changes in lifestyle. Explore nutritional habits and any appetite or weight changes. Carefully review the patient's medical and psychiatric history for any chronic disorders that commonly produce fatigue, and ask about a family history of such disorders.

Obtain a thorough drug history, noting use of any narcotic or drug with fatigue as an adverse effect. Ask about alcohol and drug use patterns. Determine the patient's risk of carbon monoxide poisoning, and ask whether the patient has a carbon monoxide detector.

Observe the patient's general appearance for overt signs of depression or organic illness. Is he unkempt or expressionless? Does he appear tired or sickly, or have a slumped posture? If warranted, evaluate his mental status, noting especially mental clouding, attention deficits, agitation, or psychomotor retardation.

MEDICAL CAUSES

◆ ***Acquired immunodeficiency syndrome.*** Besides fatigue, this syndrome may cause fever, night sweats, weight loss, diarrhea, and a cough, followed by several concurrent opportunistic infections.

◆ ***Adrenocortical insufficiency.*** Mild fatigue, the hallmark of this disorder, initially appears after exertion and stress but later becomes more severe and persistent. Weakness and weight loss typically accompany GI disturbances, such as nausea, vomiting, anorexia, abdominal pain, and chronic diarrhea; hyperpigmentation; orthostatic hypotension; and a weak, irregular pulse.

◆ ***Anemia.*** Fatigue after mild activity is commonly the first symptom of anemia. Associated findings vary but generally include pallor, tachycardia, and dyspnea.

◆ ***Anxiety.*** Chronic, unremitting anxiety invariably produces fatigue, often characterized as nervous exhaustion. Other persistent findings include apprehension, indecisiveness, restlessness, insomnia, trembling, and increased muscle tension.

◆ ***Cancer.*** Unexplained fatigue is commonly the earliest sign of cancer. Related findings reflect the type, location, and stage of the tumor and typically include pain, nausea, vomiting, anorexia, weight loss, abnormal bleeding, and a palpable mass.

◆ ***Chronic fatigue syndrome.*** This syndrome, whose cause is unknown, is characterized by incapacitating fatigue. Other findings are sore throat, myalgia, and cognitive dysfunction.

◆ ***Chronic obstructive pulmonary disease.*** The earliest and most persistent symptoms of this disease are progressive fatigue and dyspnea. The patient may also experience a chronic and usually productive cough, weight loss, barrel chest, cyanosis, slight dependent edema, and poor exercise tolerance.

◆ ***Cirrhosis.*** Severe fatigue typically occurs late in this disorder, accompanied by weight loss, bleeding tendencies, jaundice, hepatomegaly, ascites, dependent edema, severe pruritus, and decreased level of consciousness.

◆ ***Cushing's syndrome (hypercortisolism).*** This disorder typically causes fatigue, related in part to accompanying sleep disturbances. Cardinal signs include truncal obesity with slender extremities, buffalo hump, moon face, purple striae, acne, and hirsutism; increased blood pressure and muscle weakness may also occur.

◆ ***Depression.*** Persistent fatigue unrelated to exertion nearly always accompanies chronic depression. Associated somatic complaints include headache, anorexia (occasionally, increased appetite), constipation, and sexual dysfunction. The patient may also experience insomnia, slowed speech, agitation or bradykinesia, irritability, loss of concentration, feelings of worthlessness, and persistent thoughts of death.

◆ ***Diabetes mellitus.*** Fatigue, the most common symptom of this disorder, may begin insidiously or abruptly. Related findings include weight loss, blurred vision, polyuria, polydipsia, and polyphagia.

◆ ***Heart failure.*** Persistent fatigue and lethargy characterize this disorder. Left-sided heart failure produces exertional and paroxysmal nocturnal dyspnea, orthopnea, and tachycardia. Right-sided heart failure produces jugular vein distention and possibly a slight but persistent nonproductive cough. In both types, later signs and symptoms include mental status changes, nausea, anorexia, weight gain and, possibly, oliguria. Cardiopulmonary findings include tachypnea, inspiratory crackles, palpitations and chest tightness, hypotension, narrowed pulse pressure, ventricular gallop, pallor, diaphoresis, clubbing, and dependent edema.

◆ ***Hypopituitarism.*** Fatigue, lethargy, and weakness usually develop slowly. Other insidious effects may include irritability, anorexia, amenorrhea or impotence, decreased libido, hypotension, dizziness, headache, visual disturbances, and cold intolerance.

◆ ***Hypothyroidism.*** Fatigue occurs early in this disorder along with forgetfulness, cold intolerance, weight gain, metrorrhagia, and constipation.

◆ ***Infection.*** Fatigue is commonly the most prominent symptom—and sometimes the only one—in a chronic infection. Low-grade fever and weight loss may accompany signs and symptoms that reflect the type and location of the infection, such as burning on urination or swollen, painful gums. Subacute bacterial endocarditis is an example of a chronic infection that causes fatigue and acute hemodynamic decompensation.

In an acute infection, brief fatigue typically accompanies headache, anorexia, arthralgia, chills, high fever, and such infection-specific signs as a cough, vomiting, or diarrhea.

◆ ***Influenza type A H1N1 virus (swine flu).*** Influenza type A H1N1, or swine flu, is a respiratory disease of pigs caused by type A influenza virus. Swine flu viruses cause high levels of illness and low death rates in pigs. Swine flu viruses normally don't infect humans. However, sporadic human infections with swine flu have occurred. Most commonly, these cases occur in persons with direct exposure to pigs. The virus has changed slightly and is known as H1N1 flu. Outbreaks of H1N1 flu in 2009 showed that the virus can be transmitted from person to person, causing transmission across the globe. The H1N1 flu is similar to influenza, and causes illness and in some cases death. The symptoms of swine flu include fatigue, fever, nonproductive cough, myalgia, chills, headache, and vomiting. The use of antiviral drugs is recommended to treat H1N1 flu.

◆ ***Lyme disease.*** Besides fatigue and malaise, signs and symptoms of this tick-borne disease include intermittent headache, fever, chills, an expanding red rash, and muscle and joint aches. Later, patients may develop arthritis, fluctuating meningoencephalitis, and cardiac abnormalities, such as a brief, fluctuating atrioventricular heart block.

◆ ***Malnutrition.*** Easy fatigability, lethargy, and apathy are common findings in patients with protein-calorie malnutrition. Patients may also exhibit weight loss, muscle wasting, sensations of coldness, pallor, edema, and dry, flaky skin.

◆ ***Methicillin-resistant* Staphylococcus aureus *(MRSA).*** MRSA is a strain of staphylococcus that's resistant to antibiotics commonly used to treat staphylococcal infections. The incidence of MRSA has greatly increased in recent years. This increase is thought to be related to the increase in antibiotic use in hospital and outpatient settings and the widespread use of hand sanitizers and disinfectants. Older adults and patients with compromised immune systems are at greatest risk for MRSA, although it's becoming more common in community settings. Patients with MRSA may have a variety of signs and symptoms (most commonly fatigue and fever), depending on where the infection is located.

◆ ***Myasthenia gravis.*** The cardinal symptoms of this disorder are easy fatigability and muscle weakness, which worsen as the day progresses. They also worsen with exertion and abate with rest. Related findings depend on the specific muscles affected.

◆ ***Myocardial infarction.*** Fatigue can be severe but is typically overshadowed by chest pain. Related findings include dyspnea, anxiety, pallor, cold sweats, increased or decreased blood pressure, and abnormal heart sounds.

◆ ***Narcolepsy.*** One or more of the following characterizes this disorder: hypersomnia, hypnagogic hallucinations, cataplexy, sleep paralysis, and insomnia. Fatigue is a common symptom as well.

◆ ***Popcorn lung disease.*** Popcorn lung disease occurs in factory workers who experience respiratory symptoms after inhaling butter flavoring chemicals such as diacetyl, used in the manufacture of microwave popcorn. The patient typically complains of gradual onset of a nonproductive cough that worsens over time, progressive shortness of breath, and unusual fatigue. Clinical findings include wheezing, chest pain, fever, night sweats, and weight loss. Bronchiolitis fibrosa obliterans, an irreversible fixed airway obstructive lung disorder, is the most severe condition reported.

◆ ***Renal failure.*** Acute renal failure commonly causes sudden fatigue, drowsiness, and lethargy. Oliguria, an early sign, is followed by severe systemic effects: ammonia breath odor, nausea, vomiting, diarrhea or constipation, and dry skin and mucous membranes. Neurologic findings include muscle twitching, personality changes, and altered level of consciousness, which may progress to seizures and coma.

Chronic renal failure produces insidious fatigue and lethargy along with marked changes in all body systems, including GI disturbances, ammonia breath odor, Kussmaul's respirations, bleeding tendencies, poor skin turgor, severe pruritus, paresthesia, visual disturbances, confusion, seizures, and coma.

◆ ***Restrictive lung disease.*** Chronic fatigue may accompany the characteristic signs and symptoms: dyspnea, cough, and rapid, shallow respirations. Cyanosis first appears with exertion; later, even at rest.

◆ ***Rheumatoid arthritis.*** Fatigue, weakness, and anorexia precede localized articular findings: joint pain, tenderness, warmth, and swelling along with morning stiffness.

◆ ***Systemic lupus erythematosus.*** Fatigue usually occurs along with generalized aching, malaise, low-grade fever, headache, and irritability. Primary signs and symptoms include joint pain and stiffness, butterfly rash, and photosensitivity. Also common are Raynaud's phenomenon, patchy alopecia, and mucous membrane ulcers.

◆ ***Thyrotoxicosis.*** In this disorder, fatigue may accompany characteristic signs and symptoms, including an enlarged thyroid, tachycardia and palpitations, tremors, weight loss despite increased appetite, diarrhea, dyspnea, nervousness, diaphoresis, heat intolerance, amenorrhea and, possibly, exophthalmos.

◆ ***Valvular heart disease.*** All types of valvular heart disease commonly produce progressive fatigue and a cardiac murmur. Additional signs and symptoms vary but generally include exertional dyspnea, cough, and hemoptysis.

◆ ***Vancomycin-resistant enterococci (VRE) infection.*** Enterococci are bacteria naturally present in the intestinal tract of all people; however, some strains of enterococci have become resistant to vancomycin. Serious VRE infections may occur in hospitalized patients with such comorbidities as cancer, kidney disease, or immune deficiencies. Elderly patients and those hospitalized for long periods are also at risk for developing VRE infections. Symptoms of VRE infection depend on where the infection is; patients with VRE infections may have diarrhea, fever, and fatigue.

◆ ***Vancomycin-resistant* Staphylococcus aureus *(VRSA).*** VRSA is a strain of staphylococcus that's resistant to vancomycin, an antibiotic commonly used to treat staphylococcal infections. Patients most susceptible to VRSA infections include those with diabetes, kidney disease, or previous infection with MRSA, and those with I.V. catheters. VRSA can be difficult to diagnose because of the patient's overlying medical problems. Patients with VRSA commonly complain of fatigue and fever that don't respond to treatment with vancomycin. VRSA is usually diagnosed when cultures are done to see why the patient isn't responding to vancomycin; after the patient is started on a different antibiotic, the infection improves.

Other causes

◆ ***Carbon monoxide poisoning.*** Fatigue occurs along with headache, dyspnea, and confusion; apnea and unconsciousness may occur eventually.

◆ ***Drugs.*** Fatigue may result from various drugs, notably antihypertensives and sedatives. In those receiving cardiac glycoside therapy, fatigue may indicate toxicity.

◆ ***Surgery.*** Most types of surgery cause temporary fatigue, probably from the combined effects of hunger, anesthesia, and sleep deprivation.

Special considerations

If fatigue results from organic illness, help the patient determine which daily activities he may need help with and how he should pace himself to ensure sufficient rest. You can help him reduce chronic fatigue by alleviating pain, which may interfere with rest, or nausea, which may lead to malnutrition. He may benefit from referral to a community health nurse or housekeeping service. If fatigue results from a psychogenic cause, refer him for psychological counseling.

Pediatric pointers

When evaluating a child for fatigue, ask his parents if they've noticed any change in his activity level. Fatigue without an organic cause occurs normally during accelerated growth phases in preschool-age and prepubescent children. However, psychological causes of fatigue must be considered; for example, a depressed child may try to escape problems at home or school by taking refuge in sleep. In the pubescent child, consider the possibility of drug abuse, particularly of hypnotics and tranquilizers.

Geriatric pointers

Always ask older patients about fatigue because this symptom may be insidious and mask more serious underlying conditions in this age-group. Temporal arthritis, which is much more common in people older than age 60, is usually characterized by fatigue, weight loss, jaw claudication, proximal muscle weakness, headache, visual disturbances, and associated anemia.

Patient counseling

Regardless of the cause of fatigue, you may need to help the patient alter his lifestyle to achieve a balanced diet, a program of regular exercise, and adequate rest. Counsel him about setting priorities, keeping a reasonable schedule, and developing good sleep habits. Teach stress management techniques as appropriate.

Fecal incontinence

Fecal incontinence, the involuntary passage of feces, follows any loss or impairment of external anal sphincter control. It can result from various GI, neurologic, and psychological disorders; the effects of drugs; or surgery. In some patients, it may even be a purposeful manipulative behavior.

Fecal incontinence may be temporary or permanent; its onset may be gradual, as in dementia, or sudden, as in spinal cord trauma. Although usually not a sign of severe illness, it can greatly affect the patient's physical and psychological well-being.

History and physical examination

Ask the patient with fecal incontinence about its onset, duration, and severity and about any discernible pattern—for example, at night or with diarrhea. Note the frequency, consistency, and volume of stools passed within the last 24 hours and obtain a stool specimen. Focus your history taking on GI, neurologic, and psychological disorders.

Let the history guide your physical examination. If you suspect a brain or spinal cord lesion, perform a complete neurologic examination. (See *Neurologic control of defecation*.) If a GI disturbance seems likely, inspect the abdomen for distention, auscultate for bowel sounds, and percuss and palpate for a mass. Inspect the anal area for signs of excoriation or infection. If not contraindicated, check for fecal impaction, which may be associated with incontinence.

Neurologic control of defecation

Three neurologic mechanisms normally regulate defecation: the intrinsic defecation reflex in the colon, the parasympathetic defecation reflex involving sacral segments of the spinal cord, and voluntary control. Here's how they interact.

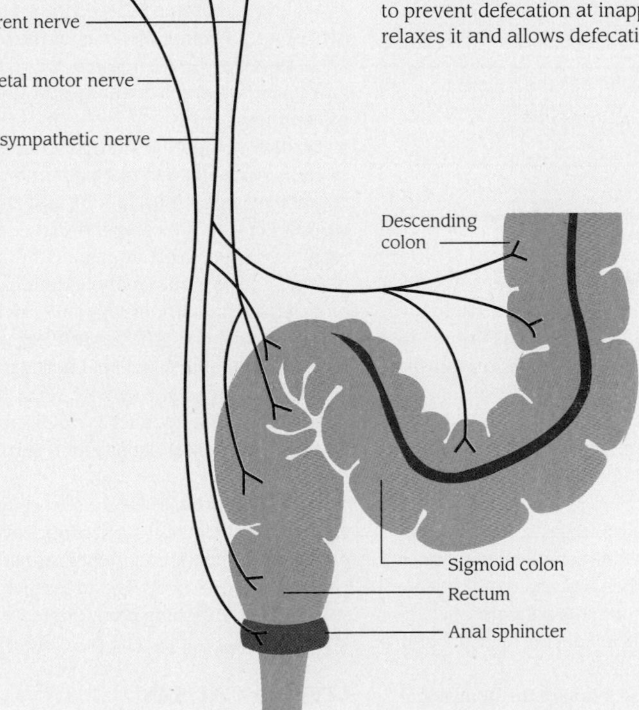

Fecal distention of the rectum activates the relatively weak intrinsic reflex, causing afferent impulses to spread through the myenteric plexus, initiating peristalsis in the descending and sigmoid colon and in the rectum. Subsequent movement of feces toward the anus causes receptive relaxation of the internal anal sphincter.

To ensure defecation, the parasympathetic reflex magnifies the intrinsic reflex. Stimulation of afferent nerves in the rectal wall propels impulses through the spinal cord and back to the descending and sigmoid colon, rectum, and anus to intensify peristalsis (see illustration).

However, fecal movement and internal sphincter relaxation cause immediate contraction of the external anal sphincter and temporary fecal retention. At this point, conscious control of the external sphincter either prevents or permits defecation. Except in infants or neurologically impaired patients, this voluntary mechanism further contracts the sphincter to prevent defecation at inappropriate times or relaxes it and allows defecation to occur.

Bowel retraining tips

You can help your patient control fecal incontinence by instituting a bowel retraining program. Here's how:

◆ Begin by establishing a specific time for defecation. A typical schedule is once a day or once every other day after a meal, usually breakfast. However, be flexible when establishing a schedule, and consider the patient's normal habits and preferences.

◆ If necessary, help ensure regularity by administering a suppository, either glycerin or bisacodyl, about 30 minutes before the scheduled defecation time. Avoid the routine use of enemas or laxatives because they can cause dependence.

◆ Provide privacy and a relaxed environment to encourage regularity. If "accidents" occur, assure the patient that they're normal and don't mean that he has failed in the program.

◆ Adjust the patient's diet to provide adequate bulk and fiber; encourage him to eat more raw fruits and vegetables and whole grains. Ensure a fluid intake of at least 1 qt (1 L)/day.

◆ If appropriate, encourage the patient to exercise regularly to help stimulate peristalsis.

◆ Be sure to keep accurate intake and elimination records.

Medical causes

◆ ***Dementia.*** Any chronic degenerative brain disease can produce fecal as well as urinary incontinence. Associated signs and symptoms include impaired judgment and abstract thinking, amnesia, emotional lability, hyperactive deep tendon reflexes (DTRs), aphasia or dysarthria and, possibly, diffuse choreoathetoid movements.

◆ ***Gastroenteritis.*** Severe gastroenteritis may result in temporary fecal incontinence manifested by explosive diarrhea. Nausea, vomiting, and colicky, peristaltic abdominal pain are typical. Other findings include headache, myalgia, and hyperactive bowel sounds.

◆ ***Head trauma.*** Disruption of the neurologic pathways that control defecation can cause fecal incontinence. Additional findings depend on the location and severity of the injury and may include decreased level of consciousness, seizures, vomiting, and a wide range of motor and sensory impairments.

◆ ***Inflammatory bowel disease.*** Nocturnal fecal incontinence occurs occasionally with diarrhea. Related findings include abdominal pain, anorexia, weight loss, blood in the stool, and hyperactive bowel sounds.

◆ ***Multiple sclerosis.*** Fecal incontinence occasionally appears as one of this disorder's extremely variable signs. Other effects depend on the area of demyelination and may include muscle weakness, ataxia, and paralysis; gait disturbances; sensory impairment, such as paresthesia and genital anesthesia; visual blurring, diplopia, or nystagmus; urinary disturbances; and emotional lability.

◆ ***Rectovaginal fistula.*** Fecal incontinence occurs in tandem with uninhibited passage of flatus.

◆ ***Spinal cord lesion.*** Any lesion that causes compression or transsection of sensorimotor spinal tracts can lead to fecal incontinence. Incontinence may be permanent, especially with severe lesions of the sacral segments. Other signs and symptoms reflect motor and sensory disturbances below the level of the lesion, such as urinary incontinence, weakness or paralysis, paresthesia, analgesia, and thermanesthesia.

◆ ***Stroke.*** Temporary fecal incontinence occasionally occurs in a stroke patient but usually disappears when muscle tone and DTRs are restored. Persistent fecal incontinence may reflect extensive neurologic damage. Other findings depend on the location and extent of damage and may include urinary incontinence, hemiplegia, dysarthria, aphasia, sensory losses, reflex changes, and visual field deficits. Typical generalized signs and symptoms include headache, vomiting, nuchal rigidity, fever, disorientation, mental impairment, seizures, and coma.

◆ ***Tabes dorsalis.*** This late sign of syphilis occasionally results in fecal incontinence. It also produces urinary incontinence, ataxic gait, paresthesia, loss of DTRs and temperature sensation, severe flashing pain, Charcot's joints, Argyll Robertson pupils, and possibly impotence.

Other causes

◆ ***Drugs.*** Chronic laxative abuse may cause insensitivity to a fecal mass or loss of the colonic defecation reflex.

◆ ***Surgery.*** Pelvic, prostate, or rectal surgery occasionally produces temporary fecal incontinence. A colostomy or an ileostomy causes permanent or temporary fecal incontinence.

Special considerations
Maintain proper hygienic care, including control of foul odors. Also, provide emotional support for the patient because he may feel deep embarrassment. For the patient with intermittent or temporary fecal incontinence, encourage Kegel exercises to strengthen abdominal and perirectal muscles. (See *How to do Kegel exercises,* page 232.) For the neurologically capable patient with chronic incontinence, provide bowel retraining. (See *Bowel retraining tips.*)

Pediatric pointers
Fecal incontinence is normal in infants and may occur temporarily in young children who experience stress-related psychological regression or a physical illness associated with diarrhea. Pediatric fecal incontinence can also result from myelomeningocele.

Geriatric pointers
Fecal incontinence is an important factor when long-term care is considered for an elderly patient. Leakage of liquid fecal material is especially common in males. Age-related changes affecting smooth-muscle cells of the colon may change GI motility and lead to fecal incontinence. Before age is determined to be the cause, however, any pathology must be ruled out.

Fetor hepaticus

Fetor hepaticus—a distinctive musty, sweet breath odor—characterizes hepatic encephalopathy, a life-threatening complication of severe liver disease. The odor results from the damaged liver's inability to metabolize and detoxify mercaptans produced by bacterial degradation of methionine, a sulfurous amino acid. These substances circulate in the blood, are expelled by the lungs, and flavor the breath.

EMERGENCY INTERVENTIONS *If you detect fetor hepaticus, quickly determine the patient's level of consciousness. If he's comatose, evaluate his respiratory status. Prepare to intubate him and provide ventilatory support if necessary. Start a peripheral I.V. catheter for fluid administration, begin cardiac monitoring, and insert an indwelling urinary catheter to monitor output. Obtain arterial and venous samples for analysis of blood gases, ammonia, and electrolytes.*

History and physical examination
If the patient is conscious, closely observe him for signs of impending coma. Evaluate deep tendon reflexes, and test for asterixis and Babinski's reflex. Be alert for signs of GI bleeding and shock, common complications of end-stage liver failure. Also, watch for increased anxiety, restlessness, tachycardia, tachypnea, hypotension, oliguria, hematemesis, melena, or cool, moist, pale skin. Place the patient in a supine position with the head of the bed at 30 degrees. Administer oxygen if necessary, and determine the patient's need for I.V. fluids for albumin replacement. Draw blood samples for liver function tests, serum electrolyte levels, hepatitis panel, blood alcohol count, a complete blood count, typing and crossmatching, a clotting profile, and ammonia level. Intubation, ventilation, or cardiopulmonary resuscitation may be necessary. Evaluate the degree of jaundice and abdominal distention, and palpate the liver to assess the degree of enlargement.

Obtain a complete medical history, relying on the patient's family if necessary. Focus on any factors that may have precipitated liver disease or coma, such as a recent severe infection; overuse of sedatives, analgesics, (especially acetaminophen), alcohol, or diuretics; excessive protein intake; or recent blood transfusion, surgery, or GI bleeding.

Medical causes
◆ ***Hepatic encephalopathy.*** Fetor hepaticus usually occurs in the final, comatose stage of this disorder but it may occur earlier. Tremors progress to asterixis in the impending stage, which is also marked by lethargy, aberrant behavior, and apraxia. Hyperventilation and stupor mark the stuporous stage, during which the patient acts agitated when aroused. Seizures and coma herald the final stage, along with decreased pulse and respiratory rates, positive Babinski's reflex, hyperactive reflexes, decerebrate posture, and opisthotonos.

Special considerations
Effective treatment of hepatic encephalopathy reduces blood ammonia levels by eliminating ammonia from the GI tract. You may have to administer neomycin or lactulose to suppress bacterial production of ammonia, give sorbitol solution to induce osmotic diarrhea, give potassium supplements to correct alkalosis, provide continuous gastric aspiration of blood, or

maintain the patient on a low-protein diet. If these methods prove unsuccessful, hemodialysis or exchange transfusions may be performed.

During treatment, closely monitor the patient's level of consciousness, intake and output, and fluid and electrolyte balance.

Pediatric pointers

A child who is slipping into a hepatic coma may cry, be disobedient, or become preoccupied with an activity.

Geriatric pointers

Along with fetor hepaticus, elderly patients with hepatic encephalopathy may exhibit disturbances of awareness and mentation, such as forgetfulness and confusion.

Patient counseling

Advise the patient to restrict his intake of dietary protein to as little as 40 g/day. Recommend that he eat vegetable protein rather than animal protein sources. Inform the patient that medications used to treat and prevent hepatic encephalopathy do so by causing diarrhea, so he shouldn't stop taking the drug when diarrhea occurs.

Fever

[Pyrexia]

Fever is a common sign that can arise from numerous disorders. Because these disorders can affect virtually any body system, fever in the absence of other signs usually has little diagnostic significance. A persistent high fever, though, represents an emergency.

Fever can be classified as low (oral reading of 99° to 100.4° F [37.2° to 38° C]), moderate (100.5° to 104° F [38.1° to 40° C]), or high (above 104° F). Fever over 106° F (41.1° C) causes unconsciousness and, if sustained, leads to permanent brain damage.

Fever may also be classified as remittent, intermittent, sustained, relapsing, or undulant. *Remittent fever,* the most common type, is characterized by daily temperature fluctuations above the normal range. *Intermittent fever* is marked by a daily temperature drop into the normal range and then a rise back to above normal. An intermittent fever that fluctuates widely, typically producing chills and sweating, is called *hectic* (or *septic*) *fever. Sustained fever* involves persistent temperature elevation with little fluctuation. *Relapsing fever* consists of alternating feverish and afebrile periods. *Undulant fever* refers to a gradual increase in temperature that stays high for a few days and then decreases gradually.

Fever can be either brief (less than 3 weeks) or prolonged. Prolonged fevers include fever of unknown origin, a classification used when careful examination fails to detect an underlying cause.

EMERGENCY INTERVENTIONS *If you detect a fever higher than 106° F (41.1° C), take the patient's other vital signs and determine his level of consciousness (LOC). Administer an antipyretic and begin rapid cooling measures: Apply ice packs to the axillae and groin, give tepid sponge baths, or apply a cooling blanket. These methods may evoke a cooling response; to prevent this, constantly monitor the patient's rectal temperature.*

History and physical examination

If the patient's fever is only mild to moderate, ask him when it began and how high his temperature reached. Did the fever disappear, only to reappear later? Did he experience any other symptoms, such as chills, fatigue, or pain?

Obtain a complete medical history, noting especially immunosuppressive treatments or disorders, infection, trauma, surgery, diagnostic testing, and use of anesthesia or other medications. Ask about recent travel because certain diseases are endemic.

Let the history findings direct your physical examination. (See *Differential diagnosis: Fever,* pages 300 and 301.) Because fever can accompany diverse disorders, the examination may range from a brief evaluation of one body system to a comprehensive review of all systems. (See *How fever develops,* page 302.)

Medical causes

◆ ***Anthrax, cutaneous.*** In this disorder, the patient may experience a fever along with lymphadenopathy, malaise, and headache. After the bacterium *Bacillus anthracis* enters a cut or abrasion on the skin, the infection begins as a small, painless or pruritic macular or papular lesion resembling an insect bite. Within 1 to 2 days, the lesion develops into a vesicle and then into a painless ulcer with a characteristic black necrotic center.

◆ ***Anthrax, GI.*** After ingesting contaminated meat from an animal infected with the bacterium *Bacillus anthracis,* the patient experiences fever, anorexia, nausea, vomiting and, possibly, abdominal pain, severe bloody diarrhea, and hematemesis.

◆ ***Anthrax, inhalation.*** This acute infectious disease initially produces flulike signs and symptoms, including fever, chills, weakness, cough, and chest pain. The disease generally occurs in two stages with a period of recovery after the initial symptoms. The second stage develops abruptly and causes rapid deterioration marked by fever, dyspnea, stridor, and hypotension; death generally results within 24 hours.

◆ ***Avian influenza.*** Avian influenza, also known as bird flu, is an infection caused by viruses that originate in the intestines of wild birds but are highly contagious to domesticated birds, such as chickens, turkeys, and geese. Infected poultry and surfaces contaminated with infected bird excretions have recently led to human infections and deaths in several Asian countries. Fever is commonly an initial symptom of these viruses along with other conventional influenza symptoms, such as muscle aches, sore throat, and cough. Individuals infected with the most virulent avian virus, influenza A (H5N1), may develop pneumonia, acute respiratory distress, and other life-threatening complications.

◆ **Escherichia coli *O157:H7.*** Fever, bloody diarrhea, nausea, vomiting, and abdominal cramps occur after eating undercooked beef or other foods contaminated with this strain of bacteria. Children younger than age 5 and elderly patients may develop hemolytic uremic syndrome, which can ultimately lead to acute renal failure.

◆ ***Immune complex dysfunction.*** When present, fever usually remains low, although moderate elevations may accompany erythema multiforme. Fever may be remittent or intermittent, as in acquired immunodeficiency syndrome (AIDS) or systemic lupus erythematosus, or sustained, as in polyarteritis. As one of several vague, prodromal complaints (such as fatigue, anorexia, and weight loss), fever produces nocturnal diaphoresis and accompanies such associated signs and symptoms as diarrhea and a persistent cough (in AIDS) or morning stiffness (in rheumatoid arthritis). Other disease-specific findings include headache and vision loss (in temporal arteritis); pain and stiffness in the neck, shoulders, back, or pelvis (in ankylosing spondylitis and polymyalgia rheumatica); skin and mucous membrane lesions (in erythema multiforme); and urethritis with urethral discharge and conjunctivitis (in Reiter's syndrome).

◆ ***Infectious and inflammatory disorders.*** Fever ranges from low (in Crohn's disease or ulcerative colitis) to extremely high (in those with bacterial pneumonia, necrotizing fasciitis, Ebola virus or *Hantavirus* pulmonary syndrome). It may be remittent, as in infectious mononucleosis or otitis media; hectic (recurring daily with sweating, chills, and flushing), as in a lung abscess, influenza, or endocarditis; sustained, as in meningitis; or relapsing, as in malaria. Fever may arise abruptly, as in toxic shock syndrome or Rocky Mountain spotted fever, or insidiously, as in mycoplasmal pneumonia. In patients with hepatitis, fever may represent a disease prodrome; in those with appendicitis, it follows the acute stage. Its sudden late appearance with tachycardia, tachypnea, and confusion heralds life-threatening septic shock in patients with peritonitis or gram-negative bacteremia.

Associated signs and symptoms involve every system. The cyclic variations of hectic fever typically produce alternating chills and diaphoresis. General systemic complaints include weakness, anorexia, and malaise.

◆ ***Influenza type A H1N1 virus (swine flu).*** Influenza type A H1N1, or swine flu, is a respiratory disease of pigs caused by type A influenza virus. Swine flu viruses cause high levels of illness and low death rates in pigs. Swine flu viruses normally don't infect humans. However, sporadic human infections with swine flu have occurred. Most commonly, these cases occur in persons with direct exposure to pigs. The virus has changed slightly and is known as H1N1 flu. Outbreaks of H1N1 flu in 2009 showed that the virus can be transmitted from person to person, causing transmission across the globe. The H1N1 flu is similar to influenza, and causes illness and in some cases death. The symptoms of swine flu include fever, nonproductive cough, fatigue, myalgia, chills, headache, and vomiting. The use of antiviral drugs is recommended to treat H1N1 flu.

◆ ***Kawasaki syndrome.*** Fever, typically high and spiking, is the primary characteristic of this acute illness. The diagnosis of Kawasaki syndrome is confirmed when fever persists for 5 or more days (or until administration of I.V. gamma globulin if given before the fifth day) and is accompanied by other clinical signs, including conjunctival injection, erythema,

Differential diagnosis: Fever

History of present illness

Focused physical examination: All systems

Common signs and symptoms

- ◆ Fatigue
- ◆ Malaise
- ◆ Anorexia

Thermoregulatory dysfunction

Additional signs and symptoms

- ◆ Sudden onset of fever that rises rapidly and remains high
- ◆ Temperature that may rise to 107° F (41.7° C)
- ◆ Vomiting
- ◆ Anhidrosis
- ◆ Decreased level of consciousness (LOC)
- ◆ Hot, flushed skin
- ◆ Tachycardia
- ◆ Tachypnea
- ◆ Hypotension

Diagnosis: Patient history with additional signs or symptoms that would indicate source of thermoregulatory dysfunction (such as heatstroke, thyroid storm, neuroleptic malignant syndrome, malignant hyperthermia, lesions of the central nervous system)

Treatment: Cooling techniques to decrease temperature, treatment of cause, antipyretics

Follow-up: As needed (depending on cause of dysfunction)

Neoplasms

Additional signs and symptoms

- ◆ Prolonged fever of varying elevations
- ◆ Nocturnal diaphoresis
- ◆ Weight loss
- ◆ Lymphadenopathy
- ◆ Palpable mass

Diagnosis: Varies depending on additional signs and symptoms but usually includes imaging studies (computed tomography scan, magnetic resonance imaging)

Treatment: Varies based on type and location of neoplasm but may include medication (antipyretics, chemotherapy), radiation therapy and, possibly, surgery

Follow-up: Referral to oncologist

lymphadenopathy, and peripheral extremity swelling. This syndrome occurs worldwide, with the highest incidence in Japan. It primarily affects children under age 5, is more prevalent in boys, and can cause serious heart damage and death without prompt treatment with I.V. gamma globulin.

◆ ***Listeriosis.*** Signs and symptoms of this infection include fever, myalgia, abdominal pain, nausea, vomiting, and diarrhea. If the infection spreads to the nervous system, it may cause meningitis, whose symptoms include fever, headache, nuchal rigidity, and change in LOC.

GENDER CUE *Listeriosis during pregnancy may lead to premature delivery, infection of the neonate, or stillbirth.*

◆ ***Methicillin-resistant* Staphylococcus aureus *(MRSA).*** MRSA is a strain of staphylococcus

Infection and inflammatory disorders

Additional signs and symptoms
- ◆ Low or extremely high temperature that may be intermittent or sustained and may rise abruptly or insidiously
- ◆ Chills
- ◆ Diaphoresis
- ◆ Weakness
- ◆ Associated signs that may involve every system

Diagnosis: Varies depending on additional signs and symptoms
Treatment: Varies depending on source of fever but usually includes antipyretics
Follow-up: As needed (depending on source of infection)

Immune complex dysfunction

Additional signs and symptoms
- ◆ Low-grade fever that may be remittent, intermittent, or sustained
- ◆ Nocturnal diaphoresis

Diagnosis: Varies depending on additional signs and symptoms
Treatment: Varies depending on specific cause of fever but usually includes antipyretics
Follow-up: As needed (depending on cause of fever)

West Nile encephalitis

Additional signs and symptoms
- ◆ Mild to moderate fever
- ◆ Headache
- ◆ Myalgia
- ◆ Rash
- ◆ Swollen lymph glands
- ◆ Neck stiffness
- ◆ Decreased LOC
- ◆ Seizures

Diagnosis: History of recent mosquito bite, West Nile activity reported in locality, blood culture
Treatment: Supportive treatment, treatment of symptoms, medication (antipyretics, analgesics)
Follow-up: As needed (depending on severity of infection)

Other causes: anticholinergics ◆ chemotherapy (especially with bleomycin, vincristine, and asparaginase) ◆ hypersensitivity to antifungals, sulfonamides, penicillins, cephalosporins, tetracyclines, barbiturates, phenytoin, quinidine, iodides, phenolphthalein, methyldopa, procainamide, and some antitoxins ◆ inhalant anesthetics ◆ monoamine oxidase inhibitors ◆ muscle relaxants ◆ phenothiazines ◆ radiographic tests that use contrast medium ◆ surgery ◆ toxic doses of salicylates, amphetamines, and tricyclic antidepressants ◆ transfusion reactions

that's resistant to antibiotics commonly used to treat staphylococcal infections. The incidence of MRSA has greatly increased in recent years. This increase is thought to be related to the increase in antibiotic use in hospital and outpatient settings and the widespread use of hand sanitizers and disinfectants. Older adults and patients with compromised immune systems are at greatest risk for MRSA, although it's becoming more common in community settings. Patients with MRSA may have a variety of signs and symptoms (most commonly fatigue and fever), depending on where the infection is located.

◆ ***Monkeypox.*** Fever is one of the initial symptoms that occurs in almost all patients infected with this rare viral disease. A papular rash that

How fever develops

Body temperature is regulated by the hypothalamic thermostat, which has a specific set point under normal conditions. Fever can result from a resetting of this set point or from an abnormality in the thermoregulatory system itself, as shown in this flowchart.

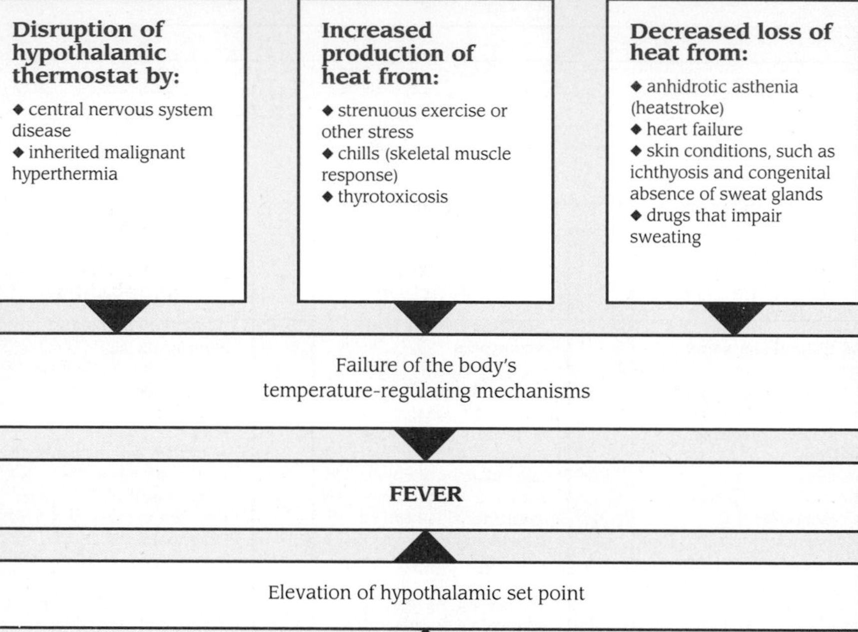
Disruption of hypothalamic thermostat by:
◆ central nervous system disease
◆ inherited malignant hyperthermia
Increased production of heat from:
◆ strenuous exercise or other stress
◆ chills (skeletal muscle response)
◆ thyrotoxicosis
Decreased loss of heat from:
◆ anhidrotic asthenia (heatstroke)
◆ heart failure
◆ skin conditions, such as ichthyosis and congenital absence of sweat glands
◆ drugs that impair sweating
Failure of the body's temperature-regulating mechanisms
FEVER
Elevation of hypothalamic set point
Production of endogenous pyrogens
Entrance of exogenous pyrogens, such as bacteria, viruses, or immune complexes, into the body

may be localized or generalized appears within 1 to 3 days after the fever begins. Additional symptoms commonly include sore throat, chills, and lymphadenopathy. There is no treatment for monkeypox, but the disease is rarely fatal in developed countries and usually lasts 2 to 4 weeks.

◆ ***Neoplasms.*** Primary neoplasms and metastases can produce prolonged fever of varying elevations. For instance, acute leukemia may manifest insidiously with a low fever, pallor, and bleeding tendencies, or more abruptly with a high fever, frank bleeding, and prostration. Occasionally, Hodgkin's disease produces undulant fever or Pel-Ebstein fever, an irregularly relapsing fever.

Besides fever and nocturnal diaphoresis, neoplastic disease commonly causes anorexia, fatigue, malaise, and weight loss. Examination may reveal lesions, lymphadenopathy, palpable masses, and hepatosplenomegaly.

◆ ***Plague.*** Caused by *Yersinia pestis,* plague is one of the most virulent bacterial infections known. The bubonic form of plague is transmitted to man from the bite of infected fleas and causes fever, chills, and swollen, inflamed, and tender lymph nodes near the site of the bite. Septicemic plague may deveop as a complication of untreated bubonic or pneumonic plague, and occurs when bacteria enter the bloodstream and multiply. Pneumonic plague manifests as a sudden onset of chills, fever, headache, and myalgia after person-to-person transmission by respiratory droplets. Other signs and symptoms of the pneumonic form include a productive cough, chest pain, tachypnea, dyspnea, hemoptysis, increasing respiratory distress, and cardiopulmonary insufficiency.

◆ ***Popcorn lung disease.*** Popcorn lung disease occurs in factory workers who experience respiratory symptoms after inhaling butter flavoring chemicals such as diacetyl, used in the manufacture of microwave popcorn. The patient typically complains of gradual onset of a nonproductive cough that worsens over time, progressive shortness of breath, and unusual fatigue. Clinical findings include wheezing, chest pain, fever, night sweats, and weight loss. Bronchiolitis fibrosa obliterans, an irreversible fixed airway obstructive lung disorder, is the most severe condition reported.

◆ ***Q fever.*** This rickettsial disease caused by *Coxiella burnetii* causes fever (which may last up to 2 weeks), chills, severe headache, malaise, chest pain, nausea, vomiting, and diarrhea. In severe cases, the patient may develop hepatitis or pneumonia.

◆ ***Respiratory syncytial virus (RSV).*** Fever is one of the initial symptoms of this common illness that affects most children by age 2. Healthy adults and children older than age 3 usually develop a low-grade fever along with other common coldlike symptoms of runny nose, cough, and wheezing. Many children less than age 3 have a high-grade fever that may be accompanied by a severe cough, rapid breathing, and high-pitched expiratory wheezing. Infants with RSV typically exhibit lethargy, poor eating, irritability, and difficulty breathing; severe cases may require hospitalization. To avoid repeated RSV infection, individuals should practice infection-control techniques, such as proper hand-washing and avoiding contact with contaminated surfaces.

◆ ***Rhabdomyolysis.*** This disorder results in muscle breakdown and release of the muscle cell contents (myoglobin) into the bloodstream. Signs and symptoms include fever, muscle weakness or pain, nausea, vomiting, malaise, and dark urine. Acute renal failure, the most common complication rhabdomyolysis, results from renal structure obstruction and injury during the kidneys' attempt to filter the myoglobin from the bloodstream.

◆ ***Rift Valley fever.*** Typical signs and symptoms of this infection include fever, myalgia, weakness, dizziness, and back pain. A small percentage of patients may develop encephalitis or may progress to hemorrhagic fever that can lead to shock and hemorrhage. Inflammation of the retina may result in some permanent vision loss.

◆ ***Severe acute respiratory syndrome (SARS).*** SARS is an acute infectious disease of unknown etiology; however, a novel coronavirus has been implicated as a possible cause. Although most cases have been reported in Asia (China, Vietnam, Singapore, Thailand), cases have cropped up in Europe and North America. After an incubation period of 2 to 7 days, the illness generally begins with a fever (usually greater than 100.4° F [38° C]). Other symptoms include headache, malaise, a nonproductive cough, and dyspnea. SARS may produce only mild symptoms, or it may progress to pneumonia and, in some cases, even respiratory failure and death.

◆ ***Smallpox (variola major).*** Initial signs and symptoms of this virus include high fever, malaise, prostration, severe headache, backache, and abdominal pain. A maculopapular rash develops on the mucosa of the mouth, pharynx, face, and forearms and then spreads to the trunk and legs. Within 2 days, the rash becomes vesicular and later pustular. The lesions develop at the same time, appear identical, and are more prominent on the face and extremities. The pustules are round, firm, and deeply embedded in the skin. After 8 or 9 days, they form a crust, which later separates from the skin, leaving a pitted scar. Death may result from encephalitis, extensive bleeding, or secondary infection.

◆ ***Thermoregulatory dysfunction.*** Sudden onset of fever that rises rapidly and remains as high as 107° F (41.7° C) occurs in life-threatening disorders, such as heatstroke, thyroid storm, neuroleptic malignant syndrome, and malignant hyperthermia, and in lesions of the central nervous system (CNS). A low or moderate fever occurs in dehydrated patients.

Prolonged high fever commonly produces vomiting, anhidrosis, decreased level of consciousness (LOC), and hot, flushed skin. Related cardiovascular effects may include tachycardia, tachypnea, and hypotension. Other disease-specific findings include skin changes (dry skin and mucous membranes, poor skin turgor) and oliguria in dehydration; mottled cyanosis in malignant hyperthermia; diarrhea in thyroid storm; and ominous signs of increased intracranial pressure (decreased LOC with bradycardia, widened pulse pressure, and increased systolic pressure) in CNS tumor, trauma, or hemorrhage.

◆ ***Tularemia.*** This infectious disease, also known as "rabbit fever," causes abrupt onset of fever, chills, headache, generalized myalgia, nonproductive cough, dyspnea, pleuritic chest pain, and empyema.

◆ ***Typhus.*** In this rickettsial disease, the patient initially experiences headache, myalgia, arthralgia, and malaise. These symptoms are followed by an abrupt onset of fever, chills, nausea, vomiting, and—in some cases—a maculopapular rash.

◆ ***Vancomycin-resistant enterococci (VRE) infection.*** Enterococci are bacteria naturally present in the intestinal tract of all people; however, some strains of enterococci have become resistant to vancomycin. Serious VRE infections may occur in hospitalized patients with such comorbidities as cancer, kidney disease, or immune deficiencies. Elderly patients and those hospitalized for long periods are also at risk for developing VRE infections. Symptoms of VRE infection depend on where the infection is; patients with VRE infections may have diarrhea, fever, and fatigue.

◆ ***Vancomycin-resistant* Staphylococcus aureus *(VRSA).*** VRSA is a strain of staphylococcus that's resistant to vancomycin, an antibiotic commonly used to treat staphylococcal infections. Patients most susceptible to VRSA infections include those with diabetes, kidney disease, or previous infection with MRSA, and those with I.V. catheters. VRSA can be difficult to diagnose because of the patient's overlying medical problems. Patients with VRSA commonly complain of fatigue and fever that don't respond to treatment with vancomycin. VRSA is usually diagnosed when cultures are done to see why the patient isn't responding to vancomycin; after the patient is started on a different antibiotic, the infection improves.

◆ ***West Nile encephalitis.*** This brain infection is caused by West Nile virus, a mosquito-borne flavivirus commonly found in Africa, West Asia, and the Middle East and rarely in North America. Most patients have mild signs and symptoms, including fever, headache, body aches, rash, and swollen lymph glands. More severe infection is marked by high fever, headache, neck stiffness, stupor, disorientation, coma, tremors and, occasionally, paralysis or seizures. Death rarely occurs.

Other causes

◆ ***Diagnostic tests.*** Immediate or delayed fever infrequently follows radiographic tests that use a contrast medium.

◆ ***Drugs.*** Fever and rash commonly result from hypersensitivity to antifungals, sulfonamides, penicillins, cephalosporins, tetracyclines, barbiturates, phenytoin, quinidine, iodides, methyldopa, procainamide, and some antitoxins. Fever can accompany chemotherapy, especially with bleomycin, vincristine, and asparaginase. It can result from drugs that impair sweating, such as anticholinergics, phenothiazines, and monoamine oxidase inhibitors. A drug-induced fever typically disappears after the drug is discontinued. Fever can also stem from toxic doses of salicylates, amphetamines, and tricyclic antidepressants.

Inhaled anesthetics and muscle relaxants can trigger malignant hyperthermia in patients with this inherited trait.

◆ ***Treatments.*** A remittent or intermittent low fever may occur for several days after surgery. Transfusion reactions characteristically produce an abrupt onset of fever and chills.

Special considerations

Regularly monitor the patient's temperature, and record it on a chart for easy follow-up of the temperature curve. Provide increased fluid and nutritional intake. When administering a prescribed antipyretic, minimize resultant chills and diaphoresis by following a regular dosage schedule. Promote patient comfort by maintaining a stable room temperature and providing frequent changes of bedding and clothing. Prepare the patient for laboratory tests, such as complete blood count and cultures of blood, urine, sputum, and wound drainage.

Pediatric pointers

Infants and young children experience higher and more prolonged fevers, more rapid temperature increases, and greater temperature fluctuations than older children and adults.

Keep in mind that seizures commonly accompany extremely high fever, so take appropriate precautions. Also, instruct parents not to give aspirin to a child with varicella or flulike symptoms because of the risk of precipitating Reye's syndrome.

Common pediatric causes of fever include varicella, croup syndrome, dehydration, meningitis, mumps, otitis media, pertussis, roseola infantum, rubella, rubeola, and tonsillitis. Fever can also occur as a reaction to immunizations and antibiotics.

GERIATRIC POINTERS

Elderly people may have an altered sweating mechanism that predisposes them to heatstroke when exposed to high temperatures; they may also have an impaired thermoregulatory mechanism, making temperature change a much less reliable measure of disease severity.

PATIENT COUNSELING

If the patient has not been admitted to the hospital, ask him to measure his oral temperature at home and record the time and value. Explain to him that fever is a response to an underlying condition and that it plays an important role in fighting infection. For this reason, advise him not to take an antipyretic until his body temperature reaches 101° F (38.3° C).

Flank pain

Pain in the flank, the area extending from the ribs to the ilium, is a leading indicator of renal and upper urinary tract disease or trauma. Depending on the cause, this symptom may vary from a dull ache to severe stabbing or throbbing pain, and may be unilateral or bilateral and constant or intermittent. It's aggravated by costovertebral angle (CVA) percussion and, in patients with renal or urinary tract obstruction, by increased fluid intake and ingestion of alcohol, caffeine, or diuretics. Unaffected by position changes, flank pain typically responds only to analgesics or, of course, to treatment of the underlying disorder. (See *Flank pain: Causes and associated findings,* pages 306 and 307.)

EMERGENCY INTERVENTIONS *If the patient has suffered trauma, quickly look for a visible or palpable flank mass, associated injuries, CVA pain, hematuria, Turner's sign, and signs of shock (such as tachycardia and cool, clammy skin). If one or more of these signs is present, insert an I.V. catheter to allow fluid or drug infusion. Insert an indwelling urinary catheter to monitor urine output and evaluate hematuria. Obtain blood samples for typing and crossmatching, complete blood count, and electrolyte levels.*

HISTORY AND PHYSICAL EXAMINATION

If the patient's condition isn't critical, take a thorough history. Ask about the pain's onset and apparent precipitating events. Have him describe the pain's location, intensity, pattern, and duration. Find out if anything aggravates or alleviates it.

Ask the patient about any changes in his normal pattern of fluid intake and urine output. Explore his history for urinary tract infection (UTI) or obstruction, renal disease, or recent streptococcal infection.

During the physical examination, palpate the patient's flank area and percuss the CVA to determine the extent of pain.

MEDICAL CAUSES

◆ ***Bladder cancer.*** Dull, constant flank pain may be unilateral or bilateral and may radiate to the leg, back, and perineum. Commonly, the first sign of bladder cancer is gross, painless, intermittent hematuria, often with clots. Related effects may include urinary frequency and urgency, nocturia, dysuria, or pyuria; bladder distention; pain in the bladder, rectum, pelvis, back, or legs; diarrhea; vomiting; and sleep disturbances.

◆ ***Calculi.*** Renal and ureteral calculi produce intense unilateral, colicky flank pain. Typically, initial CVA pain radiates to the flank, suprapubic region, and perhaps the genitalia; abdominal and low back pain are also possible. Nausea and vomiting commonly accompany severe pain. Associated findings include CVA tenderness, hematuria, hypoactive bowel sounds and, possibly, signs and symptoms of UTI (urinary frequency and urgency, dysuria, nocturia, fatigue, low-grade fever, and tenesmus).

◆ ***Cortical necrosis (acute).*** Unilateral flank pain is usually severe in this disorder. Accompanying findings include gross hematuria, anuria, leukocytosis, and fever.

◆ ***Cystitis (bacterial).*** Unilateral or bilateral flank pain occurs secondarily to an ascending UTI in bacterial cystitis. The patient may also report perineal, low back, and suprapubic pain. Other effects include dysuria, nocturia, hematuria, urinary frequency and urgency, tenesmus, fatigue, and low-grade fever.

◆ ***Glomerulonephritis (acute).*** Flank pain in patients with this disorder is bilateral, constant,

(Text continues on page 308.)

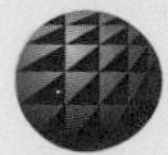

SIGNS & SYMPTOMS

Flank pain: Causes and associated findings

Major associated signs and symptoms

Common causes	Abdominal distention	Abdominal mass	Abdominal pain	Anuria	Back pain	Bladder distention	Blood pressure, decreased	Blood pressure, increased	Bowel sounds, hypoactive	Chills	Costovertebral angle tenderness
Bladder cancer					●	●					
Calculi			●						●		●
Cortical necrosis (acute)				●							
Cystitis (bacterial)					●						
Glomerulonephritis (acute)				●				●			
Obstructive uropathy	●	●	●	●		●			●		●
Pancreatitis (acute)			●		●		●		●		
Papillary necrosis (acute)			●	●					●	●	●
Perirenal abscess		●								●	●
Polycystic kidney disease					●			●			
Pyelonephritis (acute)			●							●	●
Renal cancer								●			
Renal infarction			●	●					●		●
Renal trauma	●		●						●		●
Renal vein thrombosis					●						●

	Dysuria	Edema, generalized	Fatigue	Fever	Flank mass	Groin pain	Hematuria	Leg pain	Nausea	Nocturia	Oliguria	Perineal pain	Polyuria	Pyuria	Suprapubic pain	Tenesmus	Urinary frequency	Urinary urgency	Urine retention	Vomiting
	●						●	●		●		●		●			●	●		●
	●		●	●		●	●		●	●					●	●	●	●		●
				●			●													
	●		●	●			●			●		●			●	●	●	●		
		●	●	●			●		●		●									●
						●			●		●		●							●
				●	●				●											●
				●			●				●			●						●
	●			●																
							●					●	●		●	●	●	●		
	●		●	●			●			●						●	●	●		
				●	●		●		●										●	●
				●					●		●									●
					●	●	●		●		●									●
				●			●		●		●									●

and of moderate intensity. The most common findings are moderate facial and generalized edema, hematuria, oliguria or anuria, and fatigue. Other effects include slightly increased blood pressure, low-grade fever, malaise, headache, nausea, and vomiting. Accompanying signs of pulmonary congestion include dyspnea, tachypnea, and crackles.

◆ ***Obstructive uropathy.*** In an acute obstruction, flank pain may be excruciating; in a gradual obstruction, it's typically a dull ache. In both types, the pain may also localize in the upper abdomen and radiate to the groin. Nausea and vomiting, abdominal distention, anuria alternating with periods of oliguria and polyuria, and hypoactive bowel sounds may also occur. Additional findings—a palpable abdominal mass, CVA tenderness, and bladder distention—vary with the site and cause of the obstruction.

◆ ***Pancreatitis (acute).*** Bilateral flank pain may develop as severe epigastric or left-upper-quadrant pain radiates to the back. A severe attack causes extreme pain, nausea and persistent vomiting, abdominal tenderness and rigidity, hypoactive bowel sounds and, possibly, restlessness, low-grade fever, tachycardia, hypotension, and positive Turner's and Cullen's signs.

◆ ***Papillary necrosis (acute).*** In this disorder, intense bilateral flank pain occurs along with renal colic, CVA tenderness, and abdominal pain and rigidity. Urinary signs and symptoms—oliguria or anuria, hematuria, and pyuria—are associated with high fever, chills, vomiting, and hypoactive bowel sounds.

◆ ***Perirenal abscess.*** Intense unilateral flank pain and CVA tenderness accompany dysuria, persistent high fever, chills and, in some patients, a palpable abdominal mass.

◆ ***Polycystic kidney disease.*** Dull, aching, bilateral flank pain is commonly the earliest symptom of this renal disorder. The pain can become severe and colicky if cysts rupture and clots migrate or cause an obstruction. Nonspecific early findings include polyuria, increased blood pressure, and signs and symptoms of UTI. Later findings include hematuria and perineal, low back, and suprapubic pain.

◆ ***Pyelonephritis (acute).*** Intense, constant, unilateral or bilateral flank pain develops over a few hours or days along with typical urinary features: dysuria, nocturia, hematuria, urgency, frequency, and tenesmus. Other common findings include persistent high fever, chills, anorexia, weakness, fatigue, generalized myalgia, abdominal pain, and marked CVA tenderness.

◆ ***Renal cancer.*** Unilateral flank pain, gross hematuria, and a palpable flank mass form the classic clinical triad in renal cancer. Flank pain is usually dull and vague, although severe colicky pain can occur during bleeding or passage of clots. Associated signs and symptoms include fever, increased blood pressure, and urine retention. Weight loss, leg edema, nausea, and vomiting are indications of advanced disease.

◆ ***Renal infarction.*** Unilateral, constant, severe flank pain and tenderness typically accompany persistent, severe upper abdominal pain in this disorder. The patient may also develop CVA tenderness, anorexia, nausea and vomiting, fever, hypoactive bowel sounds, hematuria, and oliguria or anuria.

◆ ***Renal trauma.*** Variable bilateral or unilateral flank pain, a visible or palpable flank mass, and CVA or abdominal pain (which may be severe and radiate to the groin) are common findings in renal trauma. Other findings include hematuria, oliguria, abdominal distention, Turner's sign, hypoactive bowel sounds, and nausea and vomiting. Severe injury may produce signs of shock, such as tachycardia and cool, clammy skin.

◆ ***Renal vein thrombosis.*** Severe unilateral flank and low back pain with CVA and epigastric tenderness typify the rapid onset of venous obstruction. Other features include fever, hematuria, and leg edema. Bilateral flank pain, oliguria, and other uremic signs and symptoms (nausea, vomiting, and uremic fetor) typify bilateral obstruction.

Special considerations

Administer pain medication. Continue to monitor the patient's vital signs, and maintain a precise record of the patient's intake and output.

Diagnostic evaluation may involve serial urine and serum analysis, excretory urography, flank ultrasonography, computed tomography scan, voiding cystourethrography, cystoscopy, and retrograde ureteropyelography, urethrography, and cystography.

Pediatric pointers

Assessment of flank pain can be difficult if a child can't describe the pain. In such cases, transillumination of the abdomen and flanks may help to detect bladder distention and identify masses. Common causes of flank pain in children include obstructive uropathy, acute poststreptococcal glomerulonephritis, infantile polycystic kidney disease, and nephroblastoma.

Flatulence

A sensation of gaseous abdominal fullness, flatulence can result from GI disorders, abdominal surgery, excessive intake of certain foods, and stress. It may be accompanied by belching, discomfort, and excessive passage of flatus.

Flatulence reflects slowed intestinal motility, which hampers the passage of gas; excessive swallowing of air (aerophagia), often brought on by stress; or increased intraluminal gas production due to an excess of fermentable substrates, such as digested, unabsorbed carbohydrates and proteins.

Although generally not considered a serious symptom, flatulence—and accompanying expulsion of flatus—may cause the patient embarrassment and discomfort.

History and physical examination

Determine how long the patient has noticed the flatulence. Find out if he passes an excessive amount of flatus. Also, ask about frequent belching or snoring, and observe for overly rapid speech. These signs are all possible clues to aerophagia.

In addition, be sure to ask the patient if he's undergoing unusual emotional stress because this can cause aerophagia or irritable bowel syndrome. Obtain a medical history, focusing on GI disorders and systemic illnesses such as scleroderma, which can cause malabsorption syndrome. Then inspect the patient's abdomen for distention, and auscultate for abnormal bowel sounds. Percuss for increased tympany due to gas accumulation, and palpate for tenderness and masses.

Medical causes

◆ ***Cirrhosis.*** Flatulence typically develops early and insidiously in cirrhosis along with anorexia, dyspepsia, nausea, vomiting, diarrhea or constipation, dull right-upper-quadrant pain, hepatomegaly, splenomegaly, fatigue, and malaise.

◆ ***Colon cancer.*** Obstruction of the colon by a tumor may cause flatulence; an acute obstruction also produces abdominal distention and tympany on percussion. Other findings may include abdominal pain, anorexia, weight loss, malaise, and altered bowel habits (constipation, diarrhea, or a change in the timing, frequency, or consistency of stools).

◆ ***Crohn's disease.*** In this disease, flatulence accompanies other acute inflammatory signs and symptoms that mimic those of appendicitis: abdominal pain, cramps, and tenderness; diarrhea; low-grade fever; nausea; and melena.

◆ ***Irritable bowel syndrome.*** The effects of this disorder include chronic flatulence, belching, and excessive flatus. Chronic constipation is typical, although the patient may also experience diurnal diarrhea. Intermittent lower abdominal pain characteristically abates with defecation or passage of flatus.

◆ ***Lactose intolerance.*** In this disorder, flatulence develops within several hours after the ingestion of dairy products. Accompanying signs and symptoms include abdominal pain and cramping and, possibly, diarrhea.

◆ ***Malabsorption syndrome.*** Findings vary considerably, depending on which dietary constituent isn't absorbed, but may include flatulence, abdominal pain, anorexia, weight loss, and passage of bulky, oily, malodorous, or slightly watery stools. Severe malabsorption may also cause muscle wasting and weakness as well as skeletal pain, edema, ecchymosis, and ulceration of the tongue.

Other causes

◆ ***Abdominal surgery.*** When peristalsis returns after postoperative paralytic ileus, gas accumulation in hypomotile areas produces flatulence.

HERB ALERT *Some herbal products, such as garlic, can cause flatulence.*

Special considerations

Prepare the patient for diagnostic studies, such as blood tests, stool analysis, upper GI series, barium enema, and endoscopy. To aid expulsion of excessive flatus, position the patient on his left side. To prevent gas buildup, encourage frequent repositioning, ambulation, and normal fluid intake, as permitted. If these measures aren't effective, try inserting a rectal tube into his anus to relieve flatus or administering an enema, a suppository, an antiflatulent, or an anticholinergic. As appropriate, provide the patient with a diet plan that excludes gaseous foods. (See *Antiflatulence diet,* page 310.)

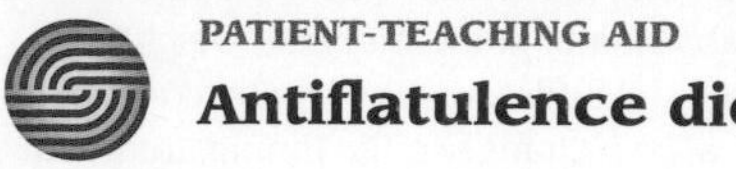

PATIENT-TEACHING AID

Antiflatulence diet

Dear Patient:
To help reduce gas, follow these dietary suggestions:

- Try to avoid such vegetables and fruits as broccoli, brussels sprouts, cabbage, cauliflower, cucumbers, dried beans, green peppers, kohlrabi, lettuce, lima beans, onions, peas, radishes, melons, prunes, and raw apples.
- Avoid all fatty foods, such as red meats, fried foods, and pastries.
- Avoid foods and beverages that contain excess air, including soufflés, carbonated drinks, and milk shakes.
- If you have lactose intolerance, avoid milk, cheese, ice cream, and all other dairy products.
- Don't overeat, eat too rapidly, or eat while under emotional stress.
- Don't drink large amounts of liquids with meals.
- Don't take laxatives.

PEDIATRIC POINTERS

The common childhood complaint of stomachache commonly results from flatulence. Children may also be more sensitive than adults to flatus-producing foods. They're also generally more prone to aerophagia, especially during eating.

GERIATRIC POINTERS

In elderly patients, increased flatulence may result from poor dentition, leading to poor mastication of food, poor dietary intake, and decreased GI motility. However, pathology must first be ruled out.

Fontanel bulging

In a normal infant, the anterior fontanel, or "soft spot," is flat, soft yet firm, and well demarcated against surrounding skull bones. The posterior fontanel shouldn't be fused at birth but may be overriding after the birthing process. This fontanel usually closes by age 3 months. (See *Locating fontanels.*) Subtle pulsations may be visible, reflecting the arterial pulse.

A bulging fontanel—widened, tense, and with marked pulsations—is a cardinal sign of meningitis associated with increased intracranial pressure (ICP), a medical emergency. It can also be an indication of encephalitis or fluid overload. Because prolonged coughing, crying, or lying down can cause transient, physiologic bulging, the infant's head should be observed and palpated while the infant is upright and relaxed to detect pathologic bulging.

EMERGENCY INTERVENTIONS *If you detect a bulging fontanel, measure fontanel size and head circumference, and note the overall shape of the head. Take vital signs, and determine level of consciousness by observing spontaneous activity, postural reflex activity, and sensory responses. Note whether the infant assumes a normal, flexed posture or one of extreme extension, opisthotonos, or hypotonia. Observe arm and leg movements; excessive tremulousness or frequent twitching may herald the onset of a seizure. Look for other signs of increased ICP: abnormal respiratory patterns and a distinctive high-pitched cry.*

Ensure airway patency, and have size-appropriate emergency equipment on hand. Provide oxygen and establish I.V. access; if the infant is having a seizure, stay with him to prevent injury and administer an anticonvulsant. Administer an antibiotic, antipyretic, and osmotic diuretic to help reduce cerebral edema and decrease ICP. If these measures fail to reduce ICP, neuromuscular blockade, intubation, mechanical ventilation and, in rare cases, a barbiturate coma and total body hypothermia may be necessary.

HISTORY AND PHYSICAL EXAMINATION

Once the infant's condition is stabilized, you can begin investigating the underlying cause of increased ICP. Obtain the child's medical history from a parent or caregiver, paying particular

Locating fontanels

The anterior fontanel lies at the junction of the sagittal, coronal, and frontal sutures. It normally measures about 2.5 × 4 to 5 cm at birth and usually closes by age 18 to 20 months.

The posterior fontanel lies at the junction of the sagittal and lambdoid sutures. It measures 1 to 2 cm and normally closes by age 3 months.

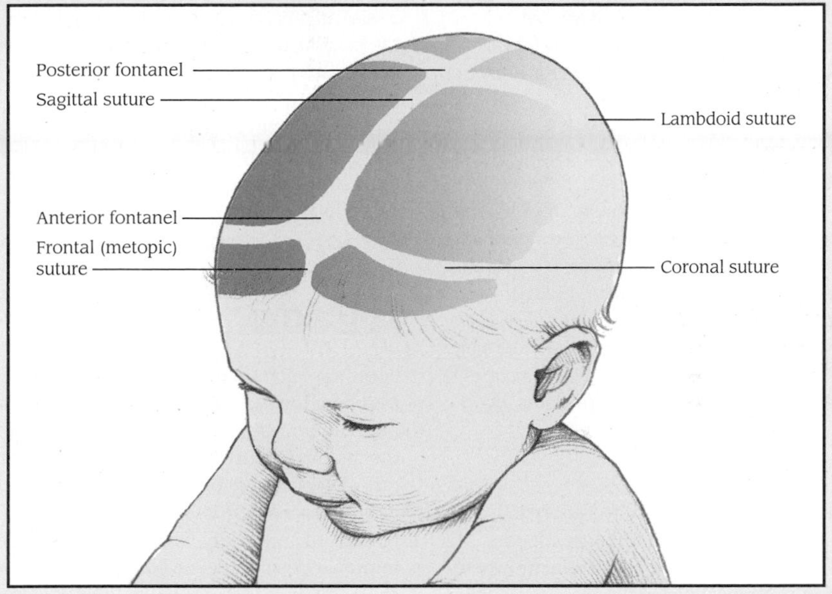

attention to any recent infection or trauma, including birth trauma. Has the infant or any family member had a recent rash or fever? Ask about any changes in the infant's behavior, such as frequent vomiting, lethargy, or disinterest in feeding.

Medical causes

◆ ***Increased ICP.*** Besides a bulging fontanel and increased head circumference, other early signs and symptoms of increased ICP are typically subtle and difficult to discern. They may include behavioral changes, irritability, fatigue, and vomiting. As ICP rises, the infant's pupils may dilate and his level of consciousness may decrease to drowsiness and eventually coma. Seizures commonly occur.

Special considerations

Closely monitor the infant's condition, including urine output (by an indwelling urinary catheter if necessary), and continue to observe the patient for seizures. Restrict fluids and place the infant in the supine position, with his body tilted 30 degrees and his head up, to enhance cerebral venous drainage and reduce intracranial blood volume.

Explain the purpose and procedure of diagnostic tests to the infant's parents or caregiver. Such tests may include intracranial computed tomography scan or skull X-ray, cerebral angiography, and a full sepsis workup, including blood studies and urine cultures.

Fontanel depression

Depression of the anterior fontanel below the surrounding bony ridges of the skull is a sign of dehydration. A common disorder of infancy and early childhood, dehydration can result from insufficient fluid intake, but it typically reflects excessive fluid loss from severe vomiting or diarrhea. It may also reflect insensible water loss, pyloric stenosis, or tracheoesophageal fistula. Assess the fontanel when the infant is in an upright position and isn't crying.

EMERGENCY INTERVENTIONS *If you detect a markedly depressed fontanel, take vital signs, weigh the infant, and check for signs of shock—tachycardia, tachypnea, and cool, clammy skin. If these signs are present, insert an I.V. catheter and administer fluids. Have size-appropriate emergency equipment on hand. Anticipate oxygen administration. Monitor urine output by weighing the wet diapers.*

HISTORY AND PHYSICAL EXAMINATION

Obtain a thorough patient history from a parent or caregiver, focusing on recent fever, vomiting, diarrhea, and behavioral changes. Monitor the infant's fluid intake and urine output over the last 24 hours, including the number of wet diapers during that time. Ask about the child's pre-illness weight, and compare it with his current weight; weight loss in an infant reflects water loss.

MEDICAL CAUSES

◆ ***Dehydration.*** In mild dehydration (5% weight loss), the anterior fontanel appears slightly depressed. Other findings include pale, dry skin and mucous membranes; decreased urine output; a normal or slightly elevated pulse rate; and possibly irritability.

Moderate dehydration (10% weight loss) causes slightly more pronounced fontanel depression along with gray skin with poor turgor, dry mucous membranes, decreased tears, and decreased urine output. The infant has normal or decreased blood pressure and an increased pulse rate; he may also be lethargic.

Severe dehydration (15% or greater weight loss) may result in a markedly sunken fontanel along with extremely poor skin turgor, parched mucous membranes, marked oliguria or anuria, lethargy, and signs of shock, such as rapid, thready pulse, very low blood pressure, and obtundation.

SPECIAL CONSIDERATIONS

Continue to monitor the infant's vital signs and intake and output, and watch for signs of worsening dehydration. Obtain serum electrolyte values to check for an increased or decreased sodium, chloride, or potassium level. If the patient has mild dehydration, provide small amounts of clear fluids frequently or provide an oral rehydration solution. If the infant can't ingest sufficient fluid, begin I.V. parenteral nutrition.

If the patient has moderate to severe dehydration, your first priority is rapid restoration of extracellular fluid volume to treat or prevent shock. Continue to administer the I.V. solution with sodium bicarbonate added to combat acidosis. As renal function improves, administer I.V. potassium replacements. Once the infant's fluid status has stabilized, begin to replace depleted fat and protein stores through diet.

Tests to evaluate dehydration include urinalysis for specific gravity and possibly blood tests to determine blood urea nitrogen and serum creatinine levels, osmolality, and acid-base status.

Footdrop

Footdrop—plantar flexion of the foot with the toes bent toward the instep—results from weakness or paralysis of the dorsiflexor muscles of the foot and ankle. A characteristic and important sign of certain peripheral nerve or motor neuron disorders, footdrop may also stem from prolonged immobility when inadequate support, improper positioning, or infrequent passive exercise produces shortening of the Achilles tendon. Unilateral footdrop can result from compression of the common peroneal nerve against the head of the fibula.

Footdrop can range in severity from slight to complete, depending on the extent of muscle weakness or paralysis. It develops slowly in progressive muscle degeneration or suddenly in spinal cord injury. (See *Footdrop: Causes and associated findings*.)

HISTORY AND PHYSICAL EXAMINATION

Ask the patient about the sign's onset, duration, and character. Does the footdrop fluctuate in severity or remain constant? Does it worsen with fatigue or improve with rest? Ask the patient if he feels weak or tires easily.

During the physical examination, assess muscle tone and strength in the patient's feet and legs, and compare findings on both sides. Assess deep tendon reflexes (DTRs) in both legs as well. Have the patient walk; inspect his shoes for wear and observe the patient for steppage gait—a compensatory response to footdrop in which the legs are raised abnormally high.

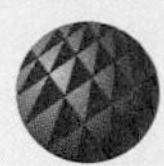

SIGNS & SYMPTOMS

Footdrop: Causes and associated findings

Common causes	Bowel and bladder dysfunction	Deep tendon reflexes, hypoactive	Gait, steppage	Level of consciousness, altered	Muscle atrophy	Muscle weakness	Pain	Paralysis	Paresthesia	Respiratory difficulty	Sensory loss	Vision disturbances
Guillain-Barré syndrome	●	●	●			●		●	●	●		
Herniated lumbar disk		●	●		●	●	●		●		●	
Multiple sclerosis	●		●			●			●		●	●
Myasthenia gravis						●		●		●		●
Peroneal muscle atrophy		●	●		●	●	●		●		●	
Peroneal nerve trauma			●		●	●					●	
Poliomyelitis	●	●	●		●	●		●	●	●		
Polyneuropathy		●	●		●	●	●	●	●		●	
Spinal cord trauma	●	●	●		●	●	●	●	●	●	●	
Stroke	●			●		●		●	●		●	●

Major associated signs and symptoms

Medical causes

◆ ***Guillain-Barré syndrome.*** In this disorder, unilateral or bilateral footdrop and steppage gait may result from profound muscle weakness, which usually begins in the legs and extends to the arms and face within 72 hours. It can progress to total motor paralysis with respiratory failure. The patient may also develop transient paresthesia, hypoactive DTRs, hypernasality, dysphagia, diaphoresis, tachycardia, orthostatic hypotension, and incontinence.

◆ ***Herniated lumbar disk.*** Footdrop and steppage gait may result from leg muscle weakness and atrophy. However, the most pronounced symptom of a herniated lumbar disk is severe low back pain that may radiate to the buttocks, legs, and feet, usually unilaterally. Sciatic pain follows, often with muscle spasms and sensorimotor loss. Paresthesia, hypoactive DTRs, and fasciculations may also occur.

◆ ***Multiple sclerosis (MS).*** Footdrop may develop suddenly or slowly in MS, producing steppage gait; like other signs and symptoms of MS, these signs are prone to periodic exacerbation and remission. Muscle weakness, usually affecting the legs, ranges from minor fatigability to paraparesis with urinary urgency and constipation. Related findings include facial pain, visual disturbances, paresthesia, lack of coordination, and loss of vibration and position sensation in the ankle and toes.

◆ ***Myasthenia gravis.*** Footdrop and related limb weakness are common manifestations of this disorder, which is commonly heralded by weak eye closure, ptosis, and diplopia. Skeletal muscle weakness and fatigability may progress to paralysis. Typically, muscle function worsens throughout the day and with exercise, and improves with rest. Involvement of respiratory muscles can cause breathing difficulty.

◆ ***Peroneal muscle atrophy.*** Bilateral footdrop, ankle instability, and steppage gait occur early in this chronic disorder along with paresthesia, aching, cramping, coldness, swelling, and cyanosis in the feet and legs. Foot, peroneal, and ankle dorsiflexor muscles are affected first. As the disease progresses, all leg muscles become weak and atrophic, and DTRs are hypoactive or absent. Later, atrophy and sensory losses spread to the hands and forearms.

◆ ***Peroneal nerve trauma.*** Footdrop may occur suddenly after this type of trauma, but it's usually temporary, resolving with the release of peroneal nerve compression. It's associated with ipsilateral steppage gait, muscle weakness, and sensory loss over the lateral surface of the calf and foot.

◆ ***Poliomyelitis.*** Unilateral or bilateral footdrop may develop after the acute stage of poliomyelitis, producing a steppage gait. This sign is usually preceded by fever, asymmetrical muscle weakness, coarse fasciculations, paresthesia, hypoactive or absent DTRs, and permanent muscle paralysis and atrophy. Dysphagia, urine retention, and respiratory difficulty may also occur.

◆ ***Polyneuropathy.*** Footdrop and steppage gait may accompany muscle weakness, which usually affects distal areas of the extremities and can progress to flaccid paralysis. Muscle atrophy and hypoactive or absent DTRs may occur along with paresthesia, hyperesthesia, or anesthesia and loss of vibration sensation in the hands and feet. Cutaneous manifestations include glossy red skin and anhidrosis.

◆ ***Spinal cord trauma.*** Unilateral or bilateral footdrop can occur suddenly and may be permanent. In the ambulatory patient, it also produces steppage gait. Other findings vary and may include neck and back pain; paresthesia, sensory loss, and muscle weakness, atrophy, or paralysis distal to the injury; asymmetrical or absent DTRs; and fecal and urinary incontinence.

◆ ***Stroke.*** Unilateral footdrop is a common sign of stroke along with arm and leg weakness or paralysis. Other effects vary according to the site and severity of vascular damage. Sensorimotor disturbances may include paresthesia, dysphagia, visual field deficits, diplopia, and bowel and bladder dysfunction. Personality changes, amnesia, aphasia, dysarthria, and decreased level of consciousness may also occur.

SPECIAL CONSIDERATIONS

Prepare the patient for electromyography to evaluate nerve function. The patient may require physical therapy for gait retraining and possibly in-shoe splints or leg braces to maintain correct foot alignment for walking and standing.

PEDIATRIC POINTERS

Common causes of footdrop in children include spinal birth defects (such as spina bifida) and degenerative disorders (such as muscular dystrophy). To aid ambulation, the child should be fitted with supportive shoes and possibly in-shoe splints or braces.

PATIENT COUNSELING

Instruct the patient in the use of assistive devices, such as canes, crutches, or walkers, as necessary. Review the importance of asking for assistance with activities to prevent falls and promote safety. Include the patient's family in this teaching.

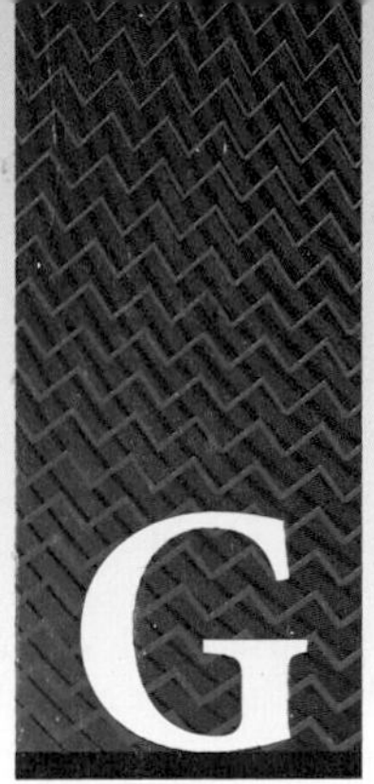

Gag reflex abnormalities

[Pharyngeal reflex abnormalities]

The gag reflex—a protective mechanism that prevents aspiration of food, fluid, and vomitus—normally can be elicited by touching the posterior wall of the oropharynx with a tongue depressor or by suctioning the throat. Prompt elevation of the palate, constriction of the pharyngeal musculature, and a sensation of gagging indicate a normal gag reflex. An abnormal gag reflex—either decreased or absent—interferes with the ability to swallow and, more important, increases susceptibility to life-threatening aspiration.

An impaired gag reflex can result from any lesion that affects its mediators—cranial nerves IX (glossopharyngeal) and X (vagus), the pons, or the medulla. It can also occur during a coma, in muscle diseases such as severe myasthenia gravis, or as a temporary result of anesthesia or drug or alcohol use.

EMERGENCY INTERVENTIONS *If you detect an abnormal gag reflex, immediately stop the patient's oral intake to prevent aspiration. Quickly evaluate his level of consciousness (LOC). If it's decreased, place him in a side-lying position to prevent aspiration; if not, place him in Fowler's position. Have suction equipment ready to use.*

History and physical examination

Ask the patient (or a family member if the patient can't communicate) about the onset and duration of swallowing difficulties, if any. Are liquids more difficult to swallow than solids? Is swallowing more difficult at certain times of the day (as occurs in the bulbar palsy associated with myasthenia gravis)? If the patient also has trouble chewing, suspect more widespread neurologic involvement because chewing involves different cranial nerves.

Explore the patient's medical history for vascular and degenerative disorders. Then assess his respiratory status for evidence of aspiration, and perform a neurologic examination.

Medical causes

◆ ***Basilar artery occlusion.*** This disorder may suddenly diminish or obliterate the gag reflex. It also causes diffuse sensory loss, dysarthria, facial weakness, extraocular muscle palsies, quadriplegia, and decreased LOC.

◆ ***Brain stem glioma.*** This lesion causes gradual loss of the gag reflex. Related symptoms reflect bilateral brain stem involvement and include diplopia and facial weakness. Involvement of the corticospinal pathways causes spasticity and paresis of the arms and legs as well as gait disturbances.

◆ ***Bulbar palsy.*** Loss of the gag reflex reflects temporary or permanent paralysis of muscles supplied by cranial nerves IX and X. Other indicators of this paralysis include jaw and facial muscle weakness, dysphagia, loss of sensation at the base of the tongue, increased salivation, fasciculations and, possibly, difficulty articulating and breathing.

◆ ***Myasthenia gravis.*** In severe myasthenia, the motor limb of the gag reflex is reduced. Weakness worsens with repetitive use and may also involve other muscles.
◆ ***Wallenberg's syndrome.*** Paresis of the palate and an impaired gag reflex usually develop within hours to days of thrombosis. The patient may experience analgesia and thermanesthesia, occurring ipsilaterally on the face and contralaterally on the body, as well as vertigo. He may also display nystagmus, ipsilateral ataxia of the arm and leg, and signs of Horner's syndrome (unilateral ptosis and miosis, hemifacial anhidrosis).

Other causes

◆ ***Alcohol.*** Excessive alcohol ingestion can lead to temporary loss of the gag reflex.
◆ ***Anesthesia.*** General and local (throat) anesthesia can produce temporary loss of the gag reflex.

Special considerations

Continually assess the patient's ability to swallow. If his gag reflex is absent, provide tube feedings; if it's merely diminished, try pureed foods. Advise the patient to take small amounts and eat slowly while sitting or in high Fowler's position. Stay with him while he eats and observe for choking. Remember to keep suction equipment handy in case of aspiration. Keep accurate intake and output records, and assess the patient's nutritional status daily.

Refer the patient to a therapist to determine his aspiration risk and develop an exercise program to strengthen specific muscles.

Prepare the patient for diagnostic studies, such as swallow studies, computed tomography scan, magnetic resonance imaging, EEG, lumbar puncture, and arteriography.

Pediatric pointers

Brain stem glioma is an important cause of abnormal gag reflex in children.

Gait, bizarre

[Hysterical gait]

A bizarre gait has no obvious organic cause; rather, it's produced unconsciously by a person with a somatoform disorder (such as hysterical neurosis) or consciously by a malingerer. The gait has no consistent pattern. It may mimic an organic impairment but characteristically has a more theatrical or bizarre quality with key elements missing, such as a spastic gait without hip circumduction, or leg "paralysis" with normal reflexes and motor strength. Its manifestations may include wild gyrations, exaggerated stepping, leg dragging, or mimicking unusual walks, such as that of a tightrope walker.

History and physical examination

If you suspect that the patient's gait impairment has no organic cause, begin to investigate other possibilities. Ask the patient when he first developed the impairment and whether it coincided with any stressful period or event, such as the death of a loved one or loss of a job. Ask about associated symptoms, and explore any reports of frequent unexplained illnesses and multiple physician's visits. Subtly try to determine if he'll gain anything from malingering, for instance, added attention or an insurance settlement.

Begin the physical examination by testing the patient's reflexes and sensorimotor function, noting any abnormal response patterns. To quickly check his reports of leg weakness or paralysis, perform a test for Hoover's sign: Place the patient in the supine position and stand at his feet. Cradle a heel in each of your palms, and rest your hands on the table. Ask the patient to raise the affected leg. In true motor weakness, the heel of the other leg will press downward; in hysteria, this movement will be absent. As a further check, observe the patient for normal movements when he's unaware of being watched.

Medical causes

◆ ***Conversion disorder.*** In this rare somatoform disorder, a bizarre gait or paralysis may develop after severe stress and is not accompanied by other symptoms. The patient typically shows indifference toward his impairment.
◆ ***Malingering.*** In this rare cause of bizarre gait, the patient may also complain of headache and chest and back pain.
◆ ***Somatization disorder.*** Bizarre gait is one of many possible somatic complaints. The patient may exhibit any combination of pseudoneurologic signs and symptoms—fainting, weakness, memory loss, dysphagia, visual problems (diplopia, vision loss, blurred vision), loss of voice, seizures, and bladder dysfunction. He may also report pain in the back, joints, and extremities (most commonly the legs) and complaints in almost any body system. For example, characteristic GI complaints include pain, bloating, nausea, and vomiting.

The patient's reflexes and motor strength remain normal, but he may exhibit peculiar contractures and arm or leg rigidity. His reputed sensory loss doesn't conform to any known sensory dermatome. He may claim that he can't stand (astasia) or walk (abasia), remaining bedridden although still able to move his legs in bed.

Special considerations

A full neurologic workup may be necessary to completely rule out an organic cause of the patient's abnormal gait. Remember, even though a bizarre gait has no organic cause, it's real to the patient (unless, of course, he's malingering). Avoid expressing judgment on the patient's actions or motives; you'll need to be supportive and reinforce positive progress. Because muscle atrophy and bone demineralization can develop in bedridden patients, encourage ambulation and resumption of normal activities. Consider a referral for psychiatric counseling as appropriate.

Pediatric pointers

Bizarre gait is rare in patients younger than age 8. More common in prepubescence, it usually results from conversion disorder.

Patient counseling

Instruct the patient in the use of assistive devices as necessary. Review the components of a safe environment, such as establishing a clear path to the bathroom and using proper footwear.

Gait, propulsive

[Festinating gait]

Propulsive gait is characterized by a stooped, rigid posture—the patient's head and neck are bent forward; his flexed, stiffened arms are held away from the body; his fingers are extended; and his knees and hips are stiffly bent. During ambulation, this posture results in a forward shifting of the body's center of gravity and consequent impairment of balance, causing increasingly rapid, short, shuffling steps with involuntary acceleration (festination) and lack of control over forward motion (propulsion) or backward motion (retropulsion).

Propulsive gait is a cardinal sign of advanced Parkinson's disease; it results from progressive degeneration of the ganglia, which are primarily responsible for smooth muscle movement. Because this sign develops gradually and its accompanying effects are often wrongly attributed to aging, propulsive gait commonly goes unnoticed or unreported until severe disability results.

History and physical examination

Ask the patient when his gait impairment first developed and whether it has recently worsened. Because he may have difficulty remembering, having attributed the gait to "old age," you may be able to gain information from family members or friends, especially those who see the patient only sporadically.

Obtain a thorough drug history, including dosages. Ask the patient if he has been taking any tranquilizers, especially phenothiazines. If he knows he has Parkinson's disease and has been taking levodopa, pay particular attention to the dosage because an overdose can cause acute exacerbation of signs and symptoms. If Parkinson's disease isn't a known or suspected diagnosis, ask the patient if he has been acutely or routinely exposed to carbon monoxide or manganese.

Begin the physical examination by testing the patient's reflexes and sensorimotor function, noting any abnormal response patterns.

Medical causes

◆ ***Parkinson's disease.*** The characteristic and permanent propulsive gait associated with Parkinson's disease begins early as a shuffle. As the disease progresses, the gait slows. Cardinal signs of the disease are progressive muscle rigidity, which may be uniform (lead-pipe rigidity) or jerky (cogwheel rigidity); akinesia; and an insidious tremor that begins in the fingers, increases during stress or anxiety, and decreases with purposeful movement and sleep. Besides the gait, akinesia also typically produces a monotone voice; drooling; masklike facies; stooped posture; and dysarthria, dysphagia, or both. Occasionally, it also causes an oculogyric crisis or blepharospasm.

Other causes

◆ ***Carbon monoxide poisoning.*** Propulsive gait commonly appears several weeks after acute carbon monoxide intoxication. Earlier effects include muscle rigidity, choreoathetoid movements, generalized seizures, myoclonic jerks, masklike facies, and dementia.

◆ ***Drugs.*** Propulsive gait and other extrapyramidal effects can result from the use of phenothiazines, other antipsychotics (notably haloperidol, thiothixene, and loxapine) and, infrequently, metoclopramide and metyrosine. Such effects are usually temporary, disappearing within a few weeks after therapy is discontinued.

◆ ***Manganese poisoning.*** Chronic overexposure to manganese can cause an insidious, usually permanent, propulsive gait. Typical early findings include fatigue, muscle weakness and rigidity, dystonia, resting tremor, choreoathetoid movements, masklike facies, and personality changes. Those at risk for manganese poisoning are welders, railroad workers, miners, steelworkers, and workers who handle pesticides.

Special considerations

Because of his gait and associated motor impairment, the patient may have problems performing activities of daily living. Assist him as appropriate, while at the same time encouraging his independence, self-reliance, and confidence. Advise the patient and his family to allow plenty of time for these activities, especially walking, because festination and poor balance make him particularly susceptible to falls. Encourage the patient to maintain ambulation; for safety reasons, remember to stay with him while he's walking, especially if he's on unfamiliar or uneven ground. You may need to refer him to a physical therapist for exercise therapy and gait retraining.

Pediatric pointers

Propulsive gait, usually with severe tremors, typically occurs in juvenile parkinsonism, a rare form. Other rare causes include Hallervorden-Spatz disease and kernicterus.

Gait, scissors

Resulting from bilateral spastic paresis (diplegia), scissors gait affects both legs and has little or no effect on the arms. The patient's legs flex slightly at the hips and knees, so he looks as if he's crouching. With each step, his thighs adduct and his knees bump together or cross in a scissorslike movement. His steps are short, regular, and laborious, as if he were wading through waist-deep water. His feet may be plantarflexed and turned inward, with a shortened Achilles tendon; as a result, he walks on his toes or on the balls of his feet and may scrape his toes on the ground.

History and physical examination

Ask the patient (or a family member if the patient can't answer) about the onset and duration of the gait. Has it progressively worsened or remained constant? Ask about a history of trauma, including birth trauma, and neurologic disorders. Thoroughly evaluate motor and sensory function and deep tendon reflexes (DTRs) in the legs.

Medical causes

◆ ***Cerebral palsy.*** In the spastic form of this disorder, patients walk on their toes with a scissors gait. Other features include hyperactive DTRs, increased stretch reflexes, rapid alternating muscle contraction and relaxation, muscle weakness, underdevelopment of affected limbs, and a tendency toward contractures.

◆ ***Cervical spondylosis with myelopathy.*** Scissors gait develops in the late stages of this degenerative disease and steadily worsens. Related findings mimic those of a herniated disk: severe low back pain, which may radiate to the buttocks, legs, and feet; muscle spasms; sensorimotor loss; and muscle weakness and atrophy.

◆ ***Hepatic failure.*** Scissors gait may appear several months before the onset of hepatic failure. Other findings may include asterixis, generalized seizures, jaundice, purpura, dementia, and fetor hepaticus.

◆ ***Multiple sclerosis.*** Progressive scissors gait usually develops gradually, with periodic remissions. Characteristic muscle weakness, usually in the legs, ranges from minor fatigability to paraparesis with urinary urgency and constipation. Related findings include facial pain, visual disturbances, paresthesia, incoordination, and loss of proprioception and vibration sensation in the ankle and toes.

◆ ***Pernicious anemia.*** Scissors gait sometimes occurs as a late sign in untreated pernicious anemia. Besides this disorder's classic triad of symptoms—weakness, sore tongue, and numbness and tingling in the extremities—the patient may exhibit pale lips, gums, and tongue; faintly jaundiced sclerae and pale to bright yellow skin; impaired proprioception; incoordination; and vision disturbances (diplopia, blurring).

◆ ***Spinal cord trauma.*** Scissors gait may develop during recovery from partial spinal cord compression, particularly with an injury below C6. Associated findings may include sensory loss or paresthesia, muscle weakness or paralysis distal to the injury, and bladder and bowel dysfunction.

◆ ***Spinal cord tumor.*** Scissors gait can develop gradually from a thoracic or lumbar tumor. Other findings reflect the location of the tumor and may include radicular, subscapular, shoulder, groin, leg, or flank pain; muscle spasms or fasciculations; muscle atrophy; sensory deficits, such as paresthesia and a girdle sensation of the abdomen and chest; hyperactive DTRs; bilateral Babinski's reflex; spastic neurogenic bladder; and sexual dysfunction.
◆ ***Stroke.*** Scissors gait occasionally develops during the late recovery stage of bilateral occlusion of the anterior cerebral artery. The patient may also display leg muscle paraparesis and atrophy, incoordination, numbness, urinary incontinence, confusion, and personality changes.
◆ ***Syphilitic meningomyelitis.*** Scissors gait appears late in this disorder and may improve with treatment. The patient may also experience sensory ataxia, changes in proprioception and vibration sensation, optic atrophy, and dementia.
◆ ***Syringomyelia.*** Scissors gait usually occurs late in this disorder along with analgesia and thermanesthesia, muscle atrophy and weakness, and Charcot's joints. Other effects may include loss of fingernails, fingers, or toes; Dupuytren's contracture of the palms; scoliosis; and clubfoot. Skin in the affected areas is typically dry, scaly, and grooved.

SPECIAL CONSIDERATIONS

Because of the sensory loss associated with scissors gait, provide meticulous skin care to prevent skin breakdown and pressure ulcer formation. Also, give the patient and his family complete skin care instructions. If appropriate, provide bladder and bowel retraining.

Promote daily active and passive range-of-motion exercises. Refer the patient to a physical therapist, if appropriate, for gait retraining and for possible application of in-shoe splints or leg braces to maintain proper foot alignment for standing and walking.

PEDIATRIC POINTERS

The major causes of scissors gait in children are cerebral palsy, hereditary spastic paraplegia, and spinal injury at birth. If spastic paraplegia is present at birth, scissors gait becomes apparent when the child begins to walk, which is usually later than normal.

Gait, spastic

[Hemiplegic gait]

Spastic gait—sometimes referred to as paretic or weak gait—is a stiff, foot-dragging walk caused by unilateral leg muscle hypertonicity. This gait indicates focal damage to the corticospinal tract. The affected leg becomes rigid, with a marked decrease in flexion at the hip and knee and possibly plantar flexion and equinovarus deformity of the foot. Because the patient's leg doesn't swing normally at the hip or knee, his foot tends to drag or shuffle, causing his toes to scrape on the ground. To compensate, the pelvis on the affected side tilts upward in an attempt to lift the toes, causing the patient's leg to abduct and circumduct. Also, arm swing is hindered on the same side as the affected leg.

Spastic gait usually develops after a period of flaccidity (hypotonicity) in the affected leg. Whatever the cause, spastic gait is usually permanent.

HISTORY AND PHYSICAL EXAMINATION

Find out when the patient first noticed the gait impairment and whether it developed suddenly or gradually. Ask him if it waxes and wanes or if it has worsened progressively. Does fatigue, hot weather, or warm baths or showers worsen the gait? Such exacerbation typically occurs in multiple sclerosis. Focus your medical history questions on neurologic disorders, recent head trauma, and degenerative diseases.

During the physical examination, test and compare strength, range of motion, and sensory function in all limbs. Also, observe and palpate for muscle flaccidity or atrophy.

MEDICAL CAUSES

◆ ***Brain abscess.*** In this disorder, spastic gait generally develops slowly after a period of muscle flaccidity and fever. Early signs and symptoms of abscess reflect increased intracranial pressure (ICP): headache, nausea, vomiting, and focal or generalized seizures. Later, site-specific features may include hemiparesis, tremors, visual disturbances, nystagmus, and pupillary inequality. The patient's level of consciousness may range from drowsiness to stupor.
◆ ***Brain tumor.*** Depending on the site and type of tumor, spastic gait usually develops gradually and worsens over time. Accompanying effects may include signs of increased ICP (headache, nausea, vomiting, and focal or generalized

seizures), papilledema, sensory loss on the affected side, dysarthria, ocular palsies, aphasia, and personality changes.

◆ ***Head trauma.*** Spastic gait typically follows the acute stage of head trauma. The patient may also experience focal or generalized seizures, personality changes, headache, and focal neurologic signs, such as aphasia and visual field deficits.

◆ ***Multiple sclerosis (MS).*** Spastic gait begins insidiously and follows this disorder's characteristic cycle of remission and exacerbation. Like other signs and symptoms of MS, the gait commonly worsens in warm weather or after a warm bath or shower. Characteristic weakness, usually affecting the legs, ranges from minor fatigability to paraparesis with urinary urgency and constipation. Other effects include vision disturbances, facial pain, paresthesia, incoordination, and loss of proprioception and vibration sensation in the ankle and toes.

◆ ***Stroke.*** Spastic gait usually appears after a period of muscle weakness and hypotonicity on the affected side. Associated effects may include unilateral muscle atrophy, sensory loss, and footdrop; aphasia; dysarthria; dysphagia; visual field deficits; diplopia; and ocular palsies.

Special considerations

Because leg muscle contractures are commonly associated with spastic gait, promote daily exercise and range of motion—both active and passive. The patient may have poor balance and a tendency to fall to the paralyzed side, so stay with him while he's walking. Provide a cane or a walker if indicated. Refer the patient to a physical therapist, if appropriate, for gait retraining and possible application of in-shoe splints or leg braces to maintain proper foot alignment for standing and walking.

Pediatric pointers

Causes of spastic gait in children include sickle cell crisis, cerebral palsy, porencephalic cysts, and arteriovenous malformation that causes hemorrhage or ischemia.

Gait, steppage

[Equine gait, paretic gait, prancing gait, weak gait]

Steppage gait typically results from footdrop caused by weakness or paralysis of pretibial and peroneal muscles, usually from lower motor neuron lesions. Footdrop causes the foot to hang with the toes pointing down, causing the toes to scrape the ground during ambulation. To compensate, the hip rotates outward and the hip and knee flex in an exaggerated fashion to lift the advancing leg off the ground. The foot is thrown forward and the toes hit the ground first, producing an audible slap. Steppage gait usually has a regular rhythm, with even steps and normal upper body posture and arm swing. It can be unilateral or bilateral and permanent or transient, depending on the site and type of neural damage.

History and physical examination

Begin by asking the patient about the onset of the gait and any recent changes in its character. Does any family member have a similar gait? Find out if the patient has had any traumatic injury to the buttocks, hips, legs, or knees. Ask about a history of chronic disorders that may be associated with polyneuropathy, such as diabetes mellitus, polyarteritis nodosa, and alcoholism. While you're taking the history, observe whether the patient crosses his legs while sitting because this may put pressure on the peroneal nerve.

Inspect and palpate the patient's calves and feet for muscle atrophy and wasting. Using a pin, test for sensory deficits along the entire length of both legs.

Medical causes

◆ ***Guillain-Barré syndrome.*** Typically occurring after recovery from the acute stage of this disorder, steppage gait can be mild or severe and unilateral or bilateral; it's invariably permanent. Muscle weakness usually begins in the legs, extends to the arms and face within 72 hours, and can progress to total motor paralysis and respiratory failure. Other effects include footdrop, transient paresthesia, hypernasality, dysphagia, diaphoresis, tachycardia, orthostatic hypotension, and incontinence.

◆ ***Herniated lumbar disk.*** Unilateral steppage gait and footdrop commonly occur with late-stage weakness and atrophy of leg muscles. However, the most pronounced symptom of a herniated lumbar disk is severe low back pain, which may radiate to the buttocks, legs, and feet, usually unilaterally. Sciatic pain follows, often accompanied by muscle spasms and sensorimotor loss. Paresthesia and fasciculations may also occur.

◆ ***Multiple sclerosis (MS).*** Like other signs and symptoms of MS, steppage gait and footdrop follow a characteristic cycle of periodic exacerbation and remission. Muscle weakness, usually affecting the legs, can range from minor fatigability to paraparesis with urinary urgency and constipation. Related findings include facial pain, visual disturbances, paresthesia, incoordination, and sensory loss in the ankle and toes.

◆ ***Peroneal muscle atrophy.*** Bilateral steppage gait and footdrop begin insidiously in this disorder. Other early signs and symptoms include paresthesia, aching, cramping, coldness, swelling, and cyanosis in the feet and legs. Foot, peroneal, and ankle dorsiflexor muscles are affected first. As the disorder progresses, all leg muscles become weak and atrophic, with hypoactive or absent deep tendon reflexes (DTRs). Later, atrophy and sensory losses spread to the hands and arms.

◆ ***Peroneal nerve trauma.*** Temporary ipsilateral steppage gait occurs suddenly but resolves with the release of peroneal nerve pressure. Steppage gait is associated with footdrop, muscle weakness, and sensory loss over the lateral surface of the calf and foot.

◆ ***Poliomyelitis.*** Steppage gait, usually permanent and unilateral, commonly develops after the acute stage of poliomyelitis. It's typically preceded by fever, asymmetrical muscle weakness, coarse fasciculations, paresthesia, hypoactive or absent DTRs, and permanent muscle paralysis and atrophy. Dysphagia, urine retention, and respiratory difficulty may also occur.

◆ ***Polyneuropathy.*** Diabetic polyneuropathy is a rare cause of bilateral steppage gait, which appears as a late but permanent effect. This sign is preceded by burning pain in the feet and is accompanied by leg weakness, sensory loss, and skin ulcers.

In polyarteritis nodosa with polyneuropathy, unilateral or bilateral steppage gait is a late finding. Related findings include vague leg pain, abdominal pain, hematuria, fever, and increased blood pressure.

In alcoholic polyneuropathy, steppage gait appears 2 to 3 months after the onset of vitamin B deficiency. The gait may be bilateral, and it resolves with treatment of the deficiency. Early findings include paresthesia in the feet, leg muscle weakness and, possibly, sensory ataxia.

◆ ***Spinal cord trauma.*** In an ambulatory patient, spinal cord trauma may cause steppage gait. Its other effects vary with the severity of injury and may include unilateral or bilateral footdrop, neck and back pain, and vertebral tenderness and deformity. Paresthesia, sensory loss, asymmetrical or absent DTRs, and muscle weakness or paralysis may occur distal to the injury. The patient may also develop fecal and urinary incontinence.

Special considerations

The patient with steppage gait may tire rapidly when walking because of the extra effort he must expend to lift his feet off the ground. When he tires, he may stub his toes, causing a fall. To prevent this, help the patient recognize his exercise limits, and encourage him to get adequate rest. Refer him to a physical therapist, if appropriate, for gait retraining and possible application of in-shoe splints or leg braces to maintain correct foot alignment.

Gait, waddling

Waddling gait, a distinctive ducklike walk, is an important sign of muscular dystrophy, spinal muscle atrophy or, rarely, congenital hip displacement. It may be present when the child begins to walk or may appear only later in life. The gait results from deterioration of the pelvic girdle muscles—primarily the gluteus medius, hip flexors, and hip extensors. Weakness in these muscles hinders stabilization of the weight-bearing hip during walking, causing the opposite hip to drop and the trunk to lean toward that side in an attempt to maintain balance.

Typically, the legs assume a wide stance and the trunk is thrown back to further improve stability, exaggerating lordosis and abdominal protrusion. In severe cases, leg and foot muscle contractures may cause equinovarus deformity of the foot combined with circumduction or bowing of the legs.

History and physical examination

Ask the patient (or a family member if the patient is a young child) when the gait first appeared and if it has recently worsened. To determine the extent of pelvic girdle and leg muscle weakness, ask if the patient falls frequently or has difficulty climbing stairs, rising from a chair, or walking. Also, find out if he was late in learning to walk or holding his head upright. Obtain a family history, focusing on problems of muscle weakness and gait and on congenital motor disorders.

Inspect and palpate leg muscles, especially in the calves, for size and tone. Check for a positive Gowers' sign (an inability to lift the trunk without using the hands and arms to brace and push), which indicates pelvic muscle weakness. Next, assess motor strength and function in the shoulders, arms, and hands, looking for weakness or asymmetrical movements.

Medical causes

◆ ***Congenital hip dysplasia.*** Bilateral hip dislocation produces a waddling gait with lordosis and pain.

◆ ***Muscular dystrophy.*** In *Duchenne's muscular dystrophy,* waddling gait becomes clinically evident by ages 3 to 5. The gait worsens as the disease progresses, until the child loses the ability to walk and needs a wheelchair, usually between ages 10 and 12. Early signs are usually subtle: delay in learning to walk, frequent falls, gait or posture abnormalities, and intermittent calf pain. Common later findings include lordosis with abdominal protrusion, a positive Gowers' sign, and equinovarus foot position. As the disease progresses, its effects become more prominent; they commonly include rapid muscle wasting beginning in the legs and spreading to the arms (although calf and upper arm muscles may become hypertrophied, firm, and rubbery), muscle contractures, limited dorsiflexion of the feet and extension of the knees and elbows, obesity and, possibly, mild mental retardation. If kyphoscoliosis develops, it may lead to respiratory dysfunction and, eventually, death from cardiac or respiratory failure.

In *Becker's muscular dystrophy,* waddling gait typically becomes apparent in late adolescence, slowly worsens during the third decade, and culminates in total loss of ambulation. Muscle weakness first appears in the pelvic and upper arm muscles. Progressive wasting with selected muscle hypertrophy produces lordosis with abdominal protrusion, poor balance, a positive Gowers' sign and, possibly, mental retardation.

In *facioscapulohumeral muscular dystrophy,* which usually occurs late in childhood or during adolescence, waddling gait appears after muscle wasting has spread downward from the face and shoulder girdle to the pelvic girdle and legs. Earlier effects include progressive weakness and atrophy of facial, shoulder, and arm muscles; slight lordosis; and pelvic instability.

◆ ***Spinal muscle atrophy.*** In Kugelberg-Welander syndrome, waddling gait occurs early (usually after age 2) and typically progresses slowly, culminating in total loss of ambulation up to 20 years later. Related findings may include muscle atrophy in the legs and pelvis, progressing to the shoulders; a positive Gowers' sign; ophthalmoplegia; and tongue fasciculations.

In Werdnig-Hoffmann disease, waddling gait typically begins when the child learns to walk. Reflexes may be absent. The gait progressively worsens, culminating in complete loss of ambulation by adolescence. Associated findings include lordosis with abdominal protrusion and muscle weakness in the hips and thighs.

Special considerations

Although there's no cure for waddling gait, daily passive and active muscle-stretching exercises should be performed for both arms and legs. If possible, have the patient walk at least 3 hours each day (with leg braces if necessary) to maintain muscle strength, reduce contractures, and delay further gait deterioration. Stay near the patient during the walk, especially if he's on unfamiliar or uneven ground. Provide a balanced diet to maintain energy levels and prevent obesity. Because of the grim prognosis associated with muscular dystrophy and spinal muscle atrophy, provide emotional support for the patient and his family.

Patient counseling

Caution the patient against long, unbroken periods of bed rest, which accelerate muscle deterioration. As indicated, refer him to a local chapter of the Muscular Dystrophy Association. Suggest genetic testing and counseling for the parents if they're considering having another child.

Gallop, atrial

[S_4]

An atrial (or presystolic) gallop is an extra heart sound (known as S_4) that's heard or commonly palpated immediately before the first heart sound, late in diastole. This low-pitched sound is heard best with the bell of the stethoscope pressed lightly against the cardiac apex. Some clinicians say that an S_4 has the cadence of the "Ten" in Tennessee (Ten = S_4; nes = S_1; see = S_2).

An atrial gallop typically results from hypertension, conduction defects, valvular disorders, or other problems such as ischemia. Occasionally, it helps differentiate angina from other causes of chest pain. It results from abnormal forceful atrial contraction caused by augmented ventricular filling or by decreased left ventricular

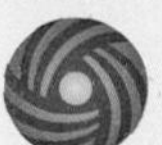

EXAMINATION TIP

Locating heart sounds

When auscultating heart sounds, remember that certain sounds are heard best in specific areas. Use the auscultatory points shown below to locate heart sounds quickly and accurately. Then expand your auscultation to nearby areas.

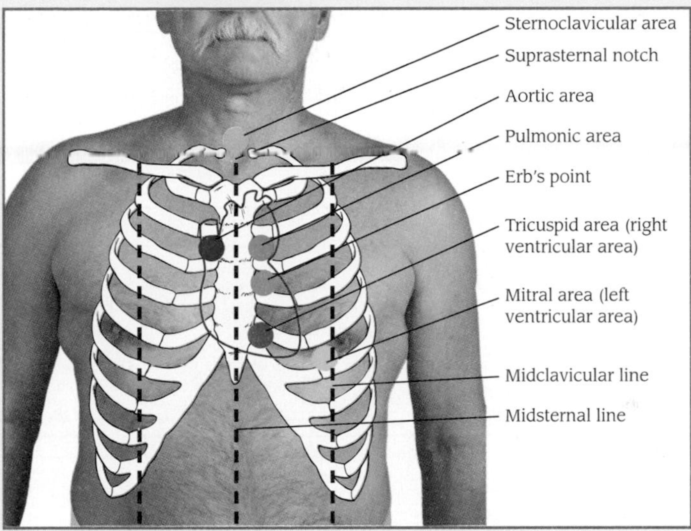

compliance. An atrial gallop usually originates from left atrial contraction, is heard at the apex, and doesn't vary with inspiration. A left-sided S_4 can occur in hypertensive heart disease, coronary artery disease, aortic stenosis, and cardiomyopathy. It may also originate from right atrial contraction. A right-sided S_4 is indicative of pulmonary hypertension and pulmonary stenosis. It's heard best at the lower left sternal border and intensifies with inspiration.

An atrial gallop seldom occurs in normal hearts; however, it may occur in elderly people and in athletes with physiologic hypertrophy of the left ventricle.

EMERGENCY INTERVENTIONS *Suspect myocardial ischemia if you auscultate an atrial gallop in a patient with chest pain. (See* Locating heart sounds. *Also see* Interpreting heart sounds, *pages 324 and 325.) Take the patient's vital signs and quickly assess for signs of heart failure, such as dyspnea, crackles, and distended jugular veins. If you detect these signs, connect the patient to a cardiac monitor and obtain an electrocardiogram. Administer an antianginal and oxygen. If the patient has dyspnea, elevate the head of the bed. Then auscultate for abnormal breath sounds. If you detect coarse crackles, ensure patent I.V. access and give oxygen and diuretics as needed. If the patient has bradycardia, he may require atropine and a pacemaker.*

History and physical examination

When the patient's condition permits, ask about a history of hypertension, angina, valvular stenosis, or cardiomyopathy. If appropriate, have him describe the frequency and severity of anginal attacks.

Medical causes

◆ ***Anemia.*** In this disorder, an atrial gallop may accompany increased cardiac output. Associated findings may include fatigue, pallor, dyspnea, tachycardia, bounding pulse, crackles, and a systolic bruit over the carotid arteries.

◆ ***Angina.*** An intermittent atrial gallop characteristically occurs during an anginal attack and disappears when angina subsides. This gallop may be accompanied by a paradoxical second heart sound (S_2) or a new murmur. Typically, the patient complains of anginal chest pain—a feeling of tightness, pressure, achiness, or burning that usually radiates from

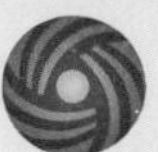

EXAMINATION TIP

Interpreting heart sounds

Detecting subtle variations in heart sounds requires both concentration and practice. Once you recognize normal heart sounds, the abnormal sounds become more obvious.

Heart sound and cause | **Timing and cadence**

First heart sound (S_1)
Vibrations associated with mitral and tricuspid valve closure

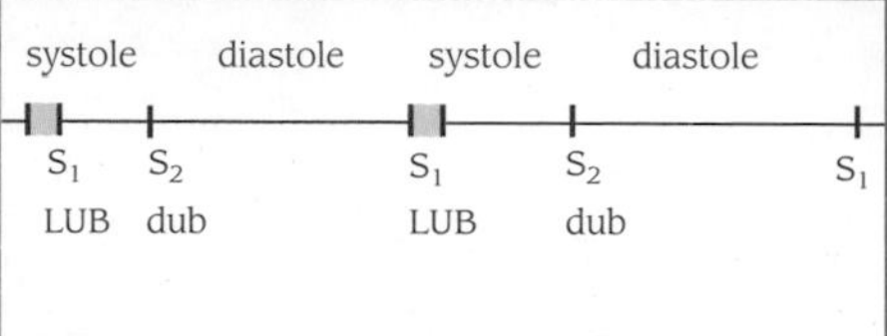

Second heart sound (S_2)
Vibrations associated with aortic and pulmonic valve closure

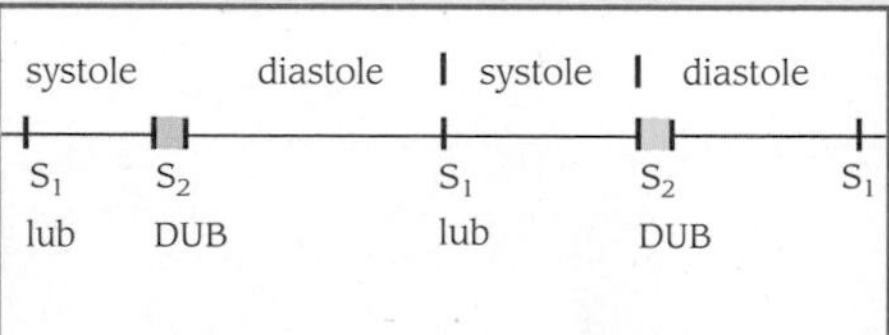

Ventricular gallop (S_3)
Vibrations produced by rapid blood flow into the ventricles

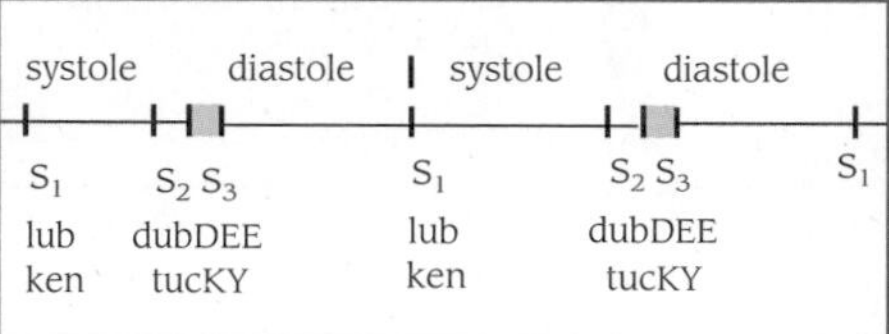

Atrial gallop (S_4)
Vibrations produced by an increased resistance to sudden, forceful ejection of atrial blood

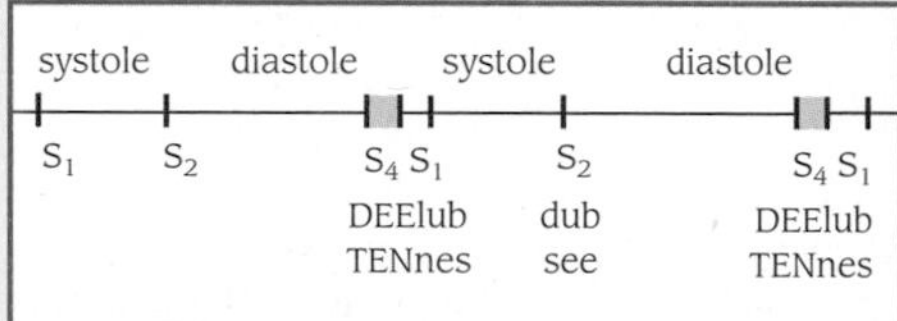

Summation gallop
Vibrations produced in middiastole by simultaneous ventricular and atrial gallops, usually caused by tachycardia

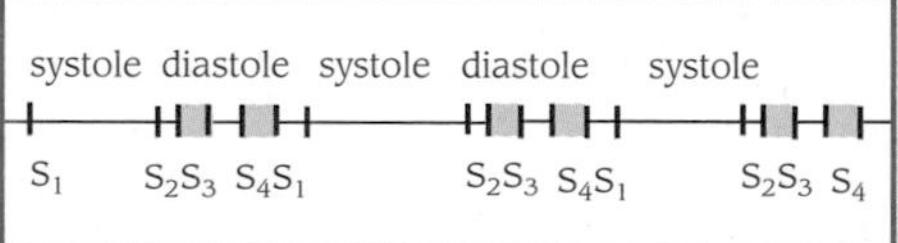

the retrosternal area to the neck, jaws, left shoulder, and arm. He may also exhibit dyspnea, tachycardia, palpitations, increased blood pressure, dizziness, diaphoresis, belching, nausea, and vomiting.

◆ ***Aortic insufficiency (acute).*** This disorder causes an atrial gallop accompanied by a soft, short diastolic murmur along the left sternal border. S_2 may be soft or absent. Sometimes a soft, short midsystolic murmur may be heard over the second right intercostal space. Related cardiopulmonary findings may include tachycardia, a ventricular gallop (S_3), dyspnea, jugular vein distention, crackles and, possibly, angina. The patient may also be fatigued and have cool extremities.

Auscultation tips

Best heard with the diaphragm of the stethoscope at the apex (mitral area).

Best heard with the diaphragm of the stethoscope in the second or third right and left parasternal intercostal spaces with the patient sitting or in a supine position.

Best heard through the bell of the stethoscope at the apex with the patient in the left lateral position. May be visible and palpable during early diastole at the midclavicular line between the fourth and fifth intercostal spaces.

Best heard through the bell of the stethoscope at the apex with the patient in the left semilateral position. May be visible in late diastole at the midclavicular line between the fourth and fifth intercostal spaces. May also be palpable in the midclavicular area with the patient in the left lateral decubitus position.

Best heard through the bell of the stethoscope at the apex with the patient in the left lateral position. May be louder than S_1 or S_2. May be visible and palpable during diastole.

◆ ***Aortic stenosis.*** This disorder usually causes an atrial gallop, especially if valvular obstruction is severe. Auscultation reveals a harsh, crescendo-decrescendo, systolic ejection murmur that's loudest at the right sternal border near the second intercostal space. Dyspnea, angina, and syncope are cardinal associated findings. The patient may also display crackles, palpitations, fatigue, and diminished carotid pulses.

◆ ***Atrioventricular (AV) block.*** First-degree AV block may cause an atrial gallop accompanied by a faint first heart sound (S_1). Although the patient may have bradycardia, he's usually asymptomatic. In second-degree AV block, an atrial gallop is easily heard. If bradycardia develops, the patient may also experience hypotension, light-headedness, dizziness, and fatigue. An atrial gallop is also common in third-degree AV block. It varies in intensity with S_1 and is loudest when atrial systole coincides with early, rapid ventricular filling during diastole. The patient with third-degree AV block may be asymptomatic or have hypotension, light-headedness, dizziness, or syncope, depending on the ventricular rate. Bradycardia may also aggravate or provoke angina or symptoms of heart failure such as dyspnea.

◆ ***Cardiomyopathy.*** An atrial gallop is a sign associated with all types of cardiomyopathy—dilated (most common), hypertrophic, or restrictive (least common). Additional findings may include dyspnea, orthopnea, crackles, fatigue, syncope, chest pain, palpitations, edema, jugular vein distention, a ventricular gallop, and transient or sustained bradycardia that's usually associated with tachycardia.

◆ ***Hypertension.*** One of the earliest findings in systemic arterial hypertension is an atrial gallop. The patient may be asymptomatic, or he may experience headache, weakness, epistaxis, tinnitus, dizziness, and fatigue.

◆ ***Mitral insufficiency.*** In acute mitral insufficiency, auscultation may reveal an atrial gallop accompanied by an S_3, a ventricular gallop that's heard best at the apex or over the precordium. This murmur radiates to the axilla and back and along the left sternal border. Other features may include fatigue, dyspnea, tachypnea, orthopnea, tachycardia, crackles, and jugular vein distention.

◆ ***Myocardial infarction (MI).*** An atrial gallop is a classic sign of life-threatening MI; in fact, it may persist even after the infarction heals. Typically, the patient reports crushing substernal chest pain that may radiate to the back, neck, jaw, shoulder, and left arm. Associated signs and symptoms include dyspnea, restlessness, anxiety, a feeling of impending doom, diaphoresis, pallor, clammy skin, nausea, vomiting, and increased or decreased blood pressure.

◆ ***Pulmonary embolism.*** This life-threatening disorder causes a right-sided atrial gallop that's usually heard along the lower left sternal border with a loud pulmonic closure sound. Other features include tachycardia, tachypnea, fever, chest pain, dyspnea, decreased breath sounds, crackles, a pleural friction rub, apprehension, diaphoresis, syncope, and cyanosis. The patient may have a productive cough with blood-tinged sputum or a nonproductive cough.

- ***Thyrotoxicosis.*** This disorder may produce atrial and ventricular gallops. Its cardinal features include an enlarged thyroid gland, tachycardia, bounding pulse, widened pulse pressure, palpitations, weight loss despite increased appetite, diarrhea, tremors, dyspnea, nervousness, difficulty concentrating, diaphoresis, heat intolerance, exophthalmos, weakness, fatigue, and muscle atrophy.

Special considerations

Prepare the patient for diagnostic tests, such as electrocardiography, echocardiography, cardiac catheterization, laboratory tests such as creatine kinase-MB and, possibly, a lung scan.

Pediatric pointers

An atrial gallop may occur normally in children, especially after exercise. However, it may also result from congenital heart defects, such as atrial septal defect, ventricular septal defect, patent ductus arteriosus, and severe pulmonary valvular stenosis.

Geriatric pointers

Because the absolute intensity of an atrial gallop doesn't decrease with age, as it does with an S_1, the relative intensity of S_4 increases compared with S_1. This explains the increased frequency of an audible S_4 in elderly patients and why this sound may be considered a normal finding in older patients.

Gallop, ventricular

[S_3]

A ventricular gallop is a heart sound (known as S_3) that's associated with rapid ventricular filling in early diastole. Usually palpable, this low-frequency sound occurs about 0.15 second after the second heart sound (S_2). It may originate in either the right or left ventricle. A right-sided S_3 usually sounds louder on inspiration and is heard best along the lower left sternal border or over the xiphoid region. A left-sided S_3 usually sounds louder on expiration and is heard best at the apex.

Ventricular gallops are easily overlooked because they're usually faint. Fortunately, certain techniques make their detection more likely. These include auscultating in a quiet environment; examining the patient in the supine, left lateral, and semi-Fowler's positions; and having the patient cough or raise his legs to augment the sound.

A physiologic ventricular gallop normally occurs in children and adults younger than age 40; however, most people lose this third heart sound by age 40. This gallop may also occur during the third trimester of pregnancy. An abnormal S_3 (in adults older than age 40) can be a sign of decreased myocardial contractility, myocardial failure, and volume overload of the ventricle, as in mitral and tricuspid valve regurgitation. Although a physiologic S_3 has the same timing as a pathologic S_3, its intensity waxes and wanes with respiration. It's also heard more faintly if the patient is sitting or standing.

A pathologic ventricular gallop may be one of the earliest signs of ventricular failure. It may result from one of two mechanisms: rapid deceleration of blood entering a stiff, noncompliant ventricle, or rapid acceleration of blood associated with increased flow into the ventricle. A gallop that persists despite therapy indicates a poor prognosis.

Patients with cardiomyopathy or heart failure may develop both a ventricular gallop and an atrial gallop—a condition known as a summation gallop. (See *Summation gallop: Two gallops in one.*)

History and physical examination

After auscultating a ventricular gallop, focus your history and examination on the cardiovascular system. Begin the history by asking the patient if he has had any chest pain. If so, have him describe its character, location, frequency, and duration as well as any alleviating or aggravating factors. Also, ask about palpitations, dizziness, or syncope. Does the patient have difficulty breathing after exertion? While lying down? At rest? Does he have a cough? Ask about a history of cardiac disorders. Is the patient currently receiving any treatment for heart failure? If so, which medications is he taking?

During the physical examination, carefully auscultate for murmurs or abnormalities in the first and second heart sounds. Then listen for pulmonary crackles. Next, assess peripheral pulses, noting an alternating strong and weak pulse. Finally, palpate the liver to detect enlargement or tenderness, and assess for jugular vein distention and peripheral edema.

MEDICAL CAUSES

◆ ***Aortic insufficiency.*** Aortic insufficiency occurs secondary to reduced ejection fraction and elevated end-systolic volume. Both the acute and chronic forms may produce a ventricular gallop. Typically, acute aortic insufficiency also causes an atrial gallop and a soft, short diastolic murmur over the left sternal border. S_2 may be soft or absent. At times, a soft, short midsystolic murmur may be heard over the second right intercostal space. Related findings include tachycardia, dyspnea, jugular vein distention, and crackles.

Chronic aortic insufficiency produces a ventricular gallop and a high-pitched, blowing, decrescendo diastolic murmur that's best heard over the second or third right intercostal space or the left sternal border. An Austin Flint murmur—an apical, rumbling, mid- to late-diastolic murmur—may also occur. Typical related findings include palpitations, tachycardia, angina, fatigue, dyspnea, orthopnea, and crackles.

◆ ***Cardiomyopathy.*** A ventricular gallop is characteristic in this disorder. When accompanied by an alternating pulse and altered first and second heart sounds, this gallop usually signals advanced heart disease. Other effects may include fatigue, dyspnea, orthopnea, chest pain, palpitations, syncope, crackles, peripheral edema, jugular vein distention, and an atrial gallop.

◆ ***Heart failure.*** A ventricular gallop is a cardinal sign of heart failure. When it's loud and accompanied by sinus tachycardia, this gallop may indicate severe heart failure. The patient with left-sided heart failure also exhibits fatigue, exertional dyspnea, paroxysmal nocturnal dyspnea, orthopnea and, possibly, a dry cough; the patient with right-sided heart failure also displays jugular vein distention. Other late features include tachypnea, chest tightness, palpitations, anorexia, nausea, dependent edema, weight gain, slowed mental response, diaphoresis, hypotension, pallor, narrowed pulse pressure and, possibly, oliguria. In some patients, inspiratory crackles, clubbing, and a tender, palpable liver may be present. As heart failure progresses, hemoptysis, cyanosis, severe pitting edema, and marked hepatomegaly may develop.

◆ ***Mitral insufficiency.*** Both acute and chronic mitral insufficiency may produce a ventricular gallop. In acute mitral insufficiency, auscultation may also reveal an early or holosystolic decrescendo murmur at the apex, an atrial gallop, and a widely split S_2. Typically, the patient displays sinus tachycardia, tachypnea, orthopnea, dyspnea, crackles, jugular vein distention, and fatigue.

In chronic mitral insufficiency, a progressively severe ventricular gallop is typical. Auscultation also reveals a holosystolic, blowing, high-pitched apical murmur. The patient may report fatigue, exertional dyspnea, and palpitations, or he may be asymptomatic.

◆ ***Thyrotoxicosis.*** This disorder may produce ventricular and atrial gallops, but its cardinal features are an enlarged thyroid gland, weight loss despite increased appetite, heat intolerance,

Summation gallop: Two gallops in one

When atrial and ventricular gallops occur simultaneously, they produce a short, low-pitched sound known as a *summation gallop*. This relatively uncommon sound occurs during mid-diastole (between S_2 and S_1) and is best heard with the bell of the stethoscope pressed lightly against the cardiac apex. It may be louder than either S_1 or S_2 and may cause visible apical movement during diastole.

Causes

A summation gallop may result from tachycardia or from delayed or blocked atrioventricular (AV) conduction. Tachycardia shortens ventricular filling time during diastole, causing it to coincide with atrial contraction. When the heart rate slows, the summation gallop is replaced by separate atrial and ventricular gallops, producing a quadruple rhythm much like the canter of a horse. Delayed AV conduction also brings atrial contraction closer to ventricular filling, creating a summation gallop.

A summation gallop usually results from heart failure or dilated congestive cardiomyopathy, but it may also accompany other cardiac disorders. Occasionally, it signals further cardiac deterioration. For example, consider the hypertensive patient with a chronic atrial gallop who develops tachycardia and a superimposed ventricular gallop. If this patient abruptly displays a summation gallop, heart failure is the likely cause.

diaphoresis, nervousness, tremors, tachycardia, palpitations, diarrhea, and dyspnea.

Special considerations

Monitor the patient with a ventricular gallop; watch for and report tachycardia, dyspnea, crackles, and jugular vein distention. Give oxygen, diuretics, and other drugs, such as digoxin and angiotensin-converting enzyme inhibitors, to prevent pulmonary edema.

Prepare the patient for electrocardiography, echocardiography, gated blood pool imaging, and cardiac catheterization.

Pediatric pointers

A ventricular gallop is normally heard in children. However, it may accompany congenital abnormalities associated with heart failure, such as a large ventricular septal defect and patent ductus arteriosus. It may also result from sickle cell anemia. Clearly, this gallop must be correlated with the patient's associated signs and symptoms to be of diagnostic value.

Genital lesions in the male

Among the diverse lesions that may affect the male genitalia are warts, papules, ulcers, scales, and pustules. These common lesions may be painful or painless, singular or multiple. They may be limited to the genitalia or may also occur elsewhere on the body. (See *Recognizing common male genital lesions*.)

Genital lesions may result from infection, neoplasms, parasites, allergy, or the effects of drugs. These lesions can profoundly affect the patient's self-image and relationships. In fact, the patient may hesitate to seek medical attention because he fears cancer or a sexually transmitted disease (STD).

Genital lesions that arise from an STD could mean that the patient is at risk for human immunodeficiency virus (HIV) infection. Genital ulcers make HIV transmission between sexual partners more likely. Unfortunately, if the patient is treating himself, he may alter the lesions, making differential diagnosis especially difficult.

History and physical examination

Begin by asking the patient when he first noticed the lesion. Did it erupt after he began taking a new drug or after a trip out of the country? Has he had similar lesions before? If so, did he get medical treatment for them? Find out if he has been treating the lesion himself. If so, how? Does the lesion itch? If so, is the itching constant or does it bother him only at night? Note whether the lesion is painful. Ask for a description of any drainage from the lesion. Next, take a complete sexual history, noting the frequency of relations, the number of sexual partners, and the pattern of condom use.

Before you examine the patient, observe his clothing. Do his pants fit properly? Tight pants or underwear, especially those made of nonabsorbent fabrics, can promote the growth of bacteria and fungi. Examine the entire skin surface, noting the location, size, color, and pattern of the lesions. Do genital lesions resemble lesions on other parts of the body? Palpate for nodules, masses, and tenderness. Also, look for bleeding, edema, or signs of infection, such as purulent drainage or erythema. Finally, take the patient's vital signs.

Medical causes

◆ ***Balanitis and balanoposthitis.*** Typically, balanitis (glans infection) and posthitis (prepuce infection) occur together (balanoposthitis), causing painful ulceration on the glans, foreskin, or penile shaft. Ulceration is usually preceded by 2 to 3 days of prepuce irritation and soreness, followed by a foul discharge and edema. The patient may then develop features of acute infection, such as fever with chills, malaise, and dysuria. Without treatment, the ulcers may deepen and multiply. Eventually, the entire penis and scrotum may become gangrenous, resulting in life-threatening sepsis.

◆ ***Bowen's disease.*** This painless, premalignant lesion usually occurs on the penis or scrotum but may appear elsewhere. It appears as a brownish red, raised, scaly, indurated, well-defined plaque, which may have an ulcerated center.

◆ ***Candidiasis.*** When this infection involves the anogenital area, it produces erythematous, weepy, circumscribed lesions, usually under the prepuce. Vesicles and pustules may also develop.

◆ ***Chancroid.*** This STD is characterized by the eruption of one or more lesions, usually on the groin, inner thigh, or penis. Within 24 hours, the lesion changes from a reddened area to a small papule. (A similar papule may erupt on the tongue, lip, breast, or umbilicus.) It then becomes an inflamed pustule that rapidly

Recognizing common male genital lesions

A wide variety of lesions may affect the male genitalia. Some of the more common ones and their causes appear below.

Penile cancer causes a painless ulcerative lesion on the glans or foreskin, possibly accompanied by a foul-smelling discharge.

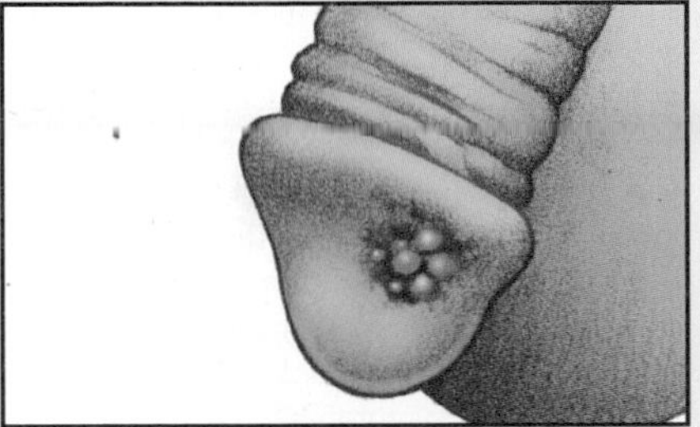

Genital herpes begins as a swollen, slightly pruritic wheal and later becomes a group of small vesicles or blisters on the foreskin, glans, or penile shaft.

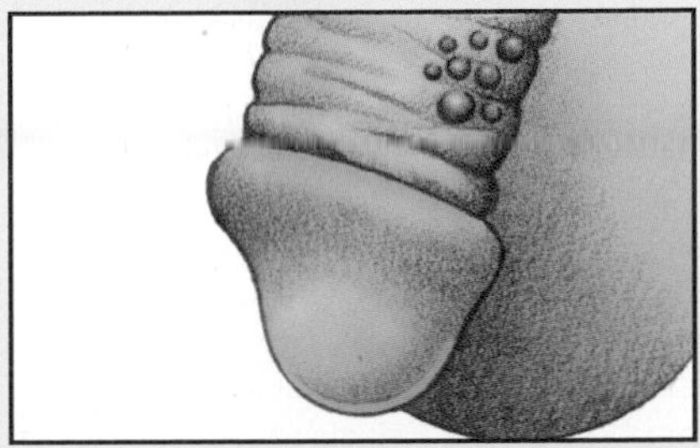

Genital warts are marked by clusters of flesh-colored papillary growths that may be barely visible or several inches in diameter.

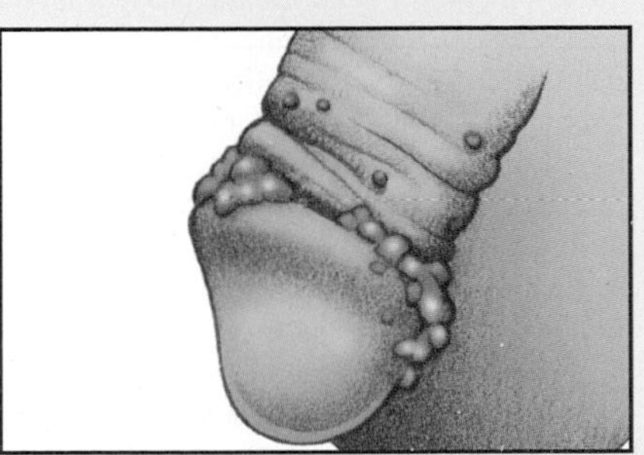

Syphilis causes a hard, round papule on the penis. When palpated, this syphilitic chancre may feel like a button. Eventually, the papule erodes into an ulcer. You may also note swollen lymph nodes in the inguinal area.

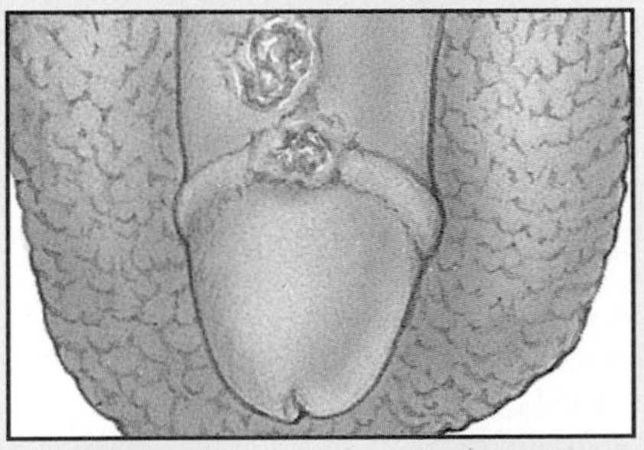

ulcerates. This painful—and usually deep—ulcer bleeds easily and commonly has a purulent gray or yellow exudate covering its base. Rarely more than 2 cm in diameter, it's typically irregular in shape. The inguinal lymph nodes also enlarge, become very tender, and may drain pus.

◆ ***Erythroplasia of Queyrat.*** This premalignant lesion is a form of Bowen's disease that appears exclusively under the foreskin of an uncircumcised penis. It typically appears as a red, raised, well-defined, velvety, indurated plaque, which may have an ulcerated center.

◆ ***Folliculitis and furunculosis.*** Hair follicle infection may cause red, sharply pointed, tender and swollen lesions with central pustules. If folliculitis progresses to furunculosis, these lesions become hard, painful nodules that may gradually enlarge and rupture, discharging pus and necrotic material. Rupture relieves the pain, but erythema and edema may persist for days or weeks.

◆ ***Fournier's gangrene.*** In this life-threatening form of cellulitis, the scrotum suddenly becomes tense, swollen, painful, red, warm, and glossy. As gangrene develops, the scrotum also becomes moist. Fever and malaise may accompany these scrotal changes.

◆ ***Genital herpes.*** Caused by herpesvirus type I or II, this STD produces fluid-filled vesicles on the glans penis, foreskin, or penile shaft and, occasionally, on the mouth or anus. Usually painless at first, these vesicles may rupture and become extensive, shallow, painful ulcers accompanied by redness, marked edema, and tender, inguinal lymph nodes. Other findings may include fever, malaise, and dysuria. If the vesicles recur in the same area, the patient usually feels localized numbness and tingling before they erupt. Associated inflammation is typically less marked.

◆ ***Genital warts.*** Most common in sexually active males, genital warts initially develop on the subpreputial sac, urethral meatus or, less commonly, the penile shaft and then spread to the perineum and the perianal area. These painless warts start as tiny red or pink swellings that may grow to 10 cm and become pedunculated. Multiple swellings are common, giving the warts a cauliflower-like appearance. Infected warts are also malodorous.

◆ ***Granuloma inguinale.*** Initially, this rare, chronic STD causes a single painless macule or papule on the external genitalia that ulcerates and becomes a raised, beefy red lesion with a granulated, friable border. Later, other painless lesions may erupt and blend together on the glans penis, foreskin, or penile shaft. Lesions may also develop on the nose, mouth, or pharynx. Eventually, these lesions become infected, malodorous, and painful and may be accompanied by fever, weight loss, malaise, and signs of anemia such as weakness. Later, they're marked by fibrosis, keloidal scarring, and depigmentation.

◆ ***Leukoplakia.*** This precancerous disorder is characterized by white, scaly patches on the glans and prepuce accompanied by skin thickening and occasionally fissures.

◆ ***Lichen planus.*** Small, shiny, polygonal, violet papules develop on the glans penis in this disorder. These papules are less than 3 cm in diameter and have white, lacy, milky striations. They may be linear or coalesce into plaques. Occasionally, oral lesions precede genital lesions; lesions may also appear on the lower back, ankles, and lower legs. Accompanying findings may include pruritus, distorted nails, and alopecia.

◆ ***Lymphogranuloma venereum.*** One to three weeks after sexual exposure, this STD may produce a penile erosion or papule that heals rapidly and spontaneously; in fact, it often goes unnoticed. A few days or weeks later, the inguinal and subinguinal nodes enlarge, becoming painful, fluctuant masses. If these nodes become infected, they rupture and form sinus tracts, discharging a thick, yellow, granular secretion. Eventually, a scar or chronic indurated mass forms in the inguinal area. Systemic signs and symptoms include a rash, fever with chills, headache, migratory joint and muscle pain, malaise, and weight loss.

◆ ***Pediculosis pubis.*** This parasitic infestation is characterized by erythematous, pruritic papules in the pubic area and around the anus, abdomen, and thigh. Inspection may detect grayish white specks (lice eggs) attached to hair shafts. Skin irritation from scratching in these areas is common.

◆ ***Penile cancer.*** This cancer usually produces a painless, enlarging wartlike lesion on the glans or foreskin. The patient may experience localized pain, however, if the foreskin becomes unretractable. Examination may reveal a foul-smelling discharge from the prepuce, a firm lump in the glans, and enlarged lymph nodes. Late signs and symptoms may include dysuria, pain, bleeding from the lesion, and urine retention and bladder distention associated with obstruction of the urinary tract.

◆ ***Psoriasis.*** Red, raised, scaly plaques typically affect the scalp, chest, knees, elbows, and lower back. When they occur on the groin or on the shaft and glans of the penis, the plaques are usually redder; on an uncircumcised penis, the characteristic silver scales are absent. The patient commonly reports itching and, possibly, pain from dry, cracked, encrusted lesions. Nail pitting and joint stiffness may also occur.

◆ ***Scabies.*** In this disorder, mites that burrow under the skin may cause crusted lesions or large papules on the glans and shaft of the penis and on the scrotum. Lesions may also occur on the wrists, elbows, axillae, and waist. They're usually raised, threadlike, and 1 to 10 cm long and have a swollen nodule or red papule that contains the mite. Nocturnal pruritus is typical and commonly causes excoriation.

◆ ***Seborrheic dermatitis.*** Initially, this disorder causes erythematous, dry or moist, greasy, scaling papules with yellow crusts that enlarge to form annular plaques. These pruritic plaques may affect the glans and shaft of the penis, scrotum, and groin as well as the scalp, chest, eyebrows, back, axillae, and umbilicus.

◆ ***Syphilis.*** Two to four weeks after exposure to the spirochete *Treponema pallidum,* one or more primary lesions, or chancres, may erupt on the genitalia; occasionally, they also erupt elsewhere on the body, typically on the mouth or perianal area. The chancre usually starts as a small, red, fluid-filled papule and then erodes to form a painless, firm, indurated, shallow ulcer with a clear base and a scant yellow serous discharge or, less commonly, a hard papule. This lesion gradually involutes and disappears. Painless, unilateral regional lymphadenopathy is also typical.

◆ ***Tinea cruris.*** Also called "jock itch," this superficial fungal infection usually causes sharply defined, slightly raised, scaling patches on the inner thigh or groin (often bilaterally) and, less commonly, on the scrotum and penis. Pruritus may be severe.

◆ ***Urticaria.*** This common allergic reaction is characterized by intensely pruritic hives, which may appear on the genitalia, especially on the foreskin or shaft of the penis. These distinct, raised, evanescent wheals are surrounded by an erythematous flare.

Other causes

◆ ***Drugs.*** Barbiturates and certain broad-spectrum antibiotics, such as tetracycline and sulfonamides, may cause a fixed drug eruption and a genital lesion.

Special considerations

Many disorders produce penile lesions that resemble those of syphilis. Expect to screen every patient with penile lesions for STDs, using the dark-field examination and the Venereal Disease Research Laboratory test. In addition, you may need to prepare the patient for a biopsy to confirm or rule out penile cancer. Provide emotional support, especially if cancer is suspected.

To prevent cross-contamination, wash your hands before and after every patient contact. Wear gloves when handling urine or performing catheter care. Dispose of all needles carefully, and double-bag all material contaminated by secretions.

Pediatric pointers

In infants, contact dermatitis ("diaper rash") may produce minor irritation or bright red, weepy, excoriated lesions. Use of disposable diapers and careful cleaning of the penis and scrotum can help reduce diaper rash.

In children, impetigo may cause pustules with thick, yellow, weepy crusts. Like adults, children may develop genital warts, but they'll need more reassurance that the treatment (excision) won't hurt or castrate them. Children with an STD must be evaluated for signs of sexual abuse.

Adolescents ages 15 to 19 have a high incidence of STDs and related genital lesions. The spirochete that causes syphilis can pass through the human placenta, producing congenital syphilis.

Geriatric pointers

Elderly adults who are sexually active with multiple partners have as high a risk of developing STDs as do younger adults. However, because of decreased immunity, poor hygiene, poor symptom reporting and, possibly, several concurrent conditions, they may present with different symptoms. Seborrheic dermatitis lasts longer and is more extensive in bedridden patients and those with Parkinson's disease.

Patient counseling

Explain to the patient how to use prescribed ointments or creams. Advise him to use a heat lamp to dry moist lesions or to take sitz baths to relieve crusting and itching. Also, instruct him to report any changes in the lesions.

Explain to male patients that condoms effectively prevent many STDs when used correctly. Advise them to use a new condom for each coitus; to avoid damaging the condom with a sharp object, such as fingernails or teeth; to put the condom on the erect penis before any genital contact; to use only water-based lubricants; to hold the condom firmly while withdrawing the penis; to always withdraw the penis while it's still erect to avoid premature condom loss; and to check the expiration date on the individual condom packet. Teach the patient that hormonal contraceptives, diaphragms, foams, and jellies don't protect against STDs.

Gum bleeding

[Gingival bleeding]

Bleeding gums usually result from dental disorders; less often, they may stem from blood dyscrasias or the effects of certain drugs. Physiologic causes of this common sign include pregnancy, which can produce gum swelling in the first or second trimester (pregnancy epulis); atmospheric pressure changes, which usually affect divers and aviators; and oral trauma. Bleeding ranges from slight oozing to life-threatening hemorrhage. It may be spontaneous or may follow trauma. Occasionally, direct pressure can control it.

EMERGENCY INTERVENTIONS *If you detect profuse, spontaneous bleeding in the oral cavity, quickly check the patient's airway* *and look for signs of cardiovascular collapse, such as tachycardia and hypotension. Suction the patient. Apply direct pressure to the bleeding site. Expect to insert an airway, administer I.V. fluids, and collect serum samples for diagnostic evaluation.*

History and physical examination

If gum bleeding isn't an emergency, obtain a history. Find out when the bleeding began. Has it been continuous or intermittent? Does it occur spontaneously or when the patient brushes his teeth or flosses? Have the patient show you the site of the bleeding if possible.

Find out if the patient or any family members have bleeding tendencies; for example, ask about easy bruising and frequent nosebleeds. How much does the patient bleed after a tooth extraction? Does he have a history of liver or spleen disease? Next, check the patient's dental history. Find out how often he brushes his teeth, flosses, and goes to the dentist, and what kind of toothbrush and floss he uses. Has he seen a dentist recently? To evaluate nutritional status, have the patient describe his normal diet and intake of alcohol. Finally, note any prescription and over-the-counter drugs he takes.

Next, perform a complete oral examination. If the patient wears dentures, have him remove them. Examine the gums to determine the site and amount of bleeding. Gums normally appear pink and rippled with their margins snugly against the teeth. Check for inflammation, pockets around the teeth, swelling, retraction, hypertrophy, discoloration, and gum hyperplasia. Note obvious decay, discoloration, foreign material such as food, and absence of any teeth.

Medical causes

◆ ***Agranulocytosis.*** Spontaneous gum bleeding and other systemic hemorrhages may occur in this hematologic disorder, which typically causes progressive fatigue and weakness, followed by signs of infection, such as fever and chills. Inspection may reveal oral and perianal lesions, which are usually rough edged with a gray or black membrane.

◆ ***Aplastic anemia.*** In this disorder, profuse or scant gum bleeding may follow trauma. Other signs of bleeding, such as epistaxis and ecchymosis, are also characteristic. The patient exhibits progressive weakness and fatigue, shortness of breath, headache, pallor and, possibly, fever. Eventually, tachycardia and signs of heart failure, such as jugular vein distention and dyspnea, also develop.

◆ ***Cirrhosis.*** A late sign of cirrhosis, gum bleeding occurs with epistaxis and other bleeding tendencies. Other late effects include ascites, hepatomegaly, pruritus, and jaundice.

◆ ***Ehlers-Danlos syndrome.*** In this congenital syndrome, gums bleed easily after toothbrushing. Easy bruising and other signs of abnormal bleeding are also typical. Skin is fragile and hyperelastic; joints are hyperextendible.

◆ ***Giant cell epulis.*** This pedunculated granuloma, which occurs on the gums or alveolar process in front of the molars, is dark red and vascular, resembling a surface ulcer. Gums bleed easily with slight trauma.

◆ ***Gingivitis.*** Reddened and edematous gums are characteristic of this disorder. The gingivae between the teeth become bulbous and bleed easily with slight trauma. However, with acute necrotizing ulcerative gingivitis, bleeding is spontaneous and the gums become so painful that the patient may be unable to eat. A characteristic grayish yellow pseudomembrane develops over punched-out gum erosions. Halitosis is typical and may be accompanied by headache, malaise, fever, and cervical adenopathy.

◆ ***Hemophilia.*** Hemorrhage occurs from many sites in the oral cavity, especially the gums. Mild hemophilia causes easy bruising, hematomas, epistaxis, bleeding gums, and prolonged bleeding during even minor surgery and for up to 8 days afterward. Moderate hemophilia produces more frequent episodes of abnormal bleeding and occasional bleeding into the joints, which may cause swelling and pain. Severe hemophilia causes spontaneous or severe bleeding after minor trauma, possibly resulting in large subcutaneous and intramuscular hematomas. Bleeding into joints and muscles causes pain, swelling, extreme tenderness and, possibly, permanent deformity. Bleeding near peripheral nerves causes peripheral neuropathies, pain, paresthesia, and muscle atrophy. Signs of anemia and fever may follow bleeding. Severe blood loss may lead to shock and death.

◆ ***Hereditary hemorrhagic telangiectasia.*** This disorder is characterized by red to violet spiderlike hemorrhagic areas on the gums, which blanch on pressure and bleed spontaneously. These telangiectases may also occur on the lips, buccal mucosa, and palate; on the face, ears, scalp, hands, arms, and feet; and under the nails. Epistaxis commonly occurs early and is difficult to control. Hemoptysis and signs of GI bleeding may develop.

◆ ***Hypofibrinogenemia.*** In this rare disorder, the patient has frequent, spontaneous episodes of severe gum bleeding. Hematomas, ecchymosis, and epistaxis are also common. Signs of GI bleeding (such as hematemesis) and of central nervous system bleeding (such as focal neurologic deficits) may also occur.

◆ ***Leukemia.*** An early sign of acute monocytic, lymphocytic, or myelocytic leukemia, easy gum bleeding is accompanied by gum swelling, necrosis, and petechiae. The soft, tender gums appear glossy and bluish. Acute leukemia causes severe prostration marked by high fever and bleeding tendencies, such as epistaxis and prolonged menses. It may also cause dyspnea, tachycardia, palpitations, and abdominal or bone pain. Later effects may include confusion, headaches, vomiting, seizures, papilledema, and nuchal rigidity.

Chronic leukemia usually develops insidiously, producing less severe bleeding tendencies. Other effects may include anorexia, weight loss, low-grade fever, chills, skin eruptions, and enlarged spleen, tonsils, and lymph nodes. Signs of anemia, such as fatigue and pallor, may occur.

◆ ***Pemphigoid (benign mucosal).*** Most common in women between ages 40 and 50, this autoimmune disorder typically causes thick-walled gum lesions that rupture, desquamate, and then bleed easily. Extensive scars form with healing, and the gums remain red for months. Lesions may also develop on other parts of the oral mucosa, the conjunctivae and, less often, the skin. Secondary fibrous bands may lead to dysphagia, hoarseness, or blindness.

◆ ***Periodontal disease.*** Gum bleeding typically occurs after chewing, toothbrushing, or gum probing but may also occur spontaneously. As gingivae separate from the bone, pus-filled pockets develop around the teeth; occasionally, pus can be expressed. Other findings include unpleasant taste with halitosis, facial pain, loose teeth, and dental calculi and plaque.

◆ ***Pernicious anemia.*** Gum bleeding and a sore tongue can make eating painful in this disorder whose other cardinal symptoms are weakness and paresthesia. The patient's lips, gums, and tongue appear markedly pale, and his sclerae and skin are jaundiced. Other features are typically widespread, affecting the GI, cardiovascular, and central nervous systems, and include altered bowel and bladder habits, personality changes, ataxia, tinnitus, dyspnea, and tachycardia.

◆ ***Polycythemia vera.*** In this disorder, engorged gums ooze blood after even a slight trauma. Polycythemia vera usually turns the oral mucosa—especially the gums and tongue—a deep red-violet. Associated findings include headache, dyspnea, dizziness, fatigue, paresthesia, tinnitus, diplopia or blurred vision, aquagenic pruritus, epigastric distress, weight loss, increased blood pressure, ruddy cyanosis, ecchymosis, and hepatosplenomegaly.

◆ ***Pyogenic granuloma.*** Commonly affecting the gums, lips, tongue, and buccal mucosa, this granuloma may ulcerate and bleed spontaneously or with slight trauma. The lesion is pedunculated with a smooth or warty surface.

◆ ***Thrombasthenia (familial).*** This hereditary blood platelet disorder causes spontaneous bleeding from the oral cavity, especially the gums. The patient commonly displays purpura, epistaxis, hemarthrosis, and signs of GI bleeding, such as hematemesis and melena.

◆ ***Thrombocytopenia.*** In this disorder, blood usually oozes between the teeth and gums; however, severe bleeding may follow minor trauma. Associated signs of hemorrhage include large blood-filled bullae in the mouth, petechiae, ecchymosis, epistaxis, and hematuria. Malaise, fatigue, weakness, and lethargy eventually develop.

◆ ***Thrombocytopenic purpura (immune).*** Profuse gum bleeding occurs in this disorder. Its classic feature, though, is spontaneous hemorrhagic skin lesions that range from pinpoint petechiae to massive hemorrhages. The patient has a tendency to bruise easily, develops petechiae on the oral mucosa, and may exhibit melena, epistaxis, or hematuria.

◆ ***Vitamin C deficiency (scurvy).*** This deficiency causes swollen, spongy, tender gums that bleed easily. The gums between the teeth are red or purple. The teeth themselves become loose and may be surrounded by pockets filled with clotted blood. Other findings include muscle and joint pain, petechiae, ecchymosis, splinter hemorrhages in the nail beds, and ocular hemorrhages. Associated effects are anorexia, dry mouth, pallor, weakness, lethargy, insomnia, scaly skin, and psychological disturbances, such as depression or hysteria.

◆ ***Vitamin K deficiency.*** The first sign of this deficiency is usually gums that bleed when the teeth are brushed. Other signs of abnormal

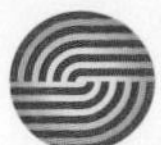

PATIENT-TEACHING AID

Preventing bleeding gums

Dear Patient:
Follow these tips to improve oral hygiene and prevent your gums from bleeding:

- Eliminate between-meal snacks and reduce carbohydrate intake to help prevent plaque formation on your teeth.
- Visit the dentist once every 6 months for thorough plaque removal.
- Avoid citrus fruits and juices, rough or spicy food, alcohol, and tobacco if they irritate mouth ulcers or sore gums and cause bleeding. Be sure to take vitamin C supplements if you can't consume citrus fruits and juices.
- Avoid using toothpicks, which may cause gum injury and infection.
- Brush your teeth gently after every meal, using a soft-bristled toothbrush held at a 45-degree angle to the gum line.
- If dentures make your gums bleed, wear them *only* during meals.
- If the dentist tells you not to brush your teeth, rinse your mouth with salt water or hydrogen peroxide and water. Avoid using commercial mouthwashes, which contain irritating alcohol.
- Floss your teeth daily to remove plaque, unless flossing causes pain or bleeding.
- Use a Water Pik on the low pressure setting to massage your gums.
- Use aspirin sparlingly for toothaches or general pain relief.
- Control gum bleeding by applying direct pressure to the area with a gauze pad soaked in ice water.

bleeding, such as ecchymosis, epistaxis, and hematuria, may also occur. GI bleeding may produce hematemesis and melena; intracranial bleeding may cause decreased level of consciousness and focal neurologic deficits.

Other causes

- ***Chemical irritants.*** Occupational exposure to benzene may irritate the gums, resulting in bleeding. Other signs of abnormal bleeding may accompany limb weakness and sensory changes.
- ***Drugs.*** Warfarin and heparin interfere with blood clotting and may cause prolonged gum bleeding. Abuse of aspirin and nonsteroidal anti-inflammatory drugs may alter platelets, producing bleeding gums. Localized gum bleeding may also occur with mucosal "aspirin burn" caused by dissolving aspirin near an aching tooth.

Special considerations

Prepare the patient for diagnostic tests, such as blood studies or facial X-rays. Prepare him for the possibility of a blood or blood product (platelets or fresh frozen plasma) transfusion if necessary. When providing mouth care, avoid using lemon-glycerin swabs, which may burn or dry the gums.

Pediatric pointers

In neonates, bleeding gums may result from vitamin K deficiency associated with a lack of normal intestinal flora or poor maternal nutrition. In infants who primarily drink cow's milk and don't receive vitamin supplements, bleeding gums can result from vitamin C deficiency.

Encourage parents to teach proper oral hygiene early. Daily brushing in the morning and before bedtime should begin with eruption of the first tooth. When the child has all of his baby teeth, he should begin receiving regular dental checkups.

Geriatric pointers

In patients who have no teeth, constant gum trauma and bleeding may result from using a dental prosthesis.

Patient counseling

Teach the patient proper mouth and gum care, including proper brushing techniques using a soft-bristled toothbrush. (See *Preventing bleeding gums.*) Make sure patients with chronic disorders that predispose them to bleeding, such as chronic leukemia, cirrhosis, or idiopathic thrombocytopenic purpura, are aware that bleeding gums may indicate a worsening of their condition, requiring immediate medical attention.

Gum swelling

Gum swelling may result from one of two mechanisms: an increase in the size of existing gum cells (hypertrophy) or an increase in their number (hyperplasia). This common sign may involve one or many papillae—the triangular bits of gum between adjacent teeth. Occasionally, the gums swell markedly, obscuring the teeth altogether. Usually, the swelling is most prominent on the labia and bucca.

Gum swelling usually results from the effects of phenytoin; less commonly, from nutritional deficiency or certain systemic disorders. Physiologic gum swelling and bleeding may occur during the first and second trimesters of pregnancy when hormonal changes make the gums highly vascular; even slight irritation causes swelling and gives the papillae a characteristic raspberry hue (pregnancy epulis). Irritating dentures may also cause swelling associated with red, soft, movable masses on the gums.

History and physical examination

After ruling out pregnancy or the use of phenytoin or similar prescription drugs as the cause of gum swelling, take a history. Have the patient fully describe the swelling. Has he had it before? Is it localized or generalized? Find out when the swelling began, and ask about any aggravating or alleviating factors. Is the swelling painful? Then explore the patient's medical history, focusing on major illnesses, bleeding disorders, and pregnancies. Also check his dental history. Does he wear dentures? If so, are they new? Ask about use of alcohol and tobacco, which are gum irritants. Then have the patient describe his diet to evaluate nutritional status. Ask about his intake of citrus fruits and vegetables.

Next, inspect the patient's mouth in a good light. If he wears dentures, ask him to remove them before you begin. As you examine the gums, characterize their color and texture, and note any ulcers, lesions, masses, lumps, or debris-filled pockets around the teeth. Then inspect the teeth for discoloration, obvious decay, and looseness.

Medical causes

◆ ***Crohn's disease.*** Granular or cobblestone gum swelling occurs in this disorder, which is characterized by cramping abdominal pain and diarrhea. In acute Crohn's disease, the patient may also have nausea, fever, tachycardia, abdominal tenderness and guarding, hyperactive bowel sounds, and abdominal distention. Chronic effects include anorexia, weight loss, a palpable lower quadrant mass, perianal lesions, skin lesions (erythema nodosum), arthritis, and occasionally constipation.

◆ ***Fibrous hyperplasia (idiopathic).*** In this disorder, the gums become diffusely enlarged and may even cover the teeth. Large, firm, painless masses of fibrous tissue that form on the gums may prevent tooth eruption and cause lip protrusion and difficulty chewing.

◆ ***Leukemia.*** Gum swelling is commonly an early sign, especially in acute monocytic, lymphocytic, or myelocytic leukemia. Usually, the swelling is localized and accompanied by necrosis. The tender gums appear blue and glossy and bleed easily.

Acute leukemia also causes severe prostration, high fever, and signs of abnormal bleeding, such as ecchymosis and prolonged menses. Sometimes it produces dyspnea, tachycardia, palpitations, and abdominal or bone pain. Late effects may include confusion, headache, vomiting, seizures, papilledema, and nuchal rigidity. In chronic leukemia, signs and symptoms develop insidiously and may include malaise, pallor, low-grade fever, chills, minor bleeding tendencies, and enlarged tonsils, lymph nodes, and spleen.

◆ ***Vitamin C deficiency (scurvy).*** In this deficiency, the gums are spongy, tender, and edematous, and the papillae appear red or purple. The gums bleed easily, and inspection may reveal pockets filled with clotted blood around loose teeth. Associated findings include anorexia, pallor, dry mouth, scaly dermatitis, weakness, lethargy, insomnia, and signs of abnormal bleeding, such as myalgia and arthralgia (possibly with swelling), from hemorrhage into joints and muscles. Occasionally, psychological changes, such as depression and hysteria, occur.

Other causes

◆ ***Drugs.*** Gum swelling is a common side effect of the anticonvulsant phenytoin. Cyclosporine, a drug used to prevent rejection of transplanted organs, also produces this sign in about 15% of patients.

Special considerations

When performing mouth care, avoid using lemon-glycerin swabs, which can irritate the gums. Instead, use a soft-bristled toothbrush or one that's padded with sponge or gauze. For phenytoin-induced swelling, expect to substitute another anticonvulsant, such as carbamazepine, and prepare the patient for surgery. Because gum swelling may affect the patient's appearance, offer emotional support and reassure him that swelling usually resolves with treatment.

Pediatric pointers

Gum swelling in children commonly results from nutritional deficiency. It may also accompany phenytoin therapy; in fact, drug-induced gum swelling is more common in children than in adults. Fortunately, this dramatic swelling is usually painless and limited to one or two papillae. Gum swelling may also result from idiopathic fibrous hyperplasia and from inflammatory gum hyperplasia, which is especially common in pubertal girls.

Good nutrition and oral hygiene help control gum swelling in children, so encourage parents to make brushing as much fun as possible.

Geriatric pointers

Always ask an elderly patient if he wears dentures and, if so, whether they're new. Also ask him when he last visited the dentist. If dentures are causing gum inflammation, the patient may require a new set. Always evaluate oral hygiene in older patients, especially bedridden ones who can't perform self-care.

Patient counseling

To prevent further swelling, teach the patient the basics of good nutrition. Remind him to eat foods high in vitamin C, such as fresh fruits and vegetables, daily. Also, encourage him to avoid gum irritants, such as commercial mouthwashes, alcohol, and tobacco. Advise him to see a periodontist at least once every 6 months.

Gynecomastia

Occurring only in males, gynecomastia refers to increased breast size due to excessive mammary gland development. This change in breast size may be barely palpable or immediately obvious. Usually bilateral, gynecomastia may be associated with breast tenderness and milk secretion.

Normally, several hormones regulate breast development. Estrogens, growth hormone, and corticosteroids stimulate ductal growth, while progesterone and prolactin stimulate growth of the alveolar lobules. Although the pathophysiology of gynecomastia isn't fully understood, a hormonal imbalance—particularly a change in the estrogen-androgen ratio and an increase in prolactin—is a likely contributing factor. This explains why gynecomastia commonly results from the effects of estrogens and other drugs. It may also result from hormone-secreting tumors and from endocrine, genetic, hepatic, or adrenal disorders. Physiologic gynecomastia may occur in neonatal, pubertal, and geriatric males because of normal fluctuations in hormone levels.

History and physical examination

Begin the history by asking the patient when he first noticed his breast enlargement. How old was he at the time? Since then, have his breasts gotten progressively larger, smaller, or stayed the same? Does he also have breast tenderness or discharge? Have him describe the discharge, if any. Ask him if he ever had his nipples pierced and, if so, if he developed any complications. Next, take a thorough drug history, including prescription, over-the-counter, herbal, and street drugs. Then explore associated signs and symptoms, such as testicular mass or pain, loss of libido, decreased potency, and loss of chest, axillary, or facial hair.

Focus the physical examination on the breasts, testicles, and penis. As you examine the breasts, note any asymmetry, dimpling, abnormal pigmentation, or ulceration. Observe the testicles for size and symmetry. Then palpate them to detect nodules, tenderness, or unusual consistency. Look for normal penile development after puberty, and note hypospadias.

Medical causes

◆ ***Adrenal carcinoma.*** Estrogen production by an adrenal tumor may produce a feminizing syndrome in males characterized by bilateral gynecomastia, loss of libido, impotence, testicular atrophy, and reduced facial hair growth. Cushingoid signs, such as moon face and purple striae, may also occur.

◆ ***Breast cancer.*** Painful unilateral gynecomastia develops rapidly in males with breast cancer. Palpation may reveal a hard or stony breast lump suggesting a malignant tumor. Breast examination may also detect changes in breast symmetry; skin changes, such as thickening, dimpling, peau d'orange, or ulceration; a warm, reddened area; and nipple changes, such as itching, burning, erosion, deviation, flattening, retraction, and a watery, bloody, or purulent discharge.

◆ ***Cirrhosis.*** A late sign of cirrhosis, bilateral gynecomastia results from failure of the liver to inactivate circulating estrogens. It's often accompanied by testicular atrophy, decreased libido, impotence, and loss of facial, chest, and axillary hair. Other late signs and symptoms include mental changes, bleeding tendencies, spider angiomas, palmar erythema, severe pruritus and dry skin, fetor hepaticus, enlarged superficial abdominal veins and, possibly, jaundice and hepatomegaly.

◆ ***Hermaphroditism.*** In true hermaphroditism, ovarian and testicular tissues coexist, resulting in external genitalia with both feminine and masculine characteristics. At puberty, the patient typically develops marked bilateral gynecomastia. About 50% of hermaphrodites also experience male menstruation in the form of cyclic hematuria.

◆ ***Hypothyroidism.*** Typically, this disorder produces bilateral gynecomastia along with bradycardia, cold intolerance, weight gain despite anorexia, and mental dullness. The patient may display periorbital edema and puffiness in the face, hands, and feet. His hair appears brittle and sparse and his skin is dry, pale, cool, and doughy.

◆ ***Klinefelter's syndrome.*** Painless bilateral gynecomastia first appears during adolescence in this genetic disorder. Before puberty, symptoms also include abnormally small testicles and slight mental deficiency; after puberty, sparse facial hair, a small penis, decreased libido, and impotence.

◆ ***Liver cancer.*** This type of cancer may produce bilateral gynecomastia and other characteristics of feminization, such as testicular atrophy, impotence, and reduced facial hair growth. The patient may complain of severe epigastric or right-upper-quadrant pain associated with a right-upper-quadrant mass. A large tumor may also produce a bruit on auscultation. Related findings may include anorexia, weight loss, dependent edema, fever, cachexia and, possibly, jaundice or ascites.

◆ ***Lung cancer.*** Bronchogenic carcinoma or metastasis to the lung from testicular choriocarcinoma may result in bilateral gynecomastia. Other effects vary according to the tumor's primary site but usually include anorexia, weight loss, fatigue, chronic cough, hemoptysis, clubbing, dyspnea, and diffuse chest pain. Fever and wheezing may occur.

◆ ***Malnutrition.*** Painful unilateral gynecomastia (known as refeeding gynecomastia) may occur when the malnourished patient begins to take nourishment again. Other effects of malnutrition include apathy, muscle wasting, weakness, limb paresthesia, anorexia, nausea, vomiting, and diarrhea. Inspection may reveal dull, sparse, dry hair; brittle nails; dark, swollen cheeks and lips; dry, flaky skin; and, occasionally, edema and hepatomegaly.

◆ ***Pituitary tumor.*** This hormone-secreting tumor causes bilateral gynecomastia accompanied by galactorrhea, impotence, and decreased libido. Other hormonal effects may include enlarged hands and feet, coarse facial features with prognathism, voice deepening, weight gain, increased blood pressure, diaphoresis, heat intolerance, hyperpigmentation, and thickened, oily skin. Paresthesia or sensory loss and muscle weakness commonly affect the limbs. If the tumor expands, it may cause blurred vision, diplopia, headache, or partial bitemporal hemianopia that may progress to blindness.

◆ ***Reifenstein's syndrome.*** This genetic disorder produces painless bilateral gynecomastia at puberty. Associated signs may include hypospadias, testicular atrophy, and an underdeveloped penis.

◆ ***Renal failure (chronic).*** This disorder may produce bilateral gynecomastia accompanied by decreased libido and impotence. Among its more characteristic features, however, are ammonia breath odor, oliguria, fatigue, decreased mental acuity, seizures, muscle cramps, and peripheral neuropathy. Common GI effects include anorexia, nausea, vomiting, and constipation or diarrhea. The patient also typically has bleeding tendencies, pruritus, yellow-brown or bronze skin and, occasionally, uremic frost and increased blood pressure.

◆ ***Testicular failure (secondary).*** Commonly associated with mumps and other infectious disorders, secondary testicular failure produces bilateral gynecomastia that appears after normal puberty. This disorder may also cause sparse facial hair, decreased libido, impotence, and testicular atrophy.

◆ ***Testicular tumor.*** Choriocarcinomas, Leydig's cell tumors, and other testicular tumors typically cause bilateral gynecomastia, nipple tenderness, and decreased libido. Because these tumors are usually painless, testicular swelling may be the patient's initial complaint. A firm mass and a heavy sensation in the scrotum may occur.

◆ ***Thyrotoxicosis.*** Bilateral gynecomastia may occur with loss of libido and impotence. Cardinal findings include an enlarged thyroid gland, tachycardia, palpitations, weight loss despite increased appetite, diarrhea, tremors, dyspnea, nervousness, diaphoresis, heat intolerance, and possibly exophthalmos. An atrial or ventricular gallop may also occur.

Other causes

◆ ***Drugs.*** When gynecomastia is an effect of drugs, it's typically painful and unilateral. Estrogens used to treat prostate cancer, including estramustine, directly affect the estrogen-androgen ratio. Drugs that have an estrogen-like effect, such as cardiac glycosides and human chorionic gonadotropin, may do the same. Regular use of alcohol, marijuana, or heroin reduces plasma testosterone levels, causing gynecomastia. Other drugs—such as flutamide, spironolactone, cimetidine, and ketoconazole—produce this sign by interfering with androgen production or action. Some common drugs, including phenothiazines, tricyclic antidepressants, and antihypertensives, produce gynecomastia in an unknown way.

◆ ***Treatments.*** Gynecomastia may develop within weeks of starting hemodialysis for chronic renal failure. It may also follow major surgery or testicular irradiation.

Special considerations

To make the patient as comfortable as possible, apply cold compresses to his breasts and administer analgesics. Prepare him for diagnostic tests, including chest and skull X-rays and blood hormone levels.

Because gynecomastia may alter the patient's body image, provide emotional support. Reassure the patient that treatment can reduce gynecomastia. Some patients are helped by tamoxifen, an antiestrogen, or by testolactone, an inhibitor of testosterone-to-estrogen conversion. Surgical removal of breast tissue may be an option if drug treatment fails.

Pediatric pointers

In neonates, gynecomastia may be associated with galactorrhea ("witch's milk"). This sign usually disappears within a few weeks but may persist until age 2.

Most males have physiologic gynecomastia at some time during adolescence, usually around age 14. This gynecomastia is usually asymmetrical and tender; it commonly resolves within 2 years and rarely persists beyond age 20.

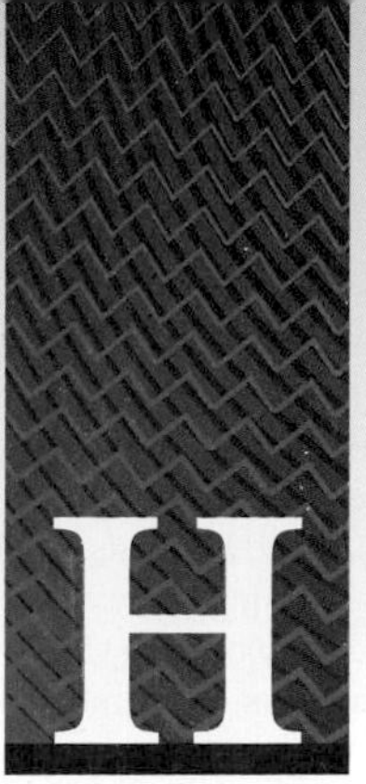

Halitosis

Halitosis describes any breath odor that's unpleasant, disagreeable, or offensive. This common sign is usually easy to detect, but an embarrassed patient may take measures to hide it. The patient may be unaware that he has halitosis, even though he may complain of a bad taste in his mouth, or he may believe that he has halitosis but that no one else can detect it (psychogenic halitosis).

Certain types of halitosis characterize specific disorders—for example, a fruity breath odor typifies ketoacidosis. (See "Breath with ammonia odor," page 120; "Breath with fecal odor," page 121; "Breath with fruity odor," page 123; and "Fetor hepaticus," page 297.) Other types of halitosis include putrid, foul, fetid, and musty breath odors.

Halitosis may result from a disorder of the oral cavity, nasal passages, sinuses, respiratory tract, or esophageal diverticula. It may also stem from a GI disorder associated with belching, regurgitation, or vomiting, or it may be an adverse effect of an oral or inhaled drug.

Other causes of halitosis include cigarette smoking, ingestion of alcohol and certain foods (such as garlic and onions), and poor oral hygiene—especially in patients with an orthodontic device, dentures, or dental caries. In addition, offensive skin odors—for example, from foot perspiration—may be absorbed locally and later expelled by the lungs, resulting in halitosis.

History and physical examination

If you detect halitosis, try to characterize the odor. Does it smell fruity, fecal, or musty? If the patient is aware of it, find out how long he has had it. Does he also have a bad taste in his mouth? Does he have difficulty swallowing or chewing? Does he have reflux or regurgitation? Does he have pain or tenderness? Ask the patient if he has a problem with flatus. Also ask him to describe the frequency of his bowel movements and the size and consistency of his stools.

Find out if the patient smokes or chews tobacco. Have him describe his diet and daily oral hygiene. Does he wear dentures? Complete the history by asking about chronic disorders and recent respiratory tract infection. If the patient reports a cough, find out if it's productive.

Begin the physical examination by examining the patient's mouth, throat, and nose. Look for lesions, bleeding, drainage, obstruction, and signs of infection, such as redness and swelling. Check for tenderness by percussing and palpating over the sinuses. Then auscultate the lungs for abnormal breath sounds. Auscultate the abdomen for bowel sounds, and percuss it, noting any tympany. Finally, take vital signs.

Medical causes

◆ ***Bowel obstruction.*** Halitosis is a late sign in both small- and large-bowel obstructions, resulting from vomiting of bilious and later fecal material. Other findings in a small-bowel obstruction include constipation, abdominal distention, and intermittent periumbilical cramping pain. In a large-bowel obstruction, abdominal pain is milder and more constant than that associated with a small-bowel obstruction and is usually located lower in the abdomen.

◆ ***Bronchiectasis.*** Bronchiectasis usually produces foul or putrid halitosis, but some patients may have a sickeningly sweet breath odor. The patient typically also has a chronic productive cough with copious, foul-smelling, mucopurulent sputum. The cough is aggravated by lying down and is most productive in the morning. Associated findings commonly include exertional dyspnea, fatigue, malaise, weakness, and weight loss. Auscultation reveals coarse or moist crackles over the affected lung areas during inspiration. Digital clubbing is a late sign.

◆ ***Common cold.*** A musty breath odor may accompany a common cold, which usually also causes a dry, hacking cough with sore throat, sneezing, nasal congestion, rhinorrhea, headache, malaise, fatigue, arthralgia, and myalgia.

◆ ***Esophageal cancer.*** In esophageal cancer, halitosis may accompany classic findings of dysphagia, hoarseness, chest pain, and weight loss. Nocturnal regurgitation and cachexia are late signs.

◆ ***Gastric cancer.*** Halitosis is a late sign in gastric cancer. Accompanying findings include chronic dyspepsia unrelieved by antacids, a vague feeling of fullness, nausea, anorexia, fatigue, pallor, weakness, altered bowel habits, weight loss, and muscle wasting. Hematemesis and melena are signs of associated gastric bleeding.

◆ ***Gastrocolic fistula.*** In this disorder, fecal vomiting is responsible for fecal breath odor, which is typically preceded by intermittent diarrhea.

◆ ***Gingivitis.*** Characterized by red, edematous gums, gingivitis may also cause halitosis. The gingivae between the teeth become bulbous and bleed easily with slight trauma.

Acute necrotizing ulcerative gingivitis also causes fetid breath, a bad taste in the mouth, and ulcers—especially between the teeth—that may become covered with a gray exudate. Severe ulceration may occur with fever, cervical adenopathy, headache, and malaise.

◆ ***Hepatic encephalopathy.*** A characteristic late sign of hepatic encephalopathy is fetor hepaticus, a musty, sweet, or mousy (new-mown hay) breath odor. Other late effects include coma, asterixis (flapping tremor), and hyperactive deep tendon reflexes.

◆ ***Ketoacidosis.*** Alcohol-induced, diabetic, and starvation forms of ketoacidosis produce a fruity breath odor. *Alcohol-induced ketoacidosis* is usually seen in poorly nourished alcoholics who have eaten very little over several days. Symptoms include sudden Kussmaul's respirations with vomiting for several days, light dehydration, abdominal pain and distention, and absent bowel sounds. The patient is alert and has a normal or slightly decreased blood glucose level.

Life-threatening *diabetic ketoacidosis* produces a rapid, thready pulse; marked hypovolemia; nausea and vomiting; and, in its early stages, the triad of polydipsia, polyphagia, and polyuria.

Also life-threatening, *starvation ketoacidosis* produces Kussmaul's respirations; weight loss; bradycardia; dry, scaly skin; sore tongue; muscle and tissue wasting; abdominal distention; and signs of dehydration, such as oliguria and poor skin turgor.

Other common effects of diabetic and starvation ketoacidosis include orthostatic hypotension, generalized weakness, anorexia, abdominal pain, and altered level of consciousness.

◆ ***Lung abscess.*** Lung abscess typically causes putrid halitosis, but its cardinal sign is a productive cough with copious, purulent, often bloody sputum. Other findings include fever with chills, dyspnea, headache, anorexia, weight loss, malaise, pleuritic chest pain, asymmetrical chest movement, and temporary clubbing.

◆ ***Necrotizing ulcerative mucositis (acute).*** A strong, putrid breath odor is characteristic of this uncommon disorder, which initially causes slight cheek inflammation that's rapidly followed by tooth loss and extensive bone sloughing in the mandible or maxilla.

◆ ***Ozena.*** This severe, chronic form of rhinitis causes a musty or fetid breath odor as well as thick green mucus and progressive anosmia.

◆ ***Periodontal disease.*** Periodontal disease causes halitosis and an unpleasant taste. Typically, the patient's gums bleed spontaneously or with slight trauma and are marked by pus-filled pockets around the teeth. Related findings include facial pain, headache, and loose teeth covered by calculi and plaque.

◆ ***Pharyngitis (gangrenous).*** Halitosis is a chief sign of gangrenous pharyngitis. The patient also complains of a foul taste in the mouth, an extremely sore throat, and a choking sensation. Examination reveals a swollen, red, ulcerated pharynx, possibly with a grayish membrane. Fever and cervical lymphadenopathy are also common.

◆ ***Renal failure (chronic).*** Renal failure produces a urinous or ammonia breath odor. Among its widespread effects are anemia, emotional lability, lethargy, irritability, decreased mental acuity, coarse muscular twitching, peripheral neuropathies, muscle wasting, anorexia, signs of GI bleeding, ecchymosis, yellow-brown or bronze skin, pruritus, anuria, and increased blood pressure.

◆ ***Sinusitis.*** Acute sinusitis causes a purulent nasal discharge that leads to halitosis. Besides a characteristic postnasal drip, the patient may exhibit nasal congestion, sore throat, cough, malaise, headache, facial pain and tenderness, and fever.

Chronic sinusitis causes a continuous mucopurulent discharge that leads to a musty breath odor, postnasal drip, nasal congestion, and a chronic nonproductive cough.

◆ ***Zenker's diverticulum.*** This esophageal disorder causes halitosis and a bad taste in the mouth associated with regurgitation. The patient may also report a chronic cough that's most pronounced at night, hoarseness, odynophagia, neck pain, and "gurgling" sounds in the throat when he swallows liquids.

OTHER CAUSES

◆ ***Drugs.*** Drugs that can cause halitosis include triamterene, inhaled anesthetics, and any drugs known to cause metabolic acidosis such as nitroprusside.

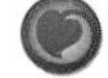

HERB ALERT *Some herbal medicines, such as garlic, may cause halitosis.*

SPECIAL CONSIDERATIONS

If examination of the mouth and sinuses doesn't reveal the cause of halitosis, prepare the patient for upper GI and chest X-rays or endoscopy.

PEDIATRIC POINTERS

In children, halitosis commonly results from physiologic causes, such as continual mouth breathing and thumb or blanket sucking. Phenylketonuria—a metabolic disorder that affects infants—may produce a musty or mousy breath odor.

GERIATRIC POINTERS

Extensive dental caries, mouth dryness, and poor oral hygiene can cause halitosis in elderly patients.

PATIENT COUNSELING

To help control halitosis, encourage good oral hygiene. If halitosis is drug induced, reassure the patient that it will disappear as soon as his body completely eliminates the drug.

Halo vision

Halo vision refers to seeing rainbowlike colored rings around lights or bright objects. The rainbowlike effect can be explained by this physical principle: As light passes through water (in the eye, through tears or the cells of various anteretinal media), it breaks up into spectral colors.

Halo vision usually develops suddenly; its duration depends on the causative disorder. This symptom may occur in disorders associated with excessive tearing and corneal epithelial edema. Among these causes, the most common and significant is acute angle-closure glaucoma, which can lead to blindness. In this ophthalmic emergency, increased intraocular pressure (IOP) forces fluid into corneal tissues anterior to Bowman's membrane, causing edema. Halo vision is also an early symptom of cataracts, resulting from dispersion of light by abnormal lens opacity.

Nonpathologic causes of excessive tearing associated with halo vision include poorly fitted or overworn contact lenses, emotional extremes, and exposure to intense light, as in snow blindness.

HISTORY AND PHYSICAL EXAMINATION

First, ask the patient how long he has been seeing halos around lights and when he usually sees them. Patients with glaucoma usually see halos in the morning, when IOP is most elevated. Ask the patient if light bothers his eyes. Does he have eye pain? If so, have him describe it. Remember that halos associated with excruciating eye pain or a severe headache may point to acute angle-closure glaucoma, an ocular emergency. Note a history of glaucoma or cataracts.

Next, examine the patient's eyes, noting conjunctival injection, excessive tearing, and lens changes. Examine pupil size, shape, and response to light. Then test visual acuity by performing an ophthalmoscopic examination.

MEDICAL CAUSES

◆ ***Cataract.*** Halo vision may be an early symptom of painless, progressive cataract formation.

The glare of headlights may blind the patient, making nighttime driving impossible. Other features include blurred vision, impaired visual acuity, and lens opacity, all of which develop gradually.

◆ ***Corneal endothelial dystrophy.*** Typically, halo vision is a late symptom of this disorder, which may also cause impaired visual acuity.

◆ ***Glaucoma.*** Halo vision characterizes all types of glaucoma. *Acute angle-closure glaucoma*—an ophthalmic emergency—also causes blurred vision, followed by a severe headache or excruciating pain in and around the affected eye. Examination reveals a moderately dilated fixed pupil that doesn't respond to light, conjunctival injection, a cloudy cornea, impaired visual acuity and, possibly, nausea and vomiting.

Chronic angle-closure glaucoma usually produces no symptoms until pain and blindness occur in advanced disease. Sometimes, halos and blurred vision develop slowly.

In *chronic open-angle glaucoma,* halo vision is a late symptom that's accompanied by mild eye ache, peripheral vision loss, and impaired visual acuity.

Special considerations

To help minimize halo vision, remind the patient not to look directly at bright lights.

Pediatric pointers

Halo vision in a child usually results from congenital cataracts or glaucoma. In a young child, limited verbal ability may make halo vision difficult to assess.

Geriatric pointers

Primary glaucoma, the most common cause of halo vision, is more common in older patients.

Headache

The most common neurologic symptom, headaches may be localized or generalized, producing mild to severe pain. About 90% of all headaches are benign and can be described as vascular, muscle-contraction, or a combination of both. (See *Comparing benign headaches.*) Occasionally, though, headaches indicate a severe neurologic disorder associated with intracranial inflammation, increased intracranial pressure (ICP), or meningeal irritation. They may also result from an ocular or sinus disorder, tests, drugs, or other treatments.

Other causes of headache include fever, eyestrain, dehydration, and systemic febrile illnesses. Headaches may occur in certain metabolic disturbances—such as hypoxemia, hypercapnia, hyperglycemia, and hypoglycemia—but they aren't a diagnostic or prominent symptom in these disorders. Some individuals get headaches after seizures or from coughing, sneezing, heavy lifting, or stooping.

History and physical examination

If the patient reports a headache, ask him to describe its characteristics and location. How often does he get a headache? How long does a typical headache last? Try to identify precipitating factors, such as eating certain foods or exposure to bright lights. Ask what helps to relieve the headache. Is the patient under stress? Has he had trouble sleeping?

Take a drug and alcohol history, and ask about head trauma within the last 4 weeks. Has the patient recently experienced nausea, vomiting, photophobia, or visual changes? Does he feel drowsy, confused, or dizzy? Has he recently developed seizures, or does he have a history of seizures?

Begin the physical examination by evaluating the patient's level of consciousness (LOC). Then check his vital signs. Be alert for signs of increased ICP—widened pulse pressure, bradycardia, altered respiratory pattern, and increased blood pressure. Check pupil size and response to light, and note any neck stiffness. (See *Differential diagnosis: Headache*, pages 344 and 345.)

Medical causes

◆ ***Anthrax, cutaneous.*** Along with a macular or papular lesion that develops into a vesicle and finally a painless ulcer, this disorder may produce a headache, lymphadenopathy, fever, and malaise.

◆ ***Brain abscess.*** In this disorder, the headache is localized to the abscess site; it usually intensifies over a few days and is aggravated by straining. Accompanying the headache may be nausea, vomiting, and focal or generalized seizures. The patient's LOC varies from drowsiness to deep stupor. Depending on the abscess site, associated signs and symptoms may include aphasia, impaired visual acuity, hemiparesis, ataxia, tremors, and personality changes. Signs of infection, such as fever and pallor, usually develop late; however, if the

Comparing benign headaches

Of the many patients who report headaches, only about 10% have an underlying medical disorder. The other 90% suffer from benign headaches, which may be classified as muscle-contraction (tension), vascular (migraine and cluster), or a combination of both.

As you review the chart below, you'll see that the two major types — muscle-contraction and vascular headaches — are quite different. In a combined headache, features of both appear; this type of headache may affect the patient with a severe muscle-contraction headache or a late-stage migraine. Treatment of a combined headache includes analgesics and sedatives.

Characteristics	Muscle-contraction headaches	Vascular headaches
Incidence	◆ Most common type, accounting for 80% of all headaches	◆ More common in women and those with a family history of migraines ◆ Onset after puberty
Precipitating factors	◆ Stress, anxiety, tension, improper posture, and body alignment ◆ Prolonged muscle contraction without structural damage ◆ Eye, ear, and paranasal sinus disorders that produce reflex muscle contractions	◆ Hormone fluctuations ◆ Alcohol ◆ Emotional upset ◆ Too little or too much sleep ◆ Foods, such as chocolate, cheese, monosodium glutamate, and cured meats; caffeine withdrawal ◆ Weather changes, such as shifts in barometric pressure
Intensity and duration	◆ Produce an aching tightness or a band of pain around the head, especially in the neck and in occipital and temporal areas ◆ Occur frequently and usually last for several hours	◆ May begin with an awareness of an impending migraine or a 5- to 15-minute prodrome of neurologic deficits, such as visual disturbances, dizziness, unsteady gait, or tingling of the face, lips, or hands ◆ Produce severe, constant, throbbing pain that is typically unilateral and may be incapacitating ◆ Last for 4 to 6 hours
Associated signs and symptoms	◆ Tense neck and facial muscles	◆ Anorexia, nausea, and vomiting ◆ Occasionally, photophobia, sensitivity to loud noises, weakness, and fatigue ◆ Depending on the type (cluster headache or classic, common, or hemiplegic migraine), possibly chills, depression, eye pain, ptosis, tearing, rhinorrhea, diaphoresis, and facial flushing
Alleviating factors	◆ Mild analgesics, muscle relaxants, or other drugs during an attack ◆ Measures to reduce stress, such as biofeedback, relaxation techniques, and counseling; posture correction to prevent attacks	◆ Methysergide and propranolol to prevent vascular headache ◆ Ergot alkaloids or serotonin-receptor drugs at the first sign of a migraine ◆ Rest in a quiet, darkened room ◆ Elimination of irritating foods from diet

Differential diagnosis: Headache

History of present illness

Focused physical examination: Neurologic and musculoskeletal systems; head, eyes, ears, nose, and throat; neck; mental health; lymph nodes

Sinusitis

Signs and symptoms
- Dull periorbital headache
- Unilateral or bilateral frontal or maxillary sinus pain that's increased by palpation or bending over
- Fever
- Malaise
- Nasal turbinate edema
- Sore throat
- Nasal discharge

Diagnosis: Physical examination, transillumination, sinus X-ray
Treatment: Medication (decongestants, analgesics, antibiotics)
Follow-up: None unless signs and symptoms worsen or recur

Brain abscess

Signs and symptoms
- Localized headache that increases over a few days
- Possible nausea and vomiting
- Focal or generalized seizures
- Drowsiness

Subdural hematoma

Signs and symptoms
- Decreased level of consciousness (LOC)
- Acute drowsiness, confusion, or agitation
- Pounding headache
- Giddiness
- Personality changes
- Dizziness
- Confusion

Encephalitis

Signs and symptoms
- Severe, generalized headache
- Deteriorating LOC within 48 hours of initial headache
- Fever
- Nuchal rigidity
- Irritability
- Seizures
- Nausea and vomiting
- Photophobia

Diagnosis: Possible history of head trauma, lumbar puncture, imaging studies (computed tomography scan, magnetic resonance imaging, arteriography)
Treatment: Medication (antibiotics if indicated; analgesics, anticonvulsants, osmotic diuretics); surgery if appropriate; chemotherapy or radiation therapy if malignancy is present
Follow-up: Referral to neurologist or neurosurgeon

abscess remains encapsulated, these signs may not appear.

◆ ***Brain tumor.*** Initially, a tumor causes a localized headache near the tumor site; as the tumor grows, the headache eventually becomes generalized. The pain is usually intermittent, deep seated, and dull and is most intense in the morning. It's aggravated by coughing, stooping, Valsalva's maneuver, and changes in head position, and it's relieved by sitting and rest.

Epidural hemorrhage	Cerebral aneurysm (ruptured)	Intracranial hemorrhage	Brain tumor
Signs and symptoms ◆ Progressively severe headache ◆ Unilateral seizures ◆ Decreased LOC ◆ Hemiparesis or hemiplegia ◆ High-grade fever	**Signs and symptoms** ◆ Sudden severe, possibly unilateral headache ◆ Possible nausea and vomiting ◆ Change in LOC ◆ Vision changes	**Signs and symptoms** ◆ Severe generalized headache ◆ Rapid, steady decrease in LOC ◆ Hemiparesis or hemiplegia ◆ Aphasia ◆ Dizziness ◆ Nausea and vomiting ◆ Irregular respirations ◆ Positive Babinski's reflex	**Signs and symptoms** ◆ Localized or generalized headache ◆ Intermittent deep pain that's more intense in the morning and increases with Valsalva's maneuver ◆ Personality changes ◆ Changes in LOC

Associated signs and symptoms include personality changes, altered LOC, motor and sensory dysfunction, and eventually signs of increased ICP, such as vomiting, increased systolic blood pressure, and widened pulse pressure.

◆ ***Cerebral aneurysm (ruptured).*** Cerebral aneurysm is a life-threatening disorder that's characterized by a sudden excruciating headache, which may be unilateral and usually peaks within minutes of the rupture. The patient may lose consciousness immediately or display a variably altered LOC. Depending on the severity and location of the bleeding, he may also exhibit nausea and vomiting; signs and symptoms of meningeal irritation, such as nuchal rigidity and blurred vision; hemiparesis; and other features.

◆ ***Ebola virus.*** A sudden headache commonly occurs on the 5th day of this deadly illness. Additionally, the patient has a history of malaise, myalgia, high fever, diarrhea, abdominal pain, dehydration, and lethargy. A maculopapular rash develops between the 5th and 7th days of the illness. Other possible findings include pleuritic chest pain; a dry, hacking cough; pronounced pharyngitis; hematemesis; melena; and bleeding from the nose, gums, and vagina. Death usually occurs in the 2nd week of the illness, preceded by massive blood loss and shock.

◆ ***Encephalitis.*** A severe, generalized headache is characteristic with this disorder. Within 48 hours, the patient's LOC typically deteriorates—perhaps from lethargy to coma. Associated signs and symptoms include fever, nuchal rigidity, irritability, seizures, nausea and vomiting, photophobia, cranial nerve palsies such as ptosis, and focal neurologic deficits, such as hemiparesis and hemiplegia.

◆ ***Epidural hemorrhage (acute).*** Head trauma and a sudden, brief loss of consciousness usually precede this hemorrhage, which causes a progressively severe headache that's accompanied by nausea and vomiting, bladder distention, confusion, and then a rapid decrease in LOC. Other signs and symptoms include unilateral seizures, hemiparesis, hemiplegia, high fever, decreased pulse rate and bounding pulse, widened pulse pressure, increased blood pressure, a positive Babinski's reflex, and decerebrate posture.

If the patient slips into a coma, his respirations deepen and become stertorous, then shallow and irregular, and eventually cease. Pupil dilation may occur on the same side as the hemorrhage.

◆ ***Glaucoma, acute angle-closure.*** This type of glaucoma is an ophthalmic emergency that may cause an excruciating headache as well as acute eye pain, blurred vision, halo vision, nausea, and vomiting. Assessment reveals conjunctival injection, a cloudy cornea, and a moderately dilated, fixed pupil.

◆ **Hantavirus *pulmonary syndrome.*** Noncardiogenic pulmonary edema distinguishes this viral disease, which was first reported in the United States in 1993. Common reasons for seeking treatment include flulike signs and symptoms—headache, myalgia, fever, nausea, vomiting, and a cough—followed by respiratory distress. Fever, hypoxia, and (in some patients) serious hypotension typify the hospital course. Other signs and symptoms include a rising respiratory rate (28 breaths/minute or more) and an increased heart rate (120 beats/minute or more).

◆ ***Hypertension.*** This disorder may cause a slightly throbbing occipital headache on awakening that decreases in severity during the day. However, if the patient's diastolic blood pressure exceeds 120 mm Hg, the headache remains constant. Associated signs and symptoms include an atrial gallop, restlessness, confusion, nausea and vomiting, blurred vision, seizures, and altered LOC.

◆ ***Influenza.*** A severe generalized or frontal headache usually begins suddenly with the flu. Accompanying signs and symptoms may last for 3 to 5 days and include stabbing retro-orbital pain, weakness, diffuse myalgia, fever, chills, coughing, rhinorrhea and, occasionally, hoarseness.

◆ ***Influenza type A H1N1 virus (swine flu).*** Influenza type A H1N1, or swine flu, is a respiratory disease of pigs caused by type A influenza virus. Swine flu viruses cause high levels of illness and low death rates in pigs. Swine flu viruses normally don't infect humans; however, sporadic human infections with swine flu have occurred. Most commonly, these cases occur in persons with direct exposure to pigs. The virus has changed slightly and is known as H1N1 flu. Recent outbreaks of H1N1 flu have shown that the virus can be transmitted from person to person, causing transmission across the globe. The H1N1 flu is similar to influenza, and causes illness and in some cases death. The symptoms of swine flu include headache, nonproductive cough, fatigue, myalgia, chills, fever, and vomiting. The use of antiviral drugs is recommended to treat H1N1 flu.

◆ ***Intracerebral hemorrhage.*** In some patients, this hemorrhage produces a severe generalized headache. Other signs and symptoms vary with the size and location of the hemorrhage. A large hemorrhage may produce a rapid, steady decrease in LOC, perhaps resulting in a coma. Other common findings include hemiplegia, hemiparesis, abnormal pupil size and response, aphasia, dizziness, nausea, vomiting, seizures, decreased sensation, irregular respirations, positive Babinski's reflex, decorticate or decerebrate posture, and increased blood pressure.

◆ ***Listeriosis.*** If this infection spreads to the nervous system, it may cause meningitis, whose signs and symptoms include headache, nuchal rigidity, fever, and change in LOC. Earlier signs and symptoms of listeriosis include fever, myalgia, abdominal pain, nausea, vomiting, and diarrhea.

GENDER CUE *Listeriosis during pregnancy may lead to premature delivery, infection of the neonate, or stillbirth.*

◆ ***Meningitis.*** This disorder is marked by the sudden onset of a severe, constant, generalized headache that worsens with movement. Fever and chills are other early signs. As meningitis progresses, it also causes nuchal rigidity, positive Kernig's and Brudzinski's signs, hyperreflexia, altered LOC, seizures, ocular palsies, facial weakness, hearing loss, vomiting and, possibly, opisthotonos and papilledema.

◆ ***Plague.*** The pneumonic form of this lethal bacterial infection causes a sudden onset of headache, chills, fever, and myalgia. Pulmonary findings include a productive cough, chest pain, tachypnea, dyspnea, hemoptysis, respiratory distress, and cardiopulmonary insufficiency.

◆ ***Postconcussion syndrome.*** A generalized or localized headache may develop 1 to 30 days after head trauma and last for 2 to 3 weeks. This characteristic symptom may be described as an aching, pounding, pressing, stabbing, or throbbing pain. The patient's neurologic examination is normal, but he may experience giddiness or dizziness, blurred vision, fatigue, insomnia, inability to concentrate, and noise and alcohol intolerance.

◆ ***Q fever.*** Signs and symptoms of this disease include severe headaches, fever, chills, malaise, chest pain, nausea, vomiting, and diarrhea. The fever may last for up to 2 weeks, and in severe cases, the patient may develop hepatitis or pneumonia.

◆ ***Severe acute respiratory syndrome (SARS).*** SARS is an acute infectious disease caused by a coronavirus. Although most cases have been reported in Asia (China, Vietnam, Singapore, Thailand), cases have cropped up in Europe and North America. After an incubation period of 2 to 7 days, the illness generally begins with a fever (usually greater than 100.4° F [38° C]). Other symptoms include headache, malaise, a nonproductive cough, and dyspnea. SARS may produce only mild symptoms, or it may progress to pneumonia and, in some cases, even respiratory failure and death.

◆ ***Sinusitis (acute).*** This disorder is usually marked by a dull periorbital headache that's usually aggravated by bending over or touching the face and is relieved by sinus drainage. Fever, sinus tenderness, nasal turbinate edema, sore throat, malaise, cough, and nasal discharge may accompany the headache.

◆ ***Smallpox (variola major).*** Initial signs and symptoms of this virus include a severe headache, backache, abdominal pain, high fever, malaise, prostration, and a maculopapular rash on the mucosa of the mouth, pharynx, face, and forearms and then on the trunk and legs. The rash becomes vesicular, then pustular. After 8 or 9 days, the pustules form a crust, which later separates from the skin, leaving a pitted scar. Death may result from encephalitis, extensive bleeding, or secondary infection.

◆ ***Subarachnoid hemorrhage.*** This hemorrhage commonly produces a sudden, violent headache along with nuchal rigidity, nausea and vomiting, seizures, dizziness, ipsilateral pupil dilation, and altered LOC that may rapidly progress to coma. The patient also exhibits positive Kernig's and Brudzinski's signs, photophobia, blurred vision and, possibly, a fever. Focal signs and symptoms (such as hemiparesis, hemiplegia, sensory or vision disturbances, and aphasia) and signs of elevated ICP (such as bradycardia and increased blood pressure) may also occur.

◆ ***Subdural hematoma.*** Typically associated with head trauma, both acute and chronic subdural hematomas may cause headache and decreased LOC. An *acute subdural hematoma* also produces drowsiness, confusion, and agitation that may progress to coma. Later findings include signs of increased ICP and focal neurologic deficits such as hemiparesis.

A *chronic subdural hematoma* produces a dull, pounding headache that fluctuates in severity and is located over the hematoma. Weeks or months after the initial head trauma, the patient may experience giddiness, personality changes, confusion, seizures, and progressively worsening LOC. Late signs may include unilateral pupil dilation, sluggish pupil reaction to light, and ptosis.

◆ ***Temporal arteritis.*** A throbbing unilateral headache in the temporal or frontotemporal region may be accompanied by vision loss, hearing loss, confusion, and fever. The temporal arteries are tender, swollen, nodular, and sometimes erythematous.

◆ ***Tularemia.*** Signs and symptoms following inhalation of the bacterium *Francisella tularensis* include abrupt onset of headache, fever, chills, generalized myalgia, a nonproductive cough, dyspnea, pleuritic chest pain, and empyema.

◆ ***Typhus.*** In typhus, initial symptoms of headache, myalgia, arthralgia, and malaise are followed by an abrupt onset of chills, fever, nausea, and vomiting. A maculopapular rash may also occur.

◆ ***West Nile encephalitis.*** This brain infection is caused by West Nile virus, a mosquito-borne flavivirus commonly found in Africa, West Asia, the Middle East and, rarely, in North America. Most patients have mild signs and symptoms, including fever, headache, body aches, rash, and swollen lymph glands. More severe infection is marked by high fever, headache, neck stiffness, stupor, disorientation, coma, tremors, and paralysis.

OTHER CAUSES

◆ ***Diagnostic tests.*** A lumbar puncture or myelogram may produce a throbbing frontal headache that worsens on standing.

◆ ***Drugs.*** A wide variety of drugs can cause headaches. For example, indomethacin produces headaches—usually in the morning—in many patients. Vasodilators and drugs with a vasodilating effect, such as nitrates, typically cause a throbbing headache. Headaches may also follow withdrawal from vasopressors, such as caffeine, ergotamine, and sympathomimetics.

HERB ALERT *Herbal remedies, such as St. John's wort, ginseng, and ephedra (ma huang), can cause various adverse reactions, including headaches. (Note: The FDA has banned the sale of dietary supplements containing ephedra because they pose an unreasonable risk of injury or illness.)*

◆ ***Traction.*** Cervical traction with pins commonly causes a headache, which may be generalized or localized to pin insertion sites.

SPECIAL CONSIDERATIONS

Continue to monitor the patient's vital signs and LOC. Watch for any change in the headache's severity or location. To help ease the headache, administer an analgesic, darken the patient's room, and minimize other stimuli. Explain the rationale of these interventions to the patient.

Prepare the patient for diagnostic tests, such as skull X-rays, computed tomography scan, lumbar puncture, or cerebral arteriography.

PEDIATRIC POINTERS

If a child is too young to describe his symptom, suspect a headache if you see him banging or holding his head. In an infant, a shrill cry or bulging fontanels may indicate increased ICP and headache. In a school-age child, ask the parents about the child's recent scholastic performance and about any problems at home that may produce a tension headache.

Twice as many young boys have migraine headaches as girls. In children older than age 3, headache is the most common symptom of a brain tumor.

Hearing loss

Affecting nearly 16 million Americans, hearing loss may be temporary or permanent and partial or complete. This common symptom may involve reception of low-, middle-, or high-frequency tones. If the hearing loss doesn't affect speech frequencies, the patient may be unaware of it.

Normally, sound waves enter the external auditory canal and travel to the middle ear's tympanic membrane and ossicles (incus, malleus, and stapes) and then into the inner ear's cochlea. The cochlear division of the eighth cranial (auditory) nerve carries the sound impulse to the brain. This type of sound transmission, called air conduction, is normally better than bone conduction—sound transmission through bone to the inner ear.

Hearing loss can be classified as conductive, sensorineural, mixed, or functional. Conductive hearing loss results from external or middle ear disorders that block sound transmission. This type of hearing loss usually responds to medical or surgical intervention (or in some cases, both). Sensorineural hearing loss results from disorders of the inner ear or of the eighth cranial nerve. Mixed hearing loss combines aspects of conductive and sensorineural hearing loss. Functional hearing loss results from psychological factors rather than identifiable organic damage.

Hearing loss may also result from trauma, infection, allergy, tumors, certain systemic and hereditary disorders, and the effects of ototoxic drugs and treatments. In most cases, though, it results from presbycusis, a type of sensorineural hearing loss that usually affects people older than age 50. Other physiologic causes of hearing loss include cerumen (earwax) impaction; barotitis media (unequal pressure on the eardrum) associated with descent in an airplane or elevator, diving, or close proximity to an explosion; and chronic exposure to noise over 90 decibels, which can occur on the job, with certain hobbies, or from listening to live or recorded music.

History and physical examination

If the patient reports hearing loss, ask him to describe it fully. Is it unilateral or bilateral? Continuous or intermittent? Ask about a family history of hearing loss. Then obtain the patient's medical history, noting chronic ear infections, ear surgery, and ear or head trauma. Has the patient recently had an upper respiratory tract infection? After taking a drug history, have the patient describe his occupation and work environment.

Next, explore associated signs and symptoms. Does the patient have ear pain? If so, is it unilateral or bilateral? Continuous or intermittent? Ask the patient if he has noticed discharge from one or both ears. If so, have him describe its color and consistency, and note when it began. Does he hear ringing, buzzing, hissing, or other noises in one or both ears? If so, are the noises constant or intermittent? Does he experience any dizziness? If so, when did he first notice it?

Begin the physical examination by inspecting the external ear for inflammation, boils, foreign bodies, and discharge. Then apply pressure to the tragus and mastoid to elicit tenderness. If you detect tenderness or external ear abnormalities, ask the physician whether an otoscopic examination should be done. (See *Using an otoscope correctly*, page 255.) During the otoscopic examination, note any color change, perforation, bulging, or retraction of the tympanic membrane, which normally looks like a shiny, pearl gray cone.

Next, evaluate the patient's hearing acuity, using the ticking watch and whispered voice tests. Then perform the Weber and Rinne tests to obtain a preliminary evaluation of the type and degree of hearing loss. (See *Differentiating conductive from sensorineural hearing loss*, page 350.)

Medical causes

◆ ***Acoustic neuroma.*** This eighth cranial nerve tumor causes unilateral, progressive, sensorineural hearing loss. The patient may also develop tinnitus, vertigo, and—with cranial nerve compression—facial paralysis.

◆ ***Adenoid hypertrophy.*** Eustachian tube dysfunction gradually causes conductive hearing loss accompanied by intermittent ear discharge. The patient also tends to breathe through his mouth and may complain of a sensation of ear fullness.

◆ ***Allergies.*** Conductive hearing loss may result when an allergy produces eustachian tube and middle ear congestion. Other features include ear pain or a feeling of fullness, nasal congestion, and conjunctivitis.

◆ ***Aural polyps.*** If a polyp occludes the external auditory canal, partial hearing loss may occur. The polyp typically bleeds easily and is covered by a purulent discharge.

◆ ***Cholesteatoma.*** Gradual hearing loss is characteristic in this disorder and may be accompanied by vertigo and, at times, facial paralysis. Examination reveals eardrum perforation, pearly white balls in the ear canal and, possibly, a discharge.

◆ ***Cyst.*** Ear canal obstruction by a sebaceous or dermoid cyst causes progressive conductive hearing loss. On inspection, the cyst looks like a soft mass.

◆ ***External ear canal tumor (malignant).*** Progressive conductive hearing loss is characteristic and is accompanied by deep, boring ear pain; a purulent discharge; and eventually facial paralysis. Examination may detect the granular, bleeding tumor.

◆ ***Furuncle.*** Reversible conductive hearing loss may occur when one of these painful, hard nodules forms in the ear. The patient may report a sense of fullness in the ear and pain on palpation of the tragus or auricle. Rupture relieves the pain and produces a purulent, necrotic discharge.

◆ ***Glomus jugulare tumor.*** Initially, this benign tumor causes mild, unilateral conductive hearing loss that becomes progressively more severe. The patient may report tinnitus that sounds like his heartbeat. Associated signs and symptoms include gradual congestion in the affected ear, throbbing or pulsating discomfort, bloody otorrhea, facial nerve paralysis, and vertigo. Although the tympanic membrane is normal, a reddened mass appears behind it.

◆ ***Glomus tympanum tumor.*** This cancerous middle ear tumor causes slowly progressive hearing loss and throbbing or pulsating tinnitus.

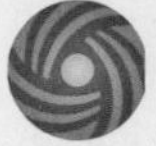

EXAMINATION TIP

Differentiating conductive from sensorineural hearing loss

The Weber and Rinne tests can help determine whether the patient's hearing loss is conductive or sensorineural. The Weber test evaluates bone conduction; the Rinne test, bone and air conduction. Using a 512-Hz tuning fork, perform these preliminary tests as described below.

Weber test

Place the base of a vibrating tuning fork firmly against the midline of the patient's skull. Ask him if he hears the tone equally well in both ears. If he does, the Weber test is graded *midline*—a normal finding. In an abnormal Weber test (graded *right* or *left*), sound is louder either in the impaired ear, suggesting a conductive hearing loss in that ear, or in the normal ear, suggesting a sensorineural loss in the opposite ear.

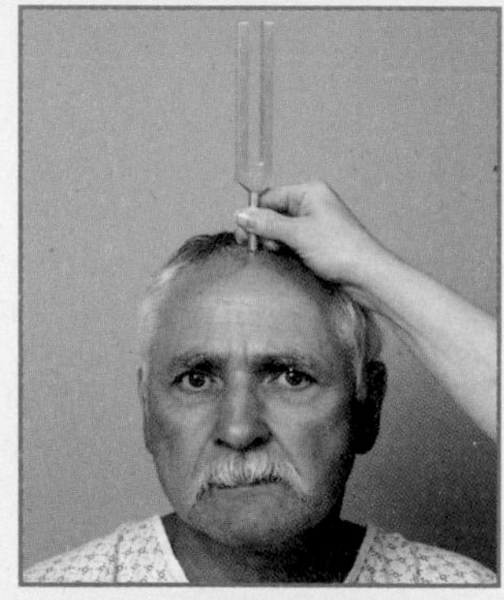

Rinne test

Hold the base of a vibrating tuning fork against the patient's mastoid process to test bone conduction (BC). Then quickly move the vibrating fork in front of his ear canal to test air conduction (AC). Ask him to tell you which location has the louder or longer sound. Repeat the procedure for the other ear. In a positive Rinne test, the AC sound lasts longer or is louder than the BC sound—a normal finding. In a negative test, the opposite is true: the BC sound lasts as long as or longer than the AC sound. In sensorineural loss, the AC sound lasts longer than the BC sound, but the BC sound is louder.

After performing both tests, correlate the results with other assessment data.

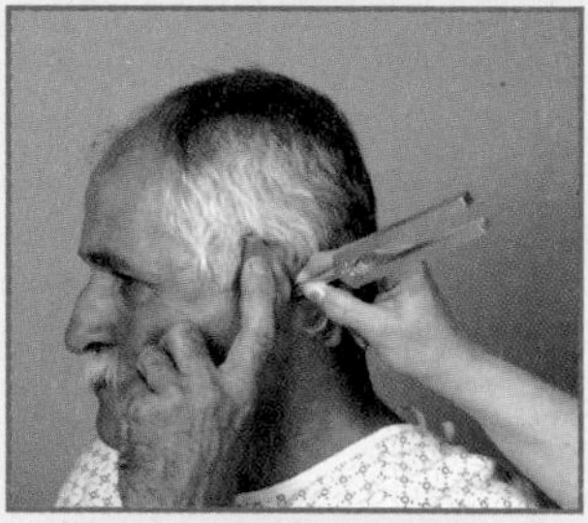

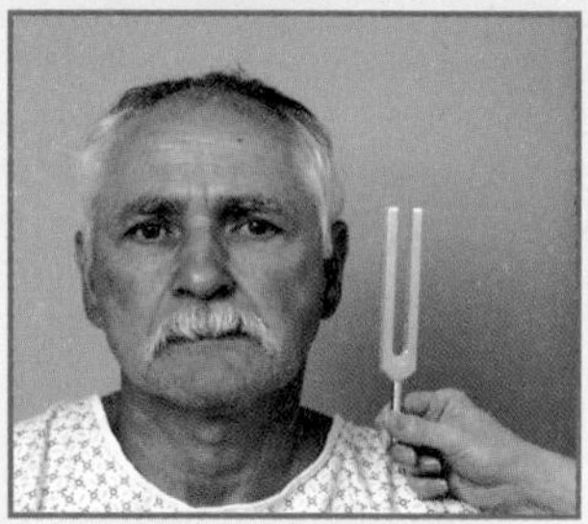

Implications of results

Conductive hearing loss produces:
- abnormal Weber test result
- negative Rinne test result
- improved hearing in noisy areas
- normal ability to discriminate sounds
- difficulty hearing when chewing
- a quiet speaking voice.

Sensorineural hearing loss produces:
- positive Rinne test
- poor hearing in noisy areas
- difficulty hearing high-frequency sounds
- complaints that others mumble or shout
- tinnitus
- loud speaking voice.

It usually bleeds easily when manipulated. Late features include ear pain, dizziness, and total unilateral deafness.

◆ ***Granuloma.*** A rare cause of conductive hearing loss, a granuloma may also produce fullness in the ear, deep-seated pain, and a bloody discharge.

◆ ***Head trauma.*** Sudden conductive or sensorineural hearing loss may result from ossicle disruption, ear canal fracture, tympanic membrane perforation, or cochlear fracture associated with head trauma. Typically, the patient reports a headache and exhibits bleeding from his ear. Neurologic features vary and may include impaired vision and altered level of consciousness.

◆ ***Herpes zoster oticus (Ramsay Hunt syndrome).*** This syndrome causes sudden severe, unilateral mixed hearing loss, which may be accompanied by vesicles in the external ear, tinnitus, vertigo, ear pain, malaise, and transient ipsilateral facial paralysis.

◆ ***Hypothyroidism.*** This disorder may produce reversible sensorineural hearing loss. Other effects include bradycardia, weight gain despite anorexia, mental dullness, cold intolerance, facial edema, brittle hair, and dry skin that's pale, cool, and doughy.

◆ ***Ménière's disease.*** Initially, this inner ear disorder produces intermittent, unilateral sensorineural hearing loss that involves only low tones. Later, hearing loss becomes constant and affects other tones. Associated signs and symptoms include intermittent severe vertigo, nausea and vomiting, a feeling of fullness in the ear, a roaring or hollow-seashell tinnitus, diaphoresis, and nystagmus.

◆ ***Multiple sclerosis.*** Rarely, this disorder causes sensorineural hearing loss associated with myelin destruction of the central auditory pathways. The hearing loss may be sudden and unilateral or intermittent and bilateral. Among other characteristics are impaired vision, paresthesia, muscle weakness, gait ataxia, intention tremor, urinary disturbances, and emotional lability.

◆ ***Myringitis.*** Rarely, acute infectious myringitis produces conductive hearing loss when fluid accumulates in the middle ear or a large bleb totally obstructs the ear canal. Small, reddened inflamed blebs may develop in the canal, on the tympanic membrane, or in the middle ear and may produce a bloody discharge if they rupture. Associated findings may include severe ear pain, mastoid tenderness, and fever.

Chronic granular myringitis produces gradual hearing loss accompanied by pruritus and a purulent discharge.

◆ ***Nasopharyngeal cancer.*** This type of cancer causes mild unilateral conductive hearing loss when it compresses the eustachian tube. Bone conduction is normal, and inspection reveals a retracted tympanic membrane backed by fluid. When this tumor obstructs the nasal airway, the patient may exhibit nasal speech and a bloody nasal and postnasal discharge. Cranial nerve involvement produces other findings, such as diplopia and rectus muscle paralysis.

◆ ***Osteoma.*** Commonly affecting women and swimmers, osteoma may cause sudden or intermittent conductive hearing loss. Typically, bony projections are visible in the ear canal, but the tympanic membrane appears normal.

◆ ***Otitis externa.*** Conductive hearing loss resulting from debris in the ear canal characterizes both acute and malignant otitis externa. In *acute otitis externa,* ear canal inflammation produces pain, itching, and a foul-smelling, sticky yellow discharge. Severe tenderness is typically elicited by chewing, opening the mouth, and pressing on the tragus or mastoid. The patient may also develop a low-grade fever, regional lymphadenopathy, a headache on the affected side, and mild to moderate pain around the ear that may later intensify. Examination may reveal greenish white debris or edema in the canal.

In *malignant otitis externa,* debris is also visible in the canal. This life-threatening disorder, which most commonly occurs in diabetics, causes sensorineural hearing loss, pruritus, tinnitus, and severe ear pain.

◆ ***Otitis media.*** This middle ear inflammation typically produces unilateral conductive hearing loss. In *acute suppurative otitis media,* the hearing loss develops gradually over a few hours and is usually accompanied by an upper respiratory tract infection with sore throat, cough, nasal discharge, and headache. Related signs and symptoms include dizziness, a sensation of fullness in the ear, intermittent or constant ear pain, fever, nausea, and vomiting. Rupture of the bulging, swollen tympanic membrane relieves the pain and produces a brief bloody and purulent discharge. Hearing returns after the infection subsides.

Hearing loss also develops gradually in patients with *chronic otitis media.* Assessment may reveal a perforated tympanic membrane, purulent ear drainage, earache, nausea, and vertigo.

Commonly associated with an upper respiratory tract infection or nasopharyngeal cancer, *serous otitis media* commonly produces a stuffy feeling in the ear and pain that worsens at night. Examination reveals a retracted—and perhaps discolored—tympanic membrane and possibly air bubbles behind the membrane.

◆ ***Otosclerosis.*** In this hereditary disorder, unilateral conductive hearing loss usually begins when the patient is in his early twenties and may gradually progress to bilateral mixed hearing loss. The patient may report tinnitus and an ability to hear better in a noisy environment.

GENDER CUE *Otosclerosis affects twice as many women as men and may worsen during pregnancy.*

◆ ***Skull fracture.*** Auditory nerve injury causes sudden unilateral sensorineural hearing loss. Accompanying signs and symptoms include ringing tinnitus, blood behind the tympanic membrane, scalp wounds, and other findings.

◆ ***Syphilis.*** In tertiary syphilis, sensorineural hearing loss may develop suddenly or gradually and usually affects one ear more than the other. It's usually accompanied by a gumma lesion—a chronic, superficial nodule or a deep, granulomatous lesion on the skin or mucous membranes. The lesion is solitary, asymmetrical, painless, and indurated. The patient may also exhibit signs of liver, respiratory, cardiovascular, or neurologic dysfunction.

◆ ***Temporal arteritis.*** This disorder may produce unilateral sensorineural hearing loss accompanied by throbbing unilateral facial pain, pain behind the eye, temporal or frontotemporal headache, and occasionally vision loss. The hearing loss is usually preceded by a prodrome of malaise, anorexia, weight loss, weakness, and myalgia that lasts for several days. Examination may reveal a nodular, swollen temporal artery. Low-grade fever, confusion, and disorientation may also occur.

◆ ***Temporal bone fracture.*** This fracture can cause sudden unilateral sensorineural hearing loss accompanied by hissing tinnitus. The tympanic membrane may be perforated, depending on the fracture's location. Loss of consciousness, Battle's sign, and facial paralysis may also occur.

◆ ***Tuberculosis.*** This pulmonary infection may spread to the ear, resulting in eardrum perforation, mild conductive hearing loss, and cervical lymphadenopathy.

◆ ***Tympanic membrane perforation.*** Commonly caused by trauma from sharp objects or rapid pressure changes, perforation of the tympanic membrane causes abrupt hearing loss along with ear pain, tinnitus, vertigo, and a sensation of fullness in the ear.

◆ ***Wegener's granulomatosis.*** Conductive hearing loss develops slowly in this rare necrotizing, granulomatous vasculitis. This multisystem disorder may also cause cough, pleuritic chest pain, epistaxis, hemorrhagic skin lesions, oliguria, and nasal discharge.

Other causes

◆ ***Drugs.*** Ototoxic drugs typically produce ringing or buzzing tinnitus and a feeling of fullness in the ear. Chloroquine, cisplatin, vancomycin, and aminoglycosides (especially neomycin, kanamycin, and amikacin) may cause irreversible hearing loss. Loop diuretics, such as furosemide, ethacrynic acid, and bumetanide, usually produce a brief, reversible hearing loss. Quinine, quinidine, and high doses of erythromycin or salicylates (such as aspirin) may also cause reversible hearing loss.

◆ ***Radiation therapy.*** Irradiation of the middle ear, thyroid, face, skull, or nasopharynx may cause eustachian tube dysfunction, resulting in hearing loss.

◆ ***Surgery.*** Myringotomy, myringoplasty, simple or radical mastoidectomy, or fenestrations may cause scarring that interferes with hearing.

Special considerations

When talking with the patient, remember to face him and speak slowly. Don't shout at the patient or smoke, eat, or chew gum when talking.

Prepare the patient for audiometry and auditory evoked-response testing. After testing, the patient may require a hearing aid or cochlear implant to improve his hearing.

Pediatric pointers

About 3,000 profoundly deaf infants are born in the United States each year. In about half of these infants, hereditary disorders (such as Paget's disease and Alport's, Hurler's, and Klippel-Feil syndromes) cause the typically sensorineural hearing loss. Nonhereditary disorders associated with congenital sensorineural hearing loss include albinism, onychodystrophy, cochlear dysplasia, and Pendred's, Usher's, Waardenburg's, and Jervell and Lange-Nielsen syndromes. Sensorineural hearing loss may also result from maternal use of ototoxic drugs, birth trauma, and anoxia during or after birth.

Mumps is the most common cause of unilateral sensorineural hearing loss in children. Other causes are meningitis, measles, influenza, and acute febrile illness.

Congenital conductive hearing loss may be caused by atresia, ossicle malformation, and other abnormalities. Serous otitis media commonly causes bilateral conductive hearing loss in children. Putting foreign objects in the ears can also cause conductive hearing loss.

Hearing disorders in children may lead to speech, language, and learning problems. Early identification and treatment of hearing loss is thus crucial to avoid incorrectly labeling the child as mentally retarded, brain damaged, or a slow learner.

When assessing an infant or a young child for hearing loss, remember that you can't use a tuning fork. Instead, test the startle reflex in infants younger than age 6 months, or have an audiologist test brain stem evoked response in neonates, infants, and young children. Also, obtain a gestational, perinatal, and family history from the parents.

Geriatric pointers

In older patients, presbycusis may be aggravated by exposure to noise as well as other factors.

Patient counseling

Instruct the patient to avoid exposure to loud noise and to use ear protection to arrest hearing loss. If the patient has an upper respiratory tract infection, tell him to avoid flying and driving.

Heat intolerance

Heat intolerance refers to the inability to withstand high temperatures or to maintain a comfortable body temperature. This symptom produces a continuous feeling of being overheated and, at times, profuse diaphoresis. It usually develops gradually and is chronic.

Most cases of heat intolerance result from thyrotoxicosis. In this disorder, excess thyroid hormone stimulates peripheral tissues, increasing basal metabolism and producing excess heat. Although rare, hypothalamic disease may also cause intolerance to heat and cold.

History and physical examination

Ask the patient when he first noticed his heat intolerance. Did he gradually use fewer blankets at night? Does he have to turn up the air conditioning to keep cool? Is it hard for him to adjust to warm weather? Does he sweat a lot in a hot environment? Find out if his appetite or weight has changed. Also, ask about unusual nervousness or other personality changes. Then take a drug history, especially noting use of amphetamines or amphetamine-like drugs. Ask the patient if he takes a thyroid drug. If so, what is the daily dosage and when did he last take it?

As you begin the examination, notice how much clothing the patient is wearing. After taking vital signs, inspect the patient's skin for flushing and diaphoresis. Also, note tremors and lid lag.

Medical causes

◆ ***Hypothalamic disease.*** In this rare disease, body temperature fluctuates dramatically, causing alternating heat and cold intolerance. Related features include amenorrhea, disturbed sleep patterns, increased thirst and urination, increased appetite with weight gain, impaired visual acuity, headache, and personality changes, such as bursts of rage or laughter. Common causes of hypothalamic disease are pituitary adenoma and hypothalamic and pineal tumors.

◆ ***Thyrotoxicosis.*** A classic symptom of thyrotoxicosis, heat intolerance may be accompanied by an enlarged thyroid gland, nervousness, weight loss despite increased appetite, diaphoresis, diarrhea, tremor, and palpitations. Although exophthalmos is characteristic, many patients don't display this sign. Associated findings may affect virtually every body system. Some common findings include irritability, difficulty concentrating, mood swings, insomnia, muscle weakness, fatigue, lid lag, tachycardia, full and bounding pulse, widened pulse pressure, dyspnea, amenorrhea, and gynecomastia. Typically, the patient's skin is warm and flushed; premature graying and alopecia occur in both sexes.

Other causes

◆ ***Drugs.*** Amphetamines, amphetamine-like appetite suppressants, and excessive doses of thyroid hormone may cause heat intolerance. Anticholinergics may interfere with sweating, resulting in heat intolerance.

Special considerations

Adjust room temperature to make the patient comfortable. If the patient is diaphoretic, change his clothing and bed linens as necessary, and encourage him to drink lots of fluids.

Pediatric pointers

Rarely, maternal thyrotoxicosis may be passed to the neonate, resulting in heat intolerance. More commonly, acquired thyrotoxicosis appears between ages 12 and 14, although this too is infrequent. Dehydration may also make a child sensitive to heat.

Heberden's nodes

Heberden's nodes are painless, irregular, cartilaginous or bony enlargements of the distal interphalangeal joints of the fingers. They reflect degeneration of articular cartilage, which irritates the bone and stimulates osteoblasts, causing bony enlargement. Approximately 2 to 3 mm in diameter, Heberden's nodes develop on one or both sides of the dorsal midline. The dominant hand usually has larger nodes, which affect one or more fingers but not the thumb. (See *Recognizing Heberden's nodes.*)

Osteoarthritis is the most common cause of Heberden's nodes; in fact, more than one-half of all osteoarthritic patients have these nodes. Less commonly, repeated fingertip trauma may lead to node formation in only one joint ("baseball finger"). Because Heberden's nodes aren't associated with joint pain or loss of function, they aren't a primary indicator of osteoarthritis; however, they're a helpful adjunct to diagnosis.

Recognizing Heberden's nodes

These painless bony enlargements of the distal interphalangeal finger joints appear in more than one-half of all patients with osteoarthritis.

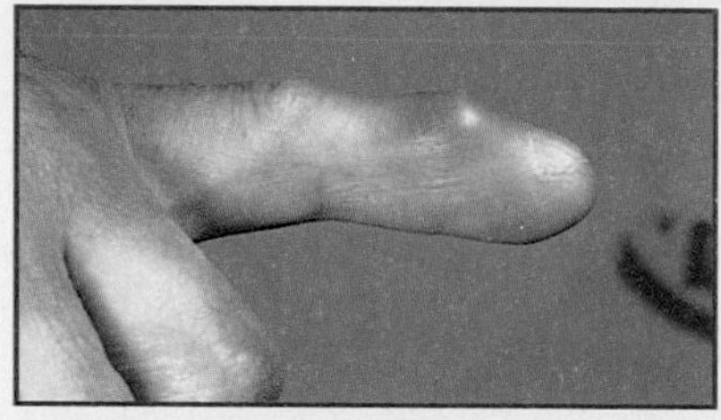

History and physical examination

Begin by asking the patient if anyone else in his family has had Heberden's nodes or osteoarthritis. Are the patient's joints stiff? Does stiffness disappear with movement? Ask him which hand is dominant. Also ask about repeated fingertip trauma associated with his job or sports.

Carefully palpate the nodes, noting any signs of inflammation, such as redness and tenderness. Then determine range of motion (ROM) in the fingers of each hand. As you do so, listen and feel for crepitation.

Medical causes

◆ ***Osteoarthritis.*** This disorder commonly causes Heberden's nodes and may also cause nodes in the proximal interphalangeal joints (Bouchard's nodes). Its chief symptom, though, is joint pain that's aggravated by movement or weight bearing. Joints may also be tender and display restricted ROM. Typically, joint stiffness is triggered by disuse and relieved by brief exercise. Stiffness may be accompanied by bony enlargement and crepitus.

Special considerations

Remind the patient to take an anti-inflammatory drug and to exercise regularly. Encourage him to avoid joint strain, for example, by maintaining a healthy body weight.

Pediatric pointers

Because children don't suffer from osteoarthritis, they don't develop Heberden's nodes.

Hematemesis

Hematemesis, the vomiting of blood, usually indicates GI bleeding above the ligament of Treitz, which suspends the duodenum at its junction with the jejunum. Bright red or blood-streaked vomitus indicates fresh or recent bleeding. Dark red, brown, or black vomitus (the color and consistency of coffee grounds) indicates that blood has been retained in the stomach and partially digested.

Although hematemesis usually results from a GI disorder, it may stem from a coagulation disorder or from a treatment that irritates the GI tract. Swallowed blood from epistaxis or oropharyngeal erosion may also cause bloody vomitus. Hematemesis may be precipitated by straining, emotional stress, and the use of anti-inflammatory drugs or alcohol. In a patient with esophageal varices, hematemesis may be due to trauma from swallowing hard or partially chewed food. (See *Rare causes of hematemesis*.)

Hematemesis is always an important sign, but its severity depends on the amount, source, and intensity of the bleeding. Massive hematemesis (vomiting of 500 to 1,000 ml of blood) may be life-threatening.

EMERGENCY INTERVENTIONS *If the patient has massive hematemesis, check his vital signs. If you detect signs of shock—such as tachypnea, hypotension, and tachycardia—place the patient in a supine position, and elevate his feet 20 to 30 degrees. Start a large-bore I.V. catheter for emergency fluid replacement. Also, obtain a blood sample for typing and crossmatching, hemoglobin level, and hematocrit, and administer oxygen. Emergency endoscopy may be necessary to locate the source of bleeding. Prepare to insert a nasogastric (NG) tube for suction or iced lavage. A Sengstaken-Blakemore tube may be used to compress esophageal varices. (See* Managing hematemesis with intubation, *page 356.)*

Rare causes of hematemesis

Two rare disorders commonly cause hematemesis. *Malaria* produces this and other GI signs, but its most characteristic effects are chills, fever, headache, muscle pain, and splenomegaly. *Yellow fever* also causes hematemesis as well as sudden fever, bradycardia, jaundice, and severe prostration.

Two relatively common disorders may cause hematemesis in rare cases. When acute diverticulitis affects the duodenum, GI bleeding and resultant hematemesis occur with abdominal pain and fever. With GI involvement, secondary syphilis can cause hematemesis; more characteristic signs and symptoms include a primary chancre, rash, fever, malaise, anorexia, weight loss, and headache.

History and physical examination

If hematemesis isn't immediately life-threatening, begin with a thorough history. First, have the patient describe the amount, color, and consistency of the vomitus. When did he first notice this sign? Has he ever had hematemesis before? Find out if he also has bloody or black tarry stools. Note whether hematemesis is usually preceded by nausea, flatulence, diarrhea, or weakness. Has he recently had bouts of retching with or without vomiting?

Next, ask about a history of ulcers or of liver or coagulation disorders. Find out how much alcohol the patient drinks, if any. Does he regularly take aspirin or another nonsteroidal anti-inflammatory drug (NSAID), such as phenylbutazone or indomethacin? These drugs may cause erosive gastritis or ulcers.

Begin the physical examination by checking for orthostatic hypotension, an early warning sign of hypovolemia. Take blood pressure and pulse with the patient in the supine, sitting, and standing positions. A decrease of 10 mm Hg or more in systolic pressure or an increase of 10 beats/minute or more in pulse rate indicates volume depletion. After obtaining other vital signs, inspect the mucous membranes, nasopharynx, and skin for any signs of bleeding or other abnormalities. Finally, palpate the abdomen for tenderness, pain, or masses. Note lymphadenopathy.

Medical causes

- ***Achalasia.*** Hematemesis is a rare effect of this disorder, which usually causes passive regurgitation and painless, progressive dysphagia. Regurgitation of undigested food may cause hoarseness, coughing, aspiration, and recurrent pulmonary infections.
- ***Anthrax, GI.*** GI anthrax is caused by eating meat contaminated with the gram-positive, spore-forming bacterium *Bacillus anthracis.* Initial signs and symptoms of anorexia, nausea, vomiting, and fever may progress to hematemesis, abdominal pain, and severe bloody diarrhea.
- ***Coagulation disorders.*** Any disorder that disrupts normal clotting, such as thrombocytopenia or hemophilia, may result in GI bleeding and moderate to severe hematemesis. Bleeding may occur in other body systems as well, resulting in such signs as epistaxis and ecchymosis. Associated effects depend on the specific coagulation disorder.
- ***Esophageal cancer.*** A late sign of this cancer, hematemesis may be accompanied by steady chest pain that radiates to the back. Other features include substernal fullness, severe dysphagia, nausea, vomiting with nocturnal regurgitation and aspiration, hemoptysis, fever, hiccups, sore throat, melena, and halitosis.

Managing hematemesis with intubation

A patient with hematemesis will need to have a GI tube inserted to allow blood drainage, to aspirate gastric contents, or to facilitate gastric lavage if necessary. Here are the most common tubes and their uses.

NASOGASTRIC TUBES

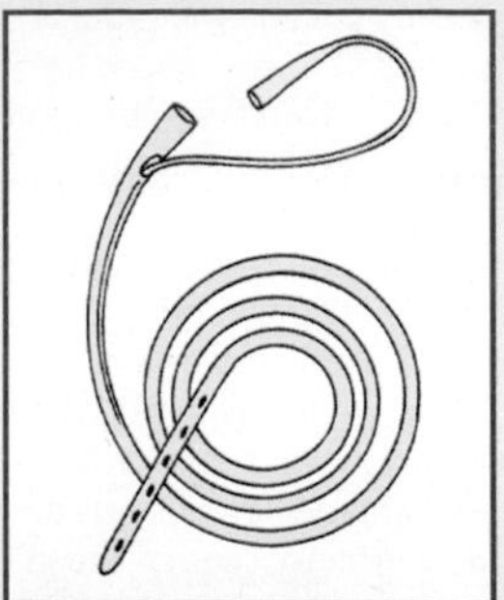

The *Salem-Sump tube* (above), a double-lumen nasogastric (NG) tube, is used to remove stomach fluid and gas or to aspirate gastric contents. It may also be used for gastric lavage, drug administration, or feeding. Its main advantage over the *Levin tube*—a single-lumen NG tube—is that it allows atmospheric air to enter the patient's stomach so the tube can float freely instead of risking adhesion and damage to the gastric mucosa.

WIDE-BORE GASTRIC TUBES

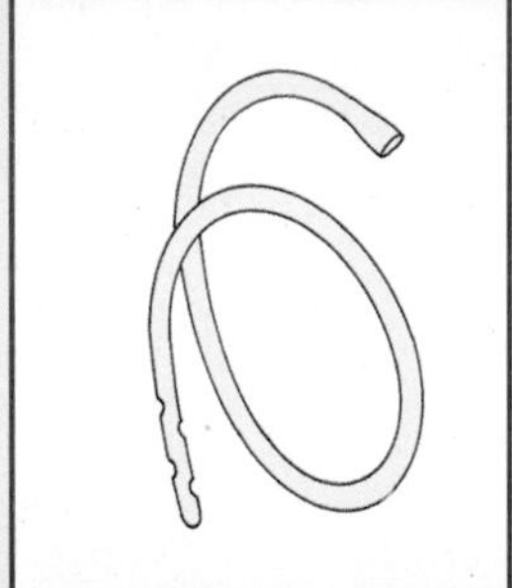

The *Edlich tube* (above) has one wide-bore lumen with four openings near the closed distal tip. A funnel or syringe can be connected at the proximal end. Like the other tubes, the Edlich can aspirate a large volume of gastric contents quickly.

The Ewald tube, a wide-bore tube that allows quick passage of a large amount of fluid and clots, is especially useful for gastric lavage in patients with profuse GI bleeding and in those who have ingested poison. Another wide-bore tube, the double-lumen Levacuator, has a large lumen for evacuation of gastric contents and a small one for lavage.

ESOPHAGEAL TUBES

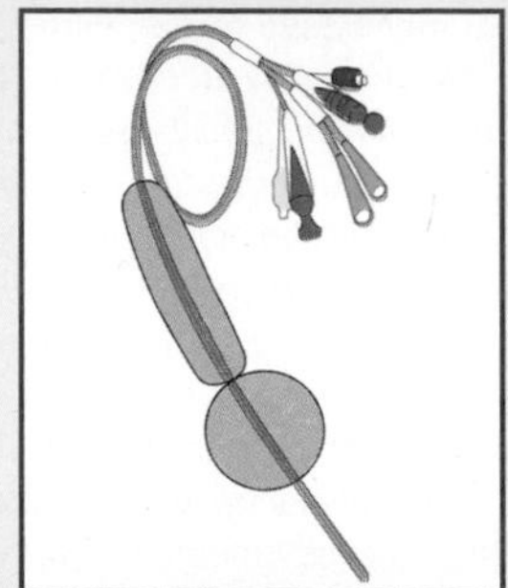

The *Sengstaken-Blakemore tube* (above), a triple-lumen double-balloon esophageal tube, provides a gastric aspiration port that allows drainage from below the gastric balloon. It can also be used to instill medication. A similar tube, the *Linton shunt,* can aspirate esophageal and gastric contents without risking necrosis because it has no esophageal balloon. The *Minnesota esophagogastric tamponade tube,* which has four lumina and two balloons, provides pressure-monitoring ports for both balloons without the need for Y-connectors.

◆ ***Esophageal injury by caustic substances.*** Ingestion of corrosive acids or alkalies produces esophageal injury associated with grossly bloody or coffee-ground vomitus. Hematemesis is accompanied by epigastric and anterior or retrosternal chest pain that's intensified by swallowing. With ingestion of alkaline agents, the oral and pharyngeal mucosa may produce a soapy white film. The mucosa becomes brown and edematous with time. Dysphagia, marked salivation, and fever may develop in 3 to 4 weeks and worsen as strictures form.

◆ ***Esophageal rupture.*** The severity of hematemesis depends on the cause of the rupture. When an instrument damages the esophagus, hematemesis is usually slight. However, rupture due to Boerhaave's syndrome (increased esophageal pressure from vomiting or retching) or other esophageal disorders typically causes more severe hematemesis. This life-threatening disorder may also produce severe retrosternal, epigastric, neck, or scapular pain accompanied by chest and neck edema. Examination reveals subcutaneous crepitation in the chest wall, supraclavicular fossa, and neck. The patient may also show signs of respiratory distress, such as dyspnea and cyanosis.

◆ ***Esophageal varices (ruptured).*** Life-threatening rupture of esophageal varices may produce coffee-ground or massive bright red vomitus. Signs of shock, such as hypotension and tachycardia, may follow or even precede hematemesis if the stomach fills with blood before vomiting occurs. Other symptoms may include abdominal distention and melena or painless hematochezia (ranging from slight oozing to massive rectal hemorrhage).

◆ ***Gastric cancer.*** Painless bright red or dark brown vomitus is a late sign of this uncommon cancer, which usually begins insidiously with upper abdominal discomfort. The patient then develops anorexia, mild nausea, and chronic dyspepsia that's unrelieved by antacids and exacerbated by food. Later symptoms may include fatigue, weakness, weight loss, feelings of fullness, melena, altered bowel habits, and signs of malnutrition, such as muscle wasting and dry skin.

◆ ***Gastritis (acute).*** Hematemesis and melena are the most common signs of acute gastritis. They may even be the only signs, although mild epigastric discomfort, nausea, fever, and malaise may also occur. Massive blood loss precipitates signs of shock. Typically, the patient has a history of alcohol abuse or has used aspirin or another NSAID. Gastritis may also occur secondary to *Helicobacter pylori* infection.

◆ ***Gastroesophageal reflux disease.*** Although rare in this disorder, hematemesis may produce significant blood loss. It's accompanied by pyrosis, flatulence, dyspepsia, and postural regurgitation that can be aggravated by lying down or stooping over. Related effects include dysphagia, retrosternal angina-like chest pain, weight loss, halitosis, and signs of aspiration, such as dyspnea and recurrent pulmonary infections.

◆ ***Leiomyoma.*** This benign tumor occasionally involves the GI tract, eroding the mucosa or vascular supply to produce hematemesis. Other features vary with the tumor's size and location. For example, esophageal involvement may cause dysphagia and weight loss.

◆ ***Mallory-Weiss syndrome.*** Characterized by a mucosal tear of the mucous membrane at the junction of the esophagus and the stomach, this syndrome may produce hematemesis and melena. It's commonly triggered by severe vomiting, retching, or straining (as from coughing), usually in alcoholics or in people whose pylorus is obstructed. Severe bleeding may precipitate signs of shock, such as tachycardia, hypotension, dyspnea, and cool, clammy skin.

◆ ***Peptic ulcer.*** Hematemesis may occur when a peptic ulcer penetrates an artery, vein, or highly vascular tissue. Massive—and possibly life-threatening—hematemesis is typical when an artery is penetrated. Other features include melena or hematochezia, chills, fever, and signs and symptoms of shock and dehydration, such as tachycardia, hypotension, poor skin turgor, and thirst. Most patients have a history of nausea, vomiting, epigastric tenderness, and epigastric pain that's relieved by foods or antacids. Some may also have a history of habitual use of tobacco, alcohol, or NSAIDs.

Other causes

◆ ***Treatments.*** Traumatic NG or endotracheal intubation may cause hematemesis associated with swallowed blood. Nose or throat surgery may also cause this sign in the same way.

Special considerations

Closely monitor the patient's vital signs, and watch for signs of shock. Check the patient's stools regularly for occult blood, and keep accurate intake and output records. Place the patient on bed rest in a low or semi-Fowler's position to prevent aspiration of vomitus. Keep suctioning equipment nearby, and use it as needed. Provide frequent oral hygiene and emotional support—the sight of bloody vomitus can be very frightening. Administer a histamine-2 blocker I.V.; vasopressin may be required for ruptured esophageal varices. As the bleeding tapers off, monitor the pH of gastric contents, and give hourly doses of antacids by NG tube as necessary.

Pediatric pointers

Hematemesis is much less common in children than in adults and may be related to foreign-body ingestion. Occasionally, neonates develop hematemesis after swallowing maternal blood during delivery or breast-feeding from a cracked nipple. Hemorrhagic disease of the neonate and esophageal erosion may also cause hematemesis in infants; such cases require immediate fluid replacement.

Geriatric pointers

In elderly patients, hematemesis may be caused by a vascular anomaly, an aortoenteric fistula, or upper GI cancer. In addition, chronic obstructive pulmonary disease, chronic hepatic or renal failure, and chronic NSAID use all predispose elderly people to hemorrhage secondary to coexisting ulcerative disorders.

Patient counseling

Explain diagnostic tests, such as endoscopy, barium swallow, and variceal banding. Explain laboratory tests, such as serum electrolyte levels, complete blood count, prothrombin time, partial thromboplastin time, and international normalized ratio.

Hematochezia

[Rectal bleeding]

The passage of bloody stools, also known as hematochezia, usually indicates—and may be the first sign of—GI bleeding below the ligament of Treitz. However, this sign—usually preceded by hematemesis—may also accompany rapid hemorrhage of 1 L or more from the upper GI tract.

Hematochezia ranges from formed, blood-streaked stools to liquid, bloody stools that may be bright red, dark mahogany, or maroon in color. This sign usually develops abruptly and is heralded by abdominal pain.

Although hematochezia is commonly associated with GI disorders, it may also result from a coagulation disorder, exposure to toxins, or certain diagnostic tests. Always a significant sign, hematochezia may precipitate life-threatening hypovolemia.

EMERGENCY INTERVENTIONS *If the patient has severe hematochezia, check his vital signs. If you detect signs of shock, such as hypotension and tachycardia, place the patient in a supine position and elevate his feet 20 to 30 degrees. Prepare to administer oxygen, and start a large-bore I.V. catheter for emergency fluid replacement. Next, obtain a blood sample for typing and crossmatching, hemoglobin level, and hematocrit. Insert a nasogastric tube. Iced lavage may be indicated to control bleeding. Endoscopy may be necessary to detect the source of the bleeding.*

History and physical examination

If the hematochezia isn't immediately life-threatening, ask the patient to fully describe the amount, color, and consistency of his bloody stools. (If possible, also inspect and characterize the stools yourself.) How long have the stools been bloody? Do they always look the same, or does the amount of blood seem to vary? Ask about associated signs and symptoms.

Next, explore the patient's medical history, focusing on GI and coagulation disorders. Ask about the use of GI irritants, such as alcohol, aspirin, and other nonsteroidal anti-inflammatory drugs.

Begin the physical examination by checking for orthostatic hypotension, an early sign of shock. Take the patient's blood pressure and pulse while he's lying down, sitting, and standing. If systolic pressure decreases by 10 mm Hg or more, or pulse rate increases by 10 beats/minute or more when he changes position, suspect volume depletion and impending shock.

Examine the skin for petechiae or spider angiomas. Palpate the abdomen for tenderness, pain, or masses. Also, note lymphadenopathy. Finally, a digital rectal examination must be done to rule out rectal masses or hemorrhoids.

Medical causes

- ***Amyloidosis.*** Hematochezia occasionally occurs when this disorder affects the GI tract. Massive, rapid hematochezia may precipitate signs of shock, such as hypotension and tachycardia. Associated signs and symptoms include hypoactive or absent bowel sounds, abdominal pain, malabsorption, diarrhea, and renal disease. The patient may also have a stiff, enlarged tongue, resulting in dysarthria.
- ***Anal fissure.*** Slight hematochezia characterizes this disorder; blood may streak the stools or appear on toilet tissue. Accompanying hematochezia is severe rectal pain that may make the patient reluctant to defecate, thereby causing constipation.
- ***Angiodysplastic lesions.*** Most common in elderly patients, these arteriovenous lesions of the ascending colon typically cause chronic, bright red rectal bleeding. Occasionally, they may result in life-threatening blood loss and signs of shock, such as tachycardia and hypotension.
- ***Anorectal fistula.*** Blood, pus, mucus, and occasionally stools may drain from this type of fistula. Other effects include rectal pain and pruritus.
- ***Coagulation disorders.*** Patients with a coagulation disorder (such as thrombocytopenia or disseminated intravascular coagulation) may experience GI bleeding marked by moderate to severe hematochezia. Bleeding may also occur

in other body systems, producing such signs as epistaxis and purpura. Associated findings vary with the specific coagulation disorder.

◆ ***Colitis.*** *Ischemic colitis* commonly causes bloody diarrhea, especially in elderly patients. Rectal bleeding may be slight or massive and is usually accompanied by severe, cramping lower abdominal pain and hypotension. Other effects include abdominal tenderness, distention, and absent bowel sounds. Severe colitis may cause life-threatening hypovolemic shock and peritonitis.

Ulcerative colitis typically causes bloody diarrhea that may also contain mucus. Blood loss may be slight or massive and is preceded by mild to severe abdominal cramps. Associated signs and symptoms include fever, tenesmus, anorexia, nausea, vomiting, hyperactive bowel sounds and, occasionally, tachycardia. Weight loss and weakness occur late.

◆ ***Colon cancer.*** Bright red rectal bleeding with or without pain is a telling sign, especially in cancer of the left colon. This type of tumor usually causes early signs of obstruction, such as rectal pressure, bleeding, and intermittent fullness or cramping. As the disease progresses, the patient also develops obstipation, diarrhea or ribbon-shaped stools, and pain that's typically relieved by passage of stools or flatus. Stools are grossly bloody.

Cancer of the right colon may initially cause melena and abdominal aching, pressure, and dull cramps. As the disease progresses, the patient may also experience diarrhea, anorexia, weight loss, anemia, weakness and fatigue, vomiting, an abdominal mass, and signs of obstruction, such as abdominal distention and abnormal bowel sounds.

◆ ***Colorectal polyps.*** These polyps are the most common cause of intermittent hematochezia in adults younger than age 60, but they don't always produce symptoms. When located high in the colon, polyps may cause blood-streaked stools that yield a positive response when tested with guaiac. If the polyps are located closer to the rectum, they may bleed freely.

◆ ***Crohn's disease.*** Hematochezia is not a common sign of this disorder unless the perineum is involved. If rectal bleeding does occur, it's likely to be massive. The chief clinical features of Crohn's disease include fever, abdominal distention and pain with guarding, diarrhea, hyperactive bowel sounds, anorexia, nausea, and fatigue. Palpation may reveal a mass in the colon.

◆ ***Diverticulitis.*** Most common in elderly patients, this disorder can suddenly cause mild to moderate rectal bleeding after the patient feels the urge to defecate. The bleeding may end abruptly or may progress to life-threatening blood loss with signs of shock. Associated signs and symptoms may include left-lower-quadrant pain that's relieved by defecation, alternating episodes of constipation and diarrhea, anorexia, nausea and vomiting, rebound tenderness, and a distended tympanic abdomen.

◆ ***Dysentery.*** Bloody diarrhea is common in infection with *Shigella, Amoeba,* and *Campylobacter*, but rare with *Salmonella*. Abdominal pain or cramps, tenesmus, fever, and nausea may also occur.

◆ ***Esophageal varices (ruptured).*** In this life-threatening disorder, hematochezia may range from slight rectal oozing to grossly bloody stools and may be accompanied by mild to severe hematemesis or melena. Signs of shock, such as tachycardia and hypotension, may follow or occasionally precede overt signs of bleeding. Typically, the patient has a history of chronic liver disease.

◆ ***Food poisoning (staphylococcal).*** The patient may have bloody diarrhea 1 to 6 hours after ingesting food toxins. Accompanying signs and symptoms, which last a few hours, include severe, cramping abdominal pain, nausea and vomiting, and prostration.

◆ ***Hemorrhoids.*** Hematochezia may accompany external hemorrhoids, which typically cause painful defecation, resulting in constipation. Less painful internal hemorrhoids usually produce more chronic bleeding with bowel movements, which may eventually lead to signs of anemia, such as weakness and fatigue.

◆ ***Leptospirosis.*** The severe form of this infection—Weil's syndrome—produces hematochezia or melena along with other signs of bleeding, such as epistaxis and hemoptysis. The bleeding is typically preceded by a sudden frontal headache, severe thigh and lumbar myalgia, cutaneous hyperesthesia, and conjunctival suffusion. Bleeding is followed by chills, a rapidly rising fever, and perhaps nausea and vomiting. Fever, headache, and myalgia usually intensify and persist for weeks. Other findings may include right-upper-quadrant tenderness, hepatomegaly, and jaundice.

◆ ***Peptic ulcer.*** Upper GI bleeding is a common complication in this disorder. The patient may display hematochezia, hematemesis, or melena, depending on the intensity and amount of bleeding. If the peptic ulcer penetrates an artery or vein, massive bleeding may precipitate signs of shock, such as hypotension and tachycardia. Other findings may include chills, fever, nausea and vomiting, and signs of dehydration, such as dry mucous membranes, poor skin turgor, and thirst. Most patients have a history of epigastric pain that's relieved by foods or antacids; some also have a history of habitual use of tobacco, alcohol, or nonsteroidal anti-inflammatory drugs.

◆ ***Rectal melanoma (malignant).*** This rare form of rectal cancer typically causes recurrent rectal bleeding that arises from a painless, asymptomatic mass.

◆ ***Small-intestine cancer.*** This disorder occasionally produces slight hematochezia or blood-streaked stools. Its characteristic features include colicky pain and postprandial vomiting. Other common signs and symptoms include anorexia, weight loss, and fever. Palpation may reveal abdominal masses.

◆ ***Typhoid fever.*** About 10% of patients with typhoid fever develop hematochezia, which is occasionally massive. However, melena is more common. Both signs of bleeding occur late and may be accompanied by marked abdominal distention, diarrhea, significant weight loss, mental dullness, and profound fatigue. Earlier signs and symptoms are pathognomonic rose spots, headache, chills, fever, constipation, dry cough, conjunctivitis, and epistaxis.

◆ ***Ulcerative proctitis.*** In this disorder, the patient typically has an intense urge to defecate but passes only bright red blood, pus, or mucus. Other common findings include acute constipation and tenesmus.

Other causes

◆ ***Heavy metal poisoning.*** Bloody diarrhea is accompanied by cramping abdominal pain, nausea, and vomiting. Other signs may include tachycardia, hypotension, seizures, paresthesia, depressed or absent deep tendon reflexes, and an altered level of consciousness.

◆ ***Tests.*** Certain procedures, especially colonoscopy, polypectomy, and proctosigmoidoscopy, may cause rectal bleeding. Bowel perforation is rare.

Special considerations

Place the patient on bed rest and check his vital signs frequently, watching for signs of shock, such as hypotension, tachycardia, weak pulse, and tachypnea. Monitor the patient's intake and output hourly. Remember to provide emotional support because hematochezia may frighten the patient.

Prepare the patient for blood tests and GI procedures, such as endoscopy and GI X-rays. Visually examine the patient's stools and test them for occult blood. If necessary, send a stool specimen to the laboratory to check for parasites.

Pediatric pointers

Hematochezia is much less common in children than in adults. It may result from structural disorders, such as intussusception and Meckel's diverticulum, and from inflammatory disorders, such as peptic ulcer disease and ulcerative colitis.

In children, ulcerative colitis typically produces chronic, rather than acute, signs and symptoms and may also cause slow growth and maturation related to malnutrition. Suspect sexual abuse in all cases of rectal bleeding in children.

Geriatric pointers

Because older people have an increased risk of colon cancer, hematochezia should be evaluated with colonoscopy after perirectal lesions have been ruled out as the cause of bleeding.

Hematuria

A cardinal sign of renal and urinary tract disorders, hematuria is the abnormal presence of blood in the urine. Strictly defined, it means three or more red blood cells (RBCs) per high-power microscopic field in the urine. Microscopic hematuria is confirmed by an occult blood test, whereas macroscopic hematuria is immediately visible. However, macroscopic hematuria must be distinguished from pseudohematuria. (See *Confirming hematuria.*) Macroscopic hematuria may be continuous or intermittent, is often accompanied by pain, and may be aggravated by prolonged standing or walking.

Hematuria may be classified by the stage of urination it predominantly affects. Bleeding at the start of urination—*initial hematuria*—usually indicates urethral pathology; bleeding at the end of urination—*terminal hematuria*—usually indicates pathology of the bladder neck, posterior urethra, or prostate; bleeding throughout urination—*total hematuria*—usually indicates pathology above the bladder neck.

Hematuria may result from one of two mechanisms: rupture or perforation of vessels in the renal system or urinary tract, or impaired glomerular filtration, which allows RBCs to seep into the urine. The color of the bloody urine provides a clue to the source of the bleeding. Generally, dark or brownish blood indicates renal or upper urinary tract bleeding, whereas bright red blood indicates lower urinary tract bleeding.

Although hematuria usually results from renal and urinary tract disorders, it may also result from certain GI, prostate, vaginal, or coagulation disorders or from the effects of certain drugs. Invasive therapy and diagnostic tests that involve manipulative instrumentation of the renal and urologic systems may also cause hematuria. Nonpathologic hematuria may result from fever and hypercatabolic states. Transient hematuria may follow strenuous exercise. (See *Hematuria: Causes and associated findings,* pages 362 to 365.)

Confirming hematuria

If the patient's urine appears blood tinged, be sure to rule out pseudohematuria, red or pink urine caused by urinary pigments. First, carefully observe the urine specimen. If it contains a red sediment, it's probably *true* hematuria.

Then check the patient's history for use of drugs associated with pseudohematuria, including rifampin, chlorzoxazone, phenazopyridine, phenothiazines, doxorubicin, phenytoin, and laxatives containing phenolphthalein.

Ask about the patient's intake of beets, berries, or foods with red dyes that may color the urine red. Be aware that porphyrinuria and excess urate excretion can also cause pseudohematuria.

Finally, test the urine using a chemical reagent strip. This test can confirm even microscopic hematuria and can also estimate the amount of blood present.

History and physical examination

After detecting hematuria, take a pertinent health history. If hematuria is macroscopic, ask the patient when he first noticed blood in his urine. Does it vary in severity between voidings? Is it worse at the beginning, middle, or end of urination? Has it occurred before? Is the patient passing any clots? To rule out artifactual hematuria, ask about bleeding hemorrhoids or the onset of menses, if appropriate. Ask if pain or burning accompanies the episodes of hematuria.

Ask about recent abdominal or flank trauma. Has the patient been exercising strenuously? Note a history of renal, urinary, prostatic, or coagulation disorders. Then obtain a drug history, noting the use of anticoagulants or aspirin.

Begin the physical examination by palpating and percussing the abdomen and flanks. Next, percuss the costovertebral angle (CVA) to elicit tenderness. Check the urinary meatus for bleeding or other abnormalities. Using a chemical reagent strip, test a urine specimen for protein. A vaginal or digital rectal examination may be necessary.

Medical causes

◆ ***Appendicitis.*** About 15% of patients with appendicitis have either microscopic or macroscopic hematuria accompanied by bladder tenderness, dysuria, and urinary urgency. More typical findings include constant right-lower-quadrant pain (especially over McBurney's point), nausea and vomiting, anorexia, abdominal rigidity, rebound tenderness, constipation, tachycardia, and low-grade fever.

◆ ***Bladder cancer.*** A primary cause of gross hematuria in men, bladder cancer may also produce pain in the bladder, rectum, pelvis, flank, back, or leg. Other common features are nocturia, dysuria, urinary frequency and urgency, vomiting, diarrhea, and insomnia.

◆ ***Bladder trauma.*** A characteristic finding in traumatic rupture or perforation of the bladder, gross hematuria is typically accompanied by lower abdominal pain. The patient may also develop anuria despite a strong urge to void; swelling of the scrotum, buttocks, or perineum; and signs of shock, such as tachycardia and hypotension.

◆ ***Calculi.*** Both bladder and renal calculi produce hematuria, which may be associated with signs of urinary tract infection, such as dysuria and urinary frequency and urgency. Bladder calculi may also cause gross hematuria, referred pain to the lower back or penile or vulvar area and, occasionally, bladder distention.

Renal calculi may produce microscopic or gross hematuria. The cardinal symptom, though, is colicky pain that travels from the CVA to the flank, suprapubic region, and external

(Text continues on page 366.)

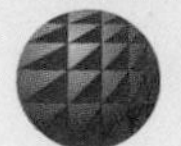

SIGNS & SYMPTOMS

Hematuria: Causes and associated findings

Common causes	Abdominal distention	Abdominal pain	Anuria	Bladder distention	Blood pressure increase	Bowel sounds, hypoactive	Colicky pain	Costovertebral angle tenderness	Dysuria	Edema, generalized	Edema of the legs	Fever
	Major associated signs and symptoms											
Appendicitis		●							●			●
Bladder cancer									●			
Bladder trauma		●	●									
Calculi (bladder)				●					●			
Calculi (renal)	●	●				●	●	●	●			●
Coagulation disorders												
Cortical necrosis (acute)			●									●
Cystitis (bacterial)									●			●
Cystitis (chronic interstitial)									●			
Cystitis (tubercular)									●			
Cystitis (viral)									●			●
Diverticulitis		●							●			●
Endocarditis (subacute infective)												●
Glomerulonephritis (acute)		●	●		●					●		●
Glomerulonephritis (chronic)					●					●		
Nephritis (acute interstitial)			●									●
Nephritis (chronic interstitial)					●							
Nephropathy (obstructive)		●	●				●	●				

	Flank mass	Flank pain	Lumbar pain	Murmurs	Nausea	Nocturia	Oliguria	Perineal pain	Polyarthralgia	Polyuria	Proteinuria	Purpura	Rash	Urethral discharge	Urinary frequency	Urinary hesitancy	Urinary stream, diminished	Urinary urgency	Vomiting
					●													●	●
		●				●		●							●			●	●
								●							●			●	
		●			●										●			●	●
												●							
		●																	
			●			●		●							●			●	
						●									●				
		●													●			●	
						●									●			●	
					●	●									●			●	
		●		●					●										
		●			●		●				●								●
											●								
							●						●						
										●									
		●					●			●									

(continued)

Hematuria: Causes and associated findings *(continued)*

Common causes	Major associated signs and symptoms: Abdominal distention	Abdominal pain	Anuria	Bladder distention	Blood pressure increase	Bowel sounds, hypoactive	Colicky pain	Costovertebral angle tenderness	Dysuria	Edema, generalized	Edema of the legs	Fever
Polycystic kidney disease		●			●		●		●			
Prostatic hyperplasia (benign)				●								
Prostatitis (acute)				●					●			●
Prostatitis (chronic)				●					●			
Pyelonephritis (acute)	●					●		●	●			●
Renal cancer					●		●	●			●	●
Renal infarction		●	●		●	●		●				●
Renal papillary necrosis (acute)		●	●			●	●	●				●
Renal trauma						●						
Renal tuberculosis		●					●		●			
Renal vein thrombosis			●					●			●	●
Schistosomiasis							●		●			
Sickle cell anemia												
Systemic lupus erythematosus												●
Urethral trauma												
Vaginitis									●			
Vasculitis			●		●							●

	Flank mass	Flank pain	Lumbar pain	Murmurs	Nausea	Nocturia	Oliguria	Perineal pain	Polyarthralgia	Polyuria	Proteinuria	Purpura	Rash	Urethral discharge	Urinary frequency	Urinary hesitancy	Urinary stream, diminished	Urinary urgency	Vomiting
			●						●	●				●				●	
						●		●						●	●	●			
			●		●			●	●					●				●	●
								●					●	●				●	
		●			●	●								●	●			●	●
	●	●			●														●
		●			●		●			●									●
		●					●												●
	●	●			●		●				●								●
			●							●				●					
		●	●				●			●									
				●					●										
										●		●							
								●											
						●		●						●				●	
									●		●	●							

genitalia when a calculus is passed. The pain may be excruciating at its peak. Other signs and symptoms may include nausea and vomiting, restlessness, fever, chills, abdominal distention and, possibly, decreased bowel sounds.

◆ ***Coagulation disorders.*** Macroscopic hematuria is commonly the first sign of hemorrhage in coagulation disorders, such as thrombocytopenia or disseminated intravascular coagulation. Among other features are epistaxis, purpura (petechiae and ecchymosis), and signs of GI bleeding.

◆ ***Cortical necrosis (acute).*** Accompanying gross hematuria in this renal disorder are intense flank pain, anuria, leukocytosis, and fever.

◆ ***Cystitis.*** Hematuria is a telling sign in all types of cystitis. *Bacterial cystitis* usually produces macroscopic hematuria with urinary urgency and frequency, dysuria, nocturia, and tenesmus. The patient complains of perineal and lumbar pain, suprapubic discomfort, and fatigue and occasionally has a low-grade fever.

More common in women, *chronic interstitial cystitis* occasionally causes gross hematuria. Associated features include urinary frequency, dysuria, nocturia, and tenesmus. Both microscopic and macroscopic hematuria may occur in *tubercular cystitis,* which may also cause urinary urgency and frequency, dysuria, tenesmus, flank pain, fatigue, and anorexia. *Viral cystitis* usually produces hematuria, urinary urgency and frequency, dysuria, nocturia, tenesmus, and fever.

◆ ***Diverticulitis.*** When this disorder involves the bladder, it usually causes microscopic hematuria, urinary frequency and urgency, dysuria, and nocturia. Characteristic findings include left-lower-quadrant pain, abdominal tenderness, constipation or diarrhea and, occasionally, a palpable, firm, fixed, and tender abdominal mass. The patient may also develop mild nausea, flatulence, and a low-grade fever.

◆ ***Endocarditis (subacute infective).*** Occasionally, this disorder produces embolization, resulting in renal infarction and microscopic or gross hematuria. Common related findings are constant fever, chills, night sweats, fatigue, pallor, anorexia, weight loss, polyarthralgia, petechiae, flank pain, severe back pain, stiff neck, cardiac murmurs, tachycardia, and splenomegaly.

◆ ***Glomerulonephritis.*** *Acute glomerulonephritis* usually begins with gross hematuria that tapers off to microscopic hematuria and RBC casts, which may persist for months. It may also produce oliguria or anuria, proteinuria, mild fever, fatigue, flank and abdominal pain, generalized edema, increased blood pressure, nausea, vomiting, and signs of lung congestion, such as crackles and a productive cough.

Chronic glomerulonephritis usually causes microscopic hematuria accompanied by proteinuria, generalized edema, and increased blood pressure. Signs and symptoms of uremia may also occur in advanced disease.

◆ ***Nephritis (interstitial).*** Typically, this infection causes microscopic hematuria. However, some patients with acute interstitial nephritis may develop gross hematuria. Other findings are fever, maculopapular rash, and oliguria or anuria. In chronic interstitial nephritis, the patient has dilute—almost colorless—urine that may be accompanied by polyuria and increased blood pressure.

◆ ***Nephropathy (obstructive).*** This disorder may cause microscopic or macroscopic hematuria, but urine is rarely grossly bloody. The patient may report colicky flank and abdominal pain, CVA tenderness, and anuria or oliguria that alternates with polyuria.

◆ ***Polycystic kidney disease.*** This hereditary disorder may cause recurrent microscopic or gross hematuria. It commonly produces no symptoms before age 40 but may cause increased blood pressure, polyuria, dull flank pain, and signs of urinary tract infection, such as dysuria and urinary frequency and urgency. Later, the patient develops a swollen, tender abdomen and lumbar pain that's aggravated by exertion and relieved by lying down. He may also have proteinuria and colicky abdominal pain from the ureteral passage of clots or calculi.

◆ ***Prostatic hyperplasia (benign).*** About 20% of patients with an enlarged prostate have macroscopic hematuria, usually when a significant obstruction is present. The hematuria is usually preceded by diminished urinary stream, tenesmus, and a feeling of incomplete voiding. It may be accompanied by urinary hesitancy, frequency, and incontinence; nocturia; perineal pain; and constipation. Inspection reveals a midline mass representing the distended bladder; rectal palpation reveals an enlarged prostate.

◆ ***Prostatitis.*** Whether acute or chronic, prostatitis may cause macroscopic hematuria, usually at the end of urination. It may also produce urinary frequency and urgency and dysuria followed by visible bladder distention.

Acute prostatitis also produces fatigue, malaise, myalgia, polyarthralgia, fever with chills, nausea, vomiting, perineal and low back pain, and decreased libido. Rectal palpation reveals a tender, swollen, boggy, firm prostate.

Chronic prostatitis commonly follows an acute attack. It may cause persistent urethral discharge, dull perineal pain, ejaculatory pain, and decreased libido.

◆ ***Pyelonephritis (acute).*** This infection typically produces microscopic or macroscopic hematuria that progresses to gross hematuria. After the infection resolves, microscopic hematuria may persist for a few months. Related signs and symptoms include persistent high fever, unilateral or bilateral flank pain, CVA tenderness, shaking chills, weakness, fatigue, dysuria, urinary frequency and urgency, nocturia, and tenesmus. The patient may also exhibit nausea, vomiting, anorexia, and signs of paralytic ileus, such as hypoactive or absent bowel sounds and abdominal distention.

◆ ***Renal cancer.*** The classic triad of signs and symptoms includes gross hematuria; dull, aching flank pain; and a smooth, firm, palpable flank mass. Colicky pain may accompany the passage of clots. Other findings include fever, CVA tenderness, and increased blood pressure. In advanced disease, the patient may develop weight loss, nausea and vomiting, and leg edema with varicoceles.

◆ ***Renal infarction.*** Typically, this disorder produces gross hematuria. The patient may complain of constant, severe flank and upper abdominal pain accompanied by CVA tenderness, anorexia, and nausea and vomiting. Other findings include oliguria or anuria, proteinuria, hypoactive bowel sounds and, a day or two after the infarction, fever and increased blood pressure.

◆ ***Renal papillary necrosis (acute).*** This disorder usually produces gross hematuria, which may be accompanied by intense flank pain, CVA tenderness, abdominal rigidity and colicky pain, oliguria or anuria, pyuria, fever, chills, vomiting, and hypoactive bowel sounds. Arthralgia and hypertension are common.

◆ ***Renal trauma.*** About 80% of patients with renal trauma have microscopic or gross hematuria. Accompanying signs and symptoms may include flank pain, a palpable flank mass, oliguria, hematoma or ecchymosis over the upper abdomen or flank, nausea and vomiting, and hypoactive bowel sounds. Severe trauma may precipitate signs of shock, such as tachycardia and hypotension.

◆ ***Renal tuberculosis.*** Gross hematuria is often the first sign of this disorder. It may be accompanied by urinary frequency, dysuria, pyuria, tenesmus, colicky abdominal pain, lumbar pain, and proteinuria.

◆ ***Renal vein thrombosis.*** Gross hematuria usually occurs in this type of thrombosis. In an abrupt venous obstruction, the patient experiences severe flank and lumbar pain as well as epigastric and CVA tenderness. Other features include fever, pallor, proteinuria, peripheral edema and, when the obstruction is bilateral, oliguria or anuria and other uremic signs. The kidneys are easily palpable. Gradual venous obstruction causes signs of nephrotic syndrome, proteinuria and, occasionally, peripheral edema.

◆ ***Schistosomiasis.*** This infection usually causes intermittent hematuria at the end of urination. It may be accompanied by dysuria, colicky renal and bladder pain, and palpable lower abdominal masses.

◆ ***Sickle cell anemia.*** In this hereditary disorder, gross hematuria may result from congestion of the renal papillae. Associated signs and symptoms may include pallor, dehydration, chronic fatigue, polyarthralgia, leg ulcers, dyspnea, chest pain, impaired growth and development, hepatomegaly and, possibly, jaundice. Auscultation reveals tachycardia and systolic and diastolic murmurs.

◆ ***Systemic lupus erythematosus.*** Gross hematuria and proteinuria may occur when this disorder involves the kidneys. Cardinal features include nondeforming joint pain and stiffness, a butterfly rash, photosensitivity, Raynaud's phenomenon, seizures or psychoses, recurrent fever, lymphadenopathy, oral or nasopharyngeal ulcers, anorexia, and weight loss.

◆ ***Urethral trauma.*** Hematuria may occur initially, possibly with blood at the urinary meatus, local pain, and penile or vulvar ecchymosis.

◆ ***Vaginitis.*** When this infection spreads to the urinary tract, it may produce macroscopic hematuria. Related signs and symptoms may include urinary frequency and urgency, dysuria, nocturia, perineal pain, pruritus, and a malodorous vaginal discharge.

◆ ***Vasculitis.*** Hematuria is usually microscopic in this disorder. Associated signs and symptoms include malaise, myalgia, polyarthralgia, fever, increased blood pressure, pallor and, occasionally, anuria. Other features, such as urticaria and purpura, may reflect the etiology of vasculitis.

Other causes

◆ ***Diagnostic tests.*** Renal biopsy is the diagnostic test most often associated with hematuria.

This sign may also result from biopsy or manipulative instrumentation of the urinary tract, as in cystoscopy.

◆ ***Drugs.*** Drugs that commonly cause hematuria are anticoagulants, aspirin (toxicity), analgesics, cyclophosphamide, metyrosine, penicillin, rifampin, and thiabendazole.

HERB ALERT *When taken with an anticoagulant, herbal medicines such as garlic and ginkgo biloba can cause excessive bleeding and hematuria.*

◆ ***Treatments.*** Any therapy that involves manipulative instrumentation of the urinary tract, such as transurethral prostatectomy, may cause microscopic or macroscopic hematuria. After a kidney transplant, a patient may experience hematuria with or without clots, which may require indwelling urinary catheter irrigation.

Special considerations

Because hematuria may frighten and upset the patient, be sure to provide emotional support. Check his vital signs at least every 4 hours and monitor intake and output, including the amount and pattern of hematuria. If the patient has an indwelling urinary catheter in place, ensure its patency and irrigate it if necessary to remove clots and tissue that may impede urine drainage. Administer prescribed analgesics, and enforce bed rest as indicated. Prepare the patient for diagnostic tests, such as blood and urine studies, cystoscopy, and renal X-rays or biopsy.

Pediatric pointers

Many of the causes described above also produce hematuria in children. However, cyclophosphamide is more likely to cause hematuria in children than in adults.

Common causes of hematuria that chiefly affect children include congenital anomalies, such as obstructive uropathy and renal dysplasia; birth trauma; hematologic disorders, such as vitamin K deficiency, hemophilia, and hemolytic-uremic syndrome; certain neoplasms, such as Wilms' tumor, bladder cancer, and rhabdomyosarcoma; allergies; and foreign bodies in the urinary tract. Artifactual hematuria may result from recent circumcision.

Geriatric pointers

Evaluation of hematuria in elderly patients should include a urine culture, excretory urography or sonography, and consultation with a urologist.

Patient counseling

Teach the patient how to collect serial urine specimens using the three-glass technique. This technique helps determine whether hematuria marks the beginning, end, or entire course of urination.

Hemianopsia

Hemianopsia is loss of vision in one-half the normal visual field (usually the right or left half) of one or both eyes. However, if the visual field defects are identical in both eyes but affect less than half the field of vision in each eye (incomplete homonymous hemianopsia), the lesion may be in the occipital lobe; otherwise, it probably involves the parietal or temporal lobe. (See *Recognizing types of hemianopsia*.)

Hemianopsia is caused by a lesion affecting the optic chiasm, the optic tract, or the optic radiation. Defects in visual perception due to cerebral lesions are usually associated with impaired color vision.

History and physical examination

Suspect a visual field defect if the patient seems startled when you approach him from one side or if he fails to see objects placed directly in front of him. To help determine the type of defect, compare the patient's visual fields with your own—assuming that yours are normal. First, ask the patient to cover his right eye while you cover your left eye. Then move a pen or similarly shaped object from the periphery of his (and your) uncovered eye into his field of vision. Ask the patient to indicate when he first sees the object. Does he see it at the same time you do? After you do? Repeat this test in each quadrant of both eyes. Then, for each eye, plot the defect by shading the area of a circle that corresponds to the area of vision loss.

Next, evaluate the patient's level of consciousness (LOC), take his vital signs, and check his pupillary reaction and motor response. Ask if he has recently experienced headache, dysarthria, or seizures. Does he have ptosis or facial or extremity weakness? Hallucinations or loss of color vision? When did his neurologic symptoms start? Obtain a medical history, noting especially eye disorders, hypertension, diabetes mellitus, and recent head trauma.

Recognizing types of hemianopsia

Lesions of the optic pathways cause visual field defects. The lesion's site determines the type of defect. For example, a lesion of the optic chiasm involving only those fibers that cross over to the opposite side causes bitemporal hemianopsia, vision loss in the temporal half of each field. However, a lesion of the optic tract or a complete lesion of the optic radiation produces vision loss in the same half of each field—either left or right homonymous hemianopsia.

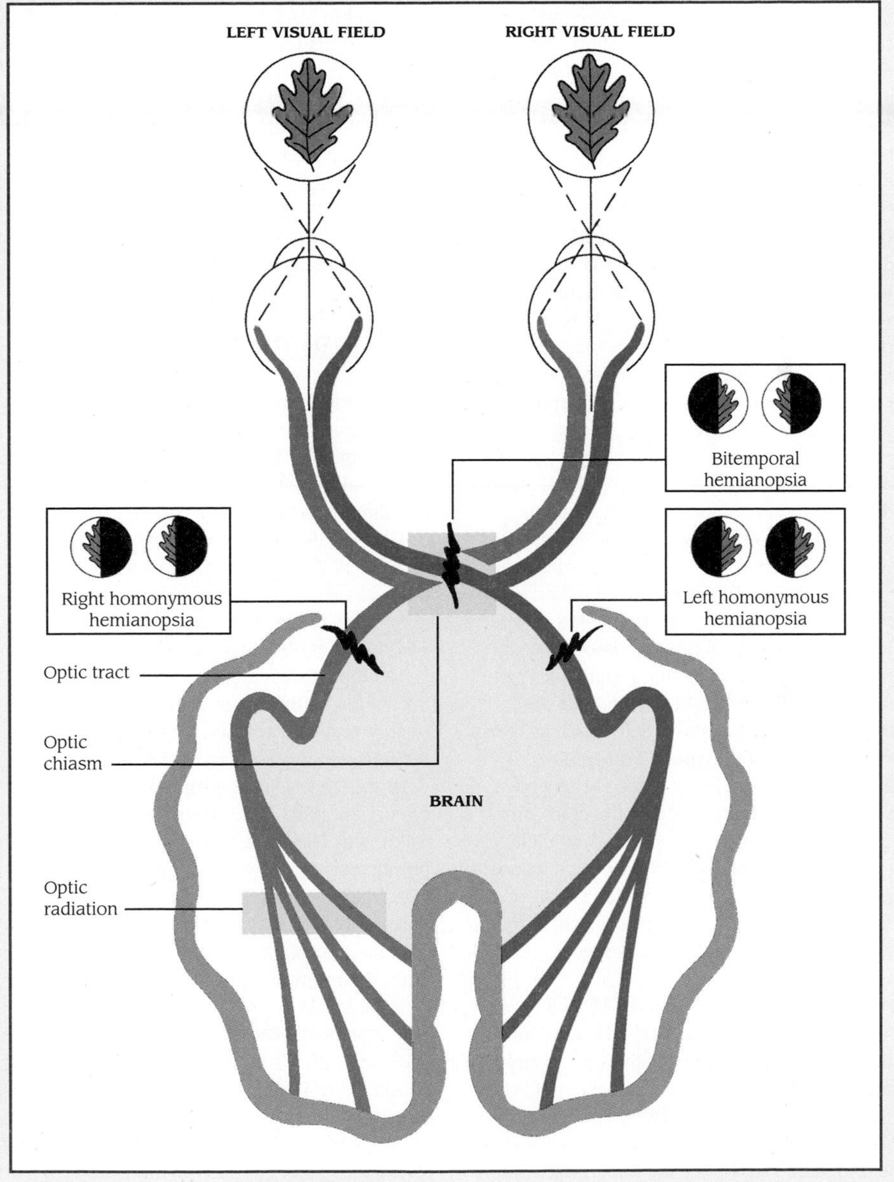

Medical causes

◆ ***Carotid artery aneurysm.*** An aneurysm in the internal carotid artery can cause contralateral or bilateral defects in the visual fields. It can also cause hemiplegia, decreased LOC, headache, aphasia, behavior disturbances, and unilateral hypoesthesia.

◆ ***Occipital lobe lesion.*** The most common symptoms arising from a lesion of one occipital lobe are incomplete homonymous hemianopsia, scotomas, and impaired color vision. The patient may also experience visual hallucinations: flashes of light or color, or visions of objects, people, animals, or geometric forms. These may appear in the defective field or may move toward it from the intact field.

◆ ***Parietal lobe lesion.*** This disorder produces homonymous hemianopsia and sensory deficits, such as an inability to perceive body position or passive movement or to localize tactile, thermal, or vibratory stimuli. It may also cause apraxia and visual or tactile agnosia.

◆ ***Pituitary tumor.*** A tumor that compresses nerve fibers supplying the nasal half of both retinas causes complete or partial bitemporal hemianopsia that first occurs in the upper visual fields but later can progress to blindness. Related findings include blurred vision, diplopia, headache, and (rarely) somnolence, hypothermia, and seizures.

◆ ***Stroke.*** Hemianopsia can result when a hemorrhagic, thrombotic, or embolic stroke affects any part of the optic pathway. Associated signs and symptoms vary according to the location and size of the stroke but may include decreased LOC; intellectual deficits, such as memory loss and poor judgment; personality changes; emotional lability; headache; and seizures. The patient may also develop contralateral hemiplegia, dysarthria, dysphagia, ataxia, unilateral sensory loss, apraxia, agnosia, aphasia, blurred vision, decreased visual acuity, and diplopia as well as urine retention or incontinence, constipation, and vomiting.

Special considerations

If the patient's visual field defect is significant, further visual field testing, such as perimetry or a tangent screen examination, may be indicated.

To avoid startling the patient, approach from the unaffected side and position his bed so that his unaffected side faces the door. If he's ambulatory, remove objects that could cause falls, and alert him to other possible hazards. Place his clock and other objects within his field of vision, and avoid putting dangerous objects (such as hot dishes) where he can't see them.

Pediatric pointers

A brain tumor is the most common cause of hemianopsia in children. To help detect this sign, look for nonverbal clues, such as the child reaching for a toy but missing it. To help the child compensate for hemianopsia, place objects within his visual field; teach his parents to do this as well.

Patient counseling

Explain to the patient the extent of his defect so that he can learn to compensate for it. Advise him to scan his surroundings frequently, turning his head in the direction of the defective visual field so that he can directly view objects he would normally notice only peripherally.

Hemoptysis

Frightening to the patient and often ominous, hemoptysis is the expectoration of blood or bloody sputum from the lungs or tracheobronchial tree. It's sometimes confused with bleeding from the mouth, throat, nasopharynx, or GI tract. (See *Identifying hemoptysis*.) Expectoration of 200 ml of blood in a single episode suggests severe bleeding; expectoration of 400 ml in 3 hours or more than 600 ml in 16 hours signals a life-threatening crisis.

Hemoptysis usually results from chronic bronchitis, lung cancer, or bronchiectasis. However, it may also result from inflammatory, infectious, cardiovascular, or coagulation disorders and, rarely, from a ruptured aortic aneurysm. In up to 15% of patients, the cause is unknown. The most common causes of massive hemoptysis are lung cancer, bronchiectasis, active tuberculosis, and cavitary pulmonary disease from necrotic infections or tuberculosis.

A number of pathophysiologic processes can cause hemoptysis. (See *What happens in hemoptysis*, page 372.)

EMERGENCY INTERVENTIONS *If the patient coughs up copious amounts of blood, endotracheal intubation may be required. Suction frequently to remove blood. Lavage may be necessary to loosen tenacious secretions or clots. Massive hemoptysis can cause airway obstruction and asphyxiation. Insert an I.V. catheter to allow fluid replacement, drug administration, and blood transfusions if needed. An emergency bronchoscopy* *should be performed to identify the bleeding site. Monitor blood pressure and pulse to detect hypotension and tachycardia, and draw an arterial blood sample for laboratory analysis to monitor respiratory status.*

History and physical examination

If the hemoptysis is mild, ask the patient when it began. Has he ever coughed up blood before? How much blood is he coughing up now and how often? Ask about a history of cardiac, pulmonary, or bleeding disorders. If he's receiving anticoagulant therapy, find out which drug, its dosage and schedule, and the duration of therapy. Is he taking other prescription drugs? Does he smoke? Ask the patient if he has recently had any infections or been exposed to tuberculosis. When was his last tine test and what were the results?

Take the patient's vital signs and examine his nose, mouth, and pharynx for sources of bleeding. Inspect the configuration of his chest and look for abnormal movement during breathing, use of accessory muscles, and retractions. Observe his respiratory rate, depth, and rhythm. Finally, examine his skin for lesions.

Next, palpate the patient's chest for diaphragm level and for tenderness, respiratory excursion, fremitus, and abnormal pulsations; then percuss for flatness, dullness, resonance, hyperresonance, and tympany. Finally, auscultate the lungs, noting especially the quality and intensity of breath sounds. Also auscultate for heart murmurs, bruits, and pleural friction rubs.

Obtain a sputum specimen and examine it for overall quantity, for the amount of blood it contains, and for its color, odor, and consistency.

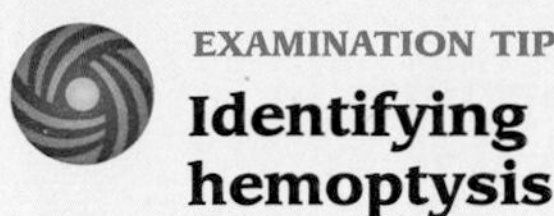

EXAMINATION TIP

Identifying hemoptysis

These guidelines will help you distinguish hemoptysis from epistaxis, hematemesis, and brown, red, or pink sputum.

Hemoptysis

Often frothy because it's mixed with air, hemoptysis typically produces bright red sputum with an alkaline pH (tested with nitrazine paper). It's strongly suggested by respiratory signs and symptoms, including a cough, a tickling sensation in the throat, and blood produced from repeated coughing episodes. (You can rule out epistaxis because the patient's nasal passages and posterior pharynx are usually clear.)

Hematemesis

Hematemesis usually originates in the GI tract; the patient vomits or regurgitates coffee-ground material that contains food particles, tests positive for occult blood, and has an acid pH. However, he may vomit bright red blood or swallowed blood from the oral cavity and nasopharynx. After an episode of hematemesis, the patient's stools may have with traces of blood. Many patients with hematemesis also complain of dyspepsia.

Brown, red, or pink sputum

Brown, red, or pink sputum can result from oxidation of inhaled bronchodilators. Sputum that looks like old blood may result from rupture of an amebic abscess into the bronchus. Red or brown sputum may occur in a patient with pneumonia caused by the enterobacterium *Serratia marcescens*. Currant-jelly sputum occurs with *Klebsiella* infections.

Medical causes

◆ ***Aortic aneurysm (ruptured).*** Rarely, an aortic aneurysm ruptures into the tracheobronchial tree, causing hemoptysis and sudden death.

◆ ***Blast lung injury.*** Although individuals with this type of injury may not have obvious external chest injuries, they sometimes show other indications of internal damage, such as hemoptysis. Health care providers should evaluate survivors of explosive detonations for other classic signs and symptoms of a blast lung injury, such as chest pain, cyanosis, dyspnea, and wheezing. Treatment includes careful administration of fluids and oxygen to ensure tissue perfusion.

◆ ***Bronchial adenoma.*** This insidious disorder causes recurring hemoptysis in up to 30% of patients along with a chronic cough and local wheezing.

◆ ***Bronchiectasis.*** Inflamed bronchial surfaces and eroded bronchial blood vessels cause hemoptysis, which can vary from blood-tinged sputum to blood (in about 20% of patients). The patient typically has a chronic cough producing copious amounts of foul-smelling, purulent sputum. He may also exhibit coarse crackles, clubbing (a late sign), fever, weight loss, fatigue, weakness, malaise, and dyspnea on exertion.

◆ ***Bronchitis (chronic).*** The first sign of this disorder is typically a productive cough that

What happens in hemoptysis

Hemoptysis results when bronchial or pulmonary vessels bleed into the respiratory tract. Bleeding reflects alterations in the vascular walls and in blood-clotting mechanisms. It can result from any of the following pathophysiologic processes:
- hemorrhage and diapedesis of red blood cells from the pulmonary microvasculature into the alveoli
- necrosis of lung tissue that causes inflammation and rupture of blood vessels or hemorrhage into the alveolar spaces
- rupture of an aortic aneurysm into the tracheobronchial tree
- rupture of distended endobronchial blood vessels from pulmonary hypertension due to mitral stenosis
- rupture of a pulmonary arteriovenous fistula, of bronchial or pulmonary artery collateral channels, or of pulmonary venous collateral channels
- sloughing of a caseous lesion into the tracheobronchial tree
- ulceration and erosion of the bronchial epithelium.

lasts at least 3 months. Eventually this leads to production of blood-streaked sputum; massive hemorrhage is unusual. Other respiratory effects include dyspnea, prolonged expirations, wheezing, scattered rhonchi, accessory muscle use, barrel chest, tachypnea, and clubbing (a late sign).

◆ ***Coagulation disorders.*** Such disorders as thrombocytopenia and disseminated intravascular coagulation can cause hemoptysis, multisystem hemorrhaging (for example, GI bleeding or epistaxis), and purpuric lesions.

◆ ***Laryngeal cancer.*** Hemoptysis occurs in this cancer, but hoarseness is usually the initial sign. Other findings may include dysphagia, dyspnea, stridor, cervical lymphadenopathy, and neck pain.

◆ ***Lung abscess.*** In about 50% of patients, this disorder produces blood-streaked sputum resulting from bronchial ulceration, necrosis, and granulation tissue. Common associated findings include a cough producing large amounts of purulent, foul-smelling sputum; fever with chills; diaphoresis; anorexia; weight loss; headache; weakness; dyspnea; pleuritic or dull chest pain; and clubbing. Auscultation reveals tubular or cavernous breath sounds and crackles. Percussion reveals dullness on the affected side.

◆ ***Lung cancer.*** Ulceration of the bronchus commonly causes recurring hemoptysis (an early sign), which can vary from blood-streaked sputum to blood. Related findings include a productive cough, dyspnea, fever, anorexia, weight loss, wheezing, and chest pain (a late symptom).

◆ ***Plague.*** The pneumonic form of this acute bacterial infection, caused by *Yersinia pestis,* can produce hemoptysis, a productive cough, chest pain, tachypnea, dyspnea, increasing respiratory distress, and cardiopulmonary insufficiency. Pneumonic plague begins abruptly with chills, fever, headache, and myalgia.

◆ ***Pneumonia.*** In up to 50% of patients, *Klebsiella* pneumonia produces dark brown or red (currant-jelly) sputum, which is so tenacious that the patient has difficulty expelling it from his mouth. This type of pneumonia begins abruptly with chills, fever, dyspnea, a productive cough, and severe pleuritic chest pain. Associated findings may include cyanosis, prostration, tachycardia, decreased breath sounds, and crackles.

Pneumococcal pneumonia causes pinkish or rusty mucoid sputum. It begins with sudden shaking chills; a rapidly rising temperature; and, in over 80% of patients, tachycardia and tachypnea. Within a few hours, the patient typically experiences a productive cough along with severe, stabbing, pleuritic pain that leads to rapid, shallow, grunting respirations with splinting. Examination reveals respiratory distress with dyspnea and accessory muscle use, crackles, and dullness on percussion over the affected lung. Malaise, weakness, myalgia, and prostration accompany a high fever.

◆ ***Pulmonary arteriovenous fistula.*** Occurring in young adults, this genetic disorder causes intermittent hemoptysis along with cyanosis, clubbing, mild dyspnea, fatigue, vertigo, syncope, confusion, and speech and visual impairments. The patient may bleed from the nose, mouth, or lips. Ruby red patches appear on the face, tongue, skin, mucous membranes, or nail beds.

◆ ***Pulmonary contusion.*** Blunt chest trauma commonly causes a cough with hemoptysis. Other signs and symptoms that appear over several hours include dyspnea, tachypnea, chest pain, tachycardia, hypotension, crackles, and decreased or absent breath sounds over the affected area. Severe respiratory distress—with oppressive dyspnea, nasal flaring, use of accessory muscles, extreme anxiety, cyanosis, and diaphoresis—may develop at any time.

◆ ***Pulmonary edema.*** Severe cardiogenic or noncardiogenic pulmonary edema commonly causes frothy, blood-tinged pink sputum, which accompanies severe dyspnea, orthopnea, gasping, anxiety, cyanosis, diffuse crackles, a ventricular gallop, and cold, clammy skin. This life-threatening condition may also cause tachycardia, lethargy, cardiac arrhythmias, tachypnea, hypotension, and a thready pulse.

◆ ***Pulmonary embolism with infarction.*** Hemoptysis is a common finding in this life-threatening disorder, although massive hemoptysis is rare. Typical initial symptoms are dyspnea and anginal or pleuritic chest pain. Other common clinical features include tachycardia, tachypnea, low-grade fever, and diaphoresis. Less common features include splinting of the chest, leg edema, and—with a large embolus—cyanosis, syncope, and jugular vein distention. Examination reveals decreased breath sounds, pleural friction rub, crackles, diffuse wheezing, dullness on percussion, and signs of circulatory collapse (weak, rapid pulse and hypotension), cerebral ischemia (transient loss of consciousness and seizures), and hypoxemia (restlessness and, particularly in elderly patients, hemiplegia and other focal neurologic deficits).

◆ ***Pulmonary hypertension (primary).*** Hemoptysis, exertional dyspnea, and fatigue generally develop late in this disorder. Angina-like pain usually occurs with exertion and may radiate to the neck but not to the arms. Other findings include arrhythmias, syncope, cough, and hoarseness.

◆ ***Pulmonary tuberculosis.*** Blood-streaked or blood-tinged sputum commonly occurs in this disorder; massive hemoptysis may occur in advanced cavitary tuberculosis. Accompanying respiratory findings include a chronic productive cough, fine crackles after coughing, dyspnea, dullness on percussion, increased tactile fremitus and, possibly, amphoric breath sounds. The patient may also develop night sweats, malaise, fatigue, fever, anorexia, weight loss, and pleuritic chest pain.

◆ ***Silicosis.*** This chronic disorder causes a productive cough with mucopurulent sputum that later becomes blood streaked. Occasionally, massive hemoptysis may occur. Other findings include fine end-inspiratory crackles at lung bases, exertional dyspnea, tachypnea, weight loss, fatigue, and weakness.

◆ ***Systemic lupus erythematosus.*** In 50% of patients with this disorder, pleuritis and pneumonitis cause hemoptysis, a cough, dyspnea, pleuritic chest pain, and crackles. Related findings are a butterfly rash in the acute phase, nondeforming joint pain and stiffness, photosensitivity, Raynaud's phenomenon, seizures or psychoses, anorexia with weight loss, and lymphadenopathy.

◆ ***Tracheal trauma.*** Torn tracheal mucosa may cause hemoptysis, hoarseness, dysphagia, neck pain, airway occlusion, and respiratory distress.

◆ ***Wegener's granulomatosis.*** Necrotizing, granulomatous vasculitis characterizes this multisystem disorder. Findings include hemoptysis, chest pain, cough, wheezing, dyspnea, epistaxis, severe sinusitis, and hemorrhagic skin lesions.

OTHER CAUSES

◆ ***Diagnostic tests.*** Lung or airway injury from bronchoscopy, laryngoscopy, mediastinoscopy, or lung biopsy can cause bleeding and hemoptysis.

SPECIAL CONSIDERATIONS

Comfort and reassure the patient, who may react to this alarming sign with anxiety and apprehension. If necessary, to protect the nonbleeding lung, place him in the lateral decubitus position, with the suspected bleeding lung facing down. Perform this maneuver with caution because hypoxemia may worsen with the healthy lung facing up.

Prepare the patient for diagnostic tests to determine the cause of bleeding. These may include a complete blood count, a sputum culture and smear, chest X-rays, coagulation studies, bronchoscopy, lung biopsy, pulmonary arteriography, and a lung scan.

PEDIATRIC POINTERS

Hemoptysis in children may stem from Goodpasture's syndrome, cystic fibrosis, or (rarely) idiopathic primary pulmonary hemosiderosis. Sometimes no cause can be found for pulmonary hemorrhage occurring within the first 2 weeks of life; in such cases, the prognosis is poor.

GERIATRIC POINTERS

If the patient is receiving anticoagulants, determine any changes that need to be made in his diet or medications (including over-the-counter drugs and natural supplements) because these factors may affect clotting.

Patient counseling

Hemoptysis usually ceases gradually during treatment of the causative disorder. Many chronic disorders, however, cause recurrent hemoptysis. Instruct the patient to report recurring episodes and to bring a sputum specimen containing blood if he returns for treatment or reevaluation.

Hepatomegaly

Hepatomegaly, an enlarged liver, indicates potentially reversible primary or secondary liver disease. This sign may stem from diverse pathophysiologic mechanisms, including dilated hepatic sinusoids (in heart failure), persistently high venous pressure leading to liver congestion (in chronic constrictive pericarditis), dysfunction and engorgement of hepatocytes (in hepatitis), fatty infiltration of parenchymal cells causing fibrous tissue (in cirrhosis), distention of liver cells with glycogen (in diabetes), and infiltration of amyloid (in amyloidosis).

Hepatomegaly may be confirmed by palpation, percussion, or radiologic tests. It may be mistaken for displacement of the liver by the diaphragm (in a respiratory disorder), by an abdominal tumor, by a spinal deformity such as kyphosis, by the gallbladder, or by fecal material or a tumor in the colon.

History and physical examination

Hepatomegaly is seldom a patient's reason for seeking care. It usually comes to light during palpation and percussion of the abdomen.

If you suspect hepatomegaly, ask the patient about his use of alcohol and exposure to hepatitis. Also ask if he's currently ill or taking any prescribed drugs. If he complains of abdominal pain, ask him to locate and describe it.

Inspect the patient's skin and sclerae for jaundice, dilated veins (suggesting generalized congestion), scars from previous surgery, and spider angiomas (common in cirrhosis). Next, inspect the contour of his abdomen. Is it protuberant over the liver or distended (possibly from ascites)? Measure his abdominal girth.

Percuss the liver, being careful to identify structures and conditions that can obscure dull percussion notes, such as the sternum, ribs, breast tissue, pleural effusions, and gas in the colon. (See *Percussing for liver size and position*.) Next, palpate the liver's edge during deep inspiration; it's tender and rounded in hepatitis and cardiac decompensation, rocklike in carcinoma, and firm in cirrhosis.

Take the patient's baseline vital signs, and assess his nutritional status. An enlarged liver that's functioning poorly causes muscle wasting, exaggerated skeletal prominences, weight loss, thin hair, and edema.

Evaluate the patient's level of consciousness. When an enlarged liver loses its ability to detoxify waste products, metabolic substances toxic to brain cells accumulate. As a result, watch for personality changes, irritability, agitation, memory loss, inability to concentrate, poor mentation, and—in a severely ill patient—a coma.

Medical causes

◆ ***Amyloidosis.*** This rare disorder can cause hepatomegaly and mild jaundice as well as renal, cardiac, and other GI effects.

◆ ***Cirrhosis.*** Late in this disorder, the liver becomes enlarged, nodular, and hard. Other late signs and symptoms affect all body systems. Respiratory findings include limited thoracic expansion due to abdominal ascites, leading to hypoxia. Central nervous system findings include signs and symptoms of hepatic encephalopathy, such as lethargy, slurred speech, asterixis, peripheral neuritis, paranoia, hallucinations, extreme obtundation, and coma. Hematologic signs include epistaxis, easy bruising, and bleeding gums. Endocrine findings include testicular atrophy, gynecomastia, loss of chest and axillary hair, and menstrual irregularities. Integumentary effects include abnormal pigmentation, jaundice, severe pruritus and dryness, poor tissue turgor, spider angiomas, and palmar erythema.

The patient may also develop fetor hepaticus, enlarged superficial abdominal veins, muscle atrophy, right-upper-quadrant pain that worsens when he sits up or leans forward, and a palpable spleen. Portal hypertension—elevated pressure in the portal vein—causes bleeding from esophageal varices.

◆ ***Diabetes mellitus.*** Poorly controlled diabetes in overweight patients commonly produces fatty infiltration of the liver, hepatomegaly, and right-upper-quadrant tenderness along with polydipsia, polyphagia, and polyuria. These features are more common in type 2 than in type 1 diabetes. A chronically enlarged fatty liver typically produces no symptoms except for slight tenderness.

◆ ***Granulomatous disorders.*** Sarcoidosis, histoplasmosis, and other granulomatous disorders commonly produce a slightly enlarged, firm liver.
◆ ***Heart failure.*** This disorder produces hepatomegaly along with jugular vein distention, cyanosis, nocturia, dependent edema of the legs and sacrum, steady weight gain, confusion and, possibly, nausea, vomiting, abdominal discomfort, and anorexia due to visceral edema. Ascites is a late sign. Massive right-sided heart failure may cause anasarca, oliguria, severe weakness, and anxiety. If left-sided heart failure precedes right-sided heart failure, the patient exhibits dyspnea, paroxysmal nocturnal dyspnea, orthopnea, tachypnea, arrhythmias, tachycardia, and fatigue.
◆ ***Hemochromatosis.*** This rare disease of iron metabolism causes hepatomegaly, altered skin pigmentation and, possibly, cardiac failure.
◆ ***Hepatic abscess.*** Hepatomegaly may accompany fever (a primary sign), nausea, vomiting, chills, weakness, diarrhea, anorexia, elevated right hemidiaphragm, and right-upper-quadrant pain and tenderness.
◆ ***Hepatitis.*** In viral hepatitis, early signs and symptoms include nausea, anorexia, vomiting, fatigue, malaise, photophobia, sore throat, cough, and headache. Hepatomegaly occurs in the icteric phase and continues during the recovery phase. Also, during the icteric phase, the early signs and symptoms diminish and others appear: liver tenderness, slight weight loss, dark urine, clay-colored stools, jaundice, pruritus, right-upper-quadrant pain, and splenomegaly.
◆ ***Leukemia and lymphomas.*** These proliferative blood cell disorders commonly cause moderate to massive hepatomegaly and splenomegaly as well as abdominal discomfort. General signs and symptoms include malaise, low-grade fever, fatigue, weakness, tachycardia, anorexia, weight loss, and bleeding disorders.
◆ ***Liver cancer.*** Primary tumors commonly cause an enlarged, irregular, nodular, firm liver with pain or tenderness in the right upper quadrant and a friction rub or bruit over the liver. Common related findings are anorexia, weight loss, cachexia, nausea, and vomiting. Peripheral edema, ascites, jaundice, and a palpable right-upper-quadrant mass may also develop. When metastatic liver tumors cause hepatomegaly, the patient's signs and symptoms reflect his primary cancer.
◆ ***Mononucleosis (infectious).*** Occasionally, this disorder causes hepatomegaly. Prodromal symptoms include headache, malaise, and fatigue. After 3 to 5 days, the patient typically develops a sore throat, cervical lymphadenopathy, and temperature fluctuations. He may also develop stomatitis, palatal petechiae, periorbital edema, splenomegaly, exudative tonsillitis, pharyngitis and, possibly, a maculopapular rash.
◆ ***Obesity.*** Hepatomegaly can result from fatty infiltration of the liver. Weight loss reduces the liver's size.
◆ ***Pancreatic cancer.*** In this disease, hepatomegaly accompanies such classic signs and

EXAMINATION TIP

Percussing for liver size and position

With your patient in a supine position, begin percussing at the right iliac crest and proceed up the right midclavicular line (MCL), as shown below. The percussion note becomes dull when you reach the liver's inferior border—usually at the costal margin but sometimes at a lower point in a patient with liver disease. Mark this point and then percuss down from the right clavicle, again along the right MCL. The liver's superior border usually lies between the fifth and seventh intercostal spaces. Mark the superior border.

The distance between the two marked points represents the approximate span of the liver's right lobe, which normally ranges from 2¼" to 4¾" (6 to 12 cm).

Next, assess the liver's left lobe similarly, percussing along the sternal midline. Again, mark the points where you hear dull percussion notes. Also, measure the span of the left lobe, which normally ranges from 1½" to 3⅛" (4 to 8 cm). Record your findings for use as a baseline.

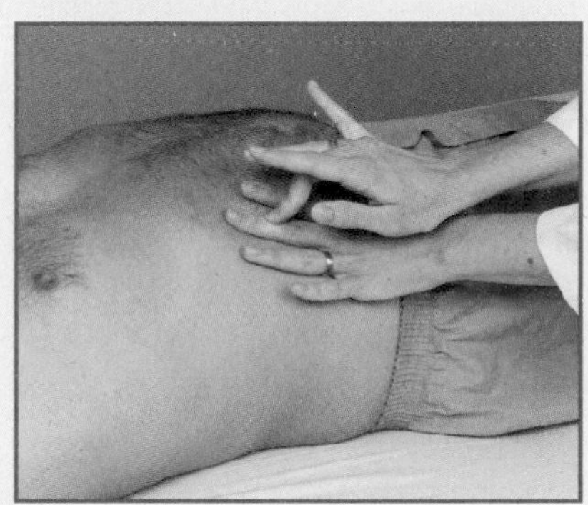

symptoms as anorexia, weight loss, abdominal or back pain, and jaundice. Other findings include nausea, vomiting, fever, fatigue, weakness, pruritus, and skin lesions (usually on the legs).

◆ ***Pericarditis.*** In chronic constrictive pericarditis, an increase in systemic venous pressure produces marked congestive hepatomegaly. Distended jugular veins (more prominent on inspiration) are a common finding. The usual signs of heart disease typically are absent; other features include peripheral edema, ascites, fatigue, and decreased muscle mass.

Other causes

◆ ***Drugs.*** Hepatomegaly is a rare but serious side effect of drugs used to treat HIV-positive hepatitis, such as tenofovir and lamivudine.

Special considerations

Prepare the patient for hepatic enzyme, alkaline phosphatase, bilirubin, albumin, and globulin studies to evaluate liver function, and for X-rays, liver scan, celiac arteriography, computed tomography scan, and ultrasonography to confirm hepatomegaly.

Bed rest, relief from stress, and adequate nutrition are important for the patient with hepatomegaly to help protect liver cells from further damage and to allow the liver to regenerate functioning cells. Dietary protein intake may need to be monitored and possibly restricted. Ammonia, a major cause of hepatic encephalopathy, is a byproduct of protein metabolism. Hepatotoxic drugs or drugs metabolized by the liver should be given in very small doses, if at all. Expalin these treatment measures to the patient.

Pediatric pointers

Assess hepatomegaly in children the same way you do in adults. Childhood hepatomegaly may stem from Reye's syndrome; biliary atresia; rare disorders, such as Wilson's disease, Gaucher's disease, and Niemann-Pick disease; or poorly controlled type 1 diabetes mellitus.

Hiccups

[Singultus]

Hiccups occur as a two-stage process: an involuntary, spasmodic contraction of the diaphragm followed by sudden closure of the glottis. Their characteristic sound reflects the vibration of closed vocal cords as air suddenly rushes into the lungs. (See *How hiccups occur.*)

Usually benign and transient, hiccups are common and usually subside spontaneously or with simple treatment. However, in a patient with a neurologic disorder, they may indicate increasing intracranial pressure or extension of a brain stem lesion. They may also occur after ingestion of hot or cold liquids or other irritants, after exposure to cold, or with irritation from a drainage tube. Persistent hiccups cause considerable distress and may lead to vomiting. Increased serum levels of carbon dioxide may inhibit hiccups; decreased levels may accentuate them.

History and physical examination

Find out when the patient's hiccups began. If he's also vomiting and unconscious, turn him on his side to prevent aspiration.

If the patient is conscious, find out if the hiccups are tiring him. Ask if he has had hiccups before, what caused them, and what made them stop. Also, note whether he has a history of abdominal or thoracic disorders.

Medical causes

◆ ***Abdominal distention.*** The most common cause of hiccups, abdominal distention also causes a feeling of fullness and, depending on the cause, abdominal pain, nausea, and vomiting.

◆ ***Brain stem lesion.*** Producing persistent hiccups, this type of lesion causes decreased level of consciousness, dysphagia, dysarthria, an absent corneal reflex on the side opposite the lesion, altered respiratory pattern, abnormal pupillary response, and ocular deviation.

◆ ***Gastric cancer.*** Persistent hiccups can be the presenting sign of this disease, which may be accompanied by dyspepsia, abdominal pain, anorexia, early satiety, and weight loss.

◆ ***Gastric dilation.*** Besides hiccups, possible signs and symptoms include a sense of fullness, epigastric pain, and regurgitation or persistent vomiting.

◆ ***Gastritis.*** This disorder can cause hiccups along with mild epigastric discomfort (sometimes the only symptom). The patient may develop upper abdominal pain, eructation, fever, malaise, nausea, vomiting, hematemesis, and melena.

◆ ***Increased intracranial pressure.*** Early findings may include hiccups, drowsiness, and

How hiccups occur

Hiccups may result from irritations in the chest or abdomen that trigger transmission of impulses through the vagus (afferent) and phrenic (efferent) nerves to the diaphragm. Upon completion of this reflex arc, the diaphragm contracts. The resulting abrupt intake of air is promptly cut off as the glottis snaps shut.

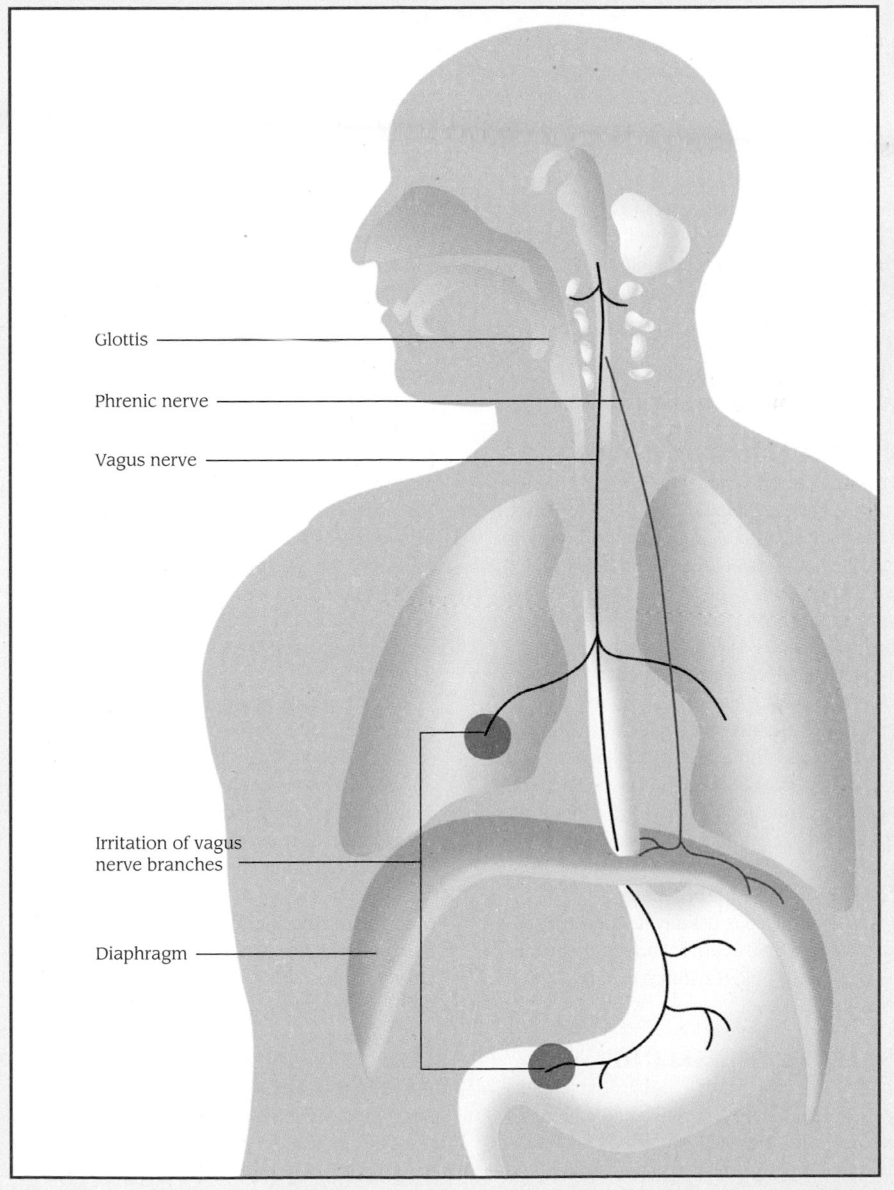

headache. Classic later signs include changes in pupillary reactions and respiratory pattern, increased systolic pressure, and bradycardia.

◆ ***Pancreatitis.*** Hiccups, vomiting, and sudden and steady epigastric pain (often radiating to the back) may occur in this disorder. A severe attack may cause persistent vomiting, extreme restlessness, fever, and abdominal tenderness and rigidity.

◆ ***Pleural irritation.*** Besides hiccups, this condition may cause cough, dyspnea, or chest pain.

◆ ***Renal failure.*** Hiccups may occur in the late stages of both chronic and acute renal failure. Associated signs and symptoms affect every body system and include fatigue, oliguria or anuria, nausea, vomiting, confusion, yellow-brown or bronze skin, uremic frost, ammonia breath odor, bleeding tendencies, gum ulcerations, asterixis, and Kussmaul's respirations.

OTHER CAUSES

◆ ***Surgery.*** Mild and transient attacks of hiccups occasionally follow abdominal surgery.

SPECIAL CONSIDERATIONS

Teach the patient simple methods of relieving hiccups, such as holding his breath repeatedly or rebreathing into a paper bag (both of which increase his serum carbon dioxide level). Other treatments for hiccups include gastric lavage or applying finger pressure on the eyeballs (through closed lids). Hiccups may also be relieved by briefly applying ice cubes to both sides of the neck at the level of the larynx. If hiccups persist, a phenothiazine (especially chlorpromazine), metoclopramide, or nasogastric intubation may provide relief. *(Caution:* The tube may cause vomiting.) If simpler methods fail, treatment may include a phrenic nerve block.

PEDIATRIC POINTERS

In an infant, hiccups usually result from rapid ingestion of liquids without adequate burping. Tell parents to hold the infant upright during feedings.

PATIENT COUNSELING

If abdominal distention is the probable cause of hiccups, teach the patient lifestyle changes, such as eating smaller, more frequent meals and avoiding large meals before bedtime. Also, advise the patient to increase fiber and fluid intake to avoid constipation.

Warn the patient with chronic renal failure that persistent hiccups, usually accompanied by nausea and vomiting, can indicate worsening or acute decompensation of renal function.

Hirsutism

Hirsutism is the excessive growth of coarse body hair in females. Excessive production of androgens (male hormones) stimulates hair growth on the pubic region, axillae, chin, upper lip, cheeks, anterior neck, sternum, linea alba, forearms, upper arms, abdomen, and back. This condition may also occur in a patient with normal levels of androgens whose skin is more sensitive to the hormones. In mild hirsutism, fine and pigmented hair appears on the sides of the face and the chin (but doesn't form a complete beard) and on the extremities, chest, abdomen, and perineum. In moderate hirsutism, coarse and pigmented hair appears on the same areas. In severe hirsutism, coarse hair also covers the whole beard area, the proximal interphalangeal joints, and the ears and nose.

Depending on the degree of excess androgen production, hirsutism may be associated with acne and increased skin oiliness, increased libido, and menstrual irregularities (including anovulation and amenorrhea). Extremely high androgen levels cause further virilization, including such signs as breast atrophy, loss of female body contour, frontal balding, and deepening of the voice. (See *Recognizing signs of virilization*.)

Hirsutism may result from endocrine abnormalities and idiopathic causes. It may also occur in pregnancy from transient androgen production by the placenta or corpus luteum, and in menopause from increased androgen and decreased estrogen production. Some patients have a strong familial predisposition to hirsutism, which may be considered normal for their genetic background, culture, and race. Although hirsutism is a female characteristic, excessive hair growth may also be present in male family members.

HISTORY AND PHYSICAL EXAMINATION

Begin by asking the patient where on her body she first noticed excessive hair. How old was she then? Where and how quickly did other hirsute areas develop? Does she use any hair removal technique? If so, how often does she use it, and when did she use it last? Next, obtain a menstrual history: the patient's age at menar-

Recognizing signs of virilization

Excessive androgen levels produce severe hirsutism and other marked signs of virilization, as shown in the figure below.

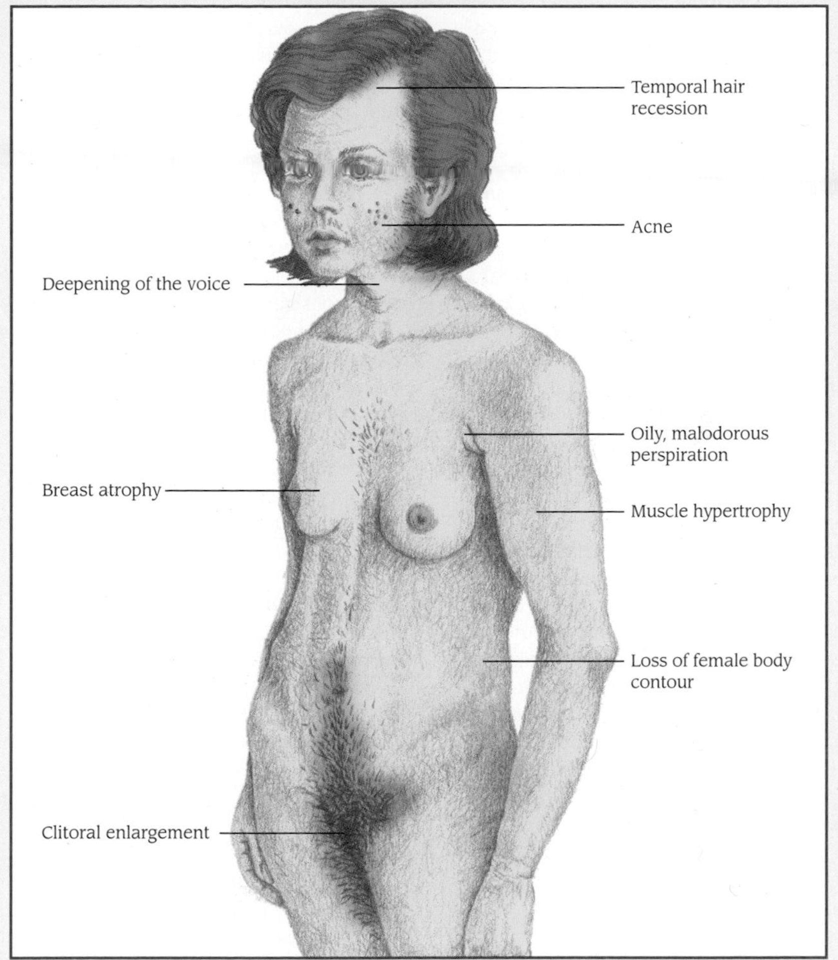

che, the duration of her periods, the usual amount of blood flow, and the number of days between periods.

Ask about medications, too. If the patient is taking a drug containing an androgen or progestin compound, or another drug that can cause hirsutism, find out its name, dosage, schedule, and therapeutic aim. Does she sometimes miss doses or take extra ones?

Next, examine the hirsute areas. Does excessive hair appear only on the upper lip or on other body parts as well? Is the hair fine and pigmented, or dense and coarse? Is the patient obese? Observe her for other signs of virilization.

Medical causes

◆ ***Acromegaly.*** About 15% of patients with this chronic, progressive disorder display hirsutism. Acromegaly also causes enlarged hands and feet, coarsened facial features, prognathism, increased diaphoresis and need for sleep, oily skin, fatigue, weight gain, heat intolerance, and lethargy.

◆ ***Adrenocortical carcinoma.*** This disorder produces rapidly progressive hirsutism along with truncal obesity, buffalo hump, moon face, oligomenorrhea, amenorrhea, muscle wasting, and thin skin with purple striae. The patient also exhibits muscle weakness, excessive diaphoresis, poor wound healing, weakness, fatigue, hypertension, hyperpigmentation, and personality changes.

◆ ***Androgen overproduction by ovaries.*** The most common cause of hirsutism, this condition is associated with anovulation that progresses slowly over several years.

◆ ***Cushing's syndrome (hypercortisolism).*** This disorder commonly causes increased hair growth on the face, abdomen, breasts, chest, or upper thighs. Other findings include truncal obesity, buffalo hump, moon face, thin skin with purple striae, ecchymosis, petechiae, muscle wasting and weakness, poor wound healing, hypertension, weakness, fatigue, excessive diaphoresis, hyperpigmentation, menstrual irregularities, and personality changes.

◆ ***Hyperprolactinemia.*** This disorder produces hirsutism, hypogonadism, galactorrhea, amenorrhea, and acne.

◆ ***Idiopathic hirsutism.*** In patients with normal-sized ovaries, normal menses, and no evidence of adrenal hyperplasia or adrenal or ovarian tumors, excess hair appears at puberty and increases into early adulthood. It's accompanied by acne, obesity, infrequent menses or anovulation, and thick, oily skin. Idiopathic hirsutism with regular ovulation and no menstrual abnormalities may be hereditary or related to certain ethnic groups who are hypersensitive to androgens.

◆ ***Ovarian tumor.*** An ovarian tumor may produce no symptoms, or it can cause rapidly progressing hirsutism (only if the tumor produces androgens) as well as amenorrhea and rapidly developing virilization.

◆ ***Polycystic ovary disease.*** Ovarian cysts, particularly chronic ones, can cause hirsutism. This hirsutism usually occurs after the onset of menstrual irregularities, which may begin at puberty. The patient may also be obese and have amenorrhea, oligomenorrhea, menometrorrhagia, infertility, insulin resistance and diabetes, and acne.

OTHER CAUSES

◆ ***Drugs.*** Hirsutism can result from drugs containing androgens or progestins or from aminoglutethimide, glucocorticoids, metoclopramide, cyclosporine, and minoxidil.

SPECIAL CONSIDERATIONS

Prepare the patient for tests to determine blood levels of luteinizing hormone, follicle-stimulating hormone, prolactin, and other hormones. Other tests may include computed tomography scan and ultrasonography.

At the patient's request, provide information on hair removal methods, such as bleaching, tweezing, hot wax treatments, chemical depilatories, shaving, and electrolysis. Inform the patient that electrolysis should be done only by a licensed professional.

PEDIATRIC POINTERS

Childhood hirsutism can stem from congenital adrenal hyperplasia. This disorder is usually detected at birth because affected infants have ambiguous genitalia. Rarely, a mild form becomes apparent after puberty when hirsutism, irregular bleeding or amenorrhea, and signs of virilization appear. Hirsutism that occurs at or after puberty often results from polycystic ovary disease.

Give the parents as well as the child emotional support and clear explanations about the cause of hirsutism. Allow the parents and child to express their concerns separately.

GERIATRIC POINTERS

Hirsutism can occur after menopause if peripheral conversion of estrogen is poor.

PATIENT COUNSELING

Help relieve the patient's anxiety by explaining the cause of excessive hair growth and by encouraging her to talk about her self-image problems or fears. Involve the family in your discussions.

Tell the patient that hormonal treatment stops further hair growth but doesn't always reverse hair growth that has already occurred. Treatment requires at least 6 to 24 months and may be lifelong.

Hoarseness

Hoarseness—a rough or harsh sound to the voice—can result from infections, inflammatory lesions, or exudates of the larynx; from laryngeal edema; and from compression or disruption of the vocal cords or recurrent laryngeal nerve. This common sign can also result from a thoracic aortic aneurysm, vocal cord paralysis, and systemic disorders, such as Sjögren's syndrome and rheumatoid arthritis. It's characteristically worsened by excessive alcohol intake, smoking, inhalation of noxious fumes, excessive talking, and shouting.

Hoarseness can be acute or chronic. For example, chronic hoarseness and laryngitis result when irritating polyps or nodules develop on the vocal cords. Gastroesophageal reflux into the larynx should also be considered as a possible cause of chronic hoarseness. Hoarseness may also result from progressive atrophy of the laryngeal muscles and mucosa caused by aging, which leads to diminished control of the vocal cords.

History and physical examination

Obtain a patient history. First, consider the patient's age and sex; laryngeal cancer is most common in men between ages 50 and 70. Be sure to ask about the onset of hoarseness. Has the patient been overusing his voice? Has he experienced shortness of breath, a sore throat, dry mouth, a cough, or difficulty swallowing dry food? In addition, ask if he has been in or near a fire within the past 48 hours. Be aware that inhalation injury can cause sudden airway obstruction.

Next, explore associated symptoms. Does the patient have a history of cancer, rheumatoid arthritis, or aortic aneurysm? Does he regularly drink alcohol or smoke?

Inspect the oral cavity and pharynx for redness or exudate, possibly indicating an upper respiratory tract infection. Palpate the neck for masses and the cervical lymph nodes and the thyroid gland for enlargement. Palpate the trachea to determine if it's midline. Ask the patient to stick out his tongue; if he can't, he may have paralysis from cranial nerve involvement. Examine the eyes for corneal ulcers and enlarged lacrimal ducts (signs of Sjögren's syndrome). Dilated neck and chest veins may indicate compression by an aortic aneurysm.

Take the patient's vital signs, noting especially fever and bradycardia. Examine him for asymmetrical chest expansion or signs of respiratory distress—nasal flaring, stridor, and intercostal retractions. Then auscultate for crackles, rhonchi, wheezing, and tubular sounds, and percuss for dullness.

Medical causes

◆ ***Gastroesophageal reflux.*** In this disorder, retrograde flow of gastric juices into the esophagus may then spill into the hypopharynx. This, in turn, irritates the larynx, resulting in hoarseness as well as a sore throat, a cough, throat clearing, and a sensation of a lump in the throat. The arytenoids and the vocal cords may appear red and swollen.

◆ ***Hypothyroidism.*** Hoarseness may be an early sign of hypothyroidism. Others include fatigue, cold intolerance, weight gain despite anorexia, and menorrhagia.

◆ ***Laryngeal cancer.*** Hoarseness is an early sign of vocal cord cancer, but it may not occur until later in cancer of other laryngeal areas. The patient usually has a long history of smoking. Other common findings include a mild, dry cough; minor throat discomfort; otalgia; and, sometimes, hemoptysis.

◆ ***Laryngeal leukoplakia.*** Leukoplakia is a common cause of hoarseness, especially in smokers. Histologic examination by direct laryngoscopy usually reveals mild, moderate, or severe dysphagia.

◆ ***Laryngitis.*** Persistent hoarseness may be the only sign of chronic laryngitis. In acute laryngitis, hoarseness or a complete loss of voice develops suddenly. Related findings include pain (especially during swallowing or speaking), a cough, fever, profuse diaphoresis, sore throat, and rhinorrhea.

◆ ***Rheumatoid arthritis.*** Hoarseness may signal laryngeal involvement. Other findings include pain, dysphagia, a sensation of fullness or tension in the throat, dyspnea on exertion, and stridor.

◆ ***Sjögren's syndrome.*** This rheumatic disorder produces hoarseness, but its cardinal signs are dry eyes, nose, and mouth. Initially, the patient complains of gritty, burning pain around the eyes and under the lids. Ocular dryness also leads to redness, photosensitivity, impaired vision, itching, and eye fatigue. Examination reveals enlarged lacrimal glands and corneal ulcers.

The patient may complain of a dry, sore mouth and difficulty chewing, talking, or swallowing. He may also exhibit nasal crusting, epistaxis, enlarged parotid and submaxillary glands, dry and scaly skin, a nonproductive cough, abdominal discomfort, and polyuria.

◆ ***Thoracic aortic aneurysm.*** Depending on the size and exact location of the aneurysm, patients may remain asymptomatic. When the aneurysm exerts pressure on surrounding structures, however, patients may experience a variety of symptoms. Hoarseness occurs when the aneurysm compresses nerves associated with the larynx. Other clinical features may include a brassy cough; dyspnea; wheezing; a substernal aching in the shoulders, lower back, or abdomen; a tracheal tug; facial and neck edema; jugular vein distention; dysphagia; prominent chest veins; stridor; penetrating pain that's especially severe when the patient is supine; and, possibly, paresthesia or neuralgia.

◆ ***Tracheal trauma.*** Torn tracheal mucosa may cause hoarseness, hemoptysis, dysphagia, neck pain, airway occlusion, and respiratory distress.

◆ ***Vocal cord nodules or polyps.*** Raspy hoarseness, the chief complaint, accompanies a chronic cough and a crackling voice.

◆ ***Vocal cord paralysis.*** Unilateral vocal cord paralysis causes hoarseness and vocal weakness. Paralysis may accompany signs of trauma, such as pain and swelling of the head and neck.

Other causes

◆ ***Inhalation injury.*** An inhalation injury from a fire or an explosion produces hoarseness and coughing, singed nasal hairs, orofacial burns, and soot-stained sputum. Subsequent signs and symptoms include crackles, rhonchi, and wheezing, which rapidly lead to respiratory distress.

◆ ***Treatments.*** Occasionally, surgical trauma to the recurrent laryngeal nerve results in temporary or permanent unilateral vocal cord paralysis, leading to hoarseness. Prolonged intubation may cause temporary hoarseness.

Special considerations

Carefully observe the patient for stridor, which may indicate bilateral vocal cord paralysis. When hoarseness lasts for longer than 2 weeks, indirect or fiber-optic laryngoscopy is indicated to observe the larynx at rest and during phonation.

Pediatric pointers

In children, hoarseness may result from congenital anomalies, such as laryngocele and dysphonia plicae ventricularis. In prepubescent boys, it can stem from juvenile papillomatosis of the upper respiratory tract.

In infants and young children, hoarseness often stems from acute laryngotracheobronchitis (croup). Acute laryngitis in children younger than age 5 may cause respiratory distress because the larynx is small and prone to spasm if irritated or infected. This may cause partial or total obstruction of the larynx. Temporary hoarseness often results from laryngeal irritation due to aspiration of liquids, foreign bodies, or stomach contents. Hoarseness may also stem from diphtheria, although immunization has made this disease rare.

Help the child with hoarseness rest his voice. Comfort an infant to minimize crying, play quiet games with him, and humidify his environment.

Patient counseling

Stress to the patient the importance of resting his voice because talking—even whispering—further traumatizes the vocal cords. Suggest other ways to communicate, such as writing or using body language. Urge the patient to avoid alcohol, smoking, and the company of smokers. If he has laryngitis, advise him to use a humidifier.

Homans' sign

Homans' sign is positive when deep calf pain results from strong and abrupt dorsiflexion of the ankle. This pain results from venous thrombosis or inflammation of the calf muscles. However, because a positive Homans' sign appears in only 35% of patients with these conditions, it's an unreliable indicator. (See *Eliciting Homans' sign.*) Even when accurate, a positive Homans' sign doesn't indicate the extent of the venous disorder.

This elicited sign may be confused with continuous calf pain, which can result from strains, contusions, cellulitis, or arterial occlusion, or with pain in the posterior ankle or Achilles tendon (for example, in a woman with Achilles tendons shortened from wearing high heels).

History and physical examination

When you detect a positive Homans' sign, focus your patient history on signs and symptoms that can accompany deep vein thrombosis or thrombophlebitis. These include throbbing, aching, heavy, or tight sensations in the calf and leg pain during or after exercise or routine activity. Also, ask about any shortness of breath or chest pain, which may indicate pulmonary embolism. Be sure to ask about predisposing events, such as leg injury, recent surgery, childbirth, use of hormonal contraceptives, associated diseases (cancer, nephrosis, hypercoagulable states), and prolonged inactivity or bed rest.

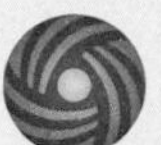

EXAMINATION TIP

Eliciting Homans' sign

To elicit Homans' sign, first support the patient's thigh with one hand and his foot with the other. Bend his leg slightly at the knee; then firmly and abruptly dorsiflex the ankle. Resulting deep calf pain indicates a positive Homans' sign. (The patient may also resist ankle dorsiflexion or flex the knee involuntarily if Homans' sign is positive.)

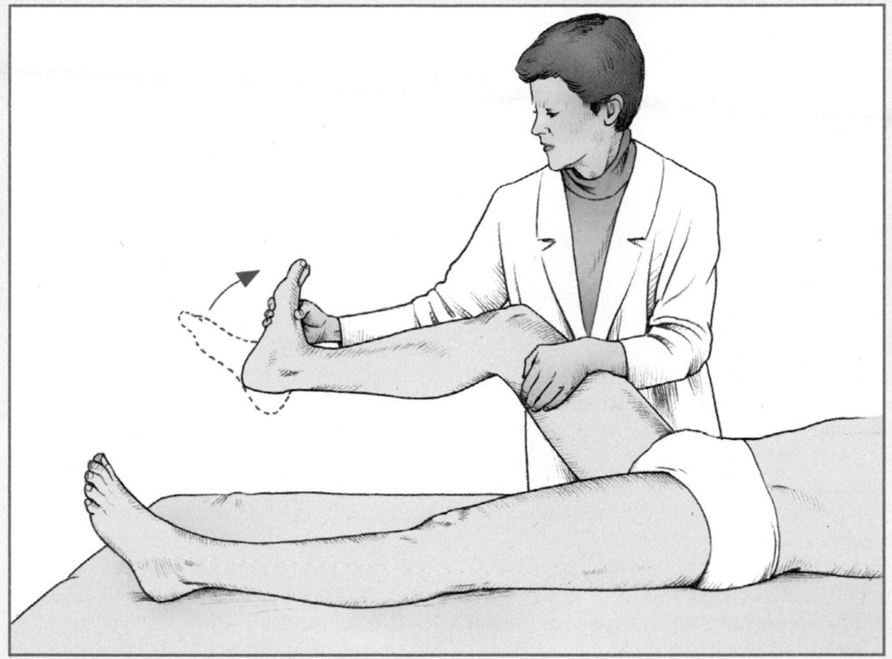

Next, inspect and palpate the patient's calf for warmth, tenderness, redness, swelling, and a palpable vein. If you strongly suspect deep vein thrombosis, elicit Homans' sign very carefully to avoid dislodging the clot, which could cause a life-threatening pulmonary embolism.

In addition, measure the circumference of both the patient's calves. The calf with the positive Homans' sign may be larger because of edema and swelling.

Medical causes

◆ ***Cellulitis (superficial).*** This disorder typically affects the legs but can also affect the arms, producing pain, redness, tenderness, and edema. Some patients also experience fever, chills, tachycardia, headache, and hypotension.

◆ ***Deep vein thrombophlebitis.*** A positive Homans' sign and calf tenderness may be the only clinical features of this disorder. However, the patient may also have severe pain, heaviness, warmth, and swelling of the affected leg; visible, engorged superficial veins or palpable, cordlike veins; and fever, chills, and malaise.

◆ ***Deep vein thrombosis (DVT).*** DVT causes a positive Homans' sign along with tenderness over the deep calf veins, slight edema of the calves and thighs, a low-grade fever, and tachycardia. If DVT affects the femoral and iliac veins, you'll notice marked local swelling and tenderness. If DVT causes venous obstruction, you'll notice cyanosis and possibly cool skin in the affected leg.

◆ ***Popliteal cyst (ruptured).*** Rupture of this synovial cyst may produce a positive Homans' sign as well as sudden onset of calf tenderness, swelling, and redness.

Special considerations

Place the patient on bed rest, with the affected leg elevated above the heart level. Apply warm, moist compresses to the affected area, and administer mild oral analgesics. In addition, prepare the patient for further diagnostic tests, such as Doppler studies and venograms.

Once the patient is ambulatory, advise him to wear elastic support stockings after his discomfort decreases (usually in 5 to 10 days) and to continue wearing them for at least 3 months. In addition, instruct the patient to keep the affected leg elevated while sitting and to avoid crossing his legs at the knees because this may impair circulation to the popliteal area. (Crossing at the ankles is acceptable.)

Pediatric pointers

Homans' sign is seldom assessed in children, who rarely have DVT or thrombophlebitis.

Patient counseling

If the patient is prescribed long-term anticoagulant therapy, instruct him to report any signs of prolonged clotting time. These include black, tarry stools; brown or red urine; bleeding gums; and bruises. Also, stress the importance of keeping follow-up appointments so that prothrombin time can be monitored.

Instruct the patient to avoid alcohol and restrict his intake of green leafy vegetables (spinach and parsley), which are high in vitamin K. Also instruct him to review all medications he's taking with his physician because some drugs may enhance or inhibit the effects of the anticoagulant. The patient should also verify with his physician that any future prescription and over-the-counter medications are safe to take.

Hyperpigmentation

[Hypermelanosis]

Hyperpigmentation, or excessive skin coloring, usually reflects overproduction, abnormal location, or maldistribution of melanin—the dominant brown or black pigment found in skin, hair, mucous membranes, nails, brain tissue, cardiac muscle, and parts of the eye. This sign can also reflect abnormalities of other skin pigments: carotenoids (yellow), oxyhemoglobin (red), and hemoglobin (blue).

Hyperpigmentation most commonly results from exposure to sunlight. However, it can also result from metabolic, endocrine, neoplastic, and inflammatory disorders; chemical poisoning; drugs; genetic defects; thermal burns; ionizing radiation; and localized activation by sunlight of certain photosensitizing chemicals on the skin.

Many types of benign hyperpigmented lesions occur normally. Some, such as acanthosis nigricans and carotenemia, may also accompany certain disorders, but their significance is unproven. Chronic nutritional insufficiency may lead to dyspigmentation—increased pigmentation in some areas and decreased pigmentation in others.

Typically asymptomatic and chronic, hyperpigmentation is a common problem that can have distressing psychological and social implications. It varies in location and intensity and may fade over time.

History and physical examination

Hyperpigmentation isn't an acute process, but an end result of another process, which should be the main target of your examination. Begin with a detailed patient history. Do any other family members have the same problem? Was the patient's hyperpigmentation present at birth? Did other signs or symptoms, such as a rash, accompany or precede it? Obtain a history of medical disorders (especially endocrine) as well as contact with or ingestion of chemicals, metals, plants, vegetables, citrus fruits, or perfumes. Is the hyperpigmentation related to exposure to sunlight or a change of season? Is the patient pregnant or taking prescription or over-the-counter drugs?

Explore other signs and symptoms, too. Ask about fatigue, weakness, muscle aches, chills, irritability, fainting, and pruritus. Does the patient have any cardiopulmonary signs or symptoms, such as cough, shortness of breath, or swelling of the ankles, hands, or other areas? Any GI complaints, such as anorexia, nausea, vomiting, weight loss, abdominal pain, diarrhea, constipation, or epigastric fullness? Also, ask about genitourinary signs and symptoms, such as dark or pink urine, increased or decreased urination, menstrual irregularities, and loss of libido.

Next, examine the patient's skin. Note the color of hyperpigmented areas: Brown suggests excess melanin in the epidermis; slate gray or a bluish tone suggests excess pigment in the dermis. Inspect for other skin changes, too—thickening and leatherlike texture as well as changes in hair distribution. Check the patient's skin and sclerae for jaundice, and note any spider angiomas, palmar erythema, or purpura.

Take the patient's vital signs, noting fever, hypotension, or pulse irregularities. Evaluate his general appearance. Does he have exophthalmos or an enlarged jaw, nose, or hands? Palpate for an enlarged thyroid gland, and auscultate for a bruit over the gland. Palpate the muscles for atrophy and the joints for swelling and tenderness. Assess the abdomen for ascites and edema, and palpate and percuss the liver and spleen to evaluate their size and position. Check the male patient for testicular atrophy and gynecomastia.

MEDICAL CAUSES

◆ ***Acanthosis nigricans.*** This soft velvety-brown verrucous pigmentation is found most commonly in the skin folds and may have associated skin tags. It typically occurs in individuals younger than age 40, may be genetically inherited, and is associated with obesity or endocrinopathies, such as hypothyroidism or hyperthyroidism, acromegaly, polycystic ovary disease, insulin-resistant diabetes, or Cushing's disease.

When seen in individuals older than age 40, this disorder is commonly associated with an internal malignancy, usually adenocarcinoma, and most commonly of the GI tract or uterus; less commonly of the lung, prostate, breast, or ovary. Acanthosis nigricans of the oral mucosa or tongue is highly suggestive of a neoplasm, especially of the GI tract. This skin condition commonly regresses with successful treatment of the neoplasm and may recur with reoccurrence of the disease.

◆ ***Acromegaly.*** This disorder results from a pituitary tumor that secretes excessive amounts of growth hormone after puberty. Hyperpigmentation (possibly acanthosis nigricans) may affect the face, neck, genitalia, axillae, palmar creases, and new scars. Skin appears oily, sweaty, thick, and leathery, with furrows and ridges formed over the face, neck, and scalp. The tongue is enlarged and furrowed; lips are thick; and the nose is large. Body hair is markedly increased. The hands are broad and spadelike. Marked prognathism interferes with chewing.

◆ ***Adrenocortical insufficiency (Addison's disease).*** This disorder produces diffuse tan, brown, or bronze-to-black hyperpigmentation of both exposed and unexposed areas of the face, knees, knuckles, elbows, antecubital areas, beltline, palmar creases, lips, gums, tongue, and buccal mucosa (where hyperpigmentation may be bluish black). Normally pigmented areas, moles, and scars become darker. Early in the disorder, hyperpigmentation occurs as persistent tanning after exposure to the sun. Some patients (usually female) lose axillary and pubic hair; about 15% have vitiligo. Patients may develop slowly progressive fatigue, weakness, anorexia, nausea, vomiting, weight loss, orthostatic hypotension, abdominal pain, irritability, weak and irregular pulse, diarrhea or constipation, decreased libido, amenorrhea, syncope and, sometimes, an enhanced sense of taste, smell, and hearing.

◆ ***Cirrhosis, biliary.*** Hyperpigmentation is a classic feature of this disorder, which primarily affects women between ages 40 and 60. A widespread and accentuated brown hyperpigmentation appears on areas exposed to sunlight, but not on the mucosa. Pruritus that worsens at bedtime may be the earliest symptom. Fatigue, weight loss, and vague abdominal pain may appear years before the onset of jaundice. Malabsorption may cause nocturnal diarrhea, frothy and bulky stools, weight loss, purpura, and osteomalacia with bone and back pain. The patient may also have hematemesis from esophageal varices, xanthomas and xanthelasmas, hepatosplenomegaly, ascites, edema, spider angiomas, and palmar erythema.

◆ ***Cirrhosis, Laënnec's.*** After about 10 years of excessive alcohol ingestion, progressive liver dysfunction causes diffuse, generalized hyperpigmentation on sun-exposed areas. Early in the disorder, the patient may complain of increasing weakness, fatigue, anorexia, slight weight loss, nausea and vomiting, indigestion, constipation or diarrhea, and a dull abdominal ache. As the disorder progresses, the patient may display major signs and symptoms in every body system resulting from hepatic insufficiency and portal hypertension.

◆ ***Cushing's syndrome (hypercortisolism).*** Most common in females, this syndrome is caused by excessive levels of adrenocortical hormones or related corticosteroids. In addition to hyperpigmentation, findings include diabetes mellitus, hypertension, left ventricular hypertrophy, capillary fragility, increased susceptibility to infection, decreased resistance to stress, suppressed inflammatory response, muscle weakness, pathologic changes from bone demineralization, gynecomastia in males, and mild virilism and amenorrhea or oligomenorrhea in females.

◆ ***Hemochromatosis.*** In this inherited disorder (also called bronzed diabetes), most common in men between ages 40 and 60, early and progressive hyperpigmentation results from melanin (and possibly iron) deposits in the skin. Hyperpigmentation develops as generalized bronzing and metallic gray areas accentuated over sun-exposed areas, genitalia, and scars. Early related effects include weakness, lassitude, weight loss, abdominal pain, loss of libido, and signs of diabetes, such as polydipsia and polyuria. Later, signs of liver and cardiac involvement become prominent.

◆ ***Malignant melanoma.*** This form of cancer causes malignant lesions of pigmented skin, commonly moles. Common sites include the head and neck in men, the legs in women, and the back in both men and women exposed to excessive sunlight. Up to 70% of these lesions arise from a preexisting nevus. Metastatic melanoma may produce generalized hyperpigmentation.

The cardinal sign of malignant melanoma is a skin lesion or nevus that enlarges, changes color, becomes inflamed, itches, ulcerates, bleeds, changes texture, or develops an associated halo nevus or vitiligo.

◆ ***Melasma.*** This light or dark brown hyperpigmentation occurs on areas exposed to sunlight, most notably on the face, and is associated with use of hormonal contraceptives or pregnancy. Some cases are idiopathic. Lesions are symmetrical and usually involve the cheeks, forehead, and upper lip. When related to pregnancy, the pigmentation may decrease after delivery. Melasma has cosmetic significance only.

◆ ***Porphyria cutanea tarda.*** Primarily affecting men between ages 40 and 60, this disorder produces generalized brownish hyperpigmentation on sun-exposed areas and extreme skin fragility (particularly on a bald scalp and on the face and hands). It also causes pink or brownish urine (from porphyrin excretion), anorexia, jaundice, and hepatomegaly.

◆ ***Scleroderma (progressive systemic sclerosis).*** Both localized and systemic scleroderma produce generalized dark brown hyperpigmentation that's unrelated to sun exposure. Other skin findings include areas of depigmentation and spider angiomas. The patient initially experiences signs and symptoms of Raynaud's phenomenon—blanching, cyanosis, and erythema of the fingers and toes when exposed to cold or stress, and possible finger shortening, fingertip ulcerations, and gangrene of the fingers and toes. Later findings include pain, stiffness, and swelling of the fingers and joints; skin thickening that progresses to taut, shiny, leathery skin over the entire hands and forearms and then over the upper arms, chest, abdomen, and back; masklike facial skin and a pinched mouth; and, possibly, contractures. Systemic scleroderma also involves the GI, cardiovascular, and other body systems.

◆ ***Thyrotoxicosis.*** This disorder can cause hyperpigmentation on the face, neck, genitalia, axillae, and palmar creases as well as in new scars. Other findings include vitiligo; warm, moist skin; erythematous palms; fine scalp hair with premature graying; and Plummer's nails.

Classic findings of Graves' disease, the most common form of thyrotoxicosis, include an enlarged thyroid gland, nervousness, heat intolerance, weight loss despite increased appetite, profuse diaphoresis, diarrhea, tremor, and palpitations. Exophthalmos, although characteristic, is absent in many patients.

◆ ***Tinea versicolor.*** This benign fungal skin infection produces raised or macular scaly lesions, usually on the upper trunk, neck, and arms, which range from hyperpigmented patches in fair-skinned patients to hypopigmented patches in dark-skinned patients.

Other causes

◆ ***Arsenic poisoning.*** Chronic arsenic poisoning can cause diffuse hyperpigmentation with scattered freckle-size areas of normal or depigmented skin. Other features may include weakness, muscle aches, peripheral neuropathy, headache, drowsiness, confusion, seizures, and mucous membrane involvement (conjunctivitis, photophobia, pharyngitis, or an irritating cough).

◆ ***Drugs.*** Hyperpigmentation can stem from use of barbiturates; salicylates; chemotherapeutic drugs, such as busulfan, cyclophosphamide, procarbazine, and nitrogen mustard; chlorpromazine; antimalarial drugs, such as hydroxychloroquine; hydantoin; minocycline; metals, such as silver (in argyria) and gold (in chrysiasis); corticotropin; and phenothiazines.

Special considerations

Wood's lamp, a special ultraviolet light, helps enhance the contrast between normal and hyperpigmented epidermis. A skin biopsy can help confirm the cause of hyperpigmentation.

Hyperpigmentation may persist even after treatment of the underlying disorder or withdrawal of the causative drug. Bleaching creams may not be effective if most of the excess melanin lies in subepidermal skin layers. Over-the-counter bleaching creams tend to be ineffective because they contain less than 2% hydroquinone.

Pediatric pointers

Most moles that are found in children are junctional nevi—flat, well demarcated, brown to black—that can appear anywhere on the skin. Although these lesions are considered benign, recent evidence suggests that some of them may become malignant in later life. Some physicians recommend removal of junctional nevi; others advise regular inspection. Congenital melanocytic nevi present at birth should be removed, especially if large (greater than 20 cm), because they become malignant in about 20% of cases. Some of these lesions may have an increased amount of hair.

Bizarre arrangements of linear or streaky hyperpigmented lesions on a child's sun-exposed lower legs suggest phytophotodermatitis. Advise parents to protect the child's skin with long pants and socks. Congenital hyperpigmented lesions include benign mongolian spots and sharply defined or diffuse lesions occurring in such disorders as neurofibromatosis, xeroderma pigmentosum, Albright's syndrome, Fanconi's syndrome, Gaucher's disease, Niemann-Pick disease, Peutz-Jeghers syndrome, phenylketonuria, and Wilson's disease.

Patient counseling

Advise the patient to use corrective cosmetics, to avoid excessive sun exposure, and to apply a sunscreen or sun blocker such as zinc oxide cream. Advise patients who stop using bleaching agents to continue using sun blockers because rebound hyperpigmentation can occur.

Warn every patient with a benign hyperpigmented area to consult his physician if the lesion's size, shape, or color changes; this may signal a developing skin cancer.

Hyperpnea

Hyperpnea indicates increased respiratory effort for a sustained period—a normal rate (at least 12 breaths/minute) with increased depth (a tidal volume greater than 7.5 ml/kg), an increased rate (more than 20 breaths/minute) with normal depth, or increased rate and depth. This sign differs from sighing (intermittent deep inspirations) and may or may not be associated with tachypnea (increased respiratory rate).

The typical patient with hyperpnea breathes at a normal or increased rate and inhales deeply, displaying marked chest expansion. He may complain of shortness of breath if a respiratory disorder is causing hypoxemia, or he may not be aware of his breathing if a metabolic, psychiatric, or neurologic disorder is causing involuntary hyperpnea. Other causes of hyperpnea include profuse diarrhea or dehydration, loss of pancreatic juice or bile from GI drainage, and ureterosigmoidostomy. All these conditions and procedures cause a loss of bicarbonate ions, resulting in metabolic acidosis. Hyperpnea may also accompany strenuous exercise, and voluntary hyperpnea can promote relaxation in patients experiencing stress or pain—for example, women in labor.

Hyperventilation, a consequence of hyperpnea, is characterized by alkalosis (arterial pH above 7.45 and partial pressure of carbon dioxide [PCO_2] below 35 mm Hg). In central neurogenic hyperventilation, brain stem dysfunction (as results from a severe cranial injury) increases the rate and depth of respirations. In acute intermittent hyperventilation, the respiratory pattern may be a response to hypoxemia, anxiety, fear, pain, or excitement. Hyperpnea may also be a compensatory mechanism in metabolic acidosis. Under these conditions, it's known as *Kussmaul's respirations.* (See *Kussmaul's respirations: A compensatory mechanism,* page 388.)

History and physical examination

If you observe hyperpnea in a patient whose other signs and symptoms signal a life-threatening emergency, you must intervene quickly and effectively. (See *Managing hyperpnea*, page 389.) However, if the patient's condition isn't grave, first determine his level of consciousness (LOC). If he's alert (and if his hyperpnea isn't interfering with speaking), ask about recent illnesses or infections; ingestion of aspirin or other drugs or chemicals; or inhalation of drugs or chemicals. Find out if the patient has diabetes mellitus, renal disease, or any pulmonary conditions. Is he excessively thirsty or hungry? Has he recently had severe diarrhea or an upper respiratory tract infection?

Next, observe the patient for clues to his abnormal breathing pattern. Is he unable to speak, or does he speak only in brief, choppy phrases?

Kussmaul's respirations: A compensatory mechanism

Kussmaul's respirations—fast, deep breathing without pauses—characteristically sound labored, with deep breaths that resemble sighs. This breathing pattern develops when respiratory centers in the medulla detect decreased blood pH, thereby triggering compensatory fast and deep breathing to remove excess carbon dioxide and restore pH balance.

Disorders (such as diabetes mellitus and renal failure), drug effects, and other conditions cause metabolic acidosis (loss of bicarbonate ions and retention of acid).

↓

Blood pH decreases.

↓

Kussmaul's respirations develop to blow off excess carbon dioxide.

↓

Blood pH rises.

↓

Respiratory rate and depth decrease (corrected pH) in effective compensation.

Is his breathing abnormally rapid? Examine the patient for cyanosis (especially of the mouth, lips, mucous membranes, and earlobes), anxiety, and restlessness—all signs of decreased tissue oxygenation, as occurs in shock. In addition, observe the patient for intercostal and abdominal retractions, use of accessory muscles, and diaphoresis, all of which may indicate deep breathing related to an insufficient supply of oxygen. Next, inspect for draining wounds or signs of infection, and ask about nausea and vomiting. Take the patient's vital signs, including oxygen saturation, noting fever. Also, examine his skin and mucous membranes for turgor, possibly indicating dehydration. Auscultate the patient's heart and lungs.

Medical causes

◆ ***Head injury.*** Hyperpnea that results from a severe head injury is called *central neurogenic hyperventilation*. Whether its onset is acute or gradual, this type of hyperpnea indicates damage to the lower midbrain or upper pons. Accompanying signs reflect the site and extent of injury and can include loss of consciousness; soft-tissue injury or bony deformity of the face, head, or neck; facial edema; clear or bloody drainage from the mouth, nose, or ears; raccoon eyes; Battle's sign; an absent doll's eye sign; and motor and sensory disturbances.

Signs of increased intracranial pressure include decreased response to painful stimulation, loss of pupillary reaction, bradycardia, increased systolic pressure, and widening pulse pressure.

◆ ***Hyperventilation syndrome.*** Acute anxiety triggers episodic hyperpnea, resulting in respiratory alkalosis. Other findings may include agitation, vertigo, syncope, pallor, circumoral and peripheral paresthesia, muscle twitching, carpopedal spasm, weakness, and arrhythmias.

◆ ***Hypoxemia.*** Many pulmonary disorders that cause hypoxemia—for example, pneumonia, pulmonary edema, chronic obstructive pulmonary disease, and pneumothorax—may cause hyperpnea and episodes of hyperventilation with chest pain, dizziness, and paresthesia. Other effects include dyspnea, cough, crackles, rhonchi, wheezing, and decreased breath sounds.

◆ ***Ketoacidosis.*** *Alcoholic ketoacidosis* (occurring most often in females with a history of alcohol abuse) typically follows cessation of drinking after a marked increase in alcohol consumption has caused severe vomiting. Kussmaul's respirations begin abruptly and are accompanied by vomiting for several days, fruity breath odor, slight dehydration, abdominal pain and distention, and absent bowel sounds. The patient is alert and has a normal blood glucose level, unlike the patient with diabetic ketoacidosis.

Diabetic ketoacidosis is potentially life-threatening and typically produces Kussmaul's respirations. The patient usually experiences polydipsia, polyphagia, and polyuria before the onset of acidosis; he may have a history of diabetes mellitus. Other clinical features include fruity breath odor; orthostatic hypotension; rapid, thready pulse; generalized weakness;

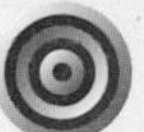

EMERGENCY INTERVENTION

Managing hyperpnea

Carefully examine the patient with hyperpnea for related signs of life-threatening conditions, such as increased intracranial pressure (ICP), metabolic acidosis, diabetic ketoacidosis, and uremia. Be prepared for rapid intervention.

Increased ICP

If you observe hyperpnea in a patient who has signs of head trauma (soft-tissue injury, edema, or ecchymosis on the face or head) from a recent accident and has lost consciousness, act quickly to prevent further brain stem injury and irreversible deterioration. Then take the patient's vital signs, noting bradycardia, increased systolic blood pressure, and widening pulse pressure—signs of increased ICP.

Examine his pupillary reaction. Elevate the head of the bed 30 degrees (unless you suspect spinal cord injury), and insert an artificial airway. Connect the patient to a cardiac monitor, and continuously observe his respiratory pattern. (Irregular respirations signal deterioration.) Start an I.V. catheter. Infuse fluids at a slow rate and prepare to administer an osmotic diuretic, such as mannitol, to decrease cerebral edema. Catheterize the patient to measure urine output, administer supplemental oxygen, and keep emergency resuscitation equipment close by. Obtain arterial blood gas measurements to help guide treatments.

Metabolic acidosis

If the patient with hyperpnea doesn't have a head injury, his increased respiratory rate probably indicates metabolic acidosis. If his level of consciousness is decreased, check his chart for history data to help you determine the cause of his metabolic acidosis, and intervene appropriately. Suspect shock if the patient has cold, clammy skin. Palpate for a rapid, thready pulse and take his blood pressure, noting hypotension. Elevate the patient's legs 30 degrees, apply pressure dressings to any obvious hemorrhage, start several large-bore I.V. catheters, and prepare to administer fluids, vasopressors, and blood transfusions.

A patient with hyperpnea who has a history of alcohol abuse, is vomiting profusely, has diarrhea or profuse abdominal drainage, has ingested an overdose of aspirin, or is cachectic and has a history of starvation may also have metabolic acidosis. Inspect his skin for dryness and poor turgor, indicating dehydration. Take his vital signs, looking for low-grade fever and hypotension. Start an I.V. catheter for fluid replacement. Draw blood for electrolyte studies, and prepare to administer sodium bicarbonate.

Diabetic ketoacidosis

If the patient has a history of diabetes mellitus, is vomiting, and has a fruity breath odor (acetone breath), suspect diabetic ketoacidosis. Catheterize him to monitor for increased urine output, and infuse saline solution. Perform a fingerstick to estimate blood glucose levels with a reagent strip. Obtain a urine specimen to test for glucose and acetone, and draw blood for glucose and ketone tests. Also, administer fluids, insulin, potassium, and sodium bicarbonate I.V.

Uremia

If the patient has a history of renal disease, an ammonia breath odor (uremic fetor), and a fine, white powder on his skin (uremic frost), suspect uremia. Start an I.V. catheter. Administer fluids at a slow rate, and prepare to administer sodium bicarbonate. Monitor his electrocardiogram for arrhythmias due to hyperkalemia. Monitor his serum electrolyte, blood urea nitrogen, and creatinine levels as well until hemodialysis or peritoneal dialysis begins.

decreased LOC (lethargy to coma); nausea; vomiting; anorexia; and abdominal pain.

Starvation ketoacidosis is also potentially life-threatening and can cause Kussmaul's respirations. Its onset is gradual; typical findings include signs of cachexia and dehydration, decreased LOC, bradycardia, and a history of severely limited food intake.

◆ ***Renal failure.*** Acute or chronic renal failure can cause life-threatening acidosis with Kussmaul's respirations. Signs and symptoms of severe renal failure include oliguria or anuria, uremic fetor, and yellow, dry, scaly skin. Other cutaneous signs include severe pruritus, uremic frost, purpura, and ecchymosis. The patient may complain of nausea and vomiting, weakness, burning pain in the legs and feet, and diarrhea or constipation.

As acidosis progresses, corresponding clinical features include frothy sputum, pleuritic chest pain, and signs of heart failure and pleural or pericardial effusion. Neurologic signs include altered LOC (lethargy to coma), twitching, and seizures. Hyperkalemia and hypertension, if present, require rapid intervention to prevent cardiovascular collapse.

◆ ***Sepsis.*** A severe infection may cause lactic acidosis, resulting in Kussmaul's respirations. Other findings include tachycardia, fever or a low temperature, chills, headache, lethargy, profuse diaphoresis, anorexia, cough, wound drainage, burning on urination, confusion or change in mental status, and other signs of local infection.

◆ ***Shock.*** Potentially life-threatening metabolic acidosis produces Kussmaul's respirations, hypotension, tachycardia, narrowed pulse pressure, weak pulse, dyspnea, oliguria, anxiety, restlessness, stupor that can progress to coma, and cool, clammy skin. Other clinical features may include external or internal bleeding (in hypovolemic shock); chest pain, arrhythmias, and signs of heart failure (in cardiogenic shock); high fever, chills and, rarely, hypothermia (in septic shock); or stridor due to laryngeal edema (in anaphylactic shock). Onset is usually acute in hypovolemic, cardiogenic, or anaphylactic shock, but it may be gradual in septic shock.

Other causes

◆ ***Drugs.*** Toxic levels of salicylates, ammonium chloride, acetazolamide, and other carbonic anhydrase inhibitors can cause Kussmaul's respirations. So can ingestion of methanol or ethylene glycol, found in antifreeze solutions.

Special considerations

Monitor vital signs, including oxygen saturation, in all patients with hyperpnea, and observe for increasing respiratory distress or an irregular respiratory pattern signaling deterioration. Prepare for immediate intervention to prevent cardiovascular collapse: Start an I.V. line for administration of fluids, blood transfusions, and vasopressors for hemodynamic stabilization, as ordered, and prepare to give ventilatory support. Prepare the patient for arterial blood gas analysis and blood chemistry studies.

Pediatric pointers

Hyperpnea in children indicates the same metabolic or neurologic causes as in adults and requires the same prompt intervention. The most common cause of metabolic acidosis in children is diarrhea, which can cause a life-threatening crisis. In infants, Kussmaul's respirations may accompany acidosis due to inborn errors of metabolism.

Hypopigmentation

[Hypomelanosis]

Hypopigmentation is a decrease in normal skin, hair, mucous membrane, or nail color resulting from deficiency, absence, or abnormal degradation of the pigment melanin. This sign may be congenital or acquired, asymptomatic or associated with other findings. Its causes include genetic disorders, nutritional deficiency, chemicals and drugs, inflammation, infection, and physical trauma. Typically chronic, hypopigmentation can be difficult to identify if the patient is light-skinned or has only slightly decreased coloring.

History and physical examination

Begin with a detailed patient history. Ask if any other family member has the same problem and if it was present from birth or developed after skin lesions or a rash. Were the lesions painful? Does the patient have any medical problems or a history of burns, physical injury, or physical contact with chemicals? Is he taking prescription or over-the-counter drugs? Find out if he has noticed other skin changes—such as erythema, scaling, ulceration, or hyperpigmentation—or if sun exposure causes unusually severe burning.

Next, examine the patient's skin, noting erythema, scaling, ulceration, areas of hyperpigmentation, and other findings.

Medical causes

◆ ***Albinism.*** This genetically inherited disease involves alterations of the melanin pigment system that affects skin, hair, and eyes. There are various forms of albinism, all of which are present at birth. Skin and hair color vary from snow white to brown, but the universal finding of iris translucency confirms the diagnosis. Associated eye findings include nystagmus, decreased visual acuity, decreased pigmentation of the retina, and strabismus.

Lifelong diligence is needed to protect the skin from sun exposure, including using sunblock with an SPF greater than 30; wearing protective clothing, hats, and sunglasses (even for infants); avoiding the sun during high solar intensity; and obtaining routine skin examinations for the development of skin cancers.

Suggest referral to a support group to assist patients with problems occurring in daily life. One such organization is the National Organization for Albinism and Hypomelanosis.

◆ ***Burns.*** Thermal and radiation burns can cause transient or permanent hypopigmentation.

◆ ***Discoid lupus erythematosus.*** This form of lupus erythematosus may produce hypopigmentation after inflammatory skin eruptions. Lesions are sharply defined, separate or fused macules, papules, or plaques; they vary from pink to purple, with a yellowish or brown crust and scaly, enlarged hair follicles. Although they may occur on other parts of the body, the lesions are typically distributed in a butterfly pattern over the cheeks and bridge of the nose. Telangiectasia may occur. After the inflammatory eruptive stage, noncontractile scarring and atrophy commonly affect the face and may also involve sun-exposed areas of the neck, ears, scalp (with possible alopecia), lips, and oral mucosa.

◆ ***Hypomelanosis (idiopathic guttate).*** Common in lightly pigmented people older than age 30, this skin disorder produces sharply marginated, angular white spots on sun-exposed extremities. In blacks, hypopigmentation occurs mainly on the upper arms.

◆ ***Inflammatory and infectious disorders.*** Skin disorders, such as psoriasis, and infectious disorders, such as viral exanthemas or syphilis, can cause transient or permanent hypopigmentation.

◆ ***Tinea versicolor.*** This benign fungal skin infection produces scaly, sharply defined lesions that usually appear on the upper trunk, neck, and arms. The lesions range from hypopigmented patches in dark-skinned patients to hyperpigmented patches in fair-skinned patients.

◆ ***Tuberculoid leprosy.*** This chronic disorder affects the skin and peripheral nervous system. Erythematous or hypopigmented macules have decreased or absent sensation for light, touch, and warmth. Because the lesions don't sweat, the skin feels dry and rough; it may be scaly. Associated effects may include very painful, palpable peripheral nerves; muscle atrophy and contractures; and ulcers of the fingers and toes.

◆ ***Vitiligo.*** This common skin disorder produces sharply defined, flat white macules and patches ranging in diameter from 1 to over 20 cm. The hypopigmented areas commonly have hyperpigmented borders. Usually bilaterally symmetrical, lesions appear on sun-exposed areas; in body folds; around the eyes, nose, mouth, and rectum; and over bony prominences. Patches of vitiligo may coalesce to form universal lack of pigment and may involve the hair, eyebrows, and eyelashes. Spontaneous repigmentation can occur. Hypopigmented patches (halo nevi) may surround pigmented moles.

Other causes

◆ ***Chemicals.*** Most phenolic compounds—for example, amylphenol (a dye) and paratertiary butylphenol, which are used in plastics and glues, and germicides used in many household and industrial products—can cause hypopigmentation.

◆ ***Drugs.*** Topical or intralesional administration of corticosteroids causes hypopigmentation at the treatment site. Chloroquine, an antimalarial drug, may cause depigmentation of hair (including eyebrows and lashes) and poor tanning 2 to 5 months after therapy begins.

Special considerations

In fair-skinned patients, a special ultraviolet (UV) light (Wood's lamp) can help differentiate hypopigmented lesions, which appear pale, from depigmented lesions, which appear white.

Advise patients to use corrective cosmetics to help hide skin lesions, and to use a sunblock because hypopigmented areas may sunburn easily. Encourage regular examinations for early detection and treatment of lesions that may become premalignant or malignant. Repigmentation therapy may be prescribed, combining a photosensitizing drug (psoralen) and UV light, wavelength A. Advise patients with associated eye problems, such as albinism, to avoid the midday sun and to wear sunglasses. Refer patients for counseling if lesions cause stress.

Pediatric pointers

In children, hypopigmentation results from genetic or acquired disorders, including albinism, phenylketonuria, and tuberous sclerosis. In neonates, hypopigmentation may indicate a metabolic or nervous system disorder.

Geriatric pointers

In elderly people, hypopigmentation is usually the result of cumulative exposure to UV light, which may also cause hyperpigmentation, telangiectasia, and purpura. These changes are known as *dermatoheliosis.*

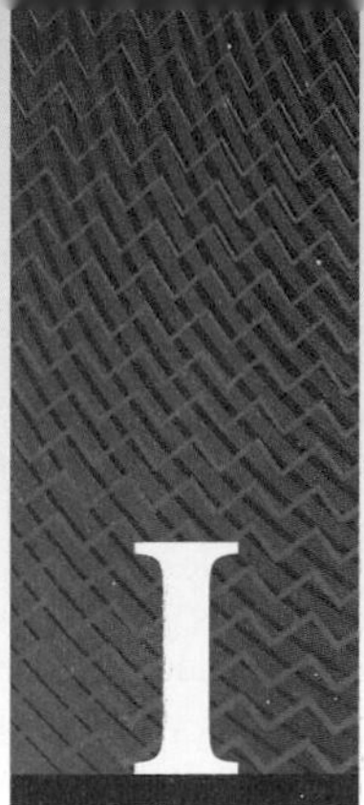

Impotence

Impotence, or erectile dysfunction, is the inability to achieve and maintain penile erection sufficient to complete satisfactory sexual intercourse; ejaculation may or may not be affected. Impotence varies from occasional and minimal to permanent and complete. Occasional impotence occurs in about one-half of adult American men, whereas chronic impotence affects about 15 million American men.

Impotence can be classified as primary or secondary. A man with primary impotence has never been potent with a sexual partner but may achieve normal erections in other situations. This uncommon condition is difficult to treat. Secondary impotence carries a more favorable prognosis because, despite his present erectile dysfunction, the patient has completed satisfactory intercourse in the past.

Penile erection involves increased arterial blood flow secondary to psychological, tactile, and other sensory stimulation. Trapping of blood within the penis produces increased length, circumference, and rigidity. Impotence results when any component of this process—psychological, vascular, neurologic, or hormonal—malfunctions.

Organic causes of impotence include vascular disease, kidney disease, diabetes mellitus, hypogonadism, a spinal cord lesion, alcohol and drug abuse, and surgical complications. (The incidence of organic impotence associated with other medical problems increases after age 50.) Psychogenic causes range from performance anxiety and marital discord to moral or religious conflicts. Fatigue, stress, poor health, age, and drugs can also disrupt normal sexual function.

History and Physical Examination

If the patient complains of impotence or of a condition that may be causing it, let him describe his problem without interruption. Then begin your examination in a systematic way, moving from less sensitive to more sensitive matters. Begin with a psychosocial history. Is the patient married, single, or widowed? How long has he been married or had a sexual relationship? What's the age and health status of his sexual partner? Find out about past marriages, if any, and ask him why he thinks they ended. If you can do so discreetly, ask about sexual activity outside marriage or his primary sexual relationship. Also ask about his job history, his typical daily activities, and his living situation. How well does he get along with others in his household?

Focus your medical history on the causes of erectile dysfunction. Does the patient have type 2 diabetes mellitus, hypertension, or heart disease? If so, ask about its onset and treatment. Also ask about neurologic diseases such as multiple sclerosis. Obtain a surgical history, emphasizing neurologic, vascular, and urologic surgery. If trauma may be causing the patient's impotence, find out the date of the injury as well as its severity, associated effects, and treatment. Ask about intake of alcohol, drug use or abuse, smoking, diet, and exercise. Obtain a urologic history, including voiding problems and past injury.

Next, ask the patient when his impotence began. How did it progress? What's its current status? Make your questions specific, but remember that many patients have difficulty discussing sexual problems, and many don't understand the physiology involved.

The following sample questions may yield helpful data: When was the first time you remember not being able to initiate or maintain an erection? How often do you wake in the morning or at night with an erection? Do you have wet dreams? Has your sexual drive changed? How often do you try to have intercourse with your partner? How often would you *like* to? Can you ejaculate with or without an erection? Do you experience orgasm with ejaculation?

Ask the patient to rate the quality of a typical erection on a scale of 0 to 10, with 0 being completely flaccid and 10 being completely erect. Using the same scale, also ask him to rate his ability to ejaculate during sexual activity, with 0 being never and 10 being always.

Next, perform a brief physical examination. Inspect and palpate the genitalia and prostate for structural abnormalities. Assess the patient's sensory function, concentrating on the perineal area. Next, test motor strength and deep tendon reflexes in all extremities, and note other neurologic deficits. Take the patient's vital signs and palpate his pulses for quality. Note any signs of peripheral vascular disease, such as cyanosis and cool extremities. Auscultate for abdominal aortic, femoral, carotid, or iliac bruits, and palpate for thyroid gland enlargement.

Medical causes

◆ ***Central nervous system disorders.*** Spinal cord lesions from trauma produce sudden impotence. A complete lesion above S_2 (upper-motor-neuron lesion) disrupts descending motor tracts to the genital area, causing loss of voluntary erectile control but not of reflex erection and reflex ejaculation. However, a complete lesion in the lumbosacral spinal cord (lower-motor-neuron lesion) causes loss of reflex ejaculation and reflex erection. Spinal cord tumors and degenerative diseases of the brain and spinal cord (such as multiple sclerosis and amyotrophic lateral sclerosis) cause progressive impotence.

◆ ***Endocrine disorders.*** Hypogonadism from testicular or pituitary dysfunction may lead to impotence from deficient secretion of androgens (primarily testosterone). Adrenocortical and thyroid dysfunction and chronic hepatic disease may also cause impotence because these organs play a role (although minor) in sex hormone regulation.

◆ ***Penile disorders.*** With Peyronie's disease, the penis is bent, making erection painful and penetration difficult and eventually impossible. Phimosis prevents erection until circumcision releases constricted foreskin. Other inflammatory, infectious, or destructive diseases of the penis may also cause impotence.

◆ ***Peripheral neuropathy.*** Systemic diseases, such as chronic renal failure and diabetes mellitus, can cause progressive impotence if the patient develops peripheral neuropathy. This condition affects about 60% of males with diabetes. Associated signs and symptoms of diabetic neuropathy include bladder distention with overflow incontinence, orthostatic hypotension, syncope, paresthesia and other sensory disturbances, muscle weakness, and leg atrophy.

◆ ***Psychological distress.*** Impotence can result from diverse psychological causes, including depression, performance anxiety, memories of previous traumatic sexual experiences, moral or religious conflicts, and troubled emotional or sexual relationships.

◆ ***Trauma.*** Traumatic injury involving the penis, urethra, prostate, perineum, or pelvis may cause sudden impotence due to structural alteration, nerve damage, or interrupted blood supply.

◆ ***Vascular disorders.*** Various vascular disorders can cause impotence. These include advanced arteriosclerosis affecting both major and peripheral blood vessels, Leriche's syndrome (slowly developing occlusion of the terminal abdominal aorta), and arteriosclerosis, thrombosis, or embolization of smaller vessels supplying the penis.

Other causes

◆ ***Alcohol and drugs.*** Alcoholism and drug abuse are associated with impotence, as are many prescription drugs, especially antihypertensives. (See *Drugs that may cause impotence.*)

◆ ***Surgery.*** Surgical injury to the penis, bladder neck, prostate, urinary sphincter, rectum, or perineum can cause impotence, as can injury to local nerves or blood vessels.

Special considerations

Care begins by ensuring privacy, confirming confidentiality, and establishing a rapport with the patient. No other medical condition affecting males is as potentially frustrating, humiliating, and devastating to self-esteem and significant relationships as impotence. Help the patient feel comfortable about discussing his sexuality. This begins with feeling comfortable about your own sexuality and adopting an accepting attitude about the sexual experiences and preferences of others.

Drugs that may cause impotence

Many commonly used drugs—especially antidepressants and antihypertensives—can cause impotence, which may be reversible if the drug is discontinued or the dosage reduced. Here are some examples.

amitriptyline	hydralazine
atenolol	imipramine
bicalutamide	methyldopa
carbamazepine	nortriptyline
cimetidine	perphenazine
clonidine	prazosin
desipramine	propranolol
digoxin	thiazide diuretics
diphenhydramine	thioridazine
finasteride	tranylcypromine

Prepare the patient for screening tests for hormonal irregularities and for Doppler studies of penile blood pressure to rule out vascular insufficiency. Other tests include voiding studies, nerve conduction tests, evaluation of nocturnal penile tumescence, and psychological screening.

Treatment of psychogenic impotence may involve counseling for the patient and his sexual partner; treatment of organic impotence focuses on reversing the cause, if possible. Other forms of treatment include surgical revascularization, drug-induced erection, surgical repair of a venous leak, and penile prostheses. Encourage the patient to maintain follow-up appointments and therapy for underlying medical disorders.

Geriatric pointers

Most people erroneously believe that sexual performance normally declines with age. Many also believe (erroneously) that elderly people are incapable of or aren't interested in sex or that they can't find elderly partners who are interested in sex. Organic disease must be ruled out in elderly people who suffer from sexual dysfunction before counseling to improve sexual performance can start.

Patient counseling

Encourage your patient to talk openly about his needs and desires, fears and anxieties, or misconceptions. Urge him to discuss these issues with his partner as well as what role both of them want sexual activity to play in their lives.

Insomnia

Insomnia is the inability to fall asleep, remain asleep, or feel refreshed by sleep. Acute and transient during periods of stress, insomnia may become chronic, causing constant fatigue, extreme anxiety as bedtime approaches, and psychiatric disorders. This common complaint is experienced occasionally by about 25% of Americans and chronically by another 10%.

Physiologic causes of insomnia include jet lag, arguing, and lack of exercise. Pathophysiologic causes range from medical and psychiatric disorders to pain, adverse effects of a drug, and idiopathic factors. Complaints of insomnia are subjective and require close investigation; for example, the patient may mistakenly attribute his fatigue from an organic cause, such as anemia, to insomnia.

History and physical examination

Take a thorough sleep and health history. Find out when the patient's insomnia began and the circumstances surrounding it. Is the patient trying to stop using a sedative? Does he take a central nervous system (CNS) stimulant, such as an amphetamine, pseudoephedrine, a theophylline derivative, phenylpropanolamine, cocaine, or a drug that contains caffeine, or does he drink caffeinated beverages?

Find out if the patient has a chronic or acute condition, the effects of which may be disturbing his sleep, particularly cardiac or respiratory disease or painful or pruritic conditions. Ask if he has an endocrine or neurologic disorder, or a history of drug or alcohol abuse. Is he a frequent traveler who suffers from jet lag? Does he use his legs a lot during the day and then feel restless at night? Ask about daytime fatigue and regular exercise. Also ask if he often finds himself gasping for air, experiencing apnea, or frequently repositioning his body. If possible, consult the patient's spouse or sleep partner because the patient may be unaware of his own behavior. Ask how many pillows the patient uses to sleep.

Assess the patient's emotional status, and try to estimate his level of self-esteem. Ask about personal and professional problems and psychological stress. Also ask if he experiences hallucinations, and note behavior that may indicate alcohol withdrawal. After reviewing any complaints that suggest an undiagnosed disorder, perform a physical examination. (See *Differential diagnosis: Insomnia*, pages 396 and 397.)

Differential diagnosis: Insomnia

History of present illness

Focused physical examination:
Mental health; respiratory, endocrine, and cardiovascular systems

Common signs and symptoms
- ◆ Diaphoresis
- ◆ Palpitations
- ◆ Shortness of breath
- ◆ Tachycardia

Generalized anxiety disorder

Additional signs and symptoms
- ◆ Fatigue
- ◆ Restlessness
- ◆ Dyspepsia
- ◆ Dry mouth
- ◆ Light-headedness
- ◆ Nausea
- ◆ Diarrhea
- ◆ Flushes or chills
- ◆ Excessive worry
- ◆ Irritability
- ◆ Difficulty concentrating

Diagnosis: Psychological evaluation
Treatment: Medication (selective serotonin reuptake inhibitors [SSRIs], antidepressants, beta-adrenergic blockers [for physical symptoms], short-term benzodiazepines), cognitive and behavioral therapies
Follow-up: Reevaluation every 2 to 3 weeks until stabilized on medication

Thyrotoxicosis

Additional signs and symptoms
- ◆ Difficulty falling asleep, then sleeping for only a brief period
- ◆ Dyspnea
- ◆ Atrial or ventricular gallop
- ◆ Inability to concentrate
- ◆ Emotional lability
- ◆ Weight loss despite increased appetite
- ◆ Tremors
- ◆ Nervousness
- ◆ Diaphoresis
- ◆ Hypersensitivity to heat
- ◆ Enlarged thyroid
- ◆ Polyuria
- ◆ Polydipsia

Diagnosis: Physical examination, laboratory tests (thyroid-stimulating hormone, T_3, T_4, thyroid resin uptake)
Treatment: Medication (antithyroid agents, therapeutic radioiodine, beta-adrenergic blockers)
Follow-up: Reevaluation of thyroid function every 6 months; reevaluation at 6 weeks and 12 weeks, and then every 6 months, if undergoing radionuclide therapy

MEDICAL CAUSES

◆ ***Alcohol withdrawal syndrome.*** Abrupt cessation of alcohol intake after long-term use causes insomnia that may persist for up to 2 years. Other early effects of this acute syndrome include excessive diaphoresis, tachycardia, hypertension, tremors, restlessness, irritability, headache, nausea, flushing, and nightmares. Progression to delirium tremens produces confusion, disorientation,

Depression

Signs and symptoms
- Chronic insomnia with difficulty falling asleep and early waking
- Dysphoria
- Decreased or increased appetite
- Psychomotor agitation or retardation
- Loss of interest in usual activities
- Feelings of worthlessness or guilt
- Fatigue
- Difficulty concentrating
- Indecisiveness
- Recurrent thoughts of death
- Tachycardia
- Possible suicidal ideation

Diagnosis: Beck Depression Inventory, Zung Self-Rating Depression Scale, Geriatric Depression Scale, laboratory tests (complete blood count, erythrocyte sedimentation rate, Venereal Disease Research Laboratory, electrolytes, thyroid profile, drug screening)
Treatment: Medication (SSRIs, tricyclic antidepressants), cognitive therapy, support groups, exercise program
Follow-up: Initial reevaluation at 2 weeks, then every 4 to 8 weeks, then every 3 months; referral to psychologist

Sleep apnea syndrome

Signs and symptoms
- Repeated episodes of obstructive apnea and hypopnea during sleep that end with a series of gasps and arousal
- Morning headache
- Daytime sleepiness
- Hypertension
- Personality changes

Diagnosis: Polysomnography in a sleep laboratory
Treatment: Treatment of underlying cause, continuous positive airway pressure at night, oral appliances, antidepressants, surgery, weight loss (if indicated), smoking and alcohol cessation, positional therapy
Follow-up: Referrals to sleep specialist and pulmonologist

Additional differential diagnoses: alcohol withdrawal syndrome ◆ mood (affective) disorders ◆ nocturnal myoclonus ◆ pain ◆ pheochromocytoma ◆ pruritus
Other causes: amphetamines ◆ caffeine-containing beverages ◆ cocaine ◆ ginseng ◆ green tea ◆ pseudoephedrine ◆ theophylline derivatives ◆ withdrawal from sedatives or hypnotics

paranoia, delusions, hallucinations, and seizures.

◆ ***Generalized anxiety disorder.*** Anxiety can cause chronic insomnia as well as symptoms of tension, such as fatigue and restlessness; signs of autonomic hyperactivity, such as diaphoresis, dyspepsia, and high resting pulse and respiratory rates; and signs of apprehension.

◆ ***Mood (affective) disorders.*** Depression commonly causes chronic insomnia with difficulty falling asleep, waking and being unable to fall back to sleep, or waking early in the morning. Related findings include dysphoria (a primary symptom), decreased appetite with weight loss or increased appetite with weight gain, and psychomotor agitation or retardation. The patient experiences loss of interest in his usual activities, feelings of worthlessness and guilt, fatigue, difficulty concentrating, indecisiveness, and recurrent thoughts of death.

Manic episodes produce a decreased need for sleep with an elevated mood and irritability. Related findings include increased energy and activity, fast speech, speeding thoughts, inflated self-esteem, easy distractibility, and involvement in high-risk activities such as reckless driving.

◆ ***Nocturnal myoclonus.*** With this seizure disorder, involuntary and fleeting muscle jerks of the legs occur every 20 to 40 seconds, disturbing sleep.

◆ ***Pain.*** Almost any condition that causes pain can cause insomnia. Related findings reflect the specific cause.

◆ ***Pheochromocytoma.*** This rare disorder causes paroxysms of acute hypermetabolic activity, which can prevent or interrupt sleep. Its cardinal sign is severe hypertension, which may be sustained between attacks. Other effects include headache, palpitations, and anxiety.

◆ ***Pruritus.*** Localized skin infections and systemic disorders, such as liver failure, can cause pruritus, resulting in insomnia.

◆ ***Sleep apnea syndrome.*** Apneic periods begin with the onset of sleep, continue for 10 to 90 seconds, and end with a series of gasps and arousal. With central sleep apnea, respiratory movement ceases for the apneic period; with obstructive sleep apnea, upper airway obstruction blocks incoming air, although breathing movements continue. Some patients display both types of apnea. Repeated possibly hundreds of times during the night, this cycle alternates with bradycardia and tachycardia. Associated findings include morning headache, daytime fatigue, hypertension, ankle edema, and personality changes, such as hostility, paranoia, and agitated depression.

◆ ***Thyrotoxicosis.*** Difficulty falling asleep and then sleeping for only a brief period is one of the characteristic symptoms of this disorder. Cardiopulmonary features include dyspnea, tachycardia, palpitations, and atrial or ventricular gallop. Other findings include weight loss despite increased appetite, diarrhea, tremors, nervousness, diaphoresis, hypersensitivity to heat, an enlarged thyroid, polyuria, and polydipsia.

OTHER CAUSES

◆ ***Drugs.*** Use of, abuse of, or withdrawal from sedatives or hypnotics may produce insomnia. CNS stimulants—including amphetamines, theophylline derivatives, pseudoephedrine, cocaine, and caffeinated beverages—may also produce insomnia.

HERB ALERT *Herbal remedies, such as ginseng and green tea, can also cause insomnia.*

SPECIAL CONSIDERATIONS

Prepare the patient for tests to evaluate his insomnia, such as blood and urine studies for 17-hydroxycorticosteroids and catecholamines, polysomnography (including an EEG, electro-oculography, and electrocardiography), and sleep EEG.

PEDIATRIC POINTERS

Insomnia in early childhood may develop along with separation anxiety at ages 2 to 3, after a stressful or tiring day, or during illness or teething. In children ages 6 to 11, insomnia usually reflects residual excitement from the day's activities; a few children continue to have bedtime fears. Sleep problems are common in foster children.

PATIENT COUNSELING

Teach the patient comfort and relaxation techniques to promote natural sleep. (See *Tips for relieving insomnia*.) Advise him to awaken and retire at the same time each day and to exercise regularly. When he can't sleep, advise him to get up but remain inactive. Urge him to use his bed only for sleeping, not for relaxation or watching television.

Advise the patient to use tranquilizers or sedatives for acute insomnia only when relaxation techniques fail. If appropriate, refer him for counseling or to a sleep disorder clinic for biofeedback training or other interventions.

Tips for relieving insomnia

Common problems	Causes	Interventions
Acroparesthesia	Improper positioning may compress superficial (ulnar, radial, and peroneal) nerves, disrupting circulation to the compressed nerve. This causes numbness, tingling and stiffness in an arm or leg.	Teach the patient to assume a comfortable position in bed, with his limbs unrestricted. If he tends to awaken with a numb arm or leg, tell him to massage and move it until sensation returns completely and then to assume an unrestricted position.
Anxiety	Physical and emotional stress produces anxiety, which causes autonomic stimulation.	Encourage the patient to discuss his fears and concerns, and teach him relaxation techniques, such as guided imagery and deep breathing. If ordered, administer a mild sedative, such as temazepam or another sedative hypnotic, before bedtime. Emphasize that these medications are to be used for the short-term only.
Dyspnea	With many cardiac and pulmonary disorders, a recumbent position and inactivity cause restricted chest expansion, secretion pooling, and pulmonary vascular congestion, leading to coughing and shortness of breath.	Elevate the head of the bed, or provide at least two pillows or a reclining chair to help the patient sleep. Suction him when he awakens, and encourage deep breathing and incentive spirometry every 2 to 4 hours. Also, provide supplementary oxygen by nasal cannula. If the patient is pregnant, encourage her to sleep on her left side at a comfortable elevation to ease dyspnea.
Pain	Chronic or acute pain from any cause can prevent or disrupt sleep.	Administer pain medication, as ordered, 20 minutes before bedtime, and teach deep, even, slow breathing to promote relaxation. If the patient has back pain, help him lie on his side with his legs flexed. If he has epigastric pain, encourage him to take an antacid before bedtime and to sleep with the head of the bed elevated. If he has incisions, instruct him to splint during coughing or movement.
Pruritus	A localized skin infection or a systemic disorder, such as liver failure, may produce intensely annoying itching, even during the night.	Wash the patient's skin with a mild soap and water, and dry the skin thoroughly. Apply moisturizing lotion on dry, unbroken skin and an antipruritic such as calamine lotion on pruritic areas. Administer diphenhydramine or hydroxyzine, as ordered, to help minimize itching.
Restless leg syndrome	Excessive exercise during the day may cause tired, aching legs at night, requiring movement for relief.	Help the patient exercise his legs gently by slowly walking with him around the room and down the hall. If ordered, administer a muscle relaxant such as diazepam.

Intermittent claudication

Most common in the legs, intermittent claudication is cramping limb pain brought on by exercise and relieved by 1 to 2 minutes of rest. This pain may be acute or chronic; when acute, it may signal acute arterial occlusion. Intermittent claudication is most common in men ages 50 to 60 with a history of diabetes mellitus, hyperlipidemia, hypertension, or tobacco use. Without treatment, it may progress to pain at rest. With chronic arterial occlusion, limb loss is uncommon because collateral circulation usually develops.

With occlusive artery disease, intermittent claudication results from an inadequate blood supply. Pain in the calf (the most common area) or foot indicates disease of the femoral or popliteal arteries; pain in the buttocks and upper thigh, disease of the aortoiliac arteries. During exercise, the pain typically results from the release of lactic acid due to anaerobic metabolism in the ischemic segment, secondary to obstruction. When exercise stops, the lactic acid clears and the pain subsides.

Intermittent claudication may also have a neurologic cause: narrowing of the vertebral column at the level of the cauda equina. This condition creates pressure on the nerve roots to the lower extremities. Walking stimulates circulation to the cauda equina, causing increased pressure on those nerves and resultant pain.

Physical findings include pallor on elevation, rubor on dependency (especially the toes and soles), loss of hair on the toes, and diminished arterial pulses.

EMERGENCY INTERVENTIONS *If the patient has sudden intermittent claudication with severe or aching leg pain at rest, check the leg's temperature and color and palpate femoral, popliteal, posterior tibial, and dorsalis pedis pulses. Ask about numbness and tingling. Suspect acute arterial occlusion if pulses are absent; if the leg feels cold and looks pale, cyanotic, or mottled; and if paresthesia and pain are present. Mark the area of pallor, cyanosis, or mottling, and reassess it frequently, noting an increase in the area.*

Don't elevate the leg. Protect it, allowing nothing to press on it. Prepare the patient for preoperative blood tests, urinalysis, electrocardiography, chest X-rays, lower-extremity Doppler studies, and angiography. Start an I.V. catheter, and administer an anticoagulant and analgesics.

History and physical examination

If the patient has chronic intermittent claudication, gather history data first. Ask how far he can walk before pain occurs and how long he must rest before it subsides. Can he walk less far now than before, or does he need to rest longer? Does the pain-rest pattern vary? Has this symptom affected his lifestyle?

Obtain a history of risk factors for atherosclerosis, such as smoking, diabetes, hypertension, and hyperlipidemia. Next, ask about associated signs and symptoms, such as paresthesia in the affected limb and visible changes in the color of the fingers (white to blue to pink) when he's smoking, exposed to cold, or under stress. If the patient is male, does he experience impotence?

Focus the physical examination on the cardiovascular system. Palpate for femoral, popliteal, dorsalis pedis, and posterior tibial pulses. Note character, amplitude, and bilateral equality. Diminished or absent popliteal and pedal pulses with the femoral pulse present may indicate atherosclerotic disease of the femoral artery. Diminished femoral and distal pulses may indicate disease of the terminal aorta or iliac branches. Absent pedal pulses with normal femoral and popliteal pulses may indicate Buerger's disease.

Listen for bruits over the major arteries. Note color and temperature differences between his legs or compared with his arms; also note where on his leg the changes in temperature and color occur. Elevate the affected leg for 2 minutes; if it becomes pale or white, blood flow is severely decreased. When the leg hangs down, how long does it take for color to return? (Thirty seconds or longer indicates severe disease.) If possible, check the patient's deep tendon reflexes after exercise; note if they're diminished in his lower extremities.

Examine his feet, toes, and fingers for ulceration, and inspect his hands and lower legs for small, tender nodules and erythema along blood vessels. Note the quality of his nails and the amount of hair on his fingers and toes.

If the patient has arm pain, inspect his arms for a change in color (to white) on elevation. Next, palpate for changes in temperature, muscle wasting, and a pulsating mass in the subclavian area. Palpate and compare the radial, ulnar, brachial, axillary, and subclavian pulses to identify obstructed areas.

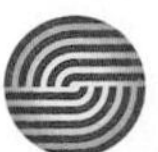

PATIENT-TEACHING AID

Improving circulation in your legs

Dear Patient:
To help stimulate circulation in your legs, perform these exercises (called *Berger's exercises*) as part of your regular exercise program. Do them four times each day or as often as your physician specifies.

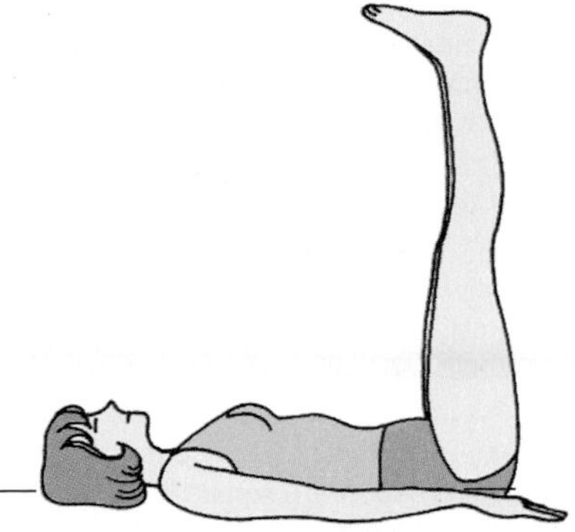

Begin by lying flat on your back; then raise your legs straight up at a 90-degree angle, and hold this position for 2 minutes.

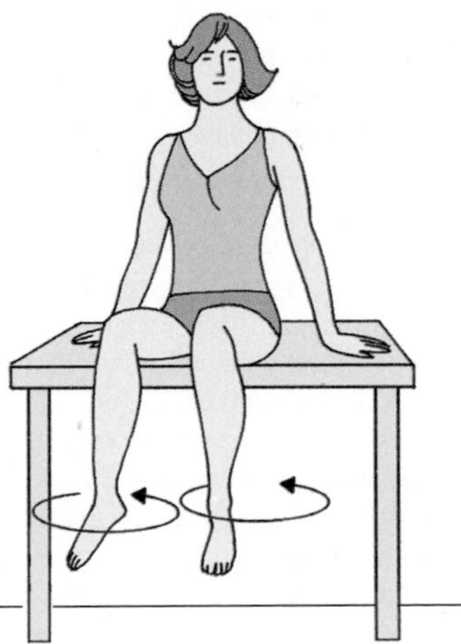

Now sit on the edge of a table or any flat surface that's high enough so that your legs don't touch the floor. Dangle your legs and swirl them in circles for 2 minutes.

Finally, lie flat for 2 minutes; then repeat the sequence twice.

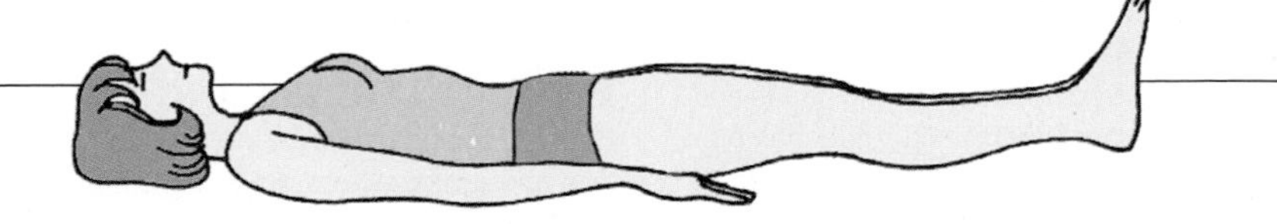

Medical causes

◆ ***Aortic arteriosclerotic occlusive disease.*** With this disorder, intermittent claudication occurs in the buttock, hip, thigh, and calf, along with absent or diminished femoral pulses. Bruits can be auscultated over the femoral and iliac arteries. Examination reveals pallor of the affected limb on elevation and profound limb weakness. The leg may be cool to the touch.

◆ ***Arterial occlusion (acute).*** This disorder produces intense intermittent claudication. A saddle embolus may affect both legs. Associated findings include paresthesia, paresis, and a sensation of cold in the affected limb. The limb is cool, pale, and cyanotic (mottled) with absent pulses below the occlusion. Capillary refill time is increased.

◆ ***Arteriosclerosis obliterans.*** This disorder usually affects the femoral and popliteal arteries, causing intermittent claudication (the most common symptom) in the calf. Typical associated findings include diminished or absent popliteal and pedal pulses, coolness in the affected limb, pallor on elevation, and profound limb weakness with continuing exercise. Other possible findings include numbness, paresthesia and, in severe disease, pain in the toes or foot while at rest, ulceration, and gangrene.

◆ ***Buerger's disease.*** This disorder typically produces intermittent claudication of the instep. Men are affected more than women; most of the affected men smoke and are between ages 20 and 40. It's common in the Orient, southeast Asia, India, and the Middle East and is rare in Blacks. Early signs include migratory superficial nodules and erythema along extremity blood vessels (nodular phlebitis) as well as migratory venous phlebitis. With exposure to cold, the feet initially become cold, cyanotic, and numb; later, they redden, become hot, and tingle. Occasionally, Buerger's disease also affects the hands and can cause painful ulcerations on the fingertips. Other characteristic findings include impaired peripheral pulses, paresthesia of the hands and feet, and migratory superficial thrombophlebitis.

◆ ***Cauda equina syndrome.*** Spinal stenosis causes pressure on nerve roots resulting in symptoms of claudication from the hip down as with Leriche's syndrome. Diagnosis can be determined by noninvasive exercise studies. With cauda equina syndrome, the pressure doesn't drop when the patient exercises on the treadmill.

◆ ***Leriche's syndrome.*** Arterial occlusion causes intermittent claudication of the hip, thigh, buttocks, and calf as well as impotence in men. Examination reveals bruits, global atrophy, absent or diminished pulses, and gangrene of the toes. The leg becomes cool and pale when elevated.

◆ ***Neurogenic claudication.*** Neurospinal disease causes pain from neurogenic intermittent claudication that requires a longer rest time than the 2 to 3 minutes needed in vascular claudication. Associated findings include paresthesia, weakness and clumsiness when walking, and hypoactive deep tendon reflexes after walking. Pulses are unaffected.

◆ ***Thoracic outlet syndrome.*** Activity that requires raising the hands above the shoulders, lifting a weight, or abducting the arm can cause intermittent pain along the ulnar distribution of the arm and forearm along with paresthesia and weakness. The pain isn't true claudication pain because it's related to position, not exercise. Signs and symptoms disappear when the arm is lowered. Other features include asymmetrical blood pressure and cool, pale skin.

Special considerations

Encourage the patient to exercise to improve collateral circulation and increase venous return, and advise him to avoid prolonged sitting or standing as well as crossing his legs at the knees. (See *Improving circulation in your legs*, page 401.) If intermittent claudication interferes with the patient's lifestyle, he may require diagnostic tests (Doppler flow studies, arteriography, and digital subtraction angiography) to determine the location and degree of occlusion.

Pediatric pointers

Intermittent claudication rarely occurs in children. Although it sometimes develops in patients with coarctation of the aorta, extensive compensatory collateral circulation typically prevents manifestation of this sign. Muscle cramps from exercise and growing pains may be mistaken for intermittent claudication in children.

Patient counseling

Counsel the patient with intermittent claudication about risk factors. Encourage him to stop smoking, and refer him to a support group, if appropriate. Teach him to inspect his legs and feet for ulcers; to keep his extremities warm, clean, and dry; and to avoid injury.

Urge the patient to immediately report skin breakdown that doesn't heal. Also urge him to report any chest discomfort when circulation is restored to his legs. Increased exercise tolerance may lead to angina if the patient has coronary artery disease that was previously asymptomatic because of exercise limitations.

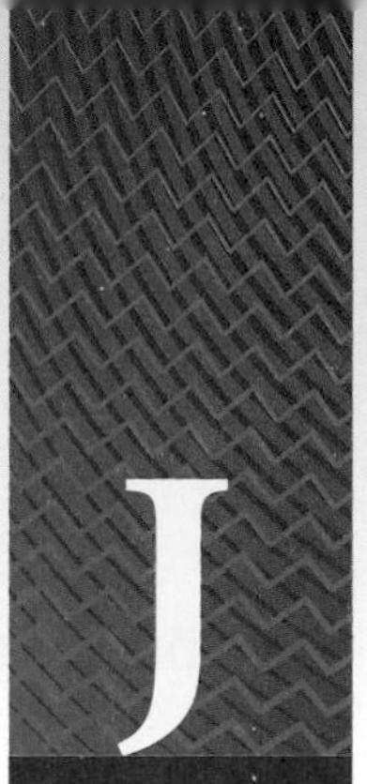

Janeway's lesions

Slightly raised but usually flat, irregular, and nontender, Janeway's lesions are small (1 to 4 mm in diameter), erythematous lesions on the palms and soles that disappear spontaneously. They blanch with pressure or elevation of the affected extremity; occasionally, they form a diffuse rash over the trunk and extremities.

Janeway's lesions were once a common finding in those with infective endocarditis, possibly reflecting an immunologic reaction to the infecting organisms (usually bacteria). These lesions are rarely seen today because the disease is now detected and managed at an earlier stage.

History and physical examination

If you observe Janeway's lesions, obtain a medical history from the patient, noting especially valvular or rheumatic heart disease. If the patient has had valvular or rheumatic heart disease, ask about recent dental procedures or invasive diagnostic tests. Does he have a prosthetic replacement valve? Find out about recent meningitis and any skin, bone, or respiratory tract infections. Does the patient have renal disease requiring an arteriovenous shunt? Has he had recent long-term I.V. therapy such as total parenteral nutrition? Ask him to describe how he feels. Does he report weakness, fatigue, chills, anorexia, or night sweats, possibly indicating an infection? Does he have other complaints?

Obtain a drug history. Find out if the patient with valvular or rheumatic heart disease has been taking a prophylactic antibiotic. Ask about I.V. drug use. Note the use of any immunosuppressant.

Next, perform a physical examination. Inspect his skin for other lesions, such as petechiae on his trunk or mucous membranes, and Osler's nodes on his palms, soles, or finger or toe pads. Inspect his fingers for clubbing and splinter hemorrhages.

Take the patient's vital signs, noting fever and tachycardia (which may indicate heart failure if it persists after fever disappears). Inspect and palpate his extremities for edema. Auscultate for gallops and murmurs. Assess other body systems for embolic complications of infective endocarditis, such as acute abdominal pain and hematuria. Examining his eyes with an ophthalmoscope may reveal Roth's spots, another sign of infective endocarditis.

Medical causes

◆ ***Acute infective endocarditis.*** Janeway's lesions are a late sign of this infectious disorder. Early signs and symptoms include a sudden onset of shaking chills and fever, peripheral edema, dyspnea, petechiae, Osler's nodes, Roth's spots, and hematuria.

◆ ***Subacute infective endocarditis.*** Janeway's lesions may appear late in this disorder, which has an insidious onset. Early findings include weakness, fatigue, weight loss, fever, night sweats, anorexia, and arthralgia. Other signs and symptoms include an elevated pulse, pale skin, Osler's nodes, splinter hemorrhages under the fingernails, petechiae, Roth's spots, clubbing of the fingers (in long-standing disease), splenomegaly, and murmurs. Embolization may produce acute signs and symptoms, such as chest, abdominal, and extremity pain; paralysis; hematuria; and blindness.

SPECIAL CONSIDERATIONS

Tell the patient that Janeway's lesions will disappear without damaging his skin. Treatment of infective endocarditis includes an antibiotic and—with complications such as heart failure—a diuretic and cardiac glycoside. Monitor the patient's intake, output, and cardiac status, and be alert for embolic complications, acute chest pain, abdominal pain, and paralysis. Prepare the patient for diagnostic tests, such as blood cultures and an echocardiogram.

PEDIATRIC POINTERS

In children, Janeway's lesions result from infective endocarditis, which commonly stems from congenital heart defects or rheumatic fever.

Jaundice

[Icterus]

A yellow discoloration of the skin, mucous membranes, or sclera of the eyes, jaundice indicates excessive levels of conjugated or unconjugated bilirubin in the blood. In fair-skinned patients, it's most noticeable on the face, trunk, and sclera; in dark-skinned patients, on the hard palate, sclera, and conjunctiva.

Jaundice is most apparent in natural sunlight. In fact, it may be undetectable in artificial or poor light. It's commonly accompanied by pruritus (because bile pigment damages sensory nerves), dark urine, and clay-colored stools.

Jaundice may result from any of three pathophysiologic processes. (See *Jaundice: Impaired bilirubin metabolism*.) It may be the only warning sign of certain disorders such as pancreatic cancer.

HISTORY AND PHYSICAL EXAMINATION

Documenting a history of the patient's jaundice is critical in determining its cause. Begin by asking the patient when he first noticed the jaundice. Does he also have pruritus, clay-colored stools, or dark urine? Ask about past episodes or a family history of jaundice. Does he have nonspecific signs or symptoms, such as fatigue, fever, or chills; GI signs or symptoms, such as anorexia, abdominal pain, nausea, weight loss, or vomiting; or cardiopulmonary symptoms, such as shortness of breath or palpitations? Ask about alcohol use and a history of cancer or liver or gallbladder disease. Has the patient lost weight recently? Also, obtain a drug history. Ask about a history of hepatitis, gallstones, or liver or pancreatic disease.

Perform the physical examination in a room with natural light. Make sure that the orange-yellow hue is jaundice and not due to hypercarotenemia, which is more prominent on the palms and soles and doesn't affect the sclera. Inspect the patient's skin for texture and dryness and for hyperpigmentation and xanthomas. Look for spider angiomas or petechiae, clubbed fingers, and gynecomastia. If the patient has heart failure, auscultate for arrhythmias, murmurs, and gallops. For all patients, auscultate for crackles and abnormal bowel sounds. Palpate the lymph nodes for swelling and the abdomen for tenderness, pain, and swelling. Palpate and percuss the liver and spleen for enlargement, and test for ascites with the shifting dullness and fluid wave techniques. Obtain baseline data on the patient's mental status: Slight changes in sensorium may be an early sign of deteriorating hepatic function. (See *Differential diagnosis: Jaundice,* pages 406 and 407.)

MEDICAL CAUSES

◆ ***Agnogenic myeloid metaplasia.*** This myeloproliferative disorder of the bone marrow may cause jaundice. Its typical effects, however, are associated with anemia, including fatigue, weakness, anorexia, massive splenomegaly, hepatomegaly, purpura, and bleeding tendencies.

◆ ***Carcinoma.*** Cancer of the ampulla of Vater initially produces fluctuating jaundice, mild abdominal pain, recurrent fever, and chills. Occult bleeding may be its first sign. Other findings include weight loss, pruritus, and back pain.

Hepatic cancer (primary liver cancer or another cancer that has metastasized to the liver) may cause jaundice by causing obstruction of the bile duct. Even advanced cancer causes nonspecific signs and symptoms, such as right-upper-quadrant discomfort and tenderness, nausea, weight loss, and slight fever. Examination may reveal irregular, nodular, firm hepatomegaly, ascites, peripheral edema, a bruit heard over the liver, and a right-upper-quadrant mass.

Jaundice: Impaired bilirubin metabolism

Jaundice occurs in three forms: prehepatic, hepatic, and posthepatic. In all three, bilirubin levels in the blood increase because of impaired metabolism.

With *prehepatic jaundice,* certain conditions and disorders, such as transfusion reactions and sickle cell anemia, cause massive hemolysis. Red blood cells rupture faster than the liver can conjugate bilirubin, so large amounts of unconjugated bilirubin pass into the blood, causing increased intestinal conversion of this bilirubin to water-soluble urobilinogen for excretion in urine and stools. (Unconjugated bilirubin is insoluble in water, so it can't be directly excreted in urine.)

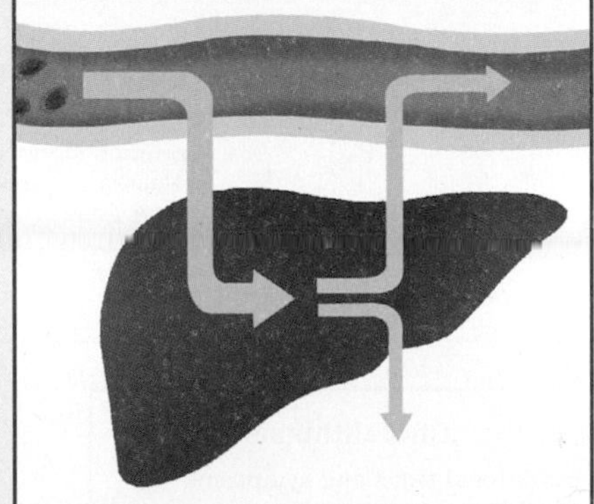

Hepatic jaundice results from the liver's inability to conjugate or excrete bilirubin, leading to increased blood levels of conjugated and unconjugated bilirubin. This occurs with such disorders as hepatitis, cirrhosis, and metastatic cancer and during the prolonged use of drugs metabolized by the liver.

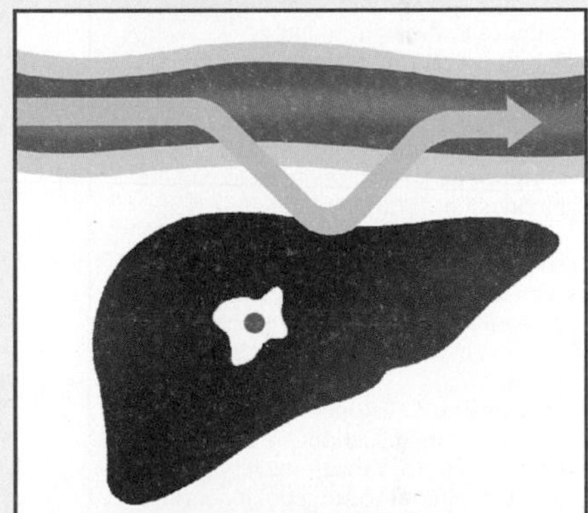

With *posthepatic jaundice,* which occurs in patients with a biliary or pancreatic disorder, bilirubin forms at its normal rate, but inflammation, scar tissue, a tumor, or gallstones block the flow of bile into the intestine. This causes an accumulation of conjugated bilirubin in the blood. Water-soluble, conjugated bilirubin is excreted in the urine.

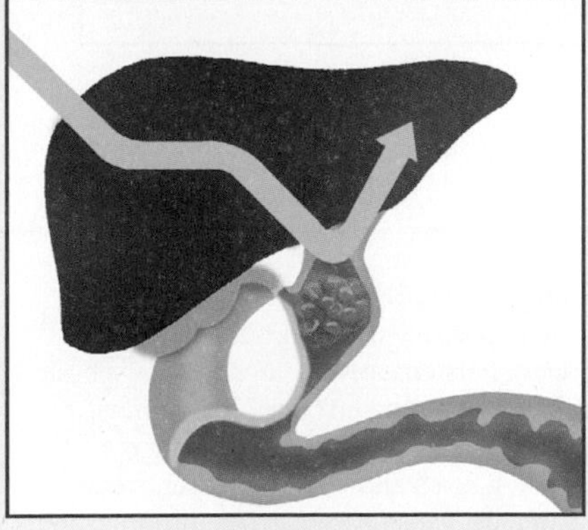

Differential diagnosis: Jaundice

History of present illness

Focused physical examination: GI system

Common signs and symptoms
- Nausea and vomiting
- Dark urine
- Clay-colored stools
- Pruritus

Cholelithiasis

Additional signs and symptoms
- Biliary colic
- Severe, steady pain in right upper quadrant (RUQ) or epigastrium that radiates to the right scapula
- Positive Murphy's sign
- Tachycardia
- Restlessness
- Dyspepsia after a fatty meal

Diagnosis: Laboratory tests (complete blood count [CBC], liver function test, electrolytes), imaging studies (ultrasound, computed tomography [CT] scan, endoscopic retrograde cholangiopancreatography [ERCP], cholecystogram, hydroxy iminodiacetic acid scan)
Treatment: Gallstone-solubilizing agent, diet modification, surgery
Follow-up: Reevaluation every 3 months; referral to surgeon, if acute

Acute hepatitis

Additional signs and symptoms
- Fatigue
- Malaise
- Arthralgia
- Myalgia
- Headache
- Anorexia
- Photophobia
- Cough
- Sore throat
- Liver and lymph node enlargement

Diagnosis: Hepatitis surface antigen or antibody based testing (A, B, C, D)
Treatment: Based on symptoms, rest, avoidance of alcohol and hepatotoxic substances, safer sex practices
Follow-up: For hepatitis A and E, reevaluation every 2 to 4 weeks; for hepatitis B, C, D, referral to hepatologist or gastroenterologist

With pancreatic cancer, progressive jaundice—possibly with pruritus—may be the only sign. Related early findings are nonspecific, such as weight loss and back or abdominal pain. Other signs and symptoms include anorexia, nausea and vomiting, fever, steatorrhea, fatigue, weakness, diarrhea, pruritus, and skin lesions (usually on the legs).

◆ ***Cholangitis.*** Obstruction and infection in the common bile duct cause Charcot's triad: jaundice, right-upper-quadrant pain, and high fever with chills.

◆ ***Cholecystitis.*** This disorder produces nonobstructive jaundice in about 25% of patients. Biliary colic typically peaks abruptly, persisting for 2 to 4 hours. The pain then localizes to the right upper quadrant and becomes constant. Local inflammation or passage of stones to the common bile duct causes jaundice. Other findings include nausea, vomiting (usually indicating

Acute pancreatitis

Signs and symptoms
- Severe relentless epigastric pain that radiates to the back
- Nausea
- Persistent vomiting
- Abdominal distention
- Turner's or Cullen's sign (possibly)
- Fever
- Tachycardia
- Hypoactive bowel sounds
- Abdominal rigidity and tenderness
- Shock (if severe)

Diagnosis: Laboratory tests (amylase, lipase, CBC, electrolytes, calcium, albumin, liver function test), imaging studies (CT scan, ultrasound)
Treatment: Based on symptoms, I.V. hydration, medication (analgesics, electrolyte replacement, insulin therapy)
Follow-up: Referral to gastroenterologist

Cholestasis

Additional signs and symptoms
- Prolonged attacks of jaundice
- Fatigue
- Weight loss
- Anorexia
- RUQ pain

Diagnosis: History, liver function tests, imaging studies (CT scan, magnetic resonance imaging, cholangiography, ultrasound, ERCP)
Treatment: Treatment of causative factor (such as certain drugs), diet modification, medication (antibacterial, phenobarbital), surgery
Follow-up: Referral to gastroenterologist

Additional differential diagnoses: agnogenic myeloid metaplasia ◆ cholangitis ◆ cholecystitis ◆ cirrhosis ◆ Dubin-Johnson syndrome ◆ glucose-6-phosphate dehydrogenase deficiency ◆ hemolytic anemia (acquired) ◆ hepatic abscess ◆ hepatic cancer ◆ leptospirosis ◆ pancreatic cancer ◆ sickle cell anemia ◆ Zieve syndrome

Other causes: androgenic steroids ◆ erythromycin estolate ◆ HMG-CoA reductase inhibitors ◆ hormonal contraceptives ◆ isoniazid ◆ I.V. tetracycline ◆ mercaptopurine ◆ niacin ◆ phenothiazines ◆ portocaval shunt ◆ sulfonamides ◆ troleandomycin ◆ upper abdominal surgery

the presence of a stone), fever, profuse diaphoresis, chills, tenderness on palpation, a positive Murphy's sign, and, possibly, abdominal distention and rigidity.

◆ ***Cholelithiasis.*** This disorder commonly causes jaundice and biliary colic. It's characterized by severe, steady pain in the right upper quadrant or epigastrium that radiates to the right scapula or shoulder and intensifies over several hours. Accompanying signs and symptoms include nausea and vomiting, tachycardia, and restlessness. Occlusion of the common bile duct causes fever, chills, jaundice, clay-colored stools, and abdominal tenderness. After consuming a fatty meal, the patient may experience vague epigastric fullness and dyspepsia.

◆ ***Cholestasis.*** With benign, recurrent intrahepatic cholestasis, the patient experiences prolonged attacks of jaundice (sometimes spaced several years apart) accompanied by pruritus.

Other signs and symptoms are similar to those of hepatitis—fatigue, nausea, weight loss, anorexia, pale stools, and right-upper-quadrant pain.

◆ ***Cirrhosis.*** With Laënnec's cirrhosis, mild to moderate jaundice with pruritus usually signals hepatocellular necrosis or progressive hepatic insufficiency. Common early findings include ascites, weakness, leg edema, nausea and vomiting, diarrhea or constipation, anorexia, weight loss, and right-upper-quadrant pain. Massive hematemesis and other bleeding tendencies may also occur. Other findings include an enlarged liver and parotid gland, clubbed fingers, Dupuytren's contracture, mental changes, asterixis, fetor hepaticus, spider angiomas, and palmar erythema. Males may exhibit gynecomastia, scanty chest and axillary hair, and testicular atrophy; females may experience menstrual irregularities.

With primary biliary cirrhosis, fluctuating jaundice may appear years after the onset of other signs and symptoms, such as pruritus that worsens at bedtime (commonly the first sign), weakness, fatigue, weight loss, and vague abdominal pain. Itching may lead to skin excoriation. Associated findings include hyperpigmentation; indications of malabsorption, such as nocturnal diarrhea, steatorrhea, purpura, and osteomalacia; hematemesis from esophageal varices; ascites; edema; xanthelasmas; xanthomas on the palms, soles, and elbows; and hepatomegaly.

◆ ***Dubin-Johnson syndrome.*** With this rare, chronic inherited syndrome, fluctuating jaundice that increases with stress is the major sign, appearing as late as age 40. Related findings include slight hepatic enlargement and tenderness, upper abdominal pain, nausea, and vomiting.

◆ ***Glucose-6-phosphate dehydrogenase deficiency.*** Acute intravascular hemolysis following ingestion of such drugs as quinine or aspirin causes jaundice, pallor, dyspnea, tachycardia, and malaise. Palpation may reveal splenomegaly and hepatomegaly.

◆ ***Heart failure.*** Jaundice due to liver dysfunction occurs in patients with severe right-sided heart failure. Other effects include jugular vein distention, cyanosis, dependent edema of the legs and sacrum, steady weight gain, confusion, hepatomegaly, nausea and vomiting, abdominal discomfort, and anorexia due to visceral edema. Ascites is a late sign. Oliguria, marked weakness, and anxiety may also occur. If left-sided heart failure develops first, other findings may include fatigue, dyspnea, orthopnea, paroxysmal nocturnal dyspnea, tachypnea, arrhythmias, and tachycardia.

◆ ***Hemolytic anemia (acquired).*** This disorder may produce prominent jaundice along with dyspnea, fatigue, pallor, tachycardia, and palpitations. Rapid hemolysis causes chills, fever, irritability, headache, and abdominal pain; severe hemolysis causes signs of shock.

◆ ***Hepatic abscess.*** Multiple abscesses may cause jaundice, but the primary effects are persistent fever with chills and sweating. Other findings include steady, severe pain in the right upper quadrant or midepigastrium that may be referred to the shoulder; nausea and vomiting; anorexia; hepatomegaly; elevated right hemidiaphragm; and ascites.

◆ ***Hepatitis.*** Dark urine and clay-colored stools usually develop before jaundice in the late stages of acute viral hepatitis. Early systemic signs and symptoms vary and include fatigue, nausea, vomiting, malaise, arthralgias, myalgias, headache, anorexia, photophobia, pharyngitis, cough, diarrhea or constipation, and a low-grade fever associated with liver and lymph node enlargement. During the icteric phase (which subsides within 2 to 3 weeks unless complications occur), systemic signs subside, but an enlarged, palpable liver may be present along with weight loss, anorexia, and right-upper-quadrant pain and tenderness.

◆ ***Leptospirosis.*** Severe leptospirosis (Weil's disease) may cause jaundice. This disorder begins suddenly with a frontal headache, severe muscle aches in the thighs and lumbar area, cutaneous hyperesthesia, abdominal pain, nausea, conjunctival suffusion, and vomiting. Chills and a rapidly rising fever follow. Signs and symptoms of meningeal irritation include drowsiness, decreased mentation, stiff neck, and positive Kernig's and Brudzinski's signs. Right-upper-quadrant tenderness, hepatomegaly, and jaundice indicate hepatic involvement; proteinuria, pyuria, and hematuria indicate renal involvement. Epistaxis, hematemesis, melena, and hemoptysis may also occur.

◆ ***Pancreatitis (acute).*** Edema of the head of the pancreas and obstruction of the common bile duct can cause jaundice; however, this disorder's primary symptom is usually severe epigastric pain that commonly radiates to the back. Lying with the knees flexed on the chest or sitting up and leaning forward brings relief. Early associated signs and symptoms include nausea, persistent vomiting, abdominal distention, and Turner's or Cullen's sign. Other findings include fever, tachycardia, abdominal rigidity and tenderness, hypoactive bowel sounds, and crackles.

Severe pancreatitis produces extreme restlessness; mottled skin; cold, diaphoretic extremities; paresthesia; and tetany—the last two being symptoms of hypocalcemia. Fulminant pancreatitis causes massive hemorrhage.

◆ ***Sickle cell anemia.*** Hemolysis produces jaundice in patients with this disorder. Other findings include impaired growth and development, increased susceptibility to infection, life-threatening thrombotic complications and, commonly, leg ulcers, (painful) swollen joints, fever, and chills. Bone aches and chest pain may also occur. Severe hemolysis may cause hematuria and pallor, chronic fatigue, weakness, dyspnea (or dyspnea on exertion), and tachycardia. The patient may also have splenomegaly. During a sickle cell crisis, the patient may have severe bone, abdominal, thoracic, and muscular pain; low-grade fever; and increased weakness, jaundice, and dyspnea.

◆ ***Zieve syndrome.*** Caused by alcohol abuse, this relatively rare disorder produces abdominal pain and a sudden onset of severe jaundice. However, spider angiomas, ascites, and other signs of advanced liver disease are absent.

Other causes

◆ ***Drugs.*** Many drugs may cause hepatic injury and resultant jaundice. Examples include acetaminophen, I.V. tetracycline, isoniazid, hormonal contraceptives, sulfonamides, mercaptopurine, erythromycin estolate, niacin, troleandomycin, androgenic steroids, HMG-CoA reductase inhibitors, phenothiazines, ethanol, methyldopa, rifampin, and phenytoin.

◆ ***Treatments.*** Upper abdominal surgery may cause postoperative jaundice, which occurs secondary to hepatocellular damage from the manipulation of organs, leading to edema and obstructed bile flow; from the administration of halothane; or from prolonged surgery resulting in shock, blood loss, or blood transfusion.

A surgical shunt used to reduce portal hypertension (such as a portacaval shunt) may also produce jaundice.

Special considerations

To help decrease pruritus, frequently bathe the patient, apply an antipruritic lotion, such as calamine, and administer diphenhydramine hydrochloride or hydroxyzine hydrochloride. Prepare the patient for diagnostic tests to evaluate biliary and hepatic function. Laboratory studies include urine and fecal urobilinogen, serum bilirubin, hepatic enzyme, and cholesterol levels; prothrombin time; and a complete blood count. Other tests include ultrasonography, cholangiography, liver biopsy, and exploratory laparotomy.

Pediatric pointers

Physiologic jaundice is common in neonates, developing 3 to 5 days after birth. In infants, obstructive jaundice usually results from congenital biliary atresia. A choledochal cyst—a congenital cystic dilation of the common bile duct—may also cause jaundice in children, particularly those of Japanese descent.

The list of other causes of jaundice is extensive and includes, but isn't limited to, Crigler-Najjar syndrome, Gilbert's disease, Rotor's syndrome, thalassemia major, hereditary spherocytosis, erythroblastosis fetalis, Hodgkin's disease, infectious mononucleosis, Wilson's disease, amyloidosis, and Reye's syndrome.

Geriatric pointers

In patients older than age 60, jaundice is usually caused by cholestasis resulting from extrahepatic obstruction.

Patient counseling

Encourage the patient with a hepatic disorder to decrease his protein intake sharply and increase his intake of carbohydrates. If he has obstructive jaundice, encourage a nutritious, balanced diet (avoiding high-fat foods) and frequent small meals.

Jaw pain

Jaw pain may arise from either of the two bones that hold the teeth in the jaw—the maxilla (upper jaw) and the mandible (lower jaw). Jaw pain also includes pain in the temporomandibular joint (TMJ), where the mandible meets the temporal bone.

Jaw pain may develop gradually or abruptly and may range from barely noticeable to excruciating, depending on its cause. It usually results from disorders of the teeth, soft tissue, or glands of the mouth or throat or from local trauma or infection. Systemic causes include musculoskeletal, neurologic, cardiovascular, endocrine, immunologic, metabolic, and infectious disorders. Life-threatening disorders, such as myocardial infarction (MI) and tetany, also produce jaw pain, as do certain drugs (especially phenothiazines) and dental or surgical procedures.

Jaw pain is seldom a primary indicator of any one disorder; however, some causes are medical emergencies.

EMERGENCY INTERVENTIONS *Ask the patient when the jaw pain began. Did it arise suddenly or gradually? Is it more severe or frequent now than when it first occurred? Sudden severe jaw pain, especially when associated with chest pain, shortness of breath, or arm pain, requires prompt evaluation because it may herald a life-threatening disorder. Perform an electrocardiogram and obtain blood samples for cardiac enzyme levels. Administer oxygen, morphine sulfate, and a vasodilator as indicated.*

History and physical examination

Begin the patient history by asking the patient to describe the pain's character, intensity, and frequency. When did he first notice the jaw pain? Where on the jaw does he feel pain? Does the pain radiate to other areas? Sharp or burning pain arises from the skin or subcutaneous tissues. Causalgia, an intense burning sensation, usually results from damage to the fifth cranial, or trigeminal, nerve. This type of superficial pain is easily localized, unlike dull, aching, boring, or throbbing pain, which originates in muscle, bone, or joints. Also ask about aggravating or alleviating factors.

Ask about recent trauma, surgery, or procedures, especially dental work. Ask about associated signs and symptoms, such as joint or chest pain, dyspnea, palpitations, fatigue, headache, malaise, anorexia, weight loss, intermittent claudication, diplopia, and hearing loss. (Keep in mind that jaw pain may accompany more characteristic signs and symptoms of life-threatening disorders, such as chest pain in a patient with an MI.)

Focus your physical examination on the jaw. Inspect the painful area for redness, and palpate for edema or warmth. Facing the patient directly, look for facial asymmetry indicating swelling. Check the TMJs by placing your fingertips just anterior to the external auditory meatus and asking the patient to open and close, and to thrust out and retract his jaw. Note the presence of crepitus, an abnormal scraping or grinding sensation in the joint. (Clicks heard when the jaw is widely spread apart are normal.) How wide can the patient open his mouth? Less than 1⅛" (3 cm) or more than 2⅜" (6 cm) between upper and lower teeth is abnormal. Next, palpate the parotid area for pain and swelling, and inspect and palpate the oral cavity for lesions, elevation of the tongue, or masses.

Medical causes

◆ ***Angina pectoris.*** Angina may produce jaw pain (usually radiating from the substernal area) and left arm pain. Angina is less severe than the pain of an MI. It's commonly triggered by exertion, emotional stress, or ingestion of a heavy meal and usually subsides with rest and the administration of nitroglycerin. Other signs and symptoms include shortness of breath, nausea and vomiting, tachycardia, dizziness, diaphoresis, belching, and palpitations.

◆ ***Arthritis.*** With osteoarthritis, which usually affects the small joints of the hand, aching jaw pain increases with activity (talking, eating) and subsides with rest. Other features are crepitus heard and felt over the TMJ, enlarged joints with a restricted range of motion, and stiffness on awakening that improves with a few minutes of activity. Redness and warmth are usually absent.

Rheumatoid arthritis causes symmetrical pain in all joints (commonly affecting proximal finger joints first), including the jaw. The joints display limited range of motion and are tender, warm, swollen, and stiff after inactivity, especially in the morning. Myalgia is common. Systemic signs and symptoms include fatigue, weight loss, malaise, anorexia, lymphadenopathy, and mild fever. Painless, movable rheumatoid nodules may appear on the elbows, knees, and knuckles. Progressive disease causes deformities, crepitation with joint rotation, muscle weakness and atrophy around the involved joint, and multiple systemic complications.

GENDER CUE *Rheumatoid arthritis usually appears in early middle age, between ages 36 and 50, and most commonly in women.*

◆ ***Head and neck cancer.*** Many types of head and neck cancer, especially of the oral cavity and nasopharynx, produce aching jaw pain of insidious onset. Other findings include a history of leukoplakia ulcers of the mucous membranes; palpable masses in the jaw, mouth, and neck; dysphagia; bloody discharge; drooling; lymphadenopathy; and trismus.

◆ ***Hypocalcemic tetany.*** Besides painful muscle contractions of the jaw and mouth, this life-threatening disorder produces paresthesia and carpopedal spasms. The patient may complain of weakness, fatigue, and palpitations. Examination reveals hyperreflexia and positive Chvostek's and Trousseau's signs. Muscle twitching, choreiform movements, and muscle cramps may also occur. With severe hypocalcemia, laryngeal spasm may occur with stridor, cyanosis, seizures, and cardiac arrhythmias.

◆ ***Ludwig's angina.*** An acute streptococcal infection of the sublingual and submandibular spaces that produces severe jaw pain in the mandibular area with tongue elevation, sublingual edema, and drooling. Fever is a common sign. Progressive disease produces dysphagia, dysphonia, and stridor and dyspnea due to laryngeal edema and obstruction by an elevated tongue.

◆ ***Myocardial infarction.*** Initially, this life-threatening disorder causes intense, crushing substernal pain that's unrelieved by rest or nitroglycerin. The pain may radiate to the lower jaw, left arm, neck, back, or shoulder blades. (Rarely, jaw pain occurs without chest pain.) Other findings include pallor, clammy skin, dyspnea, excessive diaphoresis, nausea and vomiting, anxiety, restlessness, a feeling of impending doom, low-grade fever, decreased or increased blood pressure, arrhythmias, an atrial gallop, new murmurs (in many cases from mitral insufficiency), and crackles.

◆ ***Osteomyelitis.*** Bone infection after trauma, sinus infection, dental injury, or surgery (dental or facial) may produce diffuse, aching jaw pain along with warmth, swelling, tenderness, erythema, and restricted jaw movement. Acute osteomyelitis may also cause tachycardia, sudden fever, nausea, and malaise. Chronic osteomyelitis may recur after minor trauma.

◆ ***Sialolithiasis.*** With this disorder, stones form in the salivary glands, causing painful swelling that makes chewing uncomfortable. Jaw pain occurs in the lower jaw, floor of the mouth, and TMJ. It may also radiate to the ear or neck.

◆ ***Sinusitis.*** Maxillary sinusitis produces intense boring pain in the maxilla and cheek that may radiate to the eye. This type of sinusitis also causes a feeling of fullness, increased pain on percussion of the first and second molars and, in those with nasal obstruction, the loss of the sense of smell. Sphenoid sinusitis causes scanty nasal discharge and chronic pain at the mandibular ramus and vertex of the head and in the temporal area. Other signs and symptoms of both types of sinusitis include fever, halitosis, headache, malaise, cough, sore throat, and fever.

◆ ***Suppurative parotitis.*** Bacterial infection of the parotid gland by *Staphylococcus aureus* tends to develop in debilitated patients with dry mouth or poor oral hygiene. Besides the abrupt onset of jaw pain, high fever, and chills, findings include erythema and edema of the overlying skin; a tender, swollen gland, and pus at the second top molar (Stensen's ducts). Infection may lead to disorientation; shock and death are common.

◆ ***Temporal arteritis.*** Most common in women older than age 60, this disorder produces sharp jaw pain after chewing or talking. Nonspecific signs and symptoms include low-grade fever, generalized muscle pain, malaise, fatigue, anorexia, and weight loss. Vascular lesions produce jaw pain; throbbing, unilateral headache in the frontotemporal region; swollen, nodular, tender and, possibly, pulseless temporal arteries; and, at times, erythema of the overlying skin.

◆ ***Temporomandibular joint syndrome.*** This common syndrome produces jaw pain at the TMJ; spasm and pain of the masticating muscle; clicking, popping, or crepitus of the TMJ; and restricted jaw movement. Unilateral, localized pain may radiate to other head and neck areas. The patient typically reports teeth clenching, bruxism, and emotional stress. He may also experience ear pain, headache, deviation of the jaw to the affected side upon opening the mouth, and jaw subluxation or dislocation, especially after yawning.

◆ ***Tetanus.*** A rare life-threatening disorder caused by a bacterial toxin, tetanus produces stiffness and pain in the jaw and difficulty opening the mouth. Early nonspecific signs and symptoms (commonly unnoticed or mistaken for influenza) include headache, irritability, restlessness, low-grade fever, and chills. Examination reveals tachycardia, profuse diaphoresis, and hyperreflexia. Progressive disease leads to painful, involuntary muscle spasms that spread to the abdomen, back, or face. The slightest stimulus may produce reflex spasms of any muscle group. Ultimately, laryngospasm, respiratory distress, and seizures may occur.

◆ ***Trauma.*** Injury to the face, head, or neck—particularly fracture of the maxilla or mandible—may produce jaw pain and swelling and decreased jaw mobility. Associated findings include hypotension and tachycardia (indicating shock), lacerations, ecchymoses, and hematomas. Rhinorrhea or otorrhea indicates the leakage of cerebrospinal fluid; blurred vision indicates orbital involvement.

◆ ***Trigeminal neuralgia.*** This disorder is marked by paroxysmal attacks of intense unilateral jaw pain (stopping at the facial midline) or rapid-fire shooting sensations in one division of the trigeminal nerve (usually the mandibular or maxillary division). This superficial pain, felt mainly over the lips and chin and in the teeth, lasts from 1 to 15 minutes. Mouth and nose areas may be hypersensitive. Involvement of the ophthalmic branch of the trigeminal nerve causes a diminished or absent corneal reflex on the same side. Attacks can be triggered by mild stimulation of the nerve (for example, lightly touching the cheeks), exposure to heat or cold, or consumption of hot or cold foods or beverages.

OTHER CAUSES

◆ ***Drugs.*** Some drugs, such as phenothiazines, affect the extrapyramidal tract, causing dyskinesias; others cause tetany of the jaw secondary to hypocalcemia.

SPECIAL CONSIDERATIONS

If the patient is in severe pain, withhold food, liquids, and oral medications until the diagnosis is confirmed. Administer an analgesic. Prepare the patient for diagnostic tests such as jaw X-rays. Apply an ice pack if the jaw is swollen, and discourage the patient from talking or moving his jaw.

PEDIATRIC POINTERS

Be alert for nonverbal signs of jaw pain, such as rubbing the affected area or wincing while talking or swallowing. In infants, initial signs of tetany from hypocalcemia include episodes of apnea and generalized jitteriness progressing to facial grimaces and generalized rigidity. Finally, seizures may occur.

Jaw pain in children sometimes stems from disorders uncommon in adults. Mumps, for example, causes unilateral or bilateral swelling from the lower mandible to the zygomatic arch. Parotiditis due to cystic fibrosis also causes jaw pain. When trauma causes jaw pain in children, always consider the possibility of abuse.

Jugular vein distention

Jugular vein distention is the abnormal fullness and height of the pulse waves in the internal or external jugular veins. For a patient in a supine position with his head elevated 45 degrees, a pulse wave height greater than 1 1/4″ to 1 1/2″ (3 to 4 cm) above the angle of Louis indicates distention. Engorged, distended veins reflect increased venous pressure in the right side of the heart, which in turn, indicates an increased central venous pressure. This common sign characteristically occurs in heart failure and other cardiovascular disorders, such as constrictive pericarditis, tricuspid stenosis, and obstruction of the superior vena cava.

EMERGENCY INTERVENTIONS *Evaluating jugular vein distention involves visualizing and assessing venous pulsations. (See* Evaluating jugular vein distention.*) If you detect jugular vein distention in a patient with pale, clammy skin who suddenly appears anxious and dyspneic, take his blood pressure. If you note hypotension and paradoxical pulse, suspect cardiac tamponade. Elevate the foot of the bed 20 to 30 degrees, give supplemental oxygen, and monitor cardiac status and rhythm, oxygen saturation, and mental status. Start an I.V. catheter for medication administration, and keep cardiopulmonary resuscitation equipment close by. Assemble the needed equipment for emergency pericardiocentesis (to relieve pressure on the heart.) Throughout the procedure, monitor the patient's blood pressure, heart rhythm, and respirations.*

HISTORY AND PHYSICAL EXAMINATION

If the patient isn't in severe distress, obtain a personal history. Has he recently gained weight? Does he have difficulty putting on shoes? Are his ankles swollen? Ask about chest pain, shortness of breath, paroxysmal nocturnal dyspnea, anorexia, nausea or vomiting, and a history of cancer or cardiac, pulmonary, hepatic, or renal disease. Obtain a drug history noting diuretic use and dosage. Is the patient taking drugs as prescribed? Ask the patient about his regular diet patterns, noting a high sodium intake.

Next, perform a physical examination, beginning with vital signs. Tachycardia, tachypnea, and increased blood pressure indicate fluid overload that's stressing the heart. Inspect and palpate the patient's extremities and face for

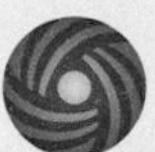

EXAMINATION TIP

Evaluating jugular vein distention

With the patient in a supine position, position him so that you can visualize jugular vein pulsations reflected from the right atrium. Elevate the head of the bed 45 to 90 degrees. (In the normal patient, veins distend only when the patient lies flat.)

Next, locate the angle of Louis (sternal notch)—the reference point for measuring venous pressure. To do so, palpate the clavicles where they join the sternum (the suprasternal notch). Place your first two fingers on the suprasternal notch. Then, without lifting them from the skin, slide them down the sternum until you feel a bony protuberance—this is the angle of Louis.

Find the internal jugular vein (which indicates venous pressure more reliably than the external jugular vein). Shine a flashlight across the patient's neck to create shadows that highlight his venous pulse. Be sure to distinguish jugular vein pulsations from carotid artery pulsations. One way to do this is to palpate the vessel: Arterial pulsations continue, whereas venous pulsations disappear with light finger pressure. Also, venous pulsations increase or decrease with changes in body position; arterial pulsations remain constant.

Next, locate the highest point along the vein where you can see pulsations. Using a centimeter ruler, measure the distance between that high point and the sternal notch. Record this finding as well as the angle at which the patient was lying. A finding greater than $1\frac{1}{4}$" to $1\frac{1}{2}$" (3 to 4 cm) above the sternal notch, with the head of the bed at a 45-degree angle, indicates jugular vein distention.

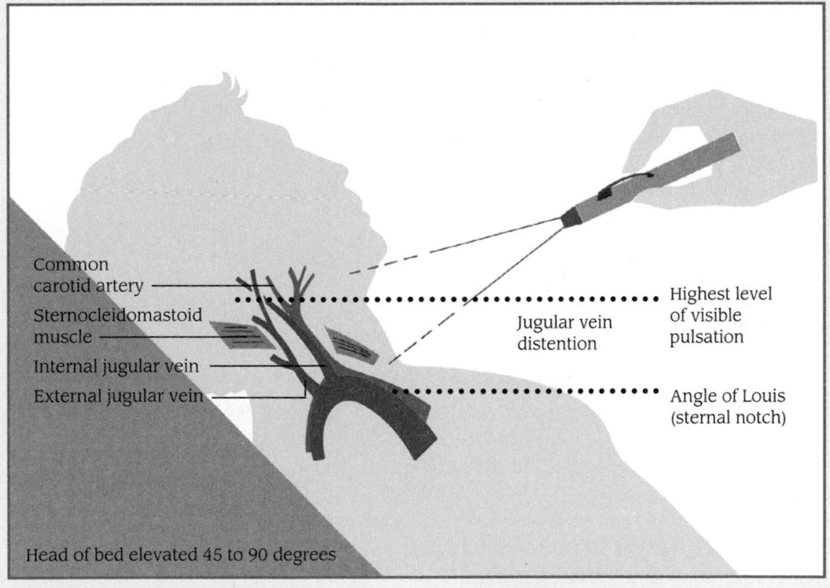

edema. Then weigh the patient and compare that weight to his baseline.

Auscultate his lungs for crackles and his heart for gallops, a pericardial friction rub, and muffled heart sounds. Inspect his abdomen for distention, and palpate and percuss for an enlarged liver. Finally monitor urine output and note any decrease.

MEDICAL CAUSES

◆ ***Cardiac tamponade.*** This life-threatening condition produces jugular vein distention along with anxiety, restlessness, cyanosis, chest pain, dyspnea, hypotension, and clammy skin. It also causes tachycardia, tachypnea, muffled heart sounds, a pericardial friction rub, weak or absent peripheral pulses or pulses that decrease during inspiration (pulsus paradoxus), and hepatomegaly. The patient may sit upright or lean forward to ease breathing.

◆ ***Heart failure.*** Sudden or gradual development of right-sided heart failure commonly causes jugular vein distention, along with weakness and anxiety, cyanosis, dependent edema of the legs and sacrum, steady weight gain, confusion, and hepatomegaly. Other findings include nausea and vomiting, abdominal discomfort, and anorexia due to visceral edema. Ascites is a late sign. Massive right-sided heart failure may produce anasarca and oliguria.

If left-sided heart failure precedes right-sided heart failure, jugular vein distention is a late sign. Other signs and symptoms include fatigue, dyspnea, orthopnea, paroxysmal nocturnal dyspnea, tachypnea, tachycardia, and arrhythmias. Auscultation reveals crackles and a ventricular gallop.

◆ ***Hypervolemia.*** Markedly increased intravascular fluid volume causes jugular vein distention, along with rapid weight gain, elevated blood pressure, bounding pulse, peripheral edema, dyspnea, and crackles.

◆ ***Pericarditis (chronic constrictive).*** Progressive signs and symptoms of restricted heart filling include jugular vein distention that's more prominent on inspiration (Kussmaul's sign). The patient usually complains of chest pain. Other signs and symptoms include fluid retention with dependent edema, hepatomegaly, ascites, and pericardial friction rub.

◆ ***Superior vena cava obstruction.*** A tumor or, rarely, thrombosis may gradually lead to jugular vein distention when the veins of the head, neck, and arms fail to empty effectively, causing facial, neck, and upper arm edema. Metastasis of a malignant tumor to the mediastinum may cause dyspnea, cough, substernal chest pain, and hoarseness.

Special considerations

If the patient has cardiac tamponade, prepare him for pericardiocentesis. If he doesn't have cardiac tamponade, restrict fluids and monitor his intake and output. Insert an indwelling urinary catheter if necessary. If the patient has heart failure, administer a diuretic. Routinely change his position to avoid skin breakdown from peripheral edema. Prepare the patient for a central venous or Swan-Ganz catheter insertion in order to measure right- and left-sided heart pressure.

Pediatric pointers

Jugular vein distention is difficult (sometimes impossible) to evaluate in most infants and toddlers because of their short, thick necks. Even in school-age children, measurement of jugular vein distention can be unreliable because the sternal angle may not be the same distance (2" to 2¾" [5 to 7 cm]) above the right atrium as it is in adults.

Patient counseling

Teach the patient with heart failure about appropriate treatments, including dietary restrictions (such as a low-sodium diet).

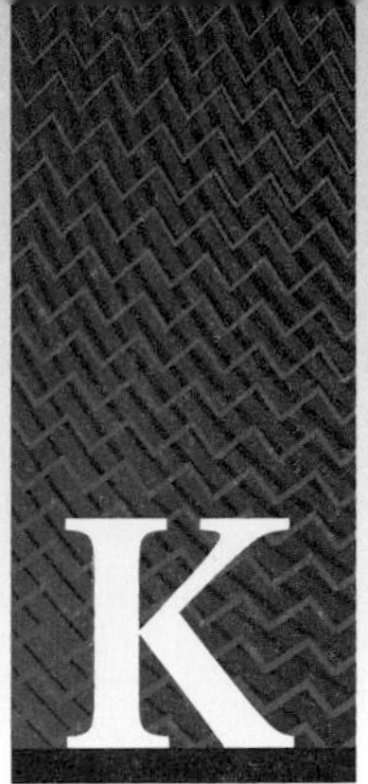

Kehr's sign

A cardinal sign of hemorrhage within the peritoneal cavity, Kehr's sign is referred left shoulder pain due to diaphragmatic irritation by intraperitoneal blood. The pain usually arises when the patient assumes the supine position or lowers his head. Such positioning increases the contact of free blood or clots with the left diaphragm, involving the phrenic nerve.

Kehr's sign usually develops right after the hemorrhage; however, its onset is sometimes delayed up to 48 hours. A classic symptom of a ruptured spleen, Kehr's sign also occurs in ruptured ectopic pregnancy.

EMERGENCY INTERVENTIONS *After you detect Kehr's sign, quickly take the patient's vital signs. If the patient shows signs of hypovolemia, elevate his feet 30 degrees. In addition, insert a large-bore I.V. catheter for fluid and blood replacement and an indwelling urinary catheter. Begin monitoring intake and output. Draw blood to determine hematocrit, and provide supplemental oxygen.*

Inspect the patient's abdomen for bruises and distention, and palpate for tenderness. Percuss for Ballance's sign—an indicator of massive perisplenic clotting and free blood in the peritoneal cavity from a ruptured spleen.

MEDICAL CAUSES

◆ ***Intra-abdominal hemorrhage.*** Kehr's sign usually accompanies intense abdominal pain, abdominal rigidity, and muscle spasm. Other findings vary with the cause of bleeding. Many patients have a history of blunt or penetrating abdominal injuries.

SPECIAL CONSIDERATIONS

In anticipation of surgery, withhold oral intake, and prepare the patient for abdominal X-rays, a computed tomography scan, an ultrasound and, possibly, paracentesis, peritoneal lavage, and culdocentesis. Give an analgesic, if needed.

PEDIATRIC POINTERS

Because a child may have difficulty describing pain, watch for nonverbal clues such as rubbing of the shoulder.

Kernig's sign

A reliable early indicator and tool used to diagnose meningeal irritation, Kernig's sign elicits both resistance and hamstring muscle pain when the examiner attempts to extend the knee while the hip and knee are both flexed 90 degrees. However, when the patient's thigh isn't flexed on the abdomen, he's usually able to completely extend his leg. (See *Eliciting Kernig's sign*, page 416.) This sign is usually elicited in meningitis or subarachnoid hemorrhage. With these potentially life-threatening disorders, hamstring muscle resistance results from stretching the blood- or exudate-irritated meninges surrounding spinal nerve roots.

Kernig's sign can also indicate a herniated disk or spinal tumor. With these disorders,

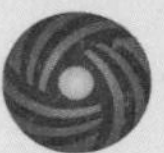

EXAMINATION TIP

Eliciting Kernig's sign

To elicit Kernig's sign, place the patient in a supine position. Flex his leg at the hip and knee, as shown here. Then try to extend the leg while you keep the hip flexed. If the patient experiences pain and possibly spasm in the hamstring muscle and resists further extension, you can assume that meningeal irritation has occurred.

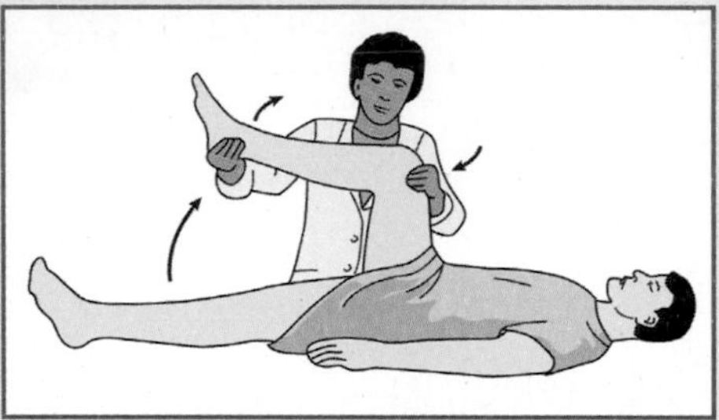

sciatic pain results from disk or tumor pressure on spinal nerve roots.

History and physical examination

If you elicit a positive Kernig's sign and suspect life-threatening meningitis or subarachnoid hemorrhage, immediately prepare for emergency intervention. (See *When Kernig's sign signals CNS crisis*.)

If you don't suspect meningeal irritation, ask the patient if he feels any back pain that radiates down one or both legs. Does he also feel leg numbness, tingling, or weakness? Ask about other signs and symptoms, and find out if he has a history of cancer or back injury. Then perform a physical examination, concentrating on motor and sensory function.

Medical causes

◆ ***Lumbosacral herniated disk.*** A positive Kernig's sign may be elicited in patients with this disorder, but the cardinal and earliest feature is sciatic pain on the affected side or on both sides. Associated findings include postural deformity (lumbar lordosis or scoliosis), paresthesia, hypoactive deep tendon reflexes in the involved leg, and dorsiflexor muscle weakness.

◆ ***Meningitis.*** A positive Kernig's sign usually occurs early with meningitis, along with fever and, possibly, chills. Other signs and symptoms of meningeal irritation include nuchal rigidity, hyperreflexia, Brudzinski's sign, and opisthotonos. As intracranial pressure (ICP) increases, headache and vomiting may occur. In severe meningitis, the patient may experience stupor, coma, and seizures. Cranial nerve involvement may produce ocular palsies, facial weakness, deafness, and photophobia. An erythematous maculopapular rash may occur in viral meningitis; a purpuric rash may be seen in those with meningococcal meningitis.

◆ ***Spinal cord tumor.*** Kernig's sign can be elicited occasionally, but the earliest symptom is typically pain felt locally or along the spinal nerve, commonly in the leg. Associated findings include weakness or paralysis distal to the tumor, paresthesia, urine retention, urinary or fecal incontinence, and sexual dysfunction.

◆ ***Subarachnoid hemorrhage.*** Kernig's sign and Brudzinski's sign can both be elicited within minutes after the initial bleed. The patient experiences a sudden onset of severe headache that begins in a localized area and then spreads, pupillary inequality, nuchal rigidity, and decreased level of consciousness. Photophobia, fever, nausea and vomiting, dizziness, and seizures are possible. Focal signs include hemiparesis or hemiplegia, aphasia, and sensory or visual disturbances. Increasing ICP may produce bradycardia, increased blood pressure, respiratory pattern change, and rapid progression to coma.

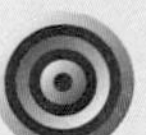

EMERGENCY INTERVENTION

When Kernig's sign signals CNS crisis

Because Kernig's sign may signal meningitis or subarachnoid hemorrhage—both life-threatening central nervous system (CNS) disorders—take the patient's vital signs at once to obtain baseline information. Then test for Brudzinski's sign to obtain further evidence of meningeal irritation. (See *Testing for Brudzinski's sign,* page 125.) Next, ask the patient or his family to describe the onset of illness. Typically, the progressive onset of headache, fever, nuchal rigidity, and confusion suggests meningitis. Conversely, the sudden onset of a severe headache, nuchal rigidity, photophobia, and, possibly, loss of consciousness usually indicates subarachnoid hemorrhage.

Meningitis

If a diagnosis of meningitis is suspected, ask about recent infections, especially tooth abscesses. Ask about exposure to infected persons or places where meningitis is endemic. Meningitis is usually a complication of another bacterial infection, so draw blood for culture studies to determine the causative organism. Prepare the patient for a lumbar puncture (if a tumor or abscess can be ruled out). Also, find out if the patient has a history of I.V. drug abuse, an open-head injury, or endocarditis. Insert an I.V. catheter, and immediately begin administering an antibiotic.

Subarachnoid hemorrhage

If subarachnoid hemorrhage is the suspected diagnosis, ask about a history of hypertension, cerebral aneurysm, head trauma, or arteriovenous malformation. Also ask about sudden withdrawal of an antihypertensive.

Check the patient's pupils for dilation, and assess him for signs of increasing intracranial pressure, such as bradycardia, increased systolic blood pressure, and widened pulse pressure. Insert an I.V. line, and administer supplemental oxygen.

Special considerations

Prepare the patient for diagnostic tests, such as a computed tomography scan, magnetic resonance imaging, spinal X-ray, myelography, and lumbar puncture. Closely monitor his vital signs, ICP, and cardiopulmonary and neurologic status. Ensure bed rest, quiet, and minimal stress.

If the patient has a subarachnoid hemorrhage, darken the room and elevate the head of the bed at least 30 degrees to reduce ICP. If he has a herniated disk or spinal tumor, he may require pelvic traction.

Pediatric pointers

Kernig's sign is considered ominous in children because of their greater potential for rapid deterioration.

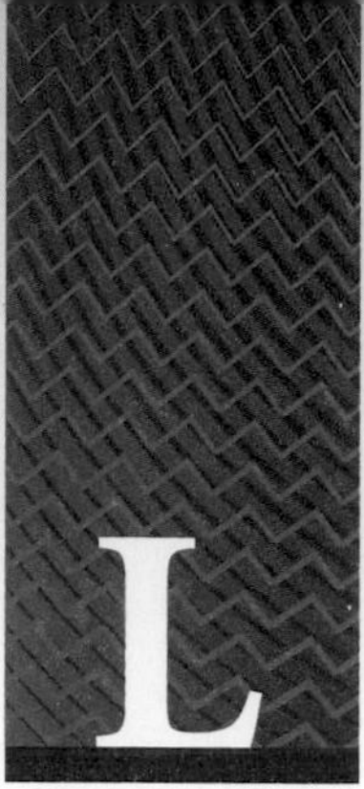

Leg pain

Although leg pain commonly signifies a musculoskeletal disorder, it can also result from a more serious vascular or neurologic disorder. The pain may arise suddenly or gradually and may be localized or affect the entire leg. Constant or intermittent, it may feel dull, burning, sharp, shooting, or tingling. Leg pain may affect locomotion, limiting weight bearing. Severe leg pain that follows cast application for a fracture may signal limb-threatening compartment syndrome. Sudden onset of severe leg pain in a patient with underlying vascular insufficiency may signal acute deterioration, possibly requiring an arterial graft or amputation. (See *Highlighting causes of local leg pain.*)

EMERGENCY INTERVENTIONS *If the patient has acute leg pain and a history of trauma, quickly take his vital signs and determine the leg's neurovascular status. Observe the patient's leg position and check for swelling, gross deformities, or abnormal rotation. Also, be sure to check distal pulses and note skin color and temperature. A pale, cool, and pulseless leg may indicate impaired circulation, which may require emergency surgery.*

History and physical examination

If the patient's condition permits, ask him when the pain began and have him describe its intensity, character, and pattern. Is the pain worse in the morning, at night, or with movement? If it doesn't prevent him from walking, must he rely on a crutch or other assistive device? Also ask him about the presence of other signs and symptoms.

Find out if the patient has a history of leg injury or surgery and if he or a family member has a history of joint, vascular, or back problems. Also ask what medications he's taking and whether they have helped to relieve his leg pain.

Begin the physical examination by watching the patient walk, if his condition permits. Observe how he holds his leg while standing and sitting. Palpate the legs, buttocks, and lower back to determine the extent of pain and tenderness. If a fracture has been ruled out, test the patient's range of motion in the hip and knee. Also, check reflexes with the patient's leg straightened and raised, noting any action that causes pain. Then compare both legs for symmetry, movement, and active range of motion. Additionally, assess sensation and strength. If the patient wears a leg cast, splint, or restrictive dressing, carefully check distal circulation, sensation, and mobility, and stretch his toes to elicit any associated pain.

Medical causes

◆ ***Bone cancer.*** Continuous deep or boring pain, commonly worse at night, may be the first symptom. Later, skin breakdown and impaired circulation may occur, along with cachexia, fever, and impaired mobility.

Highlighting causes of local leg pain

Various disorders cause hip, knee, ankle, or foot pain, which may radiate to surrounding tissues and be reported as leg pain. Local pain is commonly accompanied by tenderness, swelling, and deformity in the affected area.

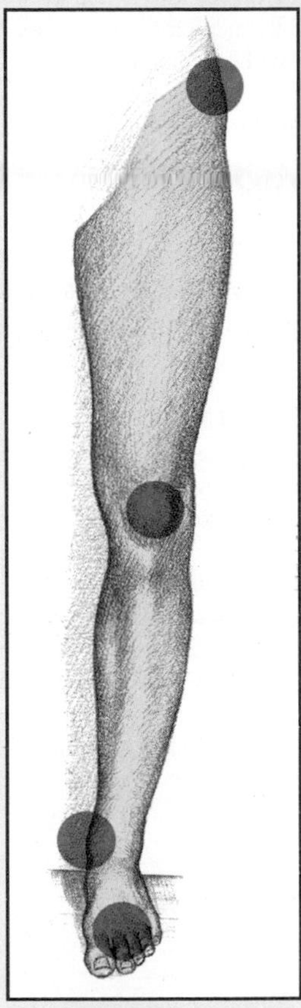

Hip pain
Arthritis
Avascular necrosis
Bursitis
Dislocation
Fracture
Sepsis
Tumor

Knee pain
Arthritis
Bursitis
Chondromalacia
Contusion
Cruciate ligament injury
Dislocation
Fracture
Meniscal injury
Osteochondritis dissecans
Phlebitis
Popliteal cyst
Radiculopathy
Ruptured extensor mechanism
Sprain

Ankle pain
Achilles tendon contracture
Arthritis
Dislocation
Fracture
Sprain
Tenosynovitis

Foot pain
Arthritis
Bunion
Callus or corn
Dislocation
Flatfoot
Fracture
Gout
Hallux rigidus
Hammer toe
Ingrown toenail
Köhler's disease
Morton's neuroma
Occlusive vascular disease
Plantar fasciitis
Plantar wart
Radiculopathy
Tabes dorsalis
Tarsal tunnel syndrome

◆ ***Compartment syndrome.*** Progressive, intense lower leg pain that increases with passive muscle stretching is a cardinal sign of this limb-threatening disorder. Restrictive dressings or traction may aggravate the pain, which typically worsens despite analgesic administration. Other findings include muscle weakness and paresthesia, but apparently normal distal circulation. With irreversible muscle ischemia, paralysis and absent pulse also occur.

◆ ***Fracture.*** Severe, acute pain accompanies swelling and ecchymosis in the affected leg. Movement produces extreme pain, and the leg may be unable to bear weight. Neurovascular status distal to the fracture may be impaired, causing paresthesia, absent pulse, mottled cyanosis, and cool skin. Deformity, muscle spasms, and bony crepitation may also occur.

◆ ***Infection.*** Local leg pain, erythema, swelling, streaking, and warmth characterize soft-tissue and bone infections. Fever and tachycardia may be present with other systemic signs.

◆ ***Multiple myeloma.*** Pain that begins in the ribs or lower back and progresses to the hips and legs may be a symptom of advanced multiple myeloma. Other signs and symptoms may include kidney problems, fatigue, and recurrent infections.

◆ ***Occlusive vascular disease.*** Continuous cramping pain in the legs and feet may worsen with walking, inducing claudication. The patient may report increased pain at night, cold feet, cold intolerance, numbness, and tingling. Examination may reveal ankle and lower leg edema, decreased or absent pulses, and increased capillary refill time. (Normal time is less than 3 seconds.)

◆ ***Sciatica.*** Pain, described as shooting, aching, or tingling that radiates down the back of the leg along the sciatic nerve. Typically, activity exacerbates the pain and rest relieves it. The patient may limp to avoid exacerbating the pain and may have difficulty moving from a sitting to a standing position.

◆ ***Strain or sprain.*** Acute strain causes sharp, transient pain and rapid swelling, followed by leg tenderness and ecchymosis. Chronic strain produces stiffness, soreness, and generalized leg tenderness several hours after the injury; active and passive motion may be painful or impossible. A sprain causes local pain, especially during joint movement; ecchymosis and, possibly, local swelling and loss of mobility develop.

◆ ***Thrombophlebitis.*** Discomfort may range from calf tenderness to severe pain accompanied by swelling, warmth, and a feeling of heaviness in the affected leg. The patient may also develop fever, chills, malaise, muscle cramps, and a positive Homans' sign. Assessment may reveal superficial veins that are visibly engorged; palpable, hard, thready, and cordlike; and sensitive to pressure.

◆ ***Varicose veins.*** Mild to severe leg symptoms may develop, including nocturnal cramping; a feeling of heaviness; diffuse, dull aching after prolonged standing or walking; and aching during menses. Assessment may reveal palpable nodules, orthostatic edema, and stasis pigmentation of the calves and ankles.

GENDER CUE *Primary varicose veins originate in the superficial system and are more common in women.*

◆ ***Venous stasis ulcers.*** Localized pain and bleeding arise from infected ulcerations on the lower extremities. Mottled, bluish pigmentation is characteristic, and local edema may occur.

Special considerations

If the patient has acute leg pain, closely monitor his neurovascular status by frequently checking distal pulses and evaluating both legs for temperature, color and sensation. Also monitor his thigh and calf circumference to evaluate bleeding into tissues from a possible fracture site. Prepare him for X-rays. Use sandbags to immobilize his leg; apply ice and, if needed, skeletal traction. If a fracture isn't suspected, prepare the patient for laboratory tests to detect an infectious agent or for venography, Doppler ultrasonography, plethysmography, or angiography to determine vascular competency. Withhold food and fluids until the need for surgery has been ruled out, and withhold analgesics until a preliminary diagnosis is made. Administer an anticoagulant and antibiotic as needed.

Pediatric pointers

Common pediatric causes of leg pain include fracture, growing pains, osteomyelitis, and bone cancer. If parents fail to give an adequate explanation for a leg fracture, consider the possibility of child abuse.

Patient counseling

If the patient has chronic leg pain, instruct him to take an anti-inflammatory and teach him to perform range-of-motion exercises and, if necessary, to use a cane, walker, or other assistive device. Discuss with the patient and his family any lifestyle changes that may be necessary until leg pain resolves. If physical therapy is necessary, stress the importance of establishing a daily exercise regimen. Based on the cause of the leg pain, discuss the appropriate positioning of the lower extremity to enhance blood flow and venous return.

Level of consciousness, decreased

A decrease in level of consciousness (LOC), from lethargy to stupor to coma, usually results from a neurologic disorder and may signal a life-threatening complication, such as hemorrhage, trauma, or cerebral edema. However, this sign can also result from a metabolic, GI, musculoskeletal, urologic, or cardiopulmonary disorder; severe nutritional deficiency; the effects of toxins; or drug use. LOC can deteriorate suddenly or gradually and can remain altered temporarily or permanently.

Consciousness is affected by the reticular activating system (RAS), an intricate network of neurons with axons extending from the brain stem, thalamus, and hypothalamus to the cerebral cortex. A disturbance in any part of this integrated system prevents the intercommunication that makes consciousness possible. Loss of consciousness can result from a bilateral cerebral disturbance, an RAS disturbance, or both. Cerebral dysfunction characteristically produces the least dramatic decrease in a patient's LOC. In contrast, dysfunction of the RAS produces the most dramatic decrease in LOC—coma.

The most sensitive indicator of decreased LOC is a change in the patient's mental status. The Glasgow Coma Scale, which measures a patient's ability to respond to verbal, sensory, and motor stimulation, can be used to quickly evaluate a patient's LOC.

EMERGENCY INTERVENTIONS *After evaluating the patient's airway, breathing, and circulation, use the Glasgow Coma Scale to quickly determine his LOC and to obtain baseline data. (See* Using the Glasgow Coma Scale, *page 422.) If the patient's score is 13 or less, emergency surgery may be necessary. Insert an artificial airway, elevate the head of the bed 30 degrees and, if spinal cord injury has been ruled out, turn the patient's head to the side. Prepare to suction the patient if necessary. You may need to hyperventilate him to reduce carbon dioxide levels and decrease intracranial pressure (ICP). Then determine the rate, rhythm, and depth of spontaneous respirations. Support his breathing with a handheld resuscitation bag, if necessary. If the patient's Glasgow Coma Scale score is 7 or less, intubation and resuscitation may be necessary.*

Continue to monitor the patient's vital signs, being alert for signs of increasing ICP, such as bradycardia and widening pulse pressure. When his airway, breathing, and circulation are stabilized, perform a neurologic examination.

HISTORY AND PHYSICAL EXAMINATION

Try to obtain history information from the patient, if he's lucid, and from his family. Did the patient complain of headache, dizziness, nausea, visual or hearing disturbances, weakness, fatigue, or any other problems before his LOC decreased? Has his family noticed any changes in the patient's behavior, personality, memory, or temperament? Also ask about a history of neurologic disease, cancer, or recent trauma or infections; drug and alcohol use; and the development of other signs and symptoms.

Because decreased LOC can result from a disorder affecting virtually any body system, tailor the remainder of your evaluation according to the patient's associated symptoms.

MEDICAL CAUSES

◆ ***Adrenal crisis.*** Decreased LOC, ranging from lethargy to coma, may develop within 8 to 12 hours of onset. Early associated findings include progressive weakness, irritability, anorexia, headache, nausea and vomiting, diarrhea, abdominal pain, and fever. Later signs and symptoms include hypotension; rapid, thready pulse; oliguria; cool, clammy skin; and flaccid extremities. The patient with chronic adrenocortical hypofunction may have hyperpigmented skin and mucous membranes.

◆ ***Brain abscess.*** Decreased LOC varies from drowsiness to deep stupor, depending on abscess size and site. Early signs and symptoms—constant intractable headache, nausea, vomiting, and seizures—reflect increasing ICP. Typical later features include ocular disturbances (nystagmus, vision loss, and pupillary inequality) and signs of infection such as fever. Other findings may include personality changes, confusion, abnormal behavior, dizziness, facial weakness, aphasia, ataxia, tremor, and hemiparesis.

◆ ***Brain tumor.*** LOC decreases slowly, from lethargy to coma. The patient may also experience apathy, behavior changes, memory loss, decreased attention span, morning headache, dizziness, vision loss, ataxia, and sensorimotor disturbances. Aphasia and seizures are possible, along with signs of hormonal imbalance, such as fluid retention or amenorrhea. Signs and symptoms vary according to the location and size of the tumor. In later stages, papilledema, vomiting, bradycardia, and widening pulse pressure also appear. In the final stages, the patient may exhibit decorticate or decerebrate posture.

◆ ***Cerebral aneurysm (ruptured).*** Somnolence, confusion and, at times, stupor characterize a moderate bleed; deep coma occurs with severe bleeding, which can be fatal. Onset is usually abrupt, with sudden, severe headache, nausea, and vomiting. Nuchal rigidity, back and leg pain, fever, restlessness, irritability, occasional seizures, and blurred vision point to meningeal irritation. The type and severity of other findings vary with the site and severity of the hemorrhage and may include hemiparesis, hemisensory defects, dysphagia, and visual defects.

◆ ***Cerebral contusion.*** Usually unconscious for a prolonged period, the patient may develop dilated, nonreactive pupils and decorticate or decerebrate posture. If he's conscious or recovers consciousness, he may be drowsy, confused,

Using the Glasgow Coma Scale

The Glasgow Coma Scale describes a patient's baseline mental status and helps to detect and interpret changes from baseline findings. When using the Glasgow Coma Scale, test the patient's ability to respond to verbal, motor, and sensory stimulation, and grade your findings according to the scale. A score of 15 indicates that the patient is alert, can follow simple commands, and is oriented to time, place, and person. A decreased score in one or more categories may signal an impending neurologic crisis. A score of 7 or less indicates severe neurologic damage.

Test	Score	Response
Eye-opening response		
Spontaneously	4	Opens eyes spontaneously
To speech	3	Opens eyes when told to
To pain	2	Opens eyes only to painful stimulus
None	1	Doesn't open eyes in response to stimuli
Motor response		
Obeys	6	Shows two fingers when asked
Localizes	5	Reaches toward painful stimulus and tries to remove it
Withdraws	4	Moves away from painful stimulus
Abnormal flexion	3	Assumes a decorticate posture (shown below) 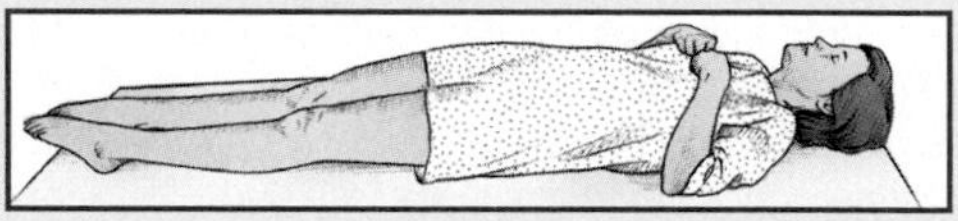
Abnormal extension	2	Assumes a decerebrate posture (shown below) 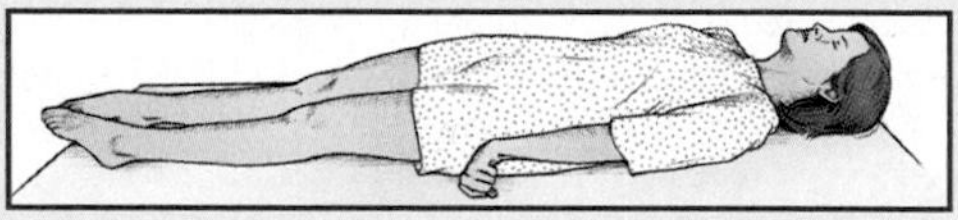
None	1	No response; just lies flaccid (an ominous sign)
Verbal response (to question, "What year is this?")		
Oriented	5	Tells correct year
Confused	4	Tells incorrect year
Inappropriate words	3	Replies randomly with incorrect words
Incomprehensible	2	Moans or screams
No response	1	No response
Total score	(3 to 15)	

disoriented, agitated, or even violent. Associated findings include blurred or double vision, fever, headache, pallor, diaphoresis, tachycardia, altered respirations, aphasia, and hemiparesis. Residual effects include seizures, impaired mental status, slight hemiparesis, and vertigo.

◆ ***Diabetic ketoacidosis.*** This disorder produces a rapid decrease in LOC, ranging from lethargy to coma, commonly preceded by polydipsia, polyphagia, and polyuria. The patient may complain of weakness, anorexia, abdominal pain, nausea, and vomiting. He may also exhibit orthostatic hypotension; fruity breath odor; Kussmaul's respirations; warm, dry skin; and a rapid, thready pulse. Untreated, this condition invariably leads to coma and death.

◆ ***Encephalitis.*** Within 24 to 48 hours after onset, the patient may develop LOC changes ranging from lethargy to coma. Other possible findings include abrupt onset of fever, headache, nuchal rigidity, nausea, vomiting, irritability, personality changes, seizures, aphasia, ataxia, hemiparesis, nystagmus, photophobia, myoclonus, and cranial nerve palsies.

◆ ***Encephalomyelitis (postvaccinal).*** This life-threatening disorder produces rapid LOC deterioration from drowsiness to coma. The patient also experiences rapid onset of fever, headache, nuchal rigidity, back pain, vomiting, and seizures.

◆ ***Encephalopathy.*** With hepatic encephalopathy, signs and symptoms develop in four stages: in the prodromal stage, slight personality changes (disorientation, forgetfulness, slurred speech) and slight tremor; in the impending stage, tremor progressing to asterixis (the hallmark of hepatic encephalopathy), lethargy, aberrant behavior, and apraxia; in the stuporous stage, stupor and hyperventilation, with the patient noisy and abusive when aroused; in the comatose stage, coma with decerebrate posture, hyperactive reflexes, positive Babinski's reflex, and fetor hepaticus.

With life-threatening hypertensive encephalopathy, LOC progressively decreases from lethargy to stupor to coma. Besides markedly elevated blood pressure, the patient may experience severe headache, vomiting, seizures, visual disturbances, transient paralysis, and eventually Cheyne-Stokes respirations.

With hypoglycemic encephalopathy, LOC rapidly deteriorates from lethargy to coma. Early signs and symptoms include nervousness, restlessness, agitation, and confusion; hunger; alternate flushing and cold sweats; and headache, trembling, and palpitations. Blurred vision progresses to motor weakness, hemiplegia, dilated pupils, pallor, decreased pulse rate, shallow respirations, and seizures. Flaccidity and decerebrate posture appear late.

Depending on its severity, hypoxic encephalopathy produces a sudden or gradual decrease in LOC, leading to coma and brain death. Early on, the patient appears confused and restless, with cyanosis and increased heart and respiratory rates and blood pressure. Later, his respiratory pattern becomes abnormal, and assessment reveals decreased pulse, blood pressure, and deep tendon reflexes (DTRs); Babinski's reflex; absent doll's eye sign; and fixed pupils.

With uremic encephalopathy, LOC decreases gradually from lethargy to coma. Early on, the patient may appear apathetic, inattentive, confused, and irritable and may complain of headache, nausea, fatigue, and anorexia. Other findings include vomiting, tremors, edema, papilledema, hypertension, cardiac arrhythmias, dyspnea, crackles, oliguria, and Kussmaul's and Cheyne-Stokes respirations.

◆ ***Epidural hemorrhage (acute).*** This life-threatening posttraumatic disorder produces momentary loss of consciousness, sometimes followed by a lucid interval. While lucid, the patient has a severe headache, nausea, vomiting, and bladder distention. Rapid deterioration in consciousness follows, possibly leading to coma. Other findings include irregular respirations, seizures, decreased and bounding pulse, increased pulse pressure, hypertension, unilateral or bilateral fixed and dilated pupils, unilateral hemiparesis or hemiplegia, decerebrate posture, and Babinski's reflex.

◆ ***Heatstroke.*** As body temperature increases, LOC gradually decreases from lethargy to coma. Early signs and symptoms include malaise, tachycardia, tachypnea, orthostatic hypotension, muscle cramps, rigidity, and syncope. The patient may be irritable, anxious, and dizzy and may report a severe headache. At the onset of heatstroke, the patient's skin is hot, flushed, and diaphoretic with blotchy cyanosis; later, when his fever exceeds 105° F (40.5° C), his skin becomes hot, flushed, and anhidrotic. Pulse and respiratory rate increase markedly, and blood pressure drops precipitously. Other findings include vomiting, diarrhea, dilated pupils, and Cheyne-Stokes respirations.

◆ ***Hypercapnia with pulmonary syndrome.*** LOC decreases gradually from lethargy to coma (usually not prolonged). The patient becomes confused or drowsy and develops asterixis and muscle twitching. He may complain of headache and exhibit mental dullness, papilledema, and small, reactive pupils.

◆ ***Hypernatremia.*** This disorder, life-threatening if acute, causes LOC to deteriorate from lethargy to coma. The patient is irritable and exhibits twitches progressing to seizures. Other associated signs and symptoms include a weak, thready pulse; nausea; malaise; fever; thirst; flushed skin; and dry mucous membranes.

◆ ***Hyperosmolar hyperglycemic nonketotic syndrome.*** LOC decreases rapidly from lethargy to coma. Early findings include polyuria, polydipsia, weight loss, and weakness. Later, the patient may develop hypotension, poor skin turgor, dry skin and mucous membranes, tachycardia, tachypnea, oliguria, and seizures.

◆ ***Hyperventilation syndrome.*** Brief episodes of unconsciousness follow stress-induced deep, rapid breathing associated with anxiety and agitation. Associated findings include dizziness, circumoral and peripheral paresthesia, twitching, carpopedal spasm, and arrhythmias.

◆ ***Hypokalemia.*** LOC gradually decreases to lethargy; coma is rare. Other findings include confusion, nausea, vomiting, diarrhea, and polyuria; weakness, decreased reflexes, and malaise; and dizziness, hypotension, arrhythmias, and abnormal electrocardiogram results.

◆ ***Hyponatremia.*** This disorder, life-threatening if acute, produces decreased LOC in late stages. Early nausea and malaise may progress to behavior changes, confusion, lethargy, incoordination and, eventually, seizures and coma.

◆ ***Hypothermia.*** With severe hypothermia (temperature below 90° F [32.2° C]), LOC decreases from lethargy to coma. DTRs disappear, and ventricular fibrillation occurs, possibly followed by cardiopulmonary arrest. With mild to moderate hypothermia, the patient may experience memory loss and slurred speech as well as shivering, weakness, fatigue, and apathy. Other early signs and symptoms include ataxia, muscle stiffness, and hyperactive DTRs; diuresis; tachycardia and decreased respiratory rate and blood pressure; and cold, pale skin. Later, muscle rigidity and decreased reflexes may develop, along with peripheral cyanosis, bradycardia, arrhythmias, severe hypotension, decreased respiratory rate with shallow respirations, and oliguria.

◆ ***Intracerebral hemorrhage.*** This life-threatening disorder produces a rapid, steady loss of consciousness within hours, commonly accompanied by severe headache, dizziness, nausea, and vomiting. Associated signs and symptoms vary and may include increased blood pressure, irregular respirations, Babinski's reflex, seizures, aphasia, decreased sensations, hemiplegia, decorticate or decerebrate posture, and dilated pupils.

◆ ***Listeriosis.*** If this serious infection spreads to the nervous system and causes meningitis, signs and symptoms include decreased LOC, fever, headache, and nuchal rigidity. Early signs and symptoms of listeriosis include fever, myalgias, abdominal pain, nausea, vomiting, and diarrhea.

GENDER CUE *Infections during pregnancy may lead to premature delivery, infection of the neonate, or stillbirth.*

◆ ***Meningitis.*** Confusion and irritability are expected; however, stupor, coma, and seizures may occur in those with severe meningitis. Fever develops early, possibly accompanied by chills. Associated findings include severe headache, nuchal rigidity, hyperreflexia and, possibly, opisthotonos. The patient exhibits Kernig's and Brudzinski's signs and, possibly, ocular palsies, photophobia, facial weakness, and hearing loss.

◆ ***Myxedema crisis.*** The patient may exhibit a swift decline in LOC. Other findings include severe hypothermia, hypoventilation, hypotension, bradycardia, hypoactive reflexes, periorbital and peripheral edema, impaired hearing and balance, and seizures.

◆ ***Pontine hemorrhage.*** A sudden, rapid decrease in LOC to the point of coma occurs within minutes and death within hours. The patient may also exhibit total paralysis, decerebrate posture, Babinski's reflex, absent doll's eye sign, and bilateral miosis (however, the pupils remain reactive to light).

◆ ***Seizure disorders.*** A complex partial seizure produces decreased LOC, manifested as a blank stare, purposeless behavior (picking at clothing, wandering, lip smacking or chewing motions), and unintelligible speech. The seizure may be heralded by an aura and followed by several minutes of mental confusion.

An absence seizure usually involves a brief change in LOC, indicated by blinking or eye rolling, blank stare, and slight mouth movements.

A generalized tonic-clonic seizure typically begins with a loud cry and sudden loss of consciousness. Muscle spasm alternates with relaxation. Tongue biting, incontinence, labored breathing, apnea, and cyanosis may also occur. Consciousness returns after the seizure, but the patient remains confused and may have difficulty talking. He may complain of drowsiness, fatigue, headache, muscle aching, and weakness and may fall into deep sleep.

An atonic seizure produces sudden unconsciousness for a few seconds.

Status epilepticus, rapidly recurring seizures without intervening periods of physiologic recovery and return of consciousness, can be life threatening.

◆ ***Shock.*** Decreased LOC—lethargy progressing to stupor and coma—occurs late in shock. Associated findings include confusion, anxiety, and restlessness; hypotension; tachycardia; weak pulse with narrowing pulse pressure; dyspnea; oliguria; and cool, clammy skin.

Hypovolemic shock is generally the result of massive or insidious bleeding, either internally or externally. Cardiogenic shock may produce chest pain or arrhythmias and signs of heart failure, such as dyspnea, cough, edema, jugular vein distention, and weight gain. Septic shock may be accompanied by high fever and chills. Anaphylactic shock usually involves stridor.

◆ ***Stroke.*** LOC changes vary in degree and onset, depending on the lesion's size and location and the presence of edema. A thrombotic stroke usually follows multiple transient ischemic attacks (TIAs). LOC changes may be abrupt or take several minutes, hours, or days. An embolic stroke occurs suddenly, and deficits reach their peak almost at once. Deficits associated with a hemorrhagic stroke usually develop over minutes or hours.

Associated findings vary with stroke type and severity and may include disorientation; intellectual deficits, such as memory loss and poor judgment; personality changes; and emotional lability. Other possible findings include dysarthria, dysphagia, ataxia, aphasia, apraxia, agnosia, unilateral sensorimotor loss, and visual disturbances. In addition, urine retention, incontinence, constipation, headache, vomiting, and seizures may occur.

◆ ***Subdural hematoma (chronic).*** LOC deteriorates slowly. Other signs and symptoms include confusion, decreased ability to concentrate, and personality changes accompanied by headache, light-headedness, seizures, and a dilated ipsilateral pupil with ptosis.

◆ ***Subdural hemorrhage (acute).*** With this potentially life-threatening disorder, agitation and confusion are followed by progressively decreasing LOC from somnolence to coma. The patient may also experience headache, fever, unilateral pupil dilation, decreased pulse and respiratory rates, widening pulse pressure, seizures, hemiparesis, and Babinski's reflex.

◆ ***Thyroid storm.*** LOC decreases suddenly and can progress to coma. Irritability, restlessness, confusion, and psychotic behavior precede the deterioration. Associated signs and symptoms include tremors and weakness; visual disturbances; tachycardia, arrhythmias, angina, and acute respiratory distress; warm, moist, flushed skin; and vomiting, diarrhea, and fever to 105° F (40.5° C).

◆ ***TIA.*** LOC decreases abruptly (with varying severity) and gradually returns to normal within 24 hours. Site-specific findings may include vision loss, nystagmus, dizziness, dysarthria, unilateral hemiparesis or hemiplegia, tinnitus, paresthesia, staggering or incoordinated gait, aphasia, or dysphagia.

◆ ***West Nile encephalitis.*** This brain infection is caused by the West Nile virus, a mosquito-borne flavivirus commonly found in Africa, West Asia, and the Middle East and, less commonly, in the United States. Mild infection is common. Signs and symptoms include fever, headache, and body aches, commonly with skin rash and swollen lymph glands. More severe infection is marked by high fever, headache, neck stiffness, stupor, disorientation, coma, tremors, occasional seizures, paralysis and, rarely, death.

Other causes

◆ ***Alcohol.*** Alcohol use causes varying degrees of sedation, irritability, and incoordination; intoxication commonly causes stupor.

◆ ***Drugs.*** Sedation and other degrees of decreased LOC can result from an overdose of a barbiturate, another central nervous system depressant, or aspirin.

◆ ***Poisoning.*** Toxins, such as lead, carbon monoxide, and snake venom, can cause varying degrees of decreased LOC. Confusion is common, as are headache, nausea, and vomiting. Other general features include hypotension, cardiac arrhythmias, dyspnea, sensorimotor loss, and seizures.

Special considerations

Reassess the patient's LOC and neurologic status at least hourly. Carefully monitor ICP and intake and output. Ensure airway patency and proper nutrition. Take precautions to help ensure the patient's safety. Keep him on bed rest with the side rails up and maintain seizure precautions. Keep emergency resuscitation equipment at the patient's bedside. Prepare the patient for a computed tomography scan of the head, magnetic resonance imaging of the brain, EEG, and lumbar puncture. Maintain an elevation of the head of the bed to at least 30 degrees. Don't administer an opioid or sedative because either may further decrease the patient's LOC and hinder an accurate, meaningful neurologic examination. Apply restraints only if necessary because their use may increase his agitation and confusion. Talk to the patient even if he appears comatose; your voice may help reorient him to reality.

Pediatric pointers

The primary cause of decreased LOC in children is head trauma, which often results from physical abuse or a motor vehicle accident. Other causes include accidental poisoning, hydrocephalus, and meningitis or brain abscess following an ear or respiratory infection. To reduce the parents' anxiety, include them in the child's care. Offer them support and realistic explanations of their child's condition.

Lid lag

[Graefe's sign]

A cardinal sign of thyrotoxicosis, lid lag is the inability of the upper eyelid to follow the eye's downward movements. Testing for lid lag involves holding a finger, penlight, or other target above the patient's eye level and then moving it downward and observing eyelid movement as his eyes follow the target. This sign is demonstrated when a rim of sclera appears between the upper lid margin and the iris when the patient lowers his eyes, when one lid closes more slowly than the other, or when both lids close slowly and incompletely with jerky movements.

History and physical examination

Because the patient isn't generally able to recognize a lid lag himself, ask a friend or family member if he has noticed it. If so, ask when he first noticed lid lag or its possible manifestation, incomplete closure of the eyelid. Explore other signs and symptoms, and ask about a history of thyroid disease. Next, perform a physical examination, focusing on the effects of thyrotoxicosis, such as an enlarged thyroid, diaphoresis, tremors, and exophthalmos.

Medical causes

◆ ***Thyrotoxicosis.*** This disorder may produce bilateral lid lag and other ocular effects, including exophthalmos, infrequent blinking, eye dryness and discomfort, conjunctival injection, and a characteristic stare. (Thyrotoxicosis is the most common cause of unilateral and bilateral exophthalmos in adults and children.) Restricted eye movement may produce diplopia. Other effects include an enlarged thyroid, nervousness, heat intolerance, weight loss despite increased appetite, diaphoresis, diarrhea, tremors, palpitations, widened pulse pressure, and silken-smooth skin texture.

Because thyrotoxicosis affects virtually every body system, it can produce many other findings. For example, central nervous system effects include clumsiness, shaky handwriting, and emotional lability. Integumentary effects include smooth, warm, flushed, and thickened skin with itchy patches; fine, soft hair with premature graying and increased loss; friable nails; and onycholysis.

Cardiopulmonary involvement causes constant dyspnea; tachycardia; full, bounding pulse; widened pulse pressure; visible point of maximal impulse; and, occasionally, systolic murmur.

Besides nausea and vomiting, GI findings include anorexia, diarrhea, and hepatomegaly. Musculoskeletal findings include weakness, fatigue, and atrophy, along with paralysis and, occasionally, acropachy. Women may report oligomenorrhea or amenorrhea; men may develop gynecomastia; both sexes may experience decreased libido.

Special considerations

If lid lag is accompanied by exophthalmos, provide privacy to ease the patient's self-consciousness. Don't cover the affected eye with a gauze pad or other object because removal could destroy the corneal epithelium. Help the patient keep his eyes lubricated with saline drops.

Pediatric pointers

Children may have lid lag associated with aberrant regeneration of cranial nerve III or, rarely, thyrotoxicosis.

Patient counseling

Stress the importance of complying with drug therapy (such as antithyroid drugs or therapeutic radioactive iodine). Subtotal thyroidectomy may be required in rare cases.

Light flashes

[Photopsias]

A cardinal symptom of vision-threatening retinal detachment, light flashes can occur locally or throughout the visual field. The patient usually reports seeing spots, stars, or lightning-type streaks. Flashes can occur suddenly or gradually and can indicate temporary or permanent vision impairment.

In most cases, light flashes signal the splitting of the posterior vitreous membrane into two layers; the inner layer detaches from the retina, and the outer layer remains fixed to it. The sensation of light flashes may result from vitreous traction on the retina, hemorrhage caused by a tear in the retinal capillary, or strands of solid vitreous floating in a local pool of liquid vitreous.

EMERGENCY INTERVENTIONS *Until retinal detachment is ruled out, restrict the patient's eye and body movement.*

History and physical examination

Ask the patient when the light flashes began. Can he pinpoint their location, or do they occur throughout the visual field? If the patient is experiencing eye pain or headache, have him describe it. Ask if the patient wears or has ever worn corrective lenses and if he or a family member has a history of eye or vision problems. Also ask if the patient has other medical problems—especially hypertension or diabetes mellitus, which can cause retinopathy and, possibly, retinal detachment. Obtain an occupational history because light flashes may be related to job stress or eye strain.

Next, perform a complete eye and vision examination, especially if trauma is apparent or suspected. Begin by inspecting the external eye, lids, lashes, and tear puncta for abnormalities and the iris and sclera for signs of bleeding. Observe pupillary size and shape; check for reaction to light, accommodation, and consensual light response. Then test visual acuity in each eye. Also test visual fields; document any light flashes that the patient reports during this test.

Medical causes

- ***Head trauma.*** A patient who has sustained minor head trauma may report "seeing stars" when the injury occurs. He may also complain of localized pain at the injury site, generalized headache, and dizziness. Later, he may develop nausea, vomiting, and decreased level of consciousness.
- ***Migraine headache.*** Light flashes—possibly accompanied by an aura—may herald a classic migraine headache. As these symptoms subside, the patient typically experiences a severe, throbbing, unilateral headache that usually lasts 1 to 12 hours and may be accompanied by paresthesia of the lips, face, or hands; slight confusion; dizziness; photophobia; nausea; and vomiting.
- ***Retinal detachment.*** Light flashes described as floaters or spots are localized in the portion of the visual field where the retina is detaching. With macular involvement, the patient may experience painless visual impairment resembling a curtain covering the visual field.
- ***Vitreous detachment.*** Visual floaters may accompany a sudden onset of light flashes. Usually, one eye is affected at a time.

Special considerations

If the patient has retinal detachment, prepare him for reattachment surgery. Explain that after surgery he may need to continue wearing bilateral eye patches and may have activity and position restrictions until the retina heals completely.

If the patient doesn't have retinal detachment, reassure him that his light flashes are temporary and don't indicate eye damage. For the patient with a migraine headache, maintain a quiet, darkened environment; encourage sleep; and administer an analgesic, as ordered.

Pediatric pointers

Children may experience light flashes after minor head trauma.

Low birth weight

Two groups of neonates are born weighing less than the normal minimum birth weight of 5½ lb (2,500 g)—those who are born prematurely (before the 37th week of gestation) and those who are small for gestational age (SGA). The premature neonate weighs an appropriate amount for his gestational age and probably would have matured normally if carried to term. Conversely, the SGA neonate weighs less than the normal amount for his age; however, his organs are mature. Differentiating between the two groups, helps direct the search for a cause.

In the premature neonate, low birth weight usually results from a disorder that prevents the uterus from retaining the fetus, interferes with the normal course of pregnancy, causes premature separation of the placenta, or stimulates uterine contractions before term. In the SGA neonate, intrauterine growth may be retarded by a disorder that interferes with placental circulation, fetal development, or maternal health. (See *Maternal causes of low birth weight.*)

Regardless of the cause, low birth weight is associated with higher neonate morbidity and mortality; in fact, these neonates are 20 times more likely to die within the first month of life. Low birth weight can also signal a life-threatening emergency.

SGA neonates who will demonstrate catch-up growth, do so by 8 to 12 months. Some SGA neonates will remain below the 10th percentile. Weights of the premature neonate should be corrected for gestational age by approximately 24 months.

EMERGENCY INTERVENTIONS *Because low birth weight may be associated with poorly developed body systems, particularly the respiratory system, your priority is to monitor the neonate's respiratory status. Be alert for signs of distress, such as apnea, grunting respirations, intercostal or xiphoid retractions, or a respiratory rate exceeding 60 breaths/minute after the first hour of life. If you detect any of these signs, prepare to provide respiratory support. Endotracheal intubation or supplemental oxygen with an oxygen hood may be needed.*

Monitor the neonate's axillary temperature. Decreased fat reserves may keep him from maintaining normal body temperature, and a drop below 97.8° F (36.5° C) exacerbates respiratory distress by increasing oxygen consumption. To maintain normal body temperature, use an overbed warmer or an Isolette. (If these are unavailable, use a wrapped rubber bottle filled with warm water, but be careful to avoid hyperthermia.) Cover neonate's head to prevent heat loss.

History and physical examination

As soon as possible, evaluate the neonate's neuromuscular and physical maturity to determine gestational age. (See *Ballard Scale for calculating gestational age,* pages 430 and 431.) Follow with a routine neonatal examination.

Medical causes

This section lists some fetal and placental causes of low birth weight as well as the associated signs and symptoms present in the neonate at birth.

◆ ***Chromosomal aberrations.*** Abnormalities in the number, size, or configuration of chromosomes can cause low birth weight and possibly multiple congenital anomalies in a premature or SGA neonate. For example, a neonate with trisomy 21 (Down syndrome) may be SGA and have prominent epicanthal folds, a flat-bridged nose, a protruding tongue, palmar simian creases, muscular hypotonia, and an umbilical hernia.

◆ ***Cytomegalovirus infection.*** Although low birth weight in this disorder is usually associated with premature birth, some neonates may be SGA. Assessment at birth may reveal these classic signs: petechiae and ecchymoses, jaundice, and hepatosplenomegaly, which increases for several days. The neonate may also have a high fever, lymphadenopathy, tachypnea, and dyspnea, along with prolonged bleeding at puncture sites.

◆ ***Placental dysfunction.*** Low birth weight and a wasted appearance occur in an SGA neonate. The neonate may be symmetrically short or may appear relatively long for his low weight. Additional findings reflect the underlying cause. For example, if maternal hyperparathyroidism caused placental dysfunction, the neonate may exhibit muscle jerking and twitching, carpopedal spasm, ankle clonus, vomiting, tachycardia, and tachypnea.

◆ ***Rubella (congenital).*** Usually, the low-birth-weight neonate with this disease is born at term but is SGA. A characteristic "blueberry muffin" rash accompanies cataracts, purpuric lesions, hepatosplenomegaly, and a large anterior fontanel. Abnormal heart sounds, if present, vary with the type of associated congenital heart defect.

◆ ***Toxoplasmosis (congenital).*** The low-birth-weight neonate may be either premature or SGA and may have hydrocephalus or microcephalus. Associated findings include fever, seizures, lymphadenopathy, hepatosplenomegaly, jaundice, and rash. Other defects, which may occur months or years later, include strabismus, blindness, epilepsy, and mental retardation.

◆ ***Varicella (congenital).*** Low birth weight is accompanied by cataracts and skin vesicles.

Special considerations

To make up for low fat and glycogen stores in the low-birth-weight neonate, initiate feedings as soon as possible and continue to feed every 2 to 3 hours. Provide gavage or I.V. feeding for sick or very premature neonates. Check abdominal girth daily or more frequently if indicated, and check stools for blood because increasing girth and bloody stools may indicate necrotizing enterocolitis. A sepsis workup may be necessary if signs of infection are associated with low birth weight.

Check the neonate's vital signs every 15 minutes for the first hour and at least once every hour thereafter until his condition stabilizes. Be alert for changes in temperature or behavior, feeding problems, respiratory distress, or periods of apnea—possible indications of infection. Also, monitor blood glucose levels and watch for signs and symptoms of hypoglycemia, such as irritability, jitteriness, tremors, seizures, irregular respirations, lethargy, and a high-pitched or weak cry. If the neonate is receiving supplemental oxygen, carefully monitor arterial blood gas values and the oxygen concentration of inspired air to prevent retinopathy.

Monitor the neonate's urine output by weighing diapers before and after voiding. Check urine color, measure specific gravity, and test for the presence of glucose, blood, or protein. Also, watch for changes in the neonate's skin color because increasing jaundice may indicate hyperbilirubinemia.

Encourage the parents to participate in their neonate's care to strengthen bonding, and allow ample time for their questions.

Maternal causes of low birth weight

If the neonate is small for gestational age, consider these possible maternal causes:
- ◆ acquired immunodeficiency syndrome
- ◆ alcohol or opioid abuse
- ◆ chronic maternal illness
- ◆ cigarette smoking
- ◆ hypertension
- ◆ hypoxemia
- ◆ malnutrition
- ◆ toxemia.

If the neonate is born prematurely, consider these common maternal causes:
- ◆ abruptio placentae
- ◆ amnionitis
- ◆ cocaine or crack use
- ◆ incompetent cervix
- ◆ placenta previa
- ◆ polyhydramnios
- ◆ preeclampsia
- ◆ premature rupture of membranes
- ◆ severe maternal illness
- ◆ urinary tract infection.

Lymphadenopathy

Lymphadenopathy—enlargement of one or more lymph nodes—may result from increased production of lymphocytes or reticuloendothelial cells, or from infiltration of cells that aren't normally present. This sign may be generalized (involving three or more node groups) or localized. Generalized lymphadenopathy may be caused by an inflammatory process, such as bacterial or viral infection, connective tissue disease, an endocrine disorder, or neoplasm. Localized lymphadenopathy most commonly results from infection or trauma affecting a specific area. (See *Areas of localized lymphadenopathy,* page 432. See also *Causes of localized lymphadenopathy,* page 433.)

Normally, lymph nodes are discrete, mobile, soft, nontender and, except in children, nonpalpable. (However, palpable nodes may be normal in adults.) Nodes that are more than 3/8" (1 cm) in diameter are cause for concern. They may be tender and the skin overlying the lymph node may be erythematous, suggesting a draining lesion. Alternatively, they may be hard and fixed, tender or nontender, suggesting a malignant tumor.

History and physical examination

Ask the patient when he first noticed the swelling, and whether it's located on one side of his body or both. Are the swollen areas sore, hard, or red? Ask the patient if he has recently had an infection or other health problem. Also ask if a biopsy has ever been done on any node because this may indicate a previously diagnosed cancer. Find out if the patient has a family history of cancer.

Palpate the entire lymph node system to determine the extent of lymphadenopathy and to detect any other areas of local enlargement. Use the pads of your index and middle fingers to

Ballard Scale for calculating gestational age

Neuromuscular maturity

NEUROMUSCULAR MATURITY SIGN	SCORE -1	0	1	2	3	4	5	RECORD SCORE HERE
POSTURE	–	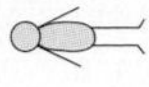	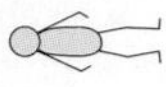	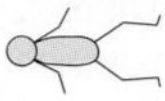	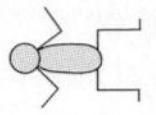	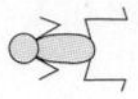	–	
SQUARE WINDOW (Wrist)	>90°	90°	60°	45°	30°	0°	–	
ARM RECOIL	–	 180°	 140° to 180°	 110° to 140°	 90° to 110°	 <90°	–	
POPLITEAL ANGLE	180°	160°	140°	120°	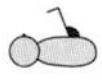 100°	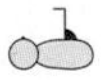 90°	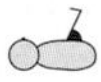 <90°	
SCARF SIGN	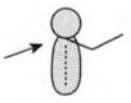	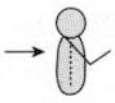	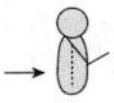	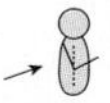	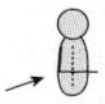	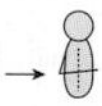	–	
HEEL TO EAR	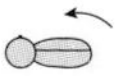	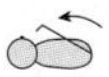	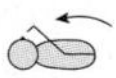	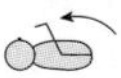	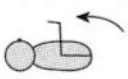	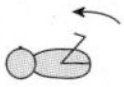	–	
							TOTAL NEUROMUSCULAR MATURITY SCORE	

Physical maturity

PHYSICAL MATURITY SIGN	SCORE -1	0	1	2	3	4	5	RECORD SCORE HERE
SKIN	Sticky, friable, transparent	Gelatinous, red, translucent	Smooth, pink; visible vessels	Superficial peeling or rash; few visible vessels	Cracking; pale areas; rare visible vessels	Parchment-like; deep cracking; no visible vessels	Leathery, cracked, wrinkled	
LANUGO	None	Sparse	Abundant	Thinning	Bald areas	Mostly bald	–	
PLANTAR SURFACE	Heel-toe 40 to 50 mm: –1; <40 mm: –2	>50 mm; no crease	Faint red marks	Anterior transverse crease only	Creases over anterior two-thirds	Creases over entire sole	–	
BREAST	Imperceptible	Barely perceptible	Flat areola, no bud	Stippled areola; 1- to 2-mm bud	Raised areola; 3- to 4-mm bud	Full areola; 5- to 10-mm bud	–	
EYE AND EAR	Lids fused, loosely: –1; tightly: –2	Lids open; pinna flat, stays folded	Slightly curved pinna; soft, slow recoil	Well-curved pinna; soft but ready recoil	Formed and firm; instant recoil	Thick cartilage; ear stiff	–	
GENITALIA, (Male)	Scrotum flat, smooth	Scrotum empty; faint rugae	Testes in upper canal; rare rugae	Testes descending; few rugae	Testes down; good rugae	Testes pendulous; deep rugae	–	
GENITALIA, (Female)	Clitoris prominent; labia flat	Prominent clitoris; small labia minora	Prominent clitoris; enlarging minora	Majora and minora equally prominent	Majora large; minora small	Majora cover clitoris and minora	–	
							TOTAL PHYSICAL MATURITY SCORE	

Adapted with permission from Ballard, J. L. "New Ballard Scale Expanded To Include Extremely Premature Infants," *Journal of Pediatrics* 119:417-23, 1991.

Score

Neuromuscular ______________________

Physical ______________________

Total ______________________

Maturity ratings

Total maturity score	Gestational age (weeks)
−10	20
−5	22
0	24
5	26
10	28
15	30
20	32
25	34
30	36
35	38
40	40
45	42
50	44

Gestestional age (weeks)

By dates ______________________

By ultrasound ______________________

By score ______________________

move the skin over underlying tissues at the nodal area. If you detect enlarged nodes, note their size in centimeters and whether they're fixed or mobile, tender or nontender, and erythematous or not. Note their texture: Is the node discrete, or does the area feel matted? If you detect tender, erythematous lymph nodes, check the area drained by that part of the lymph system for signs of infection, such as erythema and swelling. Also, palpate for and percuss the spleen.

Medical causes

◆ ***Acquired immunodeficiency syndrome.*** Besides lymphadenopathy, findings include a history of fatigue, night sweats, afternoon fevers, diarrhea, weight loss, and cough with several concurrent infections appearing soon afterward.

◆ ***Anthrax (cutaneous).*** Lymphadenopathy, malaise, headache and fever may develop along with a lesion that progresses into a painless, necrotic-centered ulcer.

◆ ***Brucellosis.*** Generalized lymphadenopathy usually affects cervical and axillary lymph nodes, making them tender. This disease usually begins insidiously with easy fatigability, malaise, headache, backache, anorexia, weight loss, and arthralgias; it may also begin abruptly with chills, fever that usually rises in the morning and subsides during the day, and diaphoresis.

◆ ***Chronic fatigue syndrome.*** Lymphadenopathy may occur with incapacitating fatigue, sore throat, low-grade fevers, myalgia, cognitive dysfunction, and sleep disturbances. The diagnosis is one of exclusion and the cause of this syndrome is unknown.

◆ ***Cytomegalovirus infection.*** Generalized lymphadenopathy occurs in the immunocompromised patient and is accompanied by fever, malaise, rash, and hepatosplenomegaly.

◆ ***Hodgkin's disease.*** The extent of lymphadenopathy reflects the stage of malignancy—from stage I involvement of a single lymph node region to stage IV generalized lymphadenopathy. Common early signs and symptoms include pruritus and, in older patients, fatigue, weakness, night sweats, malaise, weight loss, and unexplained fever (usually to 101° F [38.3° C]). Also, if mediastinal lymph nodes enlarge, tracheal and esophageal pressure produces dyspnea and dysphagia.

Areas of localized lymphadenopathy

When you detect an enlarged lymph node, palpate the entire lymph node system to determine the extent of lymphadenopathy. Include the lymph nodes indicated below in your assessment.

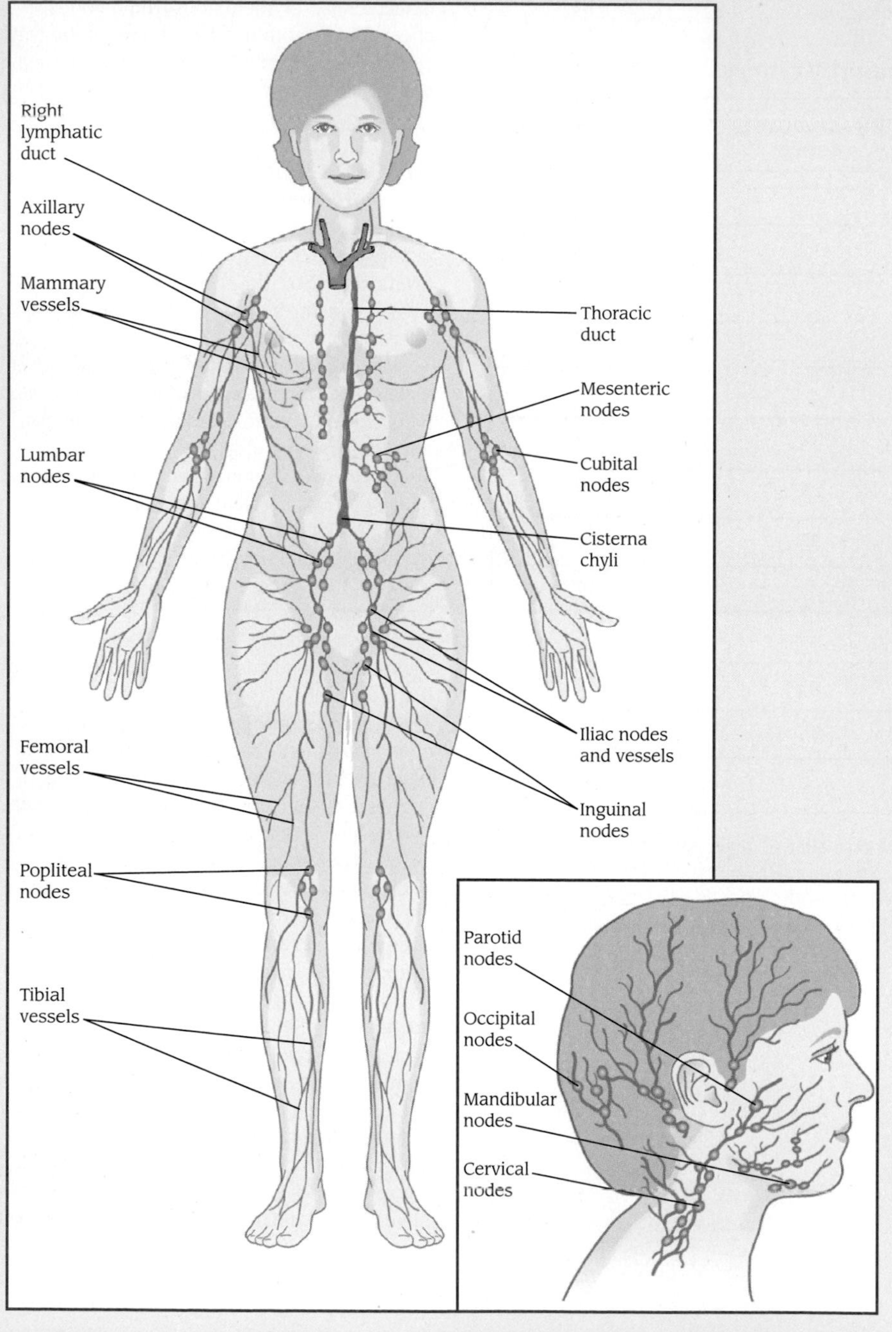

Causes of localized lymphadenopathy

Various disorders can cause localized lymphadenopathy, but this sign usually results from infection or trauma affecting the specific area. Here are some common causes of lymphadenopathy, listed according to the area affected.

Occipital
- Infection
- Roseola
- Scalp infection
- Seborrheic dermatitis
- Tick bite
- Tinea capitis

Auricular
- Erysipelas
- Herpes zoster ophthalmicus
- Infection
- Rubella
- Squamous cell carcinoma
- Styes or chalazion
- Tularemia

Supraclavicular
- Infection
- Neoplastic disease

Cervical
- Cat-scratch fever
- Facial or oral cancer
- Infection
- Mononucleosis
- Monocutaneous lymph node syndrome
- Rubella
- Rubeola
- Thyrotoxicosis
- Tonsillitis
- Tuberculosis
- Varicella

Axillary
- Breast cancer
- Infection
- Lymphoma
- Mastitis

Submaxillary and submental
- Cystic fibrosis
- Dental infection
- Gingivitis
- Glossitis
- Infection

Inguinal and femoral
- Carcinoma
- Chancroid
- Infection
- Lymphogranuloma venereum
- Syphilis

Popliteal
- Infection

◆ ***Kawasaki syndrome.*** Cervical lymphadenopathy is a characteristic sign of this potentially life-threatening illness. Affected individuals present with high, spiking fever, along with other diagnostic signs including erythema, bilateral conjunctival injection, and swelling in the peripheral extremities. Kawasaki syndrome isn't contagious, however the cause remains unknown and typically affects children under age 5. Prompt detection and treatment with I.V. gamma globulin is essential in preventing serious complications, such as coronary artery dilations and aneurysms.

◆ ***Leptospirosis.*** Lymphadenopathy occurs infrequently in this rare disease. More common findings include sudden onset of fever and chills, malaise, myalgia, headache, nausea and vomiting, and abdominal pain.

◆ ***Leukemia (acute lymphocytic).*** Generalized lymphadenopathy is accompanied by fatigue, malaise, pallor, and low fever. The patient also experiences prolonged bleeding time, swollen gums, weight loss, bone or joint pain, and hepatosplenomegaly.

◆ ***Leukemia (chronic lymphocytic).*** Generalized lymphadenopathy appears early, along with fatigue, malaise, and fever. As the disease progresses, hepatosplenomegaly, severe fatigue, and weight loss occur. Other late findings include bone tenderness, edema, pallor, dyspnea, tachycardia, palpitations, bleeding, anemia, and macular or nodular lesions.

◆ ***Lyme disease.*** Spread by the bite of certain ticks, Lyme disease begins with a skin lesion called erythema chronicum migrans. As the disease progresses, the patient may suffer from lymphadenopathy, constant malaise and fatigue, and intermittent headache, fever, chills, and aches. He may go on to develop arthralgias and, eventually, neurologic and cardiac abnormalities.

◆ ***Monkeypox.*** Lymphadenopathy is the one symptom that clearly distinguishes monkeypox from smallpox. Humans infected with monkeypox usually develop cervical or inguinal lymphadenopathy, along with other characteristic symptoms such as fever, chills, throat pain, muscle aches, and rash. This rare viral disease acquired its name after being discovered in laboratory monkeys; however, many other animals can carry this disease. Although the monkeypox virus is similar to smallpox, the smallpox vaccine is only used in limited circumstances to protect certain at-risk individuals against the disease.

◆ ***Mononucleosis (infectious).*** Characteristic, painful lymphadenopathy involves cervical, axillary, and inguinal nodes. Posterior cervical adenopathy is also common. Prodromal symptoms, such as malaise, fatigue, and headache, typically occur 3 to 5 days before the appearance of the classic triad of lymphadenopathy, sore throat, and temperature fluctuations with an evening peak of about 102° F (38.9° C). Hepatosplenomegaly may develop, along with findings of stomatitis, exudative tonsillitis, or pharyngitis.

◆ ***Mycosis fungoides.*** Lymphadenopathy occurs in stage III of this rare, chronic malignant lymphoma and is accompanied by ulcerated brownish red tumors that are painful and itchy.

◆ ***Non-Hodgkin's lymphoma.*** Painless enlargement of one or more peripheral lymph nodes is the most common sign of this disease, with generalized lymphadenopathy characterizing stage IV. Dyspnea, cough, and hepatosplenomegaly occur, along with systemic complaints of fever to 101° F (38.3° C), night sweats, fatigue, malaise, and weight loss.

◆ ***Plague* (Yersinia pestis).** Signs and symptoms of the bubonic form of this bacterial infection include lymphadenopathy, fever, and chills.

◆ ***Rheumatoid arthritis.*** Lymphadenopathy is an early, nonspecific finding associated with fatigue, malaise, continuous low fever, weight loss, and vague arthralgias and myalgias. Later, the patient develops joint tenderness, swelling, and warmth; joint stiffness after inactivity (especially in the morning); and subcutaneous nodules on the elbows. Eventually joint deformity, muscle weakness, and atrophy may occur.

◆ ***Sarcoidosis.*** Generalized, bilateral hilar and right paratracheal forms of lymphadenopathy (seen on chest X-ray) with splenomegaly are common. Initial findings are arthralgia, fatigue, malaise, weight loss, and pulmonary symptoms. Other findings vary with the site and extent of fibrosis. Typical cardiopulmonary findings include breathlessness, cough, substernal chest pain, and arrhythmias. About 90% of patients have an abnormal chest X-ray at sometime during their illness. Musculoskeletal and cutaneous features may include muscle weakness and pain, phalangeal and nasal mucosal lesions, and subcutaneous skin nodules. Common ophthalmic findings include eye pain, photophobia, and nonreactive pupils. Central nervous system involvement may produce cranial or peripheral nerve palsies and seizures.

◆ ***Sjögren's syndrome.*** Lymphadenopathy of the parotid and submaxillary nodes may occur in this rare disorder. Assessment reveals cardinal signs of dry mouth, eyes, and mucous membranes, which may be accompanied by photosensitivity, poor vision, eye fatigue, nasal crusting, and epistaxis.

◆ ***Syphilis (primary).*** Localized lymphadenopathy and a painless ulcer (canker) with an indurated border and relatively smooth base at the site of sexual exposure characterize this infection. The ulcer is usually single but more than one may be present.

◆ ***Syphilis (secondary).*** Generalized lymphadenopathy occurs in the second stage and may be accompanied by a macular, papular, pustular, or nodular rash on the arms, trunk, palms, soles, face, and scalp. A palmar rash is a significant diagnostic sign. Headache, malaise, anorexia, weight loss, nausea, vomiting, sore throat, and low fever may occur.

◆ ***Systemic lupus erythematosus.*** Generalized lymphadenopathy typically accompanies the hallmark butterfly rash, photosensitivity, Raynaud's phenomenon, and joint pain and stiffness. Pleuritic chest pain and cough may appear with systemic findings, such as fever, anorexia, and weight loss.

◆ ***Tuberculous lymphadenitis.*** Lymphadenopathy may be generalized or restricted to superficial lymph nodes. Affected lymph nodes may become fluctuant and drain to surrounding tissue. They may be accompanied by fever, chills, weakness, and fatigue.

◆ ***Waldenström's macroglobulinemia.*** Lymphadenopathy may appear along with hepatosplenomegaly. Associated findings include retinal hemorrhage, pallor, and signs of heart failure, such as jugular vein distention and crackles. The patient shows decreased level of consciousness, abnormal reflexes, and signs of peripheral neuritis. Weakness, fatigue, weight loss, epistaxis, and GI bleeding may also occur. Circulatory impairment occurs because of an increased viscosity of the blood.

OTHER CAUSES

◆ ***Drugs.*** Phenytoin may cause generalized lymphadenopathy.

◆ ***Immunizations.*** Typhoid vaccination may cause generalized lymphadenopathy.

SPECIAL CONSIDERATIONS

If the patient has fever above 101° F (38.3° C), don't automatically assume that the temperature should be lowered. A patient with a bacterial or viral infection must tolerate the fever, which may assist recovery. Provide an antipyretic if the patient is uncomfortable. Tepid sponge baths or a hypothermia blanket may also be used.

Expect to obtain blood for routine blood work, platelet and white blood cell counts, liver and renal function studies, erythrocyte sedimentation rate, and blood cultures. Prepare the patient for other scheduled diagnostic tests, such as chest X-ray, liver and spleen scan, lymph node biopsy, or lymphography, to visualize the lymphatic system. If tests reveal infection, check your facility's policy regarding infection control.

PEDIATRIC POINTERS

Infection is the most common cause of lymphadenopathy in children. The condition is commonly associated with otitis media and pharyngitis.

Provide an antipyretic if the child has a history of febrile seizures.

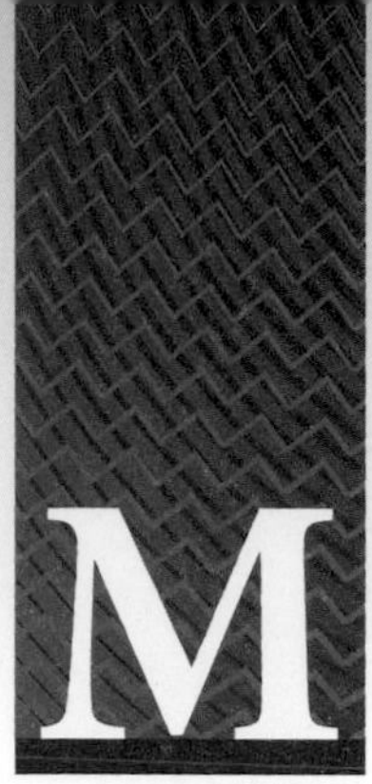

Masklike facies

A total loss of facial expression, masklike facies results from bradykinesia usually due to extrapyramidal damage. The rate of eye blinking is reduced to 1 to 4 blinks per minute, producing a characteristic "reptilian" stare. Although a neurologic disorder is the most common cause, masklike facies can also result from certain systemic diseases and the effects of drugs and toxins. The sign commonly develops insidiously, at first mistaken by the observer for depression or apathy.

History and physical examination

Ask the patient and his family or friends when they first noticed the masklike facial expression and any other signs or symptoms. Find out what medications the patient is taking, if any, and ask about any changes in dosage or schedule. Determine the degree of facial muscle weakness by asking the patient to smile and to wrinkle his forehead. Typically, the patient's responses are slowed.

Medical causes

◆ ***Dermatomyositis.*** Masklike facies reflects muscle soreness, weakness, and destruction extending from the face and neck to the shoulder and pelvic girdle. Dysphagia and dysphonia develop. Characteristic cutaneous signs involve edema and dusky lilac suffusion of the eyelid margin or periorbital tissue; an erythematous rash on the face, neck, upper back, chest, arms, and nail beds; and violet (Gottron's) papules dorsal to the interphalangeal joint.

◆ ***Facial palsy.*** Masklike facies is a hallmark of bilateral Bell's palsy and is characterized by periaural pain, hyperacusis, and disturbance of taste.

◆ ***Guillain-Barré syndrome.*** Bilateral facial weakness may occur in this disorder and is accompanied by hypoactive reflexes, paresthesia in the extremities, and limb weakness. Respiratory insufficiency may also occur, which requires pulmonary function testing and respiratory support.

◆ ***Myasthenia gravis.*** Ptosis and generalized facial muscle weakness are common in this disorder and may be accompanied by diplopia, dysarthria, dysphagia, and limb weakness. Weakness typically worsens with repetitive use of muscles, and also later in the day. Pulmonary function tests may be needed to rule out impending respiratory crisis.

◆ ***Parkinson's disease.*** Masklike facies occurs early but is commonly overlooked. This mask includes raised eyebrows and smooth facial muscles. More noticeable signs include muscle rigidity, which may be uniform (lead-pipe rigidity) or jerky (cogwheel rigidity), and an insidious tremor, which usually begins in the fingers (pill-roll tremor), increases during stress or anxiety, and decreases during purposeful movement or sleep. Typically, the patient exhibits stooped posture and propulsive gait, speaks in a monotone, and may develop drooling, dysphagia, and dysarthria.

◆ ***Scleroderma.*** A late sign, masklike facies develops along with a smooth, wrinkle-free appearance, "pinching" of the mouth and, possibly, contractures as facial skin becomes tight and inelastic. Other late features include pain, stiffness, and swelling of joints and foreshortened fingers. Skin on the fingers and then on the hands and forearms thickens and becomes taut and shiny. GI dysfunction produces frequent reflux and heartburn; weight loss; diarrhea or constipation; and malodorous floating stools.

Other causes

◆ ***Carbon monoxide poisoning.*** Masklike facies usually develops several weeks after acute poisoning. The patient may also have rigidity, dementia, impaired sensory function, choreoathetosis, generalized seizures, and myoclonus.
◆ ***Drugs.*** Phenothiazines (particularly piperazine derivatives) and other antipsychotic drugs commonly cause masklike facies as well as other extrapyramidal effects. In addition, metoclopramide and metyrosine can sometimes cause masklike facies. This sign usually improves when the drug dosage is reduced or the drug therapy discontinued.
◆ ***Manganese poisoning (chronic).*** Masklike facies develops gradually, along with a resting tremor and personality changes. The patient may also experience Huntington's disease, propulsive gait, dystonia, and rigidity. Later, extreme muscle weakness and fatigue occur.

Special considerations

If the patient's facial weakness results from Guillain-Barré syndrome or myasthenia gravis, be prepared to initiate emergency respiratory support.

Pediatric pointers

Masklike facies occurs in the juvenile form of Parkinson's disease.

Patient counseling

If the patient's masklike facies results from Parkinson's disease, explain to his family that the sign may hide facial clues to depression—a common symptom of Parkinson's disease.

McBurney's sign

A telltale indicator of localized peritoneal inflammation in acute appendicitis, McBurney's sign is tenderness elicited by palpating the right lower quadrant over McBurney's point. McBurney's point is about 2" (5 cm) above the anterior superior spine of the ilium, on the line between the spine and the umbilicus where pressure produces pain and tenderness in acute appendicitis. Before McBurney's sign is elicited, the abdomen is inspected for distention, auscultated for hypoactive or absent bowel sounds, and tested for tympany.

History and physical examination

Ask the patient to describe the abdominal pain. When did it begin? Does coughing, movement, eating, or elimination worsen or help relieve it? Also ask about the development of any other signs and symptoms such as vomiting and a low grade fever. Ask the patient to point with a finger to the spot where the pain is worst.

Continue light palpation of the patient's abdomen to detect additional tenderness, rigidity, guarding, or pain. Observe the patient's facial expression for signs of pain, such as grimacing or wincing. (See *Eliciting McBurney's sign,* page 438.) Auscultate the abdomen, noting decreased bowel sounds.

Medical causes

◆ ***Appendicitis.*** McBurney's sign appears within the first 2 to 12 hours after the onset of appendicitis, after initial pain in the epigastric and periumbilical area shifts to the right lower quadrant (McBurney's point). This persistent pain increases with walking or coughing. Nausea and vomiting may occur from the start. Boardlike abdominal rigidity and rebound tenderness that worsen as the condition progresses accompany cutaneous hyperalgia, fever, constipation or diarrhea, tachycardia, retractive respirations, anorexia, and moderate malaise.

Rupture of the appendix causes sudden cessation of pain. Then, signs and symptoms of peritonitis develop, such as severe abdominal pain, pallor, hypoactive or absent bowel sounds, diaphoresis, and high fever.

Special considerations

Draw blood for laboratory tests such as a complete blood count, including a white blood cell count, erythrocyte sedimentation rate, and blood cultures, and prepare the patient for abdominal X-rays to confirm appendicitis. Make sure the patient receives nothing by mouth, and expect to prepare the patient for an appendectomy. Administration of a cathartic or an enema

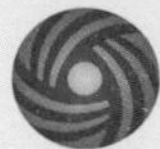

EXAMINATION TIP

Eliciting McBurney's sign

To elicit McBurney's sign, help the patient into a supine position, with his knees slightly flexed and his abdominal muscles relaxed. Then, palpate deeply and slowly in the right lower quadrant over McBurney's point—located about 2″ (5 cm) from the right anterior superior spine of the ilium, on a line between the spine and the umbilicus. Point pain and tenderness, a positive McBurney's sign, indicates appendicitis.

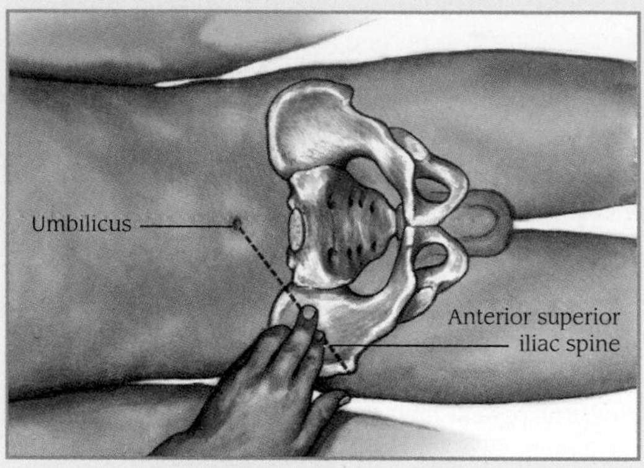

may cause the appendix to rupture and should be avoided.

Pediatric pointers

McBurney's sign is also elicited in children with appendicitis.

Geriatric pointers

In elderly patients, McBurney's sign (as well as other peritoneal signs) may be decreased or absent.

McMurray's sign

Often an indicator of medial meniscal injury, McMurray's sign is a palpable, audible click or pop elicited by rotating the tibia on the femur. It results when gentle manipulation of the leg traps torn cartilage and then lets it snap free. Because eliciting this sign forces the surface of the tibial plateau against the femoral condyles, such manipulation is contraindicated in patients with suspected fractures of the tibial plateau or femoral condyles.

A positive McMurray's sign augments other findings commonly associated with meniscal injury, such as severe joint line tenderness, locking or clicking of the joint, and decreased range of motion.

History and physical examination

After McMurray's sign has been elicited, find out if the patient is experiencing acute knee pain. Then ask him to describe any recent knee injury. For example, did his injury place twisting external or internal force on the knee, or did he experience blunt knee trauma from a fall? Also, ask about previous knee injury, surgery, prosthetic replacement, or other joint problems such as arthritis, which could have weakened the knee. Ask if anything aggravates or relieves the pain and if he needs assistance to walk.

Have the patient point to the exact area of pain. Assess the leg's range of motion, both passive and with resistance. Next, check for cruciate ligament stability by noting anterior or posterior movement of the tibia on the femur (drawer sign). Finally, measure the quadriceps muscles in both legs for symmetry. (See *Eliciting McMurray's sign*.)

Medical causes

◆ ***Meniscal tear.*** McMurray's sign can usually be elicited with this type of injury. Associated signs and symptoms include acute knee pain at the medial or lateral joint line (depending on injury site) and decreased range of motion or locking of the knee joint. Quadriceps weakening and atrophy may also occur.

Special considerations

Prepare the patient for knee X-rays, arthroscopy, and arthrography, and obtain any previous X-rays for comparison. If trauma precipitated the knee pain and McMurray's sign, an effusion or hemarthrosis may occur. Prepare the patient for aspiration of the joint. Immobilize and apply ice to the knee, and apply a cast or a knee immobilizer.

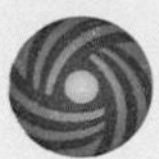

EXAMINATION TIP

Eliciting McMurray's sign

Eliciting McMurray's sign requires special training and gentle manipulation of the patient's leg to avoid extending a meniscal tear or locking the knee. If you've been trained to elicit McMurray's sign, place the patient in a supine position and flex his affected knee until his heel nearly touches his buttock. Place your thumb and index finger on either side of the knee joint space and grasp his heel with your other hand. Then rotate the foot and lower leg laterally to test the posterior aspect of the medial meniscus.

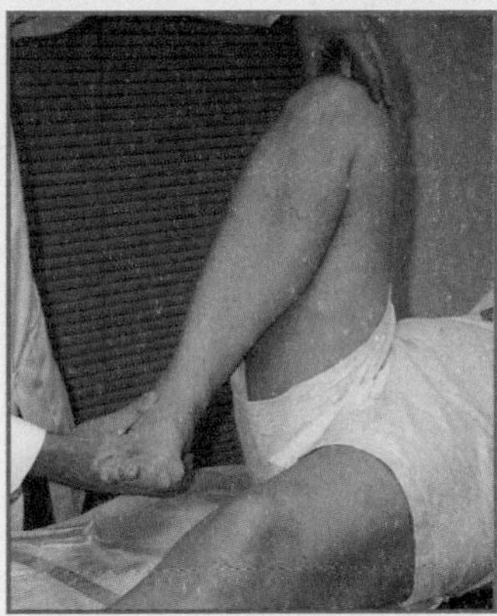

Keeping his foot in a lateral position, extend the knee to a 90-degree angle to test the anterior aspect of the medial meniscus. A palpable or audible click—a positive McMurray's sign—indicates injury to meniscal structures.

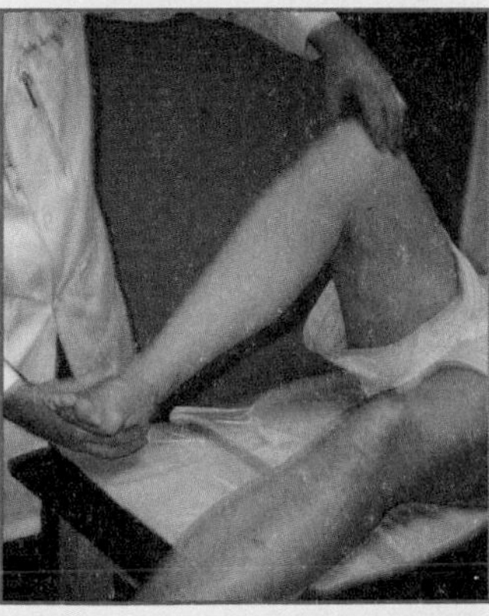

PEDIATRIC POINTERS

McMurray's sign in adolescents is usually elicited in meniscal tear caused by sports injury. It may also be elicited in children with congenital discoid meniscus.

PATIENT COUNSELING

Instruct the patient to elevate the affected leg and to perform up to 200 straight-leg raises per day. As appropriate, teach him how to use crutches. Also, tell him the prescribed dosage and schedule of any analgesics or anti-inflammatories. Help him adjust to lifestyle changes by providing support and including significant others in teaching.

Melena

A common sign of upper GI bleeding, melena is the passage of black, tarry stools containing digested blood. Characteristic color results from bacterial degradation and hydrochloric acid acting on the blood as it travels through the GI tract. At least 60 ml of blood is needed to produce this sign. (See *Comparing melena to hematochezia,* page 440.)

Severe melena can signal acute bleeding and life-threatening hypovolemic shock. Usually, melena indicates bleeding from the esophagus, stomach, or duodenum, although it can also indicate bleeding from the jejunum, ileum, or ascending colon. This sign can also result from swallowing blood, as in epistaxis; from taking certain drugs; or from ingesting alcohol. Because false melena may be caused by ingestion of lead, iron, bismuth, or licorice (which produces black stools without the presence of blood), all black stools should be tested for occult blood.

EMERGENCY INTERVENTIONS *If the patient is experiencing severe melena, quickly take orthostatic vital signs to detect hypovolemic shock. A decline of 10 mm Hg or more in systolic pressure or an increase of 10 beats/minute or more in pulse rate indicates volume depletion. Quickly examine patient for other signs of shock, such as tachycardia, tachypnea, and cool, clammy skin. Insert a large-bore I.V. catheter to administer replacement fluids and allow blood transfusion. Obtain hematocrit, prothrombin time, international normalized ratio, and partial thromboplastin time. Place the patient flat with his head turned to the side and his feet elevated. Administer supplemental oxygen as needed.*

Comparing melena to hematochezia

With GI bleeding, the site, amount, and rate of blood flow through the GI tract determine if a patient will develop melena (black, tarry stools) or hematochezia (bright red, bloody stools). Usually, melena indicates *upper* GI bleeding, and hematochezia indicates *lower* GI bleeding. However, with some disorders, melena may alternate with hematochezia. This chart helps differentiate these two commonly related signs.

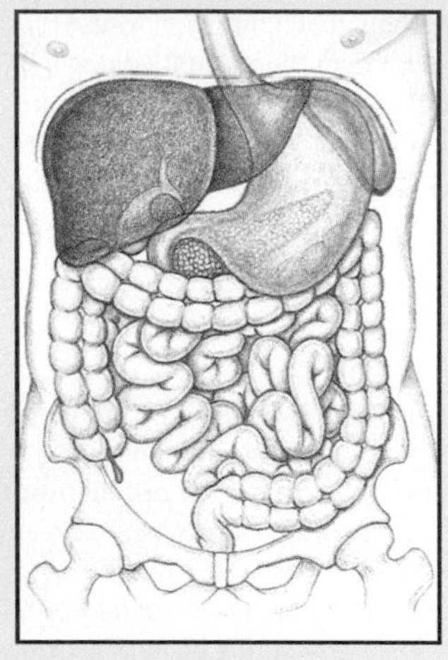

Sign	Sites	Characteristics
Melena	Esophagus, stomach, duodenum; rarely, jejunum, ileum, ascending colon.	Black, loose, tarry stools. Delayed or minimal passage of blood through GI tract.
Hematochezia	Usually distal to or affecting the colon; rapid hemorrhage of 1 L or more is associated with esophageal, stomach, or duodenal bleeding.	Bright red or dark, mahogany-colored stools; pure blood; blood mixed with formed stool; or bloody diarrhea. Reflects lower GI bleeding or rapid blood loss and passage of undigested blood through GI tract.

History and physical examination

If the patient's condition permits, ask when he discovered his stools were black and tarry. Ask about the frequency and quantity of bowel movements. Has he had melena before? Ask about other signs and symptoms, notably hematemesis or hematochezia, and about use of anti-inflammatories, alcohol, or other GI irritants. Also, find out if he has a history of GI lesions. Ask if the patient takes iron supplements, which may also cause black stools. Obtain a drug history, noting the use of warfarin or other anticoagulants.

Next, inspect the patient's mouth and nasopharynx for evidence of bleeding. Perform an abdominal examination that includes auscultation, palpation, and percussion.

Medical causes

◆ ***Colon cancer.*** On the right side of the colon, early tumor growth may cause melena accompanied by abdominal aching, pressure, or cramps. As the disease progresses, the patient develops weakness, fatigue, and anemia. Eventually, he also experiences diarrhea or obstipation, anorexia, weight loss, vomiting, and other signs and symptoms of intestinal obstruction.

With a tumor on the left side, melena is a rare sign until late in the disease. Early tumor growth commonly causes rectal bleeding with intermittent abdominal fullness or cramping and rectal pressure. As the disease progresses, the patient may develop obstipation, diarrhea, or pencil-shaped stools. At this stage, bleeding from the colon is signaled by melena or bloody stools.

◆ ***Ebola virus.*** Melena, hematemesis, and bleeding from the nose, gums, and vagina may occur later with this disorder. Patients usually report abrupt onset of headache, malaise, myalgia, high fever, diarrhea, abdominal pain, dehydration, and lethargy on the fifth day of illness. Pleuritic chest pain, dry hacking cough, and pharyngitis have also been noted. A maculopapular rash develops between days 5 and 7 of the illness.

◆ ***Esophageal cancer.*** Melena is a late sign of this malignant neoplastic disease that's three times more common in men than women. Increasing obstruction first produces painless dysphagia, then rapid weight loss. The patient may experience steady chest pain with substernal fullness, nausea, vomiting, and hematemesis. Other findings include hoarseness, persistent cough (possibly hemoptysis), hiccups, sore throat, and halitosis. In the later stages, signs and symptoms include painful dysphagia, anorexia, and regurgitation.

◆ ***Esophageal varices (ruptured).*** This life-threatening disorder can produce melena, hematochezia, and hematemesis. Melena is preceded by signs of shock, such as tachycardia, tachypnea, hypotension, and cool, clammy skin. Agitation or confusion signals developing hepatic encephalopathy.

◆ ***Gastric cancer.*** Melena and altered bowel habits may occur late with this uncommon cancer. More common findings include insidious onset of upper abdominal or retrosternal discomfort and chronic dyspepsia, which are unrelieved by antacids and exacerbated by food. Anorexia and slight nausea often occur, along with hematemesis, pallor, fatigue, weight loss, and a feeling of abdominal fullness.

◆ ***Gastritis.*** Melena and hematemesis are common. The patient may also experience mild epigastric or abdominal discomfort that's exacerbated by eating; belching; nausea; vomiting; and malaise.

◆ ***Malaria.*** Melena may accompany persistent high fever and orthostatic hypotension in severe malaria. Other features include hemoptysis, vomiting, abdominal pain, diarrhea, oliguria, and headache, seizures, delirium, or coma. These findings are interspersed throughout the malarial paroxysm—chills, then high fever, and then profuse diaphoresis.

◆ ***Mallory-Weiss syndrome.*** This condition is characterized by massive bleeding from the upper GI tract due to a tear in the mucous membrane of the esophagus or the junction of the esophagus and the stomach. Melena and hematemesis follow vomiting. Severe upper abdominal bleeding leads to signs and symptoms of shock, such as tachycardia, tachypnea, hypotension, and cool, clammy skin. The patient may also report epigastric or back pain.

◆ ***Mesenteric vascular occlusion.*** This life-threatening disorder produces slight melena with 2 to 3 days of persistent, mild abdominal pain. Later, abdominal pain becomes severe and may be accompanied by tenderness, distention, guarding, and rigidity. The patient may also experience anorexia, vomiting, fever, and profound shock.

◆ ***Peptic ulcer.*** Melena may signal life-threatening hemorrhage from vascular penetration. The patient may also develop decreased appetite, nausea, vomiting, hematemesis, hematochezia, and left epigastric pain that's gnawing, burning, or sharp and may be described as heartburn or indigestion. With hypovolemic shock come tachycardia, tachypnea, hypotension, dizziness, syncope, and cool, clammy skin.

◆ ***Small-bowel tumors.*** These tumors may bleed and produce melena. Other signs and symptoms include abdominal pain, distention, and increasing frequency and pitch of bowel sounds.

◆ ***Thrombocytopenia.*** Melena or hematochezia may accompany other manifestations of bleeding tendency: hematemesis, epistaxis, petechiae, ecchymoses, hematuria, vaginal bleeding, and characteristic blood-filled oral bullae. Typically, the patient displays malaise, fatigue, weakness, and lethargy.

◆ ***Typhoid fever.*** Melena or hematochezia occurs late in this disorder and may occur with hypotension and hypothermia. Other late findings include mental dullness or delirium, marked abdominal distention and diarrhea, marked weight loss, and profound fatigue.

◆ ***Yellow fever.*** Melena, hematochezia, and hematemesis are ominous signs of hemorrhage, a classic feature, which occurs along with jaundice. Other findings include fever, headache, nausea, vomiting, epistaxis, albuminuria, petechiae and mucosal hemorrhage, and dizziness.

Other causes

◆ ***Drugs and alcohol.*** Aspirin, other nonsteroidal anti-inflammatories, or alcohol can cause melena as a result of gastric irritation.

Special considerations

Monitor vital signs, and look closely for signs of hypovolemic shock. For general comfort, encourage bed rest, and keep the patient's perianal area clean and dry to prevent skin irritation and breakdown. A nasogastric tube may be necessary to assist with drainage of gastric contents and decompression. Prepare him for diagnostic tests, including blood studies, gastroscopy or other endoscopic studies, barium swallow, and upper GI series. Prepare the patient for blood transfusions as indicated by his hematocrit.

Pediatric pointers

Neonates may experience melena neonatorum due to extravasation of blood into the alimentary canal. In older children, melena usually results from peptic ulcer, gastritis, or Meckel's diverticulum.

Geriatric pointers

In elderly patients with recurrent intermittent GI bleeding without a clear etiology, angiography or exploratory laparotomy should be considered once the risk from continued anemia is deemed to outweigh the risk associated with the procedures.

Menorrhagia

Abnormally heavy or long menstrual bleeding, menorrhagia may occur as a single episode or a chronic sign. In menorrhagia, bleeding is heavier than the patient's normal menstrual flow; menstrual blood loss is 80 ml or more per monthly period. A form of dysfunctional uterine bleeding, menorrhagia can result from endocrine and hematologic disorders, stress, and certain drugs and procedures.

EMERGENCY INTERVENTIONS *Evaluate hemodynamic status by taking orthostatic vital signs. Insert a large-gauge I.V. catheter to begin fluid replacement if the patient shows an increase of 10 beats/minute in pulse rate, a decrease of 10 mm Hg in systolic blood pressure, or other signs of hypovolemic shock, such as pallor, tachycardia, tachypnea, and cool, clammy skin. Place the patient in a supine position with her feet elevated, and administer supplemental oxygen as needed.*

Use menstrual pads to obtain information related to the quality and quantity of bleeding. Then prepare the patient for a pelvic examination to help determine the cause of bleeding.

History and physical examination

When the patient's condition permits, obtain a history. Determine her age at menarche, the average duration of menstrual periods, and the interval between them. Establish the date of the patient's last menses, and ask about any recent changes in her normal menstrual pattern. Have the patient describe the character and amount of bleeding. For example, how many pads or tampons does the patient use? Has she noted clots or tissue in the blood? Also ask about the development of other signs and symptoms before and during the menstrual period.

Next, ask if the patient is sexually active. Does she use a method of birth control? If so, what kind? Could the patient be pregnant? Be sure to note the number of pregnancies, the outcome of each, and any pregnancy-related complications. Find out the dates of her most recent pelvic examination and Papanicolaou smear and the details of any previous gynecologic infections or neoplasms. Also, be sure to ask about any previous episodes of abnormal bleeding and the outcome of any treatment. If possible, obtain a pregnancy history of the patient's mother, and determine if the patient was exposed in utero to diethylstilbestrol. (This drug has been linked to vaginal adenosis.)

Be sure to ask the patient about her general health and medical history. Note particularly if the patient or her family has a history of thyroid, adrenal, or hepatic disease; blood dyscrasias; or tuberculosis because these may predispose the patient to menorrhagia. Also, ask about the patient's past surgical procedures and any recent emotional stress. Find out if the patient has undergone X-ray or other radiation therapy, because this may indicate prior treatment for menorrhagia. Obtain a thorough drug and alcohol history, noting the use of anticoagulants or aspirin. Perform a pelvic examination, and obtain blood and urine samples for pregnancy testing.

Medical causes

◆ ***Blood dyscrasias.*** Menorrhagia is one of several possible signs of a bleeding disorder. Other possible associated findings include epistaxis, bleeding gums, purpura, hematemesis, hematuria, and melena.

◆ ***Endometriosis.*** Menorrhagia may be a sign of this disorder, in which endometrial tissue is found outside the lining of the uterine cavity. However, the classic symptom is dysmenorrhea. Other findings depend on the location of the ectopic tissue outside the uterus but may include dyspareunia, suprapubic pain, dysuria, nausea, vomiting, abdominal cramps, cyclic pelvic pain, and infertility. Often a tender, fixed adnexal mass is palpable on bimanual examination.

◆ ***Hypothyroidism.*** Menorrhagia is a common early sign and is accompanied by such nonspecific findings as fatigue, cold intolerance, constipation, and weight gain despite anorexia. As hypothyroidism progresses, intellectual and motor activity decrease; the skin becomes dry, pale, cool, and doughy; the hair becomes dry and sparse; and the nails become thick and brittle. Myalgia, hoarseness, decreased libido, and infertility commonly occur. Eventually, the patient develops a characteristic dull, expressionless face and edema of the face, hands, and feet.

Also, deep tendon reflexes are delayed, and bradycardia and abdominal distention may occur.

◆ ***Uterine fibroids.*** Menorrhagia is the most common sign, but other forms of abnormal uterine bleeding as well as dysmenorrhea or leukorrhea, can also occur. Possible related findings include abdominal pain, a feeling of abdominal heaviness, backache, constipation, urinary urgency or frequency, and an enlarged uterus, which is usually nontender.

Other causes

◆ ***Drugs.*** Use of a hormonal contraceptive may cause sudden onset of profuse, prolonged menorrhagia. Anticoagulants have also been associated with excessive menstrual flow. Injectable or implanted contraceptives may cause menorrhagia in some women.

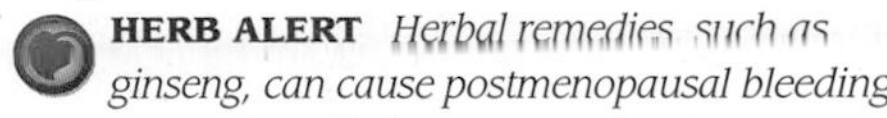

HERB ALERT *Herbal remedies, such as ginseng, can cause postmenopausal bleeding.*

◆ ***Intrauterine devices.*** Menorrhagia can result from the use of intrauterine contraceptive devices.

Special considerations

Continue to monitor the patient closely for signs of hypovolemia. Encourage the patient to maintain adequate fluid intake. Monitor intake and output, and estimate uterine blood loss by recording the number of sanitary napkins or tampons used during an abnormal period and comparing this with usage during a normal period. To help decrease blood flow, encourage the patient to rest and to avoid strenuous activities. Obtain blood samples for hematocrit, prothrombin time, partial thromboplastin time, and international normalized ratio levels.

Pediatric pointers

Irregular menstrual function in young girls may be accompanied by hemorrhage and resulting anemia.

Geriatric pointers

In postmenopausal women, menorrhagia cannot occur. In such patients, vaginal bleeding is usually caused by endometrial atrophy. Malignancy must be ruled out.

Metrorrhagia

Metrorrhagia—uterine bleeding that occurs irregularly between menstrual periods—is usually light, although it can range from staining to hemorrhage. Usually, this common sign reflects slight physiologic bleeding from the endometrium during ovulation. However, metrorrhagia may be the only indication of an underlying gynecologic disorder and can also result from stress, drugs, treatments, and intrauterine devices.

History and physical examination

Begin your evaluation by obtaining a thorough menstrual history. Ask the patient when she began menstruating and about the duration of menstrual periods, the interval between them, and the average number of tampons or pads she uses. When does metrorrhagia usually occur in relation to her period? Does she experience other signs or symptoms? Find out the date of her last menses, and ask about any other recent changes in her normal menstrual pattern. Get details of any previous gynecologic problems. If applicable, obtain a contraceptive and obstetric history. Record the dates of her last Papanicolaou smear and pelvic examination. Ask the patient when she last had sex and whether or not it was protected. Next, ask about her general health and any recent changes. Is she under emotional stress? If possible, obtain a pregnancy history of the patient's mother. Was the patient exposed in utero to diethylstilbestrol? (This drug has been linked to vaginal adenosis.)

Perform a pelvic examination if indicated, and obtain blood and urine samples for pregnancy testing.

Medical causes

◆ ***Cervicitis.*** This nonspecific infection may cause spontaneous bleeding, spotting, or posttraumatic bleeding. Assessment reveals red, granular, irregular lesions on the external cervix. Purulent vaginal discharge (with or without odor), lower abdominal pain, and fever may occur.

◆ ***Dysfunctional uterine bleeding.*** Abnormal uterine bleeding not caused by pregnancy or major gynecologic disorders usually occurs as metrorrhagia, although menorrhagia is possible. Bleeding may be profuse or scant, intermittent or constant.

◆ ***Endometrial polyps.*** In most patients, this disorder causes abnormal bleeding, usually intermenstrual or postmenopausal; however, some patients do remain asymptomatic.

◆ ***Endometriosis.*** Metrorrhagia (usually premenstrual) may be the only indication of this disorder, or it may accompany cyclical pelvic discomfort, infertility, and dyspareunia. A tender, fixed adnexal mass may be palpable on bimanual examination.

◆ ***Endometritis.*** This disorder causes metrorrhagia, purulent vaginal discharge, and enlargement of the uterus. It also produces fever, lower abdominal pain, and abdominal muscle spasm.

◆ ***Gynecologic cancer.*** Metrorrhagia is commonly an early sign of cervical or uterine cancer. Later, the patient may experience weight loss, pelvic pain, fatigue and, possibly, an abdominal mass.

◆ ***Syphilis.*** Primary- or secondary-stage syphilis may cause metrorrhagia and postcoital bleeding. In primary syphilis, one or more usually painless chancres erupt on the genitalia and possibly other areas. In secondary syphilis, generalized lymphadenopathy may appear, along with a rash on the arms, trunk, palms, soles, face, and scalp.

◆ ***Uterine leiomyomas.*** Besides metrorrhagia, these tumors may cause increasing abdominal girth and heaviness in the abdomen, constipation, and urinary frequency or urgency. The patient may report pain if the uterus attempts to expel the tumor through contractions and if the tumors twist or necrose after circulatory occlusion or infection, but many women with leiomyomas are asymptomatic.

◆ ***Vaginal adenosis.*** This disorder commonly produces metrorrhagia. Palpation reveals roughening or nodules in affected vaginal areas.

Other causes

◆ ***Drugs.*** Anticoagulants and oral, injectable, or implanted contraceptives may cause metrorrhagia.

HERB ALERT *Herbal remedies, such as ginseng, can cause postmenopausal bleeding.*

◆ ***Surgery and procedures.*** Cervical conization and cauterization may cause metrorrhagia.

Special considerations

Encourage bed rest to reduce bleeding. Give an analgesic for discomfort.

Miosis

Miosis—pupillary constriction caused by contraction of the sphincter muscle in the iris—occurs normally as a response to fatigue, increased light, or administration of a miotic; as part of the eye's accommodation reflex; and as part of the aging process (pupil size steadily decreases from adolescence to about age 60). However, it can also stem from an ocular or neurologic disorder, trauma, use of a systemic drug, or contact lens overuse. A rare form of miosis—Argyll Robertson pupils—can stem from tabes dorsalis and diverse neurologic disorders. Occurring bilaterally, these miotic (often pinpoint), unequal, and irregularly shaped pupils don't dilate properly with mydriatic use and fail to react to light, although they do constrict on accommodation.

History and physical examination

Begin by asking the patient if he has experienced other ocular symptoms, and have him describe their onset, duration, and intensity. Does he wear contact lenses? During your history, be sure to ask about trauma, serious systemic disease, and use of topical and systemic drugs.

Next, perform a thorough eye examination. Test visual acuity in each eye, with and without correction, paying particular attention to blurred or decreased vision in the miotic eye. Examine and compare both pupils for size (many persons have a normal discrepancy), color, shape, reaction to light, accommodation, and consensual light response. Examine both eyes for additional signs, and then evaluate extraocular muscle function by assessing the six cardinal fields of gaze.

Medical causes

◆ ***Cerebrovascular arteriosclerosis.*** Miosis is usually unilateral, depending on the site and extent of vascular damage. Other findings include visual blurring, slurred speech or possibly aphasia, loss of muscle tone, memory loss, vertigo, and headache.

◆ ***Cluster headache.*** Ipsilateral miosis, tearing, conjunctival injection, and ptosis commonly accompany a severe cluster headache, along with facial flushing and sweating, bradycardia, restlessness, and nasal stuffiness or rhinorrhea.

◆ ***Corneal foreign body.*** Miosis in the affected eye occurs with pain, a foreign-body sensation, slight vision loss, conjunctival injection, photophobia, and profuse tearing.

◆ ***Corneal ulcer.*** Miosis in the affected eye appears with moderate pain, visual blurring and possibly some vision loss, and diffuse conjunctival injection.

◆ ***Horner's syndrome.*** Moderate miosis is common in this neurologic syndrome and occurs ipsilaterally to the spinal cord lesion. Related ipsilateral findings include a sluggish pupillary reflex, slight enophthalmos, moderate ptosis, facial anhidrosis, transient conjunctival injection, and vascular headache. When the syndrome is congenital, the iris on the affected side may appear lighter.

◆ ***Hyphema.*** Usually the result of blunt trauma, hyphema can cause miosis with moderate pain, visual blurring, diffuse conjunctival injection, and slight eyelid swelling. The eyeball may feel harder than normal.

◆ ***Iritis (acute).*** Miosis typically occurs in the affected eye along with decreased pupillary reflex, severe eye pain, photophobia, visual blurring, conjunctival injection and, possibly, pus accumulation in the anterior chamber. The eye appears cloudy, the iris bulges, and the pupil is constricted on ophthalmic examination.

◆ ***Neuropathy.*** Two forms of neuropathy occasionally produce Argyll Robertson pupils. With diabetic neuropathy, related effects include paresthesia and other sensory disturbances, extremity pain, orthostatic hypotension, impotence, incontinence, and leg muscle weakness and atrophy.

With alcoholic neuropathy, related effects include progressive, variable muscle weakness and wasting, various sensory disturbances, and hypoactive deep tendon reflexes.

◆ ***Parry-Romberg syndrome.*** This facial hemiatrophy typically produces miosis, sluggish pupillary reflexes, enophthalmos, nystagmus, ptosis, and different-colored irises.

◆ ***Pontine hemorrhage.*** Bilateral miosis is characteristic, along with rapid onset of coma, total paralysis, decerebrate posture, absent doll's eye sign, and a positive Babinski's sign.

◆ ***Tabes dorsalis.*** This tertiary form of syphilis is marked by Argyll Robertson pupils, a wide base ataxic gait, paresthesia, loss of proprioception, analgesia, thermanesthesia, Charcot's joints, incontinence and, possibly, impotence.

◆ ***Uveitis.*** Anterior uveitis commonly produces miosis in the affected eye, moderate-to-severe eye pain, severe conjunctival injection, photophobia, and pus in the anterior chamber.

With posterior uveitis, miosis is accompanied by gradual onset of eye pain, photophobia, visual floaters, visual blurring, conjunctival injection and, commonly, distorted pupil shape.

Other causes

◆ ***Chemical burns.*** An opaque cornea may make miosis hard to detect. However, chemical burns may also cause moderate-to-severe pain, diffuse conjunctival injection, inability to keep the eye open, visual blurring, and blistering.

◆ ***Drugs.*** Such topical drugs as acetylcholine, carbachol, echothiophate iodide, and pilocarpine are used to treat eye disorders specifically for their miotic effect. Such systemic drugs as barbiturates, cholinergics, anticholinesterases, clonidine hydrochloride (overdose), opiates, and reserpine also cause miosis, as does deep anesthesia.

Special considerations

Because any ocular abnormality can be a source of fear and anxiety, reassure and support the patient. Clearly explain any diagnostic tests ordered, which may include a complete ophthalmologic examination or a neurologic workup.

Pediatric pointers

Miosis is common in neonates, simply because they're asleep or sleepy most of the time. Bilateral miosis occurs with congenital microcoria, an uncommon bilateral disease transmitted as an autosomal dominant trait and marked by the absence of the dilator muscle of the pupil. At birth, these infants have pupils less than 2 mm and seem to gaze far away.

Moon face

Moon face, a distinctive facial adiposity, usually indicates hypercortisolism resulting from ectopic or excessive pituitary production of corticotropin, adrenal adenoma or carcinoma, or long-term glucocorticoid therapy. Its typical characteristics include marked facial roundness and puffiness, a double chin, a prominent upper lip, and full supraclavicular fossae. Although the presence of moon face doesn't help differentiate causes of hypercortisolism, it does indicate a need for diagnostic testing.

History and physical examination

Ask the patient when he first noticed his facial adiposity, and try to obtain a preonset photograph to help evaluate the extent of the change.

Ask about weight gain and any personal or family history of endocrine disorders, obesity, or cancer. Has the patient noticed any fatigue, irritability, depression, or confusion? If the patient is a female of childbearing age, determine the date of her last menses and whether she's experienced any menstrual irregularities.

If the patient is receiving a glucocorticoid, ask the name of the drug, dosage and schedule, route of administration, and reason for therapy. Also ask if the dosage has ever been modified and, if so, when and why.

Take the patient's vital signs, weight, and height. Assess the patient's overall appearance for other characteristic signs of hypercortisolism, including virilism in a female or gynecomastia in a male. Also assess for purple striae on the skin, muscle weakness due to loss of muscle mass from increased catabolism, and skeletal growth retardation in children.

MEDICAL CAUSES

◆ ***Hypercortisolism.*** Moon face varies in severity, depending on the degree of cortisol excess and weight gain. The patient typically exhibits buffalo hump, truncal obesity with slender arms and legs, and thin, transparent skin with purple striae and ecchymoses. Other cushingoid features include acne, diaphoresis, fatigue, muscle wasting and weakness, poor wound healing, elevated blood pressure, and personality changes.

In addition to these findings, a woman may experience hirsutism and amenorrhea or oligomenorrhea; a man may experience gynecomastia and impotence.

OTHER CAUSES

◆ ***Drugs.*** Most cases (more than 99%) of moon face result from prolonged use of a glucocorticoid, such as cortisone, dexamethasone, hydrocortisone, or prednisone.

SPECIAL CONSIDERATIONS

Relieve the patient's concern about his body image by explaining that moon face and other disconcerting cushingoid effects can usually be corrected by treating the underlying disorder or by discontinuing or modifying glucocorticoid therapy. Explain to the patient that he should only discontinue or modify glucocorticoid therapy as directed by the physician.

Clearly explain to the patient any diagnostic tests ordered. These may include serum and urine 17-hydroxycorticosteroid studies; a 2-day, low-dose dexamethasone test followed by a 2-day, high-dose dexamethasone test; plasma corticotropin studies; and a corticotropin-releasing hormone test.

PEDIATRIC POINTERS

Moon face is rare in children. In an infant or a young child, it usually indicates adrenal adenoma or carcinoma or, rarely, cri du chat syndrome. After age 7, it usually indicates abnormal pituitary secretion of corticotropin in bilateral adrenal hyperplasia.

Mouth lesions

Mouth lesions include ulcers (the most common type), cysts, firm nodules, hemorrhagic lesions, papules, vesicles, bullae, and erythematous lesions. They may occur anywhere on the lips, cheeks, hard and soft palate, salivary glands, tongue, gingivae, or mucous membranes. Many are painful and can be readily detected. Some, however, are asymptomatic; when they occur deep in the mouth, they may be discovered only through a complete oral examination. (See *Common mouth lesions.*)

Mouth lesions can result from trauma, infection, systemic disease, drug use, or radiation therapy.

HISTORY AND PHYSICAL EXAMINATION

Begin your evaluation with a thorough history. Ask the patient when the lesions appeared and whether he has noticed any pain, odor, or drainage. Also ask about associated complaints, particularly skin lesions. Obtain a complete drug history, including drug allergies and antibiotic use, and a complete medical history. Note especially any malignancy, sexually transmitted disease, I.V. drug use, recent infection, or trauma. Ask about his dental history, including oral hygiene habits, frequency of dental examinations, and the date of his most recent dental visit.

Next, perform a complete oral examination, noting lesion sites and character. Examine the patient's lips for color and texture. Inspect and palpate the buccal mucosa and tongue for color, texture, and contour; note especially any painless ulcers on the sides or base of the tongue. Hold the tongue with a piece of gauze, lift it, and examine its underside and the floor of the mouth. Depress the tongue with a tongue blade, and examine the oropharynx. Inspect the teeth and gums, noting missing, broken, or discolored teeth; dental caries; excessive debris; and bleeding, inflamed, swollen, or discolored gums.

Palpate the neck for adenopathy, especially in patients who smoke tobacco or use alcohol excessively.

MEDICAL CAUSES

◆ ***Acquired immunodeficiency syndrome (AIDS).*** Oral lesions may be an early indication of the immunosuppression that's characteristic of this disease. Fungal infections can occur, with oral candidiasis being the most common. Bacterial or viral infections of oral mucosa,

Common mouth lesions

SQUAMOUS CELL CARCINOMA

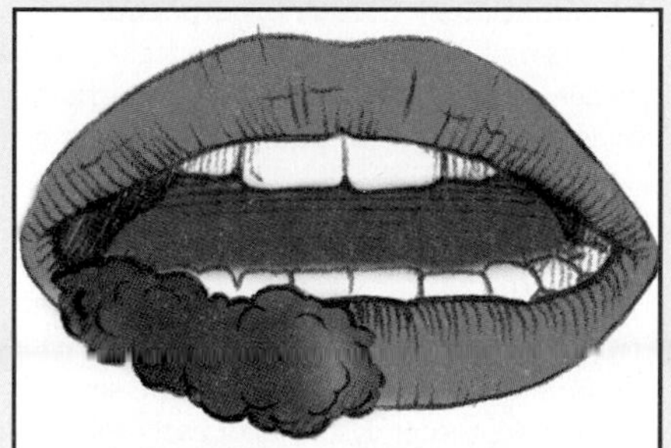

LICHEN PLANUS

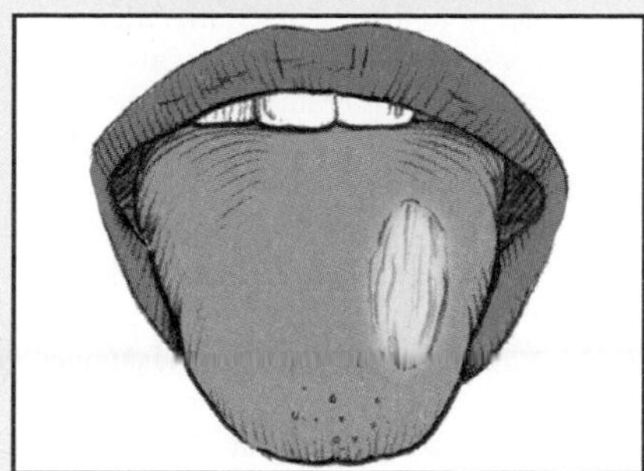

APHTHOUS STOMATITIS

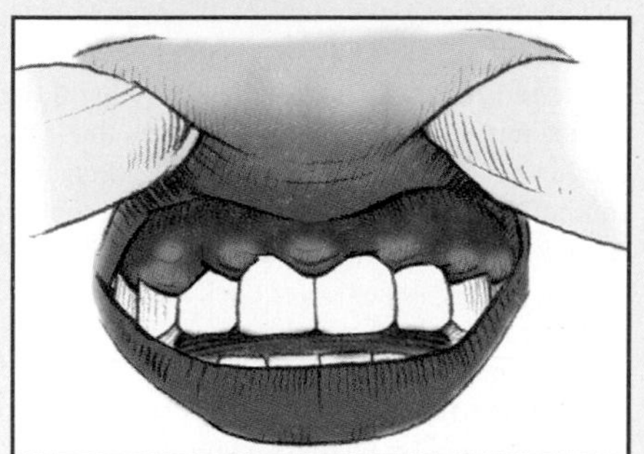

GINGIVAL HYPERPLASIA

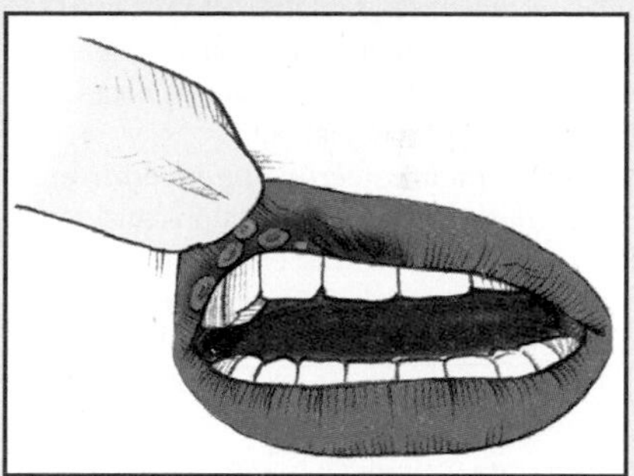

tongue, gingivae, and periodontal tissue may also occur.

The primary oral neoplasm associated with AIDS is Kaposi's sarcoma. The tumor is usually found on the hard palate and may appear initially as an asymptomatic, flat or raised lesion, ranging in color from red to blue to purple. As these tumors grow, they may ulcerate and become painful.

◆ ***Actinomycosis (cervicofacial).*** This chronic fungal infection typically produces small, firm, flat, usually painless swellings on the oral mucosa and under the skin of the jaw and neck. Swellings may indurate and abscess, producing fistulas and sinus tracts with a characteristic purulent yellow discharge.

◆ ***Behçet's syndrome.*** This chronic, progressive syndrome that generally affects young males produces small, painful ulcers on the lips, gums, buccal mucosa, and tongue. In severe cases, the ulcers also develop on the palate, pharynx, and esophagus. The ulcers typically have a reddened border and are covered with a gray or yellow exudate. Similar lesions appear on the scrotum and penis or labia majora; small pustules or papules on the trunk and limbs; and painful erythematous nodules on the shins. Ocular lesions may also develop.

◆ ***Candidiasis.*** This common fungal infection characteristically produces soft, elevated plaques on the buccal mucosa, tongue, and sometimes the palate, gingivae, and floor of the mouth; the plaques may be wiped away. The lesions of acute atrophic candidiasis are red and painful. The lesions of chronic hyperplastic candidiasis are white and firm. Localized areas of redness, pruritus, and foul odor may be present.

◆ ***Discoid lupus erythematosus.*** Oral lesions are common, typically appearing on the tongue, buccal mucosa, and palate as erythematous areas with white spots and radiating white striae. Associated findings include skin lesions on the face, possibly extending to the neck, ears, and scalp; if the scalp is involved, alopecia may result. Hair follicles are enlarged and filled with scale.

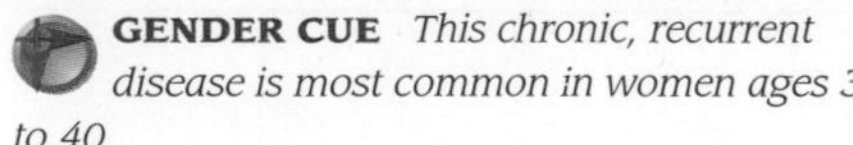

GENDER CUE *This chronic, recurrent disease is most common in women ages 30 to 40.*

◆ ***Epulis (giant cell).*** This rare tumor or growth occurs on the gingival or alveolar process, anterior to the molars. Dark red, pedunculated or sessile, and 0.5 to 1.5 cm in diameter, it commonly ulcerates to produce a concave defect in the underlying bone. Gingivae bleed easily with slight trauma.

◆ ***Erythema multiforme.*** This acute inflammatory skin disease produces sudden onset of vesicles and bullae on the lips and buccal mucosa. Also, erythematous macules and papules form symmetrically on the hands, arms, feet, legs, face, and neck and, possibly, in the eyes and on the genitalia. Lymphadenopathy may also occur. With visceral involvement, other findings include fever, malaise, cough, throat and chest pain, vomiting, diarrhea, myalgias, arthralgias, fingernail loss, blindness, hematuria, and signs of renal failure.

◆ ***Gingivitis (acute necrotizing ulcerative).*** This recurring periodontal condition causes a sudden onset of gingival ulcers covered with a grayish white pseudomembrane. Other findings include tender or painful gingivae, intermittent gingival bleeding, halitosis, enlarged lymph nodes in the neck, and fever.

◆ ***Gonorrhea.*** Painful lip ulcerations may occur, along with rough, reddened, bleeding gingivae (possibly necrotic and covered by a yellowish pseudomembrane), and a swollen, ulcerated tongue. Related effects vary. Most men develop dysuria, purulent urethral discharge, and a reddened, edematous urinary meatus. Most women remain asymptomatic, but others develop inflammation and a greenish yellow cervical discharge.

◆ ***Herpes simplex 1.*** With primary infection, a brief period of prodromal tingling and itching, which is accompanied by fever and pharyngitis, is followed by eruption of small and irritating vesicles on any part of the oral mucosa, especially the tongue, gums, and cheeks. Vesicles form on an erythematous base and then rupture, leaving a painful ulcer, followed by a yellowish crust. Other findings include submaxillary lymphadenopathy, increased salivation, halitosis, anorexia, and keratoconjunctivitis.

◆ ***Herpes zoster.*** This common viral infection may produce painful vesicles on the buccal mucosa, tongue, uvula, pharynx, and larynx. Small red nodules often erupt unilaterally around the thorax or vertically on the arms and legs, and rapidly become vesicles filled with clear fluid or pus; vesicles dry and form scabs about 10 days after eruption. Fever and general malaise accompany pruritus, paresthesia or hyperesthesia, and tenderness along the course of the involved sensory nerve.

◆ ***Inflammatory fibrous hyperplasia.*** This painless nodular swelling of the buccal mucosa typically results from cheek trauma or irritation and is characterized by pink, smooth, pedunculated areas of soft tissue.

◆ ***Leukoplakia, erythroplakia.*** Leukoplakia is a white lesion that cannot be removed simply by rubbing the mucosal surface—unlike candidiasis. It may occur in response to chronic irritation from dentures or tobacco or pipe smoking, or it may represent dysplasia or early squamous cell carcinoma.

Erythroplakia is red and edematous and has a velvety surface. About 90% of all cases of erythroplakia are either dysplasia or cancer.

◆ ***Lichen planus.*** Oral lesions develop on the buccal mucosa or, less commonly, on the tongue as painless, white or gray, velvety, threadlike papules. These precede the eruption of violet papules with white lines or spots, usually on the genitalia, lower back, ankles, and anterior lower legs; pruritus; nails with longitudinal ridges; and alopecia.

◆ ***Mucous duct obstruction.*** Obstruction produces a ranula—a painless, slow-growing mucocele on the floor of the mouth near the ducts of the submandibular and sublingual glands.

◆ ***Pemphigoid (benign mucosal).*** This rare autoimmune disease is characterized by thick-walled vesicles on the oral mucous membranes, the conjunctiva and, less often, the skin. Mouth lesions typically develop months or even years before other manifestations and may occur as desquamative patchy gingivitis or as a vesicobullous eruption. Secondary fibrous bands may lead to dysphagia, hoarseness, and blindness. Recurrent skin lesions include vesicobullous eruptions, usually on the inguinal area and extremities, and an erythematous, vesicobullous plaque on the scalp and face near the affected mucous membranes.

◆ ***Pemphigus.*** This chronic skin disease is characterized by thin-walled vesicles and bullae that appear in cycles on skin or mucous membranes that otherwise appear normal. On the oral mucosa, bullae rupture, leaving painful lesions and raw patches that bleed easily. Associated findings include bullae anywhere on the body, denudation of the skin, and pruritus.

◆ ***Pyogenic granuloma.*** Commonly the result of injury, trauma, or irritation, this soft, tender nodule, papule, or polypoid mass of excessive granulation tissue usually appears on the gingivae but can also erupt on the lips, tongue, or buccal mucosa. The lesions bleed easily because they contain many capillaries. The affected area may be smooth or have a warty surface; erythema develops in the surrounding mucosa. The lesions may ulcerate, producing a purulent exudate.

◆ ***Squamous cell carcinoma.*** This is typically a painless ulcer with an elevated, indurated border. It may erupt in areas of leukoplakia and is most common on the lower lip, but it may also occur on the edge of the tongue or the floor of the mouth. High risk factors include chronic smoking and alcohol intake.

◆ ***Stomatitis (aphthous).*** This common disease is characterized by painful ulcerations of the oral mucosa, usually on the dorsum of the tongue, gingivae, and hard palate.

With recurrent aphthous stomatitis minor, the ulcer begins as one or more erosions covered by a gray membrane and surrounded by a red halo. It's commonly found on the buccal and lip mucosa and junction, tongue, soft palate, pharynx, gingivae, and all places not bound to the periosteum.

With recurrent aphthous stomatitis major, large, painful ulcers commonly occur on the lips, cheek, tongue, and soft palate; they may last up to 6 weeks and leave a scar.

◆ ***Syphilis.*** Primary syphilis typically produces a solitary painless, red ulcer (chancre) on the lip, tongue, palate, tonsil, or gingivae. The ulcer appears as a crater with undulated, raised edges and a shiny center; lip chancres may develop a crust. Similar lesions may appear on the fingers, breasts, or genitals, and regional lymph nodes may become enlarged and tender.

During the secondary stage, multiple painless ulcers covered by a grayish white plaque may erupt on the tongue, gingivae, or buccal mucosa. A macular, papular, pustular, or nodular rash appears, usually on the arms, trunk, palms, soles, face, and scalp; genital lesions usually subside. Other findings include generalized lymphadenopathy, headache, malaise, anorexia, weight loss, nausea, vomiting, sore throat, low fever, metrorrhagia, and postcoital bleeding.

At the tertiary stage, lesions (often chronic, painless, superficial nodules or deep granulomatous lesions, called *gummas*) develop on the skin and mucous membranes, especially the tongue and palate.

◆ ***Systemic lupus erythematosus.*** Oral lesions are common and appear as erythematous areas associated with edema, petechiae, and superficial ulcers with a red halo and a tendency to bleed. Primary effects include nondeforming arthritis, butterfly rash across the nose and cheeks, and photosensitivity.

◆ ***Trauma.*** The most common cause of oral lesions, trauma can produce ulcers anywhere in the mouth, especially on the tongue and buccal mucosa.

◆ ***Tuberculosis (oral mucosal).*** This rare disorder produces a painless ulcer (usually on the tongue) and, sometimes, caseation. Other findings include lymphadenopathy, fatigue, weakness, anorexia, weight loss, cough, low fever, and night sweats.

Other causes

◆ ***Drugs.*** Various chemotherapeutic agents can directly produce stomatitis. Also, allergic reactions to penicillin, sulfonamides, gold, quinine, streptomycin, phenytoin, aspirin, and barbiturates commonly cause lesions to develop and erupt. Inhaled steroids used for pulmonary disorders can also cause oral lesions.

◆ ***Orthodontics.*** The rubbing of orthodontic equipment or prosthesis on the buccal mucosa may cause eroded, tender areas.

◆ ***Radiation therapy.*** Radiation therapy may cause oral lesions.

Special considerations

If the patient's mouth ulcers are painful, provide a topical anesthetic such as lidocaine.

Pediatric pointers

Causes of mouth ulcers in children include chickenpox, measles, scarlet fever, diphtheria, and hand-foot-and-mouth disease. In neonates, mouth ulcers can result from candidiasis or congenital syphilis.

Patient counseling

Instruct the patient to avoid irritants, such as highly seasoned foods, citrus fruits, foods that contain salt or vinegar, alcohol, and tobacco. For mouth care, warn against using lemon-glycerin swabs because these can dry and irritate the lesions.

As appropriate, teach the patient proper oral hygiene. If toothbrushing is contraindicated, instruct him to use a mouth rinse, such as normal saline solution or half-strength hydrogen peroxide, and to avoid commercial mouthwashes that contain alcohol. Stress the importance of frequently changing to a new toothbrush. If the patient uses an inhaled steroid, instruct him to rinse his mouth after each use. Also, tell him to report mouth lesions that don't heal within 2 weeks.

Murmurs

Murmurs are auscultatory sounds heard within the heart chambers or major arteries. They're classified by their timing and duration in the cardiac cycle, auscultatory location, loudness, configuration, pitch, and quality.

Timing can be characterized as systolic (between S_1 and S_2), holosystolic (continuous throughout systole), diastolic (between S_2 and S_1), or continuous throughout systole and diastole; systolic and diastolic murmurs can be further characterized as early, middle, or late.

Location refers to the area of maximum loudness, such as the apex, the lower left sternal border, or an intercostal space. *Loudness* is graded on a scale of 1 to 6. A grade 1 murmur is very faint, only detected after careful auscultation. A grade 2 murmur is a soft, evident murmur. Murmurs considered to be grade 3 are moderately loud. A grade 4 murmur is a loud murmur with a possible intermittent thrill. Grade 5 murmurs are loud and associated with a palpable precordial thrill. Grade 6 murmurs are loud and, like grade 5 murmurs, are associated with a thrill. A grade 6 murmur is audible even when the stethoscope is lifted from the thoracic wall.

Configuration, or shape, refers to the nature of loudness—crescendo (grows louder), decrescendo (grows softer), crescendo-decrescendo (first rises, then falls), decrescendo-crescendo (first falls, then rises), plateau (even intensity), or variable (uneven intensity). The murmur's *pitch* may be high or low. Its *quality* may be described as harsh, rumbling, blowing, scratching, buzzing, musical, or squeaking.

Murmurs can reflect accelerated blood flow through normal or abnormal valves; forward blood flow through a narrowed or irregular valve or into a dilated vessel; blood backflow through an incompetent valve, septal defect, or patent ductus arteriosus; or decreased blood viscosity. Commonly the result of organic heart disease, murmurs occasionally may signal an emergency situation—for example, a loud holosystolic murmur after an acute myocardial infarction (MI) may signal papillary muscle rupture or ventricular septal defect. Murmurs may also result from surgical implantation of a prosthetic valve. (See *When murmurs mean emergency*.)

Some murmurs are innocent, or functional. An *innocent systolic murmur* is generally soft, medium-pitched, and loudest along the left sternal border at the second or third intercostal space. It's exacerbated by physical activity, excitement, fever, pregnancy, anemia, or thyrotoxicosis. Examples include Still's murmur in children and mammary souffle, often heard over either breast during late pregnancy and early postpartum. (See *Detecting congenital murmurs,* pages 451 and 452.)

History and physical examination

If you discover a murmur, try to determine its type through careful auscultation. (See *Identifying common murmurs,* page 453.) Use the bell of your stethoscope for low-pitched murmurs; the diaphragm for high-pitched murmurs.

Next, obtain a patient history. Ask if the murmur is a new discovery, or if it has been known since birth or childhood. Find out if the patient has experienced any associated symptoms, particularly palpitations, dizziness, syncope, chest

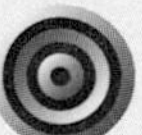

EMERGENCY INTERVENTION

When murmurs mean emergency

Although not normally a sign of an emergency, murmurs—especially newly developed ones—may signal a serious complication in patients with bacterial endocarditis or a recent acute myocardial infarction (MI).

When caring for a patient with known or suspected bacterial endocarditis, carefully auscultate for any new murmurs. Their development along with crackles, distended jugular veins, orthopnea, and dyspnea may signal heart failure.

Regular auscultation is also important in a patient who has experienced an acute MI. A loud decrescendo holosystolic murmur at the apex that radiates to the axilla and left sternal border or throughout the chest is significant, particularly in association with a widely split S_2 and an atrial gallop (S_4). This murmur, when accompanied by signs of acute pulmonary edema, usually indicates the development of acute mitral insufficiency due to rupture of the chordae tendineae—a medical emergency.

Detecting congenital murmurs

Heart defect	Type of murmur
Aortopulmonary septal defect	*Small defect:* a continuous rough or crackling murmur best heard at the upper left sternal border and below the left clavicle, possibly accompanied by a systolic ejection click. *Large defect:* a harsh systolic murmur heard at the left sternal border.
Atrial septal defect	A midsystolic, spindle-shaped murmur of grade II or III intensity heard at the upper left sternal border, with a fixed splitting of S_2. Large shunts may also produce a low- to medium-pitched early diastolic murmur over the lower left sternal border.
Bicuspid aortic valve	An early systolic, loud, high-pitched ejection sound or click that's best heard at the apex and is commonly accompanied by a soft, early or midsystolic murmur at the upper right sternal border. The aortic component of S_2 is usually accentuated at the apex. This murmur may not be recognized until early childhood.
Coarctation of the aorta	Usually a systolic ejection click at the base of the heart, at the apex, and occasionally over the carotid arteries, often accompanied by a systolic ejection murmur at the base. This disorder may also produce a blowing diastolic murmur of aortic insufficiency or an apical pansystolic murmur of unknown origin.
Common atrioventricular canal defects (endocardial cushion defect)	*With a competent mitral valve:* a midsystolic, spindle-shaped murmur of grade II or III intensity heard at the upper left sternal border, with a fixed splitting of S_2; may be accompanied by a low- to medium-pitched early diastolic murmur over the lower left sternal border. *With an incompetent mitral valve:* an early systolic or holosystolic decrescendo murmur at the apex, along with a widely split S_2 and often an S_4.
Ebstein's anomaly	A soft, high-pitched holosystolic blowing murmur that increases with inspiration (Carvallo's sign); best heard over the lower left sternal border and the xiphoid area; possibly accompanied by a low-pitched diastolic rumbling murmur at the apex. Fixed splitting of S_2 and a loud split S_4 also occur.
Left ventricular–right atrial communication	A holosystolic, decrescendo murmur of grades II to IV intensity heard along the lower left sternal border, accompanied by a normal S_2; large shunts also produce a diastolic rumbling murmur over the apex.
Mitral atresia	A nonspecific systolic murmur and a diastolic flow rumble at the lower left sternal border, with one loud S_2.
Partial anomalous pulmonary venous connection	A midsystolic, spindle-shaped grade II to III murmur at the upper left sternal border, possibly accompanied by a low- to medium-pitched early diastolic murmur over the lower left sternal border.
Patent ductus arteriosus	A continuous rough or crackling murmur best heard at the upper left sternal border and below the left clavicle. The murmur is accentuated late in systole.
Pulmonic insufficiency	An early to middiastolic, soft, medium-pitched crescendo-decrescendo murmur best heard at the second or third right intercostal space.

(continued)

Detecting congenital murmurs *(continued)*

Heart defect	Type of murmur
Pulmonic stenosis	An early systolic, harsh, crescendo-decrescendo murmur of grades IV to VI intensity heard at the second left intercostal space, possibly radiating along the left sternal border.
Single atrium	A holosystolic regurgitant murmur at the apex, accompanied by a fixed splitting of S_2.
Supravalvular aortic stenosis	A systolic ejection murmur best heard over the second right intercostal space or higher in the episternal notch or over the lower right side of the neck. The aortic closure sound is usually preserved, and no ejection clicks are heard.
Tetralogy of Fallot	A midsystolic murmur with a systolic thrill palpable at the left midsternal border; softer murmurs occurring earlier in systole generally indicate a more severe obstruction.
Tricuspid atresia	Variable, depending on associated defects.
Trilogy of Fallot	A systolic, harsh, crescendo-decrescendo murmur, best heard at the upper left sternal border with radiation toward the left clavicle. The pulmonic component of S_2 becomes progressively softer with increasing degrees of obstruction.
Ventricular septal defect	*Small defect:* usually a holosystolic (but may be limited to early or midsystole), grades II to IV decrescendo murmur heard along the lower left sternal border, accompanied by a normal S_2. *Large defect:* a holosystolic murmur at the lower left sternal border and a midsystolic rumbling murmur at the apex, accompanied by an increased S_1 at the lower left sternal border and an increased pulmonic component of S_2.

pain, dyspnea, and fatigue. (See *Differential diagnosis: Murmurs,* pages 454 and 455.) Explore the patient's medical history, noting especially any incidence of rheumatic fever, recent dental work, heart disease, or heart surgery, particularly prosthetic valve replacement.

Perform a systematic physical examination. Note especially the presence of cardiac arrhythmias, jugular vein distention, and such pulmonary signs and symptoms as dyspnea, orthopnea, and crackles. Is the patient's liver tender or palpable? Does he have peripheral edema?

MEDICAL CAUSES

◆ ***Aortic insufficiency.*** Acute aortic insufficiency typically produces a soft, short diastolic murmur over the left sternal border that's best heard when the patient sits and leans forward and at the end of a forced held expiration. S_2 may be soft or absent. Sometimes, a soft, short midsystolic murmur may also be heard over the second right intercostal space. Associated findings include tachycardia, dyspnea, jugular vein distention, crackles, increased fatigue, and pale, cool extremities.

Chronic aortic insufficiency causes a high-pitched, blowing, decrescendo diastolic murmur that's best heard over the second or third right intercostal space or the left sternal border with the patient sitting, leaning forward, and holding his breath after deep expiration. An Austin Flint murmur—a rumbling, mid-to-late diastolic murmur best heard at the apex—may also occur. Complications may not develop until ages 40 to 50; then, typical findings include palpitations, tachycardia, angina, increased fatigue, dyspnea, orthopnea, and crackles.

◆ ***Aortic stenosis.*** With this valvular disorder, the murmur is systolic, beginning after S_1 and ending at or before aortic valve closure. It's harsh and grating, medium-pitched, and crescendo-decrescendo. Loudest over the second right intercostal space when the patient is sitting and leaning forward, this murmur may also be heard at the apex, at the suprasternal notch (Erb's point), and over the carotid arteries.

Identifying common murmurs

The timing and configuration of a murmur can help you identify its underlying cause. Learn to recognize the characteristics of these common murmurs.

Aortic insufficiency (chronic)

Thickened valve leaflets fail to close correctly, permitting backflow of blood into the left ventricle.

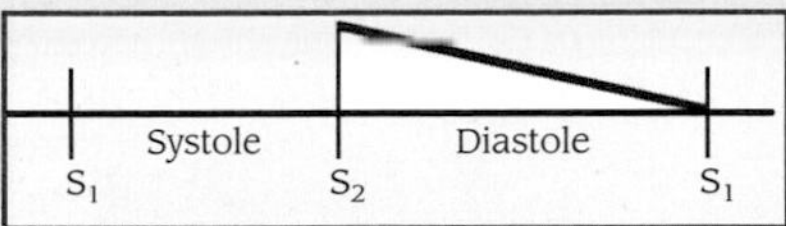

Aortic stenosis

Thickened, scarred, or calcified valve leaflets impede ventricular systolic ejection.

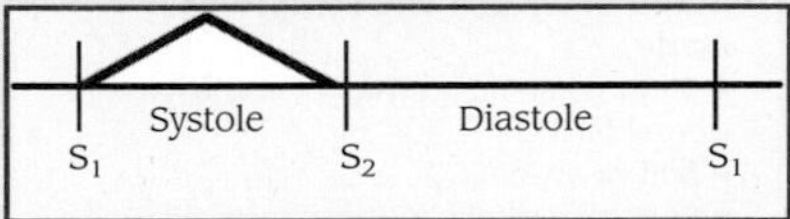

Mitral prolapse

Incompetent mitral valve bulges into the left atrium because of an enlarged posterior leaflet and elongated chordae tendineae.

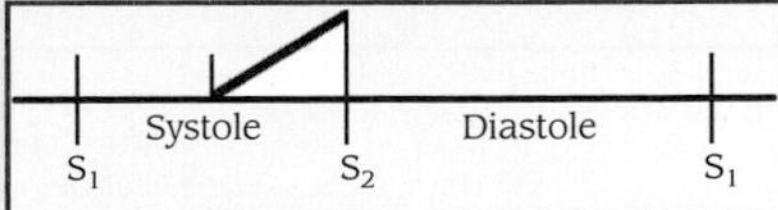

Mitral insufficiency (chronic)

Incomplete mitral valve closure permits backflow of blood into the left atrium.

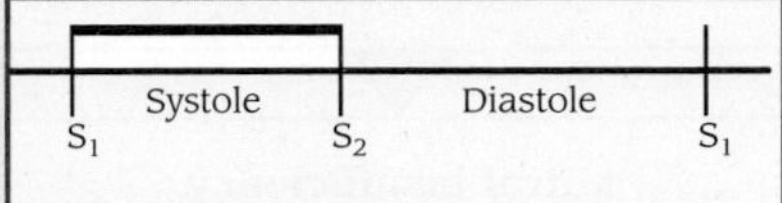

Mitral stenosis

Thickened or scarred valve leaflets cause valve stenosis and restrict blood flow.

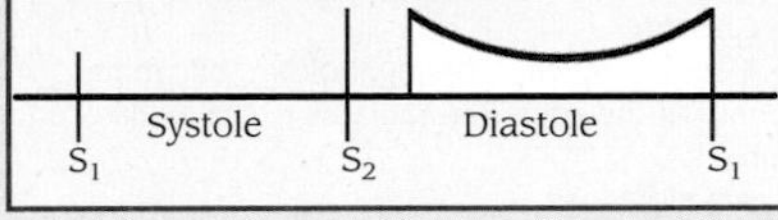

If the patient has advanced disease, S_2 may be heard as a single sound, with inaudible aortic closure. An early systolic ejection click at the apex is typical but is absent when the valve is severely calcified. Associated signs and symptoms usually don't appear until age 30 in congenital aortic stenosis, ages 30 to 65 in stenosis due to rheumatic disease, and after age 65 in calcific aortic stenosis. They may include dizziness, syncope, dyspnea on exertion, paroxysmal nocturnal dyspnea, fatigue, and angina.

◆ ***Cardiomyopathy (hypertrophic).*** This disorder generates a harsh late systolic murmur, ending at S_2. Best heard over the left sternal border and at the apex, the murmur is commonly accompanied by an audible S_3 or S_4. The murmur decreases with squatting and increases with sitting down. Major associated symptoms are dyspnea and chest pain; palpitations, dizziness, and syncope may also occur.

◆ ***Mitral insufficiency.*** Acute mitral insufficiency is characterized by a medium-pitched blowing, early systolic or holosystolic decrescendo murmur at the apex, along with a widely split S_2 and commonly an S_4. This murmur doesn't get louder on inspiration as with tricuspid insufficiency. Associated findings typically include tachycardia and signs of acute pulmonary edema.

Chronic mitral insufficiency produces a high-pitched, blowing, holosystolic plateau murmur that's loudest at the apex and usually radiates to the axilla or back. Fatigue, dyspnea, and palpitations may also occur.

◆ ***Mitral prolapse.*** This disorder generates a midsystolic to late-systolic click with a high-pitched late-systolic crescendo murmur, best heard at the apex. Occasionally, multiple clicks may be heard, with or without a systolic murmur. Associated findings include cardiac awareness, migraine headaches, dizziness, weakness, syncope, palpitations, chest pain, dyspnea, severe episodic fatigue, mood swings, and anxiety.

◆ ***Mitral stenosis.*** With this valvular disorder, the murmur is soft, low-pitched, rumbling, crescendo-decrescendo, and diastolic, accompanied by a loud S_1 or an opening snap—a cardinal sign. It's best heard at the apex with the

Differential diagnosis: Murmurs

History of present illness

Focused physical examination:
Cardiovascular and pulmonary systems

Common signs and symptoms
- Arrhythmias
- Crackles
- Fatigue
- Jugular vein distention
- Palpitations
- Shortness of breath
- Tachycardia

Mitral insufficiency

Additional signs and symptoms
Acute
- Early systolic or holosystolic decrescendo murmur at the apex
- Widely split S_2
- S_4

Chronic
- High-pitched, blowing, holosystolic murmur at the apex that radiates to the axilla or back
- Weight loss
- Nocturia

Diagnosis: Physical examination, angiography, echocardiogram
Treatment: Medication (antibiotics [if infection is present], anticoagulants [if atrial fibrillation is present], diuretics)
Follow-up: Referral to cardiologist

Aortic insufficiency

Additional signs and symptoms
Acute
- Short diastolic murmur over the left sternal border
- Soft or absent S_2
- Soft, midsystolic murmur over the second right intercostal space (possibly)

Chronic
- High-pitched, blowing, decrescendo diastolic murmur that's best heard over the second or third right intercostal space

Diagnosis: Physical examination, imaging studies (ultrasound, angiography, echocardiogram), cardiac catheterization
Treatment: As needed (based on the severity of symptoms), medications (diuretics, digoxin)
Follow-up: Referral to cardiologist

patient in the left lateral position. Mild exercise will help make this murmur audible.

With severe stenosis, the murmur of mitral insufficiency may also be heard. Other findings include hemoptysis, exertional dyspnea and fatigue, and signs of acute pulmonary edema.

◆ ***Myxomas.*** A left atrial myxoma (most common) usually produces a middiastolic murmur and a holosystolic murmur that's loudest at the apex, with an S_4, an early diastolic thudding sound (tumor plop), and a loud, widely split S_1. Related features include dyspnea, orthopnea, chest pain, fatigue, weight loss, and syncope.

A right atrial myxoma causes a late diastolic rumbling murmur, a holosystolic crescendo murmur, and tumor plop, best heard at the lower left sternal border. Other findings include fatigue, peripheral edema, ascites, and hepatomegaly.

A left ventricular myxoma (rare) produces a systolic murmur, best heard at the lower left sternal border, arrhythmias, dyspnea, and syncope.

A right ventricular myxoma commonly generates a systolic ejection murmur with delayed S_2 and a tumor plop, best heard at the left sternal border. It's accompanied by peripheral

Common signs and symptoms
- Angina
- Arrhythmias
- Dizziness
- Dyspnea
- Fatigue
- Hypotension

Aortic stenosis

Additional signs and symptoms
- Harsh, grating systolic murmur over the second right intercostal space, the apex, Erb's point, or the carotid arteries

Diagnosis: Physical examination, imaging studies (angiography, Doppler ultrasound, chest X-ray)
Treatment: Avoidance of strenuous activity, medication (diuretics, digoxin)
Follow-up: Reevaluation every 6 to 12 months

Cardiomyopathy

Additional signs and symptoms
- Harsh, late systolic murmur that ends at S_2
- Murmur located over the left sternal border and apex
- S_3 or S_4 (possibly)
- Palpitations
- Sudden cardiac death

Diagnosis: Physical examination, imaging studies (chest X-ray, computed tomography scan, magnetic resonance imaging, angiography), echocardiogram
Treatment: Symptomatic treatment, oxygen therapy
Follow-up: Referral to cardiologist

Additional differential diagnoses: mitral prolapse ◆ mitral stenosis ◆ myxomas ◆ papillary muscle rupture ◆ tricuspid insufficiency ◆ tricuspid stenosis
Other causes: prosthetic valve replacement

edema, hepatomegaly, ascites, dyspnea, and syncope.

◆ ***Papillary muscle rupture.*** With this life-threatening complication of an acute MI, a loud holosystolic murmur can be auscultated at the apex. Related findings include severe dyspnea, chest pain, syncope, hemoptysis, tachycardia, and hypotension.

◆ ***Rheumatic fever with pericarditis.*** A pericardial friction rub along with murmurs and gallops are heard best with the patient leaning forward on his hands and knees during forced expiration. The most common murmurs heard are the systolic murmur of mitral insufficiency, a midsystolic murmur due to swelling of the leaflet of the mitral valve, and the diastolic murmur of aortic insufficiency. Other signs and symptoms include fever, joint and sternal pain, edema, and tachypnea.

◆ ***Tricuspid insufficiency.*** This valvular abnormality is characterized by a soft, high-pitched, holosystolic blowing murmur that increases with inspiration (Carvallo's sign), decreases with exhalation and Valsalva's maneuver, and is best heard over the lower left sternal border and the xiphoid area. Following a lengthy asymptomatic period, exertional dyspnea and orthopnea may develop, along with jugular vein distention, ascites, peripheral cyanosis and edema, muscle wasting, fatigue, weakness, and syncope.

◆ ***Tricuspid stenosis.*** This valvular disorder produces a diastolic murmur similar to that of mitral stenosis, but louder with inspiration and decreased with exhalation and Valsalva's maneuver. S_1 may also be louder. Associated signs and symptoms include fatigue, syncope, peripheral edema, jugular vein distention, ascites, hepatomegaly, and dyspnea.

Other causes

◆ ***Treatments.*** Prosthetic valve replacement may cause variable murmurs, depending on the location, valve composition, and method of operation.

Special considerations

Prepare the patient for diagnostic tests, such as electrocardiography, echocardiography, and angiography. Administer an antibiotic and an anticoagulant as appropriate. Because any cardiac abnormality is frightening to the patient, provide emotional support.

Pediatric pointers

Innocent murmurs, such as Still's murmur, are commonly heard in young children and typically disappear in puberty. Pathognomonic heart murmurs in infants and young children usually result from congenital heart disease, such as atrial and ventricular septal defects. Other murmurs can be acquired, as with rheumatic heart disease.

Patient counseling

Instruct the patient to contact his physician before undergoing invasive procedures or dental work because prophylactic antibiotics may be necessary.

Muscle atrophy

[Muscle wasting]

Muscle atrophy results from denervation or prolonged muscle disuse. When deprived of regular exercise, muscle fibers lose both bulk and length, producing a visible loss of muscle size and contour and apparent emaciation or deformity in the affected area. Even slight atrophy usually causes some loss of motion or power.

Atrophy usually results from neuromuscular disease or injury. However, it may also stem from certain metabolic and endocrine disorders and prolonged immobility. Some muscle atrophy also occurs with aging.

History and physical examination

Ask the patient when and where he first noticed the muscle wasting and how it has progressed. Also ask about associated signs and symptoms, such as weakness, pain, loss of sensation, and recent weight loss. Review the patient's medical history for chronic illnesses; musculoskeletal or neurologic disorders, including trauma; and endocrine and metabolic disorders. Ask about his use of alcohol and drugs, particularly steroids.

Begin the physical examination by determining the location and extent of atrophy. Visually evaluate small and large muscles. Check all major muscle groups for size, tonicity, and strength. (See *Testing muscle strength,* pages 464 and 465.) Measure the circumference of all limbs, comparing sides. (See *Measuring limb circumference.*) Check for muscle contractures in all limbs by fully extending joints and noting any pain or resistance. Complete the examination by palpating peripheral pulses for quality and rate, assessing sensory function in and around the atrophied area, and testing deep tendon reflexes.

Medical causes

◆ ***Amyotrophic lateral sclerosis.*** Initial symptoms of this progressive disease include muscle weakness and atrophy that typically begin in one hand, spread to the arm, and then develop in the other hand and arm. Eventually, weakness and atrophy spread to the trunk, neck, tongue, larynx, pharynx, and legs; progressive respiratory muscle weakness leads to respiratory insufficiency. Other findings include muscle flaccidity, fasciculations, hyperactive deep tendon reflexes, slight leg muscle spasticity, dysphagia, impaired speech, excessive drooling, and depression.

◆ ***Burns.*** Fibrous scar tissue formation, pain, and loss of serum proteins from severe burns can limit muscle movement, resulting in atrophy.

◆ ***Compartment syndrome and Volkmann's ischemic contracture.*** With this acute disorder, muscle atrophy is a late sign of irreversible ischemia, along with contractures, paralysis, and loss of pulses. Earlier signs and symptoms include severe pain that increases with passive muscle movement, along with weakness and paresthesia.

◆ ***Herniated disk.*** Here, pressure on nerve roots leads to muscle weakness, disuse, and ultimately, atrophy. The primary symptom is severe lower back pain, possibly radiating to the buttocks, legs, and feet and commonly accompanied by muscle spasms. Diminished reflexes and sensory changes may also occur.

◆ ***Hypercortisolism.*** This disorder may cause limb weakness and eventually atrophy. Related cushingoid features include buffalo hump, moon face, truncal obesity, purple striae, thin skin, acne, easy bruising, poor wound healing, elevated blood pressure, fatigue, hyperpigmentation, and diaphoresis. The male patient may be impotent; the female patient may develop hirsutism and menstrual irregularities.

◆ ***Hypothyroidism.*** Reversible weakness and atrophy of proximal limb muscles may occur in hypothyroidism. Associated findings commonly include muscle cramps and stiffness; cold intolerance; weight gain despite anorexia; mental dullness; dry, pale, cool, doughy skin; puffy face, hands, and feet; and bradycardia.

◆ ***Meniscal tear.*** Quadriceps muscle atrophy, resulting from prolonged knee immobility and muscle weakness, is a classic sign of this traumatic disorder.

◆ ***Multiple sclerosis.*** This degenerative disease may produce arm and leg atrophy as a result of chronic progressive weakness; spasticity and contractures may also develop. Associated signs and symptoms typically wax and wane and include diplopia and blurred vision, nystagmus, hyperactive deep tendon reflexes, sensory loss or paresthesia, dysarthria, dysphagia, incoordination, ataxic gait, intention tremors, emotional lability, impotence, and urinary dysfunction.

◆ ***Osteoarthritis.*** This chronic disorder eventually causes atrophy proximal to involved joints as a result of progressive weakness and disuse. Other late signs and symptoms include bony joint deformities, such as Heberden's nodes on the distal interphalangeal joints, Bouchard's nodes on the proximal interphalangeal joints, crepitus and fluid accumulation, and contractures.

◆ ***Parkinson's disease.*** With this disorder, muscle rigidity, weakness, and disuse may produce muscle atrophy. The patient may exhibit insidious resting tremors that usually begin in

Measuring limb circumference

To ensure accurate and consistent limb circumference measurements, mark and use a consistent reference point each time and measure with the limb in full extension. The illustration below shows the correct reference points for arm and leg measurements.

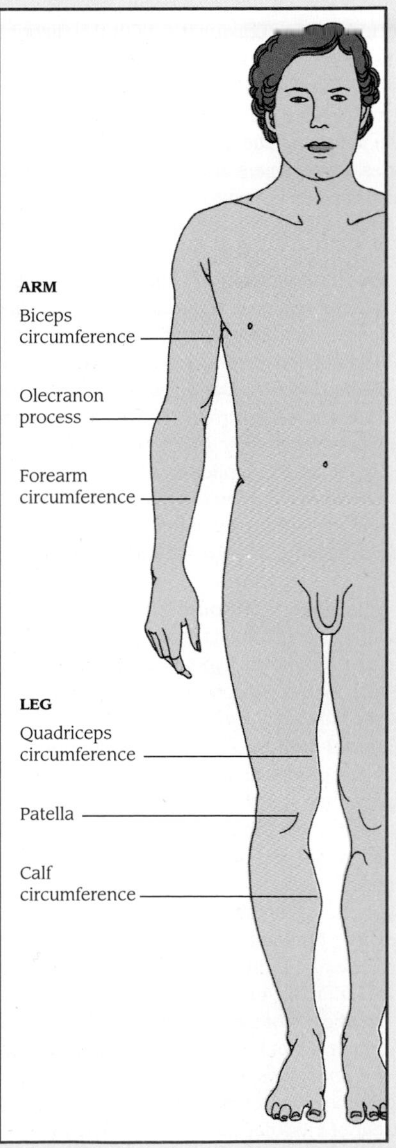

the fingers (pill-rolling tremor), worsen with stress, and ease with purposeful movement and sleep. He may also develop bradykinesia; a characteristic propulsive gait; a high-pitched, monotone voice; masklike facies; drooling; dysphagia; dysarthria; and occasionally, oculogyric crisis or blepharospasm.

◆ ***Peripheral nerve trauma.*** Injury to or prolonged pressure on a peripheral nerve leads to muscle weakness and atrophy. Associated findings include paresthesia or sensory loss, pain, and loss of reflexes supplied by the damaged nerve. Paralysis may also occur.

◆ ***Peripheral neuropathy.*** With this disorder, muscle weakness progresses slowly to flaccid paralysis and eventually atrophy. Distal extremity muscles are generally affected first. Associated findings include loss of vibration sense; paresthesia, hyperesthesia, or anesthesia in the hands and feet; mild to sharp, burning pain; anhidrosis; glossy red skin; and diminished or absent deep tendon reflexes.

◆ ***Protein deficiency.*** If chronic, this may lead to muscle weakness and atrophy. Other findings include chronic fatigue, apathy, anorexia, dry skin, peripheral edema, and dull, sparse, dry hair.

◆ ***Radiculopathy.*** Damaged spinal nerve roots can cause muscle atrophy as well as weakness, paralysis, severe pain and, at times, loss of feeling in the areas supplied by the affected nerves.

◆ ***Rheumatoid arthritis.*** Muscle atrophy occurs in the late stages of this disorder, as joint pain and stiffness decrease range of motion and discourage muscle use.

◆ ***Shy-Drager syndrome.*** This rare, progressive neurologic syndrome is characterized by muscle atrophy, orthostatic hypotension, incontinence, tremor, rigidity, incoordination, and ataxia. It's most common in young and middle-aged adults.

◆ ***Spinal cord injury.*** Trauma to the spinal cord can produce severe muscle weakness and flaccid, then spastic, paralysis, eventually leading to atrophy. Other signs and symptoms depend on the level of injury but may include respiratory insufficiency or paralysis, sensory losses, bowel and bladder dysfunction, hyperactive deep tendon reflexes, positive Babinski's reflex, sexual dysfunction, priapism, hypotension, and anhidrosis (usually unilateral).

◆ ***Stroke.*** Stroke may produce contralateral or bilateral weakness and eventually atrophy of the arms, legs, face, and tongue. Associated signs and symptoms depend on the site and extent of vascular damage and may include dysarthria, aphasia, ataxia, apraxia, agnosia, and ipsilateral paresthesia or sensory loss. The patient may develop visual disturbance, altered level of consciousness, amnesia and poor judgment, personality changes, and emotional lability. He may also report bowel and bladder dysfunction, vomiting, headache, and seizures.

◆ ***Thyrotoxicosis.*** This disorder may produce insidious, generalized muscle weakness and atrophy. Related findings include extreme anxiety, fatigue, heat intolerance, diaphoresis, tremors, tachycardia, palpitations, ventricular or atrial gallop, dyspnea, weight loss, and an enlarged thyroid. Exophthalmos may be present.

Other causes

◆ ***Drugs.*** Prolonged steroid therapy interferes with muscle metabolism and leads to atrophy, most prominently in the limbs.

◆ ***Immobility.*** Prolonged immobilization from bed rest, casts, splints, or traction may cause muscle weakness and atrophy.

Special considerations

Because contractures can occur as atrophied muscle fibers shorten, help the patient maintain muscle length by encouraging him to perform frequent, active range-of-motion exercises. If he can't actively move a joint, provide active-assistive or passive exercises, and apply splints or braces to maintain muscle length. If you find resistance to full extension during exercise, use heat, pain medication, or relaxation techniques to relax the muscle. Then slowly stretch it to full extension. (*Caution:* Don't pull or strain the muscle; you may tear muscle fibers and cause further contracture.) If these techniques fail to correct the contracture, use moist heat, a whirlpool bath, resistive exercises, or ultrasound therapy. If these techniques aren't effective, surgical release of contractures may be necessary.

Teach the patient to use necessary assistive devices properly to ensure his safety and prevent falls. Have the patient consult a physical therapist for a specialized therapy regimen.

Prepare the patient for electromyography, nerve conduction studies, muscle biopsy, and X-rays or computed tomography scans.

Pediatric pointers

In young children, profound muscle weakness and atrophy can result from muscular dystrophy. Muscle atrophy may also result from cerebral palsy and poliomyelitis, and from paralysis associated with meningocele and myelomeningocele.

Muscle flaccidity

[Muscle hypotonicity]

Flaccid muscles are profoundly weak and soft, with decreased resistance to movement, increased mobility, and greater than normal range of motion. The result of disrupted muscle innervation, flaccidity can be localized to a limb or muscle group or generalized over the entire body. Its onset may be acute, as in trauma, or chronic, as in neurologic disease.

EMERGENCY INTERVENTIONS *If the patient's muscle flaccidity results from trauma, make sure his cervical spine has been stabilized. Quickly determine his respiratory status. If you note signs and symptoms of respiratory insufficiency—dyspnea, shallow respirations, nasal flaring, cyanosis, and decreased oxygen saturation—administer oxygen by nasal cannula or mask. Intubation and mechanical ventilation may be necessary.*

History and physical examination

If the patient isn't in distress, ask about the onset and duration of muscle flaccidity and any precipitating factors. Ask about associated symptoms, notably weakness, other muscle changes, and sensory loss or paresthesia.

Examine the affected muscles for atrophy, which indicates a chronic problem. Test muscle strength, and check deep tendon reflexes in all limbs.

Medical causes

◆ ***Amyotrophic lateral sclerosis.*** Progressive muscle weakness and paralysis are accompanied by generalized flaccidity. Typically, these effects begin in one hand, spread to the arm, and then develop in the other hand and arm. Eventually, they spread to the trunk, neck, tongue, larynx, pharynx, and legs; progressive respiratory muscle weakness leads to respiratory insufficiency. Other findings include muscle cramps and coarse fasciculations, hyperactive deep tendon reflexes, slight leg muscle spasticity, dysphagia, dysarthria, excessive drooling, and depression.

◆ ***Brain lesions.*** Frontal and parietal lobe lesions may cause contralateral flaccidity, weakness or paralysis, and eventually, spasticity and possibly contractures. Other findings include hyperactive deep tendon reflexes, positive Babinski's sign, loss of proprioception, stereognosis, graphesthesia, anesthesia, and thermanesthesia.

◆ ***Cerebellar disease.*** With this disease, generalized muscle flaccidity or hypotonia is accompanied by ataxia, dysmetria, intention tremor, slight muscle weakness, fatigue, and dysarthria.

◆ ***Guillain-Barré syndrome.*** This disorder causes muscle flaccidity. Progression is typically symmetrical and ascending, moving from the feet to the arms and facial nerves within 24 to 72 hours of onset. Associated findings include sensory loss or paresthesia, absent deep tendon reflexes, tachycardia (or, less often, bradycardia), fluctuating hypertension and orthostatic hypotension, diaphoresis, incontinence, dysphagia, dysarthria, hypernasality, and facial diplegia. Weakness may progress to total motor paralysis and respiratory failure.

◆ ***Huntington's disease.*** Besides flaccidity, progressive mental status changes up to and including dementia and choreiform movements are major symptoms. Others include poor balance, hesitant or explosive speech, dysphagia, impaired respirations, and incontinence.

◆ ***Muscle disease.*** Muscle weakness and flaccidity are features of myopathies and muscular dystrophies.

◆ ***Peripheral nerve trauma.*** Flaccidity, paralysis, and loss of sensation and reflexes in the innervated area can occur.

◆ ***Peripheral neuropathy.*** Flaccidity usually occurs in the legs as a result of chronic progressive muscle weakness and paralysis. It may also cause mild-to-sharp burning pain, glossy red skin, anhidrosis, and loss of vibration sensation. Paresthesia, hyperesthesia, or anesthesia may affect the hands and feet. Deep tendon reflexes may be hypoactive or absent.

◆ ***Poliomyelitis.*** Damage to the anterior horn cells in the spinal cord and brain stem causes flaccid weakness and loss of reflexes. The large, proximal muscles of the limbs are most commonly affected.

◆ ***Seizure disorder.*** Brief periods of syncope and generalized flaccidity commonly follow a generalized tonic-clonic seizure.

◆ ***Spinal cord injury.*** Spinal shock can result in acute muscle flaccidity or spasticity below the level of injury. Associated signs and symptoms also occur below the level of injury and may include paralysis; absent deep tendon reflexes; analgesia; thermanesthesia; loss of proprioception and vibration, touch, and pressure sensation; and anhidrosis (usually unilateral). Hypotension, bowel and bladder dysfunction, and impotence or priapism may also occur. Injury in the C1 to C5 region can produce respiratory paralysis and bradycardia.

Special considerations

Provide regular, systematic, passive range-of-motion exercises to preserve joint mobility and to increase circulation. Reposition a patient with generalized flaccidity every 2 hours to protect him from skin breakdown. Pad bony prominences and other pressure points, and prevent thermal injury by testing bath water yourself before the patient bathes. Treat isolated flaccidity by supporting the affected limb in a sling or with a splint. Ensure patient safety and reduce the risk of falls by introducing assistive devices and their proper use. Consult a physician and occupational therapist to formulate a personalized therapy regimen and foster independence.

Prepare the patient for diagnostic tests, such as cranial and spinal X-rays, computed tomography scans, and electromyography.

Pediatric pointers

Pediatric causes of muscle flaccidity include myelomeningocele, Lowe's disease, Werdnig-Hoffmann disease, and muscular dystrophy. An infant or young child with generalized flaccidity may lie in a froglike position, with his hips and knees abducted.

Muscle spasms

[Muscle cramps]

Muscle spasms are strong, painful contractions. They can occur in virtually any muscle but are most common in the calf and foot. Muscle spasms typically occur from simple muscle fatigue, after exercise, and during pregnancy. However, they may also develop in electrolyte imbalances and neuromuscular disorders, or as the result of certain drugs. They're typically precipitated by movement, especially a quick or jerking movement, and can usually be relieved by slow stretching.

EMERGENCY INTERVENTIONS *If the patient complains of frequent or unrelieved spasms in many muscles, accompanied by paresthesia in his hands and feet, quickly attempt to elicit Chvostek's and Trousseau's signs. If these signs are present, suspect hypocalcemia. Evaluate respiratory function, watching for the development of laryngospasm; provide supplemental oxygen as necessary, and prepare to intubate the patient and provide mechanical ventilation. Draw blood for calcium and electrolyte levels and arterial blood gas analysis, and insert an I.V. catheter for administration of a calcium supplement. Monitor cardiac status, and prepare to begin resuscitation if necessary.*

History and physical examination

If the patient isn't in distress, ask when the spasms began. Is there any particular activity that precipitates them? How long did they last? How painful were they? Did anything worsen or lessen the pain? Ask about other symptoms, such as weakness, sensory loss, or paresthesia.

Evaluate muscle strength and tone. Then, check all major muscle groups and note whether any movements precipitate spasms. Test the presence and quality of all peripheral pulses, and examine the limbs for color and temperature changes. Test capillary refill time (normal is less than 3 seconds), and inspect for edema, especially in the involved area. Observe for signs and symptoms of dehydration such as dry mucous membranes. Obtain a thorough drug and diet history. Ask the patient if he has had recent vomiting or diarrhea. Finally, test reflexes and sensory function in all extremities.

Medical causes

◆ ***Amyotrophic lateral sclerosis.*** With this disorder, muscle spasms may accompany progressive muscle weakness and atrophy that typically begin in one hand, spread to the arm, and then spread to the other hand and arm. Eventually, muscle weakness and atrophy affect the trunk, neck, tongue, larynx, pharynx, and legs; progressive respiratory muscle weakness leads to respiratory insufficiency. Other findings include muscle flaccidity progressing to spasticity, coarse fasciculations, hyperactive deep tendon reflexes, dysphagia, impaired speech, excessive drooling, and depression.

◆ ***Arterial occlusive disease.*** Arterial occlusion typically produces spasms and intermittent claudication in the leg, with residual pain. Associated findings are usually localized to the legs and feet and include loss of peripheral pulses, pallor or cyanosis, decreased sensation, hair loss, dry or scaling skin, edema, and ulcerations.

◆ ***Cholera.*** Muscle spasms, severe water and electrolyte loss, thirst, weakness, decreased skin turgor, oliguria, tachycardia, and hypotension occur along with abrupt watery diarrhea and vomiting.

◆ ***Dehydration.*** Sodium loss may produce limb and abdominal cramps. Other findings include a slight fever, decreased skin turgor, dry mucous membranes, tachycardia, orthostatic hypotension, muscle twitching, seizures, nausea, vomiting, and oliguria.

◆ ***Fracture.*** Localized spasms and pain are mild if the fracture is nondisplaced, intense if it's severely displaced. Other findings include swelling, limited mobility and, possibly, bony crepitation.

◆ ***Hypocalcemia.*** The classic feature is tetany—a syndrome of muscle cramps and twitching, carpopedal and facial muscle spasms, and seizures, possibly with stridor. Both Chvostek's and Trousseau's signs may be elicited. Related findings include paresthesia of the lips, fingers, and toes; choreiform movements; hyperactive deep tendon reflexes; fatigue; palpitations; and cardiac arrhythmias.

◆ ***Hypothyroidism.*** Muscle involvement may produce spasms and stiffness, along with leg muscle hypertrophy or proximal limb weakness and atrophy. Other findings include forgetfulness and mental instability; fatigue; cold intolerance; dry, pale, cool, doughy skin; puffy face, hands, and feet; periorbital edema; dry, sparse, brittle hair; bradycardia; and weight gain despite anorexia.

◆ ***Muscle trauma.*** Excessive muscle strain may cause mild to severe spasms. The injured area may be painful, swollen, reddened, or warm.

◆ ***Respiratory alkalosis.*** Acute onset of muscle spasms may be accompanied by twitching and weakness, carpopedal spasms, circumoral and peripheral paresthesia, vertigo, syncope, pallor, and extreme anxiety. With severe alkalosis, cardiac arrhythmias may occur.

◆ ***Spinal injury or disease.*** Muscle spasms can result from spinal injury, such as cervical extension injury or spinous process fracture, or from spinal disease such as infection.

Other causes

◆ ***Drugs.*** Common spasm-producing drugs include diuretics, corticosteroids, and estrogens.

Special considerations

Depending on the cause, help alleviate your patient's spasms by slowly stretching the affected muscle in the direction opposite the contraction. If necessary, administer a mild analgesic.

Diagnostic studies may include serum calcium, sodium and carbon dioxide levels, thyroid function tests, and blood flow studies or arteriography.

Pediatric pointers

Muscle spasms rarely occur in children. However, their presence may indicate hypoparathyroidism, osteomalacia, rickets or, rarely, congenital torticollis.

Muscle spasticity

[Muscle hypertonicity]

Spasticity is a state of excessive muscle tone manifested by increased resistance to stretching and heightened reflexes. It's commonly detected by evaluating a muscle's response to passive movement; a spastic muscle offers more resistance when the passive movement is performed quickly. Caused by an upper-motor-neuron lesion, spasticity usually occurs in the arm and leg muscles. Long-term spasticity results in muscle fibrosis and contractures. (See *How spasticity develops,* page 462.)

History and physical examination

Once you detect spasticity, ask the patient about its onset, duration, and progression. What, if any, events precipitate onset? Has he experienced other muscular changes or related symptoms? Does his medical history reveal any incidence of trauma or degenerative or vascular disease?

Take the patient's vital signs, and perform a complete neurologic examination. Test reflexes and evaluate motor and sensory function in all limbs. Evaluate muscles for wasting and contractures.

During your examination, keep in mind that generalized spasticity and trismus in a patient with a recent skin puncture or laceration indicates tetanus. If you suspect this rare disorder, look for signs of respiratory distress. Provide ventilatory support, if necessary, and monitor the patient closely.

Medical causes

◆ ***Amyotrophic lateral sclerosis.*** This disorder commonly produces spasticity, spasms, coarse fasciculations, hyperactive deep tendon reflexes, and a positive Babinski's sign. Earlier effects include progressive muscle weakness and flaccidity that typically begin in the hands and arms and eventually spread to the trunk, neck, larynx, pharynx, and legs; progressive respiratory muscle weakness leads to respiratory insufficiency. Other findings include dysphagia, dysarthria, excessive drooling, and depression.

How spasticity develops

Motor activity is controlled by pyramidal and extrapyramidal tracts that originate in the motor cortex, basal ganglia, brain stem, and spinal cord. Nerve fibers from the various tracts converge and synapse at the anterior horn in the spinal cord. Together, they maintain segmental muscle tone by modulating the stretch reflex arc. This arc, shown in simplified form below, is basically a negative feedback loop in which muscle stretch (stimulation) causes reflexive contraction (inhibition), thus maintaining muscle length and tone.

Damage to certain tracts results in loss of inhibition and disruption of the stretch reflex arc. Uninhibited muscle stretch produces exaggerated, uncontrolled muscle activity, accentuating the reflex arc and eventually resulting in spasticity.

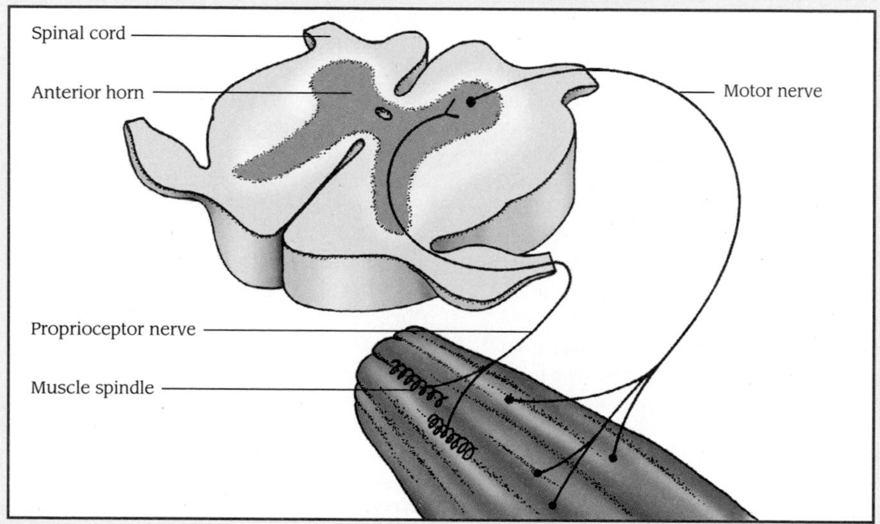

◆ ***Epidural hemorrhage.*** With this disorder, bilateral limb spasticity is a late and ominous sign. Other findings include a momentary loss of consciousness after head trauma, followed by a lucid interval and then a rapid deterioration in level of consciousness. The patient may also develop unilateral hemiparesis or hemiplegia; seizures; fixed, dilated pupils; high fever; decreased and bounding pulse; widened pulse pressure; elevated blood pressure; irregular respiratory pattern; and decerebrate posture. A positive Babinski's sign can be elicited.

◆ ***Multiple sclerosis.*** Muscle spasticity, hyperreflexia, and contractures may eventually develop; earlier muscle changes include progressive weakness and atrophy. Associated signs and symptoms typically wax and wane and may include diplopia, blurring or loss of vision, nystagmus, sensory loss or paresthesia, dysarthria, dysphagia, incoordination, ataxic gait, intention tremors, emotional lability, impotence, and urinary dysfunction.

◆ ***Spinal cord injury.*** Spasticity commonly results from cervical and high thoracic spinal cord injury, especially from incomplete lesions. Spastic paralysis in the affected limbs follows initial flaccid paralysis; typically, spasticity and muscle atrophy increase for up to 1¼ to 2 years after the injury, then gradually regress to flaccidity. Associated signs and symptoms vary with the level of injury but may include respiratory insufficiency or paralysis, sensory losses, bowel and bladder dysfunction, hyperactive deep tendon reflexes, positive Babinski's sign, sexual dysfunction, priapism, hypotension, anhidrosis, and bradycardia.

◆ ***Stroke.*** Spastic paralysis may develop on the affected side following the acute stage of a stroke. Associated findings vary with the site and extent of vascular damage and may include dysarthria, aphasia, ataxia, apraxia, agnosia, ipsilateral paresthesia or sensory loss, visual disturbance, altered level of consciousness, amnesia and poor judgment, personality changes, emotional lability, bowel and bladder dysfunction, headache, vomiting, and seizures.

◆ ***Tetanus.*** This rare, life-threatening disease produces varying degrees of spasticity. In generalized tetanus, the most common form, early signs and symptoms include painful jaw and neck stiffness, trismus, headache, irritability, restlessness, low-grade fever with chills, tachycardia, diaphoresis, and hyperactive deep tendon reflexes. As the disease progresses, painful involuntary spasms may spread and cause boardlike abdominal rigidity, opisthotonos, and a characteristic grotesque grin known as risus sardonicus. Reflex spasms may occur in any muscle group with the slightest stimulus. Glottal, pharyngeal, or respiratory muscle involvement can cause death by asphyxia or cardiac failure.

Special considerations

Prepare the patient for diagnostic tests, which may include electromyography, muscle biopsy, or intracranial or spinal magnetic resonance imaging or computed tomography. Administer pain medication and an antispasmodic. Passive range-of-motion exercises, splinting, traction, and application of heat may help relieve spasms and prevent contractures. Maintain a calm, quiet environment to help relieve spasms and prevent recurrence, and encourage bed rest. In cases of prolonged, uncontrollable spasticity, as with spastic paralysis, nerve blocks or surgical transection may be necessary for permanent relief.

Pediatric pointers

In children, muscle spasticity may be a sign of cerebral palsy.

Muscle weakness

Muscle weakness is detected by observing and measuring the strength of an individual muscle or muscle group. It can result from a malfunction in the cerebral hemispheres, brain stem, spinal cord, nerve roots, peripheral nerves, or myoneural junctions and within the muscle itself. Muscle weakness occurs with certain neurologic, musculoskeletal, metabolic, endocrine, and cardiovascular disorders; as a response to certain drugs; and after prolonged immobilization.

History and physical examination

Begin by determining the location of the patient's muscle weakness. Ask if he has difficulty with specific movements, such as rising from a chair. Find out when he first noticed the weakness; ask him whether it worsens with exercise or as the day progresses. Also ask about related symptoms, especially muscle or joint pain, altered sensory function, and fatigue.

Obtain a medical history, noting especially chronic disease such as hyperthyroidism; musculoskeletal or neurologic problems, including recent trauma; family history of chronic muscle weakness, especially in males; and alcohol and drug use.

Focus your physical examination on evaluating muscle strength. Test all major muscles bilaterally. (See *Testing muscle strength,* pages 464 and 465.) When testing, make sure the patient's effort is constant; if it isn't, suspect pain or other reluctance to make the effort. If the patient complains of pain, ease or discontinue testing and have him try the movements again. Remember that the patient's dominant arm, hand, and leg are somewhat stronger than their nondominant counterparts. Besides testing individual muscle strength, test for range of motion at all major joints (shoulder, elbow, wrist, hip, knee, and ankle). Also test sensory function in the involved areas, and test deep tendon reflexes bilaterally.

Medical causes

◆ ***Amyotrophic lateral sclerosis.*** This disorder typically begins with muscle weakness and atrophy in one hand that rapidly spread to the arm and then to the other hand and arm. Eventually, these effects spread to the trunk, neck, tongue, larynx, pharynx, and legs; progressive respiratory muscle weakness leads to respiratory insufficiency.

◆ ***Anemia.*** Varying degrees of muscle weakness and fatigue are exacerbated by exertion and temporarily relieved by rest. Other signs and symptoms include pallor, tachycardia, paresthesia, and bleeding tendencies.

◆ ***Brain tumor.*** Signs and symptoms of muscle weakness vary with the location and size of the tumor. Associated findings include headache, vomiting, diplopia, decreased visual acuity, decreased level of consciousness, pupillary changes, decreased motor strength, hemiparesis, hemiplegia, diminished sensations, ataxia, seizures, and behavioral changes.

(Text continues on page 466.)

Testing muscle strength

Obtain an overall picture of your patient's motor function by testing strength in 10 selected muscle groups. Ask the patient to attempt normal range-of-motion movements against your resistance. If the muscle group is weak, vary the amount of resistance as necessary to permit accurate assessment. If necessary, position the patient so his limbs don't have to resist gravity, and repeat the test.

Arm muscles

Biceps. With your hand on the patient's hand, have him flex his forearm against your resistance. Watch for biceps contraction.

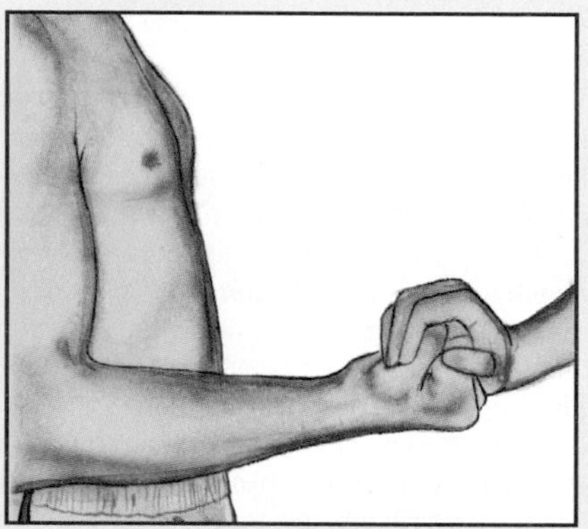

Deltoid. With the patient's arm fully extended, place one hand over his deltoid muscle and the other on his wrist. Ask him to abduct his arm to a horizontal position against your resistance; as he does so, palpate for deltoid contraction.

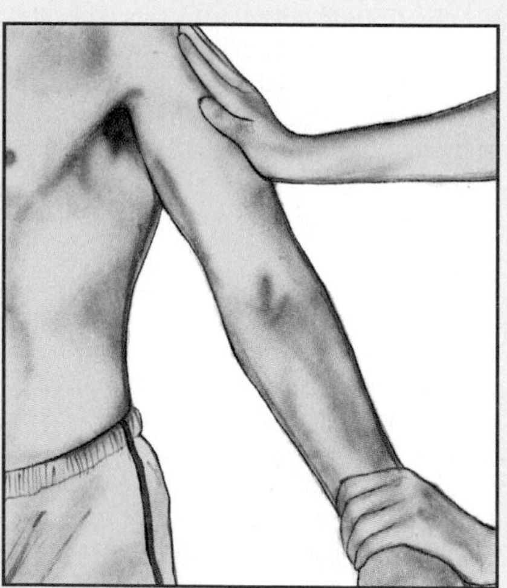

Triceps. Have the patient abduct and hold his arm midway between flexion and extension. Hold and support his arm at the wrist, and ask him to extend it against your resistance. Watch for triceps contraction.

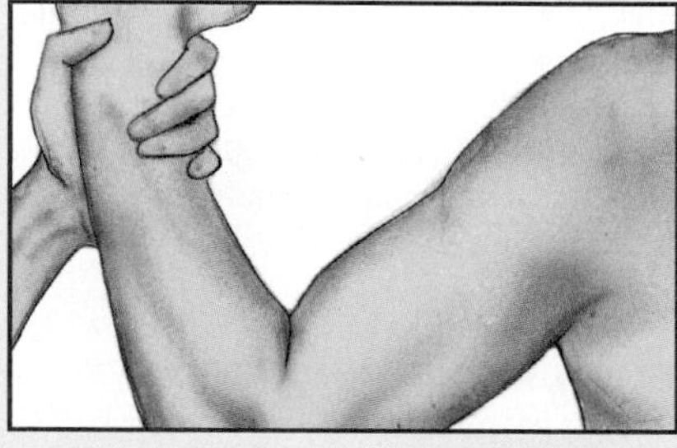

Dorsal interossei. Have the patient extend and spread his fingers, and tell him to try to resist your attempt to squeeze them together.

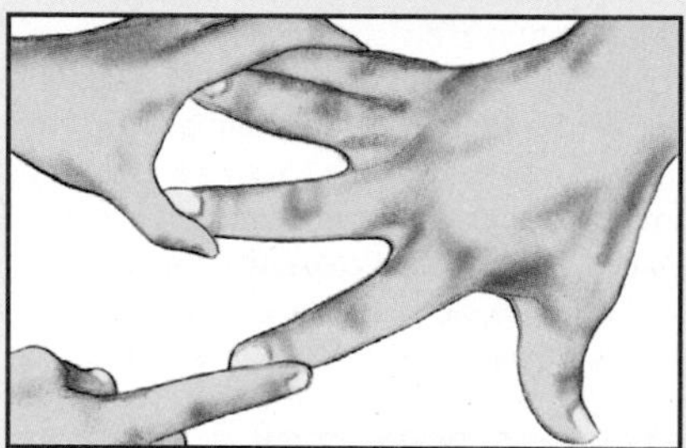

Forearm and hand (grip). Have the patient grasp your middle and index fingers and squeeze as hard as he can. To prevent pain or injury to the examiner, the examiner should cross his fingers.

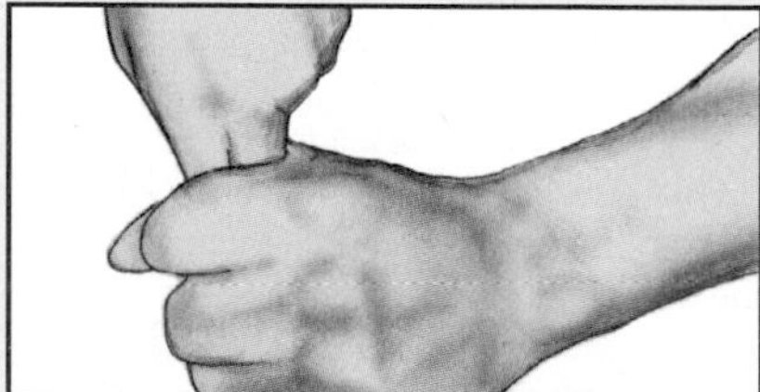

Rate muscle strength on a scale from 0 to 5:
0 = No evidence of muscle contraction; no movement
1 = Visible or palpable contraction, but no movement
2 = Full muscle movement with force of gravity eliminated
3 = Full muscle movement against gravity, but no movement against resistance
4 = Full muscle movement against gravity; partial movement against resistance
5 = Full muscle movement against both gravity and resistance—normal strength.

Leg muscles

Anterior tibial. With the patient's leg extended, place your hand on his foot and ask him to dorsiflex his ankle against your resistance. Palpate for anterior tibial contraction.

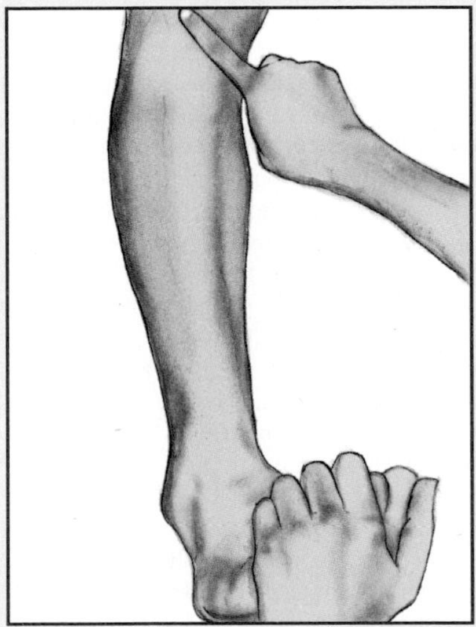

Psoas. While you support his leg, have the patient raise his knee and then flex his hip against your resistance. Watch for psoas contraction.

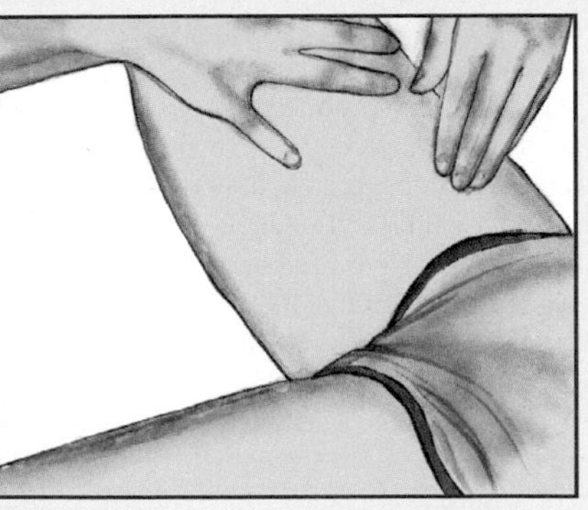

Extensor hallucis longus. With your finger on the patient's great toe, have him dorsiflex the toe against your resistance. Palpate for extensor hallucis contraction.

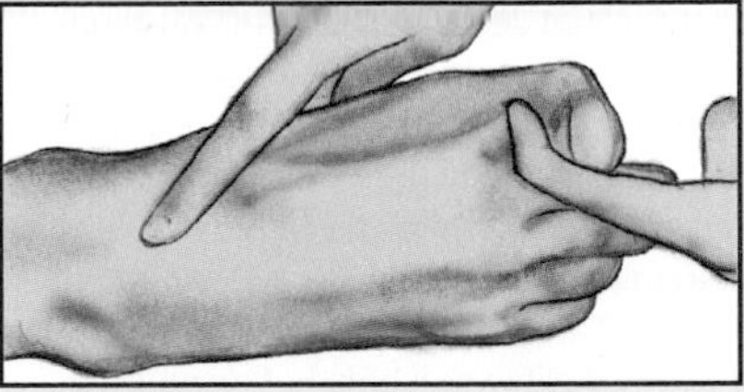

Quadriceps. Have the patient bend his knee slightly while you support his lower leg. Then ask him to extend the knee against your resistance; as he's doing so, palpate for quadriceps contraction.

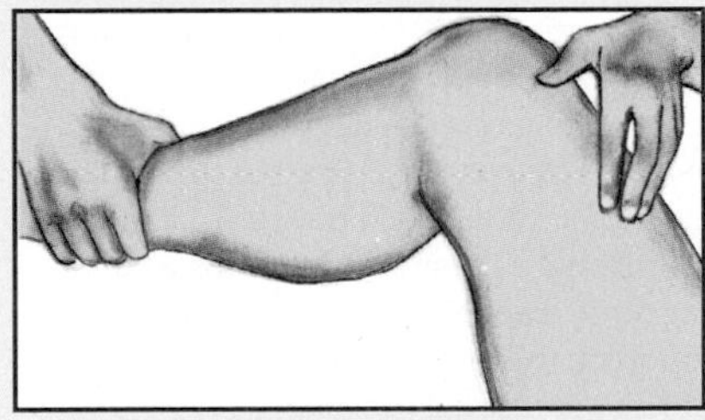

Gastrocnemius. With the patient on his side, support his foot and ask him to plantarflex his ankle against your resistance. Palpate for gastrocnemius contraction.

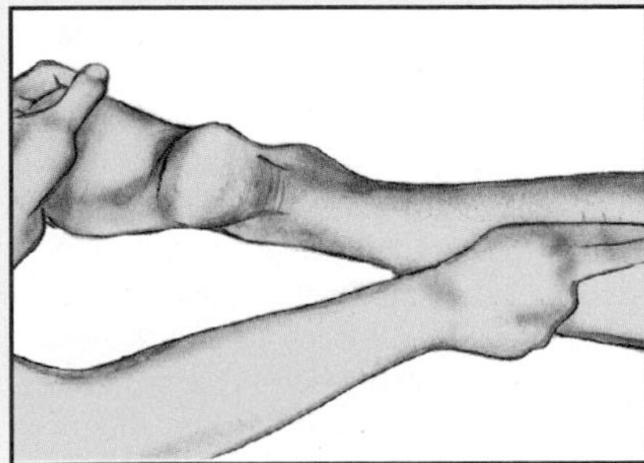

◆ ***Guillain-Barré syndrome.*** Rapidly progressive, symmetrical weakness and pain ascends from the feet to the arms and facial nerves and may progress to total motor paralysis and respiratory failure. Associated findings include sensory loss or paresthesia, muscle flaccidity, loss of deep tendon reflexes, tachycardia or bradycardia, fluctuating hypertension and orthostatic hypotension, diaphoresis, bowel and bladder incontinence, facial diplegia, dysphagia, dysarthria, and hypernasality.

◆ ***Head trauma.*** Severe head injury can cause varying degrees of muscle weakness. Other findings include decreased level of consciousness, otorrhea or rhinorrhea, raccoon eyes and Battle's sign, sensory disturbances, and signs of increased intracranial pressure.

◆ ***Herniated disk.*** Pressure on nerve roots leads to muscle weakness, disuse, and ultimately, atrophy. The primary symptom is severe low back pain, possibly radiating to the buttocks, legs, and feet—usually on one side. Diminished reflexes and sensory changes may also occur.

◆ ***Hodgkin's lymphoma.*** Muscle weakness may accompany the classic sign of painless, progressive lymphadenopathy. Other findings include paresthesia, fatigue, and weight loss.

◆ ***Hypercortisolism.*** This disorder may cause limb weakness and eventually atrophy. Related cushingoid features include buffalo hump, moon face, truncal obesity, purple striae, thin skin, acne, elevated blood pressure, fatigue, hyperpigmentation, easy bruising, poor wound healing, and diaphoresis. The male patient may be impotent; the female patient may exhibit hirsutism and menstrual irregularities.

◆ ***Hypothyroidism.*** Reversible weakness and atrophy of proximal limb muscles may occur in hypothyroidism. Accompanying findings commonly include muscle cramps; cold intolerance; weight gain despite anorexia; mental dullness; dry, pale, doughy skin; puffy face, hands, and feet; impaired hearing and balance; and bradycardia.

◆ ***Multiple sclerosis.*** Muscle weakness in one or more limbs may progress to atrophy, spasticity, and contractures. Other findings typically wax and wane and may include diplopia and blurred vision, vision loss, nystagmus, hyperactive deep tendon reflexes, sensory loss or paresthesia, dysarthria, dysphagia, incoordination, ataxic gait, intention tremors, emotional lability, impotence, and urinary dysfunction.

◆ ***Myasthenia gravis.*** Gradually progressive skeletal muscle weakness and fatigue are the cardinal symptoms of this disorder. Typically, weakness is mild upon awakening but worsens during the day. Early signs include weak eye closure, ptosis, and diplopia; a blank, masklike facies; difficulty chewing and swallowing; nasal regurgitation of fluid with hypernasality; and a hanging jaw and bobbing head. Respiratory muscle involvement may eventually lead to respiratory failure.

◆ ***Osteoarthritis.*** This chronic disorder causes progressive muscle disuse and weakness that lead to atrophy.

◆ ***Paget's disease.*** As this disease progresses, muscle weakness or paralysis may develop, along with paresthesia and pain. The patient may also have bowed tibias, frequent fractures, and kyphosis.

◆ ***Parkinson's disease.*** Muscle weakness accompanies rigidity in this degenerative disorder. Related findings include a unilateral pill-rolling tremor, propulsive gait, dysarthria, bradykinesia, drooling, dysphagia, masklike facies, and a high-pitched, monotonic voice.

◆ ***Peripheral nerve trauma.*** Prolonged pressure on or injury to a peripheral nerve causes muscle weakness and atrophy. Other findings include paresthesia or sensory loss, pain, and loss of reflexes supplied by the damaged nerve.

◆ ***Peripheral neuropathy.*** With this disorder, muscle weakness progresses slowly to flaccid paralysis, generally affecting distal extremities first. It may be accompanied by loss of vibration sense; paresthesia, hyperesthesia, or anesthesia in the hands and feet; hypoactive or absent deep tendon reflexes; mild-to-sharp burning pain; anhidrosis; and glossy red skin.

◆ ***Poliomyelitis.*** Rapidly developing asymmetrical muscle weakness, progressing to flaccid paralysis, occurs with paralytic poliomyelitis. Associated signs and symptoms include moderate fever, headache, vomiting, lethargy, irritability, and widespread pain. As the disorder progresses, it may produce loss of superficial and deep reflexes, paresthesia, hyperalgesia, urine retention, constipation, abdominal distention, nuchal rigidity, and Hoyne's, Kernig's, and Brudzinski's signs. Bulbar paralytic poliomyelitis produces symptoms of encephalitis, along with facial weakness, dysphasia, dysphagia, and respiratory abnormalities.

◆ ***Polymyositis.*** This disorder produces insidious or acute onset of symmetrical limb and trunk muscle weakness and tenderness. Weakness may progress to facial, neck, pharyngeal, and laryngeal muscles. Associated findings include hypoactive deep tendon reflexes, dysphagia, and dysphonia.

◆ ***Potassium imbalance.*** With hypokalemia, temporary generalized muscle weakness may be accompanied by nausea, vomiting, diarrhea, decreased mentation, leg cramps, diminished reflexes, malaise, polyuria, dizziness, hypotension, and arrhythmias.

With hyperkalemia, weakness may progress to flaccid paralysis accompanied by irritability and confusion, hyperreflexia, paresthesia or anesthesia, oliguria, anorexia, nausea, diarrhea, abdominal cramps, tachycardia or bradycardia, and arrhythmias.

◆ ***Protein deficiency.*** Prolonged protein deficiency may lead to muscle weakness and wasting, chronic fatigue, apathy, anorexia, lethargy, dry skin, and dull, sparse, dry hair.

◆ ***Rhabdomyolysis.*** Signs and symptoms include muscle weakness or pain, fever, nausea, vomiting, malaise, and dark urine. Acute renal failure, due to renal structure obstruction and injury from the kidneys' attempt to filter the myoglobin from the bloodstream, is a common complication.

◆ ***Rheumatoid arthritis.*** With this disease, symmetric muscle weakness may accompany increased warmth, swelling, and tenderness in involved joints; pain; and stiffness, restricting motion.

◆ ***Seizure disorder.*** Temporary generalized muscle weakness may occur after a generalized tonic-clonic seizure; other postictal findings include headache, muscle soreness, and profound fatigue.

◆ ***Spinal trauma and disease.*** Trauma can cause severe muscle weakness, leading to flaccidity or spasticity and, eventually, paralysis. Infection, tumor, and cervical spondylosis or stenosis can also cause muscle weakness.

◆ ***Stroke.*** Depending on the site and extent of damage, a stroke may produce contralateral or bilateral weakness of the arms, legs, face, and tongue, possibly progressing to hemiplegia and atrophy. Associated effects include dysarthria, aphasia, ataxia, apraxia, agnosia, ipsilateral paresthesia or sensory loss, visual disturbance, altered level of consciousness, amnesia and poor judgment, personality changes, bowel and bladder dysfunction, headache, vomiting, and seizures.

◆ ***Thyrotoxicosis.*** This disorder may produce insidious, generalized muscle weakness and atrophy. Other effects include anxiety, fatigue, heat intolerance, diaphoresis, tremors, tachycardia, palpitations, ventricular or atrial gallop, dyspnea, weight loss, an enlarged thyroid, and warm, flushed skin. Exophthalmos may be present.

OTHER CAUSES

◆ ***Drugs.*** Generalized muscle weakness can result from prolonged corticosteroid use, digoxin, and excessive doses of dantrolene sodium. Aminoglycoside antibiotics may worsen weakness in patients with myasthenia gravis.

◆ ***Immobility.*** Immobilization in a cast, a splint, or traction can lead to muscle weakness in the involved extremity; prolonged bed rest or inactivity results in generalized muscle weakness.

SPECIAL CONSIDERATIONS

Provide assistive devices as necessary, and protect the patient from injury. If he has concomitant sensory loss, guard against pressure ulcer formation and thermal injury. With chronic weakness, provide range-of-motion exercises or splint limbs as necessary. Arrange therapy sessions to allow for adequate rest periods, and administer pain medications as needed.

Prepare the patient for blood tests, muscle biopsy, electromyography, nerve conduction studies, and X-rays or computed tomography scans.

PEDIATRIC POINTERS

Muscular dystrophy, usually the Duchenne type, is a major cause of muscle weakness in children.

Mydriasis

Mydriasis—pupillary dilation caused by contraction of the dilator of the iris—is a normal response to decreased light, strong emotional stimuli, and topical administration of mydriatic and cycloplegic drugs. It can also result from ocular and neurologic disorders, eye trauma, and disorders that decrease level of consciousness. Mydriasis may be an adverse effect of antihistamines or other drugs.

HISTORY AND PHYSICAL EXAMINATION

Begin by asking the patient about any other eye problems, such as pain, blurring, diplopia, or visual field defects. Obtain a health history, focusing on eye or head trauma, glaucoma and other ocular problems, and neurologic and vascular disorders. In addition, obtain a complete drug history.

Next, perform a thorough eye and pupil examination. Inspect and compare the pupils' size, color, and shape—many people normally

Grading pupil size

To ensure accurate evaluation of pupillary size, compare your patient's pupils to the scale below. Keep in mind that maximum constriction may be less than 1 mm and maximum dilation greater than 9 mm.

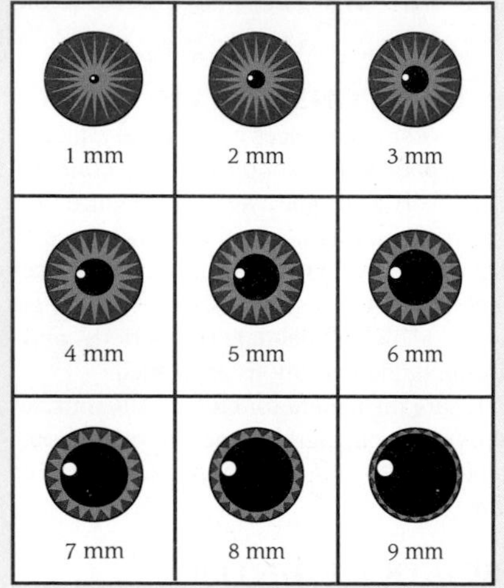

have unequal pupils. (See *Grading pupil size.*) Also, test each pupil for light reflex, consensual response, and accommodation. Perform a swinging flashlight test to evaluate a decreased response to direct light coupled with a normal consensual response (Marcus Gunn pupil). Be sure to check the eyes for ptosis, swelling, and ecchymosis. Test visual acuity in both eyes with and without correction. Evaluate extraocular muscle function by checking the six cardinal fields of gaze.

Keep in mind that mydriasis appears in two ocular emergencies: acute angle-closure glaucoma and traumatic iridoplegia.

Medical causes

◆ ***Adie's syndrome.*** This disorder is characterized by abrupt unilateral mydriasis, poor or absent pupillary reflexes, visual blurring, and cramplike eye pain. Deep tendon reflexes may be hyperactive or absent, especially the ankle and knee jerk reflexes.

◆ ***Aortic arch syndrome.*** Bilateral pupillary mydriasis commonly occurs late in this syndrome. Other ocular findings include visual blurring, transient vision loss, and diplopia. Related findings include dizziness and syncope; neck, shoulder, and chest pain; bruits; loss of radial and carotid pulses; paresthesia; and intermittent claudication. Blood pressure may be decreased in the arms.

◆ ***Botulism.*** Botulism toxin causes bilateral mydriasis, usually 12 to 36 hours after ingestion. Other early findings are loss of pupillary reflexes, visual blurring, diplopia, ptosis, strabismus and extraocular muscle palsies, anorexia, nausea, vomiting, diarrhea, and dry mouth. Vertigo, hearing loss, hoarseness, hypernasality, dysarthria, dysphagia, progressive muscle weakness, and loss of deep tendon reflexes soon follow.

◆ ***Brain stem infarction.*** This rare disorder may cause bilateral mydriatic, fixed pupils. Associated signs and symptoms vary but may include paralysis of all extremities, sudden coma, decerebrate posturing, disconjugate gaze, and respiratory pattern changes.

◆ ***Carotid artery aneurysm.*** With this disorder, unilateral mydriasis may be accompanied by bitemporal hemianopsia, decreased visual acuity, hemiplegia, decreased level of consciousness, headache, aphasia, behavioral changes, and hypoesthesia.

◆ ***Glaucoma (acute angle closure).*** This ocular emergency is characterized by moderate mydriasis and loss of pupillary reflex in the affected eye, accompanied by abrupt onset of excruciating pain, redness, decreased visual acuity, visual blurring, halo vision, conjunctival injection, and a cloudy cornea. Without treatment, permanent blindness occurs in 2 to 5 days.

◆ ***Oculomotor nerve palsy.*** Unilateral mydriasis is often the first sign of this disorder. It's soon followed by ptosis, diplopia, decreased pupillary reflexes, exotropia, and complete loss of accommodation. Focal neurologic signs may accompany signs of increased intracranial pressure.

◆ ***Traumatic iridoplegia.*** Eye trauma can paralyze the sphincter of the iris, causing mydriasis and loss of pupillary reflex; usually, this is transient. Associated findings include a quivering iris (iridodonesis), ecchymosis, pain, and swelling.

Other causes

◆ ***Drugs.*** Mydriasis can be caused by anticholinergics, antihistamines, sympathomimetics, barbiturates (in overdose), estrogens, and tricyclic antidepressants; it also commonly occurs early in anesthesia induction. Topical mydriatics and cycloplegics, such as phenylephrine, atropine, scopolamine, cyclopentolate, and tropicamide, are administered specifically for their mydriatic effects.

◆ ***Surgery.*** Traumatic mydriasis commonly results from ocular surgery.

Special considerations

Diagnostic tests may vary, depending on your findings, but may include a complete ophthalmologic examination and a thorough neurologic workup. Explain any diagnostic tests to the patient.

Pediatric pointers

Mydriasis occurs in children as a result of ocular trauma, drugs, Adie's syndrome and, most commonly, increased intracranial pressure.

Patient counseling

If the patient's mydriasis is the result of mydriatic drugs received during an eye examination, explain that he'll likely experience some photophobia and loss of accommodation. Instruct him to wear dark glasses and to avoid bright light, and reassure him that the condition is only temporary.

Myoclonus

Myoclonus—sudden, shocklike contractions of a single muscle or muscle group—occurs with various neurologic disorders and may herald onset of a seizure. These contractions may be isolated or repetitive, rhythmic or arrhythmic, symmetrical or asymmetrical, synchronous or asynchronous, and generalized or focal. They may be precipitated by bright flickering lights, a loud sound, or unexpected physical contact. One type, *intention myoclonus,* is evoked by intentional muscle movement.

Myoclonus occurs normally just before falling asleep and as a part of the natural startle reaction. It also occurs with some poisonings and, rarely, as a complication of hemodialysis.

EMERGENCY INTERVENTIONS *If you observe myoclonus, check for seizure activity. Take vital signs to rule out arrhythmias or a blocked airway. Have resuscitation equipment on hand.*

If the patient has a seizure, gently help him lie down. Place a pillow or a rolled-up towel under his head to prevent concussion. Loosen any constrictive clothing, especially around the neck, and turn his head (gently, if possible) to one side to prevent airway occlusion or aspiration of secretions.

History and physical examination

If the patient is stable, evaluate level of consciousness and mental status. Ask about the frequency, severity, location, and circumstances of the myoclonus. Has he ever had a seizure? If so, did myoclonus precede it? Is the myoclonus ever precipitated by a sensory stimulus? During the physical examination, check for muscle rigidity and wasting, and test deep tendon reflexes.

Medical causes

◆ ***Alzheimer's disease.*** Generalized myoclonus may occur in advanced stages of this slowly progressive dementia. Other late findings include mild choreoathetoid movements, muscle rigidity, bowel and bladder incontinence, delusions, and hallucinations.

◆ ***Creutzfeldt-Jakob disease.*** Diffuse myoclonic jerks appear early in this rapidly progressive dementia. Initially random, they gradually become more rhythmic and symmetrical, often occurring in response to sensory stimuli. Associated effects include ataxia, aphasia, hearing loss, muscle rigidity and wasting, fasciculations, hemiplegia, and visual disturbance, or possibly, blindness.

◆ ***Encephalitis (viral).*** With this disease, myoclonus is usually intermittent and either localized or generalized. Associated findings vary but may include rapidly decreasing level of consciousness, fever, headache, irritability, nuchal rigidity, vomiting, seizures, aphasia, ataxia, hemiparesis, facial muscle weakness, nystagmus, ocular palsies, and dysphagia.

◆ ***Encephalopathy.*** Hepatic encephalopathy occasionally produces myoclonic jerks in association with asterixis and focal or generalized seizures.

Hypoxic encephalopathy may produce generalized myoclonus or seizures almost immediately after restoration of cardiopulmonary function. The patient may also have a residual intention myoclonus.

Uremic encephalopathy commonly produces myoclonic jerks and seizures. Other signs and symptoms include apathy, fatigue, irritability, headache, confusion, gradually decreasing level of consciousness, nausea, vomiting, oliguria, edema, and papilledema. The patient may also exhibit elevated blood pressure, dyspnea, arrhythmias, and abnormal respirations.

◆ ***Epilepsy.*** With idiopathic epilepsy, localized myoclonus is usually confined to an arm or leg and occurs singly or in short bursts, usually upon awakening. It's usually more frequent and severe during the prodromal stage of a major generalized seizure, after which it diminishes in frequency and intensity.

Myoclonic jerks are usually the first signs of myoclonic epilepsy, the most common cause of progressive myoclonus. At first, myoclonus is infrequent and localized, but over a period of months, it becomes more frequent and involves the entire body, disrupting voluntary movement (intention myoclonus). As the disease progresses, myoclonus is accompanied by generalized seizures and dementia.

Other causes

- ***Drug withdrawal.*** Myoclonus may be seen in patients with alcohol, opioid, or sedative withdrawal, or delirium tremens.
- ***Poisoning.*** Acute intoxication with methyl bromide, bismuth, or strychnine may produce an acute onset of myoclonus and confusion.

Special considerations

If your patient's myoclonus is progressive, take seizure precautions. Keep an oral airway and suction equipment at his bedside, and pad the side rails. Because myoclonus may cause falls, remove potentially harmful objects from the patient's environment, and remain with him while he walks. Be sure to instruct the patient and his family about the need for safety precautions.

As needed, administer drugs that suppress myoclonus: ethosuximide, L-5-hydroxytryptophan, phenobarbital, clonazepam, or carbidopa. An EEG may be needed to evaluate myoclonus and related brain activity.

Pediatric pointers

Although myoclonus is relatively uncommon in infants and children, it can result from subacute sclerosing panencephalitis, severe meningitis, progressive poliodystrophy, childhood myoclonic epilepsy, and encephalopathies, such as Reye's syndrome.

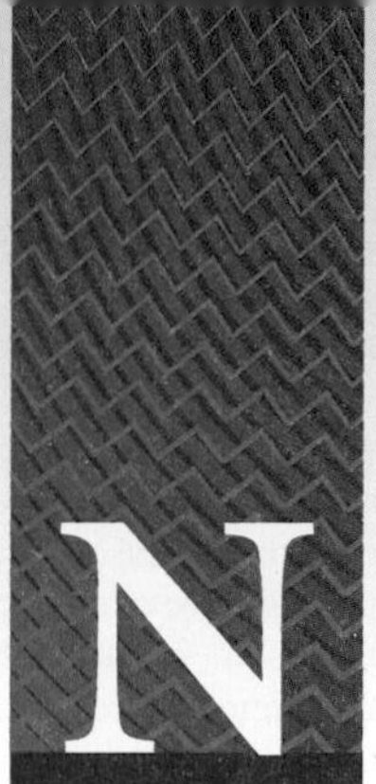

Nasal flaring

Nasal flaring is the abnormal dilation of the nostrils. Usually occurring during inspiration, nasal flaring may occasionally occur during expiration or throughout the respiratory cycle. It indicates respiratory dysfunction, ranging from mild difficulty to potentially life-threatening respiratory distress.

EMERGENCY INTERVENTIONS *If you note nasal flaring in the patient, quickly evaluate his respiratory status. Absent breath sounds, cyanosis, diaphoresis, and tachycardia point to complete airway obstruction. As necessary, deliver abdominal thrusts (Heimlich maneuver) to relieve the obstruction. If these don't clear the airway, emergency intubation or tracheostomy and mechanical ventilation may be necessary.*

If the patient's airway isn't obstructed but he displays breathing difficulty, give oxygen by nasal cannula or face mask. Intubation and mechanical ventilation may be necessary. Insert an I.V. catheter for fluid and drug access. Begin cardiac monitoring. Obtain a chest X-ray and samples for arterial blood gas and electrolyte studies.

History and physical examination

Once the patient's condition is stabilized, obtain a pertinent history. Ask about cardiac and pulmonary disorders such as asthma. Does the patient have allergies? Has he experienced a recent illness, such as a respiratory tract infection, or trauma? Does the patient smoke or have a history of smoking? Obtain a drug history.

Medical causes

◆ ***Acute respiratory distress syndrome (ARDS).*** ARDS causes increased respiratory difficulty and hypoxemia, with nasal flaring, dyspnea, tachypnea, diaphoresis, cyanosis, scattered crackles, and rhonchi. It also produces tachycardia, anxiety, and decreased level of consciousness.

◆ ***Airway obstruction.*** Complete obstruction above the tracheal bifurcation causes sudden nasal flaring, absent breath sounds despite intercostal retractions and marked accessory muscle use, tachycardia, diaphoresis, cyanosis, decreasing level of consciousness and, eventually, respiratory arrest.

Partial obstruction causes nasal flaring with inspiratory stridor, gagging, wheezing, violent cough, marked accessory muscle use, agitation, cyanosis, and hoarseness.

◆ ***Anaphylaxis.*** Severe reactions can produce respiratory distress with nasal flaring, stridor, wheezing, accessory muscle use, intercostal retractions, and dyspnea. Associated signs and symptoms include nasal congestion, sneezing, pruritus, urticaria, erythema, diaphoresis, angioedema, weakness, hoarseness, dysphagia and, rarely, vomiting, nausea, diarrhea, urinary urgency, and incontinence. Cardiac arrhythmias and signs of shock may occur late.

◆ ***Asthma (acute).*** An asthma attack can cause nasal flaring, dyspnea, tachypnea, prolonged expiratory wheezing, accessory muscle use, cyanosis, and a dry or productive cough. Auscultation may reveal rhonchi, crackles, and decreased or absent breath sounds. Other findings include anxiety, tachycardia, and increased blood pressure.

◆ ***Chronic obstructive pulmonary disease.*** This disorder can lead to acute respiratory failure secondary to pulmonary infection or edema. Nasal flaring is accompanied by prolonged pursed-lip expiration; accessory muscle use; loose, rattling, productive cough; cyanosis; reduced chest expansion; crackles; rhonchi; wheezing; and dyspnea.

◆ ***Pneumonia (bacterial).*** With this condition, nasal flaring occurs with dyspnea, tachypnea, high fever, and sudden shaking chills. An initially dry and hacking cough later becomes productive. Stabbing chest pain worsens with movement and respirations. Auscultation reveals decreased or absent breath sounds, fine crackles, and pleural friction rub. Percussion reveals dullness.

◆ ***Pneumothorax.*** This acute disorder can result in respiratory distress with nasal flaring, dyspnea, tachypnea, shallow respirations, hyperresonance or tympany on percussion, agitation, distended jugular veins, tracheal deviation, and cyanosis. Other findings typically include sharp chest pain, tachycardia, hypotension, cold and clammy skin, diaphoresis, subcutaneous crepitation, and anxiety. Breath sounds may be decreased or absent on the affected side; similarly, chest-wall motion may be decreased on the affected side.

Similar findings can occur with *hydrothorax*, *chylothorax*, or *hemothorax*, depending on the amount of fluid accumulation.

◆ ***Pulmonary edema.*** This disorder typically produces nasal flaring, severe dyspnea, wheezing, and a cough that produces frothy, pink sputum. Increased accessory muscle use may occur with tachycardia, cyanosis, hypotension, crackles, jugular vein distention, peripheral edema, and decreased level of consciousness.

◆ ***Pulmonary embolus.*** Signs of this potentially life-threatening disorder may include nasal flaring, dyspnea, tachypnea, wheezing, cyanosis, pleural friction rub, and productive cough (possibly hemoptysis). Its other effects include sudden chest tightness or pleuritic pain, tachycardia, atrial arrhythmias, hypotension, low-grade fever, syncope, marked anxiety, and restlessness.

OTHER CAUSES

◆ ***Diagnostic tests.*** Pulmonary function tests, such as vital capacity testing, can produce nasal flaring with forced inspiration or expiration.

◆ ***Treatments.*** Certain respiratory treatments, such as deep breathing, can cause nasal flaring.

SPECIAL CONSIDERATIONS

To help ease breathing, place the patient in a high Fowler's position. If he's at risk for aspirating secretions, place him in a modified Trendelenburg's or side-lying position. If necessary, suction frequently to remove oropharyngeal secretions. Administer humidified oxygen to thin secretions and decrease airway drying and irritation. Provide adequate hydration to liquefy secretions. Reposition the patient every hour, and encourage coughing and deep breathing and incentive spirometry use. Avoid administering sedatives or opiates, which can depress the cough reflex or respirations. Continually assess the patient's respiratory status, and check his vital signs and oxygen saturation every 30 minutes, or as necessary.

Prepare the patient for diagnostic tests, such as chest X-rays, lung scan, pulmonary arteriography, sputum culture, complete blood count, arterial blood gas analysis, and 12-lead electrocardiogram.

PEDIATRIC POINTERS

Nasal flaring is an important sign of respiratory distress in infants and very young children, who can't verbalize their discomfort. Common causes include airway obstruction, hyaline membrane disease, croup, and acute epiglottiditis. Use oxygen and cool humidifiers to help improve oxygenation.

Nasal obstruction

Nasal obstruction may result from an allergic, inflammatory, neoplastic, endocrine, or metabolic disorder; a structural abnormality; a traumatic injury; or a mechanical obstruction (foreign objects). It may cause discomfort, alter a person's sense of taste and smell, and cause voice changes. Although a frequent and typically benign symptom, nasal obstruction may herald certain life-threatening disorders, such as a basilar skull fracture or malignant tumor.

HISTORY AND PHYSICAL EXAMINATION

Begin the history by asking the patient about the duration and frequency of the obstruction. Did it begin suddenly or gradually? Is it intermittent or persistent? Unilateral or bilateral? Inquire about the presence and character of drainage. Is it watery, purulent, or bloody? Does the patient have nasal or sinus pain or headaches? Ask about recent travel, the use of drugs or alcohol, and previous trauma or surgery.

Examine the patient's nose; assess airflow and the condition of the turbinates and nasal septum. Evaluate the orbits for any evidence of dystopia, decreased vision, excess tearing, or abnormal appearance of the eye. Palpate over the frontal and maxillary sinuses for tenderness. Examine the ears for signs of middle ear effusions. Inspect the oral cavity, pharynx, nasopharynx, and larynx to detect inflammation, ulceration, excessive mucosal dryness, and neurologic deficits. Lastly, palpate the neck for adenopathy.

MEDICAL CAUSES

◆ ***Basilar skull fracture.*** A tear in the dura can lead to cerebrospinal rhinorrhea, which increases when the patient lowers his head. Associated findings may include epistaxis, otorrhea, and a bulging tympanic membrane from blood or fluid. A fracture may also cause headache, facial paralysis, nausea, vomiting, impaired eye movement, ocular deviation, vision and hearing loss, depressed level of consciousness, Battle's sign, and raccoon eyes.

◆ ***Common cold.*** Onset of the common cold is typified by a watery discharge along with sneezing and nasal obstruction. Edema of the nasal mucosa may lead to sinus pain and infection as well as loss of smell and taste. Related findings include sore throat, malaise, myalgia, arthralgia, and mild headache.

◆ ***Hypothyroidism.*** An underactive thyroid gland may lead to a generalized hypoactive state. This can lead to vascular dilation in the nasal mucosa, resulting in nasal obstruction. Associated findings include fatigue, weight gain despite anorexia, cold intolerance, facial edema, impaired memory, brittle hair, thick skin and tongue, bradycardia, and a hoarse voice.

◆ ***Nasal deformities.*** Deviation of the nasal septum may cause unilateral or bilateral nasal obstruction, snoring, and postnasal drip. Perforation of the nasal septum may result in a sensation of nasal congestion due to altered air flow.

◆ ***Nasal fracture.*** Nasal obstruction develops because of trauma that results in nasal mucosal swelling, epistaxis, abscess, or a septal deviation. Periorbital ecchymoses and edema, nasal deformity and pain, and crepitation of the nasal bones may occur as well.

◆ ***Nasal polyps.*** The most common signs and symptoms are nasal obstruction, anosmia, and clear, watery drainage. The patient may have a history of allergies, chronic sinusitis, trauma, cystic fibrosis, or asthma. Translucent, pear-shaped polyps that are unilateral or bilateral occur.

◆ ***Nasal tumors.*** Benign and malignant nasal tumors may cause unilateral or bilateral nasal obstruction, rhinorrhea, epistaxis, pain, foul discharge, and cheek swelling. Most of these tumors are benign papillomas and minor salivary gland tumors; malignant ones are rare. Kaposi's sarcoma of the nose may occur in acquired immunodeficiency syndrome.

◆ ***Nasopharyngeal tumors.*** Benign and malignant tumors of the nasopharynx may cause nasal obstruction, rhinorrhea, epistaxis, otitis media, and nasal speech. Tumors usually reach a considerable size before symptoms develop. Cancer of the nasopharynx is the most common malignancy of the nasopharynx and may present first with a neck mass or conductive hearing loss.

◆ ***Pregnancy.*** High levels of estrogen during pregnancy may cause vascular engorgement of the nasal mucosa, resulting in nasal obstruction. Associated findings include clear or blood-tinged drainage, sneezing, and edematous and bluish turbinates.

◆ ***Rhinitis.*** Allergic rhinitis produces intermittent watery discharge and nasal obstruction. Common signs and symptoms include sneezing, increased lacrimation, decreased sense of smell, postnasal drip, and itching of the eyes, nose, or ears. The mucosa is edematous and pale.

Vasomotor rhinitis produces a profuse watery nasal discharge in addition to nasal obstruction. Sneezing, postnasal drip, and swollen turbinates occur as well.

With atrophic rhinitis, nasal obstruction is chronic and continuous. Associated findings include intermittent, purulent drainage, foul drainage odor, and nasal crusts that bleed on removal. The mucosa is pale pink and shiny.

◆ ***Sarcoidosis.*** This systemic granulomatous disease occasionally affects the nasal tissues. Nasal membranes appear firm, woody, and erythematous, and their surfaces may be covered by foul-smelling, crusty secretions. These features may occur with a nonproductive cough, substernal pain, malaise, and weight loss.

Related findings include tachycardia, arrhythmias, parotid enlargement, cervical lymphadenopathy, skin lesions, hepatosplenomegaly, and arthritis in the ankles, knees, and wrist.

◆ ***Sinusitis.*** With acute sinusitis, the usual findings are marked nasal obstruction along with thick, purulent drainage and severe pain over the involved sinuses. Fever, inflamed nasal mucosa with purulent mucus, and facial tenderness and pressure occur.

With chronic sinusitis, nasal obstruction can be persistent or recurrent. Thick, intermittently purulent rhinorrhea and low-grade discomfort over the involved sinuses are also seen.

Chronic fungal sinusitis is clinically similar to chronic bacterial sinusitis. However, in immunocompromised patients the disease may rapidly progress to proptosis, blindness, and death.

◆ ***Wegener's granulomatosis.*** Besides nasal obstruction, other nasal findings include crusting, epistaxis, mucopurulent discharge, and cartilaginous necrosis of the septum and bridge of the nose.

Other causes

◆ ***Drugs.*** Topical nasal vasoconstrictors may cause rebound rhinorrhea and nasal obstruction if used longer than 5 days. Antihypertensives may cause nasal congestion as well.

◆ ***Surgery.*** Nasal obstruction may occur after sinus or cranial surgery, or even after rhinoplasty.

Special considerations

Prepare the patient for X-rays or computed tomography scans of the nose, sinuses, or skull. Promote fluid intake to thin secretions, as needed. Give an antihistamine, a decongestant, an analgesic, or an antipyretic.

Pediatric pointers

Acute nasal obstruction in children commonly results from the common cold. In infants and children, especially between ages 3 and 6, chronic nasal obstruction typically results from large adenoids. In neonates, choanal atresia is the most common congenital cause of nasal obstruction and can be unilateral or bilateral. Cystic fibrosis may cause nasal polyps in children, resulting in nasal obstruction. However, if the child has unilateral nasal obstruction and rhinorrhea, you should assume that a foreign body is in the nose until proven otherwise.

Patient counseling

Tell the patient not to use over-the-counter nasal vasoconstrictor sprays for more than 5 days.

Nausea

Nausea is a sensation of profound revulsion to food or of impending vomiting. Often accompanied by autonomic signs, such as hypersalivation, diaphoresis, tachycardia, pallor, and tachypnea, it's closely associated with both anorexia and vomiting.

Nausea, a common symptom of GI disorders, also occurs with fluid and electrolyte imbalance; infection; and metabolic, endocrine, labyrinthine, and cardiac disorders; and as a result of drug therapy, surgery, and radiation. Often present during the first trimester of pregnancy, nausea may also arise from severe pain, anxiety, alcohol intoxication, overeating, or ingestion of distasteful food or liquids.

History and physical examination

Begin by obtaining a complete medical history. Focus on GI, endocrine, and metabolic disorders; recent infections; and cancer and its treatment. Ask about drug use and alcohol consumption. If the patient is a female of childbearing age, ask if she is or could be pregnant. Have the patient describe the onset, duration, and intensity of the nausea, as well as what causes or relieves it. Ask about related complaints, particularly vomiting (color, amount), abdominal pain, anorexia and weight loss, changes in bowel habits or stool character, excessive belching or flatus, and a sensation of bloating.

Inspect the skin for jaundice, bruises, and spider angiomas, and assess skin turgor. Next, inspect the abdomen for distention, auscultate for bowel sounds and bruits, palpate for rigidity and tenderness, and test for rebound tenderness. Palpate and percuss the liver for enlargement. Assess other body systems as appropriate.

Medical causes

◆ ***Adrenal insufficiency.*** Common GI findings in this endocrine disorder include nausea, vomiting, anorexia, and diarrhea. Other findings include weakness; fatigue; weight loss; bronze skin; hypotension; a weak, irregular pulse; vitiligo; and depression.

◆ ***Anthrax (GI).*** Initial signs and symptoms include nausea, vomiting, loss of appetite, and fever. Signs and symptoms may progress to abdominal pain, severe bloody diarrhea, and hematemesis.

◆ ***Appendicitis.*** With acute appendicitis, a brief period of nausea may accompany onset of abdominal pain. Pain typically begins as vague epigastric or periumbilical discomfort and rapidly progresses to severe stabbing pain localized in the right lower quadrant (McBurney's sign). Associated findings usually include abdominal rigidity and tenderness, cutaneous hyperalgesia, fever, constipation or diarrhea, tachycardia, anorexia, moderate malaise, and positive psoas (increased abdominal pain occurs when the examiner places his hand above the patient's right knee and the patient flexes his right hip against resistance) and obturator signs (internal rotation of the right leg with the leg flexed to 90 degrees at the hip and knee with a resulting tightening of the internal obturator muscle that causes abdominal discomfort).

◆ ***Cholecystitis (acute).*** With this disease, nausea often follows severe right-upper-quadrant pain that may radiate to the back or shoulders, often following meals. Associated findings include mild vomiting, flatulence, abdominal tenderness and, possibly, rigidity and distention, fever with chills, diaphoresis, and a positive Murphy's sign.

◆ ***Cholelithiasis.*** With this disease, nausea accompanies attacks of severe right-upper-quadrant or epigastric pain after ingestion of fatty foods. Other associated findings include vomiting, abdominal tenderness and guarding, flatulence, belching, epigastric burning, tachycardia, and restlessness. Occlusion of the common bile duct may cause jaundice, clay-colored stools, fever, and chills.

◆ ***Cirrhosis.*** Insidious early signs and symptoms of cirrhosis typically include nausea and vomiting, anorexia, abdominal pain, and constipation or diarrhea. As the disease progresses, jaundice and hepatomegaly may occur with abdominal distention, spider angiomas, palmar erythema, severe pruritus, dry skin, fetor hepaticus, enlarged superficial abdominal veins, mental changes, and bilateral gynecomastia and testicular atrophy or menstrual irregularities.

◆ ***Diverticulitis.*** Besides nausea, diverticulitis causes intermittent crampy abdominal pain, constipation or diarrhea, low-grade fever, and often a palpable, tender, firm, fixed mass.

◆ ***Ectopic pregnancy.*** Nausea, vomiting, vaginal bleeding, and lower abdominal pain occur in this potentially life-threatening disorder. Suspect ectopic pregnancy in a female of childbearing age with a 1- to 2-month history of amenorrhea.

◆ ***Electrolyte imbalances.*** Such disturbances as hyponatremia or hypernatremia, hypokalemia, and hypercalcemia commonly cause nausea and vomiting. Other effects include cardiac arrhythmias, tremors or seizures, anorexia, malaise, and weakness.

◆ **Escherichia coli *O157:H7.*** Signs and symptoms include nausea, watery or bloody diarrhea, vomiting, fever, and abdominal cramps. In children younger than age 5 and in the elderly, hemolytic uremic syndrome may develop in which red blood cells are destroyed, which may ultimately lead to acute renal failure.

◆ ***Gastric cancer.*** This rare cancer may produce vague GI symptoms—mild nausea, anorexia, upper abdominal discomfort, and chronic dyspepsia. Fatigue, weight loss, weakness, hematemesis, melena, and altered bowel habits are also common.

◆ ***Gastritis.*** Nausea is common with this disorder, especially after ingestion of alcohol, aspirin, spicy foods, or caffeine. Vomiting of mucus or blood, epigastric pain, belching, fever, and malaise may also occur.

◆ ***Gastroenteritis.*** Usually viral, this disorder causes nausea, vomiting, diarrhea, and abdominal cramping. Fever, malaise, hyperactive bowel sounds, abdominal pain and tenderness, and possible dehydration and electrolyte imbalances may also develop.

◆ ***Heart failure.*** This disorder may produce nausea and vomiting, particularly with right-sided heart failure. Associated findings include tachycardia, ventricular gallop, profound fatigue, dyspnea, crackles, peripheral edema, jugular vein distention, ascites, nocturia, and diastolic hypertension.

◆ ***Hepatitis.*** Nausea is an insidious early symptom of viral hepatitis. Vomiting, fatigue, myalgia and arthralgia, headache, anorexia, photophobia, pharyngitis, cough, and fever also occur early in the preicteric phase.

◆ ***Hyperemesis gravidarum.*** Unremitting nausea and vomiting that persist beyond the first trimester are characteristic of this pregnancy disorder. Vomitus ranges from undigested food, mucus, and bile early in the disorder to a coffee-ground appearance in later stages. Associated findings include weight loss, signs of dehydration, headache, and delirium.

◆ ***Infection.*** Acute localized or systemic infection typically produces nausea. Other common findings include fever, headache, fatigue, and malaise.

◆ ***Inflammatory bowel disease.*** The most common symptom is recurrent diarrhea with blood, pus, and mucus. Nausea, vomiting, abdominal pain, and anorexia may also occur.

◆ ***Intestinal obstruction.*** Nausea commonly occurs, especially with high small-intestinal obstruction. Vomiting may be bilious or fecal; abdominal pain is usually episodic and colicky but can become severe and steady with strangulation. Constipation occurs early in large-intestinal obstruction and later in small-intestinal obstruction; obstipation may signal complete obstruction. Bowel sounds are typically hyperactive in partial obstruction, and hypoactive or absent in complete obstruction. Abdominal distention and tenderness occur, possibly with visible peristaltic waves and a palpable abdominal mass.

◆ ***Irritable bowel syndrome.*** Nausea, dyspepsia, and abdominal distention may occur with this syndrome especially during periods of increased stress. Other findings include lower abdominal pain and abdominal tenderness, which is generally relieved by moving the bowels; diurnal diarrhea alternating with constipation or normal bowel function; and small stools with visible mucus and a feeling of incomplete evacuation.

◆ ***Labyrinthitis.*** Nausea and vomiting commonly occur with this acute inner ear inflammation. More significant findings include severe vertigo, progressive hearing loss, nystagmus, tinnitus and, possibly, otorrhea.

◆ ***Lactose intolerance.*** Depending on the individual, signs and symptoms may include nausea, diarrhea, cramps, bloating, and gas, and they occur after eating dairy products.

◆ ***Listeriosis.*** Signs and symptoms include nausea, vomiting, diarrhea, fever, myalgias, and abdominal pain. If the infection spreads to the nervous system and causes meningitis, signs and symptoms include fever, headache, nuchal rigidity, and change in level of consciousness.

◆ ***Ménière's disease.*** This disease causes sudden, brief, recurrent attacks of nausea, vomiting, vertigo, tinnitus, diaphoresis, and nystagmus. It also causes hearing loss and ear fullness.

◆ ***Mesenteric artery ischemia.*** With this condition, nausea and vomiting may accompany severe cramping abdominal pain, especially after meals. Other findings include diarrhea or constipation, abdominal tenderness and bloating, anorexia, weight loss, and abdominal bruits.

◆ ***Mesenteric venous thrombosis.*** Insidious or acute onset of nausea, vomiting, and abdominal pain occurs, with diarrhea or constipation, abdominal distention, hematemesis, and melena.

◆ ***Metabolic acidosis.*** This acid-base imbalance may produce nausea and vomiting, anorexia, diarrhea, Kussmaul's respirations, and decreased level of consciousness.

◆ ***Migraine headache.*** Nausea and vomiting may occur in the prodromal stage, along with photophobia, light flashes, increased sensitivity to noise, light-headedness and, possibly, partial vision loss and paresthesia of the lips, face, and hands.

◆ ***Motion sickness.*** With this disorder, nausea and vomiting are brought on by motion or rhythmic movement. Headache, dizziness, fatigue, diaphoresis, hypersalivation, and dyspnea may also occur.

◆ ***Myocardial infarction.*** Nausea and vomiting may occur, but the cardinal symptom is severe substernal chest pain that may radiate to the left arm, jaw, or neck. Dyspnea, pallor, clammy skin, diaphoresis, altered blood pressure, and arrhythmias also occur.

◆ ***Norovirus infection.*** Acute gastroenteritis from noroviruses commonly causes infected individuals to experience nausea. Frequent accompanying symptoms include vomiting, diarrhea, and abdominal pain or cramping. Less commonly, individuals may develop low-grade fever, headache, chills, muscle aches, and generalized tiredness. These viruses are carried in the stool or vomit of infected individuals, and are often spread through contaminated food or water. Duration of illness is brief, with healthy individuals recovering in 24 to 60 hours.

◆ ***Pancreatitis (acute).*** Nausea, usually followed by vomiting, is an early symptom of pancreatitis. Other common findings include steady, severe pain in the epigastrium or left upper quadrant that may radiate to the back; abdominal tenderness and rigidity; anorexia; diminished bowel sounds; and fever. Tachycardia, restlessness, hypotension, skin mottling, and cold, sweaty extremities may occur in severe cases.

◆ ***Peptic ulcer.*** With this disorder, nausea and vomiting may follow attacks of sharp or gnawing, burning epigastric pain. Attacks typically occur when the stomach is empty, or after ingestion of alcohol, caffeine, or aspirin; they're relieved by eating food or taking an antacid or an antisecretory. Hematemesis or melena may also occur.

◆ ***Peritonitis.*** Nausea and vomiting usually accompany acute abdominal pain localized to the area of inflammation. Other findings include high fever with chills, tachycardia, hypoactive or absent bowel sounds; abdominal distention, rigidity, and tenderness (including rebound tenderness); positive obturator sign and obturator weakness; pale, cold skin; diaphoresis; hypotension; shallow respirations; and hiccups.

◆ ***Preeclampsia.*** Nausea and vomiting commonly occur with this disorder of pregnancy, along with rapid weight gain, epigastric pain, oliguria, severe frontal headache, hyperreflexia, and blurred or double vision. The classic diagnostic triad of signs include hypertension, proteinuria, and edema.

◆ ***Q Fever.*** Signs and symptoms include nausea, vomiting, diarrhea, fever, chills, severe headache, malaise, and chest pain. Fever may last up to 2 weeks, and in severe cases, the patient may develop hepatitis or pneumonia.

◆ ***Renal and urologic disorders.*** Cystitis, pyelonephritis, calculi, uremia, and other disorders of the renal system can cause nausea. Related findings reflect the specific disorder.

◆ ***Rhabdomyolysis.*** Signs and symptoms include nausea, vomiting, muscle weakness or pain, fever, malaise, and dark urine. Acute renal failure is the most commonly reported complication of the disorder. It results from renal structure obstruction and injury during the kidneys' attempt to filter the myoglobin from the bloodstream.

◆ ***Thyrotoxicosis.*** With this disorder, nausea and vomiting may accompany the classic findings of severe anxiety, heat intolerance, weight loss despite increased appetite, diaphoresis, diarrhea, tremor, tachycardia, and palpitations. Other signs include exophthalmos, ventricular or atrial gallop, and an enlarged thyroid gland.

◆ ***Typhus.*** An abrupt onset of nausea, vomiting, fever, and chills follows the initial symptoms of headache, myalgia, arthralgia, and malaise.

Other causes

◆ ***Drugs.*** Common nausea-producing drugs include antineoplastics, opiates, ferrous sulfate, levodopa, oral potassium chloride replacements, estrogens, sulfasalazine, antibiotics, quinidine, anesthetics, cardiac glycosides, theophylline (overdose), and nonsteroidal anti-inflammatories.

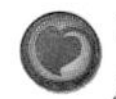
HERB ALERT *Herbal remedies, such as ginkgo biloba and St. John's wort, can produce adverse reactions, including nausea.*

◆ ***Radiation and surgery.*** Radiation therapy can cause nausea and vomiting. Postoperative nausea and vomiting are common, especially after abdominal surgery.

Special considerations

If your patient is experiencing severe nausea, prepare him for blood tests to determine fluid and electrolyte status, and acid-base balance. Have him breathe deeply to ease his nausea; keep his room air fresh and clean-smelling by removing bedpans and emesis basins promptly after use and by providing adequate ventilation. Because he could easily aspirate vomitus when in a supine position, elevate his head or position him on his side.

Because pain can precipitate or intensify nausea, administer pain medications promptly, as needed. If possible, give medications by injection or suppository to prevent exacerbating nausea. Be alert for abdominal distention and hypoactive bowel sounds when you administer an antiemetic: These signs may indicate gastric retention. If you detect these, immediately insert a nasogastric tube, as required.

Prepare the patient for such procedures as computed tomography scan, ultrasound, endoscopy, and colonoscopy. Consult the nutritionist to determine the patient's metabolic demands such as total or partial parenteral nutrition.

Pediatric pointers

Nausea, commonly described as stomachache, is one of the most common childhood complaints. Often the result of overeating, it can also occur as part of diverse disorders, ranging from acute infections to a conversion reaction caused by fear.

Geriatric pointers

Elderly patients have increased dental caries; tooth loss; decreased salivary gland function, which causes mouth dryness; reduced gastric acid output and motility; and decreased senses of taste and smell—any of which can contribute to nonpathologic nausea.

Neck pain

Neck pain may originate from any neck structure, ranging from the meninges and cervical vertebrae to its blood vessels, muscles, and lymphatic tissue. This symptom can also be referred from other areas of the body. Its location, onset, and pattern help determine its origin and underlying causes. Neck pain usually results from trauma and degenerative, congenital, inflammatory, metabolic, and neoplastic disorders.

EMERGENCY INTERVENTIONS *If the patient's neck pain is due to trauma, first ensure proper cervical spine immobilization, preferably with a long backboard and a cervical collar. Then take vital signs, and perform a quick neurologic examination. If he shows signs of respiratory distress, give oxygen. Intubation or tracheostomy and mechanical ventilation may be necessary. Ask the patient (or a family member, if the patient can't answer) how the injury occurred. Then examine the neck for abrasions, swelling, lacerations, erythema, and ecchymoses.*

History and physical examination

If the patient hasn't sustained trauma, find out the severity and onset of his neck pain. Where specifically in the neck does he feel pain? Does anything relieve or worsen the pain? Is there any particular event that precipitates the pain? Also, ask about the development of other symptoms such as headaches. Next, focus on the patient's current and past illnesses and injuries, diet, drug history, and family health history.

Thoroughly inspect the patient's neck, shoulders, and cervical spine for swelling, masses, erythema, and ecchymoses. Assess active range of motion in his neck by having him perform flexion, extension, rotation, and lateral side bending. Note the degree of pain produced by these movements. Examine his posture, and test and compare bilateral muscle strength. Check the sensation in his arms, and assess his hand grasp and arm reflexes. Attempt to elicit Brudzinski's and Kernig's signs if there is not a history of neck trauma, and palpate the cervical lymph nodes for enlargement. (See *Neck pain: Causes and associated findings,* pages 480 to 483.)

Medical causes

- ***Ankylosing spondylitis.*** Intermittent, moderate to severe neck pain and stiffness with severely restricted range of motion is characteristic of this disorder. Intermittent low back pain and stiffness and arm pain are generally worse in the morning or after periods of inactivity and are usually relieved after exercise. Related findings also include low-grade fever, limited chest expansion, malaise, anorexia, fatigue and, occasionally, iritis.
- ***Cervical extension injury.*** Anterior or posterior neck pain may develop within hours or days following a whiplash injury. Anterior pain usually diminishes within several days, but posterior pain persists and may even intensify. Associated findings include tenderness, swelling and nuchal rigidity, arm or back pain, occipital headache, muscle spasms, visual blurring, and unilateral miosis on the affected side.
- ***Cervical fibrositis.*** This disorder may produce anterior neck pain that radiates to one or both shoulders. Pain is intermittent and variable, often changing with weather patterns. Other findings are nonspecific but commonly include point tenderness over involved muscles.
- ***Cervical spine fracture.*** Fracture at C1 to C4 can cause sudden death; survivors may experience severe neck pain that restricts all movement, intense occipital headache, quadriplegia, deformity, and respiratory paralysis.
- ***Cervical spine infection (acute).*** This infection can cause neck pain that restricts motion. Other findings include fever, possible deformity, muscle spasms, local tenderness, dysphagia, paresthesia, and muscle weakness.
- ***Cervical spine tumor.*** Metastatic tumors typically produce persistent neck pain that increases with movement and isn't relieved by rest; primary tumors cause mild to severe pain along a specific nerve root. Other findings depend on the lesions and may include paresthesia, arm and leg weakness that progresses to

atrophy and paralysis, and bladder and bowel incontinence.

◆ ***Cervical spondylosis.*** This degenerative process produces posterior neck pain that restricts movement and is aggravated by it. Pain may radiate down either arm and may accompany paresthesia, weakness, and stiffness.

◆ ***Cervical stenosis.*** This progressive disorder, commonly asymptomatic, may cause nonspecific neck and arm pain, paresthesia, muscle weakness or paralysis, and decreased range of motion.

◆ ***Esophageal trauma.*** An esophageal mucosal tear or a pulsion diverticulum may produce mild neck pain, chest pain, edema, hemoptysis, and dysphagia.

◆ ***Herniated cervical disk.*** This disorder characteristically causes variable neck pain that restricts movement and is aggravated by it. It also causes referred pain along a specific dermatome, paresthesia and other sensory disturbances, and arm weakness.

◆ ***Hodgkin's lymphoma.*** This disorder may eventually result in generalized pain that may affect the neck. Lymphadenopathy, the classic sign, may accompany paresthesia, muscle weakness, fever, fatigue, weight loss, malaise, and hepatomegaly.

◆ ***Laryngeal cancer.*** Neck pain that radiates to the ear develops late in this disorder. The patient may also develop dysphagia, dyspnea, hemoptysis, stridor, hoarseness, and cervical lymphadenopathy.

◆ ***Lymphadenitis.*** With this disorder, enlarged and inflamed cervical lymph nodes cause acute pain and tenderness. Fever, chills, and malaise may also occur.

◆ ***Meningitis.*** Neck pain may accompany characteristic nuchal rigidity. Related findings include fever, headache, photophobia, positive Brudzinski's and Kernig's signs, and decreased level of consciousness.

◆ ***Neck sprain.*** Minor sprains typically produce pain, slight swelling, stiffness, and restricted range of motion. Ligament rupture causes pain, marked swelling, ecchymosis, muscle spasms, and nuchal rigidity with head tilt.

◆ ***Osteoporosis.*** Neck pain is rare with this disorder, which usually affects the thoracic or lumbar vertebrae. Cervical vertebrae involvement produces tenderness and deformity.

◆ ***Paget's disease.*** This slowly developing disease is commonly asymptomatic in its early stages. As it progresses, cervical vertebrae deformity may produce severe, persistent neck pain, along with paresthesia and arm weakness or paralysis.

◆ ***Rheumatoid arthritis.*** This disorder usually affects peripheral joints, but it can also involve the cervical vertebrae. Acute inflammation may cause moderate to severe pain that radiates along a specific nerve root; increased warmth, swelling, and tenderness in involved joints; stiffness, restricting range of motion; paresthesia and muscle weakness; low-grade fever; anorexia; malaise; fatigue; and possible neck deformity. Some pain and stiffness remain after the acute phase.

◆ ***Spinous process fracture.*** Fracture near the cervicothoracic junction produces acute pain radiating to the shoulders. Associated findings include swelling, exquisite tenderness, restricted range of motion, muscle spasms, and deformity.

◆ ***Subarachnoid hemorrhage.*** This life-threatening condition may cause moderate to severe neck pain and rigidity, headache, and a decreased level of consciousness. Kernig's and Brudzinski's signs are present. The patient may describe the headache as "the worst headache of my life."

◆ ***Thyroid trauma.*** Besides mild to moderate neck pain, thyroid trauma may cause local swelling and ecchymosis. If a hematoma forms, it can cause dyspnea.

◆ ***Torticollis.*** With this neck deformity, severe neck pain accompanies recurrent unilateral stiffness and muscle spasms that produce a characteristic head tilt.

◆ ***Tracheal trauma.*** Fracture of the tracheal cartilage, a life-threatening condition, produces moderate to severe neck pain and respiratory difficulty.

Torn tracheal mucosa produces mild to moderate pain and may result in airway occlusion, hemoptysis, hoarseness, and dysphagia.

SPECIAL CONSIDERATIONS

Promote patient comfort by giving an anti-inflammatory and an analgesic, as needed. Prepare him for diagnostic tests, such as X-rays, computed tomography scan, blood tests, and cerebrospinal fluid analysis.

PEDIATRIC POINTERS

The most common causes of neck pain in children are meningitis and trauma. A rare cause of neck pain is congenital torticollis.

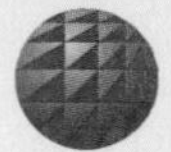

SIGNS & SYMPTOMS

Neck pain: Causes and associated findings

Major associated signs and symptoms

Common causes	Arm pain	Back pain	Brudzinski's sign	Decreased level of consciousness	Decreased range of motion	Deformity	Dysphagia	Dyspnea	Ecchymoses	Fatigue	Fever	Headache	Hemoptysis	Hoarseness
Ankylosing spondylitis	●	●			●					●	●			
Cervical extension injury	●	●										●		
Cervical fibrositis														
Cervical spine fracture					●	●						●		
Cervical spine infection (acute)					●	●	●				●			
Cervical spine tumor					●									
Cervical spondylosis	●				●									
Cervical stenosis	●				●									
Esophageal trauma							●						●	
Herniated cervical disk	●	●			●									
Hodgkin's lymphoma										●	●			
Laryngeal cancer							●	●					●	●
Lymphadenitis											●			
Meningitis			●	●							●	●		
Neck sprain					●				●					
Osteoporosis		●				●								
Paget's disease						●								

	Kernig's sign	Lymphadenopathy	Malaise	Muscle spasms	Nuchal rigidity	Paralysis	Paresthesia	Swelling	Tenderness	Weakness
			●		●					
				●	●			●		
									●	
						●				
				●			●		●	●
						●	●			●
							●			●
						●	●			●
								●		
							●			●
		●	●				●			●
		●								
		●	●						●	
	●				●					
				●	●			●		
									●	
						●	●			●

(continued)

Night blindness

[Nyctalopia]

Often difficult to identify, night blindness refers to impaired vision in the dark, especially after entering a darkened room or while driving at night. A symptom of choroidal and retinal degeneration, night blindness occurs in various ocular disorders and as an early indicator of vitamin A deficiency. In some patients, however, night blindness occurs without underlying pathology, simply reflecting poor adaptation to the dark. In these patients, it's commonly accompanied by myopia.

History and physical examination

If the patient complains of difficulty seeing at night, ask when he first noticed the problem. Is it intermittent or steadily worsening? Is it worse at certain times or in certain conditions? Also, ask about other ocular symptoms, such as eye pain, blurred or halo vision, floaters or spots, and photophobia.

Explore any history of glaucoma, cataracts, and familial degeneration of vision. If no ocular problems are apparent, briefly evaluate the patient's nutritional status for vitamin A deficiency.

Examine the eyes for ptosis, abnormal tearing, discharge, and conjunctival injection. Test visual acuity and visual fields in both eyes and, if trained and equipped, measure intraocular pressure. Check pupillary response, and evaluate extraocular muscle function by testing the six cardinal fields of gaze.

Medical causes

◆ ***Cataracts.*** Night blindness and halo vision occur early in senile-type cataract formation. As the cataract matures, it causes gradual, painless visual blurring and vision loss, sometimes with visible lens opacity.

◆ ***Choroidal dystrophies.*** Night blindness and decreased peripheral vision may occur early in choroidal dystrophies. Disease progression causes loss of central vision.

◆ ***Fundus albipunctatus.*** Night blindness is the chief complaint in this retinal and choroidal disease. Multiple small, round, yellow-white dots are present on the retina.

◆ ***Fundus flavimaculatus.*** With this disease, night blindness may be pronounced or may be an incidental finding. Irregular yellow or white lesions appear deep in the retina.

Neck pain: Causes and associated findings *(continued)*

Common causes	Major associated signs and symptoms													
	Arm pain	Back pain	Brudzinski's sign	Decreased level of consciousness	Decreased range of motion	Deformity	Dysphagia	Dyspnea	Ecchymoses	Fatigue	Fever	Headache	Hemoptysis	Hoarseness
Rheumatoid arthritis					●	●				●	●			
Spinous process fracture					●	●								
Subarachnoid hemorrhage			●	●								●		
Thyroid trauma								●	●					
Torticollis														
Tracheal trauma							●	●					●	●

◆ ***Glaucoma.*** Night blindness occurs late in chronic open-angle glaucoma, with halo vision, gradually impaired bilateral visual acuity, loss of peripheral vision and, possibly, slight eye pain.

◆ ***Goldman-Favre dystrophy.*** With this disorder, night blindness is usually the chief complaint. The retina resembles that seen in retinitis pigmentosa.

◆ ***Oguchi's disease.*** This rare, hereditary retinal and choroidal degeneration produces night blindness and a retina with a yellowish metallic sheen.

◆ ***Optic nerve atrophy.*** This disorder may cause night blindness, visual field and color vision defects, and decreased visual acuity. Pupillary reactions are sluggish, and optic disk pallor is evident.

◆ ***Retinitis pigmentosa.*** In this usually hereditary retinal degeneration, night blindness is characteristically the first symptom, usually arising in adolescence. Scattered black pigmentary bodies form in a characteristic "bone-spicule" arrangement on the retina. As the disease progresses, the visual field gradually constricts, causing tunnel or "gun barrel" vision and eventually total blindness.

◆ ***Vitamin A deficiency.*** Night blindness is typically the first symptom of vitamin A deficiency. Associated findings include xerophthalmia (conjunctival dryness) and Bitot's spots (gray-white conjunctival plaques). The patient may complain of visual blurring or vision loss. His skin may be dry and scaly. His mucous membranes may be shrunken and hardened.

Other causes

◆ ***Drugs.*** Isotretinoin, used to treat inflammatory acne, rarely causes night blindness.

Special considerations

Because any visual impairment is frightening to the patient, provide emotional support. Help decrease his anxiety and enhance cooperation by explaining scheduled diagnostic tests such as electroretinography in simple terms. Make sure the patient is safe; explain that he shouldn't drive and that he should use assistive devices at night or in darkened or dim lighting as necessary.

Pediatric pointers

Because children generally don't have adequate body reserves of vitamin A, they're especially

	Kernig's sign	Lymphadenopathy	Malaise	Muscle spasms	Nuchal rigidity	Paralysis	Paresthesia	Swelling	Tenderness	Weakness
			●				●	●	●	●
				●				●	●	
	●				●					
								●		
					●	●				

prone to deficiency and resulting night blindness.

Geriatric pointers

Night blindness due to vitamin A deficiency usually occurs in elderly and disadvantaged patients. It's also a common effect of aging.

Nipple discharge

Nipple discharge can occur spontaneously or can be elicited by nipple stimulation. It's characterized as intermittent or constant, unilateral or bilateral, and by color, consistency, and composition. Its incidence increases with age and parity. This sign rarely occurs (but is more likely to be pathologic) in men and in nulligravid, regularly menstruating women. It's relatively common and often normal in parous women. A thick, grayish discharge—benign epithelial debris from inactive ducts—can often be elicited in middle-age parous women. Colostrum, a thin, yellowish or milky discharge, often occurs in the last weeks of pregnancy.

Nipple discharge can signal serious underlying disease, particularly when accompanied by other breast changes. Significant causes include endocrine disorders, cancer, certain drugs, and blocked lactiferous ducts.

History and physical examination

Ask the patient when she first noticed the discharge, and determine its duration, extent, quantity, color, consistency, and smell, if any. Has she had other nipple and breast changes, such as pain, tenderness, itching, warmth, changes in contour, and lumps? If she reports a lump, question her about its onset, location, size, and consistency.

Obtain a complete gynecologic and obstetric history, and determine her normal menstrual cycle and the date of her last menses. Ask if she experiences breast swelling and tenderness, bloating, irritability, headaches, abdominal cramping, nausea, or diarrhea before or during menses. Note the number, date, and outcome of her pregnancies and, if she breast-fed, the approximate time of her last lactation. Also, check for any risk factors of breast cancer—family history, previous or current malignancies, nulliparity or first pregnancy after age 30, early menarche, or late menopause.

Start your physical examination by characterizing the discharge. If the discharge isn't frank, try to elicit it. (See *Eliciting nipple discharge*, page 484.) Then examine the nipples and breasts with the patient in four different positions: sitting with her arms at her sides; with her arms overhead; and with her hands pressing on her hips; and leaning forward so her breasts are suspended. Check for nipple deviation, flattening, retraction, redness, asymmetry, thickening, excoriation, erosion, or cracking. Inspect her breasts for asymmetry, irregular contours, dimpling, erythema, and peau d'orange. With the patient in a supine position, palpate the breasts and axillae for lumps, giving special attention to the areolae. Note the size, location, delineation, consistency, and mobility of any lump you find.

Is the patient taking hormones (hormonal contraceptives or hormone replacement therapy)? Is the discharge spontaneous, or does it have to be expressed?

Medical causes

◆ ***Breast abscess.*** This disorder, most common in breast-feeding women, may produce a thick, purulent discharge from a cracked nipple or infected duct. Associated findings include abrupt onset of high fever with chills; breast

Eliciting nipple discharge

If your patient has a history or evidence of nipple discharge, you can attempt to elicit it during your examination. Help the patient into a supine position, and gently squeeze her nipple between your thumb and index finger; note any discharge through the nipple. Then place your fingers on the areola, as shown, and palpate the entire areolar surface, watching for any discharge through areolar ducts.

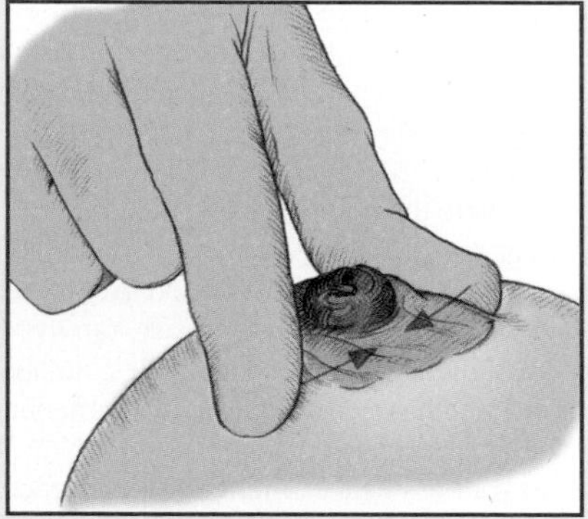

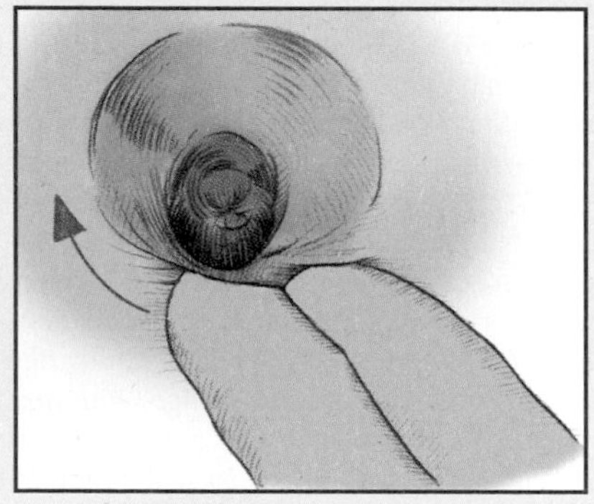

pain, tenderness, and erythema; a palpable soft nodule or generalized induration; and possibly, nipple retraction.

◆ ***Breast cancer.*** This may cause bloody, watery, or purulent discharge from a normal-appearing nipple. Characteristic findings include a hard, irregular, fixed lump; erythema; dimpling; peau d'orange; changes in contour; nipple deviation, flattening, or retraction; axillary lymphadenopathy; and possibly, breast pain.

◆ ***Choriocarcinoma.*** Galactorrhea (a white or grayish milky discharge) may result from this highly malignant neoplasm, which can follow pregnancy. Other characteristics include persistent uterine bleeding and bogginess after delivery or curettage, and vaginal masses.

◆ ***Herpes zoster.*** This virus can stimulate the thoracic nerves, causing bilateral, spontaneous, intermittent galactorrhea. Other characteristics include shooting or burning pain, eruption of small red nodules or vesicles on the thorax and possibly the arms and legs, pruritus and paresthesia or hyperesthesia in affected areas, headache, and fever and malaise.

◆ ***Hypothyroidism.*** This disorder occasionally causes galactorrhea. Related findings include bradycardia; weight gain despite anorexia; decreased mentation; periorbital edema; menorrhagia; constipation; puffy face, hands, and feet; brittle, sparse hair; and dry, doughy, pale, cool skin.

◆ ***Intraductal papilloma.*** This disorder is the primary cause of nipple discharge in the nonpregnant, non–breast-feeding woman. Unilateral serous, serosanguineous, or bloody nipple discharge—usually from only one duct—is its predominant sign. Discharge may be intermittent or profuse and constant, and can often be stimulated by gentle pressure around the areola. Subareolar nodules, breast pain, and tenderness may occur.

◆ ***Mammary duct ectasia.*** A thick, sticky, grayish discharge from multiple ducts may be the first sign of this disorder. The discharge may be bilateral and is usually spontaneous. Other findings include a rubbery, poorly delineated lump beneath the areola, with a blue-green discoloration of the overlying skin; nipple retraction; and redness, swelling, tenderness, and burning pain in the areola and nipple.

◆ ***Paget's disease.*** With this disorder, serous or bloody discharge emits from denuded skin on the nipple, which is red, intensely itchy and, possibly, eroded or excoriated. The discharge is usually unilateral.

◆ ***Prolactin-secreting pituitary tumor.*** Bilateral galactorrhea may occur with this tumor. Other findings include amenorrhea, infertility, decreased libido and vaginal secretions, headaches, and blindness.

◆ ***Proliferative (fibrocystic) breast disease.*** This benign disorder occasionally causes a bilateral clear, milky, or straw-colored discharge, which is rarely purulent or bloody. Multiple round, soft, tender nodules are usually palpable in both breasts, although they may occur singly. Usually, nodules are mobile and are located in the upper outer quadrant. Nodule size, tenderness, and discharge increase during the luteal phase of the menstrual cycle. Symptoms then regress after menses.

◆ ***Trauma.*** Bilateral galactorrhea can result from trauma to the breasts.

Other causes

◆ ***Drugs.*** Galactorrhea can be caused by psychotropic agents, particularly phenothiazines and tricyclic antidepressants; some antihypertensives (reserpine and methyldopa); hormonal contraceptives; cimetidine; metoclopramide; and verapamil.

◆ ***Surgery.*** Chest wall surgery may stimulate the thoracic nerves, causing intermittent bilateral galactorrhea.

Special considerations

Although nipple discharge is usually insignificant, it can be frightening to the patient. Help relieve the patient's anxieties by clearly explaining the nature and origin of her discharge. Apply a breast binder, which may reduce discharge by eliminating nipple stimulation.

Diagnostic tests may include tissue biopsy (if a breast lump is found), cytologic study of the discharge, mammography, ultrasonography, transillumination, and serum prolactin.

Pediatric pointers

Nipple discharge in children and adolescents is rare. When it does occur, it's almost always nonpathologic, as in the bloody discharge that sometimes accompanies onset of menarche. Infants of both sexes may experience a milky breast discharge beginning 3 days after birth and lasting up to 2 weeks due to maternal hormonal influences.

Geriatric pointers

In postmenopausal women, breast changes are considered malignant until proven otherwise.

Patient counseling

Counsel your patient to be aware of discharge characteristics—its consistency (thick or thinning), odor, origin in single or multiple ducts, and relation to the menstrual cycle. If the discharge becomes bloody, instruct the patient to seek medical evaluation. Instruct the patient to perform breast self-examinations and maintain appointments for breast examinations by a physician and mammograms as recommended.

Nipple retraction

Nipple retraction, the inward displacement of the nipple below the level of surrounding breast tissue, may indicate an inflammatory breast lesion or cancer. It results from scar tissue formation within a lesion or large mammary duct. As the scar tissue shortens, it pulls adjacent tissue inward, causing nipple deviation, flattening, and finally, retraction.

History and physical examination

Ask the patient when she first noticed retraction of the nipple. Has she experienced other nipple changes, such as itching, discoloration, discharge, or excoriation? Has she noticed breast pain, lumps, redness, swelling, or warmth? Obtain a history, noting risk factors of breast cancer, such as a family history or previous malignancy.

Carefully examine both nipples and breasts with the patient sitting upright with her arms at her sides, with her hands pressing on her hips, and with her arms overhead; and with the patient leaning forward so her breasts hang. Look for redness, excoriation, and discharge; nipple flattening and deviation; and breast asymmetry, dimpling, or contour differences. (See *Differentiating nipple retraction from inversion*, page 486.)

Try to evert the nipple by gently squeezing the areola. With the patient in a supine position, palpate both breasts for lumps, especially beneath the areola. Mold breast skin over the lump or gently pull it up toward the clavicle, looking for accentuated nipple retraction. Also, palpate axillary lymph nodes.

Medical causes

◆ ***Breast abscess.*** This disorder, most common in breast-feeding women, occasionally produces unilateral nipple retraction. More common findings include high fever with chills; breast pain, erythema, and tenderness; breast induration or soft mass; and cracked, sore nipples, possibly with purulent discharge.

◆ ***Breast cancer.*** Unilateral nipple retraction is commonly accompanied by a hard, fixed, nontender nodule beneath the areola, as well as

Differentiating nipple retraction from inversion

Nipple retraction is sometimes confused with nipple inversion, a common abnormality that's congenital in many patients and doesn't usually signal underlying disease. A *retracted* nipple appears flat and broad, whereas an *inverted* nipple can be pulled out from the sulcus where it hides.

NIPPLE RETRACTION

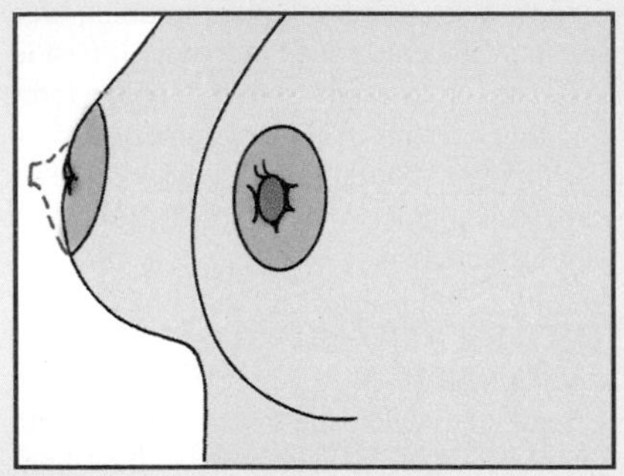

NIPPLE INVERSION

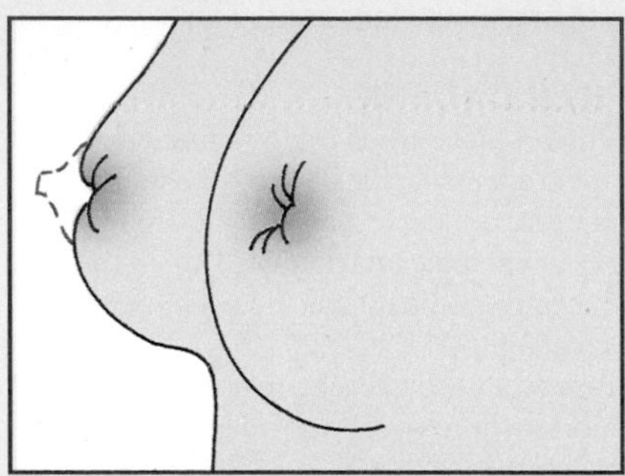

other breast nodules. Other nipple changes include itching, burning, erosion, and watery or bloody discharge. Breast changes commonly include dimpling, altered contour, peau d'orange, ulceration, tenderness (possibly pain), redness, and warmth. Axillary lymph nodes may be enlarged.

◆ ***Mammary duct ectasia.*** Nipple retraction commonly occurs along with a poorly defined, rubbery nodule beneath the areola, with a blue-green skin discoloration; areolar burning, itching, swelling, tenderness, and erythema; and nipple pain with a thick, sticky, grayish, multiductal discharge.

◆ ***Mastitis.*** Nipple retraction, deviation, cracking, or flattening may occur in this disorder with a firm and indurated or tender, flocculent, discrete breast nodule, warmth, erythema, tenderness, and edema. Fatigue, high fevers, and chills may also be present.

OTHER CAUSES

◆ ***Surgery.*** Previous breast surgery may cause underlying scarring and retraction.

SPECIAL CONSIDERATIONS

Prepare the patient for diagnostic tests, including mammography, cytology of nipple discharge, and biopsy.

PEDIATRIC POINTERS

Nipple retraction doesn't occur in prepubescent females.

PATIENT COUNSELING

Teach your patient breast self-examination and advise her to always seek medical evaluation for breast changes.

Nocturia

Nocturia—excessive urination at night—may result from disruption of the normal diurnal pattern of urine concentration or from overstimulation of the nerves and muscles that control urination. Normally, urine is more concentrated during the night than during the day. As a result, most persons excrete three to four times more urine during the day, and can sleep for 6 to 8 hours during the night without being awakened. The patient with nocturia may awaken one or more times during the night to empty his bladder and excrete 700 ml or more of urine.

Although nocturia usually results from renal and lower urinary tract disorders, it may result from certain cardiovascular, endocrine, and metabolic disorders. This common sign may also result from drugs that induce diuresis, particularly when they're taken at night, and from the ingestion of large quantities of fluids, especially caffeinated beverages or alcohol, at bedtime.

History and physical examination

Begin by exploring the history of the patient's nocturia. When did it begin? How often does it occur? Can the patient identify a specific pattern? Precipitating factors? Also, note the volume of urine voided. Ask the patient about any change in the color, odor, or consistency of his urine. Has the patient changed his usual pattern or volume of fluid intake? Next, explore associated symptoms. Ask about pain or burning on urination, difficulty initiating a urine stream, costovertebral angle tenderness, and flank, upper abdominal, or suprapubic pain.

Determine if the patient or his family has a history of renal or urinary tract disorders or endocrine and metabolic diseases, particularly diabetes. Is the patient taking a drug that increases urine output, such as a diuretic, a cardiac glycoside, or an antihypertensive?

Focus your physical examination on palpating and percussing the kidneys, the costovertebral angle, and the bladder. Carefully inspect the urinary meatus. Inspect a urine specimen for color, odor, and the presence of sediment.

Medical causes

◆ ***Benign prostatic hyperplasia.*** Common in men older than age 50, this disorder produces nocturia when significant urethral obstruction develops. Typically, it causes frequency, hesitancy, incontinence, reduced force and caliber of the urine stream and, possibly, hematuria. Oliguria may also occur. Palpation reveals a distended bladder and an enlarged prostate. The patient may also complain of lower abdominal fullness, perineal pain, and constipation. Obstruction may lead to renal failure.

◆ ***Bladder neoplasm.*** A late sign of this neoplasm, nocturia involves frequent voiding of small to moderate amounts of urine. Besides hematuria, the most common sign, associated characteristics include bladder distention; urinary frequency and urgency; dysuria; pyuria; bladder, rectal, flank, back, or leg pain; vomiting; diarrhea; and insomnia. Signs and symptoms of urinary tract infection, such as tenesmus, low-grade fever, and perineal pain, may also occur.

◆ ***Cystitis.*** All three forms of cystitis may cause nocturia marked by frequent, small voidings and accompanied by dysuria and tenesmus.

Bacterial cystitis may also cause urinary urgency; hematuria; fatigue; suprapubic, perineal, flank, and lower back pain; and occasionally, low-grade fever. Most common in women between ages 25 and 60, chronic interstitial cystitis is characterized by Hunner's ulcers—small, punctate, bleeding lesions in the bladder; it also causes gross hematuria. Because symptoms resemble bladder cancer, this must be ruled out.

Viral cystitis also causes urinary urgency, hematuria, and fever.

◆ ***Diabetes insipidus.*** The result of antidiuretic hormone deficiency, this disorder usually produces nocturia early in its course. It's characterized by periodic voiding of moderate to large amounts of urine. Diabetes insipidus can also produce polydipsia and dehydration.

◆ ***Diabetes mellitus.*** An early sign of diabetes mellitus, nocturia involves frequent, large voidings. Associated features include daytime polyuria, polydipsia, polyphagia, frequent urinary tract infections, recurrent yeast infections, vaginitis, weakness, fatigue, weight loss and, possibly, signs of dehydration, such as dry mucous membranes and poor skin turgor.

◆ ***Heart failure.*** Nocturia may develop early in this disorder—the result of increased glomerular filtration associated with movement of edematous fluid from dependent areas during recumbency. Other early effects include fatigue, jugular vein distention, dyspnea, orthopnea, tachycardia, and a dry cough with wheezing. Later, the patient may develop tachypnea, weight gain, hypotension, oliguria, cyanosis, and hepatomegaly.

◆ ***Hypercalcemic nephropathy.*** With this disorder, nocturia involves the periodic voiding of moderate to large amounts of urine. Related findings include daytime polyuria, polydipsia, and occasionally, hematuria and pyuria.

◆ ***Hypokalemic nephropathy.*** Again, nocturia involves the periodic voiding of moderate to large amounts of urine. Associated findings typically include polydipsia, daytime polyuria, muscle weakness or paralysis, hypoactive bowel sounds, and increased susceptibility to pyelonephritis.

◆ ***Prostate cancer.*** The second leading cause of cancer deaths in men, this disorder is usually asymptomatic in early stages. Later, it produces nocturia characterized by infrequent voiding of moderate amounts of urine. Other characteristic effects include dysuria (most common symptom), difficulty initiating a urine stream, interrupted urine stream, bladder distention, urinary frequency, weight loss, pallor, weakness, perineal pain, and constipation. Palpation reveals a hard, irregularly shaped, nodular prostate.

◆ ***Pyelonephritis (acute).*** Nocturia is common with this disorder and is usually characterized by infrequent voiding of moderate amounts of urine. The urine may appear cloudy. Associated signs and symptoms include a high, sustained fever with chills, fatigue, unilateral or bilateral flank pain, costovertebral angle tenderness, weakness, dysuria, hematuria, urinary frequency and urgency, and tenesmus. Occasionally, anorexia, nausea, vomiting, diarrhea, and hypoactive bowel sounds may also occur.

◆ ***Renal failure (chronic).*** Nocturia occurs relatively early in this disorder and is usually characterized by infrequent voiding of moderate amounts of urine. As the disorder progresses, oliguria or even anuria develops. Other widespread effects of chronic renal failure include fatigue, ammonia breath odor, Kussmaul's respirations, peripheral edema, elevated blood pressure, decreased level of consciousness, confusion, emotional lability, muscle twitching, anorexia, metallic taste in the mouth, constipation or diarrhea, petechiae, ecchymoses, pruritus, yellow- or bronze-tinged skin, nausea, and vomiting.

OTHER CAUSES

◆ ***Drugs.*** Any drug that mobilizes edematous fluid or produces diuresis (for example, a diuretic or a cardiac glycoside) may cause nocturia; obviously, this effect depends on when the drug is administered.

SPECIAL CONSIDERATIONS

Patient care includes maintaining fluid balance, ensuring adequate rest, and providing patient education. Monitor vital signs, intake and output, and daily weight; continue to document the frequency of nocturia, amount, and specific gravity. Plan administration of a diuretic for daytime hours, if possible. Also plan rest periods to compensate for sleep lost because of nocturia.

Prepare the patient for diagnostic tests, which may include routine urinalysis; urine concentration and dilution studies; serum blood urea nitrogen, creatinine, and electrolyte levels; and cystoscopy.

PEDIATRIC POINTERS

In children, nocturia may be voluntary or involuntary. The latter is commonly known as enuresis, or bedwetting. With the exception of prostate disorders, causes of nocturia are generally the same for children and adults.

However, children with pyelonephritis are more susceptible to sepsis, which may display as fever, irritability, and poor skin perfusion. In addition, girls may experience vaginal discharge and vulvar soreness or pruritus.

GERIATRIC POINTERS

Postmenopausal women have decreased bladder elasticity, but urine output remains constant, resulting in nocturia.

PATIENT COUNSELING

Advise patients to reduce fluid intake (especially of caffeinated and alcoholic beverages) before bedtime. Also advise them to void 15 to 20 minutes before retiring. Voiding once more just before retiring may be helpful.

Nuchal rigidity

Commonly an early sign of meningeal irritation, nuchal rigidity refers to stiffness of the neck that prevents flexion. To elicit this sign, attempt to passively flex the patient's neck and touch his chin to his chest. If nuchal rigidity is present, this maneuver triggers pain and muscle spasms. (Be sure that there is no cervical spinal misalignment, such as a fracture or dislocation, before testing for nuchal rigidity. Severe spinal cord damage could result.) The patient may also notice nuchal rigidity when he attempts to flex his neck during daily activities. This sign is not reliable in children and infants.

Nuchal rigidity may herald life-threatening subarachnoid hemorrhage or meningitis. It may also be a late sign of cervical arthritis, in which joint mobility is gradually lost.

EMERGENCY INTERVENTIONS *After eliciting nuchal rigidity, attempt to elicit Kernig's and Brudzinski's signs. Quickly evaluate level of consciousness (LOC). Take vital signs. If you note signs of increased intracranial pressure (ICP), such as increased systolic pressure, bradycardia, and widened pulse pressure, start an I.V. catheter for drug administration and deliver oxygen as necessary, and keep the head of the bed no lower than 30 degrees. Draw a specimen for routine blood studies such as a complete blood count with a white blood cell count and electrolyte levels.*

History and physical examination

Obtain a patient history, relying on family members if altered LOC prevents the patient from responding. Ask about the onset and duration of neck stiffness. Were there any precipitating factors? Also ask about associated signs and symptoms, such as headache, fever, nausea and vomiting, and motor and sensory changes. Check for a history of hypertension, head trauma, cerebral aneurysm or arteriovenous malformation, endocarditis, recent infection (such as sinusitis or pneumonia), or recent dental work. Then, obtain a complete drug history.

If the patient has no other signs of meningeal irritation, ask about a history of arthritis or neck trauma. Can the patient recall pulling a muscle in his neck? Inspect the patient's hands for swollen, tender joints, and palpate the neck for pain or tenderness.

Medical causes

◆ ***Cervical arthritis.*** With this disorder, nuchal rigidity develops gradually. Initially, the patient may complain of neck stiffness in the early morning or after a period of inactivity. Stiffness then becomes increasingly severe and frequent. Pain on movement, especially with lateral motion or head turning, is common. Typically, arthritis also affects other joints, especially those in the hands.

◆ ***Encephalitis.*** This viral infection may cause nuchal rigidity accompanied by other signs of meningeal irritation, such as positive Kernig's and Brudzinski's signs. Usually, nuchal rigidity appears abruptly and is preceded by headache, vomiting, and fever. The patient may display a rapidly decreasing LOC, progressing from lethargy to coma within 24 to 48 hours of onset. Associated features include seizures, ataxia, hemiparesis, nystagmus, and cranial nerve palsies, such as dysphagia and ptosis.

◆ ***Listeriosis.*** If this bacterial infection spreads to the nervous system, meningitis may develop. Signs and symptoms include nuchal rigidity, fever, headache, and change in LOC. Initial signs and symptoms include fever, myalgias, abdominal pain, nausea, vomiting, and diarrhea.

◆ ***Meningitis.*** Nuchal rigidity is an early sign of this disorder and is accompanied by other signs of meningeal irritation—positive Kernig's and Brudzinski's signs, hyperreflexia and, possibly, opisthotonos. Other early features include fever with chills, headache, photophobia, and vomiting. Initially, the patient is confused and irritable; later, he may become stuporous and seizure-prone or may slip into coma. Cranial nerve involvement may cause ocular palsies, facial weakness, and hearing loss. An erythematous papular rash occurs in some forms of viral meningitis; a purpuric rash may occur in meningococcal meningitis.

◆ ***Subarachnoid hemorrhage.*** Nuchal rigidity develops immediately after bleeding into the subarachnoid space. Examination may detect positive Kernig's and Brudzinski's signs. The patient may experience abrupt onset of severe headache, photophobia, fever, nausea and vomiting, dizziness, cranial nerve palsies, and focal neurologic signs, such as hemiparesis or hemiplegia. His LOC deteriorates rapidly, possibly progressing to coma. Signs of increased ICP, such as bradycardia and altered respirations, may also occur.

Special considerations

Prepare the patient for diagnostic tests, such as computed tomography scans, magnetic resonance imaging, and cervical spinal X-rays.

Monitor vital signs, intake and output, and neurologic status closely. Avoid routine administration of opioid analgesics because these may mask signs of increasing ICP. Enforce strict bed rest; keep the head of the bed elevated at least 30 degrees to help minimize ICP.

Assist the patient in finding a comfortable position to obtain adequate rest.

Pediatric pointers

Tests for nuchal rigidity are generally less reliable in children, especially infants. In younger children, move the head gently in all directions, observing for resistance. In older children, ask the child to sit upright and touch his chin to his chest. Resistance to this movement may indicate meningeal irritation.

Nystagmus

Nystagmus refers to the involuntary oscillations of one or, more commonly, both eyeballs. These oscillations are usually rhythmic and may be horizontal, vertical, rotary, or mixed. They may be transient or sustained and may occur spontaneously or on deviation or fixation of the eyes.

Minor degrees of nystagmus at the extremes of gaze are normal. Nystagmus when the eyes are stationary and looking straight ahead is always abnormal. Although nystagmus is fairly easy to identify, the patient may be unaware of it unless it affects his vision.

Nystagmus may be classified as pendular or jerk. *Pendular nystagmus* consists of horizontal (pendular) or vertical (seesaw) oscillations that are equal in rate in both directions and resemble the movements of a clock's pendulum. *Jerk nystagmus* (convergence-retraction, downbeat, and vestibular), which is more common than pendular nystagmus, has a fast component and then a slow—perhaps unequal—corrective component in the opposite direction. (See *Classifying nystagmus*.)

Nystagmus is considered a *supranuclear* ocular palsy—that is, it's caused by pathology in the visual perceptual area, vestibular system, cerebellum, or brain stem rather than in the extraocular muscles or cranial nerves III, IV, and VI. Its causes are varied and include brain stem or cerebellar lesions, multiple sclerosis, encephalitis, labyrinthine disease, and drug toxicity. Occasionally, nystagmus is entirely normal; it's also considered a normal response in the unconscious patient during the doll's eye test (oculocephalic stimulation) or the cold water caloric test (oculovestibular stimulation).

History and physical examination

Begin by asking the patient how long he has had nystagmus. Does it occur intermittently? Does it affect his vision? Ask about recent infection, especially of the ear or respiratory tract, and about head trauma and cancer. Does the patient or anyone in his family have a history of stroke? Then explore associated signs and symptoms. Ask about vertigo, dizziness, tinnitus, nausea or vomiting, numbness, weakness, bladder dysfunction, and fever.

Begin the physical examination by assessing the patient's level of consciousness (LOC) and vital signs. Be alert for signs of increased intracranial pressure (ICP), such as pupillary changes, drowsiness, elevated systolic pressure, and altered respiratory pattern. Next, assess nystagmus fully by testing extraocular muscle function: Ask the patient to focus straight ahead and then to follow your finger up, down, and in an "X" across his face. Note when nystagmus occurs, as well as its velocity and direction. Finally, test reflexes, motor and sensory function, and the cranial nerves.

Medical causes

◆ ***Brain tumor.*** Insidious onset of jerk nystagmus may occur with tumors of the brain stem and cerebellum. Associated characteristics include deafness, dysphagia, nausea and vomiting, vertigo, and ataxia. Brain stem compression by the tumor may cause signs of increased ICP, such as altered LOC, bradycardia, widening pulse pressure, and elevated systolic blood pressure.

◆ ***Encephalitis.*** With this disorder, jerk nystagmus is typically accompanied by altered LOC ranging from lethargy to coma. Usually, it's preceded by sudden onset of fever, headache, and vomiting. Among other features are nuchal rigidity, seizures, aphasia, ataxia, photophobia, and cranial nerve palsies, such as dysphagia and ptosis.

◆ ***Head trauma.*** Brain stem injury may cause jerk nystagmus, which is usually horizontal. The patient may also display pupillary changes, altered respiratory pattern, coma, and decerebrate posture.

◆ ***Labyrinthitis (acute).*** This inner ear inflammation causes sudden onset of jerk nystagmus, accompanied by dizziness, vertigo, tinnitus, nausea, and vomiting. The fast component of the nystagmus is toward the unaffected ear. Gradual sensorineural hearing loss may also occur.

◆ ***Ménière's disease.*** This inner ear disorder is characterized by acute attacks of jerk nystagmus, severe nausea and vomiting, dizziness, vertigo, progressive hearing loss, tinnitus, and diaphoresis. Typically, the direction of jerk nystagmus varies from one attack to the next. Attacks may last from 10 minutes to several hours.

◆ ***Multiple sclerosis.*** With this disorder, jerk or pendular nystagmus may occur intermittently. Usually, it's preceded by diplopia, blurred vision, and paresthesia. Related signs and symptoms may include muscle weakness or paralysis, spasticity, hyperreflexia, intention tremor, gait ataxia, dysphagia, dysarthria, impotence, and emotional instability. The patient may also develop constipation, as well as urinary frequency, urgency, and incontinence.

◆ ***Stroke.*** A stroke involving the posterior inferior cerebellar artery may cause sudden horizontal or vertical jerk nystagmus that may be gaze dependent. Other findings include

Classifying nystagmus

Jerk nystagmus

Convergence-retraction nystagmus refers to the irregular jerking of the eyes back into the orbit during upward gaze. It can indicate midbrain tegmental damage.

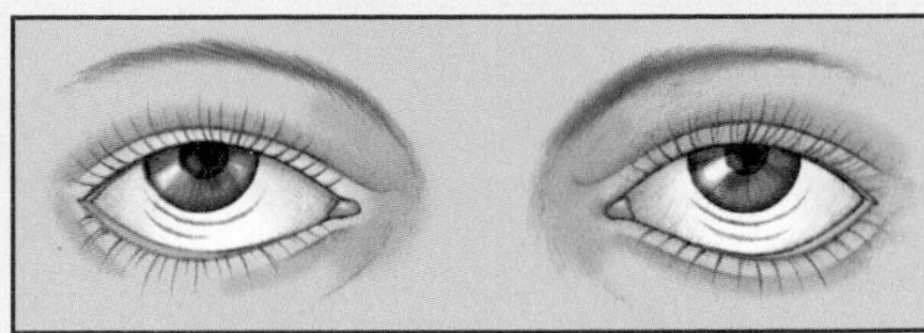

Downbeat nystagmus refers to the irregular downward jerking of the eyes during downward gaze. It can signal lower medullary damage.

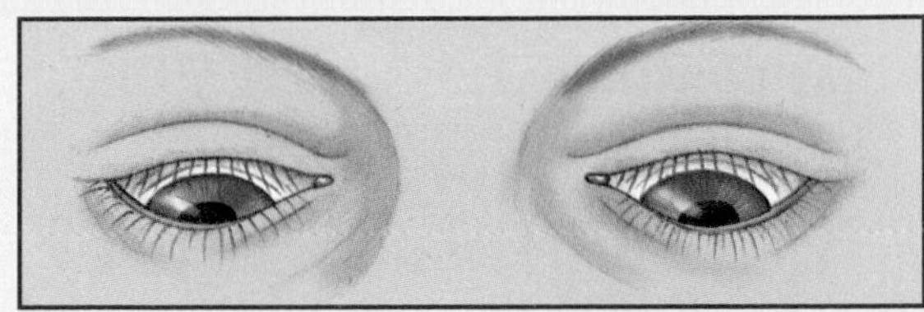

Vestibular nystagmus, the horizontal or rotary movement of the eyes, suggests vestibular disease or cochlear dysfunction.

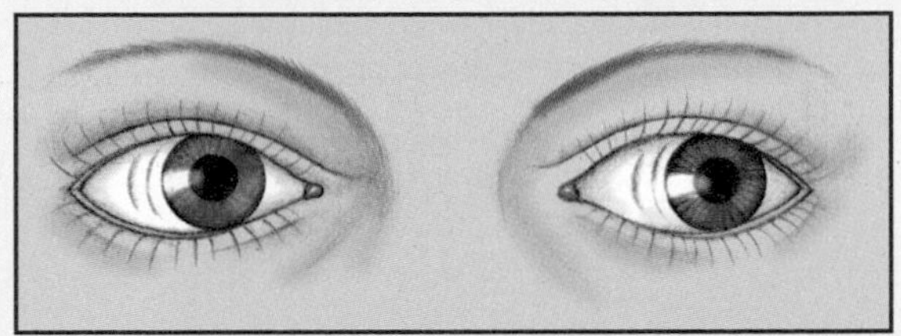

Pendular nystagmus

Horizontal, or pendular, nystagmus refers to oscillations of equal velocity around a center point. It can indicate congenital loss of visual acuity or multiple sclerosis.

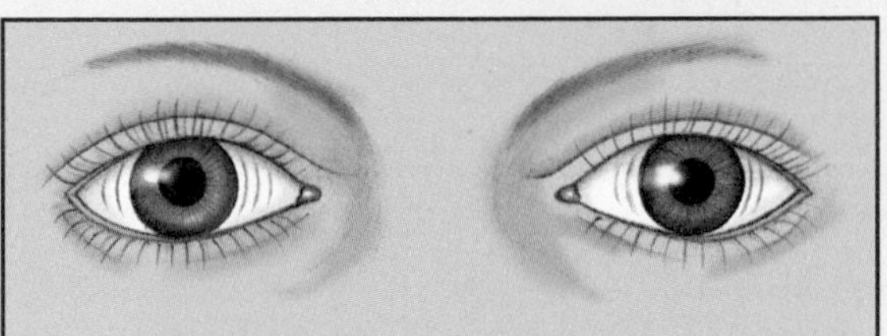

Vertical, or seesaw, nystagmus is the rapid, seesaw movement of the eyes: one eye appears to rise while the other appears to fall. It suggests an optic chiasm lesion.

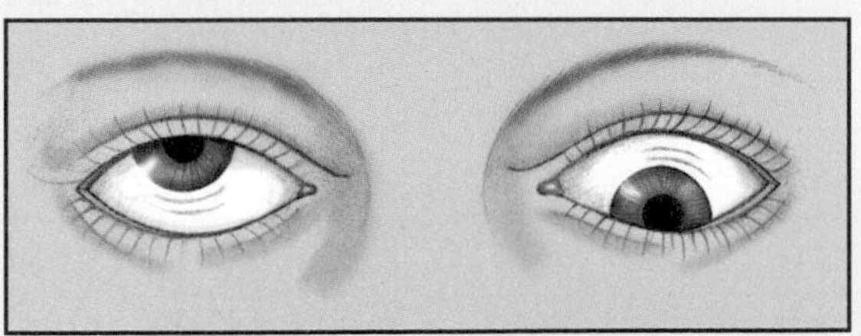

dysphagia, dysarthria, loss of pain and temperature sensation on the ipsilateral face and contralateral trunk and limbs, ipsilateral Horner's syndrome (unilateral ptosis, pupillary constriction, and facial anhidrosis), and cerebellar signs, such as ataxia and vertigo. Signs of increased intracranial pressure (such as altered LOC, bradycardia, widening pulse pressure, and elevated systolic pressure) may also occur.

Other causes

◆ ***Drugs and alcohol.*** Jerk nystagmus may result from barbiturate, phenytoin, or carbamazepine toxicity, or from alcohol intoxication.

Special considerations

Prepare the patient for diagnostic tests, such as electronystagmography and a cerebral computed tomography scan.

Pediatric pointers

In children, pendular nystagmus may be idiopathic, or it may result from early impaired vision associated with such disorders as optic atrophy, albinism, congenital cataracts, or severe astigmatism.

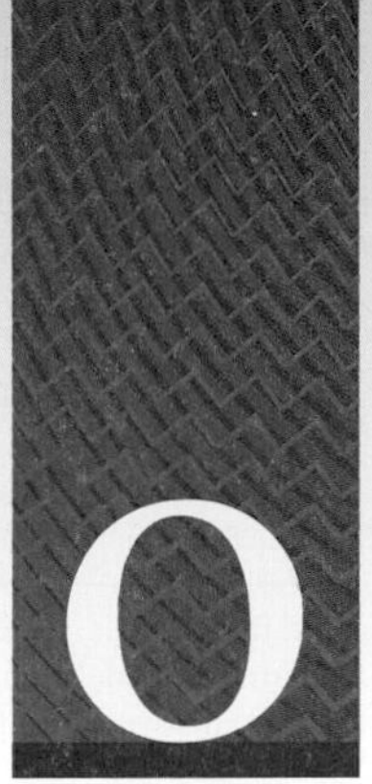

Ocular deviation

Ocular deviation refers to abnormal eye movement that may be conjugate (both eyes move together) or disconjugate (one eye moves separately from the other). This common sign may result from ocular, neurologic, endocrine, and systemic disorders that interfere with the muscles, nerves, or brain centers governing eye movement. Occasionally, it signals a life-threatening disorder such as a ruptured cerebral aneurysm. (See *Ocular deviation: Its characteristics and causes in cranial nerve damage*, page 494.)

Normally, eye movement is directly controlled by the extraocular muscles innervated by the oculomotor, trochlear, and abducens nerves (cranial nerves III, IV, and VI). Together, these muscles and nerves direct a visual stimulus to fall on corresponding parts of the retina. Disconjugate ocular deviation may result from unequal muscle tone (nonparalytic strabismus) or from muscle paralysis associated with cranial nerve damage (paralytic strabismus). Conjugate ocular deviation may result from disorders that affect the centers in the cerebral cortex and brain stem responsible for conjugate eye movement. Typically, such disorders cause gaze palsy—difficulty moving the eyes in one or more directions.

EMERGENCY INTERVENTIONS *If the patient displays ocular deviation, take his vital signs immediately and assess him for altered level of consciousness (LOC), pupil changes, motor or sensory dysfunction, and severe headache. If possible, ask the patient's family about behavioral changes. Is there a history of recent head trauma? Respiratory support may be necessary. Also, prepare the patient for emergency neurologic tests such as a computed tomography scan.*

History and physical examination

If the patient isn't in distress, find out how long he has had the ocular deviation. Is it accompanied by double vision, eye pain, or headache? Also, ask if he has noticed any associated motor or sensory changes, or fever.

Check for a history of hypertension, diabetes, allergies, and thyroid, neurologic, or muscular disorders. Then obtain a thorough ocular history. Has the patient ever had extraocular muscle imbalance, eye or head trauma, or eye surgery?

During the physical examination, observe the patient for partial or complete ptosis. Does he spontaneously tilt his head or turn his face to compensate for ocular deviation? Check for eye redness or periorbital edema. Assess visual acuity, then evaluate extraocular muscle function by testing the six cardinal fields of gaze.

Medical causes

◆ ***Brain tumor.*** The nature of ocular deviation depends on the site and extent of the tumor. Associated signs and symptoms include headaches that are most severe in the morning, behavioral changes, memory loss, dizziness, confusion, vision loss, motor and sensory dysfunction, aphasia and, possibly, signs of hormonal imbalance. The patient's LOC may slowly deteriorate from lethargy to coma. Late signs

Ocular deviation: Its characteristics and causes in cranial nerve damage

Characteristics	Cranial nerve and extraocular muscles involved	Probable causes
Inability to move the eye upward, downward, inward, and outward; drooping eyelid; and, except in diabetes, adilated pupil in the affected eye	Oculomotor nerve (III); medial rectus, superior rectus, inferior rectus, and inferior oblique muscles	Cerebral aneurysm, diabetes, temporal lobe herniation from increased intracranial pressure, brain tumor
Loss of downward and outward movement in the affected eye	Trochlear nerve (IV); superior oblique muscle	Head trauma
Loss of outward movement in the affected eye	Abducens nerve (VI); lateral rectus muscle	Brain tumor

include papilledema, vomiting, increased systolic blood pressure, widening pulse pressure, and decorticate posture.

◆ ***Cavernous sinus thrombosis.*** In this disorder, ocular deviation may be accompanied by diplopia, photophobia, exophthalmos, orbital and eyelid edema, corneal haziness, diminished or absent pupillary reflexes, and impaired visual acuity. Other features include high fever, headache, malaise, nausea and vomiting, seizures, and tachycardia. Retinal hemorrhages and papilledema are late signs.

◆ ***Cerebral aneurysm.*** When an aneurysm near the internal carotid artery compresses the oculomotor nerve, it may produce features that resemble third cranial nerve palsy. Typically, ocular deviation and diplopia are the presenting signs. Other cardinal findings include ptosis, a dilated pupil on the affected side, and a severe, unilateral headache, usually in the frontal area. Rupture of the aneurysm abruptly intensifies the pain, which may be accompanied by nausea and vomiting. Bleeding from the site causes meningeal irritation, resulting in nuchal rigidity, back and leg pain, fever, irritability, occasional seizures, and blurred vision. Other signs and symptoms associated with intracranial bleeding include hemiparesis, dysphagia, and visual defects.

◆ ***Diabetes mellitus.*** A leading cause of isolated third cranial nerve palsy, especially in the middle-age patient with long-standing mild diabetes, this disorder may cause ocular deviation and ptosis. Typically, the patient also complains of sudden onset of diplopia and pain.

◆ ***Encephalitis.*** This infection causes ocular deviation and diplopia in some patients. Typically, it begins abruptly with fever, headache, and vomiting, followed by signs of meningeal irritation (for example, nuchal rigidity) and of neuronal damage (for example, seizures, aphasia, ataxia, hemiparesis, cranial nerve palsies, and photophobia). The patient's LOC may rapidly deteriorate from lethargy to coma within 24 to 48 hours after onset.

◆ ***Head trauma.*** The nature of ocular deviation depends on the site and extent of head trauma. The patient may have visible soft-tissue injury, bony deformity, facial edema, and clear or bloody otorrhea or rhinorrhea. Besides these obvious signs of trauma, he may also develop blurred vision, diplopia, nystagmus, behavioral changes, headache, motor and sensory dysfunction, and a decreased LOC that may progress to coma. Signs of increased intracranial pressure—such as bradycardia, increased systolic pressure, and widening pulse pressure—may also occur.

◆ ***Multiple sclerosis.*** Ocular deviation may be an early sign of this disorder. Accompanying it are diplopia, blurred vision, and sensory dysfunction, such as paresthesia. Other signs and symptoms include nystagmus, constipation, muscle weakness, paralysis, spasticity, hyperreflexia, intention tremor, gait ataxia, dysphagia, dysarthria, impotence, and emotional instability. In addition, the patient may experience urinary frequency, urgency, and incontinence.

◆ ***Myasthenia gravis.*** Ocular deviation may accompany the more common presenting signs of diplopia and ptosis. This disorder may affect only the eye muscles, or it may progress to other muscle groups, causing altered facial expression, difficulty chewing, dysphagia, weakened voice, and impaired fine hand movements. Signs of respiratory distress reflect weakness of the diaphragm and other respiratory muscles.

◆ ***Ophthalmoplegic migraine.*** Most common in young adults, this disorder produces ocular deviation and diplopia that persist for days after the pain subsides. Associated signs and symptoms include unilateral headache, possibly with ptosis on the same side; temporary hemiplegia; and sensory deficits. Irritability, depression, or slight confusion may also occur.

◆ ***Orbital blowout fracture.*** In this fracture, the inferior rectus muscle may become entrapped, resulting in limited extraocular movement and ocular deviation. Typically, the patient's upward gaze is absent; other directions of gaze may be affected if edema is dramatic. The globe may also be displaced downward and inward. Associated signs and symptoms include pain, diplopia, nausea, periorbital edema, and ecchymosis.

◆ ***Orbital cellulitis.*** This disorder may cause sudden onset of ocular deviation and diplopia. Other signs and symptoms include unilateral eyelid edema and erythema, hyperemia, chemosis, and extreme orbital pain. Purulent discharge makes eyelashes matted and sticky. Proptosis is a late sign.

◆ ***Orbital tumor.*** Ocular deviation occurs as the tumor gradually enlarges. Associated findings include proptosis, diplopia and, possibly, blurred vision.

◆ ***Stroke.*** This life-threatening disorder may cause ocular deviation, depending on the site and extent of the stroke. Accompanying features are also variable and include altered LOC, contralateral hemiplegia and sensory loss, dysarthria, dysphagia, homonymous hemianopsia, blurred vision, and diplopia. In addition, the patient may develop urine retention or incontinence or both, constipation, behavioral changes, headache, vomiting, and seizures.

◆ ***Thyrotoxicosis.*** This disorder may produce exophthalmos—proptotic or protruding eyes—which, in turn, causes limited extraocular movement and ocular deviation. Usually, the patient's upward gaze weakens first, followed by diplopia. Other features are lid retraction, a wide-eyed staring gaze, excessive tearing, edematous eyelids and, sometimes, inability to close the eyes. Cardinal features of thyrotoxicosis include tachycardia, palpitations, weight loss despite increased appetite, diarrhea, tremors, an enlarged thyroid, dyspnea, nervousness, diaphoresis, heat intolerance, and an atrial or ventricular gallop.

Special considerations

Continue to monitor the patient's vital signs and neurologic status if you suspect an acute neurologic disorder. Take seizure precautions, if necessary. Also, prepare the patient for diagnostic tests, such as blood studies, orbital and skull X-rays, and computed tomography scan.

Pediatric pointers

In children, the most common cause of ocular deviation is nonparalytic strabismus. Normally, children achieve binocular vision by age 3 to 4 months. Although severe strabismus is readily apparent, mild strabismus must be confirmed by tests for misalignment, such as the corneal light reflex test and the cover test. Testing is crucial—early corrective measures help preserve binocular vision and cosmetic appearance. Also, mild strabismus may indicate retinoblastoma, a tumor that may be asymptomatic before age 2 except for a characteristic whitish reflex in the pupil.

Oligomenorrhea

In most women, menstrual bleeding occurs every 28 days plus or minus 4 days. Although some variation is normal, menstrual bleeding at intervals of greater than 36 days may indicate oligomenorrhea—abnormally infrequent menstrual bleeding characterized by three to six menstrual cycles per year. When menstrual bleeding does occur, it's usually profuse, prolonged (up to 10 days), and laden with clots and tissue. Occasionally, scant bleeding or spotting occurs between these heavy menses.

Oligomenorrhea may develop suddenly or it may follow a period of gradually lengthening cycles. Although oligomenorrhea may alternate with normal menstrual bleeding, it can progress to secondary amenorrhea.

Because oligomenorrhea is commonly associated with anovulation, it's common in infertile, early postmenarchal, and perimenopausal women. This sign usually reflects abnormalities of the hormones that govern normal endometrial function. It may result from ovarian, hypothalamic, pituitary, and other metabolic disorders, and from the effects of certain drugs. It may also result from emotional or physical stress, such as sudden weight change, debilitating illness, or rigorous physical training.

History and physical examination

After asking the patient's age, find out when menarche occurred. Has the patient ever experienced normal menstrual cycles? When did she begin having abnormal cycles? Ask her to describe the pattern of bleeding. How many days does the bleeding last, and how frequently does it occur? Are there clots and tissue fragments in her menstrual flow? Note when she last had menstrual bleeding.

Next, determine if she's having symptoms of ovulatory bleeding. Does she experience mild, cramping abdominal pain 14 days before she bleeds? Is the bleeding accompanied by premenstrual symptoms, such as breast tenderness, irritability, bloating, weight gain, nausea, and diarrhea? Does she have cramping or pain with bleeding? Also, check for a history of infertility. Does the patient have any children? Is she trying to conceive? Ask if she's currently using hormonal contraceptives or if she's ever used them in the past. If she has, find out when she stopped taking them.

Then ask about previous gynecologic disorders such as ovarian cysts. If the patient is breast-feeding, has she experienced any problems with milk production? If she hasn't been breast-feeding recently, has she noticed milk leaking from her breasts? Ask about recent weight gain or loss. Is the patient less than 80% of her ideal weight? If so, does she claim that she's overweight? Ask if she's exercising more vigorously than usual.

Screen for metabolic disorders by asking about excessive thirst, frequent urination, or fatigue. Has the patient been jittery or had palpitations? Ask about headache, dizziness, and impaired peripheral vision. Complete the history by finding out what drugs the patient is taking.

Begin the physical examination by taking the patient's vital signs and weighing her. Inspect for increased facial hair growth, sparse body hair, male distribution of fat and muscle, acne, and clitoral enlargement. Note if the skin is abnormally dry or moist, and check hair texture. Also, be alert for signs of psychological or physical stress. Rule out pregnancy by a blood or urine pregnancy test.

Medical causes

◆ ***Adrenal hyperplasia.*** In this disorder, oligomenorrhea may occur with signs of androgen excess, such as clitoral enlargement and male distribution of hair, fat, and muscle mass.

◆ ***Anorexia nervosa.*** Anorexia nervosa may cause sporadic oligomenorrhea or amenorrhea. Its cardinal symptom, however, is a morbid fear of being fat associated with weight loss of more than 20% of ideal body weight. Typically, the patient displays dramatic skeletal muscle atrophy and loss of fatty tissue; dry or sparse scalp hair; lanugo on the face and body; and blotchy or sallow, dry skin. Other symptoms include constipation, decreased libido, and sleep disturbances.

◆ ***Diabetes mellitus.*** Oligomenorrhea may be an early sign in this disorder. In juvenile-onset diabetes, the patient may have never had normal menses. Associated findings include excessive hunger, polydipsia, polyuria, weakness, fatigue, dry mucous membranes, poor skin turgor, irritability and emotional lability, and weight loss.

◆ ***Hypothyroidism.*** Besides oligomenorrhea, this disorder may result in fatigue; forgetfulness; cold intolerance; unexplained weight gain; constipation; bradycardia; decreased mental acuity; dry, flaky, inelastic skin; puffy face, hands, and feet; hoarseness; periorbital edema; ptosis; dry, sparse hair; and thick, brittle nails.

◆ ***Polycystic ovary disease.*** About 25% of women with polycystic ovary disease have oligomenorrhea; but some may have amenorrhea, menometrorrhagia, or irregular menses. Infertility, anovulation, and enlarged, palpable ovaries are also common. Other features vary but may include signs of androgen excess—male distribution of body hair and muscle mass, facial hair growth, acne and, occasionally, obesity.

◆ ***Prolactin-secreting pituitary tumor.*** Oligomenorrhea or amenorrhea may be the first sign of a prolactin-secreting pituitary tumor. Accompanying findings include unilateral or bilateral galactorrhea, infertility, loss of libido, and sparse pubic hair. Headache and visual field disturbances—such as diminished peripheral vision, blurred vision, diplopia, and hemianopsia—signal tumor expansion.

◆ ***Sheehan's syndrome.*** This pituitary necrosis usually follows severe obstetric hemorrhage. Oligomenorrhea or amenorrhea may occur with failure to lactate, sparse pubic and axillary hair, decreased libido, and fatigue.

◆ ***Thyrotoxicosis.*** This disorder may produce oligomenorrhea along with reduced fertility. Cardinal findings include irritability, weight loss despite increased appetite, dyspnea, tachycardia, palpitations, diarrhea, tremors, diaphoresis, heat intolerance, an enlarged thyroid and, possibly, exophthalmos.

Other causes

◆ ***Drugs.*** Drugs that increase androgen levels—such as corticosteroids, corticotropin, anabolic steroids, danocrine, and injectable and implanted contraceptives—may cause oligomenorrhea. Hormonal contraceptives may be associated with delayed resumption of normal menses when their use is discontinued; however, 95% of women resume normal menses within 3 months. Other drugs that may cause oligomenorrhea include phenothiazine derivatives and amphetamines, and antihypertensive drugs, which increase prolactin levels.

Special considerations

Prepare the patient for diagnostic tests, such as blood hormone levels, thyroid studies, or pelvic imaging studies.

Pediatric pointers

Teenage girls may experience oligomenorrhea associated with immature hormonal function. However, prolonged oligomenorrhea or the development of amenorrhea may signal congenital adrenal hyperplasia or Turner's syndrome.

Geriatric pointers

Oligomenorrhea in the perimenopausal woman usually indicates impending onset of menopause.

Patient counseling

Ask the patient to record her basal body temperature to determine if she's having ovulatory cycles. Provide her with blank charts, and teach her how to keep them accurately. Have the patient use a home ovulation testing or urine luteinizing hormone kit to provide evidence of ovulation. Remind the patient that she may become pregnant since ovulation may still occur even though she isn't menstruating normally. Discuss contraceptive measures, as appropriate.

Oliguria

A cardinal sign of renal and urinary tract disorders, oliguria is clinically defined as urine output of less than 400 ml/24 hours. Typically, this sign occurs abruptly and may herald serious—possibly life-threatening—hemodynamic instability. Its causes can be classified as prerenal (decreased renal blood flow), intrarenal (intrinsic renal damage), or postrenal (urinary tract obstruction); the pathophysiology differs for each classification. (See *How oliguria develops*, page 498.) Oliguria associated with a prerenal or postrenal cause is usually promptly reversible with treatment, although it may lead to intrarenal damage if untreated. However, oliguria associated with an intrarenal cause is usually more persistent and may be irreversible.

History and physical examination

Begin by asking the patient about his usual daily voiding pattern, including frequency and amount. When did he first notice changes in this pattern and in the color, odor, or consistency of his urine? Ask about pain or burning on urination. Has the patient had a fever? Note his normal daily fluid intake. Has he recently been drinking more or less than usual? Has his intake of caffeine or alcohol changed drastically? Has he had recent episodes of diarrhea or vomiting that might cause fluid loss? Next, explore associated complaints, especially fatigue, loss of appetite, thirst, dyspnea, chest pain, or recent weight gain or loss (in dehydration).

Check for a history of renal, urinary tract, or cardiovascular disorders. Note recent traumatic injury or surgery associated with significant blood loss, as well as recent blood transfusions. Was the patient exposed to nephrotoxic agents, such as heavy metals, organic solvents, anesthetics, or radiographic contrast media? Next, obtain a drug history.

Begin the physical examination by taking the patient's vital signs and weighing him. Assess his overall appearance for edema. Palpate both kidneys for tenderness and enlargement, and percuss for costovertebral angle (CVA) tenderness. Also, inspect the flank area for edema or erythema. Auscultate the heart and lungs for abnormal sounds, and the flank area for renal artery bruits. Assess the patient for edema or signs of dehydration such as dry mucous membranes.

Obtain a urine sample and inspect it for abnormal color, odor, or sediment. Use reagent strips to test for glucose, protein, and blood. Also, use a urinometer to measure specific gravity.

How oliguria develops

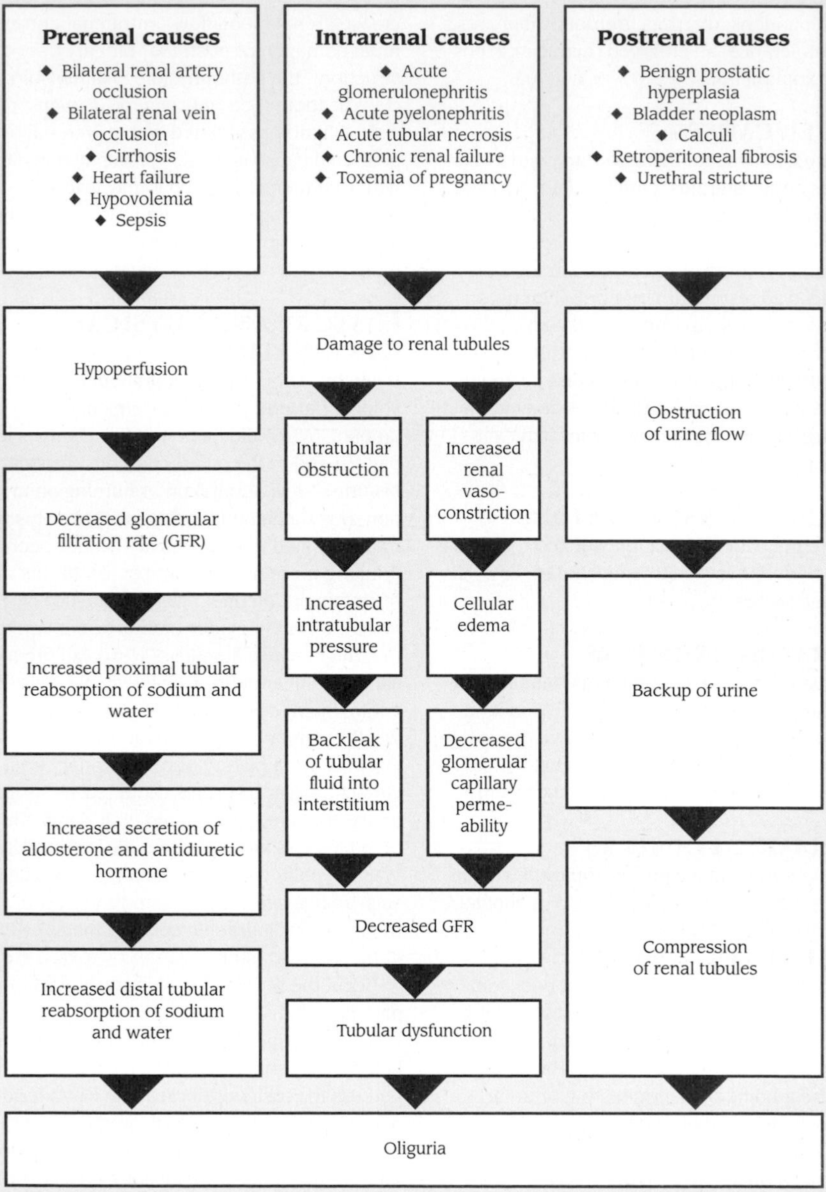

Prerenal causes
- Bilateral renal artery occlusion
- Bilateral renal vein occlusion
- Cirrhosis
- Heart failure
- Hypovolemia
- Sepsis

→ Hypoperfusion → Decreased glomerular filtration rate (GFR) → Increased proximal tubular reabsorption of sodium and water → Increased secretion of aldosterone and antidiuretic hormone → Increased distal tubular reabsorption of sodium and water → Oliguria

Intrarenal causes
- Acute glomerulonephritis
- Acute pyelonephritis
- Acute tubular necrosis
- Chronic renal failure
- Toxemia of pregnancy

→ Damage to renal tubules
- → Intratubular obstruction → Increased intratubular pressure → Backleak of tubular fluid into interstitium
- → Increased renal vaso-constriction → Cellular edema → Decreased glomerular capillary perme-ability

→ Decreased GFR → Tubular dysfunction → Oliguria

Postrenal causes
- Benign prostatic hyperplasia
- Bladder neoplasm
- Calculi
- Retroperitoneal fibrosis
- Urethral stricture

→ Obstruction of urine flow → Backup of urine → Compression of renal tubules → Oliguria

MEDICAL CAUSES

◆ ***Acute tubular necrosis (ATN).*** An early sign of ATN, oliguria may occur abruptly (in shock) or gradually (in nephrotoxicity). Usually, it persists for about 2 weeks, followed by polyuria. Related features include signs of hyperkalemia (muscle weakness and cardiac arrhythmias); uremia (anorexia, confusion, lethargy, twitching, seizures, pruritus, and Kussmaul's respirations); and heart failure (edema, jugular vein distention, crackles, and dyspnea).

◆ ***Benign prostatic hyperplasia.*** This disorder, which is common in men older than age 50, in rare cases may cause oliguria resulting from bladder outlet obstruction. More common symptoms include urinary frequency or hesitancy, urge or overflow incontinence, decrease in the force of the urine stream or inability to stop the stream, nocturia and, possibly, hematuria.

◆ ***Bladder neoplasm.*** Uncommonly, this disorder may produce oliguria if the tumor obstructs the bladder outlet. The cardinal signs of such obstruction include urinary frequency and urgency, as well as gross hematuria, which may lead to clot retention and flank pain.

◆ ***Calculi.*** Oliguria or anuria may result from stones lodging in the kidneys, ureters, bladder outlet, or urethra. Associated signs and symptoms include urinary frequency and urgency, dysuria, and hematuria or pyuria. Usually, the patient experiences renal colic—excruciating pain that radiates from the CVA to the flank, the suprapubic region, and the external genitalia. This pain may be accompanied by nausea, vomiting, hypoactive bowel sounds, abdominal distention and, occasionally, fever and chills.

◆ ***Cholera.*** In this bacterial infection, severe water and electrolyte loss lead to oliguria, thirst, weakness, muscle cramps, decreased skin turgor, tachycardia, hypotension, and abrupt watery diarrhea and vomiting. Death may occur in hours without treatment.

◆ ***Cirrhosis.*** In severe cirrhosis, hepatorenal syndrome may develop with oliguria, in addition to ascites, edema, fatigue, weakness, jaundice, hypotension, tachycardia, gynecomastia, testicular atrophy, and signs of GI bleeding such as hematemesis.

◆ ***Glomerulonephritis (acute).*** This disorder produces oliguria or anuria. Other features are mild fever, fatigue, gross hematuria, proteinuria, generalized edema, elevated blood pressure, headache, nausea and vomiting, flank and abdominal pain, and signs of pulmonary congestion (dyspnea and productive cough).

◆ ***Heart failure.*** Oliguria may occur in left ventricular failure as a result of low cardiac output and decreased renal perfusion. Accompanying signs and symptoms include dyspnea, fatigue, weakness, peripheral edema, distended jugular veins, tachycardia, tachypnea, crackles, and a dry or productive cough. In advanced heart failure, the patient may also develop orthopnea, cyanosis, clubbing, ventricular gallop, diastolic hypertension, cardiomegaly, and hemoptysis.

◆ ***Hypovolemia.*** Any disorder that decreases circulating fluid volume can produce oliguria. Associated findings include orthostatic hypotension, apathy, lethargy, fatigue, gross muscle weakness, anorexia, nausea, profound thirst, dizziness, sunken eyeballs, poor skin turgor, and dry mucous membranes.

◆ ***Pyelonephritis (acute).*** Accompanying the sudden onset of oliguria in this disorder are high fever with chills, fatigue, flank pain, CVA tenderness, weakness, nocturia, dysuria, hematuria, urinary frequency and urgency, and tenesmus. The urine may appear cloudy. Occasionally, the patient also experiences anorexia, nausea, diarrhea, and vomiting.

◆ ***Renal artery occlusion (bilateral).*** This disorder may produce oliguria or, more commonly, anuria. Other features include severe, constant upper abdominal and flank pain, nausea and vomiting, and hypoactive bowel sounds. The patient also develops a fever 1 to 2 days after the occlusion, as well as diastolic hypertension.

◆ ***Renal failure (chronic).*** Oliguria is a major sign of end-stage chronic renal failure. Associated findings reflect progressive uremia and include fatigue, weakness, irritability, uremic fetor, ecchymoses and petechiae, peripheral edema, elevated blood pressure, confusion, emotional lability, drowsiness, coarse muscle twitching, muscle cramps, peripheral neuropathies, anorexia, metallic taste in the mouth, nausea and vomiting, constipation or diarrhea, stomatitis, pruritus, pallor, and yellow- or bronze-tinged skin. Eventually, seizures, coma, and uremic frost may develop.

◆ ***Renal vein occlusion (bilateral).*** This disorder occasionally causes oliguria accompanied by acute low back and flank pain, CVA tenderness, fever, pallor, hematuria, enlarged and palpable kidneys, edema and, possibly, signs of uremia.

◆ ***Retroperitoneal fibrosis.*** Oliguria may result from bilateral ureteral obstruction by dense fibrous tissue. Other effects include hematuria, diffuse low back pain, anorexia, weight loss, nausea and vomiting, fatigue, malaise, low-grade fever, and elevated blood pressure.

◆ ***Sepsis.*** Any condition that results in sepsis may produce oliguria, along with fever, chills, restlessness, confusion, diaphoresis, anorexia, vomiting, diarrhea, pallor, hypotension, and tachycardia. The patient may exhibit signs of local infection, such as dysuria and wound drainage. In severe infection, he may develop lactic acidosis marked by Kussmaul's respirations.

◆ ***Toxemia of pregnancy.*** In severe preeclampsia, oliguria may be accompanied by elevated blood pressure, dizziness, diplopia, blurred vision, epigastric pain, nausea and vomiting, irritability, and severe frontal headache. Typically, the oliguria is preceded by generalized edema and sudden weight gain of more than 3 lb (1.4 kg) per week during the second trimester, or more than 1 lb (0.5 kg) per week during the third trimester. If preeclampsia progresses to eclampsia, the patient develops seizures and may slip into coma.

◆ ***Urethral stricture.*** This disorder produces oliguria accompanied by chronic urethral discharge, urinary frequency and urgency, dysuria, pyuria, and diminished urine stream. As obstruction worsens, urine extravasation may lead to formation of urinomas and urosepsis.

Other causes

◆ ***Diagnostic studies.*** Radiographic studies that use contrast media may cause nephrotoxicity and oliguria.

◆ ***Drugs.*** Oliguria may result from drugs that cause decreased renal perfusion (diuretics), nephrotoxicity (most notably, aminoglycosides and chemotherapeutic drugs), urine retention (adrenergics and anticholinergics), or urinary obstruction associated with precipitation of urinary crystals (sulfonamides and acyclovir).

Special considerations

Monitor vital signs, intake and output, and daily weight. Depending on the cause of the oliguria, fluids are normally restricted to between 600 ml and 1 L more than the patient's urine output for the previous day. Provide a diet low in sodium, potassium, and protein.

Laboratory tests may be necessary to determine if the oliguria is reversible. Such tests include serum blood urea nitrogen and creatinine levels, urea and creatinine clearance, urine sodium levels, and urine osmolality. Abdominal X-rays, ultrasonography, computed tomography scan, cystography, and a renal scan may be required.

Pediatric pointers

In the neonate, oliguria may result from edema or dehydration. Major causes include congenital heart disease, respiratory distress syndrome, sepsis, congenital hydronephrosis, acute tubular necrosis, and renal vein thrombosis. Common causes of oliguria in children between ages 1 and 5 are acute poststreptococcal glomerulonephritis and hemolytic-uremic syndrome. After age 5, causes of oliguria are similar to those in adults.

Geriatric pointers

In elderly patients, oliguria may result from gradual progression of an underlying disorder. It may also result from overall poor muscle tone secondary to inactivity, poor fluid intake, and infrequent voiding attempts.

Opisthotonos

A sign of severe meningeal irritation, opisthotonos is severe, prolonged spasm characterized by a strongly arched, rigid back; hyperextended neck; the heels bent back; and the arms and hands flexed at the joints. Usually, this posture occurs spontaneously and continuously; however, it may be aggravated by movement. Presumably, opisthotonos represents a protective reflex because it immobilizes the spine, alleviating the pain associated with meningeal irritation.

Usually caused by meningitis, opisthotonos may also result from subarachnoid hemorrhage, Arnold-Chiari syndrome, and tetanus. Occasionally, it occurs in achondroplastic dwarfism, although not necessarily as an indicator of meningeal irritation.

Opisthotonos is far more common in children—especially infants—than in adults. It's also more exaggerated in children because of nervous system immaturity. (See *Opisthotonos: Sign of meningeal irritation*.)

EMERGENCY INTERVENTIONS *If the patient is stuporous or comatose, immediately evaluate his vital signs. Employ resuscitative measures, as appropriate. Place the patient in a bed, with rails raised and padded, or in a crib.*

History and physical examination

If the patient's condition permits, obtain a history. Consult with a relative of the young child or infant. Ask about a history of cerebral aneurysm or arteriovenous malformation and about hypertension. Note any recent infection that may have spread to the nervous system. Explore associated findings, such as headache, chills, and vomiting.

Opisthotonos: Sign of meningeal irritation

In the characteristic posture, the back is severely arched with the neck hyperextended. The heels bend back on the legs, and the arms and hands flex rigidly at the joints, as shown.

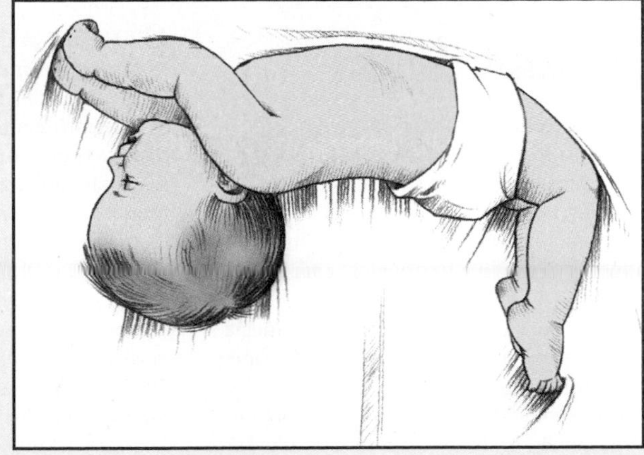

Focus the physical examination on the patient's neurologic status. Evaluate level of consciousness (LOC) and test sensorimotor and cranial nerve function. Then check for Brudzinski's and Kernig's signs and for nuchal rigidity.

Medical causes

◆ ***Arnold-Chiari syndrome.*** Here, opisthotonos typically occurs with hydrocephalus, with its characteristic, enlarged head; thin, shiny scalp with distended veins; and underdeveloped neck muscles. The infant usually also exhibits a high-pitched cry, abnormal leg muscle tone, anorexia, vomiting, nuchal rigidity, irritability, noisy respirations, and a weak sucking reflex.

◆ ***Meningitis.*** In this infection, opisthotonos accompanies other signs of meningeal irritation, including nuchal rigidity, positive Brudzinski's and Kernig's signs, and hyperreflexia. Meningitis also causes cardinal signs of infection (moderate to high fever with chills and malaise) and of increased intracranial pressure (headache, vomiting, and eventually, papilledema). Other features include irritability; photophobia; diplopia, deafness, and other cranial nerve palsies; and decreased LOC that may progress to seizures and coma.

◆ ***Subarachnoid hemorrhage.*** This disorder may produce opisthotonos along with other signs of meningeal irritation, such as nuchal rigidity and positive Kernig's and Brudzinski's signs. Focal signs of hemorrhage, such as severe headache, hemiplegia or hemiparesis, aphasia, and photophobia, along with other vision problems, may also occur. With increasing intracranial pressure, the patient may develop bradycardia, elevated blood pressure, altered respiratory pattern, seizures, and vomiting. His LOC may rapidly deteriorate, resulting in coma; then, decerebrate posture may alternate with opisthotonos.

◆ ***Tetanus.*** This life-threatening infection can cause opisthotonos. Initially, trismus occurs. Eventually, muscle spasms may affect the abdomen, producing boardlike rigidity; the back, resulting in opisthotonos; or the face, producing risus sardonicus. Spasms may affect the respiratory muscles, causing distress. Tachycardia, diaphoresis, hyperactive deep tendon reflexes, and seizures may also develop.

Other causes

◆ ***Antipsychotics.*** Phenothiazines and other antipsychotic drugs may cause opisthotonos, usually as part of an acute dystonic reaction. This usually can be treated with I.V. diphenhydramine.

Special considerations

Assess neurologic status and check vital signs frequently. Make the patient as comfortable as possible; place him in a side-lying position with pillows for support. If meningitis is suspected, institute respiratory isolation. Lumbar puncture may be ordered to identify pathogens and analyze cerebrospinal fluid. If subarachnoid hemorrhage is suspected, prepare the patient for a computed tomography scan or magnetic resonance imaging.

Orofacial dyskinesia

Orofacial dyskinesia—abnormal involuntary movements involving muscles of the face, mouth, tongue, eyes, and occasionally, the neck—may be unilateral or bilateral, and constant or intermittent. This sign occurs more commonly in women than in men, especially after age 50.

The pathophysiology of orofacial dyskinesia isn't clearly understood. Although the dyskinesia may result from hemifacial spasm and the effects of certain drugs, it's frequently idiopathic. Presumably, orofacial dyskinesia results from pressure on the facial nerves associated with an extrapyramidal lesion or from a chemical imbalance. Psychogenic factors may also play a role, as evidenced by the fact that emotional upset aggravates the dyskinesia.

History and physical examination

If the patient abruptly displays orofacial dyskinesia, review his medication regimen. If he's taking a phenothiazine or other antipsychotic, withhold the drug if possible, and prepare to give 50 mg of diphenhydramine to reverse the drug's effects. If he has difficulty swallowing, take precautions necessary to prevent aspiration and choking and have suction equipment on hand.

If the patient's dyskinesia is chronic, ask when it began. Then obtain a complete drug history. Also, note a history of seizures. Next, closely examine the patient's dyskinesia. Is it unilateral or bilateral? Does it involve the entire face or only part of it? Are neck muscles involved? Does the patient have any voluntary control over the movements? Characterize the abnormal movements. Are they constant, or repetitive and intermittent? Listen to his speech—does it sound abnormal? Can he swallow?

Medical causes

◆ ***Hemifacial spasm.*** This disorder is characterized by unilateral, intermittent spasms of muscles of the face, eye, and mouth. The patient may have some voluntary control over the spasms. Typically, the spasms are aggravated by emotional upset and disappear during sleep. Spasms may interfere with swallowing and speech.

Other causes

◆ ***Metoclopramide and metyrosine.*** Rarely, these drugs cause orofacial dyskinesia.

◆ ***Phenothiazines and other antipsychotic drugs.*** These drugs may cause orofacial dyskinesia and other extrapyramidal effects. Movements are sustained, involving the eyes, mouth, face, and neck; they occur with prolonged treatment, especially after it has been reduced. Lip retraction and dysphagia are common.

Among the phenothiazines, the piperazine derivatives (perphenazine, prochlorperazine, fluphenazine, and trifluoperazine) most commonly cause this sign. Aliphatic phenothiazines (chlorpromazine) occasionally cause it. Piperidine phenothiazines (thioridazine) rarely cause orofacial dyskinesia. Other antipsychotic drugs (haloperidol, thiothixene, and loxapine) commonly cause this sign.

Special considerations

Prepare the patient for diagnostic studies, such as blood screening for drugs and computed tomography or magnetic resonance imaging scan.

Pediatric pointers

In children, orofacial dyskinesia is usually drug-induced. These abnormal movements may also result from Tourette syndrome, seizure disorders, and dystonia musculorum deformans.

Patient counseling

If orofacial dyskinesia is drug-induced, assure the patient and his family that movements may disappear eventually, after the drug is stopped. If orofacial dyskinesia is uncontrollable, advise the patient and his family that drug therapy or psychotherapy may be beneficial.

Orthopnea

Orthopnea—difficulty breathing in the supine position—is a common symptom of cardiopulmonary disorders that produce dyspnea. It's often a subtle symptom; the patient may complain that he can't catch his breath when lying down, or he may mention that he sleeps most comfortably in a reclining chair or propped up by pillows.

Derived from this complaint is the common classification of two- or three-pillow orthopnea.

Orthopnea presumably results from increased hydrostatic pressure in the pulmonary vasculature related to gravitational effects in the supine position. It may be aggravated by obesity or pregnancy, which restricts diaphragmatic excursion. Assuming the upright position relieves orthopnea by placing much of the pulmonary vasculature above the left atrium, which reduces mean hydrostatic pressure, and by enhancing diaphragmatic excursion, which increases inspiratory volume.

History and physical examination

Begin by asking about a history of cardiopulmonary disorders, such as myocardial infarction, rheumatic heart disease, valvular disease, asthma, emphysema, or chronic bronchitis. Does the patient smoke? If so, how much? Explore associated symptoms, noting especially complaints of cough, nocturnal or exertional dyspnea, fatigue, weakness, loss of appetite, or chest pain. Does the patient use alcohol or have a history of heavy alcohol use?

When examining the patient, check for other signs of increased respiratory effort, such as accessory muscle use, shallow respirations, and tachypnea. Also note barrel chest. Inspect the patient's skin for pallor or cyanosis, and the fingers for clubbing. Observe and palpate for edema, and check for neck vein distention. Auscultate the lungs and heart. Monitor the patient's oxygen saturation.

Medical causes

◆ ***Chronic obstructive pulmonary disease.*** This disorder typically produces orthopnea and other dyspneic complaints, accompanied by accessory muscle use, tachypnea, tachycardia, and paradoxical pulse. Auscultation may reveal diminished breath sounds, rhonchi, crackles, and wheezing. The patient may also exhibit a dry or productive cough with copious sputum. Other features include anorexia, weight loss, and edema. Barrel chest, cyanosis, and clubbing are usually late signs.

◆ ***Left-sided heart failure.*** Orthopnea occurs late in this disorder. If heart failure is acute, orthopnea may begin suddenly; if chronic, it may become constant. The earliest symptom of this disorder is progressively severe dyspnea. Other common early symptoms include Cheyne-Stokes respirations, paroxysmal nocturnal dyspnea, fatigue, weakness, and a cough that may occasionally produce clear or blood-tinged sputum. Tachycardia, tachypnea, and crackles may also occur.

Other late findings include cyanosis, clubbing, ventricular gallop, and hemoptysis. Left-sided heart failure may also lead to signs of shock, such as hypotension, thready pulse, and cold, clammy skin.

◆ ***Mediastinal tumor.*** Orthopnea is an early sign of this disorder, resulting from pressure of the tumor against the trachea, bronchus, or lung when the patient lies down. However, many patients are asymptomatic until the tumor enlarges. Then, it produces retrosternal chest pain, dry cough, hoarseness, dysphagia, stertorous respirations, palpitations, and cyanosis. Examination reveals suprasternal retractions on inspiration, bulging of the chest wall, tracheal deviation, dilated jugular and superficial chest veins, and edema of the face, neck, and arms.

Special considerations

To relieve orthopnea, place the patient in semi-Fowler's or high Fowler's position; if this doesn't help, have the patient lean over a bedside table with his chest forward. If necessary, administer oxygen via nasal cannula. A diuretic may be needed to reduce lung fluid. Monitor electrolyte levels closely after administering diuretics. Angiotensin-converting enzyme inhibitors should be used for patients with left-sided heart failure, unless contraindicated. Monitor intake and output closely.

An electrocardiogram, chest X-ray, pulmonary function test, and an arterial blood gas test may be necessary for further evaluation.

A central venous access device or pulmonary artery catheter may be inserted to help measure central venous pressure and wedge and cardiac output, respectively.

Pediatric pointers

Common causes of orthopnea in children include heart failure, croup syndrome, cystic fibrosis, and asthma. Sleeping in an infant seat may improve symptoms for a young child.

Geriatric pointers

If the elderly patient is using more than one pillow at night, consider noncardiogenic pulmonary reasons for this, such as gastroesophageal reflux disease, sleep apnea, arthritis, or simply the need for greater comfort.

Patient counseling

Instruct the patient to notify the physician if he's using additional pillows regularly, or if dyspnea worsens at night.

Orthostatic hypotension

[Postural hypotension]

In orthostatic hypotension, the patient's blood pressure drops 15 to 20 mm Hg or more—with or without an increase in the heart rate of at least 20 beats/minute—when he rises from a supine to a sitting or standing position. (Blood pressure should be measured 5 minutes after the patient has changed his position.) This common sign indicates failure of compensatory vasomotor responses to adjust to position changes. It's typically associated with lightheadedness, syncope, or blurred vision, and may occur in a hypotensive, normotensive, or hypertensive patient. Although commonly a nonpathologic sign in the elderly, orthostatic hypotension may result from prolonged bed rest, fluid and electrolyte imbalance, endocrine or systemic disorders, and the effects of drugs.

To detect orthostatic hypotension, take and compare blood pressure readings with the patient supine, sitting, and then standing.

EMERGENCY INTERVENTIONS *If you detect orthostatic hypotension, quickly check for tachycardia, altered level of consciousness (LOC), and pale, clammy skin. If these signs are present, suspect hypovolemic shock. Insert a large-bore I.V. catheter for fluid or blood replacement. Take the patient's vital signs every 15 minutes, and monitor his intake and output.*

History and physical examination

If the patient is in no danger, obtain a history. Ask the patient if he frequently experiences dizziness, weakness, or fainting when he stands. Also ask about associated symptoms, particularly fatigue, orthopnea, impotence, nausea, headache, abdominal or chest discomfort, and GI bleeding. Then obtain a complete drug history.

Begin the physical examination by checking the patient's skin turgor. Palpate peripheral pulses and auscultate the heart and lungs. Finally, test muscle strength and observe the patient's gait for unsteadiness.

Medical causes

- ***Adrenal insufficiency.*** This disorder typically begins insidiously, with progressively severe signs and symptoms. Orthostatic hypotension may be accompanied by fatigue, muscle weakness, poor coordination, anorexia, nausea and vomiting, fasting hypoglycemia, weight loss, abdominal pain, irritability, and a weak, irregular pulse. Another common feature is hyperpigmentation—bronze coloring of the skin—which is especially prominent on the face, lips, gums, tongue, buccal mucosa, elbows, palms, knuckles, waist, and knees. Diarrhea, constipation, decreased libido, amenorrhea, and syncope may also occur along with enhanced taste, smell, and hearing, and cravings for salty food.
- ***Alcoholism.*** Chronic alcoholism can lead to the development of peripheral neuropathy, which can present as orthostatic hypotension. Impotence is also a major issue in these patients. Other symptoms include numbness, tingling, nausea, vomiting, changes in bowel habits, and bizarre behavior.
- ***Amyloidosis.*** Orthostatic hypotension is commonly associated with amyloid infiltration of the autonomic nerves. Associated signs and symptoms vary widely and include angina, tachycardia, dyspnea, orthopnea, fatigue, and cough.
- ***Diabetic autonomic neuropathy.*** Here, orthostatic hypotension may be accompanied by syncope, dysphagia, constipation or diarrhea, painless bladder distention with overflow incontinence, impotence, and retrograde ejaculation.
- ***Hyperaldosteronism.*** This disorder typically produces orthostatic hypotension with sustained elevated blood pressure. Most other clinical effects of hyperaldosteronism result from hypokalemia, which increases neuromuscular irritability and produces muscle weakness, intermittent flaccid paralysis, fatigue, headache, paresthesia and, possibly, tetany with positive Trousseau's and Chvostek's signs. The patient may also exhibit visual disturbance, nocturia, polydipsia, and personality changes. Diabetes mellitus is a common finding.
- ***Hyponatremia.*** In this disorder, orthostatic hypotension is typically accompanied by headache, profound thirst, tachycardia, nausea and vomiting, abdominal cramps, muscle twitching and weakness, fatigue, oliguria or anuria, cold clammy skin, poor skin turgor, irritability, seizures, and decreased LOC. Cyanosis,

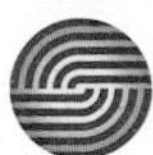

PATIENT-TEACHING AID

Performing preambulation exercises

Dear Patient:
To help minimize the effects of orthostatic hypotension, such as dizziness and blurred vision when you stand up, perform these leg exercises before getting out of bed.

Lie flat on your back, and flex one knee slightly, keeping your heel on the bed.

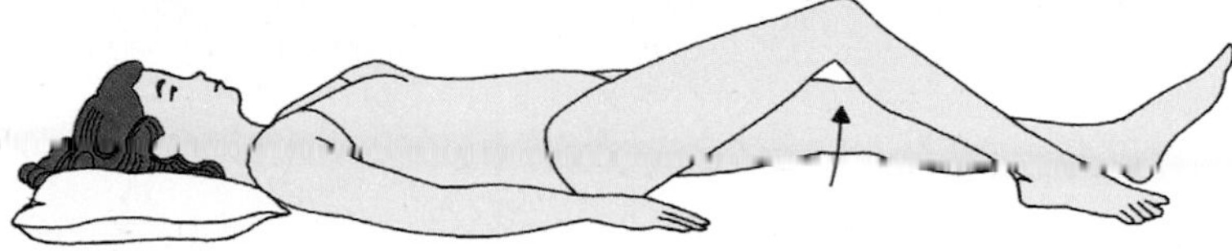

Extend your leg and raise your heel off the bed.

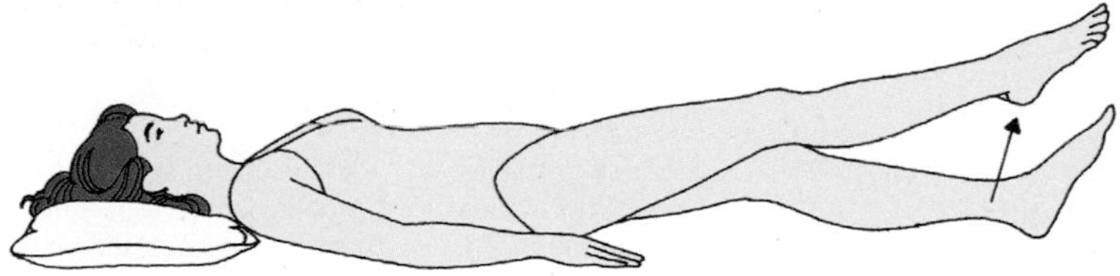

Flex your knee again, and lower your heel to the bed.

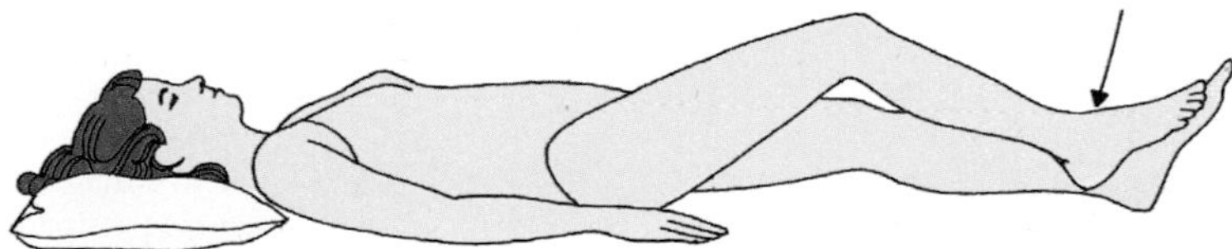

Straighten your leg.

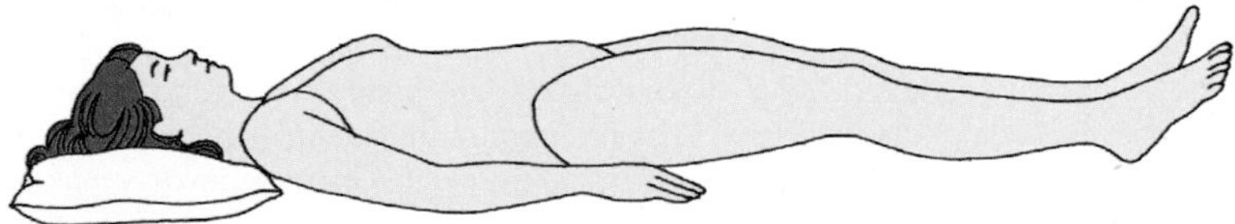

Repeat the procedure for the other leg. Alternating sides, perform the exercises six times for each leg.

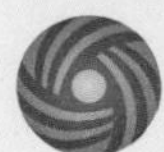

EXAMINATION TIP

Detecting developmental dysplasia of the hip

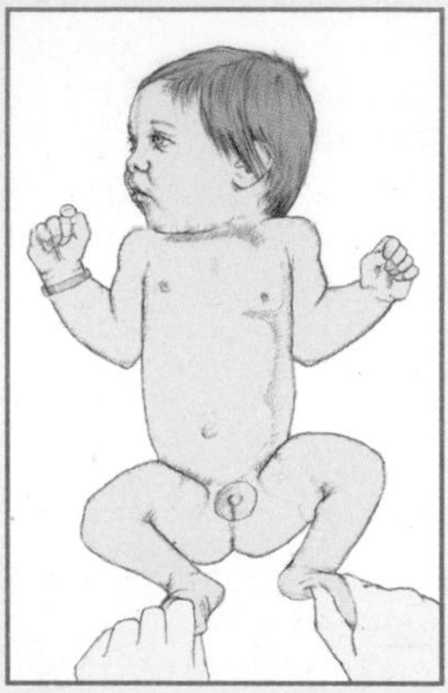

When assessing the neonate, attempt to elicit Ortolani's sign to detect developmental dysplasia of the hip (DDH). Begin by placing the infant in a supine position with his knees and hips flexed. Observe for symmetry.

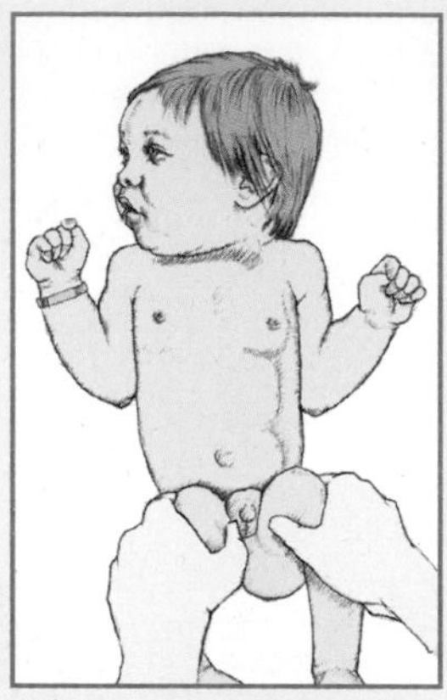

Place your hands on the infant's knees, with your index fingers along his lateral thighs on the greater trochanter. Then raise his knees to a 90-degree angle with his back.

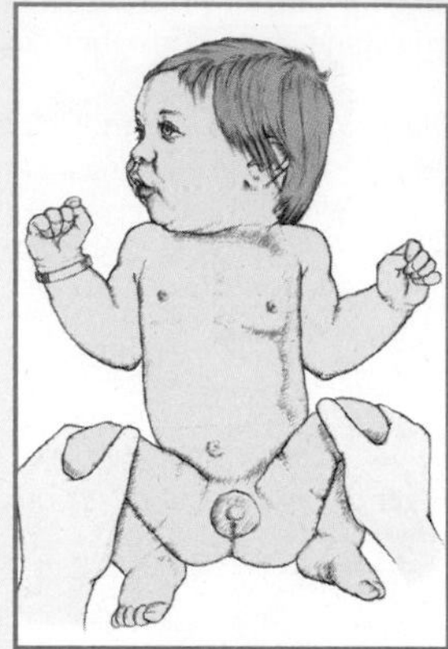

Abduct the infant's thighs so that the lateral aspect of his knees lies almost flat on the table. If the infant has a dislocated hip, you'll feel and often hear a click, clunk, or popping sensation (Ortolani's sign) as the head of the femur moves out of the acetabulum. The infant may also give a sudden cry of pain. Be sure to distinguish a positive Ortolani's sign from the normal clicks due to rotation of the hip, that do not elicit the sensation of instability, or simultaneous movement of the knee.

thready pulse, and eventually vasomotor collapse may occur in severe sodium deficit. Common causes include adrenal insufficiency, hypothyroidism, syndrome of inappropriate antidiuretic hormone secretion, and use of thiazide diuretics.

◆ ***Hypovolemia.*** Mild to moderate hypovolemia may cause orthostatic hypotension associated with apathy, fatigue, muscle weakness, anorexia, nausea, and profound thirst. The patient may also develop dizziness, oliguria, sunken eyeballs, poor skin turgor, and dry mucous membranes.

◆ ***Pheochromocytoma.*** Although this disorder may produce orthostatic hypotension, its cardinal sign is paroxysmal or sustained hypertension. Typically, the patient is pale or flushed and diaphoretic, and his extreme anxiety makes him appear panicky. Associated signs and symptoms include tachycardia, palpitations, chest and abdominal pain, paresthesia, tremors, nausea and vomiting, low-grade fever, insomnia, and headache.

◆ ***Shy-Drager syndrome.*** This neurodegenerative disorder is characterized by an insidious onset of multiple autonomic failure, manifested by orthostatic hypotension, urinary and fecal incontinence, decreased sweating, and impotence. This syndrome is most common in young and middle-age adults.

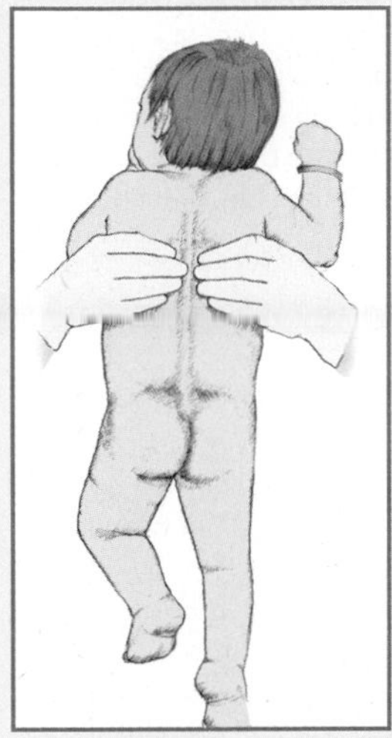

If you elicit a positive Ortolani's sign, look for other signs of DDH.

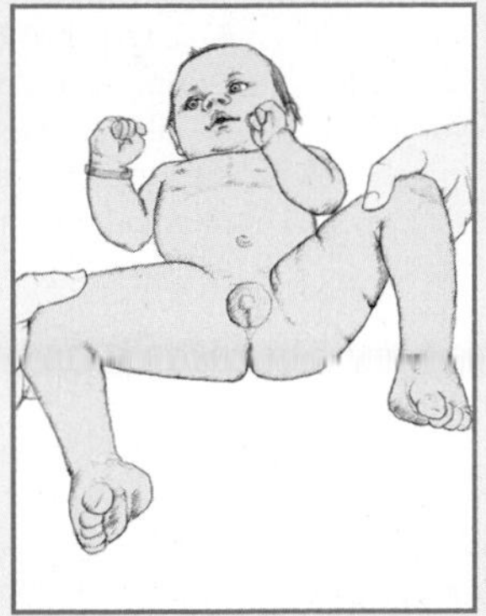

Flex the infant's hips to detect limited abduction.

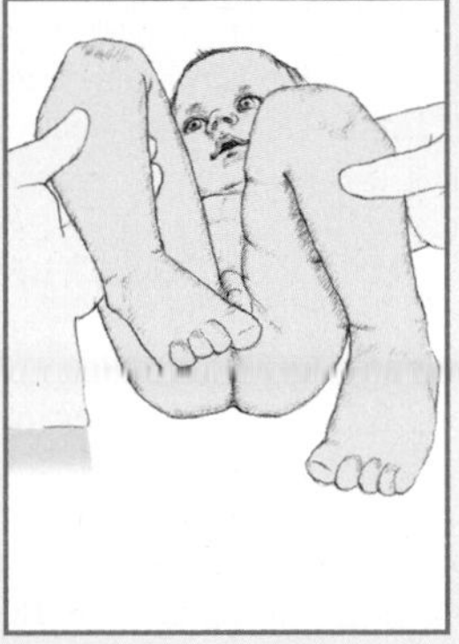

Flex the infant's knees, and observe for apparent shortening of the femur

OTHER CAUSES

◆ ***Drugs.*** Certain drugs may cause orthostatic hypotension by reducing circulating blood volume, causing blood vessel dilation, or depressing the sympathetic nervous system. These drugs include antihypertensives (especially the initial dosage of prazosin hydrochloride), tricyclic antidepressants, phenothiazines, levodopa, nitrates, monoamine oxidase inhibitors, morphine, bretylium tosylate, and spinal anesthesia. Large doses of diuretics can also cause orthostatic hypotension.

◆ ***Treatments.*** Orthostatic hypotension is commonly associated with prolonged bed rest (24 hours or longer). It may also result from sympathectomy, which disrupts normal vasoconstrictive mechanisms.

SPECIAL CONSIDERATIONS

Monitor the patient's fluid balance by carefully recording his intake and output and weighing him daily. To help minimize orthostatic hypotension, advise the patient to change his position gradually. (See *Performing preambulation exercises*, page 505.) Elevate the head of the patient's bed, and help him to a sitting position with his feet dangling over the side of the bed. If he can tolerate this position, have him sit in a chair for brief periods. Immediately return him to bed if he becomes dizzy or pale, or displays other signs of hypotension.

Always keep the patient's safety in mind. Never leave him unattended while he's sitting or walking; evaluate his need for assistive devices, such as a cane or walker.

Prepare the patient for diagnostic tests, such as hematocrit, serum electrolyte and drug levels, urinalysis, 12-lead electrocardiogram, and chest X-ray.

Pediatric pointers

Because normal blood pressure is lower in children than in adults, familiarize yourself with normal age-specific values to detect orthostatic hypotension. From birth to age 3 months, normal systolic pressure is 40 to 80 mm Hg; from age 3 months to 1 year, 80 to 100 mm Hg; and from ages 1 to 12, 100 mm Hg plus 2 mm Hg for every year over age 1. Diastolic blood pressure is first heard at about age 4; it's normally 60 mm Hg at this age and gradually increases to 70 mm Hg by age 12.

The causes of orthostatic hypotension in children may be the same as those in adults.

Geriatric pointers

Elderly patients commonly experience autonomic dysfunction, which can present as orthostatic hypotension. Postprandial hypotension occurs 45 to 60 minutes after a meal and has been documented in up to one-third of nursing home residents.

Patient counseling

Patients with conditions that can lead to autonomic dysfunction should be made aware of the acute drop in blood pressure than can occur with positional changes. This is particularly important in diabetic patients. Once the problem appears, such patients need to avoid volume depletion and perform positional changes gradually instead of suddenly.

Ortolani's sign

Ortolani's sign—a click, clunk, or popping sensation that's felt and often heard when a neonate's hip is flexed 90 degrees and abducted—is an indication of developmental dysplasia of the hip (DDH); it results when the femoral head enters or exits the acetabulum. Screening for this sign is an important part of neonate care because early detection and treatment of developmental dysplasia of the hip improves the infant's chances of growing with a correctly formed, functional joint. (See *Detecting developmental dysplasia of the hip*, pages 506 and 507.)

History and physical examination

During assessment for Ortolani's sign, the infant should be relaxed and lying supine. After eliciting Ortolani's sign, evaluate the infant for asymmetrical gluteal folds, limited hip abduction, and unequal leg length.

Medical causes

◆ ***DDH.***

GENDER CUE *Most common in females, DDH produces Ortolani's sign, which may be accompanied by limited hip abduction and unequal gluteal folds. Usually, the infant with DDH has no gross deformity or pain.*

With complete dysplasia, the affected leg may appear shorter, or the affected hip may appear more prominent.

CULTURAL CUE *A strong relationship between hip dysplasia and methods of handling the infant has been demonstrated. For instance, Inuit and Navajo Indians have a high incidence of DDH, which may be related to their practice of wrapping neonates in blankets or strapping them to cradleboards. In cultures where mothers carry infants on their backs or hips, such as in the Far East and Africa, hip dysplasia is rarely seen.*

Special considerations

Ortolani's sign can be elicited only during the first 4 to 6 weeks of life; this is also the optimum time for effective corrective treatment. If treatment is delayed, DDH may cause degenerative hip changes, lordosis, joint malformation, and soft-tissue damage. Various methods of abduction can be used to produce a stable joint. These methods include use of soft splinting devices and a plaster hip spica cast.

Osler's nodes

Osler's nodes are tender, raised, pea-size, red or purple lesions that erupt on the palms, soles, and especially the pads of the fingers and toes. They're a rare but reliable sign of infective endocarditis, and are pathognomonic of the subacute form. However, the nodes usually develop after other telling signs and symptoms and disappear spontaneously within several days. How and why they develop is uncertain; they may result from bacterial emboli caught in peripheral capillaries, or they may reflect an immunologic reaction to the causative organism. Osler's nodes must be distinguished from the even less common Janeway's lesions—small, painless, erythematous lesions that erupt on the palms and soles.

History and physical examination

If you discover Osler's nodes, explore the patient's history for clues to the cause of infective endocarditis. Has the patient had recent surgery or dental work? Invasive procedures of the urinary or gynecologic tract? Does he have a prosthetic valve or an arteriovenous fistula for hemodialysis? Note any history of cardiac disorders and murmurs, or recent upper respiratory, skin, or urinary tract infection. Also, find out if the patient has been using intravenous drugs. Then explore associated complaints, such as chills, fatigue, anorexia, and night sweats.

After taking the patient's vital signs, auscultate the heart for murmurs and gallops and the lungs for crackles. Inspect the skin and mucous membranes for petechiae and other lesions. If you suspect intravenous drug abuse, inspect the patient's arms and other areas for needle tracks.

Medical causes

◆ ***Acute infective endocarditis.*** This type of endocarditis may produce Osler's nodes. Among its more classic features are acute onset of high, intermittent fever with chills and signs of heart failure, such as dyspnea, peripheral edema, and distended jugular veins. Janeway's lesions and Roth's spots are more common in this form than in the subacute form; petechiae may also occur.

Embolization may abruptly occur, causing organ infarction or peripheral vascular occlusion with hematuria, chest or limb pain, paralysis, blindness, and other diverse effects.

◆ ***Subacute infective endocarditis.*** Osler's nodes are pathognomonic of this form of endocarditis. A suddenly changing murmur or the discovery of a new murmur is another cardinal sign. Associated signs and symptoms include intermittent fever, pallor, weakness, fatigue, arthralgia, night sweats, tachycardia, anorexia and weight loss, splenomegaly, clubbing, and petechiae. Occasionally, Janeway's lesions, subungual splinter hemorrhages, and Roth's spots also appear. Signs of heart failure may occur with extensive valvular damage.

Embolization may develop, producing signs and symptoms that vary depending on the location of the emboli.

Special considerations

Monitor the patient's vital signs to evaluate the effectiveness of antibiotic therapy against infective endocarditis. Later, discuss measures to prevent reinfection such as prophylactic antibiotic administration before dental or invasive procedures.

Prepare the patient for blood studies such as a complete blood count and procedures such as an electrocardiogram and echocardiogram.

Pediatric pointers

In children, Osler's nodes may result from infective endocarditis associated with congenital heart defects or rheumatic fever.

Otorrhea

Otorrhea—drainage from the ear—may be bloody (otorrhagia), purulent, clear, or serosanguineous. Its onset, duration, and severity provide clues to the underlying cause. This sign may result from disorders that affect the external ear canal or the middle ear, including allergy, infection, neoplasms, trauma, and collagen diseases. Otorrhea may occur alone or with other symptoms such as ear pain.

History and physical examination

Begin your evaluation by asking the patient when the otorrhea began, noting how he recognized it. Did he clean the drainage from deep within the ear canal, or did he wipe it from the auricle? Have him describe the color, consistency, and odor of the drainage. Is it clear, purulent, or bloody? Does it occur in one or both ears? Is it continuous or intermittent? If the patient wears cotton in his ear to absorb the drainage, ask how often he changes it.

Then explore associated otologic symptoms, especially pain. Is there tenderness on movement of the pinna or tragus? Ask about vertigo, which is absent in disorders of the external ear canal. Also ask about tinnitus.

Next, check the patient's medical history for recent upper respiratory infection or head trauma. Also, ask how he cleans his ears and if he's an avid swimmer. Note a history of cancer, dermatitis, or immunosuppressant therapy.

Focus the physical examination on the patient's external ear, middle ear, and tympanic membrane. (If his symptoms are unilateral, examine the uninvolved ear first as not to cross-contaminate.) Inspect the external ear, and apply pressure on the tragus and mastoid area to elicit tenderness. Then insert an otoscope, using the largest speculum that will comfortably fit into the ear canal. If necessary, clean cerumen, pus, or other debris from the canal. Observe for edema, erythema, crusts, or polyps. Inspect the tympanic membrane, which should look like a shiny, pearl-gray cone. Note color changes, perforation, absence of the normal light reflex (a cone of light appearing toward the bottom of the drum), or a bulging membrane.

Next, test hearing acuity. Have the patient occlude one ear while you whisper some common two-syllable words toward the unoccluded ear. Stand behind him so he doesn't read your lips, and ask him to repeat what he heard. Perform the test on the other ear using different words. Then use a tuning fork to perform the Weber and Rinne tests. (*See Differentiating conductive from sensorineural hearing loss,* page 350.)

Complete your assessment by palpating the patient's neck and his preauricular, parotid, and postauricular (mastoid) areas for lymphadenopathy. Also, test the function of cranial nerves VII, IX, X, and XI.

Medical causes

◆ ***Allergy.*** An allergy associated with tympanic membrane perforation may cause clear or cloudy otorrhea, rhinorrhea, and itchy, watery eyes.

◆ ***Aural polyps.*** These polyps may produce foul, purulent, and perhaps blood-streaked discharge. If they occlude the external ear canal, the polyps may cause partial hearing loss.

◆ ***Basilar skull fracture.*** With this disorder, otorrhea may be clear and watery and positive for glucose representing cerebrospinal fluid (CSF) leakage, or bloody, representing hemorrhage. Occasionally, inspection reveals blood behind the eardrum. The otorrhea may be accompanied by hearing loss, CSF or bloody rhinorrhea, periorbital ecchymosis (raccoon eyes), and mastoid ecchymosis (Battle's sign). Cranial nerve palsies, decreased level of consciousness, and headache are other common findings.

◆ ***Dermatitis of the external ear canal.*** With contact dermatitis, vesicles produce clear, watery otorrhea with edema and erythema of the external ear canal.

Infectious eczematoid dermatitis causes purulent otorrhea with erythema and crusting of the external ear canal.

With seborrheic dermatitis, otorrhea consists of greasy scales and flakes. The scalp, forehead, and cheeks are also marked by pruritic, scaly lesions.

◆ ***Epidural abscess.*** In this disorder, profuse, creamy otorrhea is accompanied by steady, throbbing ear pain; fever; and temporal or temporoparietal headache on the ipsilateral side.

◆ ***Mastoiditis.*** This disorder causes thick, purulent, yellow otorrhea that becomes increasingly profuse. Its cardinal features include low-grade fever and dull aching and tenderness in the mastoid area. Postauricular erythema and edema may push the auricle out from the head; pressure within the edematous mastoid antrum may produce swelling and obstruction of the external ear canal, causing conductive hearing loss.

◆ ***Myringitis (infectious).*** With acute infectious myringitis, small, reddened, blood-filled blebs erupt in the external ear canal, the tympanic membrane, and occasionally, the middle ear. Spontaneous rupture of these blebs causes serosanguineous otorrhea. Other features include severe ear pain, tenderness over the mastoid process, and rarely, fever and hearing loss.

Chronic infectious myringitis causes purulent otorrhea, pruritus, and gradual hearing loss.

◆ ***Otitis externa.*** Acute otitis externa, commonly known as swimmer's ear, usually causes purulent, yellow, sticky, foul-smelling otorrhea. Inspection may reveal white-green debris in the external ear canal. Associated findings include edema, erythema, pain, and itching of the auricle and external ear canal; severe tenderness with movement of the mastoid, tragus, mouth, or jaw; tenderness and swelling of surrounding nodes; and partial conductive hearing loss. The patient may also develop a low-grade fever and a headache ipsilateral to the affected ear.

Chronic otitis externa usually causes scanty, intermittent otorrhea that may be serous or purulent and possibly foul-smelling. Its primary symptom, though, is itching. Related findings include edema and slight erythema.

Life-threatening malignant otitis externa produces debris in the ear canal, which may build up against the tympanic membrane, causing severe pain that's especially acute during manipulation of the tragus or auricle. Most common in diabetics and immunosuppressed patients, this fulminant bacterial infection may also cause pruritus, tinnitus and, possibly, unilateral hearing loss.

◆ ***Otitis media.*** With acute otitis media, rupture of the tympanic membrane produces bloody, purulent otorrhea and relieves continuous or intermittent ear pain. Typically, a conductive hearing loss worsens over several hours.

With acute suppurative otitis media, the patient may also exhibit signs and symptoms of upper respiratory infection—sore throat, cough, nasal discharge, and headache. Other features include dizziness, fever, nausea, and vomiting.

Chronic otitis media causes intermittent, purulent, foul-smelling otorrhea commonly associated with perforation of the tympanic membrane. Conductive hearing loss occurs gradually and may be accompanied by pain, nausea, and vertigo.

◆ ***Perichondritis.*** In this disorder, multiple fistulas may open on the auricle or external ear canal, causing purulent otorrhea. Typically, the auricle is edematous and erythematous, with thickened skin.

◆ ***Trauma.*** Bloody otorrhea may result from trauma, such as a blow to the external ear, a foreign body in the ear, or barotrauma. Usually, the bleeding is minimal or moderate; it may be accompanied by partial hearing loss.

◆ ***Tuberculosis.*** Pulmonary tuberculosis may spread through the upper airway to the middle ear, causing chronic ear infection. The tympanic membrane thickens, ruptures, and produces a watery otorrhea and mild hearing loss. Cervical adenopathy may also occur.

◆ ***Tumor (benign).*** A benign tumor of the glomus jugulare (jugular bulb) may cause bloody otorrhea. Initially, the patient may complain of throbbing discomfort and tinnitus that resembles the sound of his heartbeat. Associated signs and symptoms include gradually progressive stuffiness in the affected ear, vertigo, conductive hearing loss and, possibly, a reddened mass behind the tympanic membrane.

◆ ***Tumor (malignant).*** Squamous cell carcinoma of the external ear causes purulent otorrhea with itching; deep, boring ear pain; hearing loss; and, in late stages, facial paralysis.

In squamous cell carcinoma of the middle ear, blood-tinged otorrhea occurs early, typically accompanied by hearing loss on the affected side. Pain and facial paralysis are late features.

◆ ***Wegener's granulomatosis.*** This rare, necrotizing granulomatous vasculitis commonly causes perforation of the tympanic membrane and serosanguineous otorrhea. The patient may report a slowly progressive hearing loss, a cough (possibly hemoptysis), wheezing, shortness of breath, pleuritic chest pain, hemorrhagic skin lesions, epistaxis, and signs of severe sinusitis.

Special considerations

Apply warm, moist compresses, heating pads, or hot water bottles to the patient's ears to relieve inflammation and pain. Use cotton wicks to gently clean the draining ear or to apply topical drugs. Keep eardrops at room temperature; instillation of cold eardrops may cause vertigo. If the patient has impaired hearing, ensure he understands everything that's explained to him, using written messages if necessary.

Pediatric pointers

When you examine or clean a child's ear, remember that the auditory canal lies horizontally and that the pinna must be pulled downward and backward. Restrain a child during an ear procedure by having him sit on a parent's lap with the ear to be examined facing you. Have him put one arm around the parent's waist and the other down at his own side, and then ask the parent to hold the child in place. Or, if you are alone with the child, ask him to lie on his abdomen with his arms at his sides and his head turned so the affected ear faces the ceiling. Bend over him, restraining his upper body with your elbows and upper arms.

Perforation of the tympanic membrane secondary to otitis media is the most common cause of otorrhea in infants and young children. Children are also likely to insert foreign bodies into their ears, resulting in infection, pain, and purulent discharge.

Patient counseling

Advise the patient with chronic ear problems to avoid forceful nose blowing when he has an upper respiratory infection so that infected secretions are not channeled into the middle ear. Instruct him to blow his nose with his mouth open. Also, remind him to cleanse his ears with a washcloth *only,* and not to stick anything in his ear (such as a hairpin or a cotton-tipped applicator) that might cause injury. If the patient is a swimmer, instruct him to wear earplugs and to wash and dry his ears thoroughly after swimming. Have him report recurring ear pain and drainage, especially in the absence of upper respiratory infection, as this may be a sign of cancer.

Tell the patient with a ruptured tympanic membrane that such a rupture usually heals spontaneously. However, warn him to avoid immersing his head in water while it heals; tell him to insert lubricated cotton balls into his ear canal before he showers or shampoos.

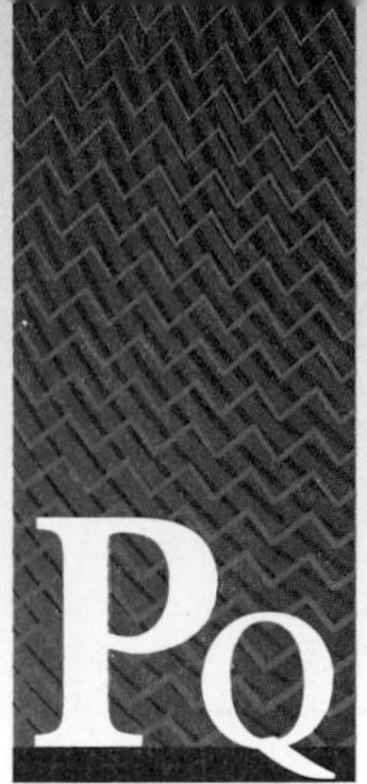

Pallor

Pallor is abnormal paleness or loss of skin color, which may develop suddenly or gradually. Although generalized pallor affects the entire body, it's most apparent on the face, conjunctiva, oral mucosa, and nail beds. Localized pallor commonly affects a single limb.

How easily pallor is detected varies with skin color and the thickness and vascularity of underlying subcutaneous tissue. At times, it's merely a subtle lightening of skin color that may be difficult to detect in dark-skinned people; sometimes it's evident only on the conjunctiva and oral mucosa.

Pallor may result from decreased peripheral oxyhemoglobin or decreased total oxyhemoglobin. The former reflects diminished peripheral blood flow associated with peripheral vasoconstriction or arterial occlusion or with low cardiac output. (Transient peripheral vasoconstriction may occur with exposure to cold, causing nonpathologic pallor.) The latter usually results from anemia, the chief cause of pallor. (See *How pallor develops*, page 514.)

EMERGENCY INTERVENTIONS *If generalized pallor suddenly develops, quickly look for signs of shock, such as tachycardia, hypotension, oliguria, and decreased level of consciousness. Prepare to rapidly infuse fluids or blood. Keep emergency resuscitation equipment nearby.*

History and physical examination

If the patient's condition permits, take a complete history. Does the patient or anyone in his family have a history of anemia or of a chronic disorder that might lead to pallor, such as renal failure, heart failure, or diabetes? Ask about the patient's diet, particularly his intake of green vegetables.

Explore the pallor more fully. Find out when the patient first noticed it. Is pallor constant or intermittent? Does it occur when he's exposed to the cold? Does it occur when he's under emotional stress? Explore associated signs and symptoms, such as dizziness, fainting, orthostasis, weakness and fatigue on exertion, dyspnea, chest pain, palpitations, menstrual irregularities, or loss of libido. If the pallor is confined to one or both legs, ask the patient if walking is painful. Do his legs feel cold or numb? If the pallor is confined to his fingers, ask about tingling and numbness.

Start the physical examination by taking the patient's vital signs. Be sure to check for orthostatic hypotension. Auscultate the heart for gallops and murmurs and the lungs for crackles. Check the patient's skin temperature—cold extremities commonly occur with vasoconstriction or arterial occlusion. Note skin ulceration. Examine the abdomen for splenomegaly. Palpate peripheral pulses. An absent pulse in a pale extremity may indicate arterial occlusion, whereas a weak pulse may indicate low cardiac output.

How pallor develops

Pallor may result from decreased peripheral oxyhemoglobin or decreased total oxyhemoglobin. The chart below illustrates the progression to pallor.

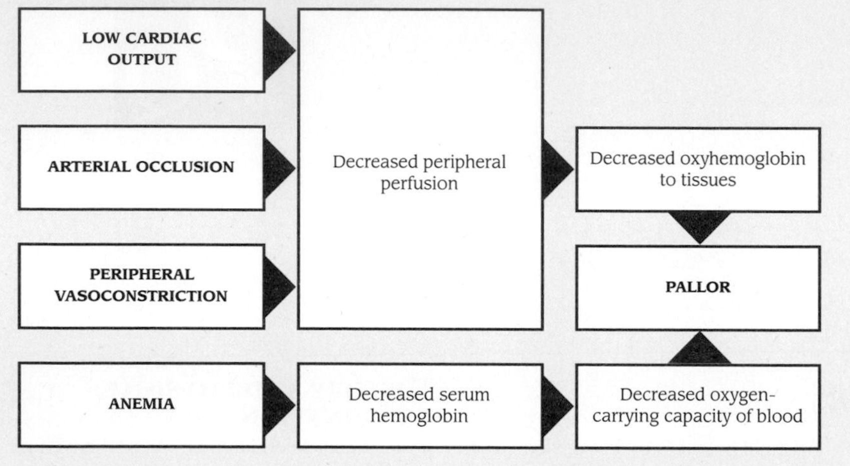

MEDICAL CAUSES

◆ ***Anemia.*** Typically, pallor develops gradually with this disorder. The patient's skin may also appear sallow or grayish. Other effects include fatigue, dyspnea, tachycardia, bounding pulse, atrial gallop, systolic bruit over the carotid arteries and, possibly, crackles and bleeding tendencies.

◆ ***Arterial occlusion (acute).*** Pallor develops abruptly in the extremity with the occlusion, which usually results from an embolus. A line of demarcation develops, separating the cool, pale, cyanotic, and mottled skin below the occlusion from the normal skin above it. Accompanying the pallor may be severe pain, intense intermittent claudication, paresthesia, and paresis in the affected extremity. Absent pulses and increased capillary refill time below the occlusion are also characteristic.

◆ ***Arterial occlusive disease (chronic).*** With this disorder, pallor is specific to an extremity—usually one leg, but occasionally, both legs or an arm. It develops gradually from obstructive arteriosclerosis or a thrombus and is aggravated by elevating the extremity. Associated findings include intermittent claudication, weakness, cool skin, diminished pulses in the extremity and, possibly, ulceration and gangrene.

◆ ***Cardiac arrhythmias.*** Cardiac arrhythmias that seriously reduce cardiac output, such as complete heart block and attacks of tachyarrhythmia, may cause acute onset of pallor. Other features include irregular, rapid, or slow pulse; dizziness; weakness and fatigue; hypotension; confusion; palpitations; diaphoresis; oliguria; and, possibly, loss of consciousness.

◆ ***Frostbite.*** Pallor is localized to the frostbitten area, such as the feet, hands, or ears. Typically, the area feels cold, waxy and, perhaps, hard in deep frostbite. The skin doesn't blanch and sensation may be absent. As the area thaws, the skin turns purplish blue. Blistering and gangrene may then follow if the frostbite was severe.

◆ ***Orthostatic hypotension.*** With this condition, pallor occurs abruptly on rising from a recumbent position to a sitting or standing position. A precipitous drop in blood pressure, an increase in heart rate, and dizziness are also characteristic. At times, the patient loses consciousness for several minutes.

◆ ***Raynaud's disease.*** Pallor of the fingers upon exposure to cold or stress is a hallmark of this vascular disease. Typically, the fingers abruptly turn pale, then cyanotic; with rewarming, they become red and paresthetic. With chronic disease, ulceration may occur.

◆ ***Shock.*** Two forms of shock initially cause acute onset of pallor and cool, clammy skin. With hypovolemic shock, other early signs and symptoms include restlessness, thirst, slight tachycardia, and tachypnea. As shock progresses, the skin becomes increasingly clammy, pulse becomes more rapid and thready, and hypotension develops with narrowing pulse pressure. Other signs and symptoms include oliguria, subnormal body temperature, and decreased level of consciousness. With cardiogenic shock, the signs and symptoms are similar, but usually more profound.

◆ ***Vasopressor syncope.*** Sudden onset of pallor immediately precedes or accompanies loss of consciousness during syncopal attacks. These common fainting spells may be triggered by emotional stress or pain and usually last only a few seconds or minutes. Before loss of consciousness, the patient may exhibit diaphoresis, nausea, yawning, hyperpnea, weakness, confusion, tachycardia, and dim vision. He then develops bradycardia, hypotension, a few clonic jerks, and dilated pupils with loss of consciousness.

Special considerations

If the patient has chronic generalized pallor, prepare him for blood studies and, possibly, bone marrow biopsy. If the patient has localized pallor, he may require arteriography or other diagnostic studies to accurately determine the cause.

When pallor results from low cardiac output, administer blood and fluids and as well as a diuretic, a cardiotonic, and an antiarrhythmic, as needed. Frequently monitor the patient's vital signs, intake and output, electrocardiogram results, and hemodynamic status.

Pediatric pointers

In children, pallor stems from the same causes as it does in adults. It can also stem from a congenital heart defect or chronic lung disease.

Palpitations

Defined as a conscious awareness of one's heartbeat, palpitations are usually felt over the precordium or in the throat or neck. The patient may describe them as pounding, jumping, turning, fluttering, or flopping, or as missing or skipping beats. Palpitations may be regular or irregular, fast or slow, paroxysmal or sustained.

Although usually insignificant, palpitations may result from a cardiac or metabolic disorder and from the effects of certain drugs. Nonpathologic palpitations may occur with a newly implanted prosthetic valve because the valve's clicking sound heightens the patient's awareness of his heartbeat. Transient palpitations may accompany emotional stress (such as fright, anger, or anxiety) or physical stress (such as exercise and fever). They can also accompany use of stimulants, such as tobacco and caffeine.

To help characterize the palpitations, ask the patient to simulate their rhythm by tapping his finger on a hard surface. An irregular "skipped beat" rhythm points to premature ventricular contractions, whereas an episodic racing rhythm that begins and ends abruptly suggests paroxysmal atrial tachycardia.

EMERGENCY INTERVENTIONS *If the patient complains of palpitations, ask him about dizziness and shortness of breath. Inspect for pale, cool, clammy skin. Take the patient's vital signs, noting hypotension and irregular or abnormal pulse. If these signs are present, suspect cardiac arrhythmia. Prepare to begin cardiac monitoring and, if necessary, synchronized cardioversion. Start an I.V. catheter to administer an antiarrhythmic, if needed.*

History and physical examination

If the patient isn't in distress, perform a complete cardiac history and physical examination. Ask if he has a cardiovascular or pulmonary disorder, which may produce arrhythmias. Does the patient have a history of hypertension or hypoglycemia? Be sure to obtain a drug history. Has the patient recently started cardiac glycoside therapy? Ask about caffeine, tobacco, and alcohol consumption.

Explore associated symptoms, such as weakness, fatigue, and angina. Auscultate for gallops, murmurs, and abnormal breath sounds.

Medical causes

◆ ***Anemia.*** Palpitations may occur with anemia, especially on exertion. Pallor, fatigue, and dyspnea are also common. Associated signs include a systolic ejection murmur, bounding pulse, tachycardia, crackles, an atrial gallop, and a systolic bruit over the carotid arteries.

◆ ***Anxiety attack (acute).*** Anxiety is the most common cause of palpitations in children and adults. With this disorder, palpitations may be accompanied by diaphoresis, facial flushing, trembling, and an impending sense of doom. Almost invariably, the patient hyperventilates, which may lead to dizziness, weakness, and syncope. Other typical findings include tachycardia, precordial pain, shortness of breath, restlessness, and insomnia.

◆ ***Cardiac arrhythmias.*** Paroxysmal or sustained palpitations may be accompanied by dizziness, weakness, and fatigue. The patient may also experience an irregular, rapid, or slow pulse rate; decreased blood pressure; confusion; pallor; oliguria; and diaphoresis.

◆ ***Hypertension.*** With this disorder, the patient may be asymptomatic or may complain of sustained palpitations alone or with headache, dizziness, tinnitus, and fatigue. His blood pressure typically exceeds 140/90 mm Hg. He may also experience nausea and vomiting, seizures, and decreased level of consciousness (LOC).

◆ ***Hypocalcemia.*** Typically, this disorder produces palpitations, weakness, and fatigue. It progresses from paresthesia to muscle tension and carpopedal spasms. The patient may also exhibit muscle twitching, hyperactive deep tendon reflexes, chorea, and positive Chvostek's and Trousseau's signs.

◆ ***Hypoglycemia.*** When blood glucose levels drop significantly, the sympathetic nervous system triggers adrenaline production. This may cause sustained palpitations, which may be accompanied by fatigue, irritability, hunger, cold sweats, tremors, tachycardia, anxiety, and headache. Eventually the patient may develop central nervous system reactions. These include blurred or double vision, muscle weakness, hemiplegia, and altered LOC.

◆ ***Mitral prolapse.*** This valvular disorder may cause paroxysmal palpitations accompanied by sharp, stabbing, or aching precordial pain. The hallmark of this disorder is a midsystolic click followed by an apical systolic murmur. Associated signs and symptoms may include dyspnea, dizziness, severe fatigue, migraine headache, anxiety, paroxysmal tachycardia, crackles, and peripheral edema.

◆ ***Mitral stenosis.*** Early features of this valvular disorder typically include sustained palpitations accompanied by exertional dyspnea and fatigue. Auscultation also reveals a loud S_1 or opening snap, and a rumbling diastolic murmur at the apex. Patients may also experience related signs and symptoms, such as an atrial gallop and, with advanced mitral stenosis, orthopnea, dyspnea at rest, paroxysmal nocturnal dyspnea, peripheral edema, jugular vein distention, ascites, hepatomegaly, and atrial fibrillations.

◆ ***Pheochromocytoma.*** This rare adrenal medulla tumor causes episodic hypermetabolism, commonly associated with paroxysmal palpitations. The cardinal sign of pheochromocytoma is dramatically elevated blood pressure, which may be sustained or paroxysmal. Associated signs and symptoms include tachycardia, headache, chest or abdominal pain, diaphoresis, warm and pale or flushed skin, paresthesia, tremors, insomnia, nausea and vomiting, and anxiety.

◆ ***Sick sinus syndrome.*** A patient with this disorder may experience palpitations, as well as bradycardia, tachycardia, chest pain, syncope, and heart failure.

◆ ***Thyrotoxicosis.*** A characteristic symptom of this disorder, sustained palpitations may be accompanied by tachycardia, dyspnea, weight loss despite increased appetite, diarrhea, tremors, nervousness, diaphoresis, heat intolerance and, possibly, exophthalmos and an enlarged thyroid. The patient may also experience an atrial or ventricular gallop.

◆ ***Wolff-Parkinson-White syndrome.*** Seen in children and adolescents, this disorder results in recurrent palpitations and frequent episodes of paroxysmal tachycardia.

OTHER CAUSES

◆ ***Drugs.*** Palpitations may result from drugs that precipitate cardiac arrhythmias or increase cardiac output, such as cardiac glycosides; sympathomimetics such as cocaine; ganglionic blockers; beta-adrenergic blockers; calcium channel blockers; atropine; and minoxidil.

◆ ***Exercise.*** Exercise can normally cause palpitations, as well as in patients with coronary heart disease, hypertension, mitral valve prolapse, and cardiomegaly.

HERB ALERT *Herbal remedies, such as ginseng and ephedra (ma huang), may cause adverse reactions, including palpitations and an irregular heartbeat. (Note: The FDA has banned the sale of dietary supplements containing ephedra because they pose an unreasonable risk of injury or illness).*

SPECIAL CONSIDERATIONS

Prepare the patient for diagnostic tests, such as an electrocardiogram and Holter monitoring. Remember that even mild palpitations can cause the patient much concern. Maintain a quiet, comfortable environment to minimize anxiety and perhaps decrease palpitations.

PEDIATRIC POINTERS

Palpitations in children commonly result from fever and congenital heart defects, such as patent ductus arteriosus and septal defects. Because many children can't describe this complaint, focus your attention on objective measurements, such as cardiac monitoring, physical examination, and laboratory tests.

Papular rash

A papular rash consists of small, raised, circumscribed—and perhaps discolored (red to purple)—lesions known as papules. It may erupt anywhere on the body in various configurations and may be acute or chronic. Papular rashes characterize many cutaneous disorders; they may also result from allergy and from infectious, neoplastic, and systemic disorders. (To compare papules with other skin lesions, see *Recognizing common skin lesions*, pages 518 and 519.)

HISTORY AND PHYSICAL EXAMINATION

Your first step is to fully evaluate the papular rash: Note its color, configuration, and location on the patient's body. Find out when it erupted. Has the patient noticed any changes in the rash since then? Is it itchy or burning, or painful or tender? Have him describe associated signs and symptoms, such as fever, headache, and GI distress.

Next, obtain a medical history, including allergies, previous rashes or skin disorders, infections, childhood diseases, sexual history, including any sexually transmitted diseases (STDs), and cancers. Has the patient recently been bitten by an insect or rodent or been exposed to anyone with an infectious disease? Finally, obtain a complete drug history.

MEDICAL CAUSES

◆ ***Acne vulgaris.*** With this disorder, rupture of enlarged comedones produces inflamed—and perhaps, painful and pruritic—papules, pustules, nodules, or cysts on the face and sometimes the shoulders, chest, and back.

◆ ***Anthrax (cutaneous).*** Anthrax is an acute infectious disease caused by the gram-positive, spore-forming bacterium *Bacillus anthracis.* The disease can occur in humans exposed to infected animals, tissue from infected animals, or biological warfare. Cutaneous anthrax occurs when the bacterium enters a cut or abrasion on the skin. The infection begins as a small, painless, or pruritic macular or papular lesion resembling an insect bite. Within 1 to 2 days it develops into a vesicle and then a painless ulcer with a characteristic black, necrotic center. Lymphadenopathy, malaise, headache, or fever may develop.

◆ ***Dermatitis (perioral).*** This inflammatory disorder causes an erythematous eruption of discrete, tiny papules and pustules on the nasolabial fold, chin, and upper lip area. The lesions may be pruritic and painful.

◆ ***Dermatomyositis.*** Gottron's papules—flat, violet-colored lesions on the dorsa of the finger joints and the nape of the neck and shoulders—are pathognomonic of this disorder, as is the dusky lilac discoloration of periorbital tissue and lid margins (heliotrope edema). These signs may be accompanied by a transient, erythematous, macular rash in a malar distribution on the face and sometimes on the scalp, forehead, neck, upper torso, and arms. This rash may be preceded by symmetrical muscle soreness and weakness in the pelvis, upper extremities, shoulders, neck and, possibly, the face (polymyositis).

◆ ***Erythema migrans.*** Transmitted through a tick bite, this systemic disorder is characterized by a papular or macular rash starting from a single lesion (usually on the leg) that spreads at the margins while clearing centrally. The rash commonly appears on the thighs, trunk, or upper arms and is the classic early sign of Lyme disease, but about 25% of patients don't develop this skin manifestation. It may be accompanied by fever, chills, headache, malaise, nausea, vomiting, fatigue, backache, knee pain, and stiff neck.

◆ ***Follicular mucinosis.*** With this cutaneous disorder, perifollicular papules or plaques are accompanied by prominent alopecia.

◆ ***Fox-Fordyce disease.*** This chronic disorder is marked by pruritic papules on the axillae, pubic area, and areolae associated with apocrine sweat gland inflammation. Sparse hair growth in these areas is also common.

◆ ***Gonococcemia.*** With this chronic STD, sporadic eruption of an erythematous macular rash is characteristic, although fistulas and petechiae may appear. The rash typically affects the distal extremities (palms and soles) and rapidly becomes maculopapular, vesiculopustular and, commonly, hemorrhagic. Bullae may form. The mature lesion is raised; has a gray, necrotic center; and is surrounded by erythema. Typically, it

Recognizing common skin lesions

MACULE

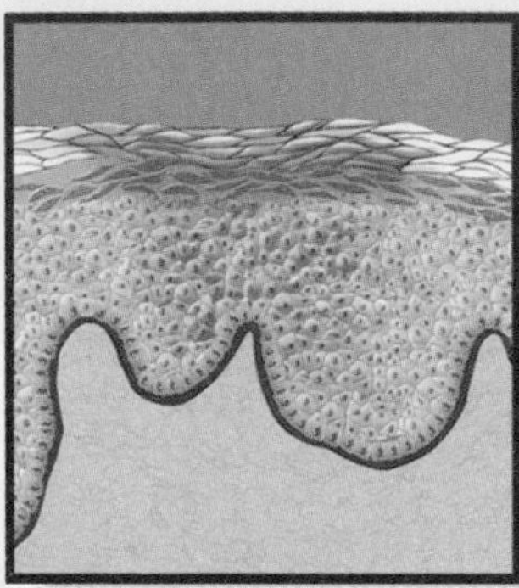

A small (usually less than 1 cm in diameter), flat blemish or discoloration that can be brown, tan, red, or white and has same texture as surrounding skin

VESICLE

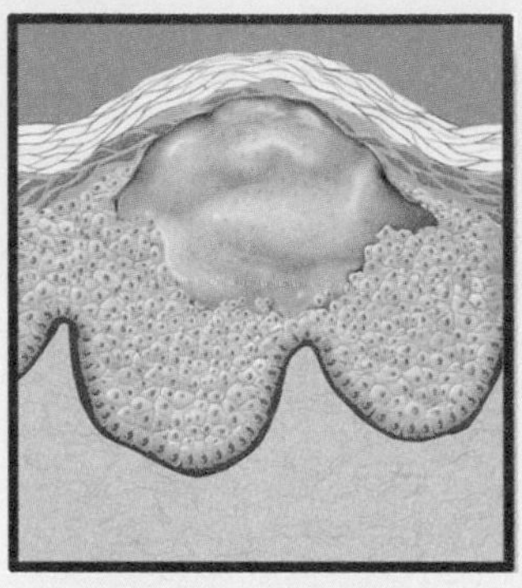

A small (less than 0.5 cm in diameter), thin-walled, raised blister containing clear, serous, purulent, or bloody fluid

BULLA

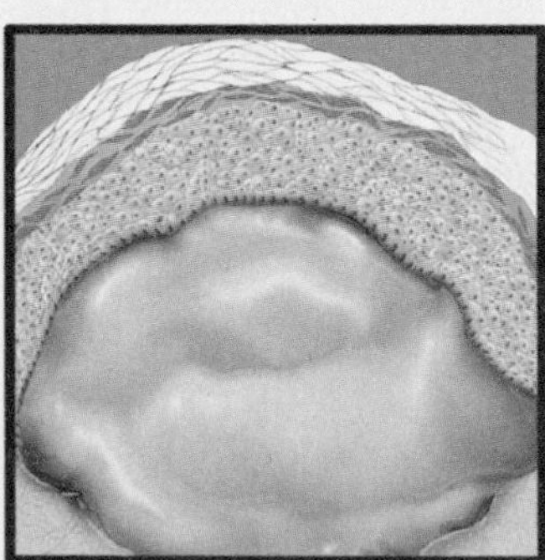

A raised, thin-walled blister greater than 0.5 cm in diameter, containing clear or serous fluid

PUSTULE

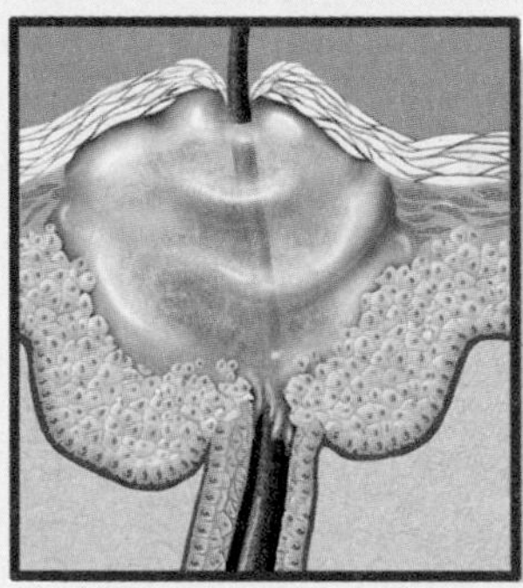

A circumscribed, pus- or lymph-filled, elevated lesion that varies in diameter and may be firm or soft, and white or yellow

heals in 3 to 4 days. Eruptions are commonly accompanied by fever and joint pain.

◆ ***Granuloma annulare.*** This benign, chronic disorder produces papules that usually coalesce to form plaques. The papules spread peripherally to form a ring with a normal or slightly depressed center. They usually appear on the feet, legs, hands, or fingers, and may be pruritic or asymptomatic.

◆ ***Human immunodeficiency virus (HIV) infection.*** Acute infection with the HIV retrovirus typically causes a generalized maculopapular rash. Other signs and symptoms include fever, malaise, sore throat, and headache. Lymphadenopathy and hepatosplenomegaly may also occur. Most patients don't recall these symptoms of acute infection.

◆ ***Insect bites.*** Salivary secretions from insect bites—especially ticks, lice, flies, and mosquitoes—may produce an allergic reaction associated with a papular, macular, or petechial rash. The rash is usually accompanied by nonspecific signs and symptoms, such as fever, myalgia, headache, lymphadenopathy, nausea, and vomiting.

◆ ***Kaposi's sarcoma.*** This neoplastic disorder is characterized by purple or blue papules or macules of vascular origin on the skin, mucous membranes, and viscera. These lesions

WHEAL

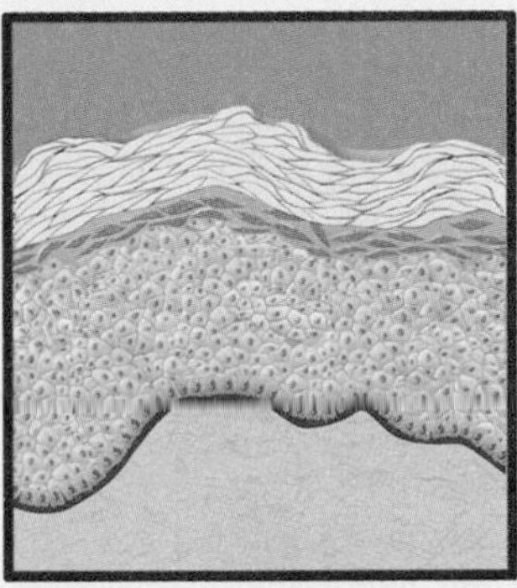

A slightly raised, firm lesion of variable size and shape, surrounded by edema; skin may be red or pale

PAPULE

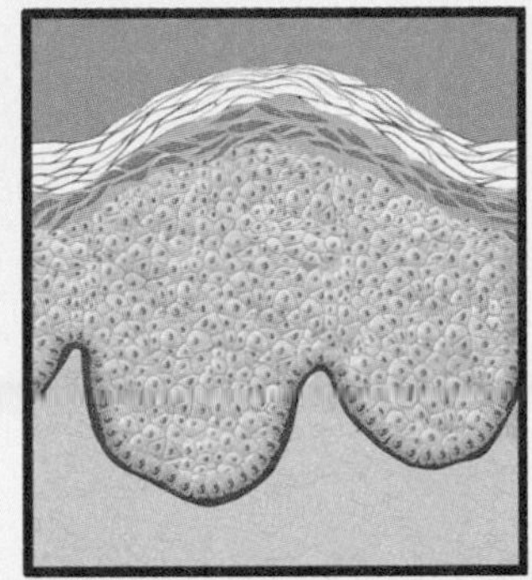

A small, solid, raised lesion less than 1 cm in diameter, with red to purple skin discoloration

NODULE

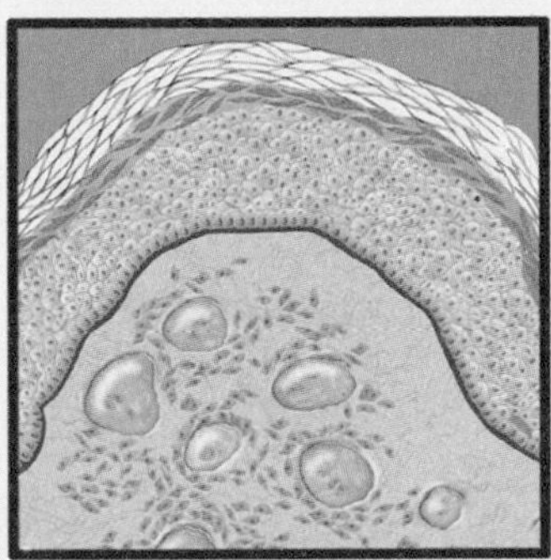

A small, firm, circumscribed, elevated lesion 1 to 2 cm in diameter with possible skin discoloration

TUMOR

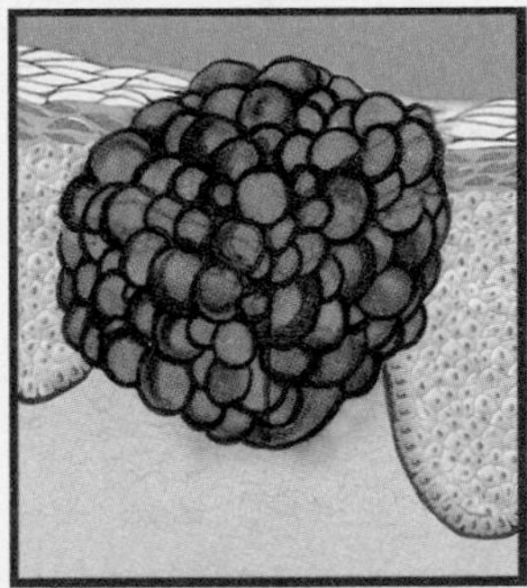

A solid, raised mass usually larger than 2 cm in diameter with possible skin discoloration

decrease in size with firm pressure and then return to their original size within 10 to 15 seconds. They may become scaly and ulcerate with bleeding.

Multiple variants of Kaposi's sarcoma are known; most individuals are immunocompromised in some way, especially those with HIV/AIDS (acquired immunodeficiency syndrome). Human herpes virus-8 (HHV-8) has been strongly implicated as a cofactor in the development of Kaposi's sarcoma.

◆ ***Leprosy.*** This chronic infectious disorder produces various skin lesions. Early papular or macular lesions are erythematous, hypopigmented, and symmetrical (with lepromatous leprosy) or asymmetrical (with tuberculoid leprosy). The lesions may spread over the entire skin surface. Later, plaques and nodules form, especially on the ear lobes, nose, eyebrows, and forehead. Associated findings include hypoesthesia or anesthesia, anhidrosis, and dry, scaly skin in affected areas; enlarged, palpable peripheral nerves with severe neuralgia; and muscle atrophy and contractures.

◆ ***Lichen amyloidosis.*** This idiopathic cutaneous disorder produces discrete, firm, hemispherical, pruritic papules on the anterior tibiae. Papules may be brown or yellow, smooth or scaly.

◆ ***Lichen planus.*** Discrete, flat, angular or polygonal, violet papules, commonly marked with white lines or spots, are characteristic of this disorder. The papules may be linear or coalesce into plaques and usually appear on the lumbar region, genitalia, ankles, anterior tibiae, and wrists. Lesions usually develop first on the buccal mucosa as a lacy network of white or gray threadlike papules or plaques. Pruritus, distorted fingernails, and atrophic alopecia commonly occur.

◆ ***Monkeypox.*** Usually preceded 1 to 3 days by a fever, a papular rash is a characteristic sign of monkeypox. The rash is often blisterlike and can follow these stages: vesiculation, postulation, umbilication, and crusting. Frequently beginning on the face and spreading to the trunk and extremities, the rash may be either localized or generalized. Other accompanying symptoms in humans include lymphadenopathy, chills, throat pain, and muscle aches. Most humans recover within 2 to 4 weeks.

◆ ***Mononucleosis (infectious).*** A maculopapular rash that resembles rubella is an early sign of this infection in 10% of patients. The rash is typically preceded by headache, malaise, and fatigue. It may be accompanied by sore throat, cervical lymphadenopathy, and fluctuating temperature with an evening peak of 101° to 102° F (38.3° to 38.9° C). Splenomegaly and hepatomegaly may also develop.

◆ ***Mycosis fungoides.*** Stage I (premycotic stage) of this rare, cutaneous T-cell lymphoma is marked by the eruption of erythematous, pruritic macules on the trunk and extremities. In stage II, these lesions coalesce into pruritic papules and plaques, and nodes become irregular. Stage III is evidenced by large, irregular, brown to red tumors that ulcerate and are painful and itchy.

◆ ***Necrotizing vasculitis.*** With this systemic disorder, crops of purpuric, but otherwise asymptomatic, papules are typical. Some patients also develop low-grade fever, headache, myalgia, arthralgia, and abdominal pain.

◆ ***Parapsoriasis (chronic).*** This disorder mimics psoriasis, producing small to moderately sized asymptomatic papules with a thin, adherent scale, primarily on the trunk, hands, and feet.

◆ ***Pityriasis rosea.*** This disorder begins with an erythematous "herald patch"—a slightly raised, oval lesion about 2 to 6 cm in diameter that may appear anywhere on the body. A few days to weeks later, yellow to tan or erythematous patches with scaly edges appear on the trunk, arms, and legs, commonly erupting along body cleavage lines in a characteristic "pine tree" pattern. These patches may be asymptomatic or slightly pruritic, are 0.5 to 1 cm in diameter, and typically improve with moderate skin exposure to sunlight. This treatment should be used cautiously, however, to avoid sunburn.

◆ ***Pityriasis rubra pilaris.*** This rare chronic disorder initially produces scaling seborrhea on the scalp that spreads to the face and ears. Scaly red patches then develop on the palms and soles; these patches thicken, become keratotic, and may develop painful fissures. Later, follicular papules erupt on the hands and forearms and then spread over wide areas of the trunk, neck, and extremities. These papules coalesce into large, scaly, erythematous plaques. Striated fingernails may appear.

◆ ***Polymorphic light eruption.*** Abnormal reactions to light may produce papular, vesicular, or nodular rashes on sun-exposed areas. Other symptoms include pruritus, headache, and malaise.

◆ ***Psoriasis.*** This common chronic disorder begins with small, erythematous papules on the scalp, chest, elbows, knees, back, buttocks, and genitalia. These papules are sometimes pruritic and painful. Eventually they enlarge and coalesce, forming elevated, red, scaly plaques covered by characteristic silver scales, except in moist areas such as the genitalia. These scales may flake off easily or thicken, covering the plaque. Associated features include pitted fingernails and arthralgia.

◆ ***Rat bite fever.*** A maculopapular or petechial rash develops on the palms and soles several weeks after a bite from an infected rodent. Other findings typically include pain, redness, and swelling at the bite site; tender regional lymph nodes; fever with chills; malaise; headache; and myalgia.

◆ ***Rosacea.*** This hyperemic disorder is characterized by persistent erythema, telangiectasia, and recurrent eruption of papules and pustules on the forehead, malar areas, nose, and chin. Eventually, eruptions occur more frequently and erythema deepens. Rhinophyma may occur in severe cases.

◆ ***Sarcoidosis.*** This multisystem granulomatous disorder may produce crops of small, erythematous or yellow-brown papules around the eyes and mouth and on the nose, nasal mucosa, and upper back. Associated findings include dyspnea with a nonproductive cough, fatigue, arthralgia, weight loss, lymphadenopathy, vision loss, and dysphagia.

◆ ***Seborrheic keratosis.*** With this cutaneous disorder, benign skin tumors begin as small, yellow-brown papules on the chest, back, or abdomen, eventually enlarging and becoming deeply pigmented. However, in blacks, these papules may remain small and affect only the malar part of the face (dermatosis papulosa nigra).

◆ ***Smallpox (variola major).*** Initial signs and symptoms include high fever, malaise, prostration, severe headache, backache, and abdominal pain. A maculopapular rash develops on the mucosa of the mouth, pharynx, face, and forearms and then spreads to the trunk and legs. Within 2 days the rash becomes vesicular and later pustular. The lesions develop at the same time, appear identical, and are more prominent on the face and extremities. The pustules are round, firm, and deeply embedded in the skin. After 8 to 9 days the pustules form a crust, and later the scab separates from the skin leaving a pitted scar. In fatal cases, death results from encephalitis, extensive bleeding, or secondary infection.

◆ ***Syphilis.*** A discrete, reddish brown, mucocutaneous rash and general lymphadenopathy herald the onset of secondary syphilis. The rash may be papular, macular, pustular, or nodular. It typically erupts between rolls of fat on the trunk and proximally on the arms, palms, soles, face, and scalp. Lesions in warm, moist areas enlarge and erode, producing highly contagious, pink or grayish white condylomata lata. The patient may also experience mild headache, malaise, anorexia, weight loss, nausea and vomiting, sore throat, low-grade fever, temporary alopecia, and brittle, pitted nails.

◆ ***Syringoma.*** With this disorder, adenoma of the sweat glands produces a yellowish or erythematous papular rash on the face (especially the eyelids), neck, and upper chest.

◆ ***Systemic lupus erythematosus (SLE).*** SLE is characterized by a "butterfly rash" of erythematous maculopapules or discoid plaques that appears in a malar distribution across the nose and cheeks. Similar rashes may appear elsewhere, especially on exposed body areas. Other cardinal features include photosensitivity and nondeforming arthritis, especially in the hands, feet, and large joints. Common effects are patchy alopecia, mucous membrane ulceration, low-grade or spiking fever, chills, lymphadenopathy, anorexia, weight loss, abdominal pain, diarrhea or constipation, dyspnea, tachycardia, hematuria, headache, and irritability.

◆ ***Typhus.*** Typhus is a rickettsial disease transmitted to humans by fleas, mites, or body louse. Initial symptoms include headache, myalgia, arthralgia, and malaise, followed by an abrupt onset of chills, fever, nausea, and vomiting. A maculopapular rash may be present in some cases.

OTHER CAUSES

◆ ***Drugs.*** Transient maculopapular rashes, usually on the trunk, may accompany reactions to many drugs, including antibiotics, such as tetracycline, ampicillin, cephalosporins, and sulfonamides; benzodiazepines such as diazepam; lithium; gold salts; allopurinol; isoniazid; and salicylates.

SPECIAL CONSIDERATIONS

Apply cool compresses or an antipruritic lotion. Administer an antihistamine for allergic reactions and an antibiotic for infection.

PEDIATRIC POINTERS

Common causes of papular rashes in children are infectious diseases, such as molluscum contagiosum and scarlet fever; scabies; insect bites; allergies and drug reactions; and miliaria, which occurs in three forms, depending on the depth of sweat gland involvement.

GERIATRIC POINTERS

In bedridden elderly patients, the first sign of pressure ulcers is commonly an erythematous area, sometimes with firm papules. If not properly managed, these lesions progress to deep ulcers and can lead to death.

PATIENT COUNSELING

Advise the patient to keep his skin clean and dry, to wear loose-fitting, nonirritating clothing, and to avoid scratching the rash. Instruct him to promptly report changes in the rash's color, size, or configuration as well as the onset of itching or bleeding. Tell him to avoid excessive exposure to direct sunlight and to apply a protective sunscreen before going outdoors.

Warn patients with chronic conditions (such as SLE, psoriasis, or sarcoidosis) about the typical skin rashes that can develop. Tell them that these rashes can be an early sign of disease flare-up and that they should seek prompt treatment to prevent serious complications.

Paralysis

Paralysis, the total loss of voluntary motor function, results from severe cortical or pyramidal tract damage. It can occur with a cerebrovascular disorder, degenerative neuromuscular disease, trauma, tumor, or central nervous system infection. Acute paralysis may be an early indicator of a life-threatening disorder, such as Guillain-Barré syndrome.

Paralysis can be local or widespread, symmetrical or asymmetrical, transient or permanent, and spastic or flaccid. It's commonly classified according to location and severity as paraplegia (sometimes transient paralysis of the legs), quadriplegia (permanent paralysis of the arms, legs, and body below the level of the spinal lesion), or hemiplegia (unilateral paralysis of varying severity and permanence). Incomplete paralysis with profound weakness (paresis) may precede total paralysis in some patients.

EMERGENCY INTERVENTIONS *If paralysis has developed suddenly, suspect trauma or an acute vascular insult. After ensuring that the patient's spine is properly immobilized, quickly determine his level of consciousness (LOC) and take his vital signs. Elevated systolic blood pressure, widening pulse pressure, and bradycardia may signal increasing intracranial pressure (ICP). If possible, elevate the patient's head 30 degrees to decrease ICP.*

Evaluate respiratory status, and be prepared to administer oxygen, insert an artificial airway, or provide intubation and mechanical ventilation, as needed. To help determine the nature of the patient's injury, ask him for an account of the precipitating events. If he's unable to respond, try to find an eyewitness.

History and physical examination

If the patient is in no immediate danger, perform a complete neurologic assessment. Start with the history, relying on family members for information if necessary. Ask about the onset, duration, intensity, and progression of paralysis and about the events preceding its development. Focus medical history questions on the incidence of degenerative neurologic or neuromuscular disease, recent infectious illness, sexually transmitted disease, cancer, or recent injury. Explore related signs and symptoms, noting fever, headache, vision disturbances, dysphagia, nausea and vomiting, bowel or bladder dysfunction, muscle pain or weakness, and fatigue.

Next, perform a complete neurologic examination, testing cranial nerve, motor, and sensory function and deep tendon reflexes. Assess strength in all major muscle groups, and note any muscle atrophy. (See *Testing muscle strength,* pages 464 and 465.) Document all findings to serve as a baseline.

Medical causes

◆ ***Amyotrophic lateral sclerosis.*** This invariably fatal disorder produces spastic or flaccid paralysis in the body's major muscle groups, eventually progressing to total paralysis. Earlier findings include progressive muscle weakness, fasciculations, and muscle atrophy, usually beginning in the arms and hands. Cramping and hyperreflexia are also common. Involvement of respiratory muscles and the brain stem produces dyspnea and possibly respiratory distress. Progressive cranial nerve paralysis causes dysarthria, dysphagia, drooling, choking, and difficulty chewing.

◆ ***Bell's palsy.*** Bell's palsy, a disease of cranial nerve VII, causes transient, unilateral facial muscle paralysis. The affected muscles sag and eyelid closure is impossible. Other signs include increased tearing, drooling, and a diminished or absent corneal reflex.

◆ ***Botulism.*** This bacterial toxin infection can cause rapidly descending muscle weakness that progresses to paralysis within 2 to 4 days after the ingestion of contaminated food. Respiratory muscle paralysis leads to dyspnea and respiratory arrest. Nausea, vomiting, diarrhea, blurred or double vision, bilateral mydriasis, dysarthria, and dysphagia are some early findings.

◆ ***Brain abscess.*** Advanced abscess in the frontal or temporal lobe can cause hemiplegia accompanied by other late findings, such as ocular disturbances, unequal pupils, decreased LOC, ataxia, tremors, and signs of infection.

◆ ***Brain tumor.*** A tumor affecting the motor cortex of the frontal lobe may cause contralateral hemiparesis that progresses to hemiplegia. Onset is gradual, but paralysis is permanent without treatment. In early stages, frontal headache and behavioral changes may be the only indicators. Eventually, seizures, aphasia, and signs of increased ICP (decreased LOC and vomiting) develop.

◆ ***Conversion disorder.*** Hysterical paralysis, a classic symptom of conversion disorder, is characterized by the loss of voluntary movement with no obvious physical cause. It can affect any muscle group, appears and disappears unpredictably, and may occur with histrionic behavior (manipulative, dramatic, vain, irrational) or a strange indifference.

◆ ***Encephalitis.*** Variable paralysis develops in the late stages of this disorder. Earlier signs and symptoms include rapidly decreasing LOC (possibly coma), fever, headache, photophobia, vomiting, signs of meningeal irritation (nuchal rigidity, positive Kernig's and Brudzinski's signs), aphasia, ataxia, nystagmus, ocular palsies, myoclonus, and seizures.

◆ ***Guillain-Barré syndrome.*** This syndrome is characterized by a rapidly developing, but reversible, ascending paralysis. It commonly begins as leg muscle weakness and progresses symmetrically, sometimes affecting even the cranial nerves, producing dysphagia, nasal speech, and dysarthria. Respiratory muscle paralysis may be life-threatening. Other effects include transient paresthesia, orthostatic hypotension, tachycardia, diaphoresis, and bowel and bladder incontinence.

◆ ***Head trauma.*** Cerebral injury can cause paralysis due to cerebral edema and increased intracranial pressure. Onset is usually sudden. Location and extent vary, depending on the injury. Associated findings also vary but include decreased LOC; sensory disturbances, such as paresthesia and loss of sensation; headache; blurred or double vision; nausea and vomiting; and focal neurologic disturbances.

◆ ***Migraine headache.*** Hemiparesis, scotomas, paresthesia, confusion, dizziness, photophobia, or other transient symptoms may precede the onset of a throbbing unilateral headache and may persist after it subsides.

◆ ***Multiple sclerosis.*** With this disorder, paralysis commonly waxes and wanes until the later stages, when it may become permanent. Its extent can range from monoplegia to quadriplegia. In most patients, vision and sensory disturbances (paresthesia) are the earliest symptoms. Later findings are widely variable and may include muscle weakness and spasticity, nystagmus, hyperreflexia, intention tremor, gait ataxia, dysphagia, dysarthria, impotence, and constipation. Urinary frequency, urgency, and incontinence may also occur.

◆ ***Myasthenia gravis.*** With this neuromuscular disease, profound muscle weakness and abnormal fatigability may produce paralysis of certain muscle groups. Paralysis is usually transient in early stages but becomes more persistent as the disease progresses. Associated findings depend on the areas of neuromuscular involvement; they include weak eye closure, ptosis, diplopia, lack of facial mobility, dysphagia, nasal speech, and frequent nasal regurgitation of fluids. Neck muscle weakness may cause the patient's jaw to drop and his head to bob. Respiratory muscle involvement can lead to respiratory distress—dyspnea, shallow respirations, and cyanosis.

◆ ***Neurosyphilis.*** Irreversible hemiplegia may occur in the late stages of neurosyphilis. Dementia, cranial nerve palsies, tremors, and abnormal reflexes are other late findings.

◆ ***Parkinson's disease.*** Tremors, bradykinesia, and lead-pipe or cogwheel rigidity are the classic signs of Parkinson's disease. Extreme rigidity can progress to paralysis, particularly in the extremities. In most cases, paralysis resolves with prompt treatment of the disease.

◆ ***Peripheral nerve trauma.*** Severe injury to a peripheral nerve or group of nerves results in the loss of motor and sensory function in the innervated area. Muscles become flaccid and atrophied, and reflexes are lost. If transection isn't complete, paralysis may be temporary.

◆ ***Peripheral neuropathy.*** Typically, this syndrome produces muscle weakness that may lead to flaccid paralysis and atrophy. Related effects include paresthesia, loss of vibration sensation, hypoactive or absent deep tendon reflexes, neuralgia, and skin changes such as anhidrosis.

◆ ***Poliomyelitis.*** This disorder can produce insidious, permanent flaccid paralysis and hyporeflexia. Sensory function remains intact, but the patient loses voluntary muscle control.

◆ ***Rabies.*** This acute disorder produces progressive flaccid paralysis, vascular collapse, coma, and death within 2 weeks of contact with an infected animal. Prodromal signs and symptoms—fever; headache; hyperesthesia; paresthesia, coldness, and itching at the bite site; photophobia; tachycardia; shallow respirations; and excessive salivation, lacrimation, and perspiration—develop almost immediately. Within 2 to 10 days, a phase of excitement begins, marked by agitation, cranial nerve dysfunction (pupil changes, hoarseness, facial weakness, ocular palsies), tachycardia or bradycardia, cyclic respirations, high fever, urine retention, drooling, and hydrophobia.

◆ ***Seizure disorders.*** Seizures, particularly focal seizures, can cause transient local paralysis (Todd's paralysis). Any part of the body may be

Understanding spinal cord syndromes

When a patient's spinal cord is incompletely severed, he experiences partial motor and sensory loss. Most incomplete cord lesions fit into one of the syndromes described below.

Anterior cord syndrome, usually resulting from a flexion injury, causes motor paralysis and loss of pain and temperature sensation below the level of injury. Touch, proprioception, and vibration sensation are usually preserved.

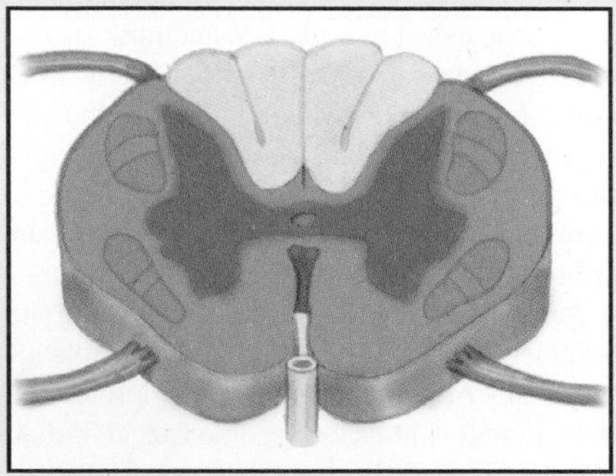

Central cord syndrome is caused by hyperextension or flexion injury. Motor loss is variable and greater in the arms than in the legs; sensory loss is usually slight.

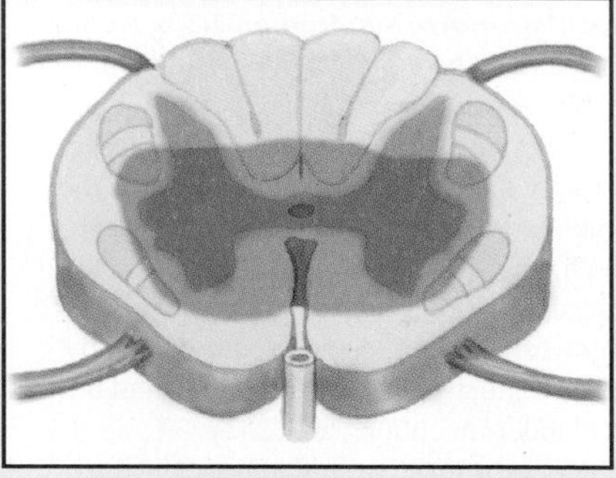

Brown-Séquard syndrome can result from flexion, rotation, or penetration injury. It's characterized by unilateral motor paralysis ipsilateral to the injury and loss of pain and temperature sensation contralateral to the injury.

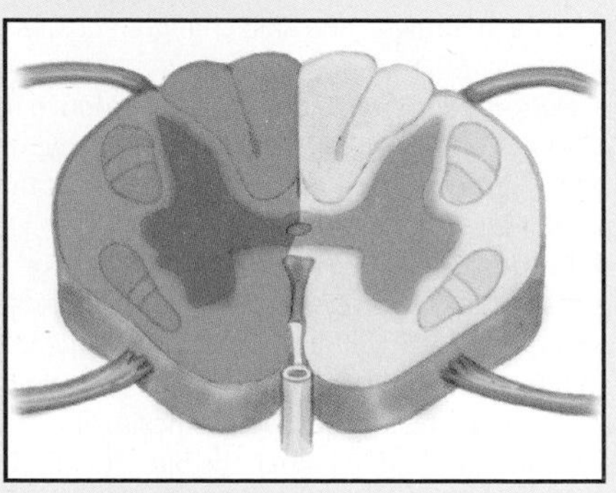

Posterior cord syndrome, produced by a cervical hyperextension injury, causes only a loss of proprioception and loss of light touch sensation. Motor function remains intact.

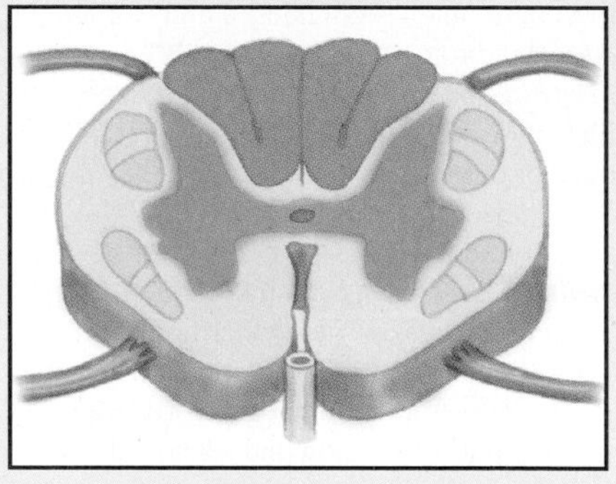

affected, although paralysis tends to occur contralateral to the side of the irritable focus.

◆ ***Spinal cord injury.*** Complete spinal cord transection results in permanent spastic paralysis below the level of injury. Reflexes may return after spinal shock resolves. Partial transection causes variable paralysis and paresthesia, depending on the location and extent of injury. (See *Understanding spinal cord syndromes*.)

◆ ***Spinal cord tumors.*** Paresis, pain, paresthesia, and variable sensory loss may occur along the nerve distribution pathway served by the affected cord segment. Eventually, these symptoms may progress to spastic paralysis with hyperactive deep tendon reflexes (unless the tumor is in the cauda equina, which produces hyporeflexia) and, perhaps, bladder and bowel incontinence. Paralysis is permanent without treatment.

◆ ***Stroke.*** A stroke involving the motor cortex can produce contralateral paresis or paralysis. Onset may be sudden or gradual, and paralysis may be transient or permanent. Associated signs and symptoms vary widely and may include headache, vomiting, seizures, decreased LOC and mental acuity, dysarthria, dysphagia, ataxia, contralateral paresthesia or sensory loss, apraxia, agnosia, aphasia, vision disturbances, emotional lability, and bowel and bladder dysfunction.

◆ ***Subarachnoid hemorrhage.*** This potentially life-threatening disorder can produce sudden paralysis. The condition may be temporary, resolving with decreasing edema, or permanent, if tissue destruction has occurred. Other acute effects are severe headache, mydriasis, photophobia, aphasia, sharply decreased LOC, nuchal rigidity, vomiting, and seizures.

◆ ***Syringomyelia.*** This degenerative spinal cord disease produces segmental paresis, leading to flaccid paralysis of the hands and arms. Reflexes are absent, and loss of pain and temperature sensation is distributed over the neck, shoulders, and arms in a capelike pattern.

◆ ***Thoracic aortic aneurysm.*** Occlusion of spinal arteries by a ruptured thoracic aortic aneurysm may cause sudden onset of transient bilateral paralysis. Severe chest pain radiating to the neck, shoulders, back, and abdomen and a sensation of tearing in the thorax are prominent symptoms. Related findings include syncope, pallor, diaphoresis, dyspnea, tachycardia, cyanosis, diastolic heart murmur, and abrupt loss of radial and femoral pulses or wide variations in pulses and blood pressure between arms and legs. Ironically, the patient appears to be in shock, and his systolic blood pressure is either normal or elevated.

◆ ***Transient ischemic attack (TIA).*** Episodic TIAs may cause transient unilateral paresis or paralysis accompanied by paresthesia, blurred or double vision, dizziness, aphasia, dysarthria, decreased LOC, and other site-dependent effects.

◆ ***West Nile encephalitis.*** This brain infection is caused by West Nile virus, a mosquito-borne flavivirus endemic to Africa, the Middle East, western Asia, and the United States. Mild infections are common and include fever, headache, and body aches, which are sometimes accompanied by skin rash and swollen lymph glands. More severe infections are marked by headache, high fever, neck stiffness, stupor, disorientation, coma, tremors, occasional convulsions, paralysis and, rarely, death.

OTHER CAUSES

◆ ***Drugs.*** Therapeutic use of neuromuscular blockers, such as pancuronium, produces paralysis.

◆ ***Electroconvulsive therapy.*** This therapy can produce acute, but transient, paralysis.

SPECIAL CONSIDERATIONS

Because a paralyzed patient is particularly susceptible to complications of prolonged immobility, provide frequent position changes, meticulous skin care, and frequent chest physiotherapy. He may benefit from passive range-of motion exercises to maintain muscle tone, application of splints to prevent contractures, and the use of footboards or other devices to prevent footdrop. If his cranial nerves are affected, the patient will have difficulty chewing and swallowing. Provide a liquid or soft diet, and keep suction equipment on hand in case aspiration occurs. Feeding tubes or total parenteral nutrition may be necessary with severe paralysis. Paralysis and accompanying vision disturbances may make ambulation hazardous; provide a call light and show the patient how to call for help. As appropriate, arrange for physical, speech, or occupational therapy.

PEDIATRIC POINTERS

Although children may develop paralysis from an obvious cause—such as trauma, infection, or tumor—they may also develop it from a hereditary or congenital disorder, such as Tay-Sachs disease, Werdnig-Hoffmann disease, spina bifida, or cerebral palsy.

Paresthesia

Paresthesia is an abnormal sensation or combination of sensations—commonly described as numbness, prickling, or tingling—felt along peripheral nerve pathways; these sensations generally aren't painful. Unpleasant or painful sensations, on the other hand, are termed *dysesthesias.* Paresthesia may develop suddenly or gradually and may be transient or permanent.

A common symptom of many neurologic disorders, paresthesia may also result from a systemic disorder or from a particular drug. It may reflect damage or irritation of the parietal lobe, thalamus, spinothalamic tract, or spinal or peripheral nerves—the neural circuit that transmits and interprets sensory stimuli.

Differential diagnosis: Paresthesia

History of present illness

Focused physical examination: Neurovascular and neurologic systems

Arterial occlusion (acute)	Transient ischemic attack	Vitamin B deficiency (chronic)
Signs and symptoms ◆ Sudden paresthesia and coldness in one or both legs ◆ Abrupt pallor of extremity ◆ Paresis ◆ Intermittent claudication ◆ Aching pain at rest ◆ Mottled skin with line of demarcation at level of occlusion ◆ Absent pulses below the occlusion **Diagnosis:** Physical examination, imaging studies (Doppler ultrasound, angiography) **Treatment:** Medication (anticoagulants, analgesics, thrombolytics), surgery **Follow-up:** Referral to vascular surgeon	**Signs and symptoms** ◆ Transient unilateral paralysis ◆ Vision disturbances ◆ Dizziness ◆ Aphasia ◆ Dysarthria ◆ Decreased level of consciousness ◆ Carotid bruit **Diagnosis:** Physical examination, imaging studies (carotid ultrasound, computed tomography scan), electrocardiogram **Treatment:** Diet modification, exercise program, reduction of risk factors for stroke, medication (anticoagulants, platelet inhibitors, antihypertensives, antiarrhythmics), surgery (if carotid stenosis is the cause) **Follow-up:** Referral to neurologist or neurosurgeon	**Signs and symptoms** ◆ Paresthesia and weakness in the arms and legs ◆ Burning leg pain ◆ Hypoactive deep tendon reflexes (DTRs) ◆ Variable sensory loss ◆ Mental changes ◆ Impaired vision **Diagnosis:** Diet history, laboratory test results (complete blood count, B_{12}, serum cobalamin levels; serum B_2 activity; 24-hour urine testing for thiamine, riboflavin, niacin, and pyridoxine) **Treatment:** Diet modification, supplementary vitamins **Follow-up**: Reevaluation of vitamin levels within 3 to 6 months

Additional differential diagnoses: arteriosclerosis obliterans ◆ arthritis ◆ brain tumor ◆ Buerger's disease ◆ diabetes mellitus ◆ Guillain-Barré syndrome ◆ head trauma ◆ heavy metal or solvent poisoning ◆ herniated disk ◆ herpes zoster ◆ hyperventilation syndrome ◆ hypocalcemia ◆ peripheral nerve trauma ◆ peripheral neuropathy ◆ rabies ◆ Raynaud's disease ◆ seizure disorders ◆ systemic lupus erythematosus ◆ spinal cord injury ◆ spinal cord tumors ◆ stroke ◆ tabes dorsalis ◆ thoracic outlet syndrome

Other causes: chemotherapeutic agents (vincristine, vinblastine, procarbazine) ◆ chloroquine ◆ isoniazid ◆ nitrofurantoin ◆ parenteral gold therapy ◆ phenytoin ◆ radiation therapy

History and physical examination

First, explore the paresthesia. When did the abnormal sensations begin? Have the patient describe their character and distribution. Ask about associated signs and symptoms, such as sensory loss and paresis or paralysis. Next, take a medical history, including neurologic, cardiovascular, metabolic, renal, and chronic inflammatory disorders, such as arthritis or lupus. Has the patient recently sustained a traumatic injury or had surgery or an invasive procedure that may have damaged peripheral nerves?

Focus the physical examination on the patient's neurologic status. (See *Differential diagnosis: Paresthesia*.) Assess his level of consciousness (LOC) and cranial nerve function. Test muscle strength and deep tendon reflexes (DTRs) in limbs affected by paresthesia. Systematically evaluate light touch, pain, temperature, vibration, and position sensation. (See *Testing for analgesia,* pages 42 and 43.) Note skin color and temperature, and palpate pulses.

Multiple sclerosis

Signs and symptoms
- Progressive muscle weakness and atrophy
- Muscle spasticity
- Hyperactive DTRs
- Dysarthria
- Dysphagia
- Waxing and waning signs and symptoms
- Vision disturbances
- Ataxic gait
- Diplopia
- Intention tremors
- Emotional lability
- Urinary and sexual dysfunction

Diagnosis: Cerebrospinal fluid analysis, magnetic resonance imaging, EEG, evoked response testing
Treatment: Symptomatic treatment; medication (antispasmotics, antidepressants, cholinergics, corticosteroids); physical, speech, and occupational therapy
Follow-up: Referral to neurologist

Migraine headache

Signs and symptoms
- Paresthesia of the lips, face, and hands
- Light flashes
- Aura
- Severe, throbbing, unilateral headache
- Dizziness
- Photophobia
- Nausea and vomiting

Diagnosis: History of headache, physical examination
Treatment: Rest during headache, cold compresses, medication (serotonin agonists, ergotamines, antiemetics, analgesics), lifestyle or diet modification (if the precipitant is identified)
Follow-up: Referral to headache clinic if uncontrolled, referral to neurologist

MEDICAL CAUSES

◆ ***Arterial occlusion (acute).*** With this disorder, sudden paresthesia and coldness may develop in one or both legs with a saddle embolus. Paresis, intermittent claudication, and aching pain at rest are also characteristic. The extremity becomes mottled with a line of temperature and color demarcation at the level of occlusion. Pulses are absent below the occlusion, and capillary refill time is increased.

◆ ***Arteriosclerosis obliterans.*** This disorder produces paresthesia, intermittent claudication (most common symptom), diminished or absent popliteal and pedal pulses, pallor, paresis, and coldness in the affected leg.

◆ ***Arthritis.*** Rheumatoid or osteoarthritic changes in the cervical spine may cause paresthesia in the neck, shoulders, and arms. The lumbar spine occasionally is affected, causing paresthesia in one or both legs and feet.

◆ ***Brain tumor.*** Tumors affecting the sensory cortex in the parietal lobe may cause progressive contralateral paresthesia accompanied by agnosia, apraxia, agraphia, homonymous hemianopsia, and loss of proprioception.

◆ ***Buerger's disease.*** With this smoking-related inflammatory occlusive disorder, exposure to cold makes the feet cold, cyanotic, and numb; later, they redden, become hot, and tingle. Intermittent claudication, which is aggravated by exercise and relieved by rest, is also common. Other findings include weak peripheral pulses, migratory superficial thrombophlebitis and, later, ulceration, muscle atrophy, and gangrene.

◆ ***Diabetes mellitus.*** Diabetic neuropathy can cause paresthesia with a burning sensation in the hands and legs. Other findings include insidious, permanent anosmia, fatigue, polyuria, polydipsia, weight loss, and polyphagia.

◆ ***Guillain-Barré syndrome.*** With this syndrome, transient paresthesia may precede muscle weakness, which usually begins in the legs and ascends to the arms and facial nerves. Weakness may progress to total paralysis. Other findings include dysarthria, dysphagia, nasal speech, orthostatic hypotension, bladder and bowel incontinence, diaphoresis, tachycardia and, possibly, signs of life-threatening respiratory muscle paralysis.

◆ ***Head trauma.*** Unilateral or bilateral paresthesia may occur when head trauma causes a concussion or contusion; however, sensory loss is more common. Other findings include variable paresis or paralysis, decreased LOC, headache, blurred or double vision, nausea and vomiting, dizziness, and seizures.

◆ ***Heavy metal or solvent poisoning.*** Exposure to industrial or household products containing lead, mercury, thallium, or organophosphates may cause paresthesia of acute or gradual onset. Mental status changes, tremors, weakness, seizures, and GI distress are also common.

◆ ***Herniated disk.*** Herniation of a lumbar or cervical disk may cause acute or gradual onset of paresthesia along the distribution pathways of affected spinal nerves. Other neuromuscular effects include severe pain, muscle spasms, and weakness that may progress to atrophy unless herniation is relieved.

◆ ***Herpes zoster.*** An early symptom of this disorder, paresthesia occurs in the dermatome supplied by the affected spinal nerve. Within several days, this dermatome is marked by a pruritic, erythematous, vesicular rash associated with sharp, shooting, or burning pain.

◆ ***Hyperventilation syndrome.*** Usually triggered by acute anxiety, this syndrome may produce transient paresthesia in the hands, feet, and perioral area, accompanied by agitation, vertigo, syncope, pallor, muscle twitching and weakness, carpopedal spasm, and cardiac arrhythmias.

◆ ***Hypocalcemia.*** Asymmetrical paresthesia usually occurs in the fingers, toes, and circumoral area early in this disorder. Other signs and symptoms are muscle weakness, twitching, or cramps; palpitations; hyperactive DTRs; carpopedal spasm; and positive Chvostek's and Trousseau's signs.

◆ ***Migraine headache.*** Paresthesia in the hands, face, and perioral area may herald an impending migraine headache. Other prodromal symptoms include scotomas, hemiparesis, confusion, dizziness, and photophobia. These effects may persist during the characteristic throbbing headache and continue after it subsides.

◆ ***Multiple sclerosis (MS).*** With this disorder, demyelination of the sensory cortex or spinothalamic tract may produce paresthesia—typically one of the earliest symptoms. Like other effects of MS, paresthesia commonly waxes and wanes until the later stages, when it may become permanent. Associated findings include muscle weakness, spasticity, and hyperreflexia.

◆ ***Peripheral nerve trauma.*** Injury to any major peripheral nerve can cause paresthesia—often dysesthesia—in the area supplied by that nerve. Paresthesia begins shortly after trauma and may be permanent. Other findings are flaccid paralysis or paresis, hyporeflexia, and variable sensory loss.

◆ ***Peripheral neuropathy.*** This syndrome can cause progressive paresthesia in all extremities. The patient also commonly displays muscle weakness, which may lead to flaccid paralysis and atrophy; loss of vibration sensation; diminished or absent DTRs; neuralgia; and cutaneous changes, such as glossy, red skin and anhidrosis.

◆ ***Rabies.*** Paresthesia, coldness, and itching at the site of an animal bite herald the prodromal stage of rabies. Other prodromal signs and symptoms are fever, headache, photophobia, hyperesthesia, tachycardia, shallow respirations, and excessive salivation, lacrimation, and perspiration.

◆ ***Raynaud's disease.*** Exposure to cold or stress makes the fingers turn pale, cold, and cyanotic; with rewarming, they become red and paresthetic. Ulceration may occur in chronic cases.

◆ ***Seizure disorders.*** Seizures originating in the parietal lobe usually cause paresthesia of the lips, fingers, and toes. The paresthesia may act as auras that precede tonic-clonic seizures.

◆ ***Spinal cord injury.*** Paresthesia may occur in partial spinal cord transection, after spinal shock resolves. It may be unilateral or bilateral, occurring at or below the level of the lesion. Associated sensory and motor loss is variable. (See *Understanding spinal cord syndromes,* page 524.) Spinal cord disorders may be associated with paresthesia on head flexion (Lhermitte's sign).

◆ ***Spinal cord tumors.*** Paresthesia, paresis, pain, and sensory loss along nerve pathways served by the affected cord segment result from such tumors. Eventually, paresis may cause spastic paralysis with hyperactive DTRs (unless the tumor is in the cauda equina, which produces hyporeflexia) and, possibly, bladder and bowel incontinence.

◆ ***Stroke.*** Although contralateral paresthesia may occur with stroke, sensory loss is more common. Associated features vary with the artery affected and may include contralateral hemiplegia, decreased LOC, and homonymous hemianopsia.

◆ ***Systemic lupus erythematosus.*** This disorder may cause paresthesia, but its primary signs and symptoms include nondeforming arthritis (usually of hands, feet, and large joints), photosensitivity, and a "butterfly rash" that appears across the nose and cheeks.

◆ ***Tabes dorsalis.*** With this disorder, paresthesia—especially of the legs—is a common, but late, symptom. Other findings include ataxia, loss of proprioception and pain and temperature sensation, absent deep tendon reflexes, Charcot's joints, Argyll Robertson pupils, incontinence, and impotence.

◆ ***Thoracic outlet syndrome.*** Paresthesia occurs suddenly in this syndrome when the affected arm is raised and abducted. The arm also becomes pale and cool with diminished pulses. Unequal blood pressure between arms may be noted.

◆ ***Transient ischemic attack (TIA).*** Paresthesia typically occurs abruptly with a TIA and is limited to one arm or another isolated part of the body. It usually lasts about 10 minutes and is accompanied by paralysis or paresis. Associated findings include decreased LOC, dizziness, unilateral vision loss, nystagmus, aphasia, dysarthria, tinnitus, facial weakness, dysphagia, and ataxic gait.

◆ ***Vitamin B deficiency.*** Chronic thiamine or vitamin B_{12} deficiency may cause paresthesia and weakness in the arms and legs. Burning leg pain, hypoactive DTRs, and variable sensory loss are common in thiamine deficiency; vitamin B_{12} deficiency also produces mental status changes and impaired vision.

OTHER CAUSES

◆ ***Drugs.*** Phenytoin, chemotherapeutic agents (such as vincristine, vinblastine, and procarbazine), D-penicillamine, isoniazid, nitrofurantoin, chloroquine, and parenteral gold therapy may produce transient paresthesia that disappears when the drug is discontinued.

◆ ***Radiation therapy.*** Long-term radiation therapy eventually may cause peripheral nerve damage, resulting in paresthesia.

SPECIAL CONSIDERATIONS

Because paresthesia is commonly accompanied by patchy sensory loss, teach the patient safety measures. For example, have him test bath water with a thermometer.

PEDIATRIC POINTERS

Although children may experience paresthesia associated with the same causes as adults, many are unable to describe this symptom. Nevertheless, hereditary polyneuropathies are usually first recognized in childhood.

Paroxysmal nocturnal dyspnea

Typically dramatic and terrifying to the patient, this sign refers to an attack of dyspnea that abruptly awakens the patient. Common findings include diaphoresis, coughing, wheezing, and chest discomfort. The attack abates after the patient sits up or stands for several minutes, but may recur every 2 to 3 hours.

Paroxysmal nocturnal dyspnea is a sign of left-sided heart failure. It may result from decreased respiratory drive, impaired left ventricular function, enhanced reabsorption of interstitial fluid, or increased thoracic blood volume. All of these pathophysiologic mechanisms cause dyspnea to worsen when the patient lies down.

HISTORY AND PHYSICAL EXAMINATION

Begin by exploring the patient's complaint of dyspnea. Does he have dyspneic attacks only at night or at other times as well, such as after exertion or while sitting down? If so, what type of activity triggers the attack? Does he experience coughing, wheezing, fatigue, or weakness during an attack? Find out if he has a history of lower extremity edema or jugular vein distention. Ask if he sleeps with his head elevated and, if so, on how many pillows or if he sleeps in a reclining chair. Obtain a cardiopulmonary history. Does the patient or a family member have a history of a myocardial infarction, coronary artery disease, or hypertension, or of chronic bronchitis, emphysema, or asthma? Has the patient had cardiac surgery?

Next perform a physical examination. Begin by taking the patient's vital signs and forming an overall impression of his appearance. Is he noticeably cyanotic or edematous? Auscultate the lungs for crackles and wheezing and the heart for gallops and arrhythmias.

MEDICAL CAUSES

◆ ***Left-sided heart failure.*** Dyspnea—on exertion, during sleep, and eventually even at rest—is an early sign of left-sided heart failure. This sign is characteristically accompanied by Cheyne-Stokes respirations, diaphoresis, weakness, wheezing, and a persistent, nonproductive cough or a cough that produces clear or blood-tinged sputum. As the patient's condition worsens, he develops tachycardia, tachypnea, alternating pulse (commonly initiated by a premature beat), a ventricular gallop, crackles, and peripheral edema.

With advanced left-sided heart failure, the patient may also exhibit severe orthopnea, cyanosis, clubbing, hemoptysis, and cardiac arrhythmias as well as signs and symptoms of shock, such as hypotension, weak pulse, and cold, clammy skin.

SPECIAL CONSIDERATIONS

Prepare the patient for diagnostic tests, such as chest X-ray, echocardiography, exercise electrocardiography, and cardiac blood pool imaging. If the hospitalized patient experiences paroxysmal nocturnal dyspnea, assist him to a sitting position or help him walk around the room. If necessary, provide supplemental oxygen. Try to calm him because anxiety can exacerbate dyspnea.

PEDIATRIC POINTERS

In a child, paroxysmal nocturnal dyspnea usually stems from a congenital heart defect that precipitates heart failure. Help relieve the child's dyspnea by elevating his head and calming him.

Peau d'orange

Usually a late sign of breast cancer, peau d'orange (orange peel skin) is the edematous thickening and pitting of breast skin. This slowly developing sign can also occur with breast or axillary lymph node infection, erysipelas, or Graves' disease. Its striking orange peel appearance stems from lymphatic edema around deepened hair follicles. (See *Recognizing peau d'orange*.)

HISTORY AND PHYSICAL EXAMINATION

Ask the patient when she first detected peau d'orange. Has she noticed any lumps, pain, or other breast changes? Does she have related signs and symptoms, such as malaise, achiness, and weight loss? Is she lactating, or has she recently weaned her infant? Has she had previous axillary surgery that might have impaired lymphatic drainage of a breast?

In a well-lit examining room, observe the patient's breasts. Estimate the extent of the peau d'orange and check for erythema. Assess the nipples for discharge, deviation, retraction, dimpling, and cracking. Gently palpate the area of peau d'orange, noting warmth or induration. Palpate the entire breast, noting any fixed or mobile lumps, and the axillary lymph nodes, noting enlargement. Take the patient's temperature.

MEDICAL CAUSES

◆ ***Breast abscess.*** Usually affecting lactating women with milk stasis, this infectious disorder causes peau d'orange, malaise, breast tenderness and erythema, and a sudden fever that may be accompanied by shaking chills. A cracked nipple may produce a purulent discharge, and an indurated or palpable soft mass may be present.

◆ ***Breast cancer.*** Advanced breast cancer is the most likely cause of peau d'orange, which usually begins in the dependent part of the breast or the areola. Palpation typically reveals a firm, immobile mass that adheres to the skin above the area of peau d'orange. Inspection of the breasts may reveal changes in contour, size, or symmetry. Inspection of the nipples may reveal deviation, erosion, retraction, and a thin and watery, bloody, or purulent discharge. The patient may report a burning and itching sensation in the nipples as well as a sensation of warmth or heat in the breast. Breast pain may occur, but it isn't a reliable indicator of cancer.

◆ ***Erysipelas.*** This streptococcal infection causes a well-demarcated erythematous elevated area, typically with a peau d'orange texture. Pain, warmth, and generalized signs and symptoms, such as fever and fatigue, also occur.

◆ ***Graves' disease.*** Patients with this thyroid disorder may exhibit raised, thickened, hyperpigmented, peau d'orange-like areas that tend to coalesce. Other common signs and symptoms of hyperthyroidism include weight loss, palpitations, anxiety, heat intolerance, tremor, and amenorrhea.

Recognizing peau d'orange

In peau d'orange, the skin appears to be pitted (as shown below). This condition usually indicates late-stage breast cancer.

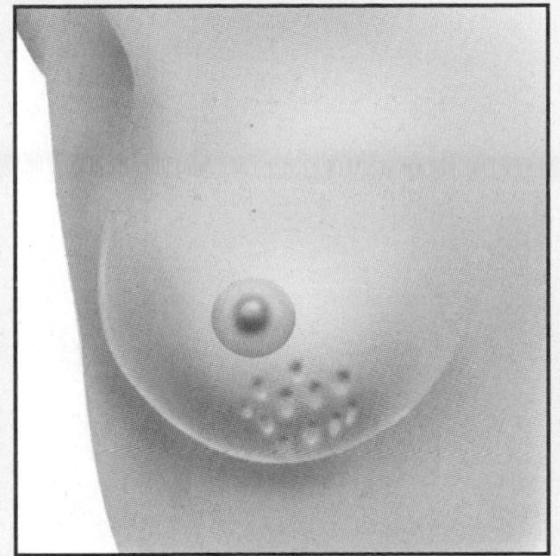

◆ ***Tuberculosis of the axillary lymph nodes.*** Peau d'orange occasionally occurs as one or more axillary lymph nodes enlarge.

SPECIAL CONSIDERATIONS

Because peau d'orange usually signals advanced breast cancer, provide emotional support for the patient. Encourage her to express her fears and concerns. Clearly explain expected diagnostic tests, such as mammography, computed tomography scan, ultrasound, and breast biopsy.

Pericardial friction rub

Commonly transient, a pericardial friction rub is a scratching, grating, or crunching sound that occurs when two inflamed layers of the pericardium slide over one another. Ranging from faint to loud, this abnormal sound is best heard along the lower left sternal border during deep inspiration. (See *Comparing auscultation findings,* pages 532 and 533.) It indicates pericarditis, which can result from acute infection, a cardiac or renal disorder, postpericardiotomy syndrome, or the use of certain drugs.

Occasionally, a pericardial friction rub can resemble a murmur (see *Pericardial friction rub or murmur?*) or a pleural friction rub. However, the classic pericardial friction rub has three components. (See *Understanding pericardial friction rubs,* page 534.)

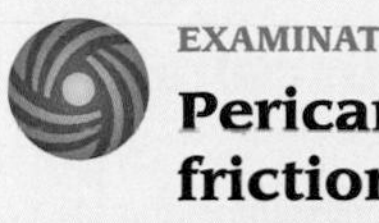

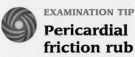

EXAMINATION TIP

Pericardial friction rub or murmur?

Is the sound you hear a pericardial friction rub or a murmur? Here's how to tell. The classic pericardial friction rub has three sound components, which are related to the phases of the cardiac cycle. In some patients, however, the rub's presystolic and early diastolic sounds may be inaudible, causing the rub to resemble the murmur of mitral insufficiency or aortic stenosis and insufficiency.

If you don't detect the classic three-component sound, you can distinguish a pericardial friction rub from a murmur by auscultating again and asking yourself these questions:

How deep is the sound?
A pericardial friction rub usually sounds superficial; a murmur sounds deeper in the chest.

Does the sound radiate?
A pericardial friction rub usually doesn't radiate; a murmur may radiate widely.

Does the sound vary with inspiration or changes in patient position?
A pericardial friction rub is usually loudest during inspiration and is best heard when the patient leans forward. A murmur varies in timing and duration with both factors.

HISTORY AND PHYSICAL EXAMINATION

Obtain a complete medical history, noting especially cardiac dysfunction. Has the patient recently had a myocardial infarction or cardiac surgery? Has he ever had pericarditis or rheumatic disorder, such as rheumatoid arthritis or systemic lupus erythematosus? Does he have chronic renal failure or an infection? If the patient complains of chest pain, ask him to describe its character and location. What relieves the pain? What worsens it?

(Text continues on page 534.)

Comparing auscultation findings

During auscultation, you may detect a pleural friction rub, a pericardial friction rub, or crackles—three abnormal sounds that are commonly confused. Use this chart to help clarify auscultation findings.

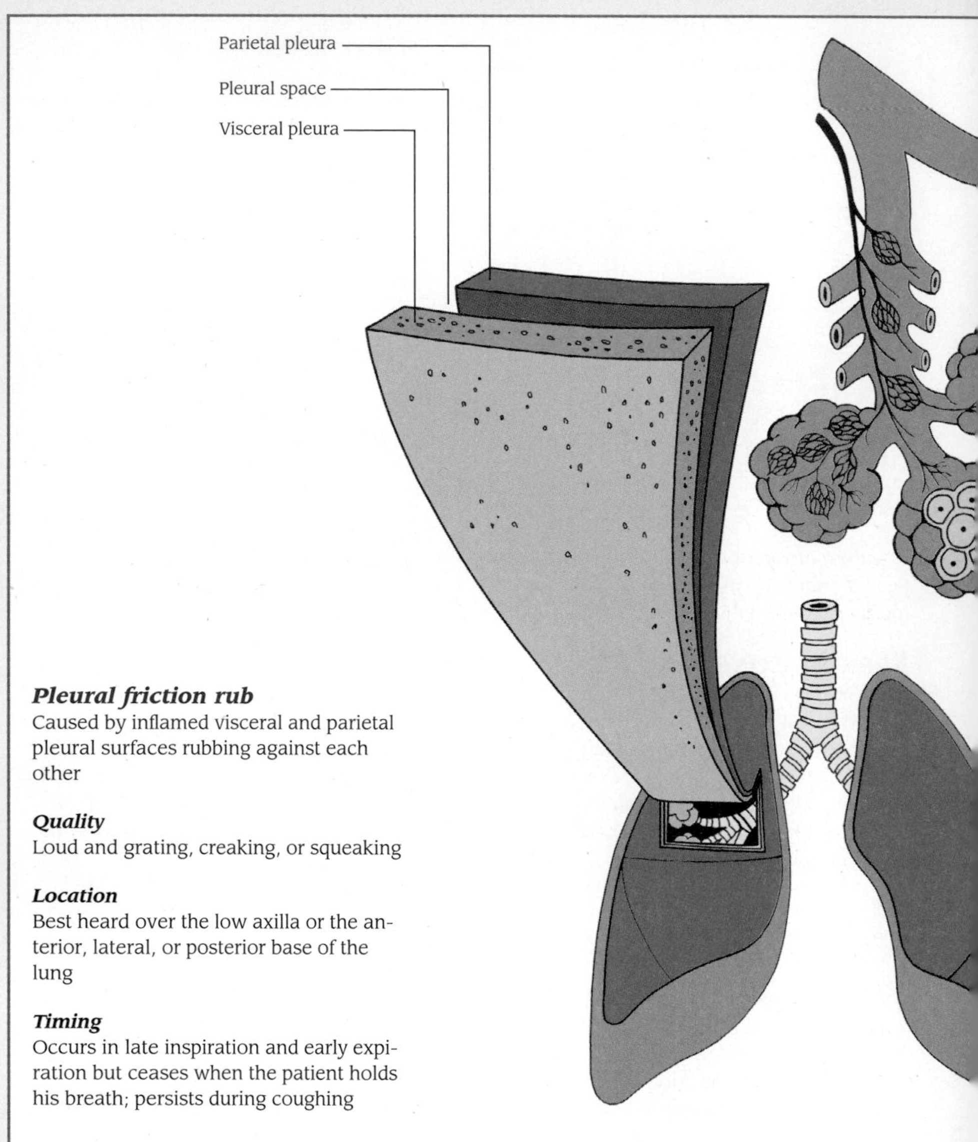

Pleural friction rub
Caused by inflamed visceral and parietal pleural surfaces rubbing against each other

Quality
Loud and grating, creaking, or squeaking

Location
Best heard over the low axilla or the anterior, lateral, or posterior base of the lung

Timing
Occurs in late inspiration and early expiration but ceases when the patient holds his breath; persists during coughing

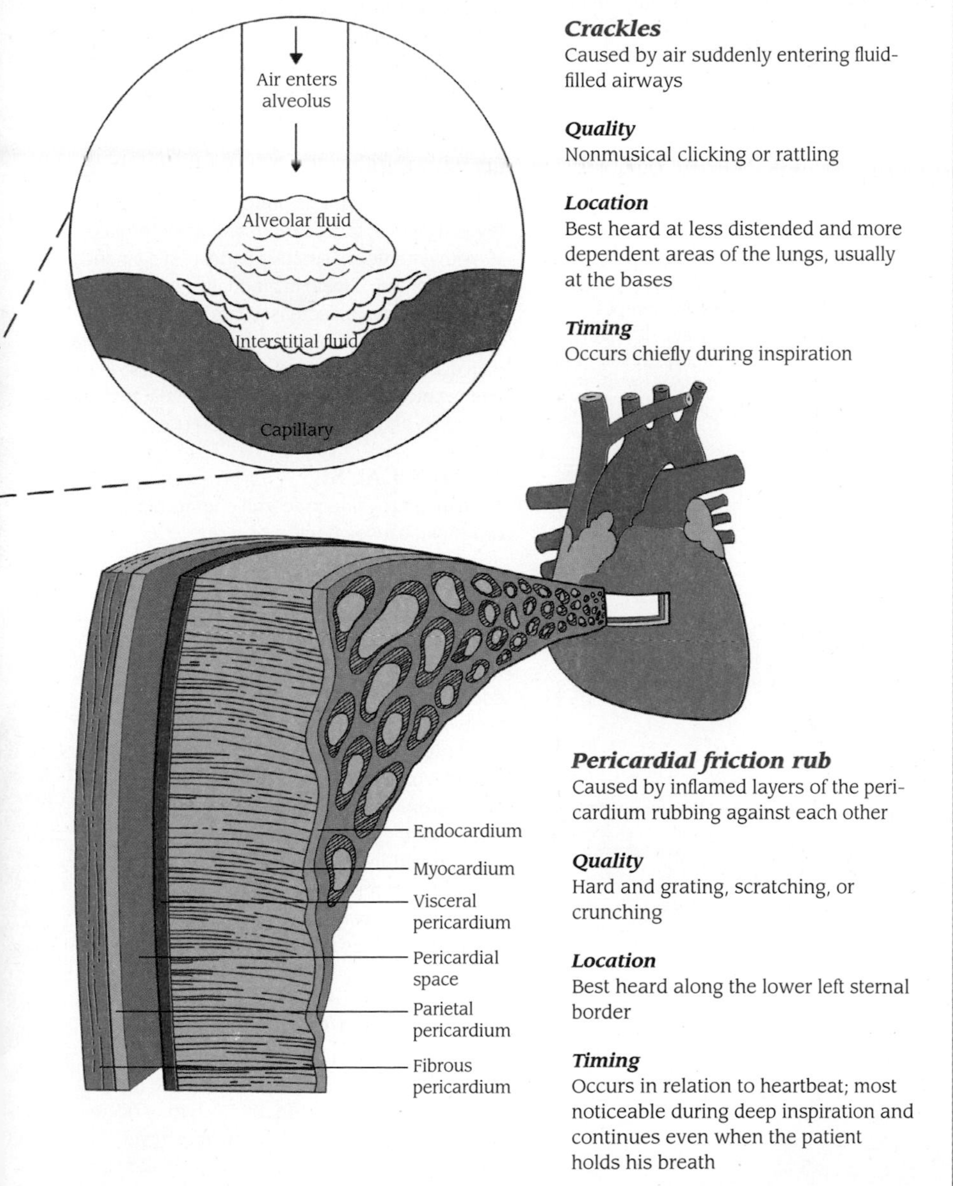

Crackles

Caused by air suddenly entering fluid-filled airways

Quality

Nonmusical clicking or rattling

Location

Best heard at less distended and more dependent areas of the lungs, usually at the bases

Timing

Occurs chiefly during inspiration

Pericardial friction rub

Caused by inflamed layers of the pericardium rubbing against each other

Quality

Hard and grating, scratching, or crunching

Location

Best heard along the lower left sternal border

Timing

Occurs in relation to heartbeat; most noticeable during deep inspiration and continues even when the patient holds his breath

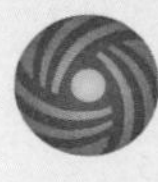

EXAMINATION TIP

Understanding pericardial friction rubs

The complete, or classic, pericardial friction rub is triphasic. Its three sound components are linked to phases of the cardiac cycle. The *presystolic* component (A) reflects atrial systole and precedes the first heart sound (S_1). The *systolic* component (B)—usually the loudest—reflects ventricular systole and occurs between the S_1 and second heart sound (S_2). The *early diastolic* component (C) reflects ventricular diastole and follows the S_2.

Sometimes, the early diastolic component merges with the presystolic component, producing a diphasic to-and-fro sound on auscultation. In other patients, auscultation may detect only one component—a monophasic rub, typically during ventricular systole.

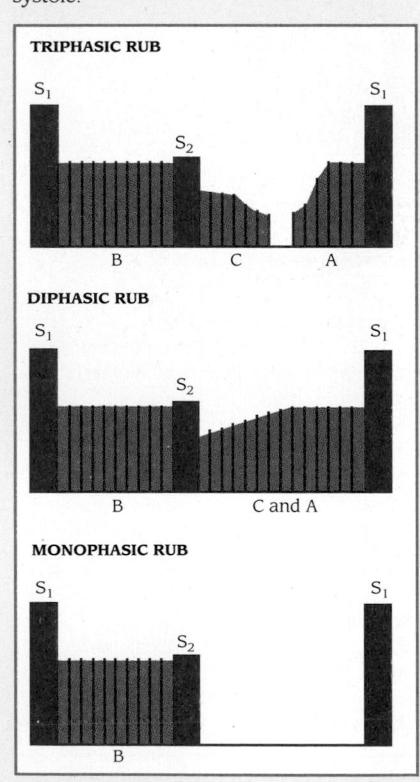

Take the patient's vital signs, noting especially hypotension, tachycardia, irregular pulse, tachypnea, and fever. Inspect for jugular vein distention, edema, ascites, and hepatomegaly. Auscultate the lungs for crackles.

MEDICAL CAUSES

◆ ***Pericarditis.*** A pericardial friction rub is the hallmark of acute pericarditis. This disorder also causes sharp precordial or retrosternal pain that usually radiates to the left shoulder, neck, and back. The pain worsens when the patient breathes deeply, coughs, or lies flat and, possibly, when he swallows. It abates when he sits up and leans forward. The patient may also develop fever, dyspnea, tachycardia, and arrhythmias.

With chronic constrictive pericarditis, a pericardial friction rub develops gradually and is accompanied by signs of decreased cardiac filling and output, such as peripheral edema, ascites, jugular vein distention on inspiration (Kussmaul's sign), and hepatomegaly. Dyspnea, orthopnea, paradoxical pulse, and chest pain may also occur.

OTHER CAUSES

◆ ***Drugs.*** Procainamide and chemotherapeutic drugs can cause pericarditis.

SPECIAL CONSIDERATIONS

Continue to monitor the patient's cardiovascular status. If the pericardial friction rub disappears, be alert for signs of cardiac tamponade: pallor; cool, clammy skin; hypotension; tachycardia; tachypnea; paradoxical pulse; and increased jugular vein distention. If these signs occur, prepare the patient for pericardiocentesis to prevent cardiovascular collapse.

Ensure that the patient gets adequate rest. Give an anti-inflammatory, antiarrhythmic, diuretic, or antimicrobial to treat the underlying cause. If necessary, prepare him for a pericardiectomy to promote adequate cardiac filling and contraction.

PEDIATRIC POINTERS

Bacterial pericarditis may develop during the first two decades of life, usually before age 6. Although a pericardial friction rub may occur, other signs and symptoms—such as fever, tachycardia, dyspnea, chest pain, jugular vein distention, and hepatomegaly—more reliably indicate this life-threatening disorder. A pericardial friction rub may also occur after surgery to correct congenital cardiac anomalies. However, it usually vanishes without development of pericarditis.

Peristaltic waves, visible

With intestinal obstruction, peristalsis temporarily increases in strength and frequency as the intestine contracts to force its contents past the obstruction. As a result, visible peristaltic waves may roll across the abdomen. Typically, these waves appear suddenly and vanish quickly, because increased peristalsis overcomes the obstruction or the GI tract becomes atonic. Peristaltic waves are best detected by stooping at the patient's side and inspecting his abdominal contour while he's in a supine position.

Visible peristaltic waves may also reflect normal stomach and intestinal contractions in thin patients or in malnourished patients with abdominal muscle atrophy.

History and physical examination

After observing peristaltic waves, collect pertinent history data. For example, ask about a history of pyloric ulcer, stomach cancer, or chronic gastritis, which can lead to pyloric obstruction. Ask about conditions leading to intestinal obstruction, such as intestinal tumors or polyps, gallstones, chronic constipation, and a hernia. Has the patient had recent abdominal surgery? Be sure to obtain a drug history.

Determine if the patient has related symptoms. Spasmodic abdominal pain, for example, accompanies small-bowel obstruction, whereas colicky pain accompanies pyloric obstruction. Is the patient experiencing nausea and vomiting? If he has vomited, ask about the consistency, amount, and color of the vomitus. Lumpy vomitus may contain undigested food particles; green or brown vomitus may contain bile or fecal matter.

Next, with the patient in a supine position, inspect the abdomen for distention, surgical scars and adhesions, or visible loops of bowel. Auscultate for bowel sounds, noting high-pitched, tinkling sounds. Then jar the patient's bed (or roll the patient from side to side) and auscultate for a succussion splash—a splashing sound in the stomach from retained secretions due to pyloric obstruction. Palpate the abdomen for rigidity and tenderness, and percuss for tympany. Check the skin and mucous membranes for dryness and poor skin turgor, indicating dehydration. Take the patient's vital signs, noting especially tachycardia and hypotension, which indicate hypovolemia.

Medical causes

◆ ***Large-bowel obstruction.*** Visible peristaltic waves in the upper abdomen are an early sign of this obstruction. Obstipation, however, may be the earliest finding. Other characteristic signs and symptoms develop more slowly than in small-bowel obstruction. These include nausea, colicky abdominal pain (milder than in small-bowel obstruction), gradual and eventually marked abdominal distention, and hyperactive bowel sounds.

◆ ***Pyloric obstruction.*** Peristaltic waves may be detected in a swollen epigastrium or in the left upper quadrant, usually beginning near the left rib margin and rolling from left to right. Related findings include vague epigastric discomfort or colicky pain after eating, nausea, vomiting, anorexia, and weight loss. Auscultation reveals a loud succussion splash.

◆ ***Small-bowel obstruction.*** Early signs of mechanical obstruction of the small bowel include peristaltic waves rolling across the upper abdomen and intermittent, cramping periumbilical pain. Associated signs and symptoms include nausea, vomiting of bilious or, later, fecal material, and constipation; in partial obstruction, diarrhea may occur. Hyperactive bowel sounds and slight abdominal distention also occur early.

Special considerations

Because visible peristaltic waves are an early sign of intestinal obstruction, monitor the patient's status and prepare him for diagnostic evaluation and treatment. Withhold food and fluids, and explain the purpose and procedure of abdominal X-rays and barium studies, which can confirm obstruction.

If tests confirm obstruction, nasogastric suctioning may be performed to decompress the stomach and small bowel. Provide frequent oral hygiene, and watch for a thick, swollen tongue and dry mucous membranes, indicating dehydration. Frequently monitor vital signs and intake and output.

Pediatric pointers

In infants, visible peristaltic waves may indicate pyloric stenosis. In small children, peristaltic waves may be visible normally because of the protuberant abdomen, or visible waves may indicate bowel obstruction stemming from congenital anomalies, volvulus, or the swallowing of a foreign body.

Geriatric pointers

In elderly patients who present with visible peristaltic waves, always check for fecal impaction, which is a common problem among those of this age-group. Obtain a detailed drug history; antidepressants and antipsychotics can predispose patients to constipation and bowel obstruction.

Patient counseling

Advise patients suffering from chronic constipation and those taking an antidepressant or antipsychotic to increase their fluid intake and eat foods high in fiber, such as cereals, fruits, and vegetables. If no improvement occurs, administer a stool softener to prevent further complications such as bowel obstruction.

Photophobia

A common symptom, photophobia is an abnormal sensitivity to light. In many patients, photophobia simply indicates increased eye sensitivity without any underlying pathology. For example, it can stem from excessive wearing of contact lenses or use of poorly fitted lenses. However, in others, this symptom can result from a systemic disorder, an ocular disorder or trauma, or the use of certain drugs. (See *Photophobia: Causes and associated findings*.)

History and physical examination

If your patient reports photophobia, find out when it began and how severe it is. Did it follow eye trauma, a chemical splash, or exposure to the rays of a sun lamp? If photophobia results from trauma, avoid manipulating the eyes. Ask the patient about eye pain and have him describe its location, duration, and intensity. Does he have a sensation of a foreign body in his eye? Does he have any other signs and symptoms, such as increased tearing and vision changes?

Next, take the patient's vital signs and assess neurologic status. Assess visual activity, unless the cause is a chemical burn. Follow this with a careful eye examination, inspecting the eyes' external structures for abnormalities. Examine the conjunctiva and sclera, noting their color. Characterize the amount and consistency of any discharge. Check pupillary reaction to light. Evaluate extraocular muscle function by testing the six cardinal fields of gaze, and test visual acuity in both eyes.

During your assessment, keep in mind that although photophobia can accompany life-threatening meningitis, it isn't a cardinal sign of meningeal irritation.

Medical causes

◆ ***Burns.*** With a chemical burn, photophobia and eye pain may be accompanied by erythema and blistering on the face and lids, miosis, diffuse conjunctival injection, and corneal changes. The patient experiences blurred vision and may be unable to keep his eyes open. With an ultraviolet radiation burn, photophobia occurs with moderate to severe eye pain. These symptoms develop about 12 hours after exposure to the rays of a welding arc or sun lamp.

◆ ***Conjunctivitis.*** When conjunctivitis affects the cornea, it causes photophobia. Other common findings include conjunctival injection, increased tearing, a foreign-body sensation, a feeling of fullness around the eyes, and eye pain, burning, and itching. Allergic conjunctivitis is distinguished by a stringy eye discharge and milky red injection. Bacterial conjunctivitis tends to cause a copious, mucopurulent, flaky eye discharge that may make the eyelids stick together, as well as brilliant red conjunctiva. Fungal conjunctivitis produces a thick, purulent discharge, extreme redness, and crusting, sticky eyelids. Viral conjunctivitis causes copious tearing with little discharge as well as enlargement of the preauricular lymph nodes.

◆ ***Corneal abrasion.*** A common finding with corneal abrasion, photophobia is usually accompanied by excessive tearing, conjunctival injection, visible corneal damage, and a foreign-body sensation in the eye. Blurred vision and eye pain may also occur.

◆ ***Corneal foreign body.*** Photophobia may occur with miosis, intense eye pain, a foreign-body sensation, slightly impaired vision, conjunctival injection, and profuse tearing. A dark speck may be visible on the cornea.

◆ ***Corneal ulcer.*** This vision-threatening disorder causes severe photophobia and eye pain that is aggravated by blinking. Impaired visual acuity may accompany blurring, eye discharge, and sticky eyelids. Conjunctival injection may occur even though the cornea appears white and opaque. A bacterial ulcer may also cause an irregularly shaped corneal ulcer and unilateral pupillary constriction. A fungal ulcer may be surrounded by progressively clearer rings.

◆ ***Dry eye syndrome.*** Although this disorder may produce photophobia, it more characteristically causes eye pain, conjunctival injection, a foreign-body sensation, itching, excessive mucus secretion and, possibly, decreased tearing and difficulty moving the eyelids.

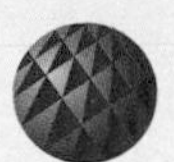

SIGNS & SYMPTOMS

Photophobia: Causes and associated findings

Major associated signs and symptoms

Common causes	Conjunctival injection	Corneal changes	Eye discharge	Eyelid edema	Eye pain	Foreign-body sensation	Nuchal rigidity	Pupillary changes	Tearing, increased	Vision changes	Visual floaters	Vomiting
Burns (chemical)	●	●			●	●		●	●	●		
Burns (ultraviolet)	●	●			●	●			●			
Conjunctivitis	●		●		●	●			●			
Corneal abrasion	●	●			●	●			●	●		
Corneal foreign body	●	●			●	●		●	●	●		
Corneal ulcer	●	●	●		●			●		●		
Dry eye syndrome	●		●		●	●						
Iritis (acute)	●				●			●		●		
Keratitis (interstitial)	●	●			●					●		
Meningitis (acute bacterial)							●	●				●
Migraine headache										●		●
Scleritis	●				●				●			
Sclerokeratitis		●			●							
Trachoma		●	●	●	●				●	●		
Uveitis (anterior)	●				●			●				
Uveitis (posterior)	●				●			●		●	●	

◆ ***Iritis (acute).*** Severe photophobia may result from this disorder, along with marked conjunctival injection, moderate to severe eye pain, and blurred vision. The pupil may be constricted and may respond poorly to light.

◆ ***Keratitis (interstitial).*** This corneal inflammation causes photophobia, eye pain, blurred vision, dramatic conjunctival injection, and grayish pink corneas.

◆ ***Meningitis (acute bacterial).*** A common symptom of this disorder, photophobia may occur with other signs of meningeal irritation, such as nuchal rigidity, hyperreflexia, and opisthotonos. Brudzinski's and Kernig's signs can be elicited. Fever, an early finding, may be accompanied by chills. Related signs and symptoms may include headache, vomiting, ocular palsies, facial weakness, pupillary abnormalities, and hearing loss. With severe meningitis, seizures may occur along with stupor progressing to coma.

◆ ***Migraine headache.*** Photophobia and noise sensitivity are prominent features of a common migraine. Typically severe, this aching or throbbing headache may also cause fatigue, blurred vision, nausea, and vomiting.

◆ ***Scleritis.*** This disorder may cause photophobia, severe eye pain, conjunctival injection, a bluish purple sclera, and profuse tearing.

◆ ***Sclerokeratitis.*** Inflammation of the sclera and cornea causes photophobia, eye pain, burning, and irritation.

◆ ***Trachoma.*** At first, trachoma resembles bacterial conjunctivitis, producing photophobia, visible conjunctival follicles, red and edematous eyelids, pain, increased tearing, and discharge. Without treatment, conjunctival follicles enlarge into inflamed papillae that later become yellow or gray; small blood vessels invade the cornea under the upper lid. Eventually, entropion may occur with corneal scarring, visual distortion and, possibly, dry eyes.

◆ ***Uveitis.*** Both anterior and posterior uveitis can cause photophobia. Typically, anterior uveitis also produces moderate to severe eye pain, severe conjunctival injection, and a small, nonreactive pupil. Posterior uveitis develops slowly, causing visual floaters, eye pain, pupil distortion, conjunctival injection, and blurred vision.

Other causes

◆ ***Drugs.*** Mydriatics—such as atropine, phenylephrine, scopolamine, cyclopentolate, and tropicamide—can cause photophobia due to ocular dilation. Cocaine, amphetamines, and ophthalmic antifungals—such as trifluridine and idoxuridine—can also cause photophobia.

Special considerations

Promote the patient's comfort by darkening the room and telling him to close both eyes. If photophobia persists at home, suggest that he wear dark glasses. Prepare the patient for diagnostic tests, such as corneal scraping and slit-lamp examination.

Pediatric pointers

Suspect photophobia in any child who squints, rubs his eyes frequently, or wears sunglasses indoors and outside. Congenital disorders, such as albinism, and childhood diseases, such as measles and rubella, can cause photophobia.

Pica

Pica refers to the craving and ingestion of normally inedible substances, such as plaster, charcoal, clay, wool, ashes, paint, or dirt, over at least 1 month. In children, the most commonly affected group, pica typically results from nutritional deficiencies. It's commonly seen in pregnant patients and may be associated with iron deficiency anemia due to increased demands for iron. However, in adults, pica may reflect a psychological disturbance. Depending on the substance eaten, pica can lead to poisoning and GI disorders.

History and physical examination

Begin by determining what substances the patient has been eating. If the patient has eaten toxic substances, such as lead, obtain a serum lead level. If the patient is a child, ask the parents to describe his eating habits and nutritional history. When did the child first display pica? Does he always crave the same substance? Is he listless or irritable?

Check the patient's vital signs, noting especially bradycardia, tachycardia, or hypotension. Then inspect the abdomen for visible peristaltic waves or other abnormalities. Observe the hair, skin, and mucous membranes for changes, such as dryness or pallor.

Medical causes

◆ ***Anemia (iron deficiency).*** Chronic, severe iron deficiency anemia may cause pica for dirt, paint, cornstarch, nails, or clay (although controversy exists over whether pica is the cause or the result of the deficiency). Pica may also cause fatigue, irritability, listlessness, and anorexia. The patient may complain of light-headedness, headache, an inability to concentrate, dysphagia, and exertional dyspnea. His muscle tone is poor, and he may experience paresthesia in his extremities. His nails are brittle and spoon shaped, his tongue is smooth, and his skin and mucous membranes are pale.

◆ ***Malnutrition.*** Severe malnutrition and starvation may cause pica for any substance, including dirt. Besides marked weight loss, the patient may develop muscle wasting and paresthesia in the extremities. He appears lethargic and apathetic. His skin is dry, thin, and flaky. His sparse, dull hair falls out easily. His nails are brittle, his cheeks are dark and swollen, and his lips are red and swollen. The patient may also experience nausea and vomiting, hepatomegaly, bradycardia, hypotension, slow and shallow respirations, and amenorrhea or gonadal atrophy.

◆ ***Psychological disorders.*** Pica can occur with psychological disorders marked by profound impairment, such as schizophrenia and autism.

CULTURAL CUE *Pica is an accepted practice in some cultures, based on presumed nutritional or therapeutic properties or on religious or superstitious beliefs.*

PEDIATRIC POINTERS

Many older homes contain lead-based paints. Children who live in older homes may be at risk for lead poisoning from eating chipped paint or even from sucking their fingers if the lead paint has infiltrated house dust. Serum lead levels of inner-city children and children in older homes should be monitored. Refer them to a dietitian for nutritional counseling.

Pleural friction rub

Commonly resulting from a pulmonary disorder or trauma, this loud, coarse, grating, creaking, or squeaking sound may be auscultated over one or both lungs during late inspiration or early expiration. It's heard best over the low axilla or the anterior, lateral, or posterior bases of the lung fields with the patient upright. Sometimes intermittent, it may resemble crackles or a pericardial friction rub. (See *Comparing auscultation findings,* pages 532 and 533.)

A pleural friction rub indicates inflammation of the visceral and parietal pleural lining, which causes congestion and edema. The resultant fibrinous exudate covers both pleural surfaces, displacing the fluid that's normally between them and causing the surfaces to rub together.

EMERGENCY INTERVENTIONS *When you detect a pleural friction rub, quickly look for signs of respiratory distress: shallow or decreased respirations; crowing, wheezing, or stridor; dyspnea; increased accessory muscle use; intercostal or suprasternal retractions; cyanosis; and nasal flaring. Check for hypotension, tachycardia, and a decreased level of consciousness.*

If you detect signs of distress, open and maintain an airway. Endotracheal intubation and supplemental oxygen may be necessary. Insert a large-bore I.V. catheter to deliver drugs and fluids. Elevate the patient's head 30 degrees. Monitor cardiac status constantly, and check vital signs frequently.

HISTORY AND PHYSICAL EXAMINATION

If the patient isn't in severe distress, explore related symptoms. Find out if he has had chest pain. If so, ask him to describe its location and severity. How long does the pain last? Does it radiate to his shoulder, neck, or upper abdomen? Does it worsen with breathing, movement, coughing, or sneezing? Does it abate if he splints his chest, holds his breath, or exerts pressure or lies on the affected side?

CULTURAL CUE *Because pain is subjective and is exacerbated by anxiety, patients who are highly emotional may complain more readily of pleuritic pain than those who are habitually stoic about symptoms of illness.*

Ask the patient about a history of rheumatoid arthritis, a respiratory or cardiovascular disorder, recent trauma, asbestos exposure, or radiation therapy. If he smokes, obtain a history in pack-years.

Characterize the pleural friction rub by auscultating the lungs with the patient sitting upright and breathing deeply and slowly through his mouth. Is the friction rub unilateral or bilateral? Listen for absent or diminished breath sounds, noting their location and timing in the respiratory cycle. Do abnormal breath sounds clear with coughing? Observe the patient for clubbing and pedal edema, which may indicate a chronic disorder. Then palpate for decreased chest motion and percuss for flatness or dullness.

MEDICAL CAUSES

◆ ***Asbestosis.*** Besides a pleural friction rub, this disorder may cause exertional dyspnea, cough, chest pain, and crackles. Clubbing is a late sign.

◆ ***Lung cancer.*** A pleural friction rub may be heard in the affected area of the lung. Other effects include a cough (with possible hemoptysis), dyspnea, chest pain, weight loss, anorexia, fatigue, clubbing, fever, and wheezing.

◆ ***Pleurisy.*** A pleural friction rub occurs early in this disorder. However, the cardinal symptom is sudden, intense chest pain that's usually unilateral and located in the lower and lateral parts of the chest. Deep breathing, coughing, or thoracic movement aggravates the pain. Decreased breath sounds and inspiratory crackles may be heard over the painful area. Other findings include dyspnea, tachypnea, tachycardia, cyanosis, fever, and fatigue.

◆ ***Pneumonia (bacterial).*** A pleural friction rub occurs with this disorder, which usually starts with a dry, painful, hacking cough that rapidly becomes productive. Related effects develop suddenly; these include shaking chills, high fever, headache, dyspnea, pleuritic chest pain, tachypnea, tachycardia, grunting respirations, nasal flaring, dullness to percussion, and cyanosis. Auscultation reveals decreased breath sounds and fine crackles.

◆ ***Pulmonary embolism.*** An embolism can cause a pleural friction rub over the affected area of the lung. Usually, the first symptom is sudden dyspnea, which may be accompanied by angina or unilateral pleuritic chest pain. Other clinical features include a nonproductive cough or a cough that produces blood-tinged sputum, tachycardia, tachypnea, low-grade fever, restlessness, and diaphoresis. Less-common findings include massive hemoptysis, chest splinting, leg edema and, with a large embolus, cyanosis, syncope, and jugular vein distention. Crackles, diffuse wheezing, decreased breath sounds, and signs of circulatory collapse may also occur.

◆ ***Rheumatoid arthritis.*** This disorder occasionally causes a unilateral pleural friction rub, but more typical early findings include fatigue, persistent low-grade fever, weight loss, and vague arthralgias and myalgias. Later findings include warm, swollen, painful joints; joint stiffness after inactivity; subcutaneous nodules on the elbows; joint deformity; and muscle weakness and atrophy.

◆ ***Systemic lupus erythematosus.*** Pulmonary involvement can cause a pleural friction rub, hemoptysis, dyspnea, pleuritic chest pain, and crackles. More characteristic effects include a butterfly rash, nondeforming joint pain and stiffness, and photosensitivity. Fever, anorexia, weight loss, and lymphadenopathy may also occur.

◆ ***Tuberculosis (pulmonary).*** With this disorder, a pleural friction rub may occur over the affected part of the lung. Early signs and symptoms include weight loss, night sweats, low-grade fever in the afternoon, malaise, dyspnea, anorexia, and easy fatigability. Progression of the disorder usually produces pleuritic pain, fine crackles over the upper lobes, and a productive cough with blood-streaked sputum. Advanced tuberculosis can cause chest retraction, tracheal deviation, and dullness to percussion.

OTHER CAUSES

◆ ***Treatments.*** Thoracic surgery and radiation therapy can cause pleural friction rub.

SPECIAL CONSIDERATIONS

Continue to monitor the patient's respiratory status and vital signs. If the patient's persistent dry, hacking cough tires him, administer an antitussive. (Avoid giving an opioid, which can further depress respirations.) Administer oxygen and an antibiotic. Prepare the patient for diagnostic tests such as chest X-rays.

PEDIATRIC POINTERS

Auscultate for a pleural friction rub in a child who has grunting respirations, reports chest pain, or protects his chest by holding it or lying on one side. A pleural friction rub in a child is usually an early sign of pleurisy.

GERIATRIC POINTERS

In elderly patients, the intensity of pleuritic chest pain may mimic that of cardiac chest pain.

PATIENT COUNSELING

Because pleuritic pain commonly accompanies a pleural friction rub, teach the patient splinting maneuvers to increase his comfort. Apply a heating pad over the affected area and administer an analgesic for pain relief. Although coughing may be painful, instruct the patient not to suppress it because coughing and deep breathing help prevent respiratory complications. Inform the patient that the pain associated with a pleural friction rub may persist even after the cause of the rub has been resolved.

Polydipsia

Polydipsia refers to excessive thirst, a common symptom associated with endocrine disorders and certain drugs. It may reflect decreased fluid intake, increased urine output, or excessive loss of water and salt.

HISTORY AND PHYSICAL EXAMINATION

Obtain a history. Find out how much fluid the patient drinks each day. How often and how much does he typically urinate? Does the need to urinate awaken him at night? Determine if he or anyone in his family has diabetes or kidney disease. What medications does he use? Has his lifestyle changed recently? If so, have these changes upset him?

If the patient has polydipsia, take his blood pressure and pulse when he's in supine and standing positions. A decrease of 10 mm Hg in systolic pressure and a pulse rate increase of 10 beats/minute from the supine position to the sitting or standing position may indicate hypovolemia. If you detect these changes, ask the patient about recent weight loss. Check for signs of dehydration, such as dry mucous membranes and decreased skin turgor. Infuse I.V. replacement fluids as needed.

MEDICAL CAUSES

◆ ***Diabetes insipidus.*** This disorder characteristically produces polydipsia and may also cause excessive voiding of dilute urine and mild to moderate nocturia. Fatigue and signs of dehydration occur in severe cases.

◆ ***Diabetes mellitus.*** Polydipsia is a classic finding with this disorder—a consequence of the hyperosmolar state. Other characteristic findings include polyuria, polyphagia, nocturia, weakness, fatigue, and weight loss. Signs of dehydration may occur.

◆ ***Hypercalcemia.*** As this disorder progresses, the patient develops polydipsia, polyuria, nocturia, constipation, paresthesia and, occasionally, hematuria and pyuria. Severe hypercalcemia can progress quickly to vomiting, decreased level of consciousness, and renal failure. Depression, mental lassitude, and increased sleep requirements are common.

◆ ***Hypokalemia.*** This electrolyte imbalance can cause nephropathy, resulting in polydipsia, polyuria, and nocturia. Related hypokalemic signs and symptoms include muscle weakness or paralysis, fatigue, decreased bowel sounds, hypoactive deep tendon reflexes, and arrhythmias.

◆ ***Psychogenic polydipsia.*** This uncommon disorder causes polydipsia and polyuria. This condition may occur with any psychiatric disorder, but more common with schizophrenia. Signs of psychiatric disturbances, such as anxiety or depression, are typical. Other findings include headache, blurred vision, weight gain, edema, elevated blood pressure and, occasionally, stupor and coma. Signs of heart failure may develop with overhydration.

◆ ***Renal disorders (chronic).*** Chronic renal disorders, such as glomerulonephritis and pyelonephritis, damage the kidneys, causing polydipsia and polyuria. Associated signs and symptoms include nocturia, weakness, elevated blood pressure, pallor and, in later stages, oliguria.

◆ ***Sheehan's syndrome.*** Polydipsia, polyuria, and nocturia occur within this syndrome of postpartum pituitary necrosis. Other features include fatigue, failure to lactate, amenorrhea, decreased pubic and axillary hair growth, and reduced libido.

◆ ***Sickle cell anemia.*** As nephropathy develops, polydipsia and polyuria occur. They may be accompanied by abdominal pain and cramps, arthralgia and, occasionally, lower extremity skin ulcers, and bone deformities, such as kyphosis and scoliosis.

◆ ***Thyrotoxicosis.*** This disorder infrequently causes polydipsia. Characteristic findings include tachycardia, palpitations, weight loss despite increased appetite, diarrhea, tremors, an enlarged thyroid, dyspnea, nervousness, diaphoresis, and heat intolerance. Exophthalmos may also occur.

OTHER CAUSES

◆ ***Drugs.*** Diuretics and demeclocycline may produce polydipsia. Phenothiazines and anticholinergics can cause dry mouth, making the patient so thirsty that he drinks compulsively.

SPECIAL CONSIDERATIONS

Carefully monitor the patient's fluid balance by recording his total intake and output. Weigh the patient at the same time each day, in the same clothing, and using the same scale. Regularly check blood pressure and pulse in the supine and standing positions to detect orthostatic hypotension, which may indicate hypovolemia. Because thirst is usually the body's way of compensating for water loss, give the patient ample liquids.

PEDIATRIC POINTERS

In children, polydipsia usually stems from diabetes insipidus or diabetes mellitus. Rare causes include pheochromocytoma, neuroblastoma, and Prader-Willi syndrome. However, some children develop habitual polydipsia that's unrelated to any disease.

Polyphagia

[Hyperphagia]

Polyphagia refers to voracious or excessive eating. This common symptom can be persistent or intermittent, resulting primarily from endocrine and psychological disorders as well as the use of certain drugs. Depending on the underlying cause, polyphagia may cause weight gain.

History and physical examination

Begin your evaluation by asking the patient what he has eaten and drunk within the last 24 hours. (If he easily recalls this information, ask about his intake for the 2 previous days, for a broader view of his dietary habits.) Note the frequency of meals and the amount and types of food eaten. Find out if the patient's eating habits have changed recently. Has he always had a large appetite? Does his overeating alternate with periods of anorexia? Ask about conditions that may trigger overeating, such as stress, depression, or menstruation. Does the patient actually feel hungry, or does he eat simply because food is available? Does he ever vomit or have a headache after overeating?

Explore related signs and symptoms. Has the patient recently gained or lost weight? Does he feel tired, nervous, or excitable? Has he experienced heat intolerance, dizziness, palpitations, diarrhea, or increased thirst or urination? Obtain a complete drug history, including the use of laxatives or enemas.

During the physical examination, weigh the patient. Tell him his current weight, and watch for any expression of disbelief or anger. Inspect the skin to detect dryness or poor turgor. Palpate the thyroid for enlargement.

Medical causes

◆ ***Anxiety.*** Polyphagia may result from mild to moderate anxiety or emotional stress. Mild anxiety typically produces restlessness, sleeplessness, irritability, repetitive questioning, and constant seeking of attention and reassurance. With moderate anxiety, selective inattention and difficulty concentrating may also occur. Other effects of anxiety may include muscle tension, diaphoresis, GI distress, palpitations, tachycardia, and urinary and sexual dysfunction.

◆ ***Bulimia.*** Most common in women ages 18 to 29, bulimia causes polyphagia that alternates with self-induced vomiting, fasting, or diarrhea. The patient typically weighs less than normal but has a morbid fear of obesity. She appears depressed, has low self-esteem, and conceals her overeating.

◆ ***Diabetes mellitus.*** With this disorder, polyphagia occurs with weight loss, polydipsia, and polyuria. It's accompanied by nocturia, weakness, fatigue, and signs of dehydration, such as dry mucous membranes and poor skin turgor.

◆ ***Migraine headache.*** Polyphagia sometimes precedes a migraine headache. The individual may experience changes in appetite or food cravings. Other prodromal signs and symptoms include fatigue, nausea, vomiting, and a visual aura. Light and noise sensitivity may also occur.

◆ ***Premenstrual syndrome.*** Appetite changes, typified by food cravings and binges, are common with this syndrome. Abdominal bloating, the most common associated finding, may occur with behavioral changes, such as depression and insomnia. Headache, paresthesia, and other neurologic symptoms may also occur. Related findings include diarrhea or constipation, edema and temporary weight gain, palpitations, back pain, breast swelling and tenderness, oliguria, and easy bruising.

◆ ***Thyrotoxicosis.*** This disorder can produce weight loss, despite constant polyphagia. Other characteristics include weakness, nervousness, diarrhea, tremors, diaphoresis, and dyspnea. The patient's hair and nails are thin and brittle, and his thyroid is enlarged. He may also exhibit palpitations, tachycardia, heat intolerance, exophthalmos, and an atrial or ventricular gallop.

Other causes

◆ ***Drugs.*** Corticosteroids, cyproheptadine, and cannabis may increase appetite, causing weight gain.

Special considerations

Offer the patient with polyphagia emotional support, and help him understand its underlying cause. As needed, refer the patient and his family for psychological counseling.

Pediatric pointers

In children, polyphagia commonly results from juvenile diabetes. In infants ages 6 to 18 months, it can result from a malabsorptive disorder such as celiac disease. However, polyphagia may occur normally in a child who is experiencing a sudden growth spurt.

Polyuria

A relatively common sign, polyuria is the daily production and excretion of more than 3 L of urine. It's usually reported by the patient as increased urination, especially when it occurs at night. Polyuria is aggravated by overhydration, consumption of caffeine or alcohol, and excessive ingestion of salt, glucose, or other hyperosmolar substances. (See *Polyuria: Causes and associated findings*, pages 544 and 545.)

Polyuria usually results from the use of certain drugs, such as a diuretic or from a psychological, neurologic, or renal disorder. It can reflect central nervous system dysfunction that diminishes or suppresses secretion of antidiuretic hormone (ADH), which regulates fluid balance. Or, when ADH levels are normal, it can reflect renal impairment. In both of these pathophysiologic mechanisms, the renal tubules fail to reabsorb sufficient water, causing polyuria.

History and physical examination

Because the patient with polyuria is at risk for developing hypovolemia, evaluate fluid status first. Take vital signs, noting increased body temperature, tachycardia, and orthostatic hypotension (a 10-mm Hg decrease in systolic blood pressure upon standing and a 10-beats per minute increase in heart rate upon standing). Inspect for dry skin and mucous membranes, decreased skin turgor and elasticity, and reduced perspiration. Is the patient unusually tired or thirsty? Has he recently lost more than 5% of his body weight? If you detect these effects of hypovolemia, you'll need to infuse replacement fluids.

If the patient doesn't display signs of hypovolemia, explore the frequency and pattern of the polyuria. When did it begin? How long has it lasted? Was it precipitated by a certain event? Ask the patient to describe the pattern and amount of his daily fluid intake. Check for a history of visual deficits, headaches, or head trauma, which may precede diabetes insipidus. Also check for a history of urinary tract obstruction, diabetes mellitus, renal disorder, chronic hypokalemia or hypercalcemia, or psychiatric disorder (both past and present). Find out the schedule and dosage of any drugs the patient is taking.

Perform a neurologic examination, noting especially any change in the patient's level of consciousness. Then palpate the bladder and inspect the urethral meatus. Obtain a urine specimen and check its specific gravity.

Medical causes

◆ ***Acute tubular necrosis.*** During the diuretic phase of this disorder, polyuria of less than 8 L/day gradually subsides after 8 to 10 days. Urine specific gravity (1.010 or less) increases as polyuria subsides. Related findings include weight loss, decreasing edema, and nocturia.

◆ ***Diabetes insipidus.*** Polyuria of about 5 L/day with a specific gravity of 1.005 or less is common, although extreme polyuria—up to 30 L/day—occasionally occurs. Polyuria is commonly accompanied by polydipsia, nocturia, fatigue, and signs of dehydration, such as poor skin turgor and dry mucous membranes.

◆ ***Diabetes mellitus.*** With this disorder, polyuria seldom exceeds 5 L/day, and urine specific gravity typically exceeds 1.020. The patient usually reports polydipsia, polyphagia, weight loss, weakness, frequent urinary tract infections and yeast vaginitis, fatigue, and nocturia. The patient may also display signs of dehydration and anorexia.

◆ ***Glomerulonephritis (chronic).*** Polyuria gradually progresses to oliguria with this disorder. Urine output is usually less than 4 L/day; specific gravity is about 1.010. Related GI findings include anorexia, nausea, and vomiting. The patient may experience drowsiness, fatigue, edema, headache, elevated blood pressure, and dyspnea. Nocturia, hematuria, frothy or malodorous urine, and mild to severe proteinuria may occur.

◆ ***Hypercalcemia.*** Elevated plasma calcium levels may lead to nephropathy, usually producing polyuria of less than 5 L/day with a specific gravity of about 1.010. Accompanying signs and symptoms include polydipsia, nocturia, constipation, paresthesia and, occasionally, hematuria, and pyuria. With severe hypercalcemia, the patient's condition worsens rapidly and he experiences anorexia, vomiting, stupor progressing to coma, and renal failure.

◆ ***Hypokalemia.*** Prolonged potassium depletion may lead to nephropathy, which results in polyuria—usually less than 5 L/day with a specific gravity of about 1.010. Associated findings include polydipsia, circumoral and foot paresthesia, hypoactive deep tendon reflexes, fatigue, hypoactive bowel sounds, nocturia, arrhythmias, and muscle cramping, weakness, or paralysis.

◆ ***Postobstructive uropathy.*** After resolution of a urinary tract obstruction, polyuria—usually more than 5 L/day with a specific gravity of less than 1.010—occurs for up to several days before gradually subsiding. Bladder distention and edema may occur with nocturia and weight loss. Occasionally, signs of dehydration appear.

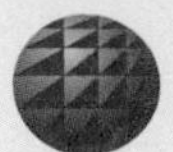

SIGNS & SYMPTOMS

Polyuria: Causes and associated findings

Major associated signs and symptoms

Common causes	Anorexia	Blood pressure increase	Constipation	Dyspnea	Dysuria	Edema	Fatigue	Fever	Flank pain	Headache	Hematuria	Level of consciousness, altered	Mucous membrane dryness
Acute tubular necrosis						●							
Diabetes insipidus							●						●
Diabetes mellitus	●						●						●
Glomerulonephritis (chronic)	●	●		●		●	●			●	●		
Hypercalcemia	●		●								●	●	
Hypokalemia	●						●						
Postobstructive uropathy						●							●
Psychogenic polydipsia		●				●				●		●	
Pyelonephritis (acute)	●				●			●	●		●		
Pyelonephritis (chronic)	●	●					●						
Sheehan's syndrome							●						
Sickle cell anemia							●						

◆ ***Psychogenic polydipsia.*** Most common in those older than age 30, this disorder usually produces dilute polyuria of 3 to 15 L/day, depending on fluid intake. The patient may appear depressed and have a headache and blurred vision. Weight gain, edema, elevated blood pressure and, occasionally, stupor or coma may develop. With severe overhydration, signs of heart failure may present.

◆ ***Pyelonephritis.*** Acute pyelonephritis usually results in polyuria of less than 5 L/day with a low but variable specific gravity. Other findings include persistent high fever, flank pain (usually unilateral), hematuria, costovertebral angle tenderness, chills, weakness, dysuria, urinary frequency and urgency, tenesmus, and nocturia. Occasionally, nausea, anorexia, vomiting, and hypoactive bowel sounds occur.

Chronic pyelonephritis produces polyuria of less than 5 L/day that declines as renal function worsens. Urine specific gravity is usually about 1.010 but may be higher if proteinuria is present. Other effects include irritability, paresthesia, fatigue, nausea, vomiting, diarrhea, drowsiness,

	Nocturia	Paresthesia	Personality changes	Polydipsia	Polyphagia	Pyuria	Vomiting	Weakness	Weight gain	Weight loss
	●									●
	●			●						
	●			●	●			●		●
	●						●			
	●	●		●		●	●			
	●	●		●				●		
	●									●
			●						●	
	●						●	●		
		●				●	●			
	●			●						
				●						

anorexia, pyuria and, in late stages, elevated blood pressure.

◆ ***Sheehan's syndrome.*** This syndrome of postpartum pituitary necrosis may cause polyuria of over 5 L/day with a specific gravity of 1.001 to 1.005. Associated findings include polydipsia, nocturia, and fatigue. Reproductive effects include failure to lactate, amenorrhea, decreased pubic and axillary hair growth, and reduced libido.

◆ ***Sickle cell anemia.*** This disorder may cause nephropathy, typically producing polyuria of less than 5 L/day with a specific gravity of about 1.020. Additional findings include polydipsia, fatigue, abdominal cramps, arthralgia, priapism and, occasionally, leg ulcers, and bony deformities.

Other causes

◆ ***Diagnostic tests.*** Transient polyuria can result from radiographic tests that use contrast media.

◆ ***Drugs.*** Diuretics characteristically produce polyuria. Cardiotonics, vitamin D, demeclocycline, phenytoin, lithium, and propoxyphene can also produce polyuria.

Special considerations

Maintaining adequate fluid balance is your primary concern when the patient has polyuria. Record intake and output accurately, and weigh him daily. Closely monitor the patient's vital signs to detect fluid imbalance, and encourage him to drink adequate fluids. Review his medications, and recommend modification where possible to help control symptoms.

Prepare the patient for serum electrolyte, osmolality, blood urea nitrogen, and creatinine studies to monitor fluid and electrolyte status, and for a fluid deprivation test to determine the cause of polyuria.

Pediatric pointers

The major causes of polyuria in children are congenital nephrogenic diabetes insipidus, medullary cystic disease, polycystic renal disease, and distal renal tubular acidosis.

Because a child's fluid balance is more delicate than an adult's, check his urine specific gravity at each voiding, and be alert for signs of dehydration. These include a decrease in body weight; decreased skin turgor; pale, mottled, or gray skin; dry mucous membranes; decreased urine output; and absence of tears when crying.

Geriatric pointers

In elderly patients, chronic pyelonephritis is commonly associated with an underlying disorder. The possibility of associated malignant disease must be investigated.

Postnasal drip

Nasal discharge, frequent throat clearing, and mucoid or mucopurulent secretions in the posterior pharynx suggest postnasal drip. This symptom

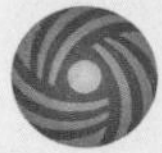

EXAMINATION TIP

Palpating the sinuses

When your patient reports postnasal drip, assess his sinuses for swelling and tenderness—telltale signs of sinusitis. To do this, carefully press up with your thumb on the areas illustrated below. Avoid placing pressure on the eyes.

Tenderness and swelling beneath the middle of the eyebrows may indicate frontal sinusitis; over the cheeks, maxillary sinusitis.

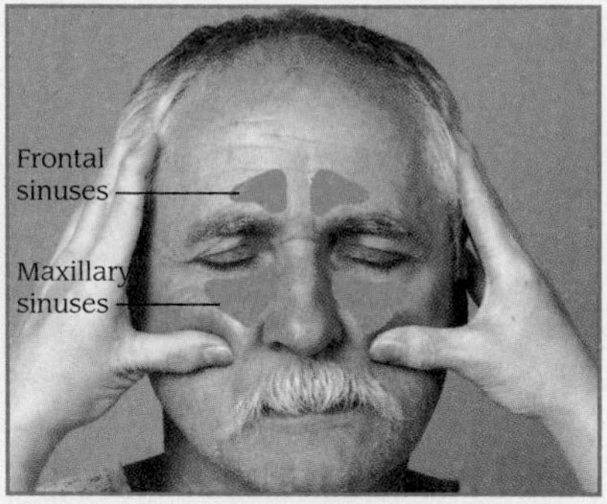

typically results from infection or allergies—a thick, tenacious, and purulent discharge suggests infection, whereas a watery discharge usually suggests an allergy. Postnasal drip may also result from environmental irritants.

History and physical examination

Ask the patient when his postnasal drip began and if it's continuous or intermittent. Does it occur during a certain season? What relieves or aggravates it? Ask about related signs and symptoms, such as cough, sinus pain, headache, and nasal congestion. Take an allergy history, and ask about occupational exposure to environmental irritants (chemical fumes, dust).

If the patient has mucosal swelling, use a vasoconstricting nasal spray before beginning the nasal examination. Then use a nasal speculum to assess the mucous membranes, which are normally pink to dull red. Observe the size and shape of the turbinates and septum, noting any abnormal structures and characterizing the secretions. If the patient wears dentures, ask him to remove them before you examine his throat. Use a tongue blade to examine the oropharynx and a size-0 indirect mirror or fiberoptic nasopharyngoscope to examine the nasopharynx for drainage. Finally, palpate the sinus areas for swelling and tenderness. (See *Palpating the sinuses*.)

Medical causes

◆ ***Rhinitis.*** Two types of rhinitis—allergic and vasomotor—can produce postnasal drip. With allergic rhinitis, symptoms can occur seasonally, as with hay fever, or year-round, as with chronic rhinitis. Nasal obstruction and edematous, pale nasal mucosa may be apparent. The mucosal surface appears smooth and shiny, and the turbinates fill the air space and press against the nasal septum. The patient has swollen, red eyelids and conjunctivae and excessive tearing. He also develops paroxysmal sneezing, a thin nasal discharge, a diminished sense of smell, frontal or temporal headache, and eye, nose and, possibly, throat itching.

A recurrent postnasal drip occurs with vasomotor rhinitis, which can be aggravated by dry air or other environmental triggers. Related findings include engorged inferior turbinates, nasal obstruction, sneezing, watery or sticky rhinorrhea, a pink nasal septum, and bluish mucosa.

◆ ***Sinusitis.*** This disorder commonly produces postnasal drip. It may also cause headache, sinus pain, purulent rhinorrhea, halitosis, fever, sore throat, cough, malaise, and red, swollen nasal mucosa and turbinates.

Other causes

◆ ***Environmental irritants.*** Exposure to environmental irritants, such as fumes, smoke, or dust, may cause postnasal drip. Other findings depend on the type of irritant and the duration of exposure but may include a cough and itching or burning eyes, nose, and throat.

Special considerations

If sinus pain accompanies postnasal drip, apply wet hot packs to the sinuses and instruct the patient to avoid nasal irritants such as tobacco smoke. Prepare the patient for diagnostic tests, such as sinus X-rays, computed tomography scan, and culture and sensitivity studies.

Pediatric pointers

If a child has postnasal drip (less common in children than a runny nose), inspect his nose by pushing its tip upward to visualize the anterior nares. If the child is younger than age 5, use a pediatric fiber-optic nasopharyngoscope to examine the nasopharynx.

PATIENT COUNSELING

Remind the patient not to use an oral decongestant for longer than 1 month at a time. If he has hypertension, advise him to avoid systemic decongestants. Warn against overuse of nasal decongestant sprays, which can produce rebound rhinitis. If he has allergic rhinitis, recommend an antihistamine.

Priapism

A urologic emergency, priapism is a persistent, painful erection that's unrelated to sexual excitation. This relatively rare sign may begin during sleep and appear to be a normal erection, but it may last for several hours or days. It's usually accompanied by a severe, constant, dull aching in the penis. Despite the pain, the patient may be too embarrassed to seek medical help and may try to achieve detumescence through continued sexual activity.

Priapism occurs when the veins of the corpora cavernosa fail to drain correctly, resulting in persistent engorgement of the tissues. Without prompt treatment, penile ischemia and thrombosis occur. In about half of all cases, priapism is idiopathic and develops without apparent predisposing factors. Secondary can priapism result from a blood disorder, neoplasm, trauma, or use of certain drugs.

EMERGENCY INTERVENTIONS *If the patient has priapism, apply an ice pack to the penis, administer an analgesic, and insert an indwelling urinary catheter to relieve urine retention. Procedures to remove blood from the corpora cavernosa, such as irrigation and surgery, may be required.*

HISTORY AND PHYSICAL EXAMINATION

If the patient's condition permits, ask him when the priapism began. Is it continuous or intermittent? Has he had a prolonged erection before? If so, what did he do to relieve it? How long did he remain detumescent? Does he have pain or tenderness when he urinates? Has he noticed any changes in sexual function?

Explore the patient's medical history. If he reports sickle cell anemia, find out about any factors that could precipitate a crisis, such as dehydration and infection. Ask if he has recently suffered genital trauma, and obtain a thorough drug history. Ask if he has had any drugs injected or objects inserted into his penis. Ask if he takes drugs to treat erectile dysfunction.

Examine the patient's penis, noting its color and temperature. Check for loss of sensation and signs of infection, such as redness or drainage. Finally, take his vital signs, particularly noting fever.

MEDICAL CAUSES

- ***Granulocytic leukemia (chronic).*** Priapism is an uncommon sign of this disorder. More characteristic signs and symptoms include fatigue, weakness, malaise, lymphadenopathy, pallor, dyspnea, tachycardia, and bleeding tendencies. Hepatosplenomegaly, bone tenderness, low-grade fever, weight loss, and anorexia may also occur.
- ***Penile cancer.*** Cancer that exerts pressure on the corpora cavernosa can cause priapism. Usually, the first sign is a painless ulcerative lesion or an enlarging warty growth on the glans or foreskin, which may be accompanied by localized pain, a foul-smelling discharge from the prepuce, a firm lump near the glans, and lymphadenopathy. Later findings include bleeding, dysuria, urine retention, and bladder distention. Phimosis and poor hygiene have been linked to the development of penile cancer.
- ***Penile trauma.*** Priapism can occur with other signs and symptoms of injury, such as bruising, abrasions, swelling, pain, and hematuria.
- ***Sickle cell anemia.*** With this congenital disorder, painful priapism can occur without warning, usually on awakening. The patient may have a history of priapism, impaired growth and development, and increased susceptibility to infection. Related findings include tachycardia, pallor, weakness, hepatomegaly, dyspnea, joint swelling, joint or bone aching, chest pain, fatigue, murmurs, leg ulcers and, possibly, jaundice and gross hematuria.

  With sickle cell crisis, signs and symptoms of sickle cell anemia may worsen and others, such as abdominal pain and low-grade fever, may appear.
- ***Spinal cord injury.*** With this condition, the patient may be unaware of the onset of priapism. Related effects depend on the extent and level of injury and may include autonomic signs, such as bradycardia.
- ***Stroke.*** A stroke may cause priapism, but sensory loss and aphasia may prevent the patient from noticing or describing it. Other

findings depend on the stroke location and extent but may include contralateral hemiplegia, seizures, headache, dysarthria, dysphagia, ataxia, apraxia, and agnosia. Visual deficits include homonymous hemianopsia, blurring, decreased acuity, and diplopia. Urine retention or incontinence, fecal incontinence, constipation, and vomiting may also occur.

◆ ***Thrombocytopenia.*** This disorder uncommonly produces priapism. More typical characteristics include blood-filled bullae in the mouth and local bleeding, such as epistaxis, ecchymosis, and hematuria. Central nervous system bleeding may cause decreased level of consciousness. Fatigue, weakness, and lethargy may occur.

Other causes

◆ ***Drugs.*** Priapism can result from the use of an erectile dysfunction treatment, phenothiazine, thioridazine, trazodone, an androgenic steroid, an anticoagulant, or an antihypertensive.

Special considerations

Prepare the patient for blood tests to help determine the cause of priapism. If he requires surgery, keep his penis flaccid postoperatively by applying a pressure dressing. At least once every 30 minutes, inspect the glans for signs of vascular compromise, such as coolness or pallor.

Pediatric pointers

In neonates, priapism can result from hypoxia but is usually resolved with oxygen therapy. Priapism is more likely to develop in children with sickle cell disease than in adults with the disease.

Patient counseling

Encourage patients with sickle cell anemia to report episodes of priapism. Quick treatment is necessary to preserve normal sexual function. Tell patients who take an erectile dysfunction drug to contact their physician if an erection that lasts longer than 4 hours occurs.

Pruritus

Commonly provoking scratching to gain relief, this unpleasant itching sensation affects the skin, certain mucous membranes, and the eyes. Most severe at night, pruritus may be exacerbated by increased skin temperature, poor skin turgor, local vasodilation, dermatoses, and stress.

The most common symptom of dermatologic disorders, pruritus may also result from a local or systemic disorder or from drug use. Physiologic pruritus, such as pruritic urticarial papules and plaques of pregnancy, may occur in primigravidas late in the third trimester. Pruritus can also stem from emotional upset or contact with skin irritants.

History and physical examination

If the patient reports pruritus, have him describe its onset, frequency, and intensity. If pruritus occurs at night, ask whether it prevents him from falling asleep or awakens him after he falls asleep. (Generally, pruritus related to dermatoses prevents—but doesn't disturb—sleep.) Is the itching localized or generalized? When is it most severe? How long does it last? Is there a relationship to activities (physical exertion, bathing, applying makeup, or use of perfumes)?

Ask the patient how he cleans his skin. In particular, look for excessive bathing, harsh soaps, contact allergy, and excessively hot water. Does he have occupational exposure to known skin irritants such as glass fiber insulation or chemicals? Ask about the patient's general health and the medications he takes (new medications are suspect). Has he recently traveled abroad? Does he have any pets? Does anyone else in the house report itching? Does exercise, stress, fear, depression, or illness seem to aggravate the itching? Ask about contact with skin irritants, previous skin disorders, and related symptoms. Obtain a complete drug history.

Examine the patient for signs of scratching, such as excoriation, purpura, scabs, scars, or lichenification. Look for primary lesions to help confirm dermatoses.

Medical causes

◆ ***Anemia (iron deficiency).*** This disorder occasionally produces pruritus. Initially asymptomatic, anemia can later cause exertional dyspnea, fatigue, listlessness, pallor, irritability, headache, tachycardia, poor muscle tone and, possibly, murmurs. Chronic anemia causes spoon-shaped (koilonychia) and brittle nails (cheilosis), cracked mouth corners, a smooth tongue (glossitis), and dysphagia.

◆ ***Anthrax (cutaneous).*** Anthrax is an acute infectious disease caused by the gram-positive, spore-forming bacterium *Bacillus anthracis*. It can occur in humans who are exposed to infected animals, tissue from infected animals, or biological warfare. Cutaneous anthrax occurs when the bacterium enters a cut or abrasion on the skin. The infection begins as a small, painless or pruritic macular or papular lesion resembling an insect bite. Within 1 to 2 days it develops into a vesicle and then a painless ulcer with a characteristic black, necrotic center. Lymphadenopathy, malaise, headache, or fever may develop.

◆ ***Conjunctivitis.*** All forms of conjunctivitis cause eye itching, burning, and pain along with photophobia, conjunctival injection, a foreign body sensation, excessive tearing, and a feeling of fullness around the eye. Allergic conjunctivitis may also cause milky redness and a stringy eye discharge. Bacterial conjunctivitis typically causes brilliant redness and a mucopurulent, discharge that may make the eyelids stick together. Fungal conjunctivitis produces a thick, purulent discharge and crusting and sticking of the eyelid. Viral conjunctivitis may cause copious tearing—but little discharge—and preauricular lymph node enlargement.

◆ ***Dermatitis.*** Several types of dermatitis can cause pruritus accompanied by a skin lesion. Atopic dermatitis begins with intense, severe pruritus and an erythematous rash on dry skin at flexion points (antecubital fossa, popliteal area, and neck). During a flare-up, scratching may produce edema, scaling, and pustules. With chronic atopic dermatitis, lesions may progress to dry, scaly skin with white dermatographia, blanching, and lichenification.

Mild irritants and allergies can cause contact dermatitis, with itchy small vesicles that may ooze and scale and are surrounded by redness. A severe reaction can produce marked localized edema.

Dermatitis herpetiformis, most common in men between ages 20 and 50, initially causes intense pruritus and stinging. Between 8 and 12 hours later, symmetrically distributed lesions form on the buttocks, shoulders, elbows, and knees. Sometimes, they also form on the neck, face, and scalp. These lesions are erythematous and papular, bullous, or pustular.

◆ ***Enterobiasis.*** Also known as pinworm or seatworm, this benign intestinal disease results from infection by *Enterobius vermicularis.* Adult worms live in the intestine; females migrate to the perianal region to deposit their eggs, causing intense perianal pruritus.

◆ ***Hemorrhoids.*** Anal pruritus may occur in patients with hemorrhoids along with rectal pain and constipation. External hemorrhoids may be seen outside the external anal sphincter; internal hemorrhoids are less obvious and less painful but more likely to cause rectal bleeding.

◆ ***Hepatobiliary disease.*** An important diagnostic clue to liver and gallbladder disease, pruritus is commonly accompanied by jaundice and may be generalized or localized to the palms and soles. Other characteristics include right-upper-quadrant pain, clay-colored stools, chills and fever, flatus, belching and a bloated feeling, epigastric burning, and bitter fluid regurgitation. Later, liver disease may produce mental changes, ascites, bleeding tendencies, spider angiomas, palmar erythema, dry skin, fetor hepaticus, enlarged superficial abdominal veins, bilateral gynecomastia, testicular atrophy or menstrual irregularities, and hepatomegaly.

◆ ***Herpes zoster.*** Within 2 to 4 days of fever and malaise, pruritus, paresthesia or hyperesthesia, and severe, deep pain from cutaneous nerve involvement develop on the trunk or the arms and legs in a dermatome distribution. Up to 2 weeks after initial symptoms, red, nodular skin eruptions appear on the painful areas and become vesicular. About 10 days later, the vesicles rupture and form scabs.

◆ ***Hodgkin's disease.*** This disease, which is most common in young adults, occasionally causes severe and unexplained itching. As the disease progresses, pruritus may become severe and unresponsive to treatment. Early nonspecific findings include persistent fever (occasionally, cyclic fever and chills), night sweats, fatigue, weight loss, malaise, and painless swelling of a cervical lymph node. Other lymph nodes may enlarge rapidly and cause pain, or they may enlarge slowly and be painless. Later findings include retroperitoneal node enlargement, hepatomegaly, splenomegaly, dyspnea, dysphagia, dry cough, hyperpigmentation, jaundice, and pallor.

◆ ***Leukemia (chronic lymphocytic).*** Pruritus is an uncommon finding in this disorder. More characteristic signs and symptoms include fatigue, malaise, generalized lymphadenopathy, fever, hepatomegaly, splenomegaly, weight loss, pallor, bleeding, and palpitations.

◆ ***Lichen planus.*** This uncommon skin disease can cause moderate to severe pruritus that's aggravated by stress. Characteristic oral lesions (white or gray, velvety, lacy, threadlike papules) develop on the buccal mucosa and may cause pain. Violet papules with white lines or spots develop later, usually on the genitalia, lower back, ankles, and shins. Nail distortion and atrophic alopecia may also occur.

◆ ***Lichen simplex chronicus.*** Persistent rubbing and scratching cause localized pruritus and a circumscribed scaling patch with sharp margins. Later, the skin thickens and papules form.

◆ ***Mastocytosis.*** With this disorder, reddish brown macules or papules (urticaria pigmentosa), along with patchy erythema and telangiectasia occur. Other signs and symptoms include pruritus, flushing, tachycardia, hypotension, and nausea.

◆ ***Multiple myeloma.*** Infrequently, this disorder produces pruritus. Other findings include severe, constant back pain that increases with exercise; achiness; joint swelling and tenderness; fever; malaise; slight peripheral neuropathy; and purpura.

◆ ***Mycosis fungoides.*** Pruritus may precede other symptoms of this neoplastic disease by 10 years. It may persist into the first, or premycotic, stage, accompanied by erythematous lesions.

◆ ***Myringitis (chronic).*** This disorder produces pruritus in the affected ear, along with a purulent discharge and gradual hearing loss.

◆ ***Pediculosis.*** A prominent symptom, pruritus occurs in the area of infestation. Pediculosis capitis (head lice) may also cause scalp excoriation from scratching, along with matted, foul-smelling, lusterless hair; occipital and cervical lymphadenopathy; and oval, gray-white nits on hair shafts.

Pediculosis corporis (body lice) initially causes small red papules (usually on the shoulders, trunk, or buttocks), which become urticarial from scratching. Later, rashes or wheals may develop. Untreated, pediculosis corporis produces dry, discolored, thickly encrusted, scaly skin with bacterial infection and scarring. In severe cases, it produces headache, fever, and malaise.

With pediculosis pubis (pubic lice), scratching commonly produces skin irritation. Nits or adult lice and erythematous, itching papules may appear in pubic hair or hair around the anus, abdomen, or thighs.

◆ ***Pityriasis rosea.*** This disorder occasionally produces mild pruritus that's aggravated by a hot bath or shower. It usually begins with an erythematous herald patch—a slightly raised, oval lesion about 2 to 6 cm in diameter. After a few days or weeks, scaly yellow-tan or erythematous patches erupt on the trunk and extremities and persist for 2 to 6 weeks. Occasionally, these patches are macular, vesicular, or urticarial.

◆ ***Polycythemia vera.*** This hematologic disorder can produce pruritus that's generalized or localized to the head, neck, face, and extremities. The itching is typically aggravated by a hot bath or shower and can last from a few minutes to an hour. The patient's oral mucosa may be deep purplish red, especially on the gingivae and tongue. His engorged gingivae ooze blood with even slight trauma.

Related findings include headache, dizziness, fatigue, dyspnea, paresthesia, impaired mentation, tinnitus, double or blurred vision, scotoma, hypotension, intermittent claudication, urticaria, ruddy cyanosis, and ecchymosis. GI effects include gastric distress, weight loss, and hepatosplenomegaly.

◆ ***Psoriasis.*** Pruritus and pain are common in psoriasis. This skin disorder typically begins with small erythematous papules that enlarge or coalesce to form red elevated plaques with silver scales on the scalp, chest, elbows, knees, back, buttocks, and genitals. Nail pitting may occur.

◆ ***Psychogenic pruritus.*** Localized or generalized pruritus occurs without symptoms of dermatologic or systemic disease. Anxiety or emotional lability may be evident.

◆ ***Renal failure (chronic).*** Pruritus may develop gradually or suddenly with this disorder. It may be accompanied by ammonia breath odor, oliguria or anuria, lassitude, fatigue, irritability, decreased mental acuity, convulsions, coarse muscular twitching, muscle cramps, peripheral neuropathies, and coma. Renal failure also causes diverse GI signs and symptoms, such as anorexia, constipation or diarrhea, nausea, and vomiting.

◆ ***Scabies.*** Typically, scabies causes localized pruritus that awakens the patient. It may become generalized and persist up to 2 weeks after treatment. Threadlike lesions several millimeters long appear with a swollen nodule or red papule.

GENDER CUE *In males, crusty lesions may form on the glans penis, penile shaft, and scrotum. In females, lesions may also be found on or around nipples. In both sexes the lesions have a predilection for skin folds. Crusty excoriated lesions form on the wrists, elbows, axillae, waistline, behind the knees and ankles. Excoriation from scratching is common.*

◆ ***Thyrotoxicosis.*** Generalized pruritus may precede or accompany the characteristic signs and symptoms of this disorder: tachycardia, palpitations, weight loss despite increased appetite, diarrhea, tremors, an enlarged thyroid, dyspnea, nervousness, diaphoresis, heat intolerance and, possibly, exophthalmos.
◆ ***Tinea pedis.*** This fungal infection causes severe foot pruritus, pain with walking, scales and blisters between the toes, and a dry, scaly squamous inflammation on the entire sole.
◆ ***Urticaria.*** Extreme pruritus and stinging occur as transient erythematous or whitish wheals form on the skin or mucous membranes. Prickly sensations typically precede the wheals, which may affect any part of the body and may range from pinpoint to palm-sized or larger.
◆ ***Vaginitis.*** This disorder commonly causes localized pruritus and foul-smelling vaginal discharge that may be purulent, white or gray, and curdlike. Perineal pain and urinary dysfunction may also occur.

Other causes

◆ ***Bedbug bites.*** Typically, bedbug bites produce itching and burning over the ankles and lower legs, along with clusters of purpuric spots.
◆ ***Drug hypersensitivity.*** When mild and localized, an allergic reaction to such drugs as penicillin and sulfonamides can cause pruritus, erythema, an urticarial rash, and edema. However, with a severe drug reaction, anaphylaxis may occur.

HERB ALERT *Ingestion of fruit pulp from the ginkgo tree can cause rapid formation of vesicles, resulting in severe itching.*

Special considerations

Administer a topical or oral corticosteroid, an antihistamine, or a tranquilizer, as ordered. If the patient doesn't have a localized infection or skin lesions, suspect a systemic disease and prepare him for a complete blood count and differential, erythrocyte sedimentation rate, protein electrophoresis, and radiologic studies.

Pediatric pointers

Many adult disorders also cause pruritus in children, but they may affect different parts of the body. For instance, scabies may affect the head in infants, but not in adults. Pityriasis rosea may affect the face, hands, and feet of adolescents.

Some childhood diseases, such as measles and chickenpox, can cause pruritus.

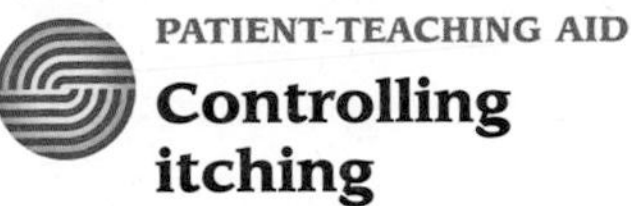

PATIENT-TEACHING AID

Controlling itching

Dear Patient:
To reduce itching and increase comfort, follow these simple steps:
◆ Avoid scratching or rubbing the itchy areas. Ask your family to let you know if you're scratching because you may be unaware of it. Keep your fingernails short to avoid skin damage from any unconscious scratching.
◆ Wear cool, light, loose bedclothes. Avoid wearing rough clothing—particularly wool—over the itchy area.
◆ Take tepid baths, using little soap and rinsing thoroughly. Try a skin-soothing oatmeal or cornstarch bath for a change.
◆ Apply an emollient lotion after bathing to soften and cool the skin.
◆ Apply cold compresses to the itchy area.
◆ Use topical ointments and take prescribed medications as directed.
◆ Avoid prolonged exposure to excessive heat and humidity. For maximum comfort, keep room temperatures at 68° to 70° F (20° to 21.1° C) and humidity at 30% to 40%.
◆ Take up an enjoyable hobby that distracts you from the itching during the day and leaves you tired enough to sleep at night.

Patient counseling

Suggest ways to control pruritus. (See *Controlling itching.*)

Psoas sign

A positive psoas sign—increased abdominal pain when the patient moves his leg against resistance—indicates direct or reflexive irritation of the psoas muscles. This sign, which can be elicited on the right or left side, usually indicates appendicitis but may also occur with localized abscesses. It's elicited in a patient with abdominal or lower back pain *after* completion of an abdominal examination to prevent spurious assessment findings. (See *Eliciting a psoas sign*, page 552.)

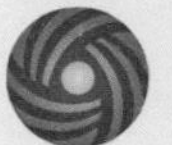

EXAMINATION TIP

Eliciting a psoas sign

You can use two techniques to elicit a psoas sign in an adult with abdominal pain. With either technique, increased abdominal pain is a positive result, indicating psoas muscle irritation from an inflamed appendix or a localized abscess.

With the patient in a supine position, instruct her to move her flexed left leg against your hand to test for a left psoas sign. Then perform this maneuver on the right leg to test for a right psoas sign.

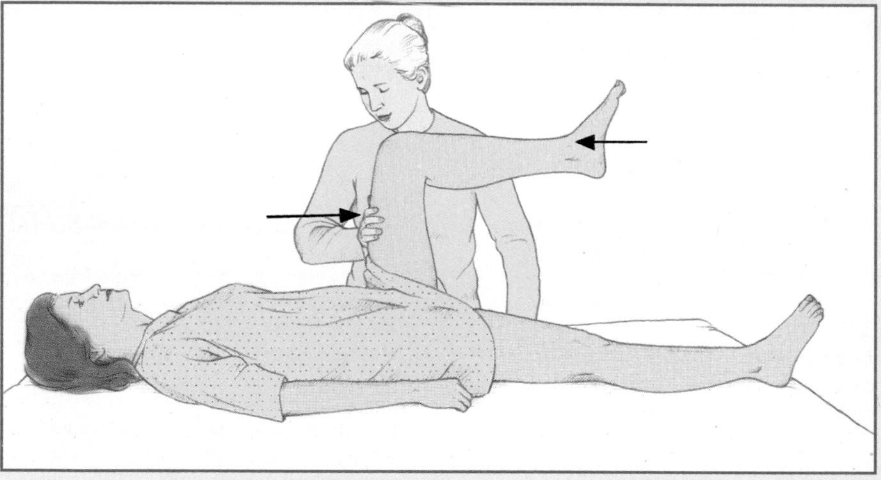

To test for a left psoas sign, turn the patient onto her right side. Then instruct her to push her left leg upward from the hip against your hand. Next, turn the patient onto her left side and repeat this maneuver to test for a right psoas sign.

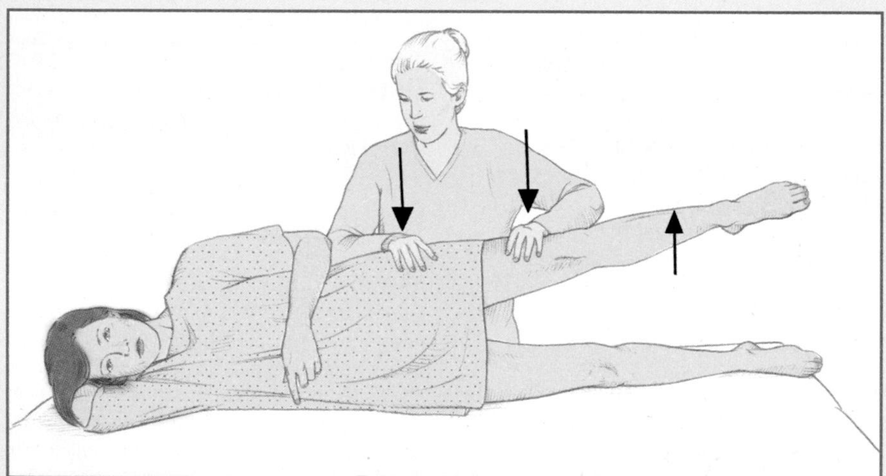

EMERGENCY INTERVENTIONS *If you elicit a positive psoas sign in a patient with abdominal pain, suspect appendicitis. Quickly check the patient's vital signs, and prepare him for surgery: Explain the procedure, restrict food and fluids, and withhold analgesics, which can mask symptoms. Administer I.V. fluids to prevent dehydration, but don't give a cathartic or an enema because it can cause a ruptured appendix and lead to peritonitis.*

Check for Rovsing's sign by deeply palpating the patient's left lower quadrant. If he reports pain in the right lower quadrant, the sign is positive, indicating peritoneal irritation.

MEDICAL CAUSES

◆ ***Appendicitis.*** An inflamed retrocecal appendix can cause a positive right psoas sign. Early epigastric and periumbilical pain disappears only to worsen and localize in the right lower quadrant. This pain also worsens with walking or coughing. Related findings include nausea and vomiting, abdominal rigidity and rebound tenderness, and constipation or diarrhea. Fever, tachycardia, retractive respirations, anorexia, and malaise may also occur. If the appendix ruptures, additional findings may include sudden, severe pain, followed by signs of peritonitis, such as hypoactive or absent bowel sounds, high fever, and boardlike abdominal rigidity. A positive obturator sign may also be evident.

◆ ***Retroperitoneal abscess.*** After a lower retroperitoneal infection, an iliac or lumbar abscess can produce a positive right or left psoas sign and fever. An iliac abscess causes iliac or inguinal pain that may radiate to the hip, thigh, flank, or knee; a tender mass in the lower abdomen or groin may be palpable. A lumbar abscess usually produces back tenderness and spasms on the affected side with a palpable lumbar mass; a tender abdominal mass without back pain may occur instead.

SPECIAL CONSIDERATIONS

Monitor vital signs to detect complications, such as pain extension along fascial planes in the abdomen, thigh, hip, subphrenic spaces, mediastinum, and pleural cavities, and peritonitis. Promote patient comfort by helping with position changes. For example, have the patient lie down and flex his right leg. Then have him sit upright.

Prepare the patient for diagnostic tests, such as electrolyte studies and abdominal X-rays.

PEDIATRIC POINTERS

Elicit a psoas sign by asking the child to raise his head while you exert pressure on his forehead. Resulting right-lower-quadrant pain usually indicates appendicitis.

GERIATRIC POINTERS

In elderly patients, the psoas sign and other peritoneal signs may be decreased or absent. Be sure to differentiate pain elicited through psoas maneuvers from musculoskeletal or degenerative joint pain.

Psychotic behavior

Psychotic behavior reflects an inability or unwillingness to recognize and acknowledge reality and to relate with others. It may begin suddenly or insidiously, progressing from vague complaints of fatigue, insomnia, or headache to withdrawal, social isolation, and preoccupation with certain issues resulting in gross impairment in functioning.

Various behaviors together or separately can constitute psychotic behavior. These include delusions, illusions, hallucinations, bizarre language, and perseveration. Delusions are persistent beliefs that have no basis in reality or in the patient's knowledge or experience, such as delusions of grandeur. Illusions are misinterpretations of external sensory stimuli such as a mirage in the desert. In contrast, hallucinations are sensory perceptions that don't result from external stimuli. Bizarre language reflects a communication disruption. It can range from echolalia (purposeless repetition of a word or phrase) and clang association (repetition of words or phrases that sound similar) to neologisms (creation and use of words whose meaning only the patient knows). Perseveration, a persistent verbal or motor response, may indicate organic brain disease. Motor changes include inactivity, excessive activity, and repetitive movements.

HISTORY AND PHYSICAL EXAMINATION

Because the patient's behavior can make it difficult—or potentially dangerous—to obtain pertinent information, conduct the interview in a calm, safe, and well-lit room. Provide enough personal space to avoid threatening or agitating the patient. Ask him to describe his problem and any circumstances that may have precipitated it. Obtain a drug history, noting especially use of an antipsychotic, and explore his use of alcohol and other drugs such as cocaine, indicating duration of use and amount. Ask about any recent illnesses or accidents.

Psychotic behavior: An adverse drug effect

Certain drugs can cause psychotic behavior and other psychiatric signs and symptoms, ranging from depression to violent behavior. Usually, these effects occur during therapy and resolve when the drug is discontinued. If your patient is receiving one of these common drugs and exhibits the behavior described below, the dosage may have to be changed or another drug may have to be substituted.

Drug	Psychiatric signs and symptoms
albuterol	Hallucinations, paranoia
alprazolam	Anger, hostility
amantadine	Visual hallucinations, nightmares
asparaginase	Confusion, depression, paranoia
atropine and anticholinergics	Auditory, visual, and tactile hallucinations; memory loss; delirium; fear; paranoia
bromocriptine	Mania, delusions, sudden relapse of schizophrenia, paranoia, aggressive behavior
cardiac glycosides	Paranoia, euphoria, amnesia, visual hallucinations
cimetidine	Hallucinations, paranoia, confusion, depression, delirium
clonidine	Delirium, hallucinations, depression
corticosteroids (prednisone, corticotropin, cortisone)	Mania, catatonia, depression, confusion, paranoia, hallucinations
cycloserine	Anxiety, depression, confusion, paranoia, hallucinations
dapsone	Insomnia, agitation, hallucinations
diazepam	Suicidal thoughts, rage, hallucinations, depression
disopyramide	Agitation, paranoia, auditory and visual hallucinations, panic
disulfiram	Delirium, auditory hallucinations, paranoia, depression
indomethacin	Hostility, depression, paranoia, hallucinations
lidocaine	Disorientation, hallucinations, paranoia
methyldopa	Severe depression, amnesia, paranoia, hallucinations
propranolol	Severe depression, hallucinations, paranoia, confusion
thyroid hormones	Mania, hallucinations, paranoia
vincristine	Hallucinations

As the patient talks, watch for cognitive, linguistic, or perceptual abnormalities such as delusions. Do thoughts and actions seem to match? Look for unusual gestures, posture, gait, tone of voice, and mannerisms. Does the patient appear to be responding to stimuli? For example, is he looking around the room?

Interview the patient's family. Which family members does he seem closest to? How does the family describe the patient's relationships, communication patterns, and role? Has any family member ever been hospitalized for psychiatric or emotional illness? Ask about the patient's compliance with his drug regimen.

Finally, evaluate the patient's environment, educational and employment history, and socioeconomic status. Are community services available? How does the patient spend his leisure time? Does he have friends? Has he ever had a close emotional relationship?

Medical causes

◆ ***Organic disorders.*** Various disorders, such as alcohol withdrawal syndrome, cocaine or amphetamine intoxication, cerebral hypoxia, and nutritional disorders, can produce psychotic behavior. Endocrine disorders, such as adrenal dysfunction, and severe infections, such as encephalitis, can also cause psychotic behavior. Neurologic causes include Alzheimer's disease and other dementias.

◆ ***Psychiatric disorders.*** Psychotic behavior usually occurs with bipolar disorder, personality disorder, schizophrenia, and some pervasive developmental disorders.

Other causes

◆ ***Drugs.*** Certain drugs can cause psychotic behavior. (See *Psychotic behavior: An adverse drug effect.*) However, almost any drug can provoke

Controlling psychotic behavior

A patient who displays psychotic behavior may be terrified and unable to differentiate between himself and his environment. To control his behavior and to prevent injury to the patient, staff, and others, follow these guidelines.

- Remove potentially dangerous objects, such as belts or metal utensils, from the patient's environment.
- Help the patient discern what is real and unreal in an honest and genuine way.
- Be straightforward, concise, and nonthreatening when speaking to the patient. Discuss simple, concrete subjects and avoid theories or philosophical issues.
- Positively reinforce the patient's perceptions of reality, and correct his misperceptions in a matter-of-fact way.
- *Never* argue with the patient, but also don't support his misperceptions.
- If the patient is frightened, stay with him.
- Touch the patient to provide reassurance *only* if you've done this before and know that it's safe.
- Move the patient to a safer, less-stimulating environment.
- Provide one-on-one care if the patient's behavior is extremely bizarre, disturbing to other patients, or dangerous to himself.
- Medicate the patient appropriately.

psychotic behavior as a rare, severe adverse or idiosyncratic reaction.

- ***Surgery.*** Postoperative delirium and depression may produce psychotic behavior.

Special considerations

Continuously evaluate the patient's orientation to reality. Help him develop a conception of reality by calling him by his preferred name, telling him your name, describing where he is, and using clocks and calendars. (See *Controlling psychotic behavior*.)

Encourage the patient to become involved in structured activities. However, if he's nonverbal or incoherent, be sure to spend time with him. For example, sit or walk with him, or talk about the day, the season, the weather, or other concrete topics. Avoid making time commitments that you can't keep: This will only upset the patient and cause him to withdraw more.

Refer the patient for psychiatric evaluation. Administer an antipsychotic or other drugs, as needed, and prepare him for transfer to a mental health center, if necessary.

Don't overlook the patient's physiologic needs. Check his eating habits to avoid dehydration and malnutrition, and monitor his elimination patterns, especially if he's receiving an antipsychotic, which can cause constipation.

Pediatric pointers

In children, psychotic behavior may result from early infantile autism, symbiotic infantile psychosis, or childhood schizophrenia—any of which can retard development of language, abstract thinking, and socialization. An adolescent patient who exhibits psychotic behavior may have a history of several days' drug use or lack of sleep or food, which must be evaluated and corrected before therapy can begin.

Ptosis

Ptosis is the excessive drooping of one or both upper eyelids. This sign can be constant, progressive, or intermittent, and unilateral or bilateral. When it's unilateral, it's easy to detect by comparing the eyelids' relative positions. When it's bilateral or mild, it's difficult to detect—the eyelids may be abnormally low, covering the upper part of the iris or even part of the pupil instead of overlapping the iris slightly. Other clues include a furrowed forehead or a tipped-back head—both of these help the patient see under his drooping lids. With severe ptosis, the patient may not be able to raise his eyelids voluntarily. Because ptosis can resemble enophthalmos, exophthalmometry may be required. (See *Differentiating enophthalmos from ptosis,* page 266.)

Ptosis can be classified as congenital or acquired. Classification is important for proper treatment. Congenital ptosis results from levator muscle underdevelopment or disorders of the third cranial (oculomotor) nerve. Acquired ptosis may result from trauma to or inflammation of these muscles and nerves, or from certain drugs, a systemic disease, an intracranial lesion, or a life-threatening aneurysm. However, the most common cause is advanced age, which reduces muscle elasticity and produces senile ptosis.

History and physical examination

Ask the patient when he first noticed his drooping eyelid and whether it has worsened or improved. Find out if he has recently suffered a traumatic eye injury. (If he has, avoid manipulating the eye to prevent further damage.) Ask about eye pain or headache, and determine its location and severity. Has the patient experienced any vision changes? If so, have him describe them. Obtain a drug history, noting especially use of a chemotherapeutic drug.

Assess the degree of ptosis, and check for eyelid edema, exophthalmos, deviation, and conjunctival injection. Evaluate extraocular muscle function by testing the six cardinal fields of gaze. Carefully examine the pupils' size, color, shape, and reaction to light, and test visual acuity.

Keep in mind that ptosis occasionally indicates a life-threatening condition. For example, sudden unilateral ptosis can herald a cerebral aneurysm.

Medical causes

◆ ***Alcoholism.*** Long-term alcohol abuse can cause ptosis and such complications as severe weight loss, jaundice, ascites, and mental disturbances.

◆ ***Botulism.*** Acute cranial nerve dysfunction causes hallmark signs of ptosis, dysarthria, dysphagia, and diplopia. Other findings include dry mouth, sore throat, weakness, vomiting, diarrhea, hyporeflexia, and dyspnea.

◆ ***Cerebral aneurysm.*** An aneurysm that compresses the oculomotor nerve can cause sudden ptosis, along with diplopia, a dilated pupil, and inability to rotate the eye. These may be the first signs of this life-threatening disorder. A ruptured aneurysm typically produces sudden severe headache, nausea, vomiting, and decreased level of consciousness (LOC). Other findings include nuchal rigidity, back and leg pain, fever, restlessness, irritability, occasional seizures, blurred vision, hemiparesis, sensory deficits, dysphagia, and visual defects.

◆ ***Dacryoadenitis.*** Ptosis may accompany unilateral exophthalmos, limited extraocular movements, eyelid edema and erythema, conjunctival injection, eye pain, and diplopia.

◆ ***Hemangioma.*** This orbital tumor can produce ptosis, exophthalmos, limited extraocular movement, and blurred vision.

◆ ***Horner's syndrome.*** This disorder causes moderate unilateral ptosis that almost disappears when the patient opens his eyes widely. Common accompanying findings include unilateral miosis and ipsilateral anhidrosis of the face and neck, which may spread to the entire body. Other signs and symptoms include transient conjunctival injection, vascular headache on the affected side, and vertigo.

◆ ***Lacrimal gland tumor.*** This disorder commonly produces mild to severe ptosis, depending on the tumor's size and location. It may also cause brow elevation, exophthalmos, eye deviation and, possibly, eye pain.

◆ ***Levator muscle maldevelopment.*** Ptosis from maldevelopment of the levator muscle of the upper eyelid—formerly classified as true congenital ptosis—is the result of an isolated dystrophy of the levator muscle affecting its contraction and relaxation. Lid lag on downgaze is an important clue to diagnosis.

◆ ***Myasthenia gravis.*** Commonly the first sign of this disorder, gradual bilateral ptosis may be mild to severe and is accompanied by weak eye closure and diplopia. Other characteristics include muscle weakness and fatigue, which eventually may lead to paralysis. Depending on the muscles affected, other findings may include masklike facies, difficulty chewing or swallowing, dyspnea, cyanosis, and others.

◆ ***Myotonic dystrophy.*** This disorder may cause mild to severe bilateral ptosis. Distinctive cataracts with iridescent dots in the cortex, miosis, diplopia, decreased tearing, and muscular and testicular atrophy may also occur.

◆ ***Ocular muscle dystrophy.*** With this disorder, bilateral ptosis progresses slowly to complete eyelid closure. Related signs and symptoms include progressive external ophthalmoplegia and muscle weakness and atrophy of the upper face, neck, trunk, and limbs.

◆ ***Ocular trauma.*** Trauma to the nerve or muscles that control the eyelids can cause mild to severe ptosis. Depending on the damage, eye pain, lid swelling, ecchymosis, and decreased visual acuity may also occur.

◆ ***Parinaud's syndrome.*** This form of ophthalmoplegia can cause ptosis, enophthalmos, nystagmus, lid retraction, dilated pupils with absent or poor light response, and papilledema. The patient's ocular muscles fail to move voluntarily.

◆ ***Parry-Romberg syndrome.*** Unilateral ptosis and facial hemiatrophy occur with this disorder. Other signs include miosis, sluggish pupil reaction to light, enophthalmos, different-colored irises, ocular muscle paralysis, nystagmus, and neck, shoulder, trunk, and extremity atrophy.

◆ ***Subdural hematoma (chronic).*** Ptosis may be a late sign, along with unilateral pupillary dilation and sluggishness. Headache, behavioral changes, and decreased LOC commonly occur.

Other causes

◆ ***Drugs.*** Vinca alkaloids can produce ptosis.
◆ ***Lead poisoning.*** With this disorder, ptosis usually develops over 3 to 6 months. Other findings include anorexia, nausea, vomiting, diarrhea, colicky abdominal pain, a lead line in the gums, decreased LOC, tachycardia, hypotension and, possibly, irritability and peripheral nerve weakness.

Special considerations

If the patient has decreased visual acuity, orient him to his surroundings. Provide special spectacle frames that suspend the eyelid by traction with a wire crutch. These frames are usually used to help patients with temporary paresis or those who aren't good candidates for surgery.

Prepare the patient for diagnostic studies, such as the Tensilon test and slit-lamp examination. If he needs surgery to correct levator muscle dysfunction, explain the procedure to him.

Pediatric pointers

Astigmatism and myopia may be associated with childhood ptosis. Parents typically discover congenital ptosis when their child is an infant. Usually, the ptosis is unilateral, constant, and accompanied by lagophthalmos, which causes the infant to sleep with his eyes open. If this occurs, teach proper eye care to prevent drying.

Pulse, absent or weak

An absent or weak pulse may be generalized or affect only one extremity. When generalized, this sign is an important indicator of such life-threatening conditions as shock and arrhythmia. Localized loss or weakness of a pulse that's normally present and strong may indicate acute arterial occlusion, which could require emergency surgery. However, the pressure of palpation may temporarily diminish or obliterate superficial pulses, such as the posterior tibial or the dorsal pedal. Thus, bilateral weakness or absence of these pulses doesn't necessarily indicate underlying pathology. (See *Evaluating peripheral pulses.*)

Evaluating peripheral pulses

The rate, amplitude, and symmetry of peripheral pulses provide important clues to cardiac function and the quality of peripheral perfusion. To gather these clues, palpate peripheral pulses lightly with the pads of your index, middle, and ring fingers, as space permits.

Rate

Count all pulses for at least 30 seconds (60 seconds when recording vital signs). The normal rate is between 60 and 100 beats/minute.

Amplitude

Palpate the blood vessel during ventricular systole. Describe pulse amplitude by using a scale such as the one below:

4+ = bounding
3+ = increased
2+ = normal
1+ = weak, thready
0 = absent.

Use a stick figure to easily document the location and amplitude of all pulses.

Symmetry

Simultaneously palpate pulses (except for the carotid pulse) on both sides of the patient's body, and note any inequality. Always assess peripheral pulses methodically, moving from the arms to the legs.

History and physical examination

If you detect an absent or weak pulse, quickly palpate the remaining arterial pulses to distinguish between localized or generalized loss or weakness. Then quickly check other vital signs, evaluate cardiopulmonary status, and obtain a brief history. Based on your findings, proceed with emergency interventions. (See *Managing an absent or weak pulse*, pages 558 and 559.)

Medical causes

◆ ***Aortic aneurysm (dissecting).*** When a dissecting aneurysm affects circulation to the innominate, left common carotid, subclavian, or femoral artery, it causes weak or absent arterial pulses distal to the affected area. Absent or

(Text continues on page 560.)

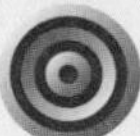

EMERGENCY INTERVENTION

Managing an absent or weak pulse

An absent or weak pulse can result from any one of several life-threatening disorders. Your evaluation and interventions will vary, depending on whether the weak or absent pulse is generalized or localized to one extremity. They'll also depend on associated signs and symptoms. Use the flowchart below to help you establish priorities for successfully managing this emergency.

Absent or weak pulse

Localized to one extremity

Generalized.

Patient is confused and restless; has hypotension and cool, pale, clammy skin.

Patient has a history of trauma, possibly with external bleeding, and reports thirst.

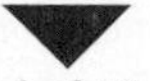

Check for flat jugular veins, low urine output, and narrowed pulse pressure.

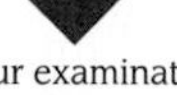

If your examination reveals these findings, suspect hypovolemic shock.

Patient has a history of myocardial infarction (MI) or heart failure.

Check for jugular vein distention, ventricular gallop (S_3), crackles, and narrowed pulse pressure.

If your examination reveals these findings, suspect cardiogenic shock.

Patient has a history of recent cardiac surgery or catheterization, chest trauma, pericardial effusion, or anticoagulant therapy.

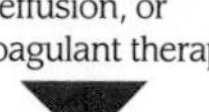

Check for jugular vein distention, pulsus paradoxus, and muffled heart sounds.

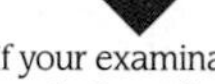

If your examination reveals these findings, suspect cardiac tamponade.

Patient has a history of MI or chronic heart or lung disease.

Check for irregular heart rate, severe tachycardia, and bradycardia.

If your examination reveals these findings, suspect an arrhythmia.

Administer oxygen by nasal cannula, and insert an I.V. catheter for fluid infusion. Begin cardiac monitoring, and check vital signs every 5 to 15 minutes. A central venous pressure catheter, an arterial catheter, or a pulmonary artery catheter may have to be inserted. Be prepared for emergency resuscitation, if necessary.

Anticipate colloid or crystalloid replacement, as well as the need for transfusion.

Anticipate administering nitroprusside, dopamine, and dobutamine.

Anticipate pericardiocentesis.

Anticipate administering antiarrhythmics or delivering cardiac electroshock therapy, or both.

Examine affected extremity for cool, mottled skin and pain.

If your examination reveals these findings, suspect arterial occlusive disease.

Prepare the patient for diagnostic tests to confirm or rule out arterial occlusion, such as arteriography, aortography, or Doppler ultrasonography. Don't elevate the affected extremity. Start an I.V. catheter in an unaffected arm or leg, and administer heparin or thrombotic, as required. Anticipate preparing the patient for emergency embolectomy or peripheral angioplasty.

Patient has a history of trauma, congenital heart disease, or hypertension and reports severe, tearing chest pain.

Check for pulse quality and blood pressure variation between extremities.

If your examination reveals these findings, suspect dissecting aortic aneurysm or aortic coarctation.

Patient has a history of severe infection—frequently gram-negative, urinary, or respiratory tract infection.

Check for fever, chills, and widened pulse pressure.

If your examination reveals these findings, suspect septic shock.

Patient has a history of an insect sting, drug ingestion, or exposure to another possible allergen.

Check for urticaria, wheezing or stridor, and dyspnea.

If your examination reveals these findings, suspect anaphylactic shock.

Patient has a history of venous stasis or deep vein thrombosis and reports sharp, substernal chest pain.

Check for dyspnea, crackles, pleural friction rub, and hemoptysis.

If your examination reveals these findings, suspect pulmonary embolism.

Administer oxygen by nasal cannula, and insert an I.V. catheter for fluid infusion. Begin cardiac monitoring, and check vital signs every 5 to 15 minutes. A central venous pressure catheter, an arterial catheter, or a pulmonary artery catheter may have to be inserted. Be prepared for emergency resuscitation, if necessary.

Anticipate preparing the patient for surgery and administering an antihypertensive or nitroprusside.

Anticipate administering antibiotics and vasopressors.

Anticipate emergency endotracheal intubation or cricothyrotomy and administration of epinephrine.

Anticipate possible endotracheal intubation and anticoagulant or thrombolytic therapy.

diminished pulses occur in 50% of patients with proximal dissection and usually involve the brachiocephalic vessels. Pulse deficits are much less common in patients with distal dissection and tend to involve the left subclavian and femoral arteries. Tearing pain usually develops suddenly in the chest and neck and may radiate to the upper and lower back and abdomen. Other findings include syncope, loss of consciousness, weakness or transient paralysis of the legs or arms, the diastolic murmur of aortic insufficiency, systemic hypotension, and mottled skin below the waist.

◆ ***Aortic arch syndrome (Takayasu's arteritis).*** This syndrome produces weak or abruptly absent carotid pulses and unequal or absent radial pulses. These signs are usually preceded by malaise, night sweats, pallor, nausea, anorexia, weight loss, arthralgia, and Raynaud's phenomenon. Other findings include neck, shoulder, and chest pain; paresthesia; intermittent claudication; bruits; vision disturbances; dizziness; and syncope. If the carotid artery is involved, diplopia and transient blindness may occur.

◆ ***Aortic bifurcation occlusion (acute).*** This rare disorder produces abrupt absence of all leg pulses. The patient reports moderate to severe pain in the legs and, less commonly, in the abdomen, lumbosacral area, or perineum. Also, his legs are cold, pale, numb, and flaccid.

◆ ***Aortic stenosis.*** With this disorder, the carotid pulse is sustained but weak. Dyspnea (especially on exertion or paroxysmal nocturnal), chest pain, and syncope dominate the clinical picture. The patient commonly has an atrial gallop. Other findings include a harsh systolic ejection murmur, crackles, palpitations, fatigue, and narrowed pulse pressure.

◆ ***Arrhythmias.*** Cardiac arrhythmias may produce generalized weak pulses accompanied by cool, clammy skin. Other findings reflect the arrhythmia's severity and may include hypotension, chest pain, dyspnea, dizziness, and decreased level of consciousness.

◆ ***Arterial occlusion.*** With acute occlusion, arterial pulses distal to the obstruction are unilaterally weak and then absent. The affected limb is cool, pale, and cyanotic, with increased capillary refill time, and the patient complains of moderate to severe pain and paresthesia. A line of color and temperature demarcation develops at the level of obstruction. Varying degrees of limb paralysis may also occur, along with intense intermittent claudication. With chronic occlusion, occurring with disorders such as arteriosclerosis and Buerger's disease, pulses in the affected limb weaken gradually.

◆ ***Cardiac tamponade.*** Life-threatening cardiac tamponade causes a weak, rapid pulse accompanied by these classic findings: paradoxical pulse, jugular vein distention, hypotension, and muffled heart sounds. Narrowed pulse pressure, pericardial friction rub, and hepatomegaly may also occur. The patient may appear anxious, restless, and cyanotic and may have chest pain, clammy skin, dyspnea, and tachypnea.

◆ ***Coarctation of the aorta.*** Findings of this disorder include bounding pulses in the arms and neck, with decreased pulsations and systolic pulse pressure in the lower extremities.

◆ ***Peripheral vascular disease.*** This disorder causes a weakening and loss of peripheral pulses. The patient complains of aching pain distal to the occlusion that worsens with exercise and abates with rest. The skin feels cool and shows decreased hair growth. Impotence may occur in male patients with occlusion in the descending aorta or femoral areas.

◆ ***Pulmonary embolism.*** This disorder causes a generalized weak, rapid pulse. It may also cause abrupt onset of chest pain, tachycardia, dyspnea, apprehension, syncope, diaphoresis, and cyanosis. Acute respiratory findings include tachypnea, dyspnea, decreased breath sounds, crackles, a pleural friction rub, and a cough—possibly with blood-tinged sputum.

◆ ***Shock.*** With anaphylactic shock, pulses become rapid and weak and then uniformly absent within seconds or minutes after exposure to an allergen. This is preceded by hypotension, anxiety, restlessness, feelings of doom, intense itching, a pounding headache and, possibly, urticaria.

With cardiogenic shock, peripheral pulses are absent and central pulses are weak, depending on the degree of vascular collapse. Pulse pressure is narrow. A drop in systolic blood pressure to 30 mm Hg below baseline, or a sustained reading below 80 mm Hg, produces poor tissue perfusion. Resulting signs include cold, pale, clammy skin; tachycardia; rapid, shallow respirations; oliguria; restlessness; confusion; and obtundation.

With hypovolemic shock, all pulses in the extremities become weak and then uniformly absent, depending on the severity of hypovolemia. As shock progresses, remaining pulses become thready and more rapid. Early signs of hypovolemic shock include restlessness, thirst, tachypnea, and cool, pale skin. Late signs include hypotension with narrowing pulse pressure, clammy skin, a drop in urine output to less than 25 ml/hour, confusion, decreased level of consciousness and, possibly, hypothermia.

With septic shock, all pulses in the extremities first become weak. Depending on the degree of vascular collapse, pulses may then become uniformly absent. Shock is heralded by chills, sudden fever and, possibly, nausea, vomiting, and diarrhea. Typically, the patient experiences tachycardia, tachypnea, and flushed, warm, and dry skin. As shock progresses, he develops thirst, hypotension, anxiety, restlessness, and confusion. Then pulse pressure narrows and the skin becomes cold, clammy, and cyanotic. The patient experiences severe hypotension, oliguria or anuria, respiratory failure, and coma.

◆ ***Thoracic outlet syndrome.*** A patient with this syndrome may develop gradual or abrupt weakness or loss of the pulses in the arms, depending on how quickly vessels in the neck compress. These pulse changes commonly occur after the patient works with his hands above his shoulders, lifts a weight, or abducts his arm. Paresthesia and pain occur along the ulnar distribution of the arm and disappear as soon as the patient returns his arm to a neutral position. The patient may also have asymmetrical blood pressure and cool, pale skin.

Other causes

◆ ***Treatments.*** Localized absent pulse may occur distal to arteriovenous shunts for dialysis.

Special considerations

Continue to monitor the patient's vital signs to detect untoward changes in his condition. Monitor hemodynamic status by measuring daily weight and hourly or daily intake and output and by assessing central venous pressure.

Pediatric pointers

Radial, dorsal pedal, and posterior tibial pulses aren't easily palpable in infants and small children, so be careful not to mistake these normally hard-to-find pulses for weak or absent pulses. Instead, palpate the brachial, popliteal, or femoral pulses to evaluate arterial circulation to the extremities. In children and young adults, weak or absent femoral and more distal pulses may indicate coarctation of the aorta.

Pulse, bounding

Produced by large waves of pressure as blood ejects from the left ventricle with each contraction, a bounding pulse is strong and easily palpable and may be visible over superficial peripheral arteries. It's characterized by regular, recurrent expansion and contraction of the arterial walls and isn't obliterated by the pressure of palpation. A healthy person develops a bounding pulse during exercise, pregnancy, and periods of anxiety. However, this sign also results from fever and certain endocrine, hematologic, and cardiovascular disorders that increase the basal metabolic rate.

History and physical examination

After you detect a bounding pulse, check other vital signs, and then auscultate the heart and lungs for any abnormal sounds, rates, or rhythms. Ask the patient if he has noticed any weakness, fatigue, shortness of breath, or other health changes. Review his medical history for hyperthyroidism, anemia, or a cardiovascular disorder, and ask about his use of alcohol.

Medical causes

◆ ***Alcoholism (acute).*** Vasodilation produces a rapid, bounding pulse and flushed face. An odor of alcohol on the breath and an ataxic gait are common. Other findings include hypothermia, bradypnea, labored and loud respirations, nausea, vomiting, diuresis, decreased level of consciousness, and seizures.

◆ ***Anemia.*** With this disorder, bounding pulse may be accompanied by capillary pulsations, a systolic ejection murmur, tachycardia, an atrial gallop (S_4), a ventricular gallop (S_3), and a systolic bruit over the carotid artery. Other findings include fatigue, pallor, dyspnea and, possibly, bleeding tendencies.

◆ ***Aortic insufficiency.*** Sometimes called a *water-hammer pulse,* the bounding pulse associated with this condition is characterized by rapid, forceful expansion of the arterial pulse followed by rapid contraction. Widened pulse pressure also occurs. Acute aortic insufficiency may produce findings associated with left-sided heart failure and cardiovascular collapse, such as weakness, severe dyspnea, hypotension, an S_3, and tachycardia. Additional findings include pallor, chest pain, palpitations, or strong, abrupt carotid pulsations. The patient may also experience pulsus bisferiens, an early systolic murmur, a murmur heard over the femoral artery during systole and diastole, and a high-pitched diastolic murmur that starts with the second heart sound. An apical diastolic rumble (Austin Flint murmur) may also occur, especially with heart failure. Most patients with chronic aortic insufficiency remain asymptomatic until their 40s or 50s, when exertional dyspnea, increased fatigue, orthopnea and, eventually, paroxysmal nocturnal dyspnea, angina, and syncope may develop.

◆ ***Febrile disorder.*** Fever can cause a bounding pulse. Accompanying findings reflect the specific disorder.

◆ ***Thyrotoxicosis.*** This disorder produces a rapid, full, bounding pulse. Associated findings include tachycardia, palpitations, an S_3 or S_4 gallop, weight loss despite increased appetite, and heat intolerance. The patient may also develop diarrhea, an enlarged thyroid, dyspnea, tremors, nervousness, chest pain, exophthalmos, and signs of cardiovascular collapse. His skin will be warm, moist, and diaphoretic, and he may be hypersensitive to heat.

Special considerations

Prepare the patient for diagnostic laboratory and radiographic studies. If bounding pulse is accompanied by rapid or irregular heartbeat, you may need to connect the patient to a cardiac monitor for further evaluation.

Pediatric pointers

A bounding pulse can be normal in infants or children because arteries lie close to the skin surface. It can also result from patent ductus arteriosus if the left-to-right shunt is large.

Pulse pressure, narrowed

Pulse pressure, the difference between systolic and diastolic blood pressures, is measured by sphygmomanometry or intra-arterial monitoring. Normally, systolic pressure exceeds diastolic by about 40 mm Hg. Narrowed pressure—a difference of less than 30 mm Hg—occurs when peripheral vascular resistance increases, cardiac output declines, or intravascular volume markedly decreases.

With conditions that cause mechanical obstruction, such as aortic stenosis, pulse pressure is directly related to the severity of the underlying condition. Usually a late sign, narrowed pulse pressure alone doesn't signal an emergency, even though it commonly occurs with shock and other life-threatening disorders.

History and physical examination

After you detect a narrowed pulse pressure, check for other signs of heart failure, such as hypotension, tachycardia, dyspnea, jugular vein distention, pulmonary crackles, and decreased urine output. Check for changes in skin temperature or color, strength of peripheral pulses, and level of consciousness (LOC). Auscultate the heart for murmurs. Ask about a history of chest pain, dizziness, or syncope.

Medical causes

◆ ***Aortic stenosis.*** Narrowed pulse pressure occurs late in significant stenosis. This disorder also produces an atrial or ventricular gallop; chest pain; a harsh, systolic ejection murmur; angina; dyspnea; paroxysmal nocturnal dyspnea; and syncope. Crackles, palpitations, fatigue, and diminished carotid pulses may also occur.

◆ ***Cardiac tamponade.*** With this life-threatening disorder, pulse pressure narrows by 10 to 20 mm Hg. Paradoxical pulse, jugular vein distention, hypotension, and muffled heart sounds are classic. The patient may be anxious, restless, and cyanotic, with clammy skin and chest pain. He may exhibit dyspnea, tachypnea, decreased LOC, and a weak, rapid pulse. Pericardial friction rub and hepatomegaly may also occur.

◆ ***Heart failure.*** Narrowed pulse pressure occurs relatively late and may accompany tachypnea, palpitations, dependent edema, steady weight gain despite nausea and anorexia, chest tightness, slowed mental response, hypotension, diaphoresis, pallor, and oliguria. Assessment reveals a ventricular gallop, inspiratory crackles and, possibly, a tender, palpable liver. Later, dullness develops over the lung bases, and hemoptysis, cyanosis, marked hepatomegaly, and marked pitting edema may occur.

◆ ***Shock.*** With anaphylactic shock, narrowed pulse pressure occurs late, preceded by a rapid, weak pulse that soon becomes uniformly absent. Within seconds or minutes after exposure to an allergen, the patient experiences hypotension, anxiety, restlessness, and feelings of doom, along with intense itching, a pounding headache and, possibly, urticaria. Other findings include dyspnea, stridor, and hoarseness; chest or throat tightness; skin flushing; nausea, abdominal cramps, and urinary incontinence; and seizures.

With cardiogenic shock, narrowed pulse pressure occurs relatively late. Typically, peripheral pulses are absent and central pulses are weak. A drop in systolic pressure to 30 mm Hg below baseline, or a sustained reading below 80 mm Hg not attributable to medication, produces poor tissue perfusion. Poor perfusion produces tachycardia; tachypnea; cold, pale, clammy skin; cyanosis; oliguria; restlessness; confusion; and obtundation.

With hypovolemic shock, narrowed pulse pressure occurs as a late sign. All peripheral pulses become first weak and then uniformly absent. Deepening shock leads to hypotension, urine output of less than 25 ml/hour, confusion, decreased LOC and, possibly, hypothermia.

With septic shock, narrowed pulse pressure is a relatively late sign. All peripheral pulses become first weak and then uniformly absent. As shock progresses, the patient exhibits oliguria, thirst, anxiety, restlessness, confusion, and hypotension. Extremities become cool and cyanotic; the skin becomes cold and clammy. In time, he develops severe hypotension, persistent oliguria or anuria, respiratory failure, and coma.

Special considerations

Monitor closely for changes in pulse rate or quality and for hypotension or diminished LOC. Prepare the patient for diagnostic studies, such as echocardiography, to detect valvular heart disease or cardiac tamponade secondary to a pericardial effusion.

Pediatric pointers

In children, narrowed pulse pressure can result from congenital aortic stenosis as well as from disorders that affect adults.

Pulse pressure, widened

Pulse pressure is the difference between systolic and diastolic blood pressures. Normally, systolic pressure is about 40 mm Hg higher than diastolic pressure. Widened pulse pressure—a difference of more than 50 mm Hg—commonly occurs as a physiologic response to fever, hot weather, exercise, anxiety, anemia, or pregnancy. However, it can also result from certain neurologic disorders—especially life-threatening increased intracranial pressure (ICP)—or from cardiovascular disorders that cause backflow of blood into the heart with each contraction, such as aortic insufficiency. Widened pulse pressure can easily be identified by monitoring of arterial blood pressure and is commonly detected during routine sphygmomanometric recordings.

EMERGENCY INTERVENTIONS *If the patient's level of consciousness (LOC) is decreased, and you suspect that his widened pulse pressure results from increased ICP, check his vital signs and oxygen saturation. Maintain a patent airway. Provide supplemental oxygen and ventilatory support to keep the patient's partial pressure of arterial oxygen above 90 mm Hg or his oxygen saturation above 95%. Give osmotic diuretics, such as mannitol, by I.V. infusion to decrease ICP. Insert an indwelling urinary catheter; monitor intake and output during mannitol therapy. Start ICP monitoring. Administer analgesics as ordered. Hyperventilation therapy to decrease the patient's partial pressure of arterial carbon dioxide and to treat ICP remains controversial but may be needed for short intervals when ICP and neurologic deterioration increase. Perform a neurologic examination. Use the Glasgow Coma Scale (see page 480) to evaluate LOC. Check cranial nerve function—especially cranial nerves III, IV, and VI—and assess papillary reactions, reflexes, and muscle tone. Continue ICP monitoring. If you don't suspect increased ICP, ask about associated symptoms, such as chest pain, shortness of breath, weakness, fatigue, or syncope. Check for edema and auscultate for murmurs.*

Medical causes

◆ ***Aortic insufficiency.*** With acute aortic insufficiency, pulse pressure widens progressively as the valve deteriorates, and a bounding pulse and an atrial gallop or ventricular gallop develop. These signs may be accompanied by chest pain; palpitations; pallor; strong, abrupt carotid pulsations; pulsus bisferiens; and signs of heart failure, such as crackles, dyspnea, and jugular vein distention. Auscultation may reveal several murmurs, such as an early diastolic murmur (common) and an apical diastolic rumble (Austin Flint murmur).

◆ ***Arteriosclerosis.*** With this disorder, reduced arterial compliance causes progressive widening of pulse pressure, which becomes permanent without treatment of the underlying disorder. This sign is preceded by moderate hypertension and accompanied by signs of vascular insufficiency, such as claudication, angina, and speech and vision disturbances.

◆ ***Febrile disorders.*** Fever can cause widened pulse pressure. Accompanying symptoms vary depending on the specific disorder.

◆ ***Increased intracranial pressure.*** Widening pulse pressure is an intermediate to late sign of increased ICP. Although decreased LOC is the earliest and most sensitive indicator of this life-threatening condition, the onset and progression of widening pulse pressure also parallel rising ICP. (Even a gap of only 50 mm Hg can signal a rapid deterioration in the patient's condition.) Assessment reveals Cushing's triad: bradycardia, hypertension, and respiratory pattern changes. Other findings include headache, vomiting, and impaired or unequal motor movement. The patient may also exhibit vision disturbances, such as blurring or photophobia, and pupillary changes.

Special considerations

If the patient displays increased ICP, continually reevaluate his neurologic status and compare your findings carefully with those of previous evaluations. Be alert for restlessness, confusion, unresponsiveness, or decreased LOC. Keep in mind, however, that increasing ICP is commonly signaled by subtle changes in the patient's condition, rather than the abrupt development of any one sign or symptom.

Pediatric pointers

Increased ICP causes widened pulse pressure in children. Patent ductus arteriosus (PDA) can also cause it, but this sign may not be evident at birth. The older child with PDA experiences exertional dyspnea, with pulse pressure that widens even further on exertion.

Geriatric pointers

Recently, widened pulse pressure has been found to be a more powerful predictor of cardiovascular events in elderly patients than either increased systolic or diastolic blood pressure.

Pulse rhythm abnormality

An abnormal pulse rhythm is an irregular expansion and contraction of the peripheral arterial walls. It may be persistent or sporadic, and rhythmic or arrhythmic. Detected by palpating the radial or carotid pulse, an abnormal rhythm is typically reported first by the patient, who complains of feeling palpitations. This important finding reflects an underlying cardiac arrhythmia, which may range from benign to life-threatening. Arrhythmias are commonly associated with cardiovascular, renal, respiratory, metabolic, and neurologic disorders as well as the effects of drugs, diagnostic tests, and treatments. (See *Abnormal pulse rhythm: A clue to cardiac arrhythmias*, pages 566 to 569.)

EMERGENCY INTERVENTIONS *Quickly look for signs of reduced cardiac output, such as decreased level of consciousness (LOC), hypotension, or dizziness. Promptly obtain an electrocardiogram (ECG) and possibly a chest X-ray, and begin cardiac monitoring. Insert an I.V. catheter for administration of emergency cardiac drugs, and give oxygen by nasal cannula or mask. Closely monitor vital signs, pulse quality, and cardiac rhythm because accompanying bradycardia or tachycardia may result in poor tolerance of the abnormal rhythm and cause further deterioration of cardiac output. Keep emergency intubation, cardioversion, and suction equipment handy.*

History and physical examination

If the patient's condition permits, ask if he's experiencing pain. If so, find out about onset and location. Does the pain radiate? Ask about a history of heart disease and treatments for arrhythmias. Obtain a drug history and check compliance. Also, ask about any caffeine or alcohol intake. Digoxin toxicity, cessation of an antiarrhythmic, and use of quinidine, a sympathomimetic (such as epinephrine), caffeine, or alcohol may cause arrhythmias.

Next, check the patient's apical and peripheral arterial pulses. An apical rate exceeding a peripheral arterial rate indicates a pulse deficit, which may also cause associated signs and symptoms of low cardiac output. Evaluate heart sounds: A long pause between S_1 (*lub*) and S_2 (*dub*) may indicate a conduction defect. A faint or absent S_1 and an easily audible S_2 may indicate atrial fibrillation or flutter. You may hear the two heart sounds close together on certain beats—possibly indicating premature atrial contractions—or other variations in heart rate or rhythm. Take the patient's apical and radial pulses while you listen for heart sounds. With some arrhythmias, such as premature ventricular contractions, you may hear the beat with your stethoscope but not feel it over the radial artery. This indicates an ineffective contraction that failed to produce a peripheral pulse. Next, count the apical pulse for 60 seconds, noting the frequency of skipped peripheral beats. Report your findings to the physician.

Medical causes

◆ ***Arrhythmias.*** An abnormal pulse rhythm may be the only sign of a cardiac arrhythmia. The patient may complain of palpitations, a fluttering heartbeat, or weak and skipped beats. Pulses may be weak and rapid or slow. Depending on the specific arrhythmia, dull chest pain or discomfort and hypotension may occur. Associated findings, if any, reflect decreased cardiac output. Neurologic findings, for example, include confusion, dizziness, light-headedness, decreased LOC and, sometimes, seizures. Other findings include decreased urine output, dyspnea, tachypnea, pallor, and diaphoresis.

Special considerations

The patient may require cardioversion therapy, before which he may need to be sedated. Prepare the patient for transfer to a cardiac or intensive care unit. If the patient remains in your care, he may require bed rest or help with ambulation, depending on his condition. To prevent falls and injury, raise the side rails of his bed and don't leave him unattended while he's sitting or walking. Check vital signs frequently to detect bradycardia, tachycardia, hypertension or hypotension, tachypnea, and dyspnea. Also, monitor intake, output, and daily weight.

Collect blood samples for serum electrolyte, cardiac enzyme, and drug level studies. Prepare the patient for a chest X-ray and a 12-lead ECG. If possible, obtain a previous ECG with which to compare current findings. Prepare the patient for 24-hour Holter monitoring. Explain to the patient the importance of keeping a diary of his activities and any symptoms that develop to correlate with the incidence of arrhythmias.

Instruct the patient to avoid tobacco and caffeine, both of which increase arrhythmias. If he has a history of failing to comply with prescribed antiarrhythmic therapy, help him develop strategies to overcome this.

Pediatric pointers

Arrhythmias also produce pulse rhythm abnormalities in children.

Pulsus alternans

A sign of severe left-sided heart failure, pulsus alternans (alternating pulse) is a beat-to-beat change in the size and intensity of a peripheral pulse. Although pulse rhythm remains regular, strong and weak contractions alternate. (See *Identifying pulse waveforms,* page 570.) An alternation in the intensity of heart sounds and of existing heart murmurs may accompany this sign.

Pulsus alternans is thought to result from the change in stroke volume that occurs with beat-to-beat alteration in the left ventricle's contractility. Recumbency or exercise increases venous return and reduces the abnormal pulse, which typically disappears with treatment for heart failure. Rarely, a patient with normal left ventricular function has pulsus alternans, but the abnormal pulse seldom persists for more than 10 to 12 beats.

Although most easily detected by sphygmomanometry, pulsus alternans can be detected by palpating the brachial, radial, or femoral artery when systolic pressure varies from beat to beat by more than 20 mm Hg. Because the small changes in arterial pressure that occur during normal respirations may obscure this abnormal pulse, you'll need to have the patient hold his breath during palpation. Apply *light* pressure to avoid obliterating the weaker pulse.

When using a sphygmomanometer to detect pulsus alternans, inflate the cuff 10 to 20 mm Hg above the systolic pressure as determined by palpation, and then slowly deflate it. At first, you'll hear only the strong beats. With further deflation, all beats will become audible and palpable, and then equally intense. (The difference between this point and the peak systolic level is commonly used to determine the degree of pulsus alternans.) When the cuff is removed, pulsus alternans returns.

Occasionally, the weak beat is so small that no palpable pulse is detected at the periphery. This produces total pulsus alternans, an apparent halving of the pulse rate.

EMERGENCY INTERVENTIONS *Pulsus alternans indicates a critical change in the patient's status. When you detect it, be sure to quickly check other vital signs. Closely evaluate the patient's heart rate, respiratory pattern, and blood pressure. Auscultate for a ventricular gallop and increased crackles.*

Medical causes

◆ ***Left-sided heart failure.*** With this disorder, pulsus alternans is commonly initiated by a

(Text continues on page 568.)

Abnormal pulse rhythm: A clue to cardiac arrhythmias

An abnormal pulse rhythm may be your only clue that the patient has a cardiac arrhythmia, but this sign doesn't help you pinpoint the specific type of arrhythmia. For that, you need a cardiac monitor or an electrocardiogram (ECG) machine. These devices record the electrical current generated by the heart's conduction system and display this information on an oscilloscope

Arrhythmia

SINUS ARRHYTHMIA

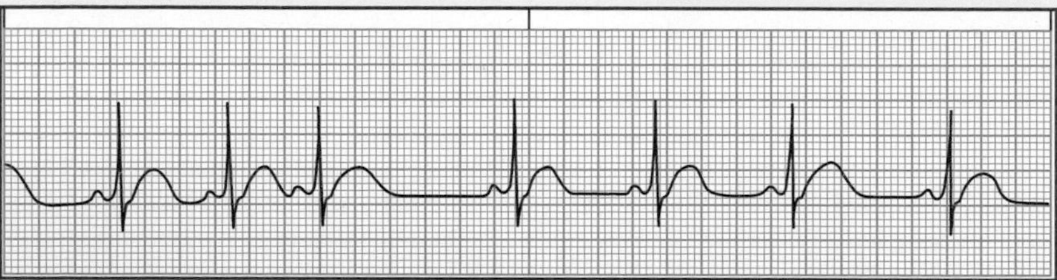

PREMATURE ATRIAL CONTRACTIONS (PACS)

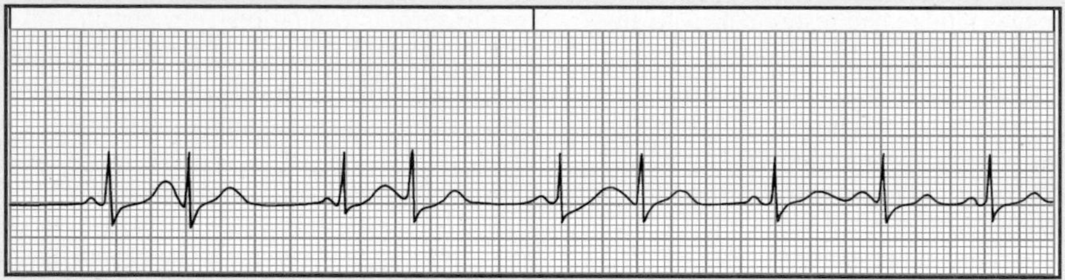

PAROXYSMAL ATRIAL TACHYCARDIA

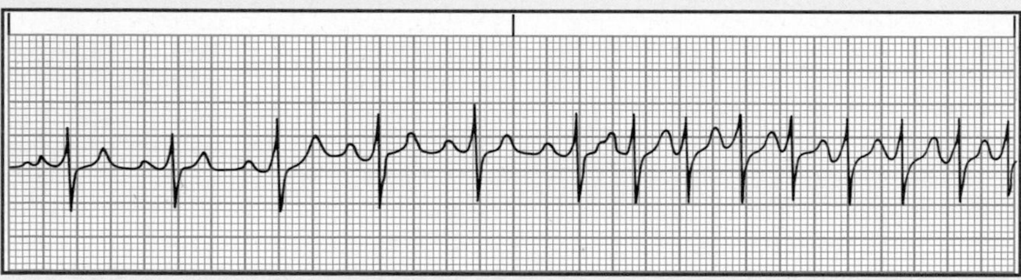

ATRIAL FIBRILLATION

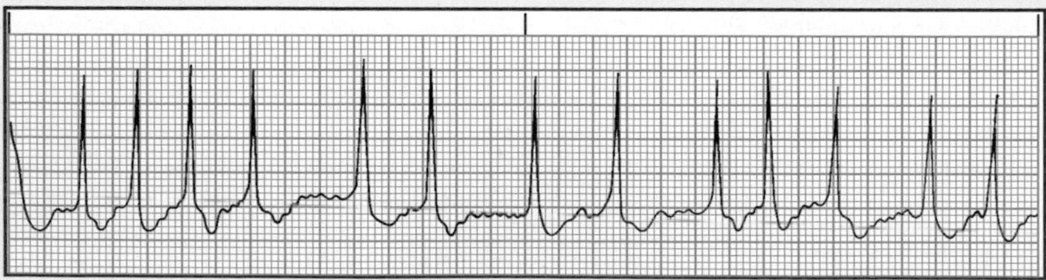

screen or a strip-chart recorder. Besides rhythm disturbances, they can identify conduction defects and electrolyte imbalances.

The ECG strips below show some common cardiac arrhythmias that can cause abnormal pulse rhythms.

Pulse rhythm and rate	Clinical implications
Irregular rhythm; fast, slow, or normal rate	◆ Reflex vagal tone inhibition (heart rate increases with inspiration and decreases with expiration) related to normal respiratory cycle. ◆ May result from drugs, as in digoxin toxicity ◆ Occurs most often in children and young adults
Irregular rhythm during PACs; fast, slow, or normal rate	◆ Occasional PAC may be normal ◆ Isolated PACs indicate atrial irritation — for example, from anxiety or excessive caffeine intake. Increasing PACs may herald other atrial arrhythmias. ◆ May result from heart failure, chronic obstructive pulmonary disease (COPD), or use of cardiac glycosides, aminophylline, or adrenergic
Regular rhythm with abrupt onset and termination of arrhythmia; heart rate exceeding 140 beats/minute	◆ May occur in otherwise normal, healthy persons who are suffering from physical or psychological stress, hypoxia, or digoxin toxicity; who use marijuana; or who consume excessive amounts of caffeine or other stimulants ◆ May precipitate angina or heart failure
Irregular rhythm; atrial rate exceeding 400 beats/minute; ventricular rate varies	◆ May result from heart failure, COPD, hypertension, sepsis, pulmonary embolus, mitral valve disease, digoxin toxicity (rarely), atrial irritation, postcoronary bypass, or valve replacement surgery ◆ Because atria don't contract, preload isn't consistent, so cardiac output changes with each beat. Emboli may also result.

(continued)

Abnormal pulse rhythm: A clue to cardiac arrhythmias *(continued)*

Arrhythmia

PREMATURE JUNCTIONAL CONTRACTIONS (PJCS)

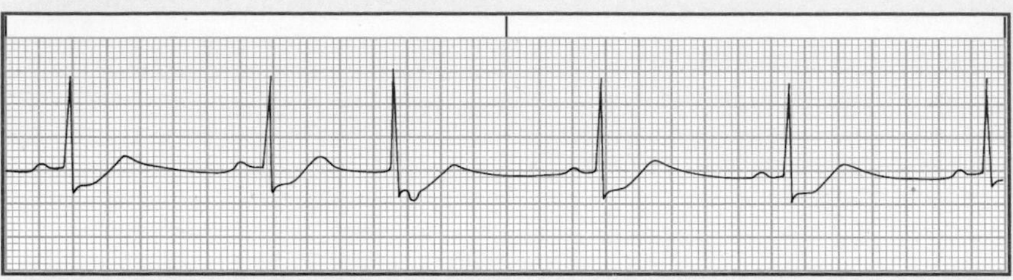

SECOND-DEGREE ATRIOVENTRICULAR HEART BLOCK, MOBITZ TYPE I (WENCKEBACH)

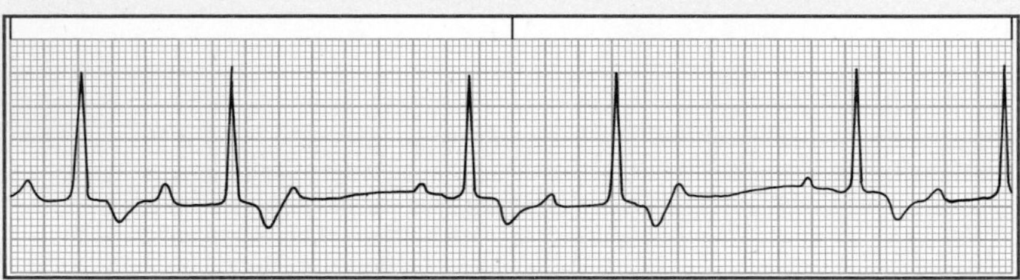

SECOND-DEGREE ATRIOVENTRICULAR HEART BLOCK, MOBITZ TYPE II

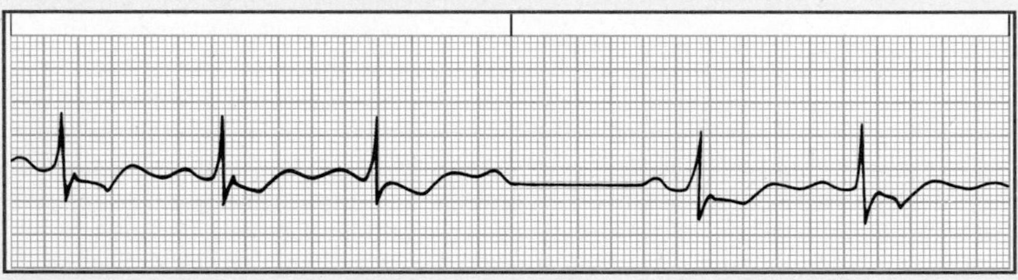

PREMATURE VENTRICULAR CONTRACTIONS (MULTIFOCAL)

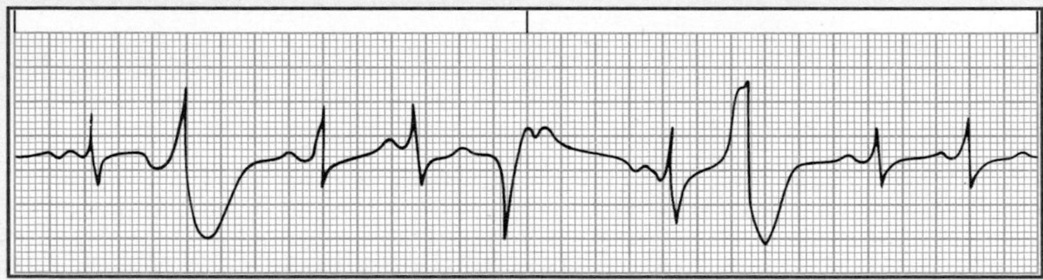

premature beat and is almost always associated with a ventricular gallop. Other findings include hypotension and cyanosis. Possible respiratory findings include exertional and paroxysmal nocturnal dyspnea, orthopnea, tachypnea, Cheyne-Stokes respirations, hemoptysis, and crackles. Fatigue and weakness are common.

SPECIAL CONSIDERATIONS

If left-sided heart failure develops suddenly, prepare the patient for transfer to an intensive

Pulse rhythm and rate	Clinical implications
Irregular rhythm during PJCs; fast, slow, or normal rate	◆ May result from myocardial infarction (MI) or ischemia, excessive caffeine intake, and most commonly digoxin toxicity (from enhanced automaticity)
Irregular ventricular rhythm; fast, slow, or normal rate	◆ Commonly transient; may progress to complete heart block ◆ May result from inferior wall MI, digoxin or quinidine toxicity, vagal stimulation, electrolyte imbalance, or arteriosclerotic heart disease
Irregular ventricular rhythm; slow or normal rate	◆ May progress to complete heart block ◆ May result from degenerative disease of conduction system, ischemia of AV node in an anterior MI, anteroseptal infarction, electrolyte imbalance, or digoxin or quinidine toxicity
Usually irregular rhythm with a long pause after the premature beat; fast, slow, or normal rate	◆ Arise from different ventricular sites or from the same site with changing patterns of conduction ◆ May result from caffeine or stress, alcohol ingestion, myocardial ischemia or infarction, myocardial irritation by pacemaker electrodes, hypocalcemia, hypercalcemia, digoxin toxicity, or exercise

or cardiac care unit. Meanwhile, elevate the head of his bed to promote respiratory excursion and increase oxygenation. Adjust the patient's current treatment plan to improve cardiac output, reduce the heart's workload, and promote diuresis.

Pediatric pointers

Pulsus alternans, which also occurs in a child with heart failure, may be difficult to assess if the child is crying or restless. Try to quiet the child by holding him, if his condition permits.

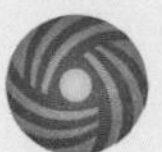

EXAMINATION TIP

Identifying pulse waveforms

To identify abnormal arterial pulses, check the waveforms below and see which one matches the patient's peripheral pulse.

NORMAL ARTERIAL PULSE

The percussion wave in a normal arterial pulse reflects ejection of blood into the aorta (early systole). The tidal wave is the peak of the pulse wave (later systole), and the dicrotic notch marks the beginning of diastole.

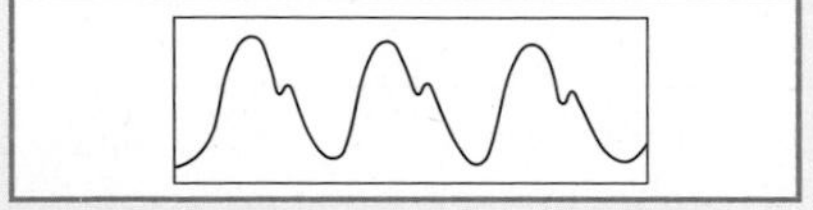

WEAK PULSE

A weak pulse has a decreased amplitude with a slower upstroke and downstroke. Possible causes of a weak pulse include increased peripheral vascular resistance, such as happens in cold weather or severe heart failure; and decreased stroke volume, as with hypovolemia or aortic stenosis.

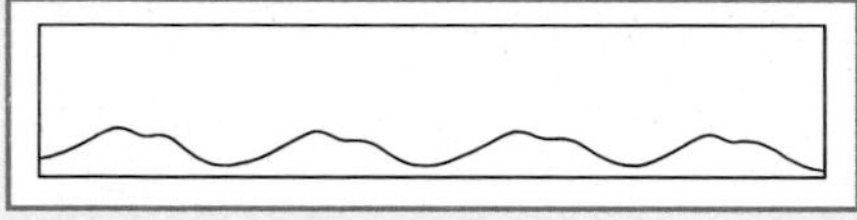

BOUNDING PULSE

A bounding pulse has a sharp upstroke and downstroke with a pointed peak. The amplitude is elevated. Possible causes of a bounding pulse include increased stroke volume, as with aortic insufficiency; or stiffness of arterial walls, as with aging.

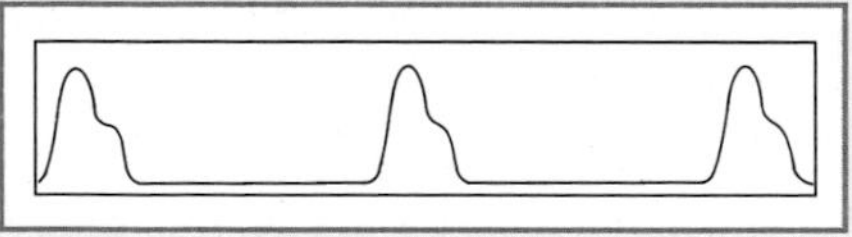

PULSUS ALTERNANS

Pulsus alternans has a regular, alternating pattern of a weak and a strong pulse. This pulse is associated with left-sided heart failure.

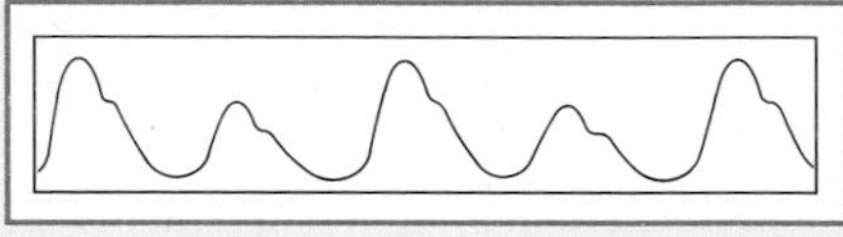

PULSUS BIGEMINUS

Pulsus bigeminus is similar to alternating pulse but occurs at irregular intervals. It is caused by premature atrial or ventricular beats.

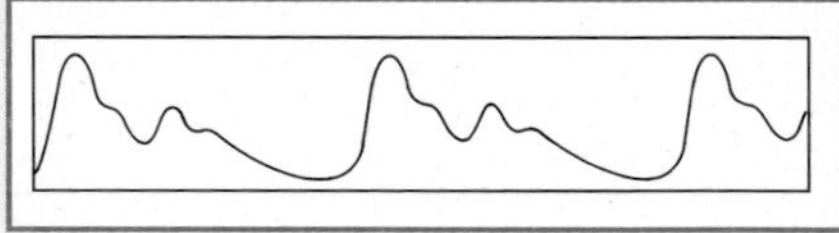

PULSUS PARADOXUS

Pulsus paradoxus has increases and decreases in amplitude associated with the respiratory cycle. Marked decreases occur when the patient inhales. Pulsus paradoxus is associated with pericardial tamponade, advanced heart failure, and constrictive pericarditis.

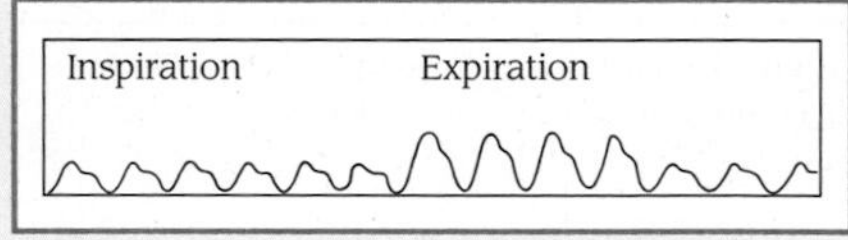

PULSUS BISFERIENS

Pulsus bisferiens shows an initial upstroke, a subsequent downstroke, and then another upstroke during systole. Pulsus bisferiens is caused by aortic stenosis and aortic insufficiency.

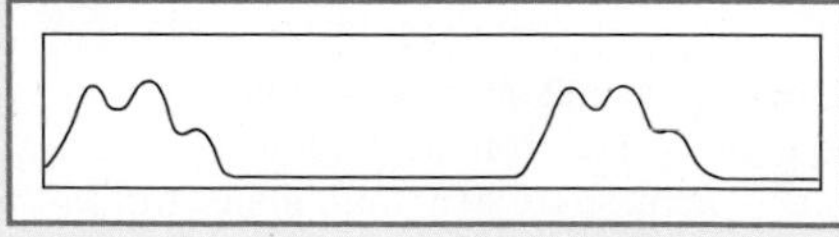

Pulsus bisferiens

A bisferious pulse is a hyperdynamic, double-beating pulse characterized by two systolic peaks separated by a midsystolic dip. Both peaks may be equal or either may be larger; usually, however, the first peak is taller or more forceful than the second. The first peak (percussion wave) is believed to be the pulse pressure and the second (tidal wave), reverberation from the periphery. Pulsus bisferiens occurs in conditions, such as aortic insufficiency, in which a large volume of blood is rapidly ejected from the left ventricle. The pulse can be palpated in peripheral arteries or observed on an arterial pressure wave recording.

To detect pulsus bisferiens, *lightly* palpate the carotid, brachial, radial, or femoral artery. (The pulse is easiest to palpate in the carotid artery.) At the same time, listen to the patient's heart sounds to determine if the two palpable peaks occur during systole. If they do, you'll feel the double pulse between the first and second heart sounds.

History and physical examination

After you detect a bisferiens pulse, review the patient's history for cardiac disorders. Next, find out what medication he's taking, if any, and ask if he has any other illnesses. Ask about the development of any associated signs and symptoms, such as dyspnea, chest pain, or fatigue. Find out how long he has had these symptoms and if they change with activity or rest. Take his vital signs and auscultate for abnormal heart or breath sounds.

Medical causes

◆ ***Aortic insufficiency.*** This heart defect is the most common organic cause of bisferiens pulse. Most patients with chronic aortic insufficiency are asymptomatic until ages 40 to 50. However, exertional dyspnea, worsening fatigue, orthopnea and, eventually, paroxysmal nocturnal dyspnea may develop.

Acute aortic insufficiency may produce signs and symptoms of left-sided heart failure and cardiovascular collapse, such as weakness, severe dyspnea, hypotension, ventricular gallop, and tachycardia. Additional findings include chest pain, palpitations, pallor, and strong, abrupt carotid pulsations. The patient may also exhibit widened pulse pressure and one or more murmurs, especially an apical diastolic rumble (Austin Flint murmur).

◆ ***Aortic stenosis with aortic insufficiency.*** A bisferiens pulse is commonly seen in aortic stenosis that is accompanied by moderately severe aortic insufficiency. In aortic stenosis, the pulse rises slowly and the second wave of the double beat is the more forceful one. This disorder is commonly accompanied by dyspnea and fatigue. Chest pain and syncope aren't specific in the combined lesion, but they do suggest predominant aortic stenosis.

◆ ***High cardiac output states.*** Pulsus bisferiens commonly occurs with high output states, such as anemia, thyrotoxicosis, fever, and exercise. Associated findings vary with the underlying cause and may include moderate tachycardia, a cervical venous hum, and widened pulse pressure.

◆ ***Hypertrophic obstructive cardiomyopathy.*** About 40% of patients with this disorder have pulsus bisferiens because of a pressure gradient in the left ventricular outflow tract. Recorded more often than it's palpated, the pulse rises rapidly, and the first wave is the more forceful one. Associated findings include a systolic murmur, dyspnea, angina, fatigue, and syncope.

Special considerations

Prepare the patient for diagnostic tests, such as an electrocardiogram, chest X-ray, cardiac catheterization, or angiography, to help determine the underlying cause of the abnormal pulse.

Pediatric pointers

Pulsus bisferiens may be palpated in children with a large patent ductus arteriosus as well as those with congenital aortic stenosis and insufficiency.

Pulsus paradoxus

Pulsus paradoxus, or paradoxical pulse, is an exaggerated decline in blood pressure during inspiration. Normally, systolic pressure falls less than 10 mm Hg during inspiration. In pulsus paradoxus, it falls more than 10 mm Hg. (See *Identifying pulse waveforms*.) When systolic pressure falls more than 20 mm Hg, the peripheral pulses may be barely palpable or may disappear during inspiration.

Pulsus paradoxus is thought to result from an exaggerated inspirational increase in negative intrathoracic pressure. Normally, systolic pressure drops during inspiration because of blood pooling in the pulmonary system. This, in turn, reduces left ventricular filling and stroke volume and transmits negative intrathoracic pressure to the aorta. Conditions associated with large intrapleural pressure swings, such as asthma, or those that reduce left-sided heart filling, such as pericardial tamponade, produce pulsus paradoxus.

To accurately detect and measure pulsus paradoxus, use a sphygmomanometer or an intra-arterial monitoring device. Inflate the blood pressure cuff 10 to 20 mm Hg beyond the peak systolic pressure. Then deflate the cuff at a rate of 2 mm Hg/second until you hear the first Korotkoff sound during expiration. Note the systolic pressure. As you continue to slowly deflate the cuff, observe the patient's respiratory pattern. If a pulsus paradoxus is present, the Korotkoff sounds will disappear with inspiration and return with expiration. Continue to deflate the cuff until you hear Korotkoff sounds during both inspiration and expiration and, again, note the systolic pressure. Subtract this reading from the first one to determine the degree of pulsus paradoxus. A difference of more than 10 mm Hg is abnormal.

You can also detect pulsus paradoxus by palpating the radial pulse over several cycles of slow inspiration and expiration. Marked pulse diminution during inspiration indicates pulsus paradoxus. When you check for pulsus paradoxus, remember that irregular heart rhythms and tachycardia cause variations in pulse amplitude and must be ruled out before a true pulsus paradoxus can be identified.

EMERGENCY INTERVENTIONS *A pulsus paradoxus may signal cardiac tamponade—a life-threatening complication of pericardial effusion that occurs when sufficient blood or fluid accumulates to compress the heart. When you detect pulsus paradoxus, quickly check the patient's other vital signs. Check for additional signs and symptoms of cardiac tamponade, such as dyspnea, tachypnea, diaphoresis, jugular vein distention, tachycardia, narrowed pulse pressure, and hypotension. Emergency pericardiocentesis to aspirate blood or fluid from the pericardial sac may be necessary. Then evaluate the effectiveness of pericardiocentesis by measuring the degree of pulsus paradoxus; it should decrease after aspiration.*

History and physical examination

If the patient doesn't have cardiac tamponade, find out if he has a history of chronic cardiac or pulmonary disease. Ask about the development of associated signs and symptoms, such as a cough or chest pain. Auscultate for abnormal breath sounds.

Medical causes

◆ ***Cardiac tamponade.*** Pulsus paradoxus commonly occurs with this disorder, but it may be difficult to detect if intrapericardial pressure rises abruptly and profound hypotension occurs. With severe tamponade, assessment also reveals these classic findings: hypotension, diminished or muffled heart sounds, and jugular vein distention. Related findings include chest pain, pericardial friction rub, narrowed pulse pressure, anxiety, restlessness, clammy skin, and hepatomegaly. Characteristic respiratory signs and symptoms include dyspnea, tachypnea, and cyanosis; the patient typically sits up and leans forward to facilitate breathing.

If cardiac tamponade develops gradually, pulsus paradoxus may be accompanied by weakness, anorexia, and weight loss. The patient may also report chest pain, but he won't have muffled heart sounds or severe hypotension.

◆ ***Chronic obstructive pulmonary disease (COPD).*** The wide fluctuations in intrathoracic pressure that characterize this disorder produce pulsus paradoxus and possibly tachycardia. Other findings vary but may include dyspnea, tachypnea, wheezing, productive or nonproductive cough, accessory muscle use, barrel chest, and clubbing. The patient may show labored, pursed-lip breathing after exertion or even at rest. He typically sits up and leans forward to facilitate breathing. Auscultation reveals decreased breath sounds, rhonchi, and crackles. Weight loss, cyanosis, and edema may occur.

◆ ***Pericarditis (chronic constrictive).*** Pulsus paradoxus can occur in up to 50% of patients with this disorder. Other findings include pericardial friction rub, chest pain, exertional dyspnea, orthopnea, hepatomegaly, and ascites. The patient also exhibits peripheral edema and Kussmaul's sign—jugular vein distention that becomes more prominent on inspiration.

◆ ***Pulmonary embolism (massive).*** Decreased left ventricular filling and stroke volume in massive pulmonary embolism produce pulsus paradoxus, as well as syncope and severe apprehension, dyspnea, tachypnea, and pleuritic chest pain. The patient appears cyanotic, with jugular vein distention. He may succumb to circulatory collapse, with hypotension and a weak, rapid pulse. Pulmonary infarction may produce hemoptysis along with decreased breath sounds and a pleural friction rub over the affected area.

◆ ***Right ventricular infarction.*** This infarction may produce pulsus paradoxus and elevated jugular venous or central venous pressure. Other findings are similar to those of myocardial infarction.

Special considerations

Prepare the patient for an echocardiogram to visualize cardiac motion and to help determine the causative disorder. Also, monitor his vital signs and frequently check the degree of paradox. An increase in the degree of paradox may indicate recurring or worsening cardiac tamponade or impending respiratory arrest in severe COPD. Vigorous respiratory treatment, such as chest physiotherapy, may avert the need for endotracheal intubation.

Pediatric pointers

Pulsus paradoxus commonly occurs in children with chronic pulmonary disease, especially during an acute asthma attack. Children with pericarditis may also develop pulsus paradoxus due to cardiac tamponade, although this disorder more commonly affects adults. A pulsus paradoxus above 20 mm Hg is a reliable indicator of cardiac tamponade in children; a change of 10 to 20 mm Hg is equivocal.

Pupils, nonreactive

Nonreactive (fixed) pupils fail to constrict in response to light or to dilate when the light is removed. The development of a unilateral or bilateral nonreactive response indicates an important change in the patient's condition and may signal a life-threatening emergency and possibly brain death. (See *Understanding pupillary changes*, page 574.) It also occurs with use of certain optic drugs.

To evaluate pupillary reaction to light, first test the patient's direct light reflex. Darken the room, and cover one of the patient's eyes while you hold open the opposite eyelid. Using a bright penlight, bring the light toward the patient from the side and shine it directly into his opened eye. If normal, the pupil will promptly constrict. Next, test the consensual light reflex. Hold the patient's eyelids open and shine the light into one eye while watching the pupil of the opposite eye. If normal, both pupils will promptly constrict. Repeat both procedures in the opposite eye. A unilateral or bilateral nonreactive response indicates dysfunction of cranial nerves II and III, which mediate the pupillary light reflex. (See *Innervation of direct and consensual light reflexes,* page 575.)

EMERGENCY INTERVENTIONS *If the patient is unconscious and develops unilateral or bilateral nonreactive pupils, quickly take his vital signs. Be alert for decerebrate or decorticate posture, bradycardia, elevated systolic blood pressure, widened pulse pressure, and the development of other untoward changes in the patient's condition. Remember, a unilateral dilated, nonreactive pupil may be an early sign of uncal brain herniation. Emergency surgery to decrease intracranial pressure (ICP) may be necessary. If the patient isn't already being treated for increased ICP, insert an I.V. catheter to administer a diuretic, an osmotic, or a corticosteroid. You may also need to start the patient on controlled hyperventilation.*

History and physical examination

If the patient is conscious, obtain a brief history. Ask him what type of eyedrops he's using, if any, and when they were last instilled. Ask if he's experiencing any pain and, if so, try to determine its location, intensity, and duration. Check the patient's visual acuity in both eyes. Then test the pupillary reaction to accommodation: Normally, both pupils constrict equally as the patient shifts his glance from a distant to a near object.

Next, hold a penlight at the side of each eye and examine the cornea and iris for any abnormalities. Measure intraocular pressure (IOP) with a tonometer, or estimate IOP by placing your second and third fingers over the patient's closed eyelid. If the eyeball feels rock-hard, suspect elevated IOP. Ophthalmoscopic and slit-lamp examinations of the eye will need to be performed. If the patient has experienced ocular trauma, don't manipulate the affected eye. After the examination, be sure to cover the affected eye with a protective metal shield, but don't let the shield rest on the globe.

Medical causes

◆ ***Adie's syndrome.*** This syndrome produces abrupt onset of unilateral mydriasis along with a sluggish or nonreactive pupillary response. It may also produce blurred vision and cramplike eye pain. Eventually, both eyes may be affected. Musculoskeletal assessment reveals hypoactive or absent deep tendon reflexes (DTRs) in the arms and legs.

Understanding pupillary changes

Use this chart as a guide when observing your patient for pupillary changes.

Pupillary change	Possible causes
Unilateral, dilated (4 mm), fixed, and nonreactive 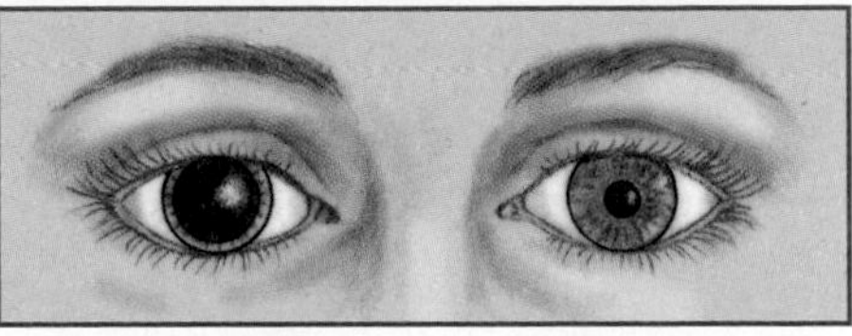	◆ Uncal herniation with oculomotor nerve damage ◆ Brain stem compression ◆ Increased intracranial pressure ◆ Tentorial herniation ◆ Head trauma with subdural or epidural hematoma ◆ May be normal in some people
Bilateral, dilated (4 mm), fixed, and nonreactive 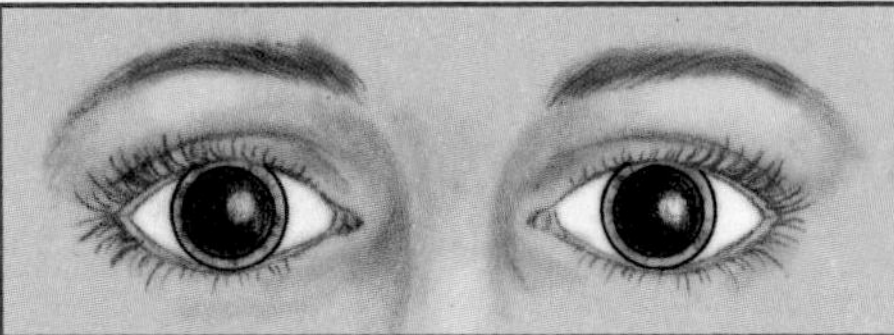	◆ Severe midbrain damage ◆ Cardiopulmonary arrest (hypoxia) ◆ Anticholinergic poisoning
Bilateral, midsize (2 mm), fixed, and nonreactive 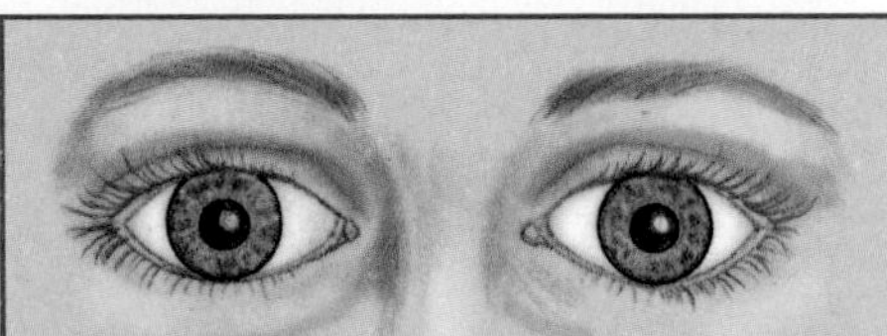	◆ Midbrain involvement caused by edema, hemorrhage, infarctions, lacerations, or contusions
Unilateral, small (1.5 mm), and nonreactive 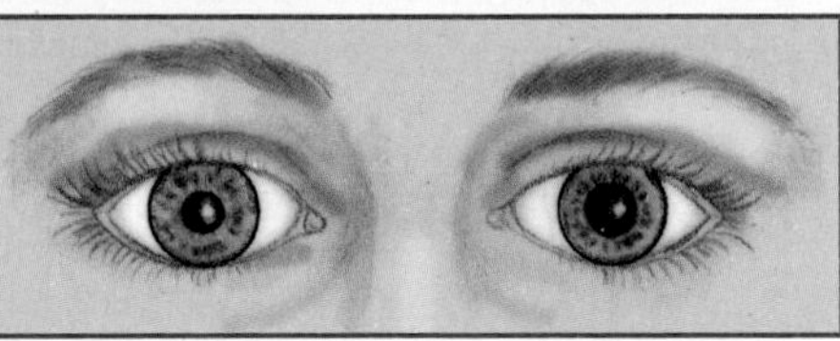	◆ Disruption of sympathetic nerve supply to the head caused by spinal cord lesion above T1
Bilateral, pinpoint (<1 mm), and usually nonreactive 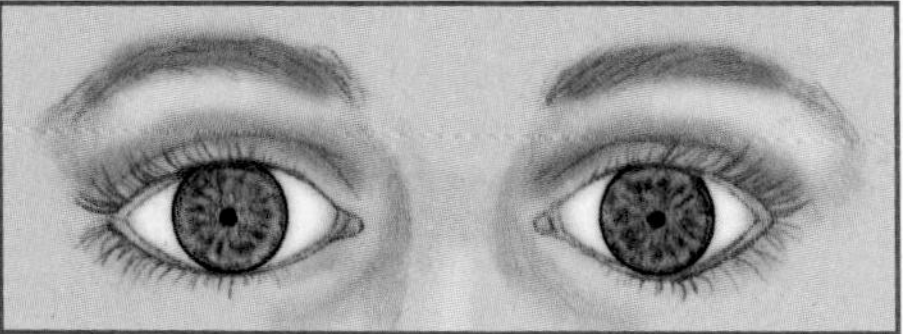	◆ Lesions of the pons, usually after hemorrhage

Innervation of direct and consensual light reflexes

Two reactions—direct and consensual—constitute the pupillary light reflex. Normally, when a light is shined directly onto the retina of one eye, the parasympathetic nerves are stimulated to cause brisk constriction of that pupil—the *direct light reflex*. The pupil of the opposite eye also constricts—the *consensual light reflex*.

The optic nerve (cranial nerve [CN] II) mediates the afferent arc of this reflex from each eye, whereas the oculomotor nerve (CN III) mediates the efferent arc to both eyes. A nonreactive or sluggish response in one or both pupils indicates dysfunction of these cranial nerves, usually from degenerative disease of the central nervous system.

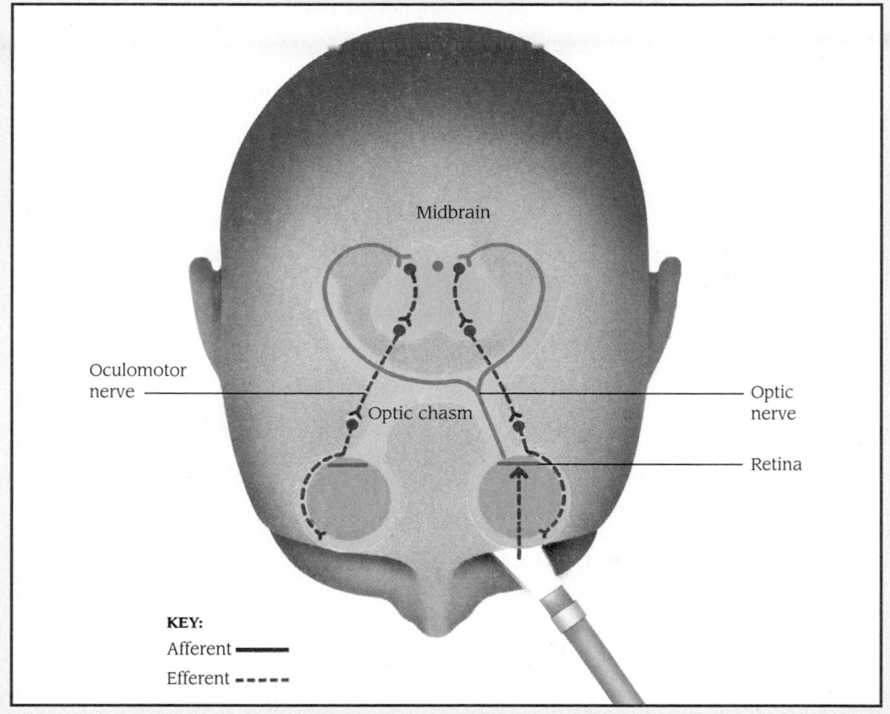

◆ ***Botulism.*** Bilateral mydriasis and nonreactive pupils usually appear 12 to 36 hours after ingestion of tainted food. Other early findings include blurred vision, diplopia, ptosis, strabismus, and extraocular muscle palsies, along with anorexia, nausea, vomiting, diarrhea, and dry mouth. Vertigo, deafness, hoarseness, nasal voice, dysarthria, and dysphagia follow. Progressive muscle weakness and absent DTRs usually evolve over 2 to 4 days, resulting in severe constipation and paralysis of respiratory muscles with respiratory distress.

◆ ***Encephalitis.*** As this disorder progresses, initially sluggish pupils become dilated and nonreactive. Decreased accommodation and other symptoms of cranial nerve palsies, such as dysphagia, develop. Within 48 hours after onset, encephalitis causes a decreased level of consciousness, high fever, headache, vomiting, and nuchal rigidity. Aphasia, ataxia, nystagmus, hemiparesis, and photophobia may occur with seizures.

◆ ***Familial amyloid polyneuropathy.*** This disorder produces sluggish or nonreactive pupils and miosis. Corneal opacities may affect visual acuity. The patient may also experience anhidrosis, orthostatic hypotension, alternating diarrhea and constipation, and impotence. Initially, he'll experience paresthesia and possibly pain in the feet and lower legs; later, absent DTRs and thinning legs.

◆ ***Glaucoma (acute angle-closure).*** With this ophthalmic emergency, examination reveals a moderately dilated, nonreactive pupil in the affected eye. Conjunctival injection, corneal clouding, and decreased visual acuity also occur. The patient experiences sudden onset of blurred vision, followed by excruciating pain in and around the affected eye. He commonly reports seeing halos around white lights at night. Severely elevated IOP commonly induces nausea and vomiting.

◆ ***Iris disease (degenerative* or *inflammatory).*** This disease causes pupillary nonreactivity in the affected eyes. Visual acuity may also decrease.

◆ ***Midbrain lesions.*** Although rare, these lesions produce bilateral midposition nonreactive pupils. Other findings include loss of upward gaze, coma, central neurogenic hyperventilation, bradycardia, hemiparesis or hemiplegia, and decorticate or decerebrate posture.

◆ ***Ocular trauma.*** Severe damage to the iris or optic nerve may produce a nonreactive, dilated pupil in the affected eye (traumatic iridoplegia). This sign is usually transitory but can be permanent. Slit-lamp examination commonly reveals a V-shaped notch in the pupillary rim, indicating a tear in the iris sphincter muscle. The patient usually experiences eye pain and may also develop eye edema and ecchymoses.

◆ ***Oculomotor nerve palsy.*** Commonly, the first signs of this oculomotor ophthalmoplegia are a dilated, nonreactive pupil and loss of the accommodation reaction. These findings may occur in one eye or both, depending on whether the palsy is unilateral or bilateral. Among the causes of total third cranial nerve palsy is life-threatening brain herniation. Central herniation causes bilateral midposition nonreactive pupils, whereas uncal herniation initially causes a unilateral dilated, nonreactive pupil. Other common findings include diplopia, ptosis, outward deviation of the eye, and inability to elevate or adduct the eye. Additional findings depend on the underlying cause of the palsy.

◆ ***Uveitis.*** A small, nonreactive pupil that appears suddenly with severe eye pain, conjunctival injection, and photophobia typifies anterior uveitis. With posterior uveitis, similar features develop insidiously, along with blurred vision and distorted pupil shape.

◆ ***Wernicke's disease.*** Nonreactive pupils are a late sign in this disease, which initially produces an intention tremor accompanied by a sluggish pupillary reaction. Other ocular findings include diplopia, gaze paralysis, nystagmus, ptosis, decreased visual acuity, and conjunctival injection. The patient may also exhibit orthostatic hypotension, tachycardia, ataxia, apathy, and confusion.

OTHER CAUSES

◆ ***Drugs.*** Instillation of a topical mydriatic and a cycloplegic may induce a temporarily nonreactive pupil in the affected eye. Opiates, such as heroin and morphine, cause pinpoint pupils with a minimal light response that can be seen only with a magnifying glass. Atropine poisoning produces widely dilated, nonreactive pupils.

SPECIAL CONSIDERATIONS

If the patient is conscious, monitor his pupillary light reflex to detect changes. If he's unconscious, close his eyes to prevent corneal exposure. (Use tape to secure the eyelids, if needed.)

PEDIATRIC POINTERS

Children have nonreactive pupils for the same reasons as adults. The most common cause is oculomotor nerve palsy from increased ICP.

Pupils, sluggish

A sluggish pupillary reaction is an abnormally slow pupillary response to light. It can occur in one pupil or both, unlike the normal reaction, which is always bilateral. A sluggish reaction accompanies degenerative disease of the central nervous system and diabetic neuropathy. It can occur normally in the elderly, whose pupils become smaller and less responsive with age.

To assess pupillary reaction to light, first test the patient's direct light reflex. Darken the room, and cover one of the patient's eyes while you hold open the opposite eyelid. Using a bright penlight, bring the light toward the patient from the side and shine it directly into his opened eye. If normal, the pupil will promptly constrict. Next, test the consensual light reflex. Hold both of the patient's eyelids open, and shine the light into one eye while watching the pupil of the opposite eye. If normal, both pupils will promptly constrict. Repeat both procedures to test light reflexes in the opposite eye. A sluggish reaction in one or both pupils indicates dysfunction of cranial nerves II and III, which mediate the pupillary light reflex. (See *Innervation of direct and consensual light reflexes,* page 575.)

History and physical examination

If you detect a sluggish pupillary reaction, determine the patient's visual function. Start by testing visual acuity in both eyes. Then test the pupillary reaction to accommodation; the pupils should constrict equally as the patient shifts his glance from a distant to a near object.

Next, hold a penlight at the side of each eye and examine the cornea and iris for irregularities, scars, and foreign bodies. Measure intraocular pressure (IOP) with a tonometer, or estimate IOP by placing your fingers over the patient's closed eyelid. If the eyeball feels rock-hard, suspect elevated IOP. Also, ophthalmoscopic and slit-lamp examinations of the eye will need to be performed.

Medical causes

◆ ***Adie's syndrome.*** This syndrome produces abrupt onset of unilateral mydriasis and a sluggish pupillary response that may progress to a nonreactive response. The patient may complain of blurred vision and cramplike eye pain. Eventually, both eyes may be affected. Musculoskeletal assessment also reveals hypoactive or absent deep tendon reflexes (DTRs) in the arms and legs.

◆ ***Diabetic neuropathy.*** A patient with long-standing diabetes mellitus may have a sluggish pupillary response. Additional findings include orthostatic hypotension, syncope, dysphagia, episodic constipation or diarrhea, painless bladder distention with overflow incontinence, retrograde ejaculation, and impotence.

◆ ***Encephalitis.*** This disorder initially produces a bilateral sluggish pupillary response. Later, pupils become dilated and nonreactive, and decreased accommodation may occur, along with other cranial nerve palsies, such as dysphagia and facial weakness. Within 24 to 48 hours after onset, encephalitis causes a decreased level of consciousness, headache, high fever, vomiting, and nuchal rigidity. Aphasia, ataxia, nystagmus, hemiparesis, and photophobia may also occur. The patient may exhibit seizure activity and myoclonic jerks.

◆ ***Familial amyloid polyneuropathy.*** A patient with this disorder exhibits sluggish or nonreactive pupils, miosis, and corneal opacities that may affect visual acuity. He may also develop anhidrosis, orthostatic hypotension, alternating diarrhea and constipation, and impotence. Initially, he'll experience paresthesia and possibly pain in the feet and lower legs. Later, absent DTRs and thinning legs may hamper walking.

◆ ***Herpes zoster.*** The patient with herpes zoster affecting the nasociliary nerve may have a sluggish pupillary response. Examination of the conjunctiva reveals follicles. Additional ocular findings include a serous discharge, absence of tears, ptosis, and extraocular muscle palsy.

◆ ***Iritis (acute).*** With this disorder, the affected eye exhibits a sluggish pupillary response and conjunctival injection. The pupil may remain constricted; if posterior synechiae have formed, the pupil will also be irregularly shaped. The patient reports sudden onset of eye pain and photophobia and may also have blurred vision.

◆ ***Multiple sclerosis.*** This disorder may produce small, irregularly shaped pupils that react better to accommodation than to light. Additional ocular findings may include ptosis, nystagmus, diplopia, and blurred vision. In most patients, vision problems and sensory impairment, such as paresthesia, are the earliest indications. Later, various features may develop, including muscle weakness and paralysis; intention tremor, spasticity, hyperreflexia, and gait ataxia; dysphagia and dysarthria; constipation; urinary urgency, frequency, and incontinence; impotence; and emotional instability.

◆ ***Myotonic dystrophy.*** With this disorder, sluggish pupillary reaction may be accompanied by lid lag, ptosis, miosis and, possibly, diplopia. The patient may develop decreased visual acuity from cataract formation. Muscular weakness and atrophy and testicular atrophy may occur.

◆ ***Tertiary syphilis.*** A sluggish pupillary reaction (especially in Argyll Robertson pupils) occurs in the late stage of neurosyphilis, along with marked weakness of the extraocular muscles, visual field defects and, possibly, cataractous changes in the lens. The patient may complain of orbital rim pain, which worsens at night. He may also exhibit lid edema, decreased visual acuity, and exophthalmos. Tertiary lesions appear on the skin and mucous membranes. Liver, respiratory, cardiovascular, and additional neurologic dysfunction may also occur.

◆ ***Wernicke's disease.*** Initially, this disorder produces an intention tremor accompanied by a sluggish pupillary reaction. Later, pupils may become nonreactive. Additional ocular findings include diplopia, gaze paralysis, nystagmus, ptosis, decreased visual acuity, and conjunctival injection. The patient may also exhibit orthostatic hypotension, tachycardia, ataxia, apathy, and confusion.

Special considerations

A sluggish pupillary reaction isn't diagnostically significant, although it occurs with various disorders.

Pediatric pointers

Children experience sluggish pupillary reactions for the same reasons as adults.

Purple striae

Purple striae—thin, purple streaks on the skin—characteristically occur in hypercortisolism along with other cushingoid signs, such as a buffalo hump and moon face. Although hypercortisolism can be caused by adrenocortical carcinoma, adrenal adenoma, and pituitary adenoma, it usually results from excessive use of glucocorticoids.

The catabolic action of excess glucocorticoids on skin, fat, and muscle produces purple striae by inhibiting fibroblast activity, resulting in loss of collagen and connective tissue. This causes extreme thinning of the skin, which, along with erythrocytosis, is responsible for the striae's purple color. Although purple striae are most common over the abdominal area, they may also occur over the breasts, hips, buttocks, thighs, and axillae. They develop gradually and, with treatment, may gradually fade or decrease in size.

History and physical examination

Ask the patient when—and on what part of his body—he first noticed purple striae. To help determine the rate of progression, find out if he has photographs of himself before and over the course of striae development. Next, obtain a complete drug history. If the patient is receiving glucocorticoid therapy, find out the drug's name, the daily dose and schedule, and the reason for treatment. Ask if the dosage has been altered recently and if the drug is given intramuscularly. Find out if the patient uses a topical corticosteroid, especially a fluorinated product; ask about concomitant use of occlusive dressings and, with large skin surface areas, the amount of corticosteroid applied.

Examine the patient and note all areas where purple striae appear. When checking for striae, remember that the patient's skin is extremely thin and susceptible to bruising.

Medical causes

◆ ***Hypercortisolism.*** With this disorder, purple striae—usually more than 1 cm wide—develop gradually over the abdomen and possibly the breasts, hips, buttocks, thighs, and axillae. Inspection also reveals the cardinal signs of moon face, buffalo hump, and truncal obesity. Other findings include acne, ecchymoses, petechiae, muscle weakness and wasting, poor wound healing, excessive perspiration, hypertension, fatigue, and personality changes. Women may develop hirsutism, menstrual irregularities, and inability to achieve orgasm. Men may become impotent.

Other causes

◆ ***Drugs.*** Excessive use of a glucocorticoid can cause purple striae and other cushingoid effects.

Special considerations

Help the patient cope with changes in his body image by clearly explaining the disease process and allowing him to openly express his concerns. Prepare him for diagnostic tests to confirm hypercortisolism and determine its cause. Expect to collect 24-hour urine specimens before and during the 2-day low-dose and 2-day high-dose dexamethasone tests. Explain that follow-up tests may be performed.

Pediatric pointers

Although relatively rare in children, hypercortisolism may occur at any age. In infancy and early childhood, it usually results from adrenal tumor, systemic absorption of a topical corticosteroid applied excessively, or oral administration of a glucocorticoid. After age 7, it usually stems from inappropriate pituitary secretion of corticotropin, with bilateral adrenal hyperplasia.

Purpura

Purpura is the extravasation of red blood cells from the blood vessels into the skin, subcutaneous tissue, or mucous membranes. It's characterized by discoloration that's easily visible through the epidermis, usually purplish or brownish red. Purpuric lesions include petechiae, ecchymoses, and hematomas. (See *Identifying purpuric lesions*.) Purpura differs from erythema in that it doesn't blanch with pressure because it involves blood in the tissues, not just dilated vessels.

Identifying purpuric lesions

Purpuric lesions fall into three categories: petechiae, ecchymoses, and hematomas.

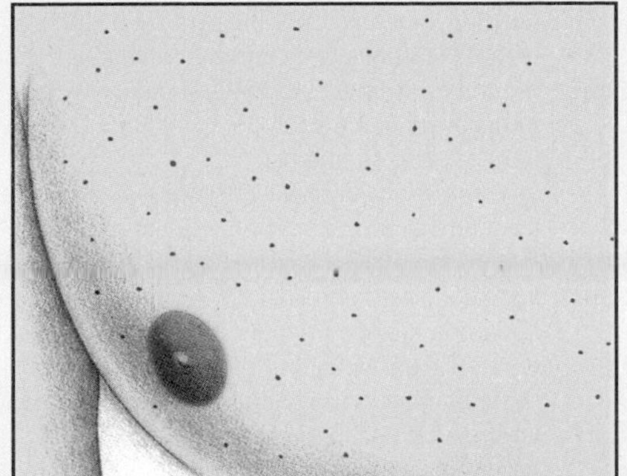

Petechiae

Petechiae are painless, round, pinpoint lesions, 1 to 3 mm in diameter. Caused by extravasation of red blood cells into cutaneous tissue, these red or brown lesions usually arise on dependent portions of the body. They appear and fade in crops and can group to form ecchymoses.

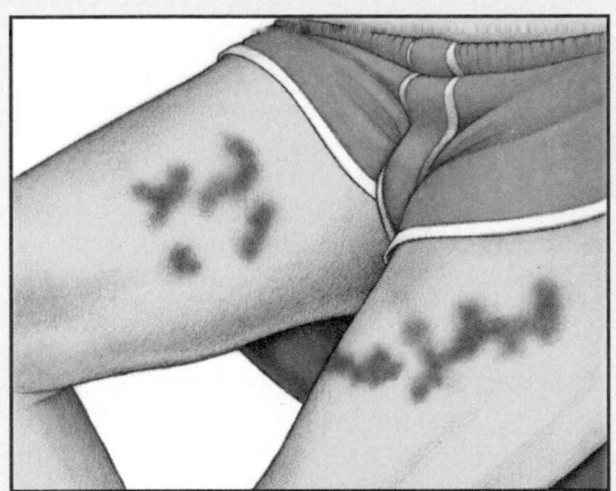

Ecchymoses

Ecchymoses, another form of blood extravasation, are larger than petechiae. These purple, blue, or yellow-green bruises vary in size and shape and can arise anywhere on the body as a result of trauma. Ecchymoses usually appear on the arms and legs of patients with bleeding disorders.

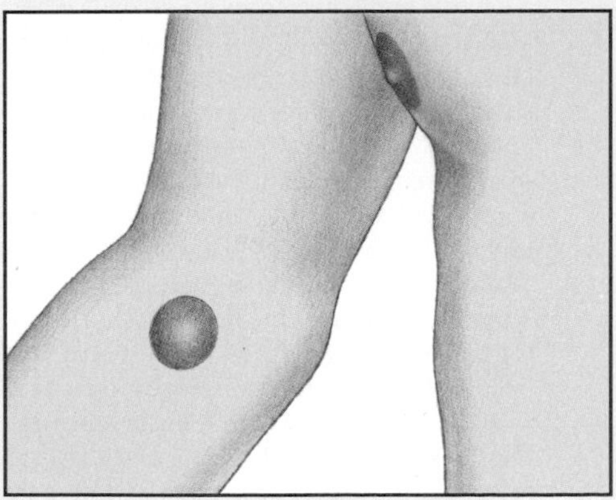

Hematomas

Hematomas are palpable ecchymoses that are painful and swollen. Usually the result of trauma, superficial hematomas are red, whereas deep hematomas are blue. Hematomas commonly exceed 1 cm in diameter, but their size varies widely.

Purpura results from damage to the endothelium of small blood vessels, a coagulation defect, ineffective perivascular support, capillary fragility and permeability, or a combination of these factors. These faulty hemostatic factors, in turn, can result from thrombocytopenia or another hematologic disorder, an invasive procedure, or the use of an anticoagulant.

Additional causes are nonpathologic. Purpura can be a consequence of aging, when loss of collagen decreases connective tissue support of upper skin blood vessels. In an elderly or cachectic person, skin atrophy and inelasticity and loss of subcutaneous fat increase susceptibility to minor trauma, causing purpura to appear along the veins of the forearms, hands, legs, and feet. Prolonged coughing or vomiting can produce crops of petechiae in loose face and neck tissue. Violent muscle contraction, as occurs in seizures or weight lifting, sometimes results in localized ecchymoses from increased intraluminal pressure and rupture. High fever, which increases capillary fragility, can also produce purpura.

GENDER CUE *This condition is more common in women and particularly in individuals with large areas of subcutaneous fat, such as the breasts, abdomen, buttocks, thighs, and calves.*

History and physical examination

Ask the patient when he first noticed the lesion and whether he has noticed other lesions on his body. Does he or his family have a history of a bleeding disorder or easy bruising? Find out what medications he's taking, if any, and ask him to describe his diet. Ask about recent trauma or transfusions and the development of associated signs, such as epistaxis, bleeding gums, hematuria, and hematochezia. Ask about systemic complaints that may suggest infection, such as fever. If the patient is female, ask about heavy menstrual flow.

Inspect the patient's entire skin surface to determine the type, size, location, distribution, and severity of purpuric lesions. Inspect the mucous membranes. Remember that the same mechanisms that cause purpura can also cause internal hemorrhage, although purpura isn't a cardinal indicator of this condition.

Medical causes

◆ ***Amyloidosis.*** This disorder produces purpura that appears either spontaneously on dependent areas of the skin or following minor trauma, coughing, or straining. The eyelids and mucous membranes are commonly affected.

◆ ***Autoerythrocyte sensitivity.*** With this syndrome, painful ecchymoses appear either singly or in groups, usually preceded by local itching, burning, or pain. Common associated findings include epistaxis, hematuria, hematemesis, and menometrorrhagia. Abdominal pain, diarrhea, nausea, vomiting, syncope, headache, and chest pain are also common.

◆ ***Cholesterol emboli.*** Purpura due to cholesterol emboli are most commonly found in the lower extremities of patient with atherosclerotic vascular disease and usually occur after anticoagulation therapy or an invasive arterial procedure such as angiogram or cardiac catheterization but may occur spontaneously. Associated findings include livedo reticularis, cyanosis, gangrene, nodules and ulceration of the skin.

◆ ***Dermatoses (pigmented).*** This group of disorders, thought to result from chronic stasis, produces benign, chronic purpura, mainly on dependent areas.

◆ ***Disseminated intravascular coagulation.*** This disorder can cause varying degrees of purpura, depending on its severity and underlying cause. Rarely, the patient develops life-threatening purpura fulminans, with symmetrical cutaneous and subcutaneous lesions on the arms and legs, or he may have cutaneous oozing, hematemesis, or bleeding from incision or needle insertion sites. Other findings include acrocyanosis; nausea; dyspnea; seizures; severe muscle, back, and abdominal pain; and signs of acute tubular necrosis, such as oliguria.

◆ ***Dysproteinemias.*** With multiple myeloma, petechiae and ecchymoses accompany other bleeding tendencies: hematemesis, epistaxis, gum bleeding, and excessive bleeding after surgery. Similar findings occur with cryoglobulinemia, which may also produce malignant maculopapular purpura. Hyperglobulinemia typically begins insidiously with occasional outbreaks of purpura over the lower legs and feet. These outbreaks eventually become more frequent and extensive, involving the entire lower leg and possibly the trunk. The purpura usually occurs after prolonged standing or exercise and may be heralded by skin burning or stinging. Leg edema, knee or ankle pain, and low-grade fever may precede or accompany the purpura, which gradually fades over 1 to 2 weeks. Persistent pigmentation develops after repeated outbreaks.

◆ ***Easy bruising syndrome.*** This syndrome is characterized by recurrent bruising on the legs, arms, and trunk, either spontaneously or following minor trauma. Bruising may be preceded by pain and is more common in women than in men, especially during menses.

◆ ***Ehlers-Danlos syndrome (EDS).*** Besides petechiae, this syndrome is marked by easy bruising, epistaxis, gum bleeding, hematuria, melena, menorrhagia, and excessive bleeding after surgery. EDS characteristically produces soft, velvety, hyperelastic skin; hyperextensible joints; increased skin and blood vessel fragility; and repeated dislocations of the temporomandibular joint.

◆ ***Fat emboli.*** Petechiae that occur on the upper body a few days after a major injury are caused by fat emboli.

◆ ***Idiopathic thrombocytopenic purpura (ITP).*** Chronic ITP typically begins insidiously, with scattered petechiae that are usually found on the distal arms and legs. Deep-lying ecchymoses may also occur. Other findings include epistaxis, easy bruising, hematuria, hematemesis, and menorrhagia.

◆ ***Leukemia.*** This disease produces widespread petechiae on the skin, mucous membranes, retina, and serosal surfaces that persist throughout the course of the disease. Confluent ecchymoses are uncommon. The patient may also exhibit swollen and bleeding gums, epistaxis, and other bleeding tendencies. Lymphadenopathy and splenomegaly are common.

Acute leukemias also produce severe prostration and high fever and may cause dyspnea, tachycardia, palpitations, and abdominal or bone pain. Confusion, headache, seizures, vomiting, papilledema, and nuchal rigidity may occur late in the disease. Chronic leukemias begin insidiously with minor bleeding tendencies, malaise, fatigue, pallor, low-grade fever, anorexia, and weight loss.

◆ ***Liver disease.*** Liver disease may cause purpura, particularly ecchymoses, and other bleeding tendencies. Associated findings include hepatomegaly, ascites, right-upper-quadrant pain, jaundice, nausea, vomiting, and anorexia.

◆ ***Lymphomas.*** T-cell (Hodgkin's) lymphomas initially may produce erythematous patches with some scaling. These lesions, which may be psoriasiform or parapsoriasiform, then become interspersed with nodules. Pruritus and discomfort are common. Later, tumors and ulcerations form, and nontender lymphadenopathy develops.

B-cell (non-Hodgkin's) lymphoma may produce a scaling dermatitis with pruritus, which usually begins on the legs and then affects the entire body. Small pink-to-brown nodules and diffuse pigmentation also occur. B-cell lymphomas typically produce painless peripheral lymphadenopathy, usually affecting the cervical nodes first. Other findings in both types of lymphoma include fever, fatigue, malaise, weight loss, and hepatosplenomegaly.

◆ ***Meningococcemia.*** Transmitted by droplet inhalation, it's most common in children and caused by *Neisseria meningitidis.* Cutaneous and oropharyngeal petechia and purpura are initially discrete but become confluent, developing into hemorrhagic bullae and ulcerations. Fulminant infection results in extensive purpura and ecchymosis with irregular borders (purpura fulminans) most notably on the extremities. These lesions may develop necrotic centers. This disease is usually fatal if not recognized and treated early. Prognosis is poor when purpura or ecchymosis is present at the time of diagnosis. Associated symptoms include spiking fevers, chills, myalgia and arthralgia, and recent upper respiratory tract infection. Rapid progression of symptoms leads to headache, neck stiffness and nuchal rigidity. Septic shock ensues within hours on onset of symptoms with altered mental status and hypotension.

◆ ***Myeloproliferative disorders.*** These disorders, which include polycythemia vera, paradoxically can cause hemorrhage accompanied by ecchymoses and ruddy cyanosis. The oral mucosa takes on a deep purplish red hue, and slight trauma causes swollen gums to bleed. Other findings include pruritus, urticaria, and such nonspecific signs and symptoms as lethargy, weakness, fatigue, and weight loss. The patient typically complains of headache, a sensation of fullness in the head, and rushing in the ears; dizziness and vertigo; dyspnea; paresthesia of the fingers; double or blurred vision and scotoma; and epigastric distress. He may also experience intermittent claudication, hypertension, hepatosplenomegaly, and impaired mentation.

◆ ***Nutritional deficiencies.*** With vitamin C deficiency (scurvy), the characteristic pattern of purpura is perifollicular petechiae, which coalesce to form ecchymoses, in the "saddle area" of the thighs and buttocks. Additional hemorrhaging occurs in arm and leg muscles (with phlebothrombosis), viscera, joints (with limb and joint pain), and nail beds. Related findings include scaly dermatitis; pallor; tender, swollen, bleeding gums and loosened teeth; dry mouth; and poor wound healing. Nonspecific symptoms include weakness, lethargy, and anorexia. Irritability, depression, insomnia, and hysteria may also develop.

Vitamin K deficiency produces abnormal bleeding tendencies, such as ecchymosis, gum bleeding, epistaxis, hematuria, and GI and intracranial bleeding.

Vitamin B_{12} deficiency can cause varying degrees of purpura. GI findings include anorexia, nausea, vomiting, weight loss, abdominal discomfort, and jaundice. Dyspnea, peripheral neuropathies, ataxia, glossitis and, occasionally, depression also occur.

Folic acid deficiency also can cause varying degrees of purpura. The patient may be irritable and forgetful and complain of fatigue, weakness, dyspnea, palpitations, nausea, anorexia, headaches, and fainting spells. Additional findings include pallor, slight jaundice, and glossitis.

◆ ***Rocky Mountain spotted fever.*** This illness is contracted through the bite of an infected tick and is most common among children between ages 5 and 10. Initial skin lesions are small pink macules that evolve into blatant petechia and palpable purpura. Hemorrhagic macules may develop. The palms and soles are particularly affected. Extensive cutaneous necrosis occurs due to disseminated intravascular coagulation in a small percentage of patients experiencing gangrene of the extremities, necessitating amputation. Associated signs and symptoms include fever, severe headache, generalized myalgia, photophobia, nausea and vomiting. Late in the course of the illness, shock and death may occur.

◆ ***Septicemia.*** Thrombocytopenia or the effects of toxins in acute infection can lead to purpura, especially in the form of petechiae. Associated findings include fever, chills, headache, tachycardia, lethargy, diaphoresis, and anorexia. Signs and symptoms specific to the area of infection—for example, cough, wound drainage, and urinary burning—also occur.

◆ ***Stasis.*** Chronic stasis usually affects the elderly, producing dusky reddish purpura on the legs after prolonged standing.

◆ ***Systemic lupus erythematosus.*** This chronic inflammatory disorder may produce purpura accompanied by other cutaneous findings, such as scaly patches on the scalp, face, neck, and arms; diffuse alopecia; telangiectasia; urticaria; and ulceration. The characteristic butterfly rash appears in the disorder's acute phase. Common associated signs and symptoms include nondeforming joint pain and stiffness, Raynaud's phenomenon, seizures, psychotic behavior, photosensitivity, fever, anorexia, weight loss, and lymphadenopathy.

◆ ***Thrombotic thrombocytopenic purpura.*** Generalized purpura, hematuria, vaginal bleeding, jaundice, and pallor are among the usual presenting signs and symptoms in this disorder. Most patients have fever, and some also experience fatigue, weakness, headache, nausea, abdominal pain, arthralgias, and hepatosplenomegaly. Possible neurologic effects include seizures, paresthesia, cranial nerve palsies, vertigo, and altered level of consciousness. Renal failure may also occur.

◆ ***Trauma.*** Traumatic injury can cause local or widespread purpura.

◆ ***Vasculitis.*** Palpable purpura is commonly caused by allergic vasculitis (leukocytoclastic vasculitis) of which Henoch-Schönlein purpura is one subtype. Most common in adolescents and children, lesions can be found anywhere on the body but are most prevalent on the lower extremities and buttocks. The purpura tends to be smooth, bordered, and circular in nature. Systemic signs and symptoms include fever, arthralgias, abdominal pain, GI bleeding and nephritis.

Other causes

◆ ***Diagnostic tests.*** Invasive procedures, such as venipuncture and arterial catheterization, may produce local ecchymoses and hematomas due to extravasated blood.

◆ ***Drugs.*** The anticoagulants heparin and warfarin can produce purpura. Administration of warfarin can result in painful areas of erythema that become purpuric then necrotic with an adherent black eschar. The lesions develop between the 3rd and 10th day of drug administration.

◆ ***Surgery and other procedures.*** Any procedure that disrupts circulation, coagulation, or platelet activity or production can cause purpura. These include pulmonary and cardiac surgery, radiation therapy, chemotherapy, hemodialysis, multiple blood transfusions with platelet-poor blood, and use of plasma expanders such as dextran.

Special considerations

Reassure the patient that purpuric lesions aren't permanent and will fade if the underlying cause can be successfully treated. Warn him not to use cosmetic fade creams or other products in an attempt to reduce pigmentation. If he has a hematoma, apply pressure and cold compresses initially to help reduce bleeding and swelling. After the first 24 hours, apply hot compresses to help speed absorption of blood.

Prepare the patient for diagnostic tests. These may include a peripheral blood smear, bone marrow examination, and blood tests to determine platelet count, bleeding and coagulation times, capillary fragility, clot retraction, one-stage prothrombin time, activated partial thromboplastin time, and fibrinogen levels.

Pediatric pointers

Neonates commonly exhibit petechiae, particularly on the head, neck, and shoulders, after vertex deliveries. Thought to result from the trauma of birth, these petechiae disappear within a few days. Other causes in infants include thrombocytopenia, vitamin K deficiency, and infantile scurvy.

The most common type of purpura in children is allergic purpura. Other causes in children include trauma, hemophilia, autoimmune hemolytic anemia, Gaucher's disease, thrombasthenia, congenital factor deficiencies, Wiskott-Aldrich syndrome, acute ITP, von Willebrand's disease, and the rare but life-threatening purpura fulminans, which usually follows bacterial or viral infection.

As a child grows and tests his motor skills, the risk of accidents multiplies, and ecchymoses and hematomas commonly occur. However, when you assess a child with purpura, be alert for signs of possible child abuse: bruises in different stages of resolution, from repeated beatings; bruise patterns resembling a familiar object, such as a belt, hand, or thumb and finger; and bruises on the face, buttocks, or genitalia, areas unlikely to be injured accidentally.

Pustular rash

A pustular rash is made up of crops of pustules—a visible collection of pus within or beneath the epidermis, commonly in a hair follicle or sweat pore. These lesions vary greatly in size and shape and can be generalized or localized to the hair follicles or sweat glands. (See *Recognizing common skin lesions*, pages 518 and 519.) Pustules can result from a skin or systemic disorder, the use of certain drugs, or exposure to a skin irritant. For example, people who've been swimming in salt water commonly develop a papulopustular rash under the bathing suit or elsewhere on the body from irritation by sea organisms. Although many pustular lesions are sterile, a pustular rash usually indicates infection. Any vesicular eruption, or even acute contact dermatitis, can become pustular if secondary infection occurs.

History and physical examination

Have the patient describe the appearance, location, and onset of the first pustular lesion. Did another type of skin lesion precede the pustule? Find out how the lesions spread. Ask what medications the patient takes and if he has applied any topical medication to his rash. If so, what type and when did he last apply it? Find out if he has a family history of a skin disorder.

Examine the entire skin surface, noting if it's dry, oily, moist, or greasy. Record the exact location and distribution of the skin lesions and their color, shape, and size.

Medical causes

◆ ***Acne vulgaris.*** Pustules typify inflammatory lesions of this disorder, which is accompanied by papules, nodules, cysts, open comedones (blackheads) and closed (whiteheads) comedones. Lesions commonly appear on the face, shoulders, back, and chest. Other findings include pain on pressure, pruritus, and burning. Chronic recurrent lesions produce scars.

◆ ***Blastomycosis.*** This fungal infection produces small, painless, nonpruritic macules or papules that can enlarge to well-circumscribed, verrucous, crusted, or ulcerated lesions edged by pustules. Localized infection may cause only one lesion; systemic infection may cause many lesions on the hands, feet, face, and wrists. Blastomycosis also produces signs of pulmonary infection, such as pleuritic chest pain and a dry, hacking or productive cough with occasional hemoptysis.

◆ ***Folliculitis.*** This bacterial infection of hair follicles produces individual pustules, each pierced by a hair and possibly accompanied by pruritus. "Hot tub" folliculitis produces pustules on areas covered by a bathing suit.

◆ ***Furunculosis.*** A furnicle is an acute, deep-seated, red, hot, tender abscess that evolves from a staphylococcus folliculitis. Furuncles usually begin as small, tender red pustules at the base of hair follicles. They're likely to occur on the face, neck, forearm, groin, axillae, buttocks, and legs; areas that are prone to repeated friction. The pustules usually remain tense for 2 to 4 days and then become fluctuant. Rupture discharges pus and necrotic material. Then pain subsides, but erythema and edema may persist.

◆ ***Gonococcemia.*** This disorder produces a rash of scanty, pinpoint erythematous macules that rapidly become vesiculopustular, maculopapular and, frequently, hemorrhagic. Bullae may form. Mature lesions are elevated, with dirty gray necrotic centers and surrounding erythema. The rash appears on the distal part of the arms and legs, usually during the 1st day that other findings, such as fever and joint pain, occur. The rash disappears after 3 to 4 days but may recur with each episode of fever.

◆ ***Impetigo contagiosa.*** This vesiculopustular eruptive disorder, which occurs in nonbullous and bullous forms, is usually caused by streptococci or staphylococci. Vesicles form and break, and a crust forms from the exudate: a thick, yellow crust in streptococcal impetigo and a thin, clear crust in staphylococcal impetigo. Both forms usually produce painless itching.

◆ ***Nummular or annular dermatitis.*** With this disorder, numerous coinlike (nummular) or ringed (annular) pustular lesions appear, usually on the extensor surfaces of the extremities, posterior trunk, buttocks, and lower legs; a few lesions may appear on the hands. The lesions commonly ooze a purulent exudate, itch severely, and rapidly become crusted and scaly. A few small, scaling patches may remain for some time.

◆ ***Pustular miliaria.*** This anhidrotic disorder causes pustular lesions that begin as tiny erythematous papulovesicles located at sweat pores. Diffuse erythema may radiate from the lesion. The rash and associated burning and pruritus worsen with sweating.

◆ ***Pustular psoriasis.*** Small vesicles form and eventually become pustules in this disorder. The patient may report pruritus, burning, and pain. Localized pustular psoriasis usually affects the hands and feet. Generalized pustular psoriasis may erupt suddenly in patients with psoriasis, psoriatic arthritis, or exfoliative psoriasis; although rare, this form of psoriasis can occasionally be fatal.

◆ ***Rosacea.*** This chronic hyperemic disorder commonly produces telangiectasia with acute episodes of pustules, papules, and edema. Characterized by persistent erythema, rosacea may begin as a flush covering the forehead, malar region, nose, and chin. Intermittent episodes gradually become more persistent, and the skin—instead of returning to its normal color—develops varying degrees of erythema.

◆ ***Scabies.*** Threadlike channels or burrows under the skin characterize this disorder, which can also produce pustules, vesicles, and excoriations. The lesions are a few millimeters long, with a swollen nodule or red papule that contains the itch mite.

GENDER CUE *In men, crusted lesions commonly develop on the glans, shaft, and scrotum. In women, lesions may form on the nipples. In both sexes these lesions have a predilection for skin folds. Crusty excoriated lesions also develop on wrists, elbows, axillae, waistline, behind the knees and ankles. Related pruritus worsens with inactivity and warmth.*

◆ ***Smallpox (variola major).*** Initial signs and symptoms include high fever, malaise, prostration, severe headache, backache, and abdominal pain. A maculopapular rash develops on the mucosa of the mouth, pharynx, face and forearms and then spreads to the trunk and legs. Within 2 days the rash becomes vesicular and later pustular. The lesions develop at the same time, appear identical and are more prominent on the face and extremities. The pustules are round, firm, and deeply embedded in the skin. After 8 to 9 days, the pustules form a crust and later the scab separates from the skin leaving a pitted scar. In fatal cases, death results from encephalitis, extensive bleeding or secondary infection.

◆ ***Varicella zoster.*** When immunity to varicella declines, the virus reactivates along a dermatome, producing extremely painful and pruritic vesicles and pustules (herpes zoster, or shingles). Even with resolution of the rash, patients may experience chronic pain (postherpetic neuralgia) that may persist for months.

OTHER CAUSES

◆ ***Drugs.*** Bromides and iodides commonly cause a pustular rash. Other drug causes include corticotropin, corticosteroids, dactinomycin, trimethadione, lithium, phenytoin, phenobarbital, isoniazid, hormonal contraceptives, androgens, and anabolic steroids.

SPECIAL CONSIDERATIONS

Observe wound and skin isolation procedures until infection is ruled out by a Gram stain or culture and sensitivity test of the pustule's contents. If the organism is infectious, don't allow any drainage to touch unaffected skin. Instruct the patient to keep his bathroom articles and linens separate from those of other family members. Associated pain and itching, altered body image, and the stress of isolation may result in loss of sleep, anxiety, and depression. Give medications to relieve pain and itching, and encourage the patient to express his feelings.

Pediatric pointers

Among the various disorders that produce pustular rash in children are varicella, erythema toxicum neonatorum, candidiasis, impetigo, infantile acropustulosis, and acrodermatitis enteropathica.

Pyrosis

Caused by reflux of gastric contents into the esophagus, pyrosis (heartburn) is a substernal burning sensation that rises in the chest and may radiate to the neck or throat. It's commonly accompanied by regurgitation, which also results from gastric reflux. Because increased intra-abdominal pressure contributes to reflux, pyrosis commonly occurs with pregnancy, ascites, or obesity. It also accompanies various GI disorders, connective tissue diseases, and the use of numerous drugs. Pyrosis usually develops after meals or when the patient lies down (especially on his right side), bends over, lifts heavy objects, or exercises vigorously. (See *How pyrosis occurs*, page 586.) It typically worsens with swallowing and improves when the patient sits upright or takes an antacid.

A patient experiencing a myocardial infarction (MI) may mistake chest pain for pyrosis. However, he'll probably develop other signs and symptoms—such as dyspnea, tachycardia, palpitations, nausea, and vomiting—that will help distinguish an MI from pyrosis. His chest pain won't be relieved by an antacid.

History and Physical Examination

Ask the patient if he has experienced heartburn before. Do certain foods or beverages trigger it? Does stress or fatigue aggravate his discomfort? Does movement, a certain body position, or ingestion of very hot or cold liquids worsen or help relieve the heartburn? Ask where the pain is located and whether it radiates to other areas. Find out if the patient regurgitates sour- or bitter-tasting fluids. (See *Regurgitation: Mechanism and causes,* page 587.) Does the patient have any associated signs and symptoms?

Medical causes

◆ ***Esophageal cancer.*** Pyrosis may be a sign of this cancer, depending on tumor size and location. The first and most common symptom is painless dysphagia that progressively worsens. Regurgitation and aspiration commonly occur at night. Eventually, partial obstruction and rapid weight loss occur, and the patient may complain of steady pain in the front and back of the chest. He may also experience hoarseness, sore throat, nausea, vomiting, and a feeling of substernal fullness.

◆ ***Esophageal diverticula.*** Although usually asymptomatic, this disorder may cause pyrosis, regurgitation, and dysphagia. Other findings include chronic cough, halitosis, and a gurgling in the esophagus when liquids are swallowed. The patient may also complain of chest pain and a bad taste in the mouth.

◆ ***Gastroesophageal reflux disease.*** Pyrosis, which is typically severe, is the most common symptom of this disorder. The pyrosis tends to be chronic, usually occurs 30 to 60 minutes after eating, and may be triggered by certain foods or beverages. It worsens when the patient lies down or bends and abates when he sits or stands upright or takes an antacid. Other findings include postural regurgitation, dysphagia, flatulent dyspepsia, and dull retrosternal pain that may radiate.

◆ ***Hiatal hernia.*** With this disorder, eructation occurs after eating and is accompanied by heartburn, regurgitation of sour-tasting fluid, and abdominal distention. The patient complains of dull substernal or epigastric pain that may radiate to the shoulder. Other features include dysphagia, nausea, weight loss, dyspnea, tachypnea, a cough, and halitosis.

◆ ***Obesity.*** Increased intra-abdominal pressure can contribute to reflux and resulting pyrosis.

◆ ***Peptic ulcer disease.*** Pyrosis and indigestion usually signal the start of a peptic ulcer attack. Most patients experience gnawing, burning pain in the left epigastrium, although some may report sharp pain. Typically, the pain arises 2 to 3 hours after eating or when the stomach is empty (usually at night), and is relieved by eating or taking an antacid or antisecretory drug. The pain may also occur after ingestion of coffee, aspirin, alcohol or, possibly, citrus juice.

◆ ***Scleroderma.*** This connective tissue disease may cause esophageal dysfunction resulting in

How pyrosis occurs

Serving as a barrier to reflux, the lower esophageal sphincter (LES) normally relaxes only to allow food to pass from the esophagus into the stomach. However, hormonal fluctuations, mechanical stress, and the effects of certain foods and drugs can lower LES pressure. When LES pressure falls and intra-abdominal or intragastric pressure rises, the normally contracted LES relaxes inappropriately and allows reflux of gastric acid or bile secretions into the lower esophagus. There, the acids or secretions irritate and inflame the esophageal mucosa, producing pyrosis.

Persistent inflammation can cause LES pressure to decrease even more and may trigger a recurrent cycle of reflux and pyrosis.

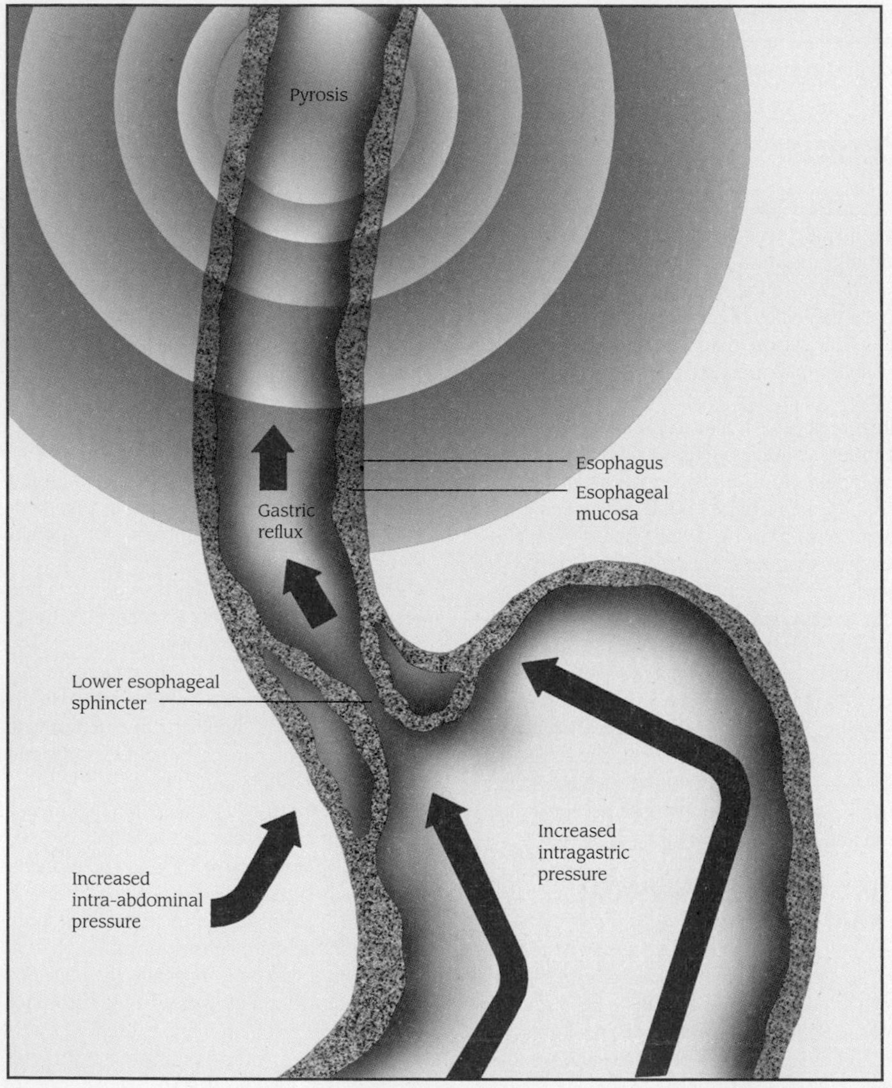

reflux with pyrosis, the sensation of food sticking behind the breastbone, odynophagia, bloating after meals, and weight loss. Other GI effects include abdominal distention, constipation or diarrhea, and malodorous floating stools. Early signs of scleroderma include blanching, pruritus, cyanosis, and stress- or cold-induced erythema of the fingers and toes. Later developments include finger and joint pain, stiffness, and swelling; skin thickening on the hands and forearms; masklike facies; and possibly flexion contractures. With advanced disease, cardiac and renal involvement may produce arrhythmias, dyspnea, cough, malignant hypertension, and signs of renal failure such as oliguria.

OTHER CAUSES

◆ ***Drugs.*** Various drugs may cause or aggravate pyrosis, including acetohexamide, tolbutamide, aspirin, anticholinergics, and drugs that have anticholinergic effects.

Both large meals and pregnancy may cause or aggravate pyrosis.

SPECIAL CONSIDERATIONS

Prepare the patient for diagnostic tests, such as barium swallow, upper GI series, esophagoscopy, and laboratory studies, to test esophageal motility and acidity.

PEDIATRIC POINTERS

A child may have difficulty distinguishing esophageal pain from pyrosis. To gain information, help him describe the sensation.

GERIATRIC POINTERS

Elderly patients with peptic ulcer disease commonly present with nonspecific abdominal discomfort or weight loss. Elderly patients are also at greater risk for complications from nonsteroidal anti-inflammatories, and many of them develop pyrosis due to intolerance to spicy foods.

PATIENT COUNSELING

After the causative disorder is determined, teach the patient how to avoid a recurrence of pyrosis. Advise him to eat frequent small meals, to sit upright (especially after a meal), and to avoid lying down for at least 2 hours after a meal. Instruct him to avoid highly seasoned foods, caffeine, acidic juices, carbonated beverages, alcohol, bedtime snacks, and foods high in fat or carbohydrates, which reduce lower esophageal sphincter (LES) pressure.

To prevent increased intra-abdominal pressure, instruct him to avoid bending, coughing, engaging in vigorous exercise, wearing tight clothing, or gaining weight. Advise him to refrain from smoking and using drugs that reduce sphincter control.

If the patient's pyrosis is severe, instruct him to sleep with extra pillows or with 6 wooden blocks under the head of the bed to reduce reflux by gravity. Tell him to take antacids (usually 1 hour after meals and at bedtime) or a histamine blocker, as ordered. Medications that increase LES contraction, such as bethanechol, may be required.

Regurgitation: Mechanism and causes

When gastric reflux moves up the esophagus and passes through the upper esophageal sphincter, regurgitation occurs. Unlike vomiting, regurgitation is effortless and unaccompanied by nausea. It usually happens when the patient is lying down or bending over and commonly accompanies pyrosis. Aspiration of regurgitated gastric contents can lead to recurrent pulmonary infections.

In adults, regurgitation usually results from esophageal disorders such as achalasia. However, it can also occur when the gag reflex is absent, as in bulbar palsy, or when the patient has an overfilled stomach or esophagus.

In infants, regurgitation can signal pyloric stenosis or dysphagia lusoria. Usually, however, infants "spit up" because their esophageal sphincters aren't fully developed during the first year of life. To help reduce regurgitation in an infant, teach the parents to handle the infant gently during feeding and to burp him frequently. After feeding, they should place the infant on his back with his head slightly elevated to avoid gravitational regurgitation and to help prevent aspiration.

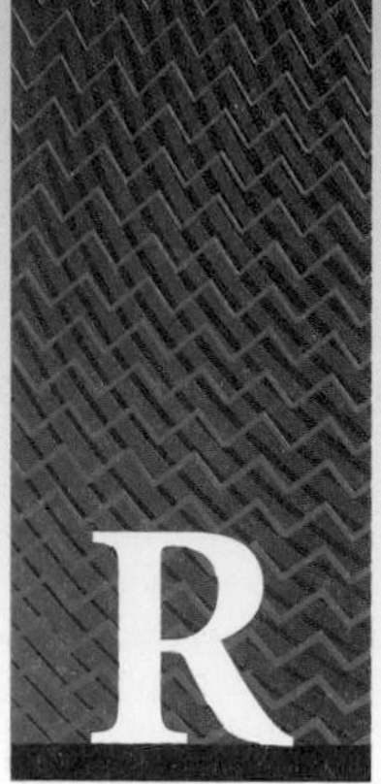

Raccoon eyes

Raccoon eyes are bilateral periorbital ecchymoses that don't result from facial soft-tissue trauma. Usually an indicator of basilar skull fracture, this sign develops when damage at the time of fracture tears the meninges and causes the venous sinuses to bleed into the arachnoid villi and the cranial sinuses. Raccoon eyes may be the only indicator of a basilar skull fracture, which isn't always visible on skull X-rays. Their appearance signals the need for careful assessment to detect any underlying trauma because a basilar skull fracture can injure cranial nerves, blood vessels, and the brain stem. Raccoon eyes can also occur after a craniotomy if the surgery causes a meningeal tear.

History and physical examination

After raccoon eyes are detected, check the patient's vital signs and try to find out when the head injury occurred and the nature of the head injury. (See *Recognizing raccoon eyes*.) Then evaluate the extent of underlying trauma.

Start by evaluating the patient's level of consciousness (LOC) using the Glasgow Coma Scale. (See *Using the Glasgow Coma Scale,* page 422.) Next, evaluate function of the cranial nerves, especially the first (olfactory), third (oculomotor), fourth (trochlear), sixth (abducens), and seventh (facial). If the patient's condition permits, test his visual acuity and gross hearing. Note any irregularities in the facial or skull bones, as well as any swelling, localized pain, a Battle's sign, or lacerations of the face or scalp. Check for ecchymoses over the mastoid bone. Inspect for hemorrhage or cerebrospinal fluid (CSF) leakage from the nose or ears.

Test any drainage with a gauze pad, and note whether you find a halo sign—a circle of clear fluid that surrounds a bloody center, indicating CSF. Use a glucose reagent stick to test any clear drainage for glucose. A positive test result indicates CSF, because mucus doesn't contain glucose.

Medical causes

◆ ***Basilar skull fracture.*** This injury produces raccoon eyes after head trauma that doesn't involve the orbital area. Associated signs and symptoms vary with the fracture site and may include pharyngeal hemorrhage, epistaxis, rhinorrhea, otorrhea, and a bulging tympanic membrane from blood or CSF. The patient may experience difficulty hearing, headache, nausea, vomiting, cranial nerve palsies, and altered LOC. He may also exhibit a positive Battle's sign.

Other causes

◆ ***Surgery.*** Raccoon eyes occurring after craniotomy may indicate a meningeal tear and bleeding into the sinuses.

Special considerations

Keep the patient on complete bed rest. Perform frequent neurologic evaluations to reevaluate

Recognizing raccoon eyes

It's usually easy to differentiate raccoon eyes from the "black eye" associated with facial trauma. Raccoon eyes (shown below) are always bilateral. They develop 2 to 3 days after a closed-head injury that results in basilar skull fracture. In contrast, the periorbital ecchymosis that occurs with facial trauma can affect one eye or both. It usually develops within hours of injury.

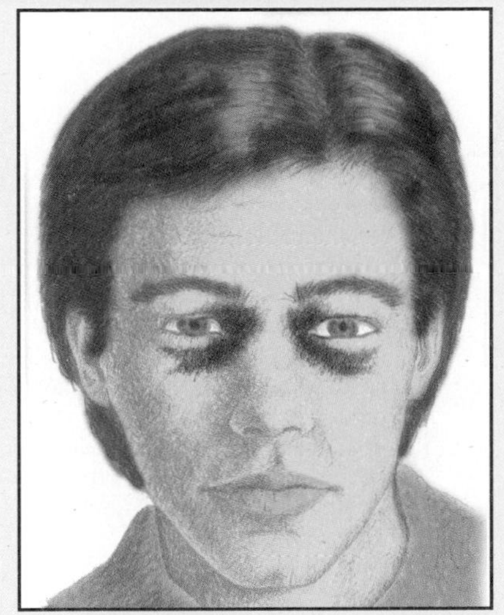

his LOC. Check vital signs hourly; be alert for such changes as bradypnea, bradycardia, hypertension, and fever. To avoid worsening a dural tear, instruct the patient not to blow his nose, cough vigorously, or strain. If otorrhea or rhinorrhea is present, don't attempt to stop the flow. Instead, place a sterile, loose gauze pad under the nose or ear to absorb the drainage. Monitor the amount and test it with a glucose reagent strip to confirm or rule out CSF leakage.

To prevent further tearing of the mucous membranes and infection, never suction or pass a nasogastric tube through the patient's nose. Observe the patient for signs and symptoms of meningitis, such as fever and nuchal rigidity, and expect to administer a prophylactic antibiotic.

Prepare the patient for diagnostic tests, such as a computed tomography scan. If the dural tear doesn't heal spontaneously, contrast cisternography may be performed to locate the tear, possibly followed by corrective surgery.

PEDIATRIC POINTERS

Raccoon eyes in children are usually caused by a basilar skull fracture after a fall.

Rebound tenderness

[Blumberg's sign]

A reliable indicator of peritonitis, rebound tenderness is intense, elicited abdominal pain caused by rebound of palpated tissue. The tenderness may be localized, as in an abscess, or generalized, as in perforation of an intra-abdominal organ. Rebound tenderness usually occurs with abdominal pain, tenderness, and rigidity. When a patient has sudden, severe abdominal pain, this symptom is usually elicited to detect peritoneal inflammation.

EMERGENCY INTERVENTIONS *If you elicit rebound tenderness in a patient who's experiencing constant, severe abdominal pain, quickly take his vital signs. Insert a large-bore I.V. catheter, and begin administering I.V. fluids. Also insert an indwelling urinary catheter, and monitor intake and output. Give supplemental oxygen as needed, and continue to monitor the patient for signs of shock, such as hypotension and tachycardia.*

HISTORY AND PHYSICAL EXAMINATION

If the patient's condition permits, ask him to describe the events that led up to the tenderness. Does movement, exertion, or any other activity relieve or aggravate the tenderness? Also, ask about other signs and symptoms, such as nausea and vomiting, fever, or abdominal bloating or distention. Inspect the abdomen for distention, visible peristaltic waves, and scars. Then auscultate for bowel sounds and characterize their motility. Palpate for associated rigidity or guarding and percuss the abdomen noting any tympany. (See *Eliciting rebound tenderness*, page 590.)

MEDICAL CAUSES

◆ ***Peritonitis.*** With this life-threatening disorder, rebound tenderness is accompanied by sudden and severe abdominal pain, which may be either diffuse or localized. Because movement worsens the patient's pain, he'll usually lie still on his back with his knees flexed. Typically, he'll display weakness, pallor, excessive sweating, and cold skin. He may

Eliciting rebound tenderness

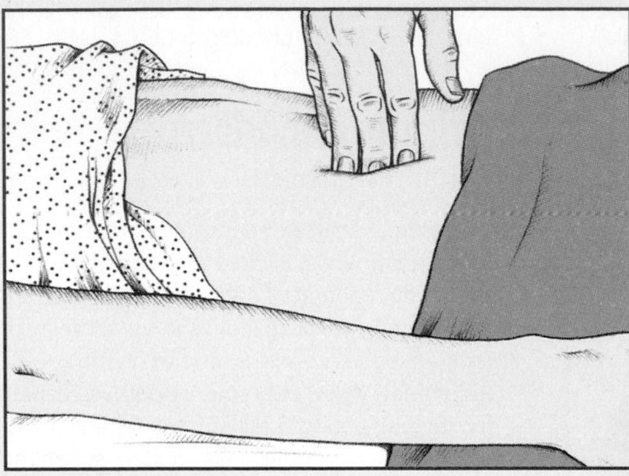

To elicit rebound tenderness, help the patient into a supine position and push your fingers deeply and steadily into his abdomen (as shown). Then quickly release the pressure. Pain that results from the rebound of palpated tissue—rebound tenderness—indicates peritoneal inflammation or peritonitis.

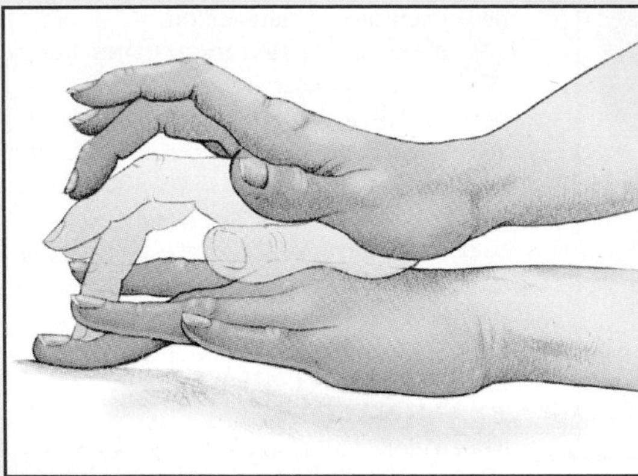

You can also elicit this symptom on a miniature scale by percussing the patient's abdomen lightly and indirectly (as shown). Better still, simply ask the patient to cough. This allows you to elicit rebound tenderness without having to touch the patient's abdomen and may also increase his cooperation because he won't associate exacerbation of his pain with your actions.

also display hypoactive or absent bowel sounds; tachypnea; nausea and vomiting; abdominal distention, rigidity and guarding; positive psoas and obturator signs; and a fever of 103° F (39.4° C) or higher. Inflammation of the diaphragmatic peritoneum may cause shoulder pain and hiccups.

Special considerations

Promote comfort by having the patient flex his knees or assume semi-Fowler's position. You may administer an analgesic, an antiemetic, and an antipyretic. However, because of decreased intestinal motility and the probability that the patient will have surgery, don't give oral drugs or fluids. Obtain samples of blood, urine, and feces for laboratory testing, and prepare the patient for chest and abdominal X-rays, ultrasounds and computed tomography scans. Perform a rectal or pelvic examination. Prepare the patient to receive an antibiotic, have a nasogastric tube inserted, to maintain a nothing-by-mouth status and to receive continuous parenteral fluid or nutrition.

Pediatric pointers

Eliciting rebound tenderness may be difficult in young children. Be alert for such clues as an anguished facial expression or intensified crying. When you elicit this symptom, use assessment techniques that produce minimal tenderness. For example, have the child hop or jump to allow tissue to rebound gently and watch as the child clutches at the furniture in pain.

GERIATRIC POINTERS

Rebound tenderness may be diminished or absent in elderly patients.

Rectal pain

A common symptom of anorectal disorders, rectal pain is discomfort that arises in the anorectal area. Although the anal canal is separated from the rest of the rectum by the internal sphincter, the patient may refer to all local pain as rectal pain.

Because the mucocutaneous border of the anal canal and the perianal skin contains somatic nerve fibers, lesions in this area are especially painful. This pain may result from or be aggravated by diarrhea, constipation, or passage of hardened stools. It may also be aggravated by intense pruritus and continued scratching associated with drainage of mucus, blood, or fecal matter that irritates the skin and nerve endings.

HISTORY AND PHYSICAL EXAMINATION

If your patient reports rectal pain, inspect the area for bleeding; abnormal drainage such as pus; or protrusions, such as skin tags or thrombosed hemorrhoids. Check for inflammation and other lesions. A rectal examination may be necessary.

After examination, proceed with your evaluation by taking the patient's history. Ask the patient to describe the pain. Is it sharp or dull, burning or knifelike? How often does it occur? Ask if the pain is worse during or immediately after defecation. Does the patient avoid having bowel movements because of anticipated pain? Find out what alleviates the pain.

Be sure to ask appropriate questions about the development of any associated signs and symptoms. For example, does the patient experience bleeding along with rectal pain? If so, find out how frequently this occurs and whether the blood appears on the toilet tissue, on the surface of the stool, or in the toilet bowl. Is the blood bright or dark red? Ask whether the patient has noticed other drainage, such as mucus or pus, and whether he's experiencing constipation or diarrhea. Ask when he last had a bowel movement. Obtain a dietary history.

MEDICAL CAUSES

◆ ***Abscess (perirectal).*** This abscess can occur in various locations in the rectum and anus, causing pain in the perianal area. Typically, a superficial abscess produces constant, throbbing local pain that's exacerbated by sitting or walking. The local pain associated with a deeper abscess may begin insidiously, often high in the rectum or even in the lower abdomen, and is accompanied by an indurated anal mass. The patient may also develop associated signs and symptoms, such as fever, malaise, anal swelling and inflammation, purulent drainage, and local tenderness.

◆ ***Abscess (prostatic).*** This disorder occasionally produces rectal pain. Common associated findings include urine retention and frequency, dysuria, and fever. A rectal examination may reveal prostatic tenderness and gas.

◆ ***Anal fissure.*** This longitudinal crack in the anal lining causes sharp rectal pain on defecation. The patient typically experiences a burning sensation and gnawing pain that can continue up to 4 hours after defecation. Fear of provoking this pain may lead to acute constipation. The patient may also develop anal pruritus and extreme tenderness and may report finding spots of blood on the toilet tissue after defecation.

◆ ***Anorectal fistula.*** Pain develops when a tract formed between the anal canal and skin temporarily seals. It persists until drainage resumes. Other chief complaints include pruritus and drainage of pus, blood, mucus, and occasionally stool.

◆ ***Cryptitis.*** This disorder results when particles of stool that are lodged in the anal folds decay and cause infection, which may produce dull anal pain or discomfort and anal pruritus.

◆ ***Hemorrhoids.*** Thrombosed or prolapsed hemorrhoids cause rectal pain that may worsen during defecation and abate after it. The patient's fear of provoking the pain may lead to constipation. Usually, rectal pain is accompanied by severe itching. Internal hemorrhoids may also produce mild, intermittent bleeding that characteristically occurs as spotting on the toilet tissue or on the stool surface. External hemorrhoids are visible outside the anal sphincter.

◆ ***Proctalgia fugax.*** With this disorder, muscle spasms of the rectum and pelvic floor produce sudden, severe episodes of rectal pain that last up to several minutes and then disappear. The patient may report being awakened by the pain, which is sometimes associated with stress or anxiety and relieved by food and drink.

◆ ***Rectal cancer.*** Rectal pain, bleeding, tenesmus, and a hard, nontender mass are typical findings in this rare form of cancer.

OTHER CAUSES

◆ ***Anal intercourse.*** Shearing forces may cause inflammation or tearing of the mucous membranes and discomfort.

SPECIAL CONSIDERATIONS

Apply analgesic ointment or suppositories, and administer a stool softener if needed. If the rectal pain results from prolapsed hemorrhoids, apply cold compresses to help shrink protruding hemorrhoids, prevent thrombosis, and reduce pain. If the patient's condition permits, place him in Trendelenburg's position with his buttocks elevated to further relieve pain.

You may have to prepare the patient for an anoscopic examination and proctosigmoidoscopy to determine the cause of rectal pain. He may also need to provide a stool sample. Because the patient may feel embarrassed by treatments and diagnostic tests involving the rectum, provide emotional support and as much privacy as possible.

PEDIATRIC POINTERS

Observe any child with rectal pain for associated bleeding, drainage, and signs of infection (fever and irritability). Acute anal fissure is a common cause of rectal pain and bleeding in children, whose fear of provoking the pain may lead to constipation. Infants who seem to have pain on defecation should be evaluated for congenital anomalies of the rectum. Consider the possibility of sexual abuse in all children who complain of rectal pain.

GERIATRIC POINTERS

Because elderly people typically underreport their symptoms and have an increased risk of neoplastic disorders, they should always be thoroughly evaluated.

PATIENT COUNSELING

Teach the patient how to apply hot, moist compresses. Teach him how to give himself a sitz bath; this will ease his discomfort by helping to relieve the sphincter spasm associated with most anorectal disorders. Stress the importance of following a high-fiber diet and drinking plenty of fluids to maintain soft stools and thus avoid aggravating pain during defecation.

Respirations, grunting

Characterized by a deep, low-pitched grunting sound at the end of each breath, grunting respirations are a chief sign of respiratory distress in infants and children. They may be soft and heard only on auscultation, or loud and clearly audible without a stethoscope. Typically, the intensity of grunting respirations reflects the severity of respiratory distress. The grunting sound coincides with closure of the glottis, an effort to increase end-expiratory pressure in the lungs and prolong alveolar gas exchange, thereby enhancing ventilation and perfusion.

Grunting respirations indicate intrathoracic disease with lower respiratory involvement. Though most common in children, they sometimes occur in adults who are in severe respiratory distress. Whether they occur in children or adults, grunting respirations demand immediate medical attention. (See *Positioning an infant for chest physical therapy,* pages 594 and 595.)

EMERGENCY INTERVENTIONS *If the patient exhibits grunting respirations, quickly place him in a comfortable position and check for signs of respiratory distress: wheezing; tachypnea (a minimum respiratory rate of 60 breaths/minute in infants, 40 breaths/minute in children ages 1 to 5, 30 breaths/minute in children older than age 5, or 20 breaths/minute in adults); accessory muscle use; substernal, subcostal, or intercostal retractions; nasal flaring; tachycardia (a minimum of 160 beats/minute in infants, 120 to 140 beats/minute in children ages 1 to 5, 120 beats/minute in children older age 5, or 100 beats/minute in adults); cyanotic lips or nail beds; hypotension (less than 80/40 mm Hg in infants, less than 80/50 mm Hg in children ages 1 to 5, less than 90/55 mm Hg in children older than age 5, or less than 90/60 mm Hg in adults); and decreased level of consciousness.*

If you detect any of these signs, monitor oxygen saturation, and administer oxygen and prescribed medications such as a bronchodilator. Have emergency equipment available and prepare to intubate the patient if necessary. Obtain arterial blood gas analysis to determine oxygenation status.

HISTORY AND PHYSICAL EXAMINATION

After addressing the child's respiratory status, ask his parents when the grunting respirations began. If the patient is a premature infant, find out his gestational age. Ask the parents if anyone in the home has recently had an upper respiratory tract infection. Has the child had signs and symptoms of such an infection, such as a runny nose, cough, low-grade fever, or anorexia? Does he have a history of frequent colds or upper respiratory tract infections? Does he have a history of respiratory syncytial virus? Ask the parents to describe changes in the child's activity level or feeding pattern to determine if the child is lethargic or less alert than usual.

Begin the physical examination by auscultating the lungs, especially the lower lobes. Note diminished or abnormal sounds, such as crackles or sibilant rhonchi, which may indicate mucus or fluid buildup. Characterize the color, amount, and consistency of any discharge or sputum. Note the characteristics of the cough, if any.

Medical causes

◆ ***Asthma.*** Grunting respirations may be apparent during a severe asthma exacerbation, usually triggered by an upper respiratory tract infection or an allergic response. As the attack progresses, dyspnea, audible wheezing, chest tightness, and coughing occur. Patients may have a silent chest if air movement is poor. Immediate bronchodilator therapy is needed.

◆ ***Heart failure.*** A late sign of left-sided heart failure, grunting respirations accompany increasing pulmonary edema. Associated features include a productive cough, crackles, jugular vein distention, and chest wall retractions. Cyanosis may also be evident, depending on the underlying congenital cardiac defect.

◆ ***Pneumonia.*** Life-threatening bacterial pneumonia is common after an upper respiratory tract infection or cold. *Pneumocystis carinii* pneumonia commonly affects children infected with human immunodeficiency virus. It causes grunting respirations accompanied by high fever, tachypnea, a productive cough, anorexia, and lethargy. Auscultation reveals diminished breath sounds, scattered crackles, and sibilant rhonchi over the affected lung. As the disorder progresses, the patient may also develop severe dyspnea, substernal and subcostal retractions, nasal flaring, cyanosis, and increasing lethargy. Some infants display GI signs, such as vomiting, diarrhea, and abdominal distention.

◆ ***Respiratory distress syndrome.*** The result of lung immaturity in a premature infant (less than 37 weeks' gestation) usually of low birth weight, this syndrome initially causes audible expiratory grunting along with intercostal, subcostal, or substernal retractions; tachycardia; and tachypnea. Later, as respiratory distress tires the infant, apnea or irregular respirations replace the grunting. Severe respiratory distress is characterized by cyanosis, frothy sputum, dramatic nasal flaring, lethargy, bradycardia, and hypotension. Eventually, the infant becomes unresponsive. Auscultation reveals harsh, diminished breath sounds and crackles over the base of the lungs on deep inspiration. Oliguria and peripheral edema may also occur.

Special considerations

Closely monitor the patient's condition. Keep emergency equipment nearby in case respiratory distress worsens. Prepare to administer oxygen using a nasal cannula or face mask. Continually monitor oxygen saturation levels and deliver the minimum amount of oxygen possible, to avoid causing retinopathy of prematurity from excessively high oxygen levels.

Begin inhalation therapy with a bronchodilator, and administer an I.V. antimicrobial if the patient has pneumonia (or, in some cases, status asthmaticus). Follow these measures with chest physical therapy as necessary.

Prepare the patient for chest X-rays. Because sedatives are contraindicated during respiratory distress, the restless child must be restrained during testing, as necessary. To prevent exposure to radiation, wear a lead apron and cover the child's genital area with a lead shield. If a blood culture is ordered, be sure to record on the laboratory slip any current antibiotic use.

Remember to explain all procedures to the patient's parents and to provide emotional support.

Respirations, shallow

Respirations are shallow when a diminished volume of air enters the lungs during inspiration. In an effort to obtain enough air, the patient with shallow respirations usually breathes at an accelerated rate. However, as he tires or as his muscles weaken, this compensatory increase in respirations diminishes, leading to inadequate gas exchange and such signs as dyspnea, cyanosis, confusion, agitation, loss of consciousness, and tachycardia.

Shallow respirations may develop suddenly or gradually and may last briefly or become chronic. They're a key sign of respiratory distress and neurologic deterioration. Causes include inadequate central respiratory control

(Text continues on page 596.)

Positioning an infant for chest physical therapy

An infant with grunting respirations may need chest physical therapy to mobilize and drain excess lung secretions. Auscultate first to locate congested areas, and determine the best drainage position. Review the illustrations here, which show the various drainage positions and where to place your hands for percussion. When you percuss the infant, use the fingers of one hand. Vibrate these fingers and move them toward the infant's head to facilitate drainage.

Hold the infant upright and about 30 degrees forward to percuss and drain the apical segments of the upper lobes.

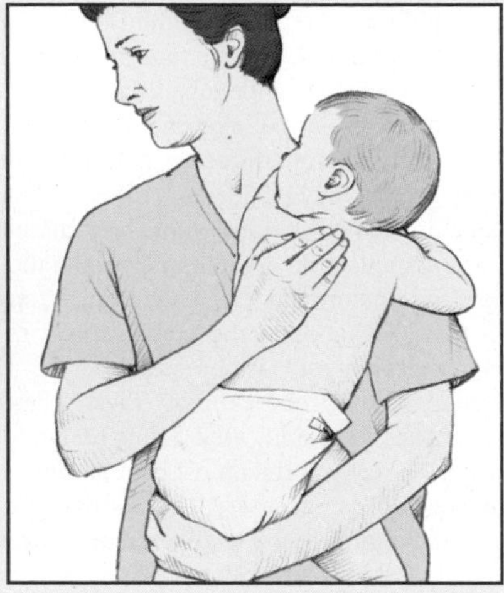

Place the infant in a supine position to percuss and drain the anterior segments of the upper lobes.

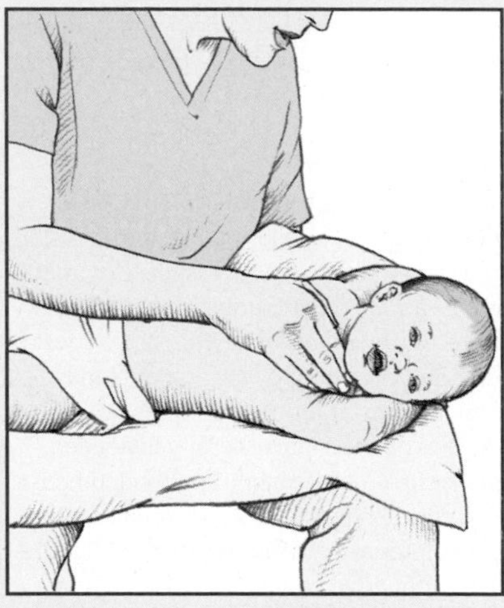

Use this position to percuss and drain the posterior segments of the upper lobes.

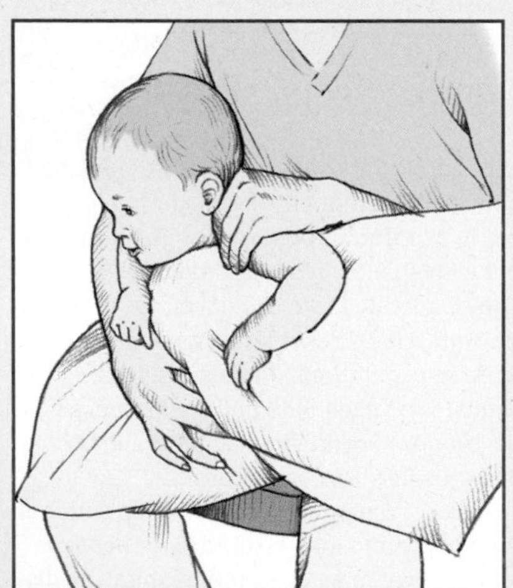

Hold the infant at a 45-degree angle on his side with his head down about 15 degrees to percuss and drain the right middle lobe.

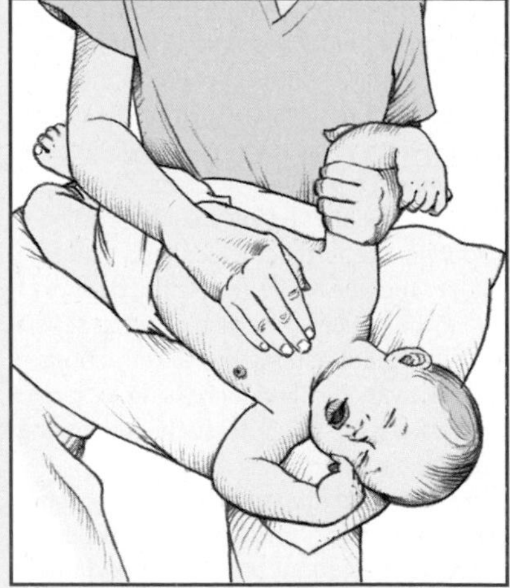

Place the infant in a supine position with his head 30 degrees lower than his feet to percuss and drain the anterior segments of the lower lobes.

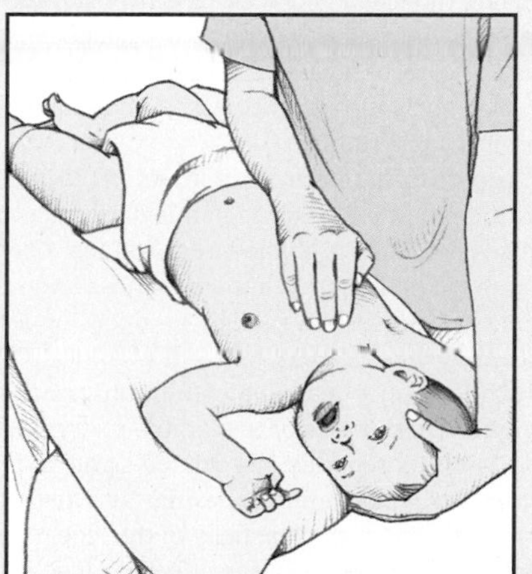

Place the infant in a prone position with his head down 30 degrees to percuss and drain the posterior basal segments of the lower lobes.

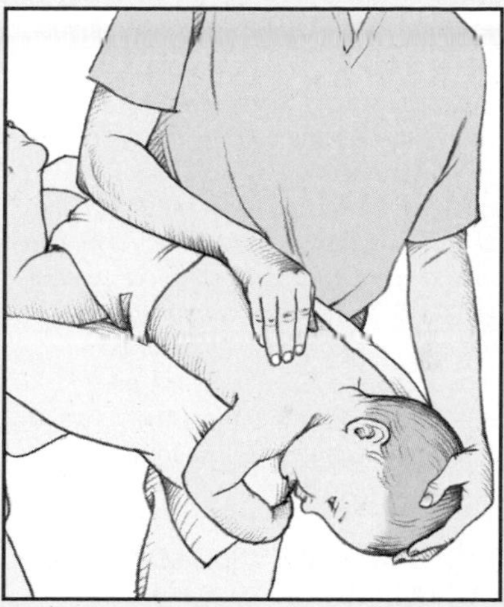

Place the infant on his side with his head down 30 degrees to percuss and drain the lateral basal segments of the lower lobes. Repeat this on the other side.

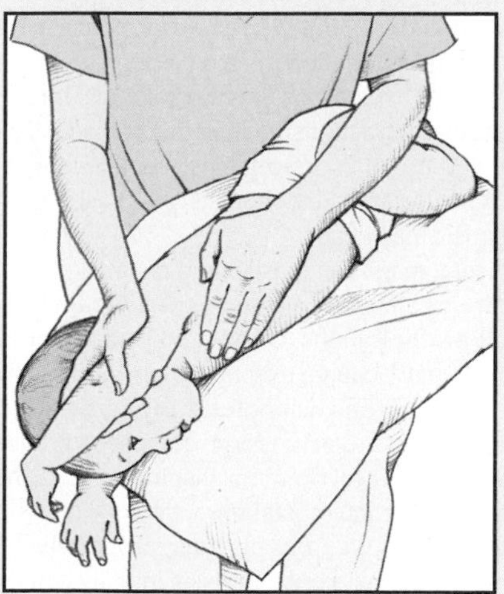

Use a prone position to percuss and drain the superior segments of the lower lobes.

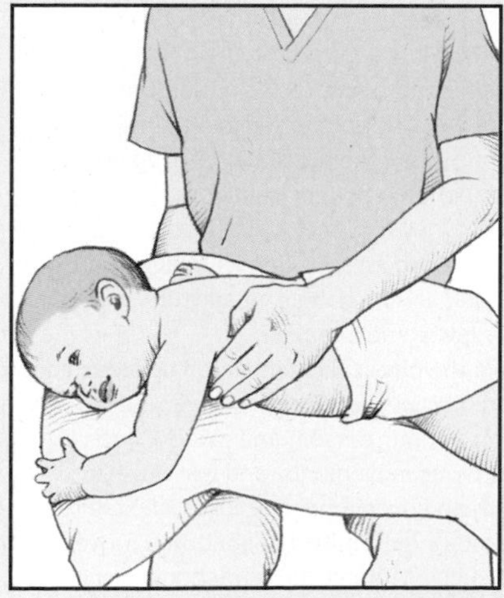

over breathing, neuromuscular disorders, increased resistance to airflow into the lungs, respiratory muscle fatigue or weakness, voluntary alterations in breathing, decreased activity from prolonged bed rest, and pain.

EMERGENCY INTERVENTIONS *If you observe shallow respirations, be alert for impending respiratory failure or arrest. Is the patient severely dyspneic? Agitated or frightened? Look for signs of airway obstruction. If the patient is choking, perform abdominal thrusts to try to expel the foreign object. Use suction if secretions occlude the patient's airway.*

If the patient is also wheezing, check for stridor, nasal flaring, and use of accessory muscles. Administer oxygen with a face mask or a handheld resuscitation bag. Attempt to calm the patient. Administer epinephrine I.V.

If the patient loses consciousness, insert an artificial airway and prepare for endotracheal intubation and ventilatory support. Check arterial blood gas (ABG) levels, heart rate, blood pressure, and oxygen saturation. Tachycardia, increased or decreased blood pressure, poor minute volume, and deteriorating ABG levels or oxygen saturation signal the need for intubation and mechanical ventilation.

History and physical examination

If the patient isn't in severe respiratory distress, begin with the history. Ask about chronic illness and any surgery or trauma. Has he had a tetanus booster in the past 10 years? Does he have asthma, allergies, or a history of heart failure or vascular disease? Does he have a chronic respiratory disorder or respiratory tract infection, tuberculosis, or a neurologic or neuromuscular disease? Does he smoke? Obtain a drug history, too, and explore the possibility of drug abuse.

Ask about the patient's shallow respirations: When did they begin? How long do they last? What makes them subside? What aggravates them? Ask about changes in appetite, weight, activity level, and behavior.

Begin the physical examination by assessing the patient's level of consciousness and his orientation to time, person, and place. Observe spontaneous movements, and test muscle strength and deep tendon reflexes. Next, inspect the chest for deformities or abnormal movements such as intercostal retractions. Inspect the extremities for cyanosis and digital clubbing.

Palpate for expansion and diaphragmatic tactile fremitus, and percuss for hyperresonance or dullness. Auscultate for diminished, absent, or adventitious breath sounds and for abnormal or distant heart sounds. Do you note any peripheral edema? Finally, examine the abdomen for distention, tenderness, or masses.

Medical causes

- ***Acute respiratory distress syndrome.*** Initially, this life-threatening syndrome produces rapid, shallow respirations and dyspnea. Hypoxemia leads to intercostal and suprasternal retractions, diaphoresis, and fluid accumulation, causing rhonchi and crackles. As hypoxemia worsens, the patient exhibits more difficulty breathing, restlessness, apprehension, decreased level of consciousness, cyanosis and, possibly, tachycardia.
- ***Amyotrophic lateral sclerosis (ALS).*** Respiratory muscle weakness in this disorder causes progressive shallow respirations. Exertion may result in increased weakness and respiratory distress. ALS initially produces upper extremity muscle weakness and wasting, which in several years affect the trunk, neck, tongue, and muscles of the larynx, pharynx, and lower extremities. Associated signs and symptoms include muscle cramps and atrophy, hyperreflexia, slight spasticity of the legs, coarse fasciculations of the affected muscle, impaired speech, and difficulty chewing and swallowing.
- ***Asthma.*** With this disorder, bronchospasm and hyperinflation of the lungs cause rapid, shallow respirations. In adults, mild persistent signs and symptoms may worsen during severe exacerbations. Related respiratory effects include wheezing, rhonchi, a dry cough, dyspnea, prolonged expirations, intercostal and supraclavicular retractions on inspiration, nasal flaring, and use of accessory muscles. Chest tightness, tachycardia, diaphoresis, and flushing or cyanosis may occur.
- ***Atelectasis.*** Decreased lung expansion or pleuritic pain causes sudden onset of rapid, shallow respirations. Other signs and symptoms include a dry cough, dyspnea, tachycardia, anxiety, cyanosis, and diaphoresis. Examination reveals dullness to percussion, decreased breath sounds and vocal fremitus, inspiratory lag, and substernal or intercostal retractions.
- ***Botulism.*** With this disorder, progressive muscle weakness and paralysis initially cause shallow respirations. Within 4 days, the patient develops respiratory distress from respiratory muscle paralysis. Early signs and symptoms

include bilateral mydriasis and nonreactive pupils, anorexia, nausea, vomiting, diarrhea, dry mouth, blurred vision, diplopia, ptosis, strabismus, and extraocular muscle palsies. Others quickly follow, including vertigo, deafness, hoarseness, constipation, nasal voice, dysarthria, and dysphagia.

◆ ***Bronchiectasis.*** Increased secretions obstruct airflow in the lungs, leading to shallow respirations and a productive cough with copious, foul-smelling, mucopurulent sputum (a classic finding). Other findings include hemoptysis, wheezing, rhonchi, coarse crackles during inspiration, and late-stage clubbing. The patient may complain of weight loss, fatigue, exertional weakness and dyspnea on, fever, malaise, and halitosis.

◆ ***Chronic bronchitis.*** Airway obstruction causes chronic shallow respirations. This disorder may begin with a nonproductive, hacking cough that later becomes productive. It may also cause prolonged expirations, wheezing, dyspnea, accessory muscle use, barrel chest, cyanosis, tachypnea, scattered rhonchi, coarse crackles, and clubbing (a late sign).

◆ ***Coma.*** Rapid, shallow respirations result from neurologic dysfunction or restricted chest movement.

◆ ***Emphysema.*** Increased breathing effort causes muscle fatigue, leading to chronic shallow respirations. The patient may also display dyspnea, anorexia, malaise, tachypnea, diminished breath sounds, cyanosis, pursed-lip breathing, accessory muscle use, barrel chest, chronic productive cough, and clubbing (a late sign).

◆ ***Flail chest.*** With this disorder, decreased air movement results in rapid, shallow respirations, paradoxical chest wall motion from rib instability, tachycardia, hypotension, ecchymoses, cyanosis, and pain over the affected area.

◆ ***Fractured ribs.*** Pain on inspiration and possibly expiration may cause shallow respirations.

◆ ***Guillain-Barré syndrome.*** Progressive ascending paralysis causes rapid or progressive onset of shallow respirations. Muscle weakness begins in the lower limbs and extends finally to the face. Associated findings include paresthesia, dysarthria, diminished or absent corneal reflex, nasal speech, dysphagia, ipsilateral loss of facial muscle control, and flaccid paralysis.

◆ ***Kyphoscoliosis.*** Skeletal cage distortion can eventually cause rapid, shallow respirations from reduced lung capacity. It also causes back pain, fatigue, tracheal deviation, and dyspnea.

◆ ***Multiple sclerosis.*** Muscle weakness causes progressive shallow respirations. Early features include diplopia, blurred vision, and paresthesia. Other possible findings are nystagmus, constipation, paralysis, spasticity, hyperreflexia, intention tremor, ataxic gait, dysphagia, dysarthria, urinary dysfunction, impotence, and emotional lability.

◆ ***Muscular dystrophy.*** With progressive thoracic deformity and muscle weakness, shallow respirations may occur along with waddling gait, contractures, scoliosis, lordosis, and muscle atrophy or hypertrophy.

◆ ***Myasthenia gravis.*** Progression of this disorder causes respiratory muscle weakness marked by shallow respirations, dyspnea, and cyanosis. Other effects include fatigue, weak eye closure, ptosis, diplopia, and difficulty chewing and swallowing.

◆ ***Obesity.*** Morbid obesity may cause shallow respirations due to the work of breathing associated with movement of the chest wall. Heart and breath sounds may be distant.

◆ ***Parkinson's disease.*** Fatigue and weakness lead to progressive shallow respirations. Typically, this disorder slowly progresses to increased rigidity (lead-pipe or cogwheel), masklike facies, stooped posture, shuffling gait, dysphagia, drooling, dysarthria, and pill-rolling tremor.

◆ ***Pleural effusion.*** With this disorder, restricted lung expansion causes shallow respirations, beginning suddenly or gradually. Other findings include nonproductive cough, weight loss, dyspnea, and pleuritic chest pain. Examination reveals pleural friction rub, tachycardia, tachypnea, decreased chest motion, flatness to percussion, egophony, decreased or absent breath sounds, and decreased tactile fremitus.

◆ ***Pneumonia.*** Pulmonary consolidation results in rapid, shallow respirations. The patient may experience dyspnea, fever, shaking chills, chest pain, cough, tachycardia, decreased breath sounds, crackles, and rhonchi. He may also develop myalgias, fatigue, anorexia, headache, abdominal pain, cyanosis, and diaphoresis.

◆ ***Pneumothorax.*** This disorder causes sudden onset of shallow respirations and dyspnea. Related effects include tachycardia; tachypnea; sudden sharp, severe chest pain (commonly unilateral) worsening with movement; nonproductive cough; cyanosis; accessory muscle use;

asymmetrical chest expansion; anxiety; restlessness; hyperresonance or tympany on the affected side; subcutaneous crepitation; decreased vocal fremitus; and diminished or absent breath sounds on the affected side.

◆ ***Pulmonary edema.*** Pulmonary vascular congestion causes rapid, shallow respirations. Early signs and symptoms include exertional dyspnea, paroxysmal nocturnal dyspnea, nonproductive cough, tachycardia, tachypnea, dependent crackles, and a ventricular gallop. Severe pulmonary edema produces more rapid, labored respirations; widespread crackles; a productive cough with frothy, bloody sputum; worsening tachycardia; arrhythmias; cold, clammy skin; cyanosis; hypotension; and thready pulse.

◆ ***Pulmonary embolism.*** This disorder causes sudden, rapid, shallow respirations and severe dyspnea with angina or pleuritic chest pain. Other clinical features include tachycardia, tachypnea, a nonproductive cough or a productive cough with blood-tinged sputum, low-grade fever, restlessness, diaphoresis, pleural friction rub, crackles, diffuse wheezing, dullness to percussion, decreased breath sounds, and signs of circulatory collapse. Less-common findings are massive hemoptysis, chest splinting, leg edema, and (with a large embolism) cyanosis, syncope, and jugular vein distention.

◆ ***Spinal cord injury.*** Diaphragmatic breathing and shallow respirations may occur in injury to the C5 to C8 area. Other findings include quadriplegia with flaccidity followed by spastic paralysis, areflexia, hypotension, sensory loss below the level of injury, and bowel and bladder incontinence.

◆ ***Tetanus.*** With this now-rare disorder, spasm of the intercostal muscles and the diaphragm causes shallow respirations. Late findings typically include jaw pain and stiffening, difficulty opening the mouth, tachycardia, profuse diaphoresis, hyperactive deep tendon reflexes, and opisthotonos.

◆ ***Upper airway obstruction.*** Partial airway obstruction causes acute shallow respirations with sudden gagging and dry, paroxysmal coughing; hoarseness; stridor; and tachycardia. Other findings include dyspnea, decreased breath sounds, wheezing, and cyanosis.

Other causes

◆ ***Drugs.*** Opioids, sedatives and hypnotics, tranquilizers, neuromuscular blockers, magnesium sulfate, and anesthetics can produce slow, shallow respirations.

◆ ***Surgery.*** After abdominal or thoracic surgery, pain associated with chest splinting and decreased chest wall motion may cause shallow respirations.

Special considerations

Prepare the patient for diagnostic tests: ABG analysis, pulmonary function tests, chest X-rays, or bronchoscopy.

Position the patient as nearly upright as possible to ease his breathing. (Help a postoperative patient splint his incision while coughing.) If he's taking a drug that depresses respirations, follow all precautions, and monitor him closely. Ensure adequate hydration, and use humidification as needed to thin secretions and to relieve inflamed, dry, or irritated airway mucosa. Administer humidified oxygen, a bronchodilator, a mucolytic, an expectorant, or an antibiotic, as ordered.

Turn the patient frequently. He may require chest physiotherapy, incentive spirometry, or continuous positive-pressure breathing. Monitor the patient for increasing lethargy, which may indicate rising carbon dioxide levels. Have emergency equipment at the patient's bedside.

Pediatric pointers

In children, shallow respirations commonly indicate a life-threatening condition. Airway obstruction can occur rapidly because of the narrow passageways; if it does, administer back blows or chest thrusts but not abdominal thrusts, which can damage internal organs.

Causes of shallow respirations in infants and children include idiopathic (infant) respiratory distress syndrome, acute epiglottiditis, diphtheria, aspiration of a foreign body, croup, acute bronchiolitis, cystic fibrosis, and bacterial pneumonia.

Observe the child to detect apnea. As needed, use humidification and suction, and administer supplemental oxygen. Give parenteral fluids to ensure adequate hydration. Chest physiotherapy may be required.

Geriatric pointers

Stiffness or deformity of the chest wall associated with aging may cause shallow respirations.

Patient counseling

Have the patient cough and deep-breathe and use an incentive spirometer every hour to clear secretions and to counteract possible hypoventilation. Provide assistance with tracheal suctioning as needed.

Respirations, stertorous

Characterized by a harsh, rattling, or snoring sound, stertorous respirations usually result from the vibration of relaxed oropharyngeal structures during sleep or coma, causing partial airway obstruction. Less often, these respirations result from retained mucus in the upper airway.

This common sign occurs in about 10% of normal individuals, especially middle-age, obese men. It may be aggravated by use of alcohol or a sedative before bed, which increases oropharyngeal flaccidity, and by sleeping in the supine position, which allows the relaxed tongue to slip back into the airway. The major pathologic causes of stertorous respirations are obstructive sleep apnea and life-threatening upper airway obstruction associated with an oropharyngeal tumor or with uvular or palatal edema. This obstruction may also occur during the postictal phase of a generalized seizure when mucous secretions or a relaxed tongue blocks the airway.

Occasionally, stertorous respirations are mistaken for stridor, which is another sign of upper airway obstruction. However, stridor indicates laryngeal or tracheal obstruction, whereas stertorous respirations signal higher airway obstruction.

EMERGENCY INTERVENTIONS *If you detect stertorous respirations, check the patient's mouth and throat for edema, redness, masses, or foreign objects. If edema is marked, quickly take vital signs including oxygen saturation. Observe the patient for signs and symptoms of respiratory distress, such as dyspnea, tachypnea, use of accessory muscles, intercostal muscle retractions, and cyanosis. Elevate the head of the bed 30 degrees to help ease breathing and reduce the edema. Then administer supplemental oxygen by nasal cannula or face mask, and prepare to intubate the patient, perform a tracheostomy, or provide mechanical ventilation. Insert an I.V. catheter for fluid and drug access, and begin cardiac monitoring.*

If you detect stertorous respirations while the patient is sleeping, observe his breathing pattern for 3 to 4 minutes. Do noisy respirations cease when he turns on his side and recur when he assumes a supine position? Watch carefully for periods of apnea and note their length. When possible, question the patient's partner about his snoring habits. Is she frequently awakened by the patient's snoring? Does the snoring improve if the patient sleeps with the window open? Has she also observed the patient talk in his sleep or sleepwalk? Ask about signs of sleep deprivation, such as personality changes, headaches, daytime somnolence, or decreased mental acuity.

Medical causes

◆ ***Airway obstruction.*** Regardless of its cause, partial airway obstruction may lead to stertorous respirations accompanied by wheezing, dyspnea, tachypnea and, later, intercostal retractions and nasal flaring. If the obstruction becomes complete, the patient abruptly loses his ability to talk and displays diaphoresis, tachycardia, and inspiratory chest movement but absent breath sounds. Severe hypoxemia rapidly ensues, resulting in cyanosis, loss of consciousness, and cardiopulmonary collapse.

◆ ***Obstructive sleep apnea.*** Loud and disruptive snoring is a major characteristic of this syndrome, which commonly affects the obese. Typically, the snoring alternates with periods of sleep apnea, which usually end with loud gasping sounds. Alternating tachycardia and bradycardia may occur.

Episodes of snoring and apnea recur in a cyclic pattern throughout the night. Sleep disturbances, such as somnambulism and talking during sleep, may also occur. Some patients display hypertension and ankle edema. Most awaken in the morning with a generalized headache, feeling tired and unrefreshed. The most common complaint is excessive daytime sleepiness. Lack of sleep may cause depression, hostility, and decreased mental acuity.

Other causes

◆ ***Endotracheal intubation, suction, or surgery.*** These procedures may cause significant palatal or uvular edema, resulting in stertorous respirations.

Special considerations

Continue to monitor the patient's respiratory status carefully. Administer a corticosteroid or an antibiotic and cool, humidified oxygen to reduce palatal and uvular inflammation and edema.

Laryngoscopy and bronchoscopy (to rule out airway obstruction) or formal sleep studies may be necessary.

Pediatric pointers

In children, the most common cause of stertorous respirations is nasal or pharyngeal obstruction secondary to tonsillar or adenoid hypertrophy or the presence of a foreign body.

Geriatric pointers

Encourage the patient to seek treatment for sleep apnea or significant hypertrophy of the tonsils or adenoids.

Retractions, costal and sternal

A cardinal sign of respiratory distress in infants and children, retractions are visible indentations of the soft tissue covering the chest wall. They may be suprasternal (directly above the sternum and clavicles), intercostal (between the ribs), subcostal (below the lower costal margin of the rib cage), or substernal (just below the xiphoid process). Retractions may be mild or severe, producing barely visible to deep indentations.

Normally, infants and young children use abdominal muscles for breathing, unlike older children and adults, who use the diaphragm. When breathing requires extra effort, accessory muscles assist respiration, especially inspiration. Retractions typically accompany accessory muscle use.

EMERGENCY INTERVENTIONS *If you detect retractions in a child, check quickly for other signs of respiratory distress, such as cyanosis, tachypnea, tachycardia, and decreased oxygen saturation. Also, prepare the child for suctioning, insertion of an artificial airway, and administration of oxygen.*

Observe the depth and location of retractions. Also, note the rate, depth, and quality of respirations. Look for accessory muscle use, nasal flaring during inspiration, or grunting during expiration. If the child has a cough, record the color, consistency, and odor of any sputum. Note whether the child appears restless or lethargic. Finally, auscultate the child's lungs to detect abnormal breath sounds. (*See* Observing retractions.)

History and physical examination

If the child's condition permits, ask his parents about his medical history. Was he born prematurely? Was he born with a low birth weight? Was the delivery complicated? Ask about recent signs of an upper respiratory tract infection, such as a runny nose, cough, and a low-grade fever. How often has the child had respiratory problems during the past year? Has he been in contact with anyone who has had a cold, the flu, or other respiratory ailments? Did he ever have respiratory syncytial virus? Did he aspirate any food, liquid, or foreign body? Inquire about any personal or family history of allergies or asthma.

Medical causes

◆ ***Asthma.*** Intercostal and suprasternal retractions may accompany an asthma exacerbation. They're preceded by dyspnea, wheezing, a hacking cough, and pallor. Related features include cyanosis or flushing, diaphoresis, tachycardia, tachypnea, a frightened, anxious expression and, in patients with severe distress, nasal flaring.

◆ ***Bronchiolitis.*** Most common in children younger than age 2, this acute lower respiratory tract infection may cause intercostal and subcostal retractions, nasal flaring, tachypnea, dyspnea, cough, restlessness and a slight fever. Periodic apnea may occur in infants younger than age 6 months.

◆ ***Croup (spasmodic).*** This disorder causes attacks of a barking cough, hoarseness, dyspnea, and restlessness. As distress worsens, the child may display suprasternal, substernal, and intercostal retractions; nasal flaring; tachycardia; cyanosis; and an anxious, frantic expression. Croup attacks usually subside within a few hours but tend to recur.

◆ ***Epiglottiditis.*** This life-threatening bacterial infection may precipitate severe respiratory distress with suprasternal, substernal, and intercostal retractions; stridor; nasal flaring; cyanosis; and tachycardia. Early features include sudden onset of a barking cough and high fever, sore throat, hoarseness, dysphagia, drooling, dyspnea, and restlessness. The child becomes panicky as edema makes breathing difficult. Total airway occlusion may occur in 2 to 5 hours.

◆ ***Heart failure.*** Usually linked to a congenital heart defect in children, this disorder may cause intercostal and substernal retractions along with nasal flaring, progressive tachypnea, and—in severe respiratory distress—grunting respirations, edema, and cyanosis. Other findings include productive cough, crackles, jugular vein distention, tachycardia, right-upper-quadrant pain, anorexia, and fatigue.

◆ ***Laryngotracheobronchitis (acute).*** With this viral infection, substernal and intercostal retractions typically follow a low to moderate fever, runny nose, poor appetite, a barking cough, hoarseness, and inspiratory stridor. Associated signs and symptoms include tachycardia;

Observing retractions

When you observe retractions in infants and children, be sure to note their exact location—an important clue to the cause and severity of respiratory distress. For example, subcostal and substernal retractions usually result from lower respiratory tract disorders; suprasternal retractions, from upper respiratory tract disorders.

Mild intercostal retractions alone may be normal. However, intercostal retractions accompanied by subcostal and substernal retractions may indicate moderate respiratory distress. Deep suprasternal retractions typically indicate severe distress.

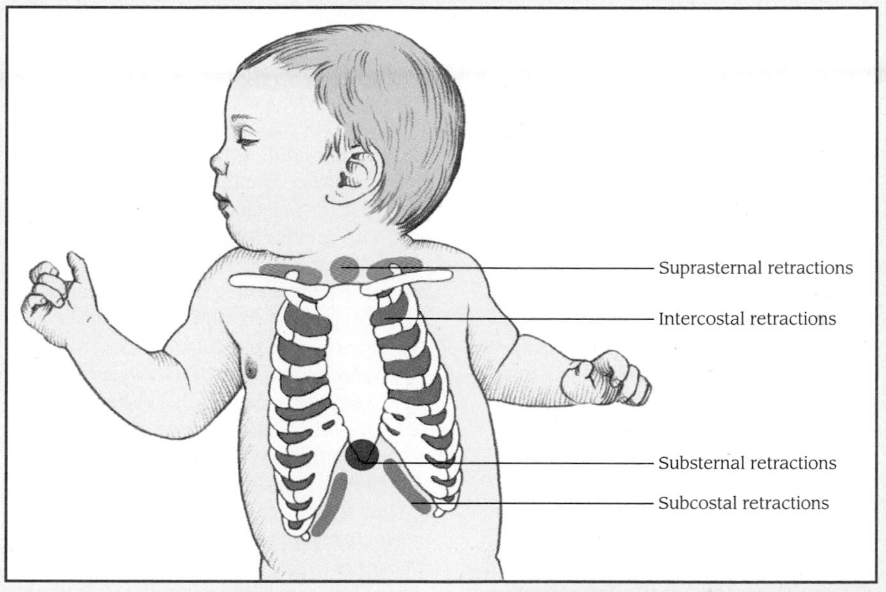

shallow, rapid respirations; restlessness; irritability; and pale, cyanotic skin.

◆ ***Pneumonia (bacterial).*** This disorder begins with signs and symptoms of acute infection, such as high fever and lethargy, which are followed by subcostal and intercostal retractions, nasal flaring, dyspnea, tachypnea, grunting respirations, cyanosis, and a productive cough. Auscultation may reveal diminished breath sounds, scattered crackles, and sibilant rhonchi over the affected lung. GI effects may include vomiting, diarrhea, and abdominal distention.

◆ ***Respiratory distress syndrome.*** Substernal and subcostal retractions are an early sign of this life-threatening syndrome, which affects premature infants shortly after birth. Associated early signs include tachypnea, tachycardia, and expiratory grunting. As respiratory distress worsens, intercostal and suprasternal retractions typically occur, and apnea or irregular respirations replace grunting. Other effects include nasal flaring, cyanosis, lethargy, and eventual unresponsiveness as well as bradycardia and hypotension. Auscultation may detect crackles over the lung bases on deep inspiration and harsh, diminished breath sounds. Oliguria and peripheral edema may occur.

Special considerations

Continue to monitor the child's vital signs. Keep suction equipment and an appropriate-sized airway at the bedside. If the infant weighs less than 15 lb (6.8 kg), place him in an oxygen hood. If he weighs more, place him in a cool mist tent instead. Perform chest physical therapy with postural drainage to help mobilize and drain excess lung secretions. (See *Positioning an infant for chest physical therapy,* pages 594 and 595.) A bronchodilator or, occasionally, a steroid may also be used.

Prepare the child for chest X-rays, cultures, pulmonary function tests, and arterial blood gas analysis. Explain the procedures to his parents, too, and have them calm and comfort the child.

Pediatric pointers

When examining a child for retractions, know that crying may accentuate the contractions.

Geriatric pointers

Although retractions may occur at any age, they're more difficult to assess in an older patient who's obese or who has chronic chest wall stiffness or deformity.

Rhinorrhea

Common but rarely serious, rhinorrhea is the free discharge of thin nasal mucus. It can be self-limiting or chronic, resulting from a nasal, sinus, or systemic disorder or from a basilar skull fracture. Rhinorrhea can also result from sinus or cranial surgery, excessive use of vasoconstricting nose drops or sprays, or inhalation of an irritant, such as tobacco smoke, dust, and fumes. Depending on the cause, the discharge may be clear, purulent, bloody, or serosanguineous.

History and physical examination

Begin the history by asking the patient if the discharge runs from both nostrils. Is the discharge intermittent or persistent? Did it begin suddenly or gradually? Does the position of his head affect the discharge?

Next, ask the patient to characterize the discharge. Is it watery, bloody, purulent, or foul smelling? Is it copious or scanty? Does the discharge worsen or improve with the time of day? Find out if the patient is using any medications, especially nose drops or nasal sprays. Has he been exposed to nasal irritants at home or at work? Does he experience seasonal allergies? Did he recently experience a head injury?

Examine the patient's nose, checking airflow from each nostril. Evaluate the size, color, and condition of the turbinate mucosa (normally pale pink). Note if the mucosa is red, unusually palc, bluc, or gray. Then examine the area beneath each turbinate. (See *Using a nasal speculum*.) Be sure to palpate over the frontal, ethmoid, and maxillary sinuses for tenderness.

To differentiate nasal mucus from cerebrospinal fluid (CSF), collect a small amount of drainage on a glucose test strip. If CSF (which contains glucose) is present, the test result will be abnormal. Finally, using a nonirritating substance, be sure to test for anosmia.

Medical causes

- ***Basilar skull fracture.*** A tear in the dura can lead to cerebrospinal rhinorrhea, which increases when the patient lowers his head. Other findings include epistaxis, otorrhea, and a bulging tympanum from blood or fluid. A basilar fracture may also cause headache, facial paralysis, nausea and vomiting, impaired eye movement, ocular deviation, vision and hearing loss, depressed level of consciousness, Battle's sign, and raccoon eyes.
- ***Common cold.*** An initially watery nasal discharge may become thicker and mucopurulent. Related findings include sneezing, nasal congestion, a dry and hacking cough, sore throat, mouth breathing, and transient loss of smell and taste. The patient may also experience malaise, fatigue, myalgia, arthralgia, a slight headache, dry lips, and a red upper lip and nose.
- ***Headache (cluster).*** Rhinorrhea can accompany a severe, unilateral cluster headache. Related ocular effects include miosis, ipsilateral tearing, conjunctival injection, and ptosis. The patient may also experience flushing, facial diaphoresis, bradycardia, and restlessness.
- ***Mucormycosis.*** Rhinocerebral mucormycosis causes a thin, serosanguineous nasal discharge. Other initial findings include dull nasal pain; black, dusky red, or necrotic turbinates; low-grade fever; periorbital and facial edema; and erythema of the skin on the cheeks. This rare fungal infection is a surgical emergency, requiring surgical debridement and an I.V. antibiotic because it may spread to the eye, lower respiratory tract, and other organs.
- ***Nasal or sinus tumors.*** Nasal tumors can produce an intermittent, unilateral bloody or serosanguineous discharge that may be purulent and foul smelling. Nasal congestion, postnasal drip, and headache may also occur. In advanced stages, paranasal sinus tumors may cause a cheek mass or eye displacement, facial paresthesia or pain, and nasal obstruction.
- ***Rhinitis.*** Allergic rhinitis produces an episodic, profuse watery discharge. (A mucopurulent discharge indicates infection.) Typical associated signs and symptoms include increased lacrimation; nasal congestion; itchy eyes, nose, and throat; postnasal drip; recurrent sneezing; mouth breathing; impaired sense of smell; and

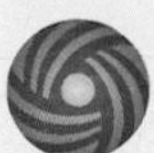

EXAMINATION TIP

Using a nasal speculum

To visualize the interior of the nares, use a nasal speculum and a good light source, such as a penlight. Hold the speculum in the palm of one hand and the penlight in the other hand. Have the patient tilt her head back slightly and rest it against a wall or other firm support, if possible. Insert the speculum blades about ½" (1.3 cm) into the nasal vestibule, as shown.

Place your index finger on the tip of the patient's nose for stability. Carefully open the speculum blades. Shine the light source in the direction of the nares. Inspect the nares, as shown. The mucosa should be deep pink. Note any discharge, masses, lesions, or mucosal swellings. Check the nasal septum for perforation, bleeding, or crusting. Bluish turbinates suggest allergy. A rounded, elongated projection suggests a polyp.

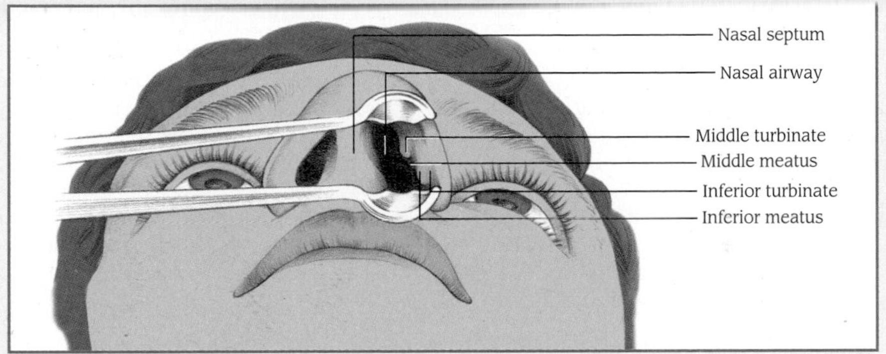

frontal or temporal headache. The turbinates are pale and engorged; the mucosa, pale and boggy.

With atrophic rhinitis, the nasal discharge is scanty, purulent, and foul smelling. Nasal obstruction is common, and the crusts may bleed on removal. The mucosa is pale pink and shiny.

With vasomotor rhinitis, a profuse and watery nasal discharge accompanies chronic nasal obstruction, sneezing, recurrent postnasal drip, and pale, swollen turbinates. The nasal septum is pink; the mucosa, blue.

◆ ***Rhinoscleroma.*** This rare, progressive condition produces watery nasal discharge that later becomes foul smelling and encrusted. It also causes firm, bluish red nodules on the mucous membranes that can develop into scars and cause stenosis.

◆ ***Sinusitis.*** With *acute sinusitis,* a thick and purulent nasal discharge leads to a purulent postnasal drip that results in throat pain and halitosis. The patient may also experience nasal congestion, severe pain and tenderness over the involved sinuses, fever, headache, and malaise.

With *chronic sinusitis,* the nasal discharge is usually scanty, thick, and intermittently purulent. Nasal congestion and low-grade discomfort or pressure over the involved sinuses can be persistent or recurrent. The patient may also be suffering from a chronic sore throat and nasal polyps.

With *chronic fungal sinusitis,* the clinical picture resembles that of chronic bacterial sinusitis. However, some cases—especially in immunocompromised patients—may progress rapidly to exophthalmos, blindness, intracranial extension and, eventually, death.

◆ ***Wegener's granulomatosis.*** Besides a bloody, mucopurulent nasal discharge, this disorder causes conductive hearing loss, crusting and tissue necrosis of the nose, and epistaxis. Less-common findings include sore throat, cough (possibly hemoptysis), wheezing, dyspnea, pleuritic chest pain, hemorrhagic skin lesions, and oliguria.

Other causes

◆ ***Drugs.*** Nasal sprays or nose drops containing vasoconstrictors may cause rebound rhinorrhea (rhinitis medicamentosa) if used longer than 5 days.

◆ ***Surgery.*** Cerebrospinal rhinorrhea may occur after sinus or cranial surgery.

SPECIAL CONSIDERATIONS

You may have to prepare the patient for X-rays of the sinuses or a computed tomography scan. You may also need to administer an antihistamine, a decongestant, an analgesic, or an antipyretic. Advise the patient to drink plenty of fluids to thin secretions.

Pregnancy causes physiologic changes that may aggravate rhinorrhea.

PEDIATRIC POINTERS

Be aware that rhinorrhea in children may stem from choanal atresia, allergic or chronic rhinitis, acute ethmoiditis, or congenital syphilis. Assume that unilateral rhinorrhea and nasal obstruction is caused by a foreign body in the nose until proven otherwise.

GERIATRIC POINTERS

Elderly patients may suffer increased adverse reactions to drugs used to treat rhinorrhea such as elevated blood pressure or confusion.

PATIENT COUNSELING

Warn the patient to avoid using over-the-counter nasal sprays for longer than 5 days.

Rhonchi

Rhonchi are continuous adventitious breath sounds detected by auscultation. They're usually louder and lower-pitched than crackles—more like a hoarse moan or a deep snore—though they may be described as rattling, sonorous, bubbling, rumbling, or musical. However, sibilant rhonchi, or wheezes, are high pitched.

Rhonchi are heard over large airways such as the trachea. They can occur in a patient with a pulmonary disorder when air flows through passages that have been narrowed by secretions, a tumor or foreign body, bronchospasm, or mucosal thickening. The resulting vibration of airway walls produces the rhonchi.

HISTORY AND PHYSICAL EXAMINATION

If you auscultate rhonchi, take the patient's vital signs, including oxygen saturation, and be alert for signs of respiratory distress. (See *Differential diagnosis: Rhonchi,* pages 606 and 607.) Characterize the patient's respirations as rapid or slow, shallow or deep, and regular or irregular. Inspect the chest, noting the use of accessory muscles. Is the patient audibly wheezing or gurgling? Auscultate for other abnormal breath sounds, such as crackles and a pleural friction rub. If you detect these sounds, note their location. Are breath sounds diminished or absent? Next, percuss the chest. If the patient has a cough, note its frequency and characterize its sound. If it's productive, examine the sputum for color, odor, consistency, and blood.

Ask related questions: Does the patient smoke? If so, obtain a history in pack-years. Has he recently lost weight or felt tired or weak? Does he have asthma or other a pulmonary disorder? Is he taking any prescribed or over-the-counter drugs?

During the examination, keep in mind that thick or excessive secretions, bronchospasm, or inflammation of mucous membranes may lead to airway obstruction. If necessary, suction the patient and keep equipment available for inserting an artificial airway. Keep a bronchodilator available to treat bronchospasm.

MEDICAL CAUSES

◆ ***Acute respiratory distress syndrome.*** Fluid accumulation with this life-threatening disorder produces rhonchi and crackles. Initial features include rapid, shallow respirations and dyspnea, sometimes after the patient's condition appears stable. Developing hypoxemia leads to intercostal and suprasternal retractions, diaphoresis, and fluid accumulation. As hypoxemia worsens, the patient displays increased difficulty breathing, restlessness, apprehension, decreased level of consciousness, cyanosis, motor dysfunction, and tachycardia.

◆ ***Aspiration of a foreign body.*** A retained foreign body in the bronchi can cause inspiratory and expiratory rhonchi and wheezing due to increased secretions. Diminished breath sounds may be auscultated over the obstructed area. Fever, pain, and cough may also occur.

◆ ***Asthma.*** An asthma exacerbation can cause rhonchi, crackles and, commonly, wheezing. Other features include apprehension, a dry cough that later becomes productive, prolonged expirations, and intercostal and supraclavicular retractions on inspiration. The patient may also exhibit increased accessory muscle use, nasal flaring, tachypnea, tachycardia, diaphoresis, and flushing or cyanosis.

◆ ***Bronchiectasis.*** This disorder causes lower-lobe rhonchi and crackles, which coughing may help relieve. Its classic sign is a cough that produces mucopurulent, foul-smelling and, possibly, bloody sputum. Other findings include fever, weight loss, exertional dyspnea, fatigue, malaise, halitosis, weakness, and late-stage clubbing.

◆ ***Bronchitis.*** Acute tracheobronchitis produces sonorous rhonchi and wheezing due to bronchospasm or increased mucus in the airways. Related findings include chills, sore throat, a low-grade fever (rising up to 102° F [38.9° C] in those with severe illness), muscle and back pain, and substernal tightness. A cough becomes productive as secretions increase.

With chronic bronchitis, auscultation may reveal scattered rhonchi, coarse crackles, wheezing, high-pitched piping sounds, and prolonged expirations. An early hacking cough later becomes productive. The patient also displays exertional dyspnea, increased accessory muscle use, barrel chest, cyanosis, tachypnea, and clubbing (a late sign).

◆ ***Emphysema.*** This disorder may cause sonorous rhonchi, but faint, high-pitched wheezing is more typical, together with weight loss; a mild, chronic, productive cough with scant sputum; exertional dyspnea; accessory muscle use on inspiration; tachypnea; and grunting expirations. Other features include anorexia, malaise, barrel chest, peripheral cyanosis, and late-stage clubbing.

◆ ***Pneumonia.*** Bacterial pneumonias can cause rhonchi and a dry cough that later becomes productive. Related signs and symptoms—shaking chills, high fever, myalgias, headache, pleuritic chest pain, tachypnea, tachycardia, dyspnea, cyanosis, diaphoresis, decreased breath sounds, and fine crackles—develop suddenly.

◆ ***Pulmonary coccidioidomycosis.*** This disorder causes rhonchi and wheezing. Other features include a cough with fever, occasional chills, pleuritic chest pain, sore throat, headache, backache, malaise, marked weakness, anorexia, hemoptysis, and an itchy macular rash.

Other causes

◆ ***Diagnostic tests.*** Pulmonary function tests or bronchoscopy can loosen secretions and mucus, causing rhonchi.

◆ ***Respiratory therapy.*** This may produce rhonchi from loosened secretions and mucus.

Special considerations

To ease the patient's breathing, place him in semi-Fowler's position, and reposition him every 2 hours. Administer an antibiotic, a bronchodilator, and an expectorant. Provide humidification to thin secretions, to relieve inflammation, and to prevent drying. Pulmonary physiotherapy with postural drainage and percussion can also help loosen secretions. Use tracheal suctioning, if necessary, to help the patient clear secretions and to promote oxygenation and comfort. Promote coughing and deep breathing and incentive spirometry.

Prepare the patient for diagnostic tests, such as arterial blood gas analysis, pulmonary function studies, sputum analysis, and chest X-rays.

Pediatric pointers

Rhonchi in children can result from bacterial pneumonia, cystic fibrosis, and croup syndrome.

Because a respiratory tract disorder may begin abruptly and progress rapidly in an infant or a child, observe closely for signs of airway obstruction.

Patient counseling

If appropriate, encourage increased activity to promote drainage of secretions. Teach deep-breathing and coughing techniques and splinting, if necessary. Encourage the patient to drink plenty of fluids to help liquefy secretions and prevent dehydration. Advise him not to suppress a moist cough.

Romberg's sign

A positive Romberg's sign refers to a patient's inability to maintain balance when standing erect with his feet together and his eyes closed. Normally (a negative Romberg's sign) the patient should be able to stand with his feet together and his eyes closed with minimal swaying for about 20 seconds.

If positive, Romberg's sign indicates a vestibular or proprioceptive disorder, or a disorder of the spinal tracts (the posterior columns) that carry proprioceptive information—the perception of one's position in space, of joint movements, and of pressure sensations—to the brain. Insufficient vestibular or proprioceptive information causes an inability to execute precise movements and maintain balance without visual cues. Difficulty performing this maneuver with eyes open or closed may indicate a cerebellar disorder.

(Text continues on page 608.)

Differential diagnosis: Rhonchi

History of present illness

Focused physical examination: Pulmonary system

Acute respiratory distress syndrome

Signs and symptoms
- Crackles
- Rapid, shallow respirations
- Dyspnea
- Intercostal and suprasternal retractions
- Diaphoresis
- Fluid accumulation

Diagnosis: Physical examination, arterial blood gases (ABGs), chest X-ray
Treatment: Oxygen therapy, treatment of underlying cause
Follow-up: Referral to pulmonologist

Common signs and symptoms
- Wheezing
- Exertional dyspnea
- Barrel chest
- Tachypnea
- Clubbing
- Decreased breath sounds

Bronchitis

Additional signs and symptoms

Acute
- Chills
- Sore throat
- Low-grade fever
- Muscle and back pain
- Substernal tightness

Chronic
- Coarse crackles
- Prolonged expiration
- Chronic productive cough
- Increased accessory muscle use
- Cyanosis
- Fluid retention

Diagnosis: Physical examination, ABGs, chest X-ray, pulmonary function test (PFT)
Treatment: Smoking cessation; antibiotics, if indicated; nebulizer treatment; oxygen therapy; chest physiotherapy
Follow-up: Referral to pulmonologist

Emphysema

Additional signs and symptoms
- Weight loss
- Mild, chronic productive cough
- Barrel chest
- Accessory muscle use on inspiration
- Grunting expirations

Diagnosis: Physical examination, ABGs, serum alpha$_1$-antitrypsin level, chest X-ray, PFT
Treatment: Smoking-cessation program, medication (diuretics, bronchodilators, corticosteroids)
Follow-up: Referral to pulmonologist

Additional differential diagnosis: asthma ◆ bronchiectasis ◆ pulmonary coccidioidomycosis
Other causes: bronchoscopy ◆ foreign body aspiration ◆ PFTs ◆ respiratory therapy

Common signs and symptoms
- ◆ Tachycardia
- ◆ Tachypnea
- ◆ Dyspnea
- ◆ Cyanosis

Pneumonia

Additional signs and symptoms
- ◆ Productive cough
- ◆ Shaking chills
- ◆ Fever
- ◆ Myalgia
- ◆ Headache
- ◆ Pleuritic chest pain
- ◆ Diaphoresis
- ◆ Decreased breath sounds
- ◆ Fine crackles

Diagnosis: Physical examination, complete blood count, ABGs, sputum Gram stain, chest X-ray
Treatment: Antibiotics, oxygen therapy
Follow-up: Reevaluation after 7 days

Pulmonary edema

Additional signs and symptoms
- ◆ Anxiety
- ◆ Paroxysmal nocturnal dyspnea
- ◆ Nonproductive cough
- ◆ Dependent crackles
- ◆ S_3

Diagnosis: Physical examination, ABGs, chest X-ray, computed tomography scan, magnetic resonance imaging
Treatment: Oxygen therapy, medication (diuretics, morphine)
Follow-up: Referral to cardiologist

History and physical examination

Once you've detected a positive Romberg's sign, perform other neurologic screening tests. A positive Romberg's sign only indicates the presence of a defect; it doesn't pinpoint its cause or location. First, test proprioception. If the patient can't maintain his balance with his eyes open, ask him to hop on one foot and then on the other. Next, ask him to do a knee bend and to walk a straight line, placing heel to toe. Lastly, ask him to walk a short distance so you can evaluate his gait.

Test the patient's awareness of body part position by changing the position of one of his fingers, or any other joint, while his eyes are closed. Ask him to describe the change you've made.

Next, test the patient's direction of movement. Ask him to close his eyes and to touch his nose with the index finger of one hand and then with the other. Ask him to repeat this movement several times, gradually increasing his speed. Then test the accuracy of his movement by having him rapidly touch each finger of one hand to the thumb. Next, test sensation in all dermatomes, using a pin to assess sharp/dull differentiation. Also test two-point discrimination by touching two pins (one in each hand) to his skin simultaneously. Does he feel one or two pinpricks? Finally, test and characterize the patient's deep tendon reflexes (DTRs).

To test the patient's vibratory sense, ask him to close his eyes; then apply a mildly vibrating tuning fork to a bony prominence such as the medial malleolus. If the patient doesn't feel the stimulus initially, increase the vibration, and then test the knee or hip. This procedure can also be done to test the fingers, the elbow, and the shoulder.

Record and compare all test results. Ask the patient if he has noticed sensory changes, such as numbness and tingling in his limbs. If so, when did these changes begin?

Medical causes

◆ ***Multiple sclerosis.*** Early features may include vision changes, diplopia, and paresthesia. Other findings include a positive Romberg's sign, nystagmus, constipation, muscle weakness and spasticity, and hyperreflexia. The patient may also have dysphagia, dysarthria, incontinence, urinary frequency and urgency, impotence, and emotional instability.

◆ ***Peripheral nerve disease.*** Besides a positive Romberg's sign, advanced disease may produce impotence, fatigue, and paresthesia, hyperesthesia, or anesthesia in the hands and feet. Related findings include incoordination, ataxia, burning pain in the affected area, progressive muscle weakness and atrophy, and loss of vibration sense. DTRs may be hypoactive.

◆ ***Pernicious anemia.*** A positive Romberg's sign and loss of proprioception in the lower limbs reflect peripheral nerve and spinal cord damage. Gait changes (usually ataxia), muscle weakness, impaired coordination, paresthesia, and sensory loss may be present. DTRs may be hypoactive or hyperactive. Other findings include a sore tongue, a positive Babinski's reflex, fatigue, blurred vision, diplopia, and lightheadedness.

◆ ***Spinal cerebellar degeneration.*** With this disorder, a positive Romberg's sign accompanies decreased visual acuity, fatigue, paresthesia, loss of vibration sense, incoordination, ataxic gait, and muscle weakness and atrophy. DTRs may be hypoactive.

◆ ***Spinal cord disease.*** A positive Romberg's sign may accompany pain, fasciculations, muscle weakness and atrophy, loss of sphincter tone, and loss of proprioception, vibration, and other senses. DTRs may be hypoactive at the level of the lesion and hyperactive above it.

◆ ***Tabes dorsalis.*** A positive Romberg's sign may occur, but burning extremity pain is this disorder's classic symptom. Other findings include a wide-based ataxic gait, loss of proprioception in the lower limbs (common), and loss of pain and temperature sensation. As the disease progresses, DTRs in the legs become hypoactive or absent, muscle tone decreases, and muscles atrophy. The patient may also develop Charcot's joints and Argyll Robertson pupils.

◆ ***Vestibular disorders.*** Besides a positive Romberg's sign, these disorders commonly cause vertigo. Nystagmus, nausea, and vomiting may also occur.

Special considerations

Help the patient with ambulation, especially in poorly lit areas. Also, keep a night-light on in his room, and raise the side rails of the bed. Encourage him to ask for assistance and to use visual cues to maintain his balance. Instruct him in the use of assistive devices if necessary.

Pediatric pointers

Romberg's sign can't be tested in children until they can stand without support and follow commands. However, a positive sign in children commonly results from spinal cord disease.

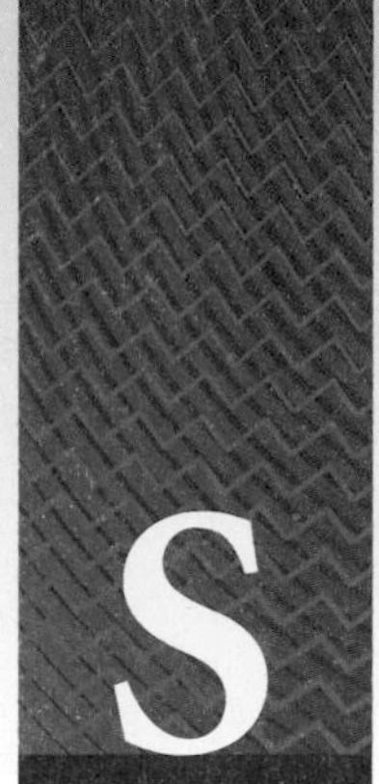

Salivation, decreased

[Xerostomia]

Typically a common but minor complaint, diminished production or excretion of saliva (dry mouth) usually results from mouth breathing. However, this symptom can also result from salivary duct obstruction, Sjögren's syndrome, the use of an anticholinergic other drug, and the effects of radiation. It can even result from vigorous exercise or autonomic stimulation—for example, as the result of fear.

History and physical examination

Evaluate the patient's complaint of dry mouth by asking pertinent history questions: When did he first notice the symptom? Was he exercising at the time? Is he currently taking any medications? Is his sensation of dry mouth intermittent or continuous? Is it related to or relieved by a particular activity? Ask about related symptoms, such as burning or itching eyes, or changes sense of smell in or taste.

Next, inspect the patient's mouth, including the mucous membranes, for any abnormalities. Observe his eyes for conjunctival irritation, matted lids, and corneal epithelial thickening. Perform simple tests of smell and taste to detect impairment of these senses. Check for enlarged parotid and submaxillary glands. (See *Examining salivary glands and ductal openings,* page 610.) Palpate for tender or enlarged areas along the neck, too.

Medical causes

◆ ***Dehydration.*** Decreased saliva production causes dry oral mucous membranes. Skin turgor is also decreased, and urine output may be low.

◆ ***Facial nerve paralysis.*** A diminished saliva production occurs along with decreased sense of taste and facial muscle movement.

◆ ***Salivary duct obstruction.*** Usually associated with a salivary stone, this obstruction causes reduced salivation and local pain and swelling.

◆ ***Sjögren's syndrome.*** Diminished secretions from the lacrimal, parotid, and submaxillary glands produce the hallmarks of this disorder: decreased or absent salivation and dry eyes with a persistent burning, gritty sensation. The patient may also experience dryness that involves the nose, respiratory tract, vagina, and skin.

Related oral signs and symptoms include difficulty chewing, talking, and swallowing as well as ulcers and soreness of the lips and mucosa. The parotid and submaxillary glands may be enlarged. Nasal crusting, epistaxis, fatigue, lethargy, nonproductive cough, abdominal discomfort, and polyuria may be present. These signs and symptoms may occur alone or with rheumatoid arthritis or another connective tissue disorder.

Other causes

◆ ***Drugs.*** Anticholinergics, antihistamines, tricyclic antidepressants, phenothiazines, clonidine, and opioid analgesics can cause decreased salivation, which disappears after discontinuation of therapy.

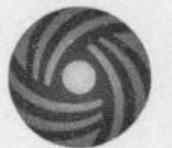

EXAMINATION TIP

Examining salivary glands and ductal openings

When a patient reports decreased salivation, assess the parotid and submaxillary glands for enlargement and the ductal openings for salivary flow.

To detect an enlarged parotid gland, ask the patient to clench his teeth, thereby tensing the masseter muscle. Then palpate the parotid duct (about 2" [5 cm] long); you should be able to feel it against the tensed muscle, on the cheek just below the zygomatic arch. Next, check the ductal orifice, opposite the second molar. Using a gloved finger, palpate the orifice for enlargement, and observe for drainage.

Palpate the submaxillary gland. About the size of a walnut, this gland is located under the mandible, anterior to the angle of the jaw. Using a gloved finger, palpate the floor of the mouth for enlargement of the submaxillary ductal orifice.

Finally, test both ductal openings for salivary flow. Place cotton under the patient's tongue, have him sip pure lemon juice, and then remove the cotton and observe salivary flow from each opening. Document your findings.

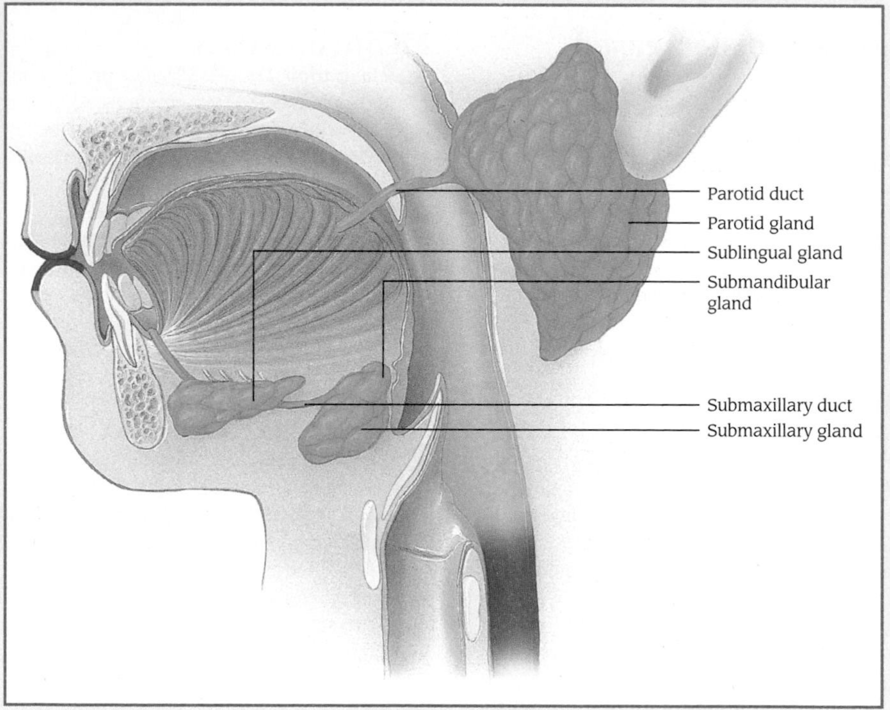

◆ ***Radiation.*** Excessive irradiation of the mouth or face from chemotherapeutic treatments or dental X-rays may cause transient decreased salivation due to salivary gland atrophy, which can lead to difficulty swallowing, discomfort, and gum disease.

Special considerations

If markedly reduced salivation interferes with speaking, eating, or swallowing, allow the patient extra time for these activities.

Pediatric pointers

Mouth breathing and anticholinergic therapy are the primary causes of decreased salivation in children.

PATIENT COUNSELING

To relieve dry mouth, encourage the patient to increase his fluid intake during meals and to chew gum or tart sugarless mints between meals. To reduce the risk of cavities, advise him to brush his teeth, floss, use mouthwash, and avoid sugary desserts, candies, and drinks. Routine dental visits and fluoride treatments may also be beneficial.

Pilocarpine hydrochloride (5 to 10 mg orally three times daily) can relieve symptoms of dry mouth, but it must be used regularly.

Salivation, increased

[Polysialia, ptyalism]

Increased salivation is an uncommon symptom that can result from a GI disorder, especially of the mouth. It also accompanies certain systemic disorders and may result from the use of certain drugs or from exposure to toxins. Saliva may also accumulate because of difficulty swallowing. (See "Dysphagia," page 235.)

HISTORY AND PHYSICAL EXAMINATION

A patient who complains of increased salivation may have overproductive salivary glands or difficulty swallowing. To distinguish these, first test for a gag reflex and observe the patient's ability to swallow and chew. Is he drooling? Is his chewing uncoordinated? An impaired gag reflex, drooling, and chewing incoordination suggest difficulty swallowing. Does he have related signs and symptoms, such as fatigue, fever, headache, or a sore throat? Ask about exposure to industrial toxins, such as mercury. Is the patient taking any medications? Note especially use of iodides, cholinergics, and miotics.

Inspect the mouth and mucous membranes for lesions. If present, are they painful? Put on gloves and palpate the lesions, which may be suppurative or infectious. Describe them in your notes. Next, inspect the uvula, gingivae, and pharynx. Palpate the lymph nodes, and determine if the parotid glands are swollen or sore.

MEDICAL CAUSES

◆ ***Bell's palsy.*** Paralysis of the facial nerve causes an inability to control salivation or close the eye on the affected side.

◆ ***Pregnancy.*** In the early months of pregnancy, many women experience increased salivation, nausea, and breast tenderness.

◆ ***Stomatitis.*** Mucosal ulcers may be accompanied by moderately increased salivation, mouth pain, fever, and erythema. Spontaneous healing usually occurs in 7 to 10 days, but scarring and recurrence are possible.

◆ ***Syphilis.*** With secondary syphilis, mucosal ulcers cause increased salivation that may persist up to a year. Related findings include fever, malaise, headache, anorexia, weight loss, nausea, vomiting, sore throat, and generalized lymphadenopathy. A bilaterally symmetrical rash appears on the arms, trunk, palms, soles, face, and scalp. Condylomata develop in the genital and perianal areas.

◆ ***Tuberculosis.*** Certain forms of tuberculosis may produce solitary, irregularly shaped mouth or tongue ulcers, covered with exudate, that cause increased salivation. Other findings include weight loss, anorexia, fever, fatigue, malaise, dyspnea, cough, night sweats (a common sign), and hemoptysis.

OTHER CAUSES

◆ ***Arsenic poisoning.*** Common effects of arsenic poisoning are diarrhea, diffuse skin hyperpigmentation, and edema of the eyelids, face, and ankles; increased salivation occurs infrequently. The patient may also exhibit garlicky breath odor, pruritus, alopecia, irritated mucous membranes, headache, drowsiness, and confusion. He may also develop muscle aching, weakness, seizures, and paresthesia in a stocking-glove distribution pattern.

◆ ***Drugs.*** Increased salivation may occur with iodide toxicity, but the earliest symptoms are a brassy taste and a burning sensation in the mouth and throat. Associated findings include sneezing, irritated eyelids, and (commonly) pain in the frontal sinus.

Pilocarpine and other miotics used to treat glaucoma may be absorbed systemically, increasing salivation. Cholinergics, such as bethanechol, may also cause this symptom.

◆ ***Mercury poisoning.*** Stomatitis, characterized by increased salivation and a metallic taste, commonly occurs in those with mercury poisoning. The patient's teeth may be loose and his gums are painful, swollen, and prone to bleeding. A blue line appears on the gingivae. The patient may also experience personality changes, memory loss, abdominal cramps, diarrhea, paresthesia, and tremors of the eyelids, lips, tongue, and fingers.

SPECIAL CONSIDERATIONS

Though annoying to the patient, increased salivation doesn't require treatments beyond those needed to correct the underlying disorder.

Pediatric pointers

Besides stemming from conditions that affect adults, increased salivation in children may also stem from congenital esophageal atresia. With this disorder, the infant is unable to swallow seemingly excessive saliva and frothy mucus.

Geriatric pointers

Drooling is common in elderly people with Parkinson's disease. It's caused by a reduction in automatic or conscious swallowing rather than by excessive salivation.

Salt craving

Craving salty foods is a compensatory response to the body's failure to adequately conserve sodium. Normally, the renal tubules reabsorb almost all sodium, allowing less than 1% of it to be excreted in the urine. This reabsorption is regulated by aldosterone, a hormone synthesized in the adrenal gland. However, adrenal dysfunction can reduce aldosterone levels, thereby impairing reabsorption and increasing excretion of sodium.

EMERGENCY INTERVENTIONS *Sudden or rapidly worsening salt craving may indicate adrenal crisis. Adrenal crisis produces profound weakness, fatigue, nausea, vomiting, hypotension, dehydration and, occasionally, high fever. If untreated, this condition can ultimately lead to vascular collapse, renal shutdown, coma, and death. It requires prompt I.V. bolus administration of hydrocortisone. Later, doses may be given I.M. or may be diluted with dextrose in saline solution and given I.V. until the patient's condition stabilizes.*

History and physical examination

Because normal salt intake varies widely, depending on dietary preferences and cultural differences, find out how much salt the patient typically uses. Has he increased this amount recently? Has he also experienced weakness, fatigue, anorexia, or weight loss? Has he fainted or felt dizzy? Check for a history of adrenal insufficiency or diabetes mellitus and for recent onset of polydipsia or polyuria. Inspect the patient's skin for hyperpigmentation or hypopigmentation. Take his vital signs, too, noting orthostatic hypotension.

Medical causes

- ***Adrenal insufficiency (primary).*** Commonly called *Addison's disease,* this disorder reduces aldosterone secretion. As a result, the patient may exhibit an intense craving for salty food. He may display diffuse brown, tan, or bronze-to-black hyperpigmentation of exposed areas (such as the face, knees, and knuckles) and of nonexposed areas (such as the tongue, buccal mucosa, or palmar creases) as well as darkening of normally pigmented areas, moles, and scars. Related findings include weakness, anorexia, nausea, irritability, vomiting, decreased cold tolerance, dizziness, low blood pressure, weight loss, abdominal pain, and slowly progressive fatigue.

Special considerations

Prepare the patient for laboratory tests, such as plasma renin activity and serum aldosterone, serum electrolyte, plasma cortisol and glucose, urine 17-ketogenic steroids and 17-hydroxycorticosteroid, and corticotropin levels. Special provocative studies may include the metyrapone test and the rapid corticotropin test. Collect a urine specimen, and use a reagent strip to test for glucose and acetone.

To check for volume depletion, monitor and record the patient's blood pressure, weight, intake and output, and skin turgor. Encourage the patient to drink plenty of fluids, and arrange for a diet that helps maintain adequate sodium and potassium levels. Be alert for signs of hyponatremia, such as hypotension, muscle twitching and weakness, and abdominal cramps. Look for signs and symptoms of hyperkalemia, such as muscle weakness, tachycardia, nausea, vomiting, and characteristic ECG changes, including tented and elevated T waves, widened QRS complex, prolonged PR interval, flattened or absent P waves, and depressed ST segment.

If diagnostic tests confirm primary adrenal insufficiency, emphasize the importance of complying with lifelong steroid (glucocorticoid or mineralocorticoid) therapy.

Pediatric pointers

Salt craving in children may stem from decompensated congenital adrenal hyperplasia; although this disorder usually responds adequately to steroid replacement. Adrenal insufficiency can also develop with surgery or acute illness. Salt craving may signal a change in condition requiring increased steroid dosage.

Patient counseling

If the patient will be taking a steroid (usually hydrocortisone), explain why he needs to take the drug. Explain to him the adverse effects of the drug and the signs and symptoms of steroid toxicity and underdosage. Instruct the patient not to decrease the dose or discontinue the drug without a physician's order. Explain that his dosage may need to be increased during times of stress (infection, injury, even profuse sweating) to prevent adrenal crisis. Tell him that he'll need lifelong medical supervision to monitor the steroid therapy.

Instruct the patient to wear a medical identification bracelet at all times, indicating his condition and the name and dosage of the drug he takes. Teach him how to self-administer the drug parenterally in emergency situations such as traveling in remote areas away from medical help. Urge him to keep a prepared syringe of the drug available for emergency use.

Scotoma

A scotoma is an area of partial or complete blindness within an otherwise normal or slightly impaired visual field. Usually located within the central 30-degree area, the defect ranges from absolute blindness to a barely detectable loss of visual acuity. Typically, the patient can pinpoint the scotoma's location in the visual field. (See *Locating scotomas,* page 614.)

A scotoma can result from a retinal, choroid, or optic nerve disorder. It can be classified as absolute, relative, or scintillating. An absolute scotoma refers to the total inability to see all sizes of test objects used in mapping the visual field. A relative scotoma, in contrast, refers to the ability to see only large test objects. A scintillating scotoma refers to the flashes or bursts of light commonly seen during a migraine headache.

History and physical examination

First, identify and characterize the scotoma, using such visual field tests as the tangent screen examination, the Goldmann perimeter test, and the automated perimetry test. Two other visual field tests—confrontation testing and the Amsler grid—may also help in identifying a scotoma.

Next, test the patient's visual acuity and inspect his pupils for size, equality, and reaction to light. An ophthalmoscopic examination and measurement of intraocular pressure (IOP) are necessary.

Explore the patient's medical history, noting especially any eye disorders, vision problems, or chronic systemic disorders. Find out if he takes medications or uses eyedrops.

Medical causes

◆ ***Chorioretinitis.*** Inflammation of the choroid and retina produces a paracentral scotoma. Ophthalmoscopic examination reveals clouding and cells in the vitreous, subretinal hemorrhage, and neovascularization. The patient may have photophobia along with blurred vision.

◆ ***Glaucoma.*** Prolonged elevation of IOP can cause an arcuate scotoma. Poorly controlled glaucoma can also cause cupping of the optic disk, loss of peripheral vision, and reduced visual acuity. The patient may also see rainbow-colored halos around lights.

◆ ***Macular degeneration.*** Any degenerative process or disorder affecting the fovea centralis results in a central scotoma. Ophthalmoscopic examination reveals changes in the macular area. The patient may notice subtle changes in visual acuity, in color perception, and in the size and shape of objects.

◆ ***Migraine headache.*** Transient scintillating scotomas, usually bilateral and often homonymous, can occur during a classic migraine aura. Besides pain, characteristic associated symptoms include paresthesia of the lips, face, or hands; slight confusion; dizziness; and photophobia.

◆ ***Optic neuritis.*** Inflammation, degeneration, or demyelination of the optic nerve produces a central, circular, or centrocecal scotoma. The scotoma may be unilateral with involvement of one nerve, or bilateral with involvement of both nerves. It can vary in size, density, and symmetry. The patient may report severe visual loss or blurring, lasting up to 3 weeks, and pain—especially with eye movement. Common ophthalmoscopic findings include hyperemia of the optic disk, retinal vein distention, blurred disk margins, and filling of the physiologic cup.

◆ ***Retinal pigmentary degenerations.*** These disorders cause premature retinal cell changes leading to cell death. One disorder, retinitis pigmentosa, initially involves loss of peripheral rods; the resulting annular scotoma progresses concentrically until only a central field of vision (tunnel vision) remains. The earliest symptom—impaired night vision—appears during adolescence. Associated signs include narrowing of the retinal blood vessels and pallor of the optic disk. Eventually, with invasion of the macula, blindness may occur.

Locating scotomas

Scotomas, or "blind spots," are classified according to the affected area of the visual field. The normal scotoma—shown in the temporal region of the right eye—appears in black in all the illustrations.

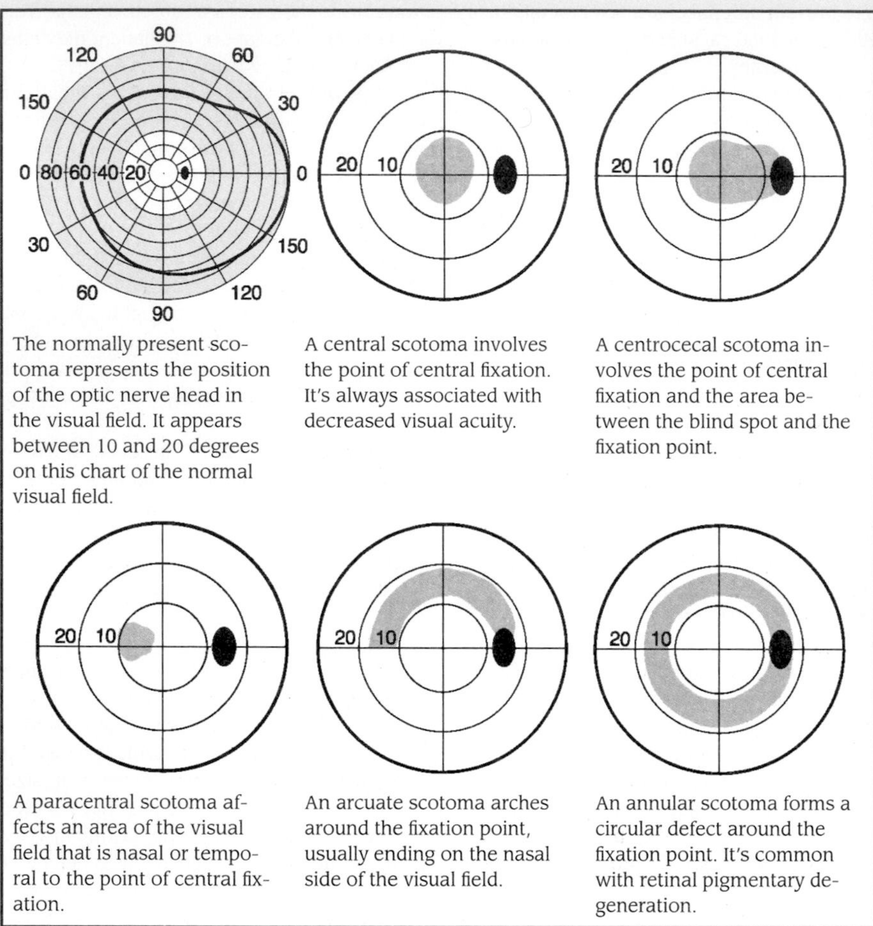

The normally present scotoma represents the position of the optic nerve head in the visual field. It appears between 10 and 20 degrees on this chart of the normal visual field.

A central scotoma involves the point of central fixation. It's always associated with decreased visual acuity.

A centrocecal scotoma involves the point of central fixation and the area between the blind spot and the fixation point.

A paracentral scotoma affects an area of the visual field that is nasal or temporal to the point of central fixation.

An arcuate scotoma arches around the fixation point, usually ending on the nasal side of the visual field.

An annular scotoma forms a circular defect around the fixation point. It's common with retinal pigmentary degeneration.

SPECIAL CONSIDERATIONS

For the patient with an arcuate scotoma associated with glaucoma, emphasize regular testing of IOP and visual fields. For the patient with a disorder involving the fovea centralis (or the area surrounding it), teach him to periodically use the Amsler grid to detect progression of macular degeneration.

PEDIATRIC POINTERS

In young children, visual field testing is difficult and requires patience. Confrontation testing is the method of choice.

Scrotal swelling

Scrotal swelling occurs when a condition affecting the testicles, epididymis, or scrotal skin produces edema or a mass; the penis may be involved. Scrotal swelling can affect males of any age. It can be unilateral or bilateral and painful or painless.

The sudden onset of painful scrotal swelling suggests torsion of a testicle or testicular appendages, especially in a prepubescent male. This emergency requires immediate surgery to untwist and stabilize the spermatic cord or to remove the appendage.

EMERGENCY INTERVENTIONS *If severe pain accompanies scrotal swelling, ask when the swelling began. Using a Doppler stethoscope, evaluate blood flow to the testicle. If it's decreased or absent, suspect testicular torsion and prepare the patient for surgery. Withhold food and fluids, insert an I.V. catheter, and apply an ice pack to the scrotum to reduce pain and swelling. An attempt may be made to untwist the cord manually, but even if this is successful, the patient may still require surgery for stabilization.*

History and physical examination

If the patient isn't in distress, proceed with the history. Ask about injury to the scrotum, urethral discharge, cloudy urine, increased urinary frequency, and dysuria. Is the patient sexually active? When was his last sexual contact? Does he have a history of sexually transmitted disease? Find out about recent illnesses, particularly mumps. Does he have a history of prostate surgery or prolonged catheterization? Does changing his body position or level of activity affect the swelling?

Take the patient's vital signs, especially noting fever, and palpate his abdomen for tenderness. Then examine the entire genital area. Assess the scrotum with the patient in supine and standing positions. Note its size and color. Is the swelling unilateral or bilateral? Do you see signs of trauma or bruising? Are there rashes or lesions present? Gently palpate the scrotum for a cyst or a lump. Note especially tenderness or increased firmness. Check the testicles' position in the scrotum. Finally, transilluminate the scrotum to distinguish a fluid-filled cyst from a solid mass. (A solid mass can't be transilluminated.)

Medical causes

◆ ***Elephantiasis of the scrotum.*** With this disorder (common in some tropical countries), infection by a filaria worm obstructs lymphatic drainage, causing chronic gross scrotal edema and pain. Associated findings include other areas of pitting and, eventually, brawny edema (especially the legs), thickened subcutaneous tissue, hyperkeratosis, and skin fissures.

◆ ***Epididymal cysts.*** Located in the head of the epididymis, these cysts produce painless scrotal swelling.

◆ ***Epididymal tuberculosis.*** This disorder produces an enlarged scrotal mass separated from the testicle. Other findings include palpable beading along the vas deferens, induration of the prostate or seminal vesicles, and pus or tubercle bacilli in the urine.

◆ ***Epididymitis.*** Key features of inflammation are pain, extreme tenderness, and swelling in the groin and scrotum. The patient waddles to avoid pressure on the groin and scrotum during walking. He may have high fever, malaise, urethral discharge and cloudy urine, and lower abdominal pain on the affected side. His scrotal skin may be hot, red, dry, flaky, and thin.

◆ ***Gumma.*** This rare, painless nodule—usually associated with benign tertiary syphilis—can affect any bone or organ. If it affects the testicle, it causes edema.

◆ ***Hernia.*** Herniation of bowel into the scrotum can cause swelling and a soft or unusually firm scrotum. Occasionally, bowel sounds can be auscultated in the scrotum.

◆ ***Hydrocele.*** Fluid accumulation produces gradual scrotal swelling that's usually painless. The scrotum may be soft and cystic or firm and tense. Palpation reveals a round, nontender scrotal mass.

◆ ***Idiopathic scrotal edema.*** Swelling occurs quickly with this disorder and usually disappears within 24 hours. The affected testicle is pink.

◆ ***Orchitis (acute).*** Mumps, syphilis, or tuberculosis may precipitate this disorder, which causes sudden painful swelling of one or, at times, both testicles. Related findings include a hot, reddened scrotum; fever of up to 104° F (40° C); chills; lower abdominal pain; nausea; vomiting; and extreme weakness. Urinary signs are usually absent.

◆ ***Scrotal burns.*** Burns cause swelling within 24 hours of injury. Depending on the burn's severity, associated findings may include severe pain, erythema, chafing, tissue sloughing, and maceration with a weeping exudate.

◆ ***Scrotal trauma.*** Blunt trauma causes scrotal swelling with bruising and severe pain. The scrotum may appear dark or bluish.

◆ ***Spermatocele.*** This usually painless cystic mass lies above and behind the testicle and contains opaque fluid and sperm. Its onset may be acute or gradual. Less than 1 cm in diameter, it's movable and may be transilluminated.

◆ ***Testicular torsion.*** Most common before puberty, this urologic emergency causes scrotal swelling; sudden, severe pain; and, possibly, elevation of the affected testicle within the scrotum. It may also cause nausea and vomiting.

◆ ***Testicular tumor.*** Typically painless, smooth, and firm, a testicular tumor produces swelling and a sensation of excessive weight in the scrotum.

◆ ***Torsion of a hydatid of Morgagni.*** Torsion of this small, pea-sized cyst severs its blood supply, causing a hard, painful swelling on the testicle's upper pole.

Other causes

◆ ***Surgery.*** An effusion of blood from surgery can produce a hematocele, leading to scrotal swelling.

Special considerations

Keep the patient on bed rest and administer an antibiotic. Provide adequate fluids, fiber, and stool softeners. Place a rolled towel between the patient's legs and under the scrotum to help reduce severe swelling. If the patient has mild or moderate swelling, advise him to wear a loose-fitting athletic supporter lined with a soft cotton dressing. For several days, administer an analgesic to relieve his pain. Encourage sitz baths, and apply heat or ice packs to decrease inflammation.

Prepare the patient for needle aspiration of fluid-filled cysts and other diagnostic tests, such as lung tomography and computed tomography scan of the abdomen, to rule out malignant tumors.

Pediatric pointers

A thorough physical assessment is especially important for children with scrotal swelling, who may be unable to provide history data. In children up to age 1, a hernia or hydrocele of the spermatic cord may stem from abnormal fetal development. In infants, scrotal swelling may stem from ammonia-related dermatitis, if diapers aren't changed often enough. In prepubescent males, it usually results from torsion of the spermatic cord.

Other disorders that can produce scrotal swelling in children include epididymitis (rare before age 10), traumatic orchitis from contact sports, and mumps, which usually occurs after puberty.

Patient counseling

Encourage the patient to perform testicular self-examinations at home. (See *How to examine your testicles.*)

Seizures, absence

Absence seizures are benign, generalized seizures thought to originate subcortically. These brief episodes of unconsciousness usually last 3 to 20 seconds and can occur 100 or more times a day, causing periods of inattention. Absence seizures usually begin between ages 4 and 12. Their first sign may be deteriorating school work and behavior. The cause of these seizures is unknown.

Absence seizures occur without warning. The patient suddenly stops all purposeful activity and stares blankly ahead, as if he were daydreaming. Absence seizures may produce automatisms, such as repetitive lip smacking, or mild clonic or myoclonic movements, including mild jerking of the eyelids. The patient may drop an object that he's holding, and muscle relaxation may cause him to drop his head or arms or to slump. After the attack, the patient resumes activity, typically unaware of the episode.

Absence status, a rare form of absence seizure, occurs as a prolonged absence seizure or as repeated episodes of these seizures. Usually not life-threatening, it occurs most commonly in patients who have previously experienced absence seizures.

History and physical examination

If you suspect a patient is having an absence seizure, evaluate its occurrence and duration by reciting a series of numbers and then asking him to repeat them after the attack ends. If the patient has had an absence seizure, he'll be unable to do this. Alternatively, if the seizures are occurring within minutes of each other, ask the patient to count for about 5 minutes. He'll stop counting during a seizure and resume when it's over. Look for accompanying automatisms. Find out if the family has noticed a change in behavior or deteriorating schoolwork.

Medical causes

◆ ***Idiopathic epilepsy.*** Some forms of absence seizure are accompanied by learning disabilities.

Patient counseling

Explain the purpose of any diagnostic tests, such as computed tomography scans, magnetic resonance imaging, and EEGs. Teach the patient and his family about these seizures and how to recognize their onset, pattern, and

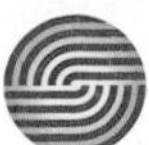

PATIENT-TEACHING AID

How to examine your testicles

Dear Patient:

To help detect abnormalities early, you should examine your testicles once a month. (Perform this examination on the same date every month.) The best time to examine your testicles is during or after a hot bath or shower. The heat causes the testicles to descend and relaxes the scrotum; this makes finding abnormalities easier.

Follow these simple instructions for performing a self-examination, using the illustration (upper right) to locate anatomic landmarks.

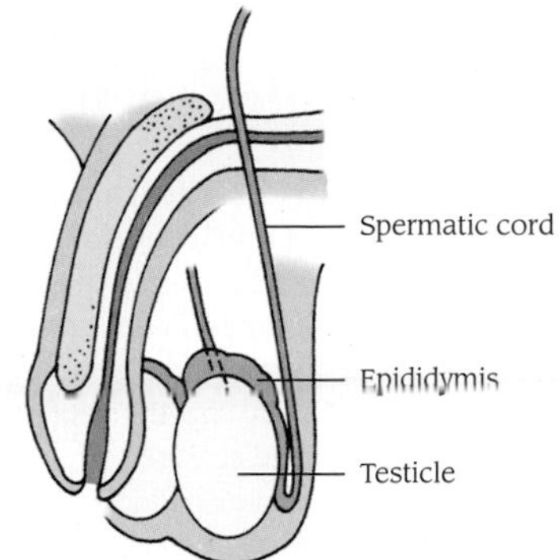

Check the scrotum

With one hand, lift your penis and check your scrotum (the pouch of skin containing the testicles and parts of the spermatic cords) for any change in shape or size and for reddened, distended veins. Expect the scrotum's left side to hang slightly lower than the right.

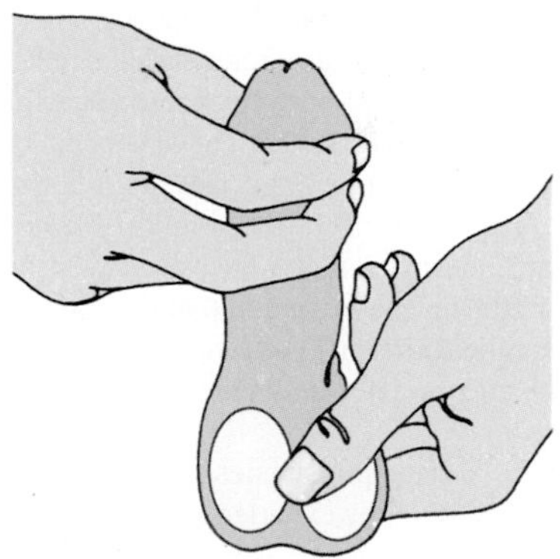

Check each testicle

Place your left thumb on the front of your left testicle and your index and middle fingers behind it (as shown middle right). Gently but firmly roll the testicle between your thumb and fingers. Then use your right hand to examine your right testicle in the same manner. Your testicles should feel smooth, rubbery, slightly tender, and movable within the scrotum.

If you notice any lumps, masses, or other changes, notify your physician.

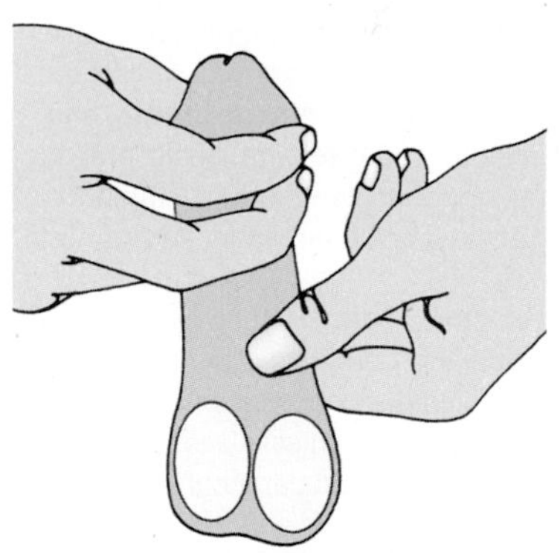

Check each spermatic cord

Locate the epididymis, the cordlike structure at the back of your testicles. Then locate the spermatic cord extending upward from it (as shown bottom right).

Gently squeeze the spermatic cord above your left testicle between your thumb and the first two fingers of your left hand. Then repeat on the right side, using your right hand. Check for lumps and masses along the entire length of the cords.

duration. Include the child's teacher and school nurse in the teaching process, if possible. If the seizures are being controlled with drug therapy, emphasize the importance of strict compliance.

Seizures, complex partial

A complex partial seizure occurs when a focal seizure begins in the temporal lobe and causes a partial alteration of consciousness—usually confusion. Psychomotor seizures can occur at any age, but incidence usually increases during adolescence and adulthood. Two-thirds of patients also have generalized seizures.

An aura—usually a complex hallucination, illusion, or sensation—typically precedes a psychomotor seizure. The hallucination may be audiovisual (images with sounds), auditory (abnormal or normal sounds or voices from the patient's past), or olfactory (unpleasant smells, such as rotten eggs or burning materials). Other types of auras include sensations of déjà vu, unfamiliarity with surroundings, or depersonalization. Some patients become fearful or anxious, experience lip smacking, or have an unpleasant feeling in the epigastric region that rises toward the chest and throat. The patient usually recognizes the aura and lies down before losing consciousness.

A period of unresponsiveness follows the aura. The patient may experience automatisms, appear dazed and wander aimlessly, perform inappropriate acts (such as undressing in public), be unresponsive, utter incoherent phrases, or (rarely) go into a rage or tantrum. After the seizure, the patient is confused, drowsy, and doesn't remember the seizure. Behavioral automatisms rarely last longer than 5 minutes, but postseizure confusion, agitation, and amnesia may persist.

Between attacks, the patient may exhibit slow and rigid thinking, outbursts of anger and aggressiveness, tedious conversation, a preoccupation with naive philosophical ideas, diminished libido, mood swings, and paranoid tendencies.

History and physical examination

If you witness a complex partial seizure, never attempt to restrain the patient. Instead, lead him gently to a safe area. *(Exception:* Don't approach him if he's angry or violent.) Calmly encourage him to sit down, and remain with him until he's fully alert. After the seizure, ask him if he experienced an aura. Record all observations and findings.

Medical causes

◆ ***Brain abscess.*** If the brain abscess is in the temporal lobe, complex partial seizures commonly occur after the abscess disappears. Related problems may include headache, nausea, vomiting, generalized seizures, and a decreased level of consciousness (LOC). The patient may also develop central facial weakness, auditory receptive aphasia, hemiparesis, and ocular disturbances.

◆ ***Head trauma.*** Severe trauma to the temporal lobe (especially from a penetrating injury) can produce complex partial seizures months or years later. The seizures may decrease in frequency and eventually stop. Head trauma also causes generalized seizures and behavior and personality changes.

◆ ***Herpes simplex encephalitis.*** The herpes simplex virus commonly attacks the temporal lobe, resulting in complex partial seizures. Other features include fever, headache, coma, and generalized seizures.

◆ ***Temporal lobe tumor.*** Complex partial seizures may be the first sign of this disorder. Other signs and symptoms include headache, pupillary changes, and mental dullness. Increased intracranial pressure may cause a decreased LOC, vomiting and, possibly, papilledema.

Special considerations

After the seizure, remain with the patient to reorient him to his surroundings and to protect him from injury. Keep him in bed until he's fully alert, and remove harmful objects from the area. Offer emotional support to the patient and his family, and teach them how to cope with seizures.

Prepare the patient for diagnostic tests, such as EEG, computed tomography scans, or magnetic resonance imaging.

Pediatric pointers

Complex partial seizures in children may resemble absence seizures. They can result from birth injury, abuse, infection, or cancer. In about one-third of patients, their cause is unknown.

Repeated complex partial seizures commonly lead to generalized seizures. The child may experience a slight aura, which is rarely as clearly defined as that seen with generalized tonic-clonic seizures.

Seizures, generalized tonic-clonic

Like other types of seizures, generalized tonic-clonic seizures are caused by the paroxysmal, uncontrolled discharge of central nervous system (CNS) neurons, leading to neurologic dysfunction. Unlike most other types of seizures, however, this cerebral hyperactivity isn't confined to the original focus or to a localized area but extends to the entire brain.

A generalized tonic-clonic seizure may begin with or without an aura. As seizure activity spreads to the subcortical structures, the patient loses consciousness, falls to the ground, and may utter a loud cry that's precipitated by air rushing from the lungs through the vocal cords. His body stiffens (tonic phase), then undergoes rapid, synchronous muscle jerking and hyperventilation (clonic phase). Tongue biting, incontinence, diaphoresis, profuse salivation, and signs of respiratory distress may also occur. The seizure usually stops after 2 to 5 minutes. The patient then regains consciousness but displays confusion. He may complain of headache, fatigue, muscle soreness, and arm and leg weakness.

Generalized tonic-clonic seizures usually occur singly. The patient may be asleep or awake and active. (See *What happens during a generalized tonic-clonic seizure*, page 620.) Possible complications include respiratory arrest due to airway obstruction from secretions, status epilepticus (occurring in 5% to 8% of patients), head or spinal injuries and bruises, Todd's paralysis and, rarely, cardiac arrest. Life-threatening status epilepticus is marked by prolonged seizure activity or by rapidly recurring seizures with no intervening periods of recovery. It's most commonly triggered by abrupt discontinuation of anticonvulsant therapy.

Generalized seizures may be caused by a brain tumor, vascular disorder, head trauma, infection, metabolic defect, drug or alcohol withdrawal syndrome, exposure to toxins, or a genetic defect. Generalized seizures may also result from a focal seizure. With recurring seizures, or epilepsy, the cause may be unknown.

EMERGENCY INTERVENTIONS *If you witness the beginning of the seizure, first check the patient's airway, breathing, and circulation, and ensure that the cause isn't asystole or a blocked airway. Stay with the patient and ensure a patent airway. Focus your care on observing the seizure and protecting the patient. Place a towel under his head to prevent injury, loosen his clothing, and move any sharp or hard objects out of his way. Never try to restrain the patient or force a hard object into his mouth; you might chip his teeth or fracture his jaw. Only at the start of the ictal phase can you safely insert a soft object into his mouth.*

If possible, turn the patient to one side during the seizure to allow secretions to drain and to prevent aspiration. Otherwise, do this at the end of the clonic phase when respirations return. (If they fail to return, check for airway obstruction and suction the patient if necessary. Cardiopulmonary resuscitation, intubation, and mechanical ventilation may be needed.)

Protect the patient after the seizure by providing a safe area in which he can rest. As he awakens, reassure and reorient him. Check his vital signs and neurologic status. Be sure to carefully record these data and your observations during the seizure.

If the seizure lasts longer than 4 minutes or if a second seizure occurs before full recovery from the first, suspect status epilepticus. Establish an airway, insert an I.V. catheter, give supplemental oxygen, and begin cardiac monitoring. Draw blood for appropriate studies. Turn the patient on his side, with his head in a semi-dependent position, to drain secretions and prevent aspiration. Periodically turn him to the opposite side, check his arterial blood gas levels for hypoxemia, and administer oxygen by mask, increasing the flow rate if necessary. Administer diazepam or lorazepam by slow I.V. push, repeated two or three times at 10- to 20-minute intervals, to stop the seizures. If the patient isn't known to have epilepsy, an I.V. bolus of dextrose 50% (50 ml) with thiamine (100 mg) may be ordered. Dextrose may stop the seizures if the patient has hypoglycemia. If his thiamine level is low, also give thiamine to guard against further damage.

If the patient is intubated, expect to insert a nasogastric (NG) tube to prevent vomiting and aspiration. Be aware that if the patient hasn't been intubated, the NG tube itself can trigger the gag reflex and cause vomiting. Be sure to record your observations and the intervals between seizures.

HISTORY AND PHYSICAL EXAMINATION

If you didn't witness the seizure, obtain a description from the patient's companion. Ask when the seizure started and how long it lasted. Did the patient report any unusual sensations before the seizure began? Did the seizure start

What happens during a generalized tonic-clonic seizure

Before the seizure

Prodromal signs and symptoms, such as myoclonic jerks, throbbing headache, and mood changes, may occur over several hours or days. The patient may have premonitions of the seizure. For example, he may report an *aura,* such as seeing a flashing light or smelling a characteristic odor.

During the seizure

If a generalized seizure begins with an aura, this indicates that irritability in a specific area of the brain quickly became widespread. Common auras include palpitations, epigastric distress rapidly rising to the throat, head or eye turning, and sensory hallucinations.

Next, *loss of consciousness* occurs as a sudden discharge of intense electrical activity overwhelms the brain's subcortical center. The patient falls and experiences brief, bilateral myoclonic contractures. Air forced through spasmodic vocal cords may produce a birdlike, piercing cry.

During the *tonic phase,* skeletal muscles contract for 10 to 20 seconds. The patient's eyelids are drawn up, his arms are flexed, and his legs are extended. His mouth opens wide, then snaps shut; he may bite his tongue. His respirations cease because of respiratory muscle spasm, and initial pallor of the skin and mucous membranes (the result of impaired venous return) changes to cyanosis secondary to apnea. The patient arches his back and slowly lowers his arms (as shown below). Other effects include dilated, nonreactive pupils; greatly increased heart rate and blood pressure; increased salivation and tracheobronchial secretions; and profuse diaphoresis.

During the *clonic phase*, lasting about 60 seconds, mild trembling progresses to violent contractures or jerks. Other motor activity includes facial grimaces (with possible tongue biting) and violent expiration of bloody, foamy saliva from clonic contractures of thoracic cage muscles. Clonic jerks slowly decrease in intensity and frequency. The patient is still apneic.

After the seizure

The patient's movements gradually cease, and he becomes unresponsive to external stimuli. Other postseizure features include stertorous respirations from increased tracheobronchial secretions, equal or unequal pupils (but becoming reactive), and urinary incontinence due to brief muscle relaxation. After about 5 minutes, the patient's level of consciousness increases, and he appears confused and disoriented. His muscle tone, heart rate, and blood pressure return to normal.

After several hours' sleep, the patient awakens exhausted and may have a headache, sore muscles, and amnesia about the seizure.

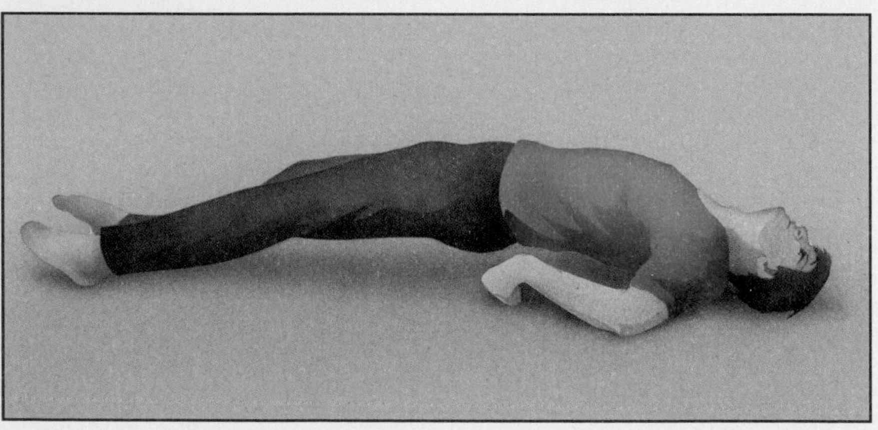

in one area of the body and spread, or did it affect the entire body right away? Did the patient fall on a hard surface? Did his eyes or head turn? Did he turn blue? Did he lose bladder control? Did he have any other seizures before recovering?

If the patient may have sustained a head injury, observe him closely for loss of consciousness, unequal or nonreactive pupils, and focal neurologic signs. Does he complain of headache and muscle soreness? Is he increasingly difficult to arouse when you check on him at 20-minute intervals? Examine his arms, legs, and face (including tongue) for injury, residual paralysis, or limb weakness.

Next, obtain a history. Has the patient ever had generalized or focal seizures before? If so, do they occur frequently? Do other family members also have them? Is the patient receiving drug therapy? Is he compliant? Ask about sleep deprivation and emotional or physical stress at the time the seizure occurred.

MEDICAL CAUSES

◆ ***Alcohol withdrawal syndrome.*** Sudden withdrawal from alcohol dependence may cause seizures 7 to 48 hours later as well as status epilepticus. The patient may also be restless and exhibit hallucinations, profuse diaphoresis, and tachycardia.

◆ ***Brain abscess.*** Generalized seizures may occur in the acute stage of abscess formation or after the abscess disappears. Depending on the size and location of the abscess, decreased level of consciousness (LOC) varies from drowsiness to deep stupor. Early signs and symptoms reflect increased intracranial pressure (ICP) and include constant headache, nausea, vomiting, and focal seizures. Typical later features include ocular disturbances, such as nystagmus, impaired vision, and unequal pupils. Other findings vary with the abscess site but may include aphasia, hemiparesis, abnormal behavior, and personality changes.

◆ ***Brain tumor.*** Generalized seizures may occur, depending on the tumor's location and type. Other findings include a slowly decreasing LOC, morning headache, dizziness, confusion, focal seizures, vision loss, motor and sensory disturbances, aphasia, and ataxia. Later findings include papilledema, vomiting, increased systolic blood pressure, widening pulse pressure, and (eventually) decorticate posture.

◆ ***Cerebral aneurysm.*** Occasionally, generalized seizures may occur with an aneurysmal rupture. Premonitory signs and symptoms may last several days, but onset is typically abrupt with severe headache, nausea, vomiting, and decreased LOC. Depending on the site and amount of bleeding, related signs and symptoms vary but may include nuchal rigidity, irritability, hemiparesis, hemisensory defects, dysphagia, photophobia, diplopia, ptosis, and unilateral pupil dilation.

◆ ***Chronic renal failure.*** End-stage renal failure produces rapid onset of twitching, trembling, myoclonic jerks, and generalized seizures. Related signs and symptoms include anuria or oliguria, fatigue, malaise, irritability, decreased mental acuity, muscle cramps, peripheral neuropathies, anorexia, and constipation or diarrhea. Integumentary effects include skin color changes (yellow, brown, or bronze), pruritus, and uremic frost. Other effects include ammonia breath odor, nausea and vomiting, ecchymoses, petechiae, GI bleeding, mouth and gum ulcers, hypertension, and Kussmaul's respirations.

◆ ***Eclampsia.*** Generalized seizures are a hallmark of this disorder. Related findings include severe frontal headache, nausea and vomiting, vision disturbances, increased blood pressure, fever of up to 104° F (40° C), peripheral edema, and sudden weight gain. The patient may also exhibit oliguria, irritability, hyperactive deep tendon reflexes (DTRs), and decreased LOC.

◆ ***Encephalitis.*** Seizures are an early sign of this disorder, indicating a poor prognosis; they may also occur after recovery as a result of residual damage. Other findings include fever, headache, photophobia, nuchal rigidity, neck pain, vomiting, aphasia, ataxia, hemiparesis, nystagmus, irritability, cranial nerve palsies (causing facial weakness, ptosis, dysphagia), and myoclonic jerks.

◆ ***Epilepsy (idiopathic).*** In most cases, the cause of recurrent seizures is unknown.

◆ ***Head trauma.*** In severe cases, generalized seizures may occur at the time of injury. (Months later, focal seizures may occur.) Severe head trauma may also cause a decreased LOC, leading to coma; soft-tissue injury of the face, head, or neck; clear or bloody drainage from the mouth, nose, or ears; facial edema; bony deformity of the face, head, or neck; Battle's sign; and lack of response to oculocephalic and oculovestibular stimulation. Motor and sensory deficits may occur along with altered respirations. Examination may reveal signs of increasing ICP, such as decreased response to painful stimuli, nonreactive pupils, bradycardia, increased systolic pressure, and widening pulse pressure. If the patient is conscious, he may exhibit visual deficits, behavioral changes, and headache.

◆ ***Hepatic encephalopathy.*** Generalized seizures may occur late in this disorder. Associated late-stage findings in the comatose patient include fetor hepaticus, asterixis, hyperactive DTRs, and a positive Babinski's sign.

◆ ***Hypertensive encephalopathy.*** This life-threatening disorder may cause seizures along with severely increased blood pressure, decreased LOC, intense headache, vomiting, transient blindness, paralysis, and (eventually) Cheyne-Stokes respirations.

◆ ***Hypoglycemia.*** Generalized seizures usually occur with severe hypoglycemia, accompanied by blurred or double vision, motor weakness, hemiplegia, trembling, excessive diaphoresis, tachycardia, myoclonic twitching, and decreased LOC.

◆ ***Hyponatremia.*** Seizures develop when serum sodium levels fall below 125 mEq/L, especially if the decrease is rapid. Hyponatremia also causes orthostatic hypotension, headache, muscle twitching and weakness, fatigue, oliguria or anuria, cold and clammy skin, decreased skin turgor, irritability, lethargy, confusion, and stupor or coma. Excessive thirst, tachycardia, nausea, vomiting, and abdominal cramps may also occur. Severe hyponatremia may cause cyanosis and vasomotor collapse, with a thready pulse.

◆ ***Hypoparathyroidism.*** Worsening tetany causes generalized seizures. Chronic hypoparathyroidism produces neuromuscular irritability and hyperactive DTRs.

◆ ***Hypoxic encephalopathy.*** Besides generalized seizures, this disorder may produce myoclonic jerks and coma. Later, if the patient has recovered, dementia, visual agnosia, choreoathetosis, and ataxia may occur.

◆ ***Multiple sclerosis.*** This disorder rarely produces generalized seizures. Characteristic findings include vision deficits, paresthesia, constipation, muscle weakness, paralysis, spasticity, hyperreflexia, intention tremor, ataxic gait, dysphagia, dysarthria, impotence, and emotional lability. Urinary frequency, urgency, and incontinence may also occur.

◆ ***Neurofibromatosis.*** Multiple brain lesions from this disorder cause focal and generalized seizures. Inspection reveals café-au-lait spots, multiple skin tumors, scoliosis, and kyphoscoliosis. Related findings include dizziness, ataxia, monocular blindness, and nystagmus.

◆ ***Porphyria (intermittent acute).*** Generalized seizures are a late sign of this disorder, indicating severe CNS involvement. Acute porphyria also causes severe abdominal pain, tachycardia, psychotic behavior, muscle weakness, and sensory loss in the trunk.

◆ ***Sarcoidosis.*** Lesions may affect the brain, causing generalized and focal seizures. Associated findings include a nonproductive cough with dyspnea, substernal pain, malaise, fatigue, arthralgia, myalgia, weight loss, tachypnea, dysphagia, skin lesions, and impaired vision.

◆ ***Stroke.*** Seizures (focal more often than generalized) may occur within 6 months of an ischemic stroke. Associated signs and symptoms vary with the location and extent of brain damage. They include decreased LOC, contralateral hemiplegia, dysarthria, dysphagia, ataxia, unilateral sensory loss, apraxia, agnosia, and aphasia. The patient may also develop visual deficits, memory loss, poor judgment, personality changes, emotional lability, urine retention or urinary incontinence, constipation, headache, and vomiting.

Other causes

◆ ***Arsenic poisoning.*** Besides generalized seizures, arsenic poisoning may cause a garlicky breath odor, increased salivation, and generalized pruritus. GI effects include diarrhea, nausea, vomiting, and severe abdominal pain. Related effects include diffuse hyperpigmentation; sharply defined edema of the eyelids, face, and ankles; paresthesia of the extremities; alopecia; irritated mucous membranes; weakness; muscle aches; and peripheral neuropathy.

◆ ***Barbiturate withdrawal.*** In chronically intoxicated patients, barbiturate withdrawal may produce generalized seizures 2 to 4 days after the last dose. Status epilepticus is possible.

◆ ***Diagnostic tests.*** Contrast agents used in radiologic tests may cause generalized seizures.

◆ ***Drugs.*** Toxic blood levels of some drugs, such as theophylline, lidocaine, meperidine, penicillins, and cimetidine, may cause generalized seizures. Phenothiazines, tricyclic antidepressants, amphetamines, isoniazid, and vincristine may cause seizures in patients with preexisting epilepsy.

Special considerations

Closely monitor the patient after the seizure for recurring seizure activity. Prepare him for a computed tomography scan or magnetic resonance imaging and EEG.

Pediatric pointers

Generalized seizures are common in children. In fact, between 75% and 90% of epileptic patients experience their first seizure before age 20. Many children between ages 3 months and 3 years experience generalized seizures associated with fever; some of these children later develop seizures without fever. Generalized seizures may also stem from inborn errors of metabolism, perinatal injury, brain infection, Reye's syndrome, Sturge-Weber syndrome, arteriovenous malformation, lead poisoning, hypoglycemia, and idiopathic causes. The pertussis component of the DPT vaccine may cause seizures; although this is rare.

Patient counseling

Advise the patient's family to observe and record his seizure activity to ensure proper treatment. Emphasize the importance of strict compliance with the drug regimen, and warn the patient about adverse reactions. Stress the importance of regular follow-up appointments for blood studies.

Seizures, simple partial

Resulting from an irritable focus in the cerebral cortex, simple partial seizures typically last about 30 seconds and don't alter the patient's level of consciousness (LOC). The type and pattern reflect the location of the irritable focus. Simple partial seizures may be classified as motor (including both jacksonian seizures and epilepsia partialis continua) or somatosensory (including visual, olfactory, and auditory seizures).

A focal motor seizure is a series of unilateral clonic (muscle jerking) and tonic (muscle stiffening) movements of one part of the body. The patient's head and eyes characteristically turn away from the hemispheric focus—usually the frontal lobe near the motor strip. A tonic-clonic contraction of the trunk or extremities may follow.

A jacksonian motor seizure typically begins with a tonic contraction of a finger, the corner of the mouth, or one foot. Clonic movements follow, spreading to other muscles on the same side of the body, moving up the arm or leg, and eventually involving the whole side. Alternatively, clonic movements may spread to the opposite side, becoming generalized and leading to loss of consciousness. In the postictal phase, the patient may experience paralysis (Todd's paralysis) in the affected limbs, usually resolving within 24 hours.

Epilepsia partialis continua causes clonic twitching of one muscle group, usually in the face, arm, or leg. Twitching occurs every few seconds and persists for hours, days, or months without spreading. Spasms usually affect the distal arm and leg muscles more than the proximal ones; in the face, they affect the corner of the mouth, one or both eyelids and, occasionally, the neck or trunk muscles unilaterally.

A focal somatosensory seizure affects a localized body area on one side. Usually, this type of seizure initially causes numbness, tingling, or crawling or "electric" sensations; occasionally, it causes pain or burning sensations in the lips, fingers, or toes. A *visual seizure* involves sensations of darkness or of stationary or moving lights or spots, usually red at first, then blue, green, and yellow. It can affect both visual fields or the visual field on the side opposite the lesion. The irritable focus is in the occipital lobe. In contrast, the irritable focus in an *auditory* or *olfactory seizure* is in the temporal lobe. (See *Body functions affected by focal seizures*, page 624.)

History and physical examination

Be sure to record the patient's seizure activity in detail; your data may be critical in locating the lesion in the brain. Does the patient turn his head and eyes? If so, to what side? Where does movement first start? Does it spread? Because a partial seizure may become generalized, you'll need to watch closely for loss of consciousness, bilateral tonicity and clonicity, cyanosis, tongue biting, and urinary incontinence. (See "Seizures, generalized tonic-clonic," page 619.)

After the seizure, ask the patient to describe exactly what he remembers, if anything, about the seizure. Check the patient's LOC, and test for residual deficits (such as weakness in the involved extremity) and sensory disturbances.

Then obtain a history. Ask the patient what happened before the seizure. Can he describe an aura or did he recognize its onset? If so, how—by a smell, a visual disturbance, or a sound or visceral phenomenon, such as an unusual sensation in his stomach? How does this seizure compare with others he has had?

Body functions affected by focal seizures

The site of the irritable focus determines which body functions are affected by a focal seizure, as shown in the illustration below.

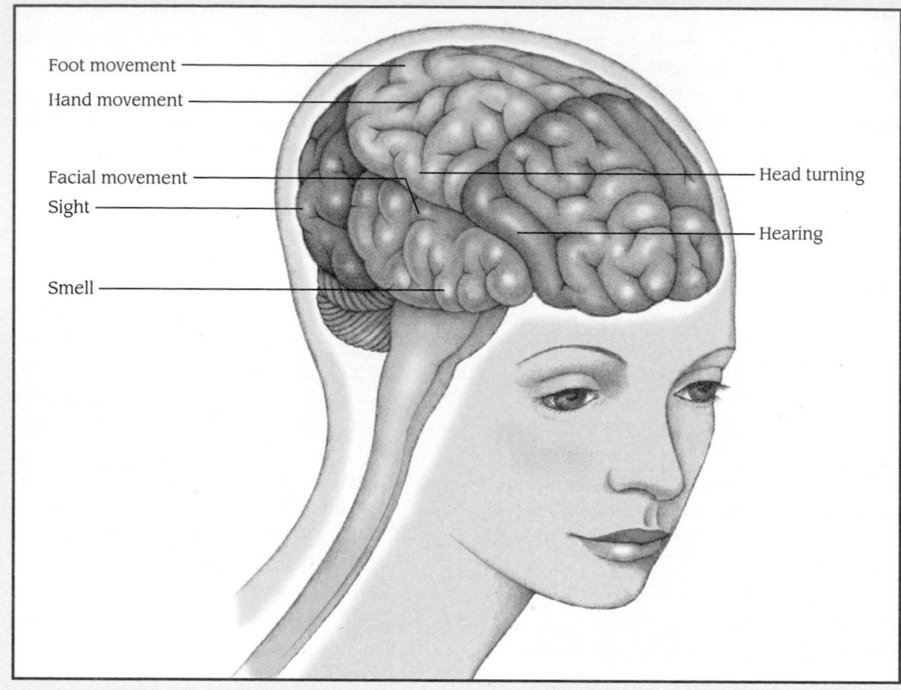

Explore fully any history, recent or remote, of head trauma. Check for a history of stroke or recent infection, especially with fever, headache, or a stiff neck.

Medical causes

◆ ***Brain abscess.*** Seizures can occur in the acute stage of abscess formation or after resolution of the abscess. Decreased LOC varies from drowsiness to deep stupor. Early signs and symptoms reflect increased intracranial pressure and include a constant, intractable headache, nausea, and vomiting. Later signs and symptoms include ocular disturbances, such as nystagmus, decreased visual acuity, and unequal pupils. Other findings vary according to the abscess site and may include aphasia, hemiparesis, and personality changes.

◆ ***Brain tumor.*** Focal seizures are commonly the earliest indicators of a brain tumor. The patient may report morning headache, dizziness, confusion, vision loss, and motor and sensory disturbances. He may also develop aphasia, generalized seizures, ataxia, decreased LOC, papilledema, vomiting, increased systolic blood pressure, and widening pulse pressure. Eventually, he may assume a decorticate posture.

◆ ***Head trauma.*** Any head injury can cause seizures, but penetrating wounds are characteristically associated with focal seizures. The seizures usually begin 3 to 15 months after injury, decrease in frequency after several years, and eventually stop. The patient may develop generalized seizures and a decreased LOC that may progress to coma.

◆ ***Multiple sclerosis.*** Focal or generalized seizures may occur with this disorder, usually during the late stages. Other findings include visual deficits, paresthesia, constipation, muscle weakness, spasticity, paralysis, hyperreflexia, intention tremor, gait ataxia, dysphagia, dysarthria, emotional lability, impotence, and urinary frequency, urgency, and incontinence.

◆ ***Neurofibromatosis.*** Multiple brain lesions cause focal seizures and, at times, generalized seizures. Inspection reveals café-au-lait spots, multiple skin tumors, scoliosis, and kyphoscoliosis. Related findings include dizziness, ataxia, progressive monocular blindness, nystagmus, and endocrine abnormalities.

◆ ***Sarcoidosis.*** Multiple lesions from this disorder affect the brain, producing focal and generalized seizures. Associated findings include a nonproductive cough with dyspnea, substernal pain, malaise, fatigue, arthralgia, myalgia, weight loss, tachypnea, dysphagia, skin lesions, and impaired vision.

◆ ***Stroke.*** A major cause of seizures in patients older than age 50, a stroke may induce focal seizures up to 6 months after its onset. Related effects depend on the type and extent of the stroke but may include decreased LOC, contralateral hemiplegia, dysarthria, dysphagia, ataxia, unilateral sensory loss, apraxia, agnosia, and aphasia. A stroke may also cause visual deficits, memory loss, poor judgment, personality changes, emotional lability, headache, urinary incontinence or retention, and vomiting. It may result in generalized seizures.

Special considerations

No emergency care is necessary during a focal seizure, unless it progresses to a generalized seizure. (See "Seizures, generalized tonic-clonic," page 619.) However, to ensure patient safety you should remain with the patient during the seizure, and reassure him.

Prepare the patient for such diagnostic tests as a computed tomography scan and EEG.

Pediatric pointers

Affecting more children than adults, focal seizures are likely to spread and become generalized. They typically cause the child's eyes, or his head and eyes, to turn to the side; in neonates, they cause mouth twitching, staring, or both.

Focal seizures in children can result from hemiplegic cerebral palsy, head trauma, child abuse, arteriovenous malformation, or Sturge-Weber syndrome. About 25% of febrile seizures present as focal seizures.

Patient counseling

After the seizure, instruct the patient to record his seizures. Also, emphasize the importance of complying with the prescribed drug regimen and maintaining a safe environment.

Setting-sun sign

[Sunset eyes]

Setting-sun sign refers to the downward deviation of an infant's or young child's eyes as a result of pressure on cranial nerves III, IV, and VI. With this late and ominous sign of increased intracranial pressure (ICP), both eyes are rotated downward, typically revealing an area of sclera above the irises; occasionally, the irises appear to be forced outward. Pupils are sluggish, responding to light unequally.

The infant with increased ICP is typically irritable and lethargic, and feeds poorly. Changes in level of consciousness (LOC), lower-extremity spasticity, and opisthotonos may also be obvious. Increased ICP typically results from space-occupying lesions—such as tumors—or from an accumulation of fluid in the brain's ventricular system, as occurs with hydrocephalus. It also results from intracranial bleeding or cerebral edema. Other signs include a globular appearance of the head (light bulb sign), a loss of upgaze, and distended scalp veins.

Setting-sun sign may be intermittent—for example, it may disappear when the infant is upright because this position slightly reduces ICP. The sign may be elicited in a normal infant younger than age 4 weeks by suddenly changing his head position, and in a normal infant up to age 9 months by shining a bright light into his eyes and removing it quickly.

History and physical examination

If you observe the setting-sun sign in an infant, evaluate his neurologic status; then obtain a brief history from his parents. Has the infant experienced a fall or even a minor trauma? When did this sign appear? Ask about early nonspecific signs of increasing ICP: Has the infant's sucking reflex diminished? Is he irritable, restless, or unusually tired? Does he cry when moved? Is his cry high pitched? Has he vomited recently?

Next, perform a physical examination, keeping in mind that neurologic responses are primarily reflexive during early infancy. Assess the infant's LOC. Is he awake, irritable, or lethargic? Keeping in mind his age and level of development, try to determine his ability to reach for a bright object or turn toward the sound of a music box. Observe his posture for normal flexion and extension or opisthotonos. Examine muscle tone, and observe for seizure automatisms.

Examine the infant's anterior fontanel for bulging, measure his head circumference and compare it with previous results, and observe his breathing pattern. (Cheyne-Stokes respirations may accompany increased ICP.) Check his pupillary response to light: Unilateral or bilateral dilation occurs as ICP rises. Finally, elicit reflexes that are diminished in increased ICP, especially Moro's reflex. Keep endotracheal intubation equipment available.

Medical causes

◆ ***Increased ICP.*** Transient or intermittent setting-sun sign often occurs late in patients with increased ICP. The infant may have bulging, widened fontanels, increased head circumference, and widened sutures. He may also exhibit a decreased level of consciousness, behavioral changes, a high-pitched cry, pupillary abnormalities, and impaired motor movement as ICP increases. Other findings include increased systolic pressure, widened pulse pressure, bradycardia, changes in breathing pattern, vomiting, and seizures as ICP increases.

Special considerations

Care of the infant with setting-sun sign includes monitoring of vital signs and neurologic status. Elevate the head of the crib to at least 30 degrees, and monitor intake and output. Monitor ICP, restrict fluids, and insert an I.V. catheter to administer a diuretic. For severely increased ICP, endotracheal intubation and mechanical hyperventilation may be required to reduce serum carbon dioxide levels and constrict cerebral vessels. Therapy to induce a barbiturate coma or hypothermia therapy may be required to lower the metabolic rate.

Try to maintain a calm environment and, when the infant cries, offer comfort to help prevent stress-related ICP elevations. Perform nursing duties judiciously because procedures may further increase ICP. Prepare the child and family for surgical management of increased ICP and hydrocephalus as appropriate. Encourage the parents' help, and offer them emotional support.

Skin, bronze

The result of excessive circulating melanin, a bronze skin tone tends to appear at pressure points—such as the knuckles, elbows, toes, and knees—and in creases on the palms and soles. Eventually, this hyperpigmentation may extend to the buccal mucosa and gums before covering the entire body. Because bronzing develops gradually, it's sometimes mistaken for a suntan. However, the hyperpigmentation can affect the entire body, not just sun-exposed areas: Sun exposure deepens the bronze color of exposed areas, but this effect fades. In fair-skinned patients, the bronze tone can range from light to dark. The tone also varies with the disorder.

History and physical examination

Begin by asking the patient when the hyperpigmentation first appeared. Has its hue changed? When was he last exposed to the sun or artificial tanning source? Also, ask about a history of infection, illness, surgery, or trauma. Does he have abdominal pain, weakness, fatigue, diarrhea, or constipation? Has he recently lost weight? If the patient is receiving maintenance therapy for adrenal insufficiency, has his dosage been increased?

Examine the mucosa, gums, and scars for hyperpigmentation. Check for signs of dehydration and for abdominal distention, loss of body hair, and tissue and muscle wasting. Palpate for hepatosplenomegaly.

Medical causes

◆ ***Adrenal hyperplasia.*** The skin assumes a dark bronze tone within a few months. Other findings include visual field deficits and headache (from an expanding pituitary lesion), and signs of masculinization in females.

◆ ***Biliary cirrhosis.*** This disorder causes bronze skin from melanosis of exposed areas of jaundiced skin: eyelids, palms, neck, and chest or back. The patient may also experience generalized pruritus, weakness, fatigue, jaundice, dark urine, pale stools with steatorrhea, decreased appetite with weight loss, and hepatomegaly.

◆ ***Chronic renal failure.*** The skin becomes pallid, yellowish bronze, dry, and scaly. Other findings include ammonia breath odor, oliguria, fatigue, decreased mental acuity, seizures, muscle cramps, peripheral neuropathy, bleeding tendencies, pruritus and, occasionally, uremic frost and hypertension.

◆ ***Hemochromatosis.*** An early sign is progressive, generalized bronzing accentuated by metallic gray-bronze skin on sun-exposed areas, genitalia, and scars. Mucous membranes are affected less often. Early associated effects include weakness, lethargy, weight loss, abdominal pain, loss of libido, polydipsia, and polyuria.

◆ ***Malnutrition.*** As weight loss depletes body nutrients, bronzing develops along with apathy, lethargy, anorexia, weakness, and slow pulse and respiratory rates. Patients may develop paresthesia in the extremities; dull, sparse, dry hair; brittle nails; dark, swollen cheeks; dry, flaky skin; red, swollen lips; muscle wasting; and gonadal atrophy in males.

◆ ***Primary adrenal insufficiency.*** Bronze skin is a classic sign. Other findings include axillary and pubic hair loss, vitiligo, progressive fatigue, weakness, anorexia, nausea and vomiting, weight loss, orthostatic hypotension, weak and irregular pulse, abdominal pain, irritability, diarrhea or constipation, amenorrhea, and syncope.

◆ ***Wilson's disease.*** Kayser-Fleischer rings—rusty brown rings of pigment around the corneas—characterize this disease, which may cause skin bronzing. Other effects include incoordination, dysarthria, chorea, ataxia, muscle spasms and rigidity, abdominal distress, fatigue, personality changes, hypotension, syncope, and seizures.

OTHER CAUSES

◆ ***Drugs.*** Prolonged therapy with high doses of a phenothiazine may cause gradual bronzing of the skin.

SPECIAL CONSIDERATIONS

Prepare the patient for the adrenocorticotropic stimulation test, thyroid function studies, complete blood count, electrolyte analysis, electrocardiography, and a computed tomography scan of the pituitary gland.

PEDIATRIC POINTERS

Celiac disease can cause bronze skin in young children. Bronzing begins with the introduction of cereals and usually subsides later in childhood or adolescence. It also stems from adrenoleukodystrophy, a rare but life-threatening X-linked recessive disorder that affects boys and young men.

Skin, clammy

Clammy skin—moist, cool, and usually pale—is a sympathetic response to stress, which triggers release of the hormones epinephrine and norepinephrine. These hormones cause cutaneous vasoconstriction and secretion of cold sweat from eccrine glands, particularly on the palms, forehead, and soles.

Clammy skin typically accompanies shock, acute hypoglycemia, anxiety reactions, arrhythmias, and heat exhaustion. It also occurs as a vasovagal reaction to severe pain associated with nausea, anorexia, epigastric distress, hyperpnea, tachypnea, weakness, confusion, tachycardia, and pupillary dilation or a combination of these findings. Marked bradycardia and syncope may follow.

HISTORY AND PHYSICAL EXAMINATION

If you detect clammy skin, remember that rapid evaluation and intervention are paramount. (See *Clammy skin: A key finding*, page 628) Ask the patient if he has a history of type 1 diabetes mellitus or a cardiac disorder. Is the patient taking any medications, especially an antiarrhythmic? Is he experiencing pain, chest pressure, nausea, or epigastric distress? Does he feel weak? Does he have a dry mouth? Does he have diarrhea or increased urination?

Next, examine the pupils for dilation. Check for abdominal distention and increased muscle tension.

MEDICAL CAUSES

◆ ***Anxiety.*** An acute anxiety attack commonly produces cold, clammy skin on the forehead, palms, and soles. Other features include pallor, dry mouth, tachycardia or bradycardia, palpitations, and hypertension or hypotension. The patient may also develop tremors, breathlessness, headache, muscle tension, nausea, vomiting, abdominal distention, diarrhea, increased urination, and sharp chest pain.

◆ ***Arrhythmias.*** Cardiac arrhythmias may produce generalized cool, clammy skin along with mental status changes, dizziness, and hypotension.

◆ ***Cardiogenic shock.*** Generalized cool, moist, pale skin accompanies confusion, restlessness, hypotension, tachycardia, tachypnea, narrowing pulse pressure, cyanosis, and oliguria.

◆ ***Heat exhaustion.*** In the acute stage of heat exhaustion, generalized cold, clammy skin accompanies an ashen appearance, headache, confusion, syncope, giddiness and, possibly, a subnormal temperature, with mild heat exhaustion. The patient may exhibit a rapid and thready pulse, nausea, vomiting, tachypnea, oliguria, thirst, muscle cramps, and hypotension.

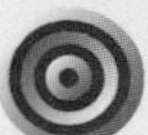

EMERGENCY INTERVENTION

Clammy skin: A key finding

Be alert for clammy skin. Why? Because it commonly accompanies emergency conditions, such as shock, acute hypoglycemia, and arrhythmias. To know what to do, review these typical clinical situations.

You detect clammy skin in a patient who appears anxious and restless.

Quickly take his vital signs, noting tachypnea, hypotension, and a weak, irregular pulse. If present:

Suspect *shock*.

Place the patient in a supine position in bed. Elevate his legs 20 to 30 degrees to promote perfusion to vital organs.

Insert an I.V. catheter for administration of drugs, fluids, or blood. Give supplemental oxygen and begin cardiac monitoring.

You detect clammy skin and possible tremors in a patient who appears irritable, anxious, confused, and possibly difficult to arouse and reports persistent hunger.

Quickly take his vital signs, which will typically be normal. A vagal reaction to the stress of hypoglycemia may cause hypotension and tachycardia.

Suspect *acute hypoglycemia*.

Immediately draw blood for glucose studies, and test a drop with a glucose reagent strip. Insert an I.V. catheter, and give a 50-ml bolus of dextrose 50%. Begin cardiac monitoring.

You detect clammy skin in a patient with changes in mental status such as confusion.

Quickly take his vital signs, noting hypotension and changes in pulse rate and rhythm. If present:

Suspect an *arrhythmia*.

Insert an I.V. catheter and administer an antiarrhythmic. Give supplemental oxygen and begin cardiac monitoring.

◆ ***Hypoglycemia (acute).*** Generalized cool, clammy skin or diaphoresis may accompany irritability, tremors, palpitations, hunger, headache, tachycardia, and anxiety. Central nervous system disturbances include blurred vision, diplopia, confusion, motor weakness, hemiplegia, and coma. These signs and symptoms typically resolve after the patient is given glucose.

◆ ***Hypovolemic shock.*** With this common form of shock, generalized pale, cold, clammy skin accompanies subnormal body temperature, hypotension with narrowing pulse pressure, tachycardia, tachypnea, and rapid, thready pulse. Other findings are flat neck veins, increased capillary refill time, decreased urine output, confusion, and decreased level of consciousness.

◆ ***Septic shock.*** The cold shock stage causes generalized cold, clammy skin. Associated findings include rapid and thready pulse, severe hypotension, persistent oliguria or anuria, and respiratory failure.

Special considerations

Take the patient's vital signs frequently, and monitor urine output. If clammy skin occurs with an anxiety reaction or pain, offer the patient emotional support, administer pain medication, and provide a quiet environment.

Pediatric pointers

Infants in shock don't have clammy skin because of their immature sweat glands.

GERIATRIC POINTERS

Elderly patients develop clammy skin easily because of decreased tissue perfusion. Always consider bowel ischemia in the differential diagnosis of older patients who present with cool, clammy skin—especially if abdominal pain or bloody stools occur.

Skin, mottled

Mottled skin is patchy discoloration indicating primary or secondary changes of the deep, middle, or superficial dermal blood vessels. It can result from a hematologic, immune, or connective tissue disorder; chronic occlusive arterial disease; dysproteinemia; immobility; exposure to heat or cold; or shock. Mottled skin can be a normal reaction, such as the diffuse mottling that occurs when exposure to cold causes venous stasis in cutaneous blood vessels (cutis marmorata).

Mottling that occurs with other signs and symptoms usually affects the extremities, typically indicating restricted blood flow. For example, livedo reticularis, a characteristic network pattern of reddish blue discoloration, occurs when vasospasm of the middermal blood vessels slows local blood flow in dilated superficial capillaries and small veins. Shock causes mottling from systemic vasoconstriction.

HISTORY AND PHYSICAL EXAMINATION

Mottled skin may indicate an emergency condition requiring rapid evaluation and intervention. (See *Mottled skin: Knowing what to do*, page 630) However, if the patient isn't in distress, obtain a history. Ask if the mottling began suddenly or gradually. What precipitated it? How long has he had it? Does anything make it go away? Does the patient have other symptoms, such as pain, numbness, or tingling in an extremity? If so, do they disappear with temperature changes?

Observe the patient's skin color, and palpate his arms and legs for skin texture, swelling, and temperature differences between extremities. Check capillary refill. Palpate for the presence (or absence) of pulses and for their quality. Note breaks in the skin, muscle appearance, and hair distribution. Assess motor and sensory function.

MEDICAL CAUSES

◆ ***Acrocyanosis.*** With this rare disorder, anxiety or exposure to cold can cause vasospasm in small cutaneous arterioles. This results in persistent symmetrical blue and red mottling of the affected hands, feet, and nose.

◆ ***Arterial occlusion (acute).*** Initial signs include temperature and color changes. Pallor may change to blotchy cyanosis and livedo reticularis. Color and temperature demarcation develop at the level of obstruction. Other effects include sudden onset of pain in the extremity and possibly paresthesia, paresis, and a sensation of cold in the affected area. Examination reveals diminished or absent pulses, cool extremities, increased capillary refill time, pallor, and diminished reflexes.

◆ ***Arteriosclerosis obliterans.*** Atherosclerotic buildup narrows intra-arterial lumina, resulting in reduced blood flow through the affected artery. Obstructed blood flow to the extremities (most commonly the lower) produces such peripheral signs and symptoms as leg pallor, cyanosis, blotchy erythema, and livedo reticularis. Related findings include intermittent claudication (most common symptom), diminished or absent pedal pulses, and leg coolness. Other symptoms include coldness and paresthesia.

◆ ***Buerger's disease.*** This form of vasculitis produces unilateral or asymmetrical color changes and mottling, particularly livedo networking in the lower extremities. It also typically causes intermittent claudication and erythema along extremity blood vessels. During exposure to cold, the feet are cold, cyanotic, and numb; later they're hot, red, and tingling. Other findings include impaired peripheral pulses and peripheral neuropathy. Buerger's disease is typically exacerbated by smoking.

◆ ***Cryoglobulinemia.*** This necrotizing disorder causes patchy livedo reticularis, petechiae, and ecchymoses. Other findings include fever, chills, urticaria, melena, skin ulcers, epistaxis, Raynaud's phenomenon, eye hemorrhages, hematuria, and gangrene.

◆ ***Hypovolemic shock.*** Vasoconstriction from shock commonly produces skin mottling, initially in the knees and elbows. As shock worsens, mottling becomes generalized. Early signs include sudden onset of pallor, cool skin, restlessness, thirst, tachypnea, and slight tachycardia. As shock progresses, associated findings include cool, clammy skin; rapid, thready pulse; hypotension; narrowed pulse pressure; decreased urine output; subnormal temperature; confusion; and decreased level of consciousness.

◆ ***Livedo reticularis (idiopathic or primary).*** Symmetrical, diffuse mottling can involve the hands, feet, arms, legs, buttocks, and trunk.

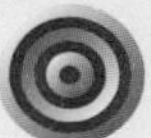

EMERGENCY INTERVENTION

Mottled skin: Knowing what to do

If your patient's skin is pale, cool, clammy, and mottled at the elbows and knees or all over, he may be developing *hypovolemic shock.* Quickly take his vital signs, and be sure to note tachycardia or a weak, thready pulse. Observe the neck for flattened veins. Does the patient appear anxious? If you detect these signs and symptoms, place the patient in a supine position in bed with his legs elevated 20 to 30 degrees. Administer oxygen by nasal cannula or face mask, and begin cardiac monitoring. Insert a large-bore I.V. catheter for rapid fluid or blood product administration, and prepare to insert a central venous access device or a pulmonary artery catheter. Prepare to insert an indwelling urinary catheter to monitor urine output.

Localized mottling in a pale, cool extremity that the patient says feels painful, numb, and tingling may signal acute arterial occlusion. Immediately check the patient's distal pulses: If they're absent or diminished, you'll need to insert an I.V. catheter in an unaffected extremity, and prepare the patient for arteriography or immediate surgery.

Initially, networking is intermittent and most pronounced on exposure to cold or stress; eventually, mottling persists even with warming.

◆ ***Periarteritis nodosa.*** Skin findings include asymmetrical, patchy livedo reticularis, palpable nodules along the path of medium-sized arteries, erythema, purpura, muscle wasting, ulcers, gangrene, peripheral neuropathy, fever, weight loss, and malaise.

◆ ***Polycythemia vera.*** This hematologic disorder produces livedo reticularis, hemangiomas, purpura, rubor, ulcerative nodules, and scleroderma-like lesions. Other symptoms include headache, a vague feeling of fullness in the head, dizziness, vertigo, vision disturbances, dyspnea, and aquagenic pruritus.

◆ ***Rheumatoid arthritis.*** This disorder may cause skin mottling. Early nonspecific signs and symptoms progress to joint pain and stiffness with subcutaneous nodules, usually on the elbows.

◆ ***Systemic lupus erythematosus.*** This connective tissue disorder can cause livedo reticularis, most commonly on the outer arms. Other signs and symptoms include a butterfly rash, nondeforming joint pain and stiffness, photosensitivity, Raynaud's phenomenon, patchy alopecia, seizures, fever, anorexia, weight loss, lymphadenopathy, and emotional lability.

OTHER CAUSES

◆ ***Immobility.*** Prolonged immobility may cause bluish mottling, most noticeably in dependent extremities.

◆ ***Thermal exposure.*** Prolonged thermal exposure, as from a heating pad or hot water bottle, may cause erythema Ab Igne—a localized, reticulated, brown-to-red mottling.

SPECIAL CONSIDERATIONS

Mottled skin typically results from a chronic condition. Teach patients to avoid tight clothing and overexposure to cold or to heating devices, such as hot water bottles and heating pads.

PEDIATRIC POINTERS

A common cause of mottled skin in children is systemic vasoconstriction from shock. Other causes are the same as those for adults.

GERIATRIC POINTERS

In elderly patients, decreased tissue perfusion can easily cause mottled skin. Besides arterial occlusion and polycythemia vera, conditions that commonly affect patients in this age-group, bowel ischemia is common in elderly patients who present with livedo reticularis, especially if they also have abdominal pain or bloody stools.

PATIENT COUNSELING

If the patient has a chronic condition, such as systemic lupus erythematosus, periarteritis nodosa, or cryoglobulinemia, advise him to watch for mottled skin because it may indicate a flare-up of his disorder.

Skin, scaly

Scaly skin results when cells of the uppermost skin layer (stratum corneum) desiccate and shed, causing excessive accumulation of loosely adherent flakes of normal or abnormal keratin. Normally, skin cell loss is imperceptible; the appearance of scale indicates increased cell proliferation secondary to altered keratinization.

Scaly skin varies in texture from fine and delicate to branlike, coarse, or stratified. Scales are typically dry, brittle, and shiny, but they can be greasy and dull. Their color ranges from whitish gray, yellow, or brown to a silvery sheen.

Usually benign, scaly skin occurs with fungal, bacterial, and viral infections (cutaneous or systemic), lymphomas, and lupus erythematosus; it's also common in those with inflammatory skin disease. A form of scaly skin—generalized fine desquamation—commonly follows prolonged febrile illness, sunburn, and thermal burns. Red patches of scaly skin that appear or worsen in winter may result from dry skin (or from actinic keratosis, common in elderly patients). Certain drugs also cause scaly skin. Aggravating factors include cold, heat, immobility, and frequent bathing.

History and physical examination

Begin the history by asking how long the patient has had scaly skin and whether he has had it before. Where did it first appear? Did a lesion or skin eruption, such as erythema, precede it? Has the patient used a new or different topical skin product recently? How often does he bathe? Has he had recent joint pain, illness, or malaise? Ask the patient about work exposure to chemicals, use of prescribed drugs, and a family history of skin disorders. Find out what kinds of soap, cosmetics, skin lotion, and hair preparations he uses.

Next, examine the entire skin surface. Is it dry, oily, moist, or greasy? Observe the general pattern of skin lesions, and record their location. Note their color, shape, and size. Are they thick or fine? Do they itch? Does the patient have other lesions besides scaly skin? Examine the mucous membranes of his mouth, lips, and nose, and inspect his ears, hair, and nails.

Medical causes

◆ ***Bowen's disease.*** This common form of intraepidermal carcinoma causes painless, erythematous plaques that are raised and indurated with a thick, hyperkeratotic scale and, possibly, ulcerated centers.

◆ ***Dermatitis.*** Exfoliative dermatitis begins with rapidly developing generalized erythema. Desquamation with fine scales or thick sheets of all or most of the skin surface may cause life-threatening hypothermia. Other possible complications include cardiac output failure and septicemia. Systemic signs and symptoms include low-grade fever, chills, malaise, lymphadenopathy, and gynecomastia.

With nummular dermatitis, round, pustular lesions commonly ooze purulent exudate, itch severely, and rapidly become encrusted and scaly. Lesions appear on the extensor surfaces of the limbs, posterior trunk, and buttocks.

Seborrheic dermatitis begins with erythematous, scaly papules that progress to larger, dry or moist, greasy scales with yellowish crusts. This disorder primarily involves the center of the face, the chest and scalp and, possibly, the genitalia, axillae, and perianal regions. Pruritus occurs with scaling.

◆ ***Dermatophytosis.*** Tinea capitis produces lesions with reddened, slightly elevated borders and a central area of dense scaling; these lesions may become inflamed and pus-filled (kerions). Patchy alopecia and itching may also occur. Tinea pedis causes scaling and blisters between the toes. The squamous type produces diffuse, fine, branlike scales. Adherent and silvery white, they're most prominent in skin creases and may affect the entire dorsum of the foot. Tinea corporis produces crusty lesions. As they enlarge, their centers heal, causing the classic ringworm shape.

◆ ***Discoid lupus erythematosus.*** This cutaneous form of lupus may occur without systemic signs and symptoms. Separate or coalescing lesions (macules, papules, or plaques), ranging from pink to purple, are covered with a yellow or brown crust. Enlarged hair follicles are filled with scales, and telangiectasia may be present. After this inflammatory stage, the lesions heal and hypopigmentation or hyperpigmentation and noncontractile scarring and atrophy may occur. Discoid lupus commonly involves the face or sun-exposed areas of the neck, ears, scalp, lips, and oral mucosa. Alopecia may also occur.

◆ ***Lichen planus.*** With this disorder, small, flat, violet lesions with a fine scale and gray lines on the surface usually affect the lumbar region, genitalia, wrists, ankles, and anterior lower legs.

◆ ***Lymphoma.*** Hodgkin's disease and non-Hodgkin's lymphoma commonly cause scaly rashes. Hodgkin's disease may cause pruritic scaling dermatitis that begins in the legs and spreads to the entire body. Remissions and recurrences are common. Small nodules and diffuse pigmentation are related signs. This disease typically produces painless enlargement of the peripheral lymph nodes. Other signs and symptoms include fever, fatigue, weight loss, malaise, and hepatosplenomegaly.

Non-Hodgkin's lymphoma initially produces erythematous patches with some scaling that later become interspersed with nodules. Pruritus and discomfort are common; later, tumors and ulcers form. Progression produces nontender lymphadenopathy.

◆ ***Parapsoriasis (chronic).*** This disorder produces small or moderate-sized maculopapular, erythematous eruption, with a thin, adherent scale on the trunk, hands, and feet. Removal of the scale reveals a shiny brown surface.

◆ ***Pityriasis.*** Pityriasis rosea, an acute, benign, and self-limiting disorder, produces widespread scales. It begins with an erythematous, raised, oval herald patch anywhere on the body. A few days or weeks later, yellow-tan or erythematous patches with scaly edges erupt on the trunk and limbs and sometimes on the face, hands, and feet. Pruritus also occurs.

Pityriasis rubra pilaris, an uncommon disorder, initially produces seborrheic scaling on the scalp, progressing to the face and ears. Later, scaly red patches develop on the palms and soles, becoming diffuse, thick, fissured, hyperkeratotic, and painful. Lesions also appear on the hands, fingers, wrists, and forearms and then on wide areas of the trunk, neck, and limbs.

◆ ***Psoriasis.*** Silvery white, micaceous scales cover erythematous plaques that have sharply defined borders. Psoriasis usually appears on the scalp, chest, elbows, knees, back, buttocks, and genitalia. Associated signs and symptoms include nail pitting, pruritus, arthritis, and sometimes pain from dry, cracked, encrusted lesions.

◆ ***Syphilis (secondary).*** Papulosquamous, slightly scaly eruptions characterize this disorder. A ring-shaped pattern of copper-red papules usually forms on the face, arms, palms, soles, chest, back, and abdomen. Annular papules may occur. Systemic findings include lymphadenopathy, malaise, weight loss, anorexia, nausea, vomiting, headache, sore throat, and low-grade fever.

◆ ***Systemic lupus erythematosus.*** This disorder produces a bright-red maculopapular eruption, sometimes with scaling. Patches are sharply defined and involve the nose and malar regions of the face in a butterfly pattern—a primary sign. Similar characteristic rashes appear on other body surfaces; scaling occurs along the lower lip or anterior hair line. Other primary signs and symptoms include photosensitivity and joint pain and stiffness. Vasculitis (leading to infarctive lesions, necrotic leg ulcers, or digital gangrene), Raynaud's phenomenon, patchy alopecia, and mucous membrane ulcers also can occur.

◆ ***Tinea versicolor.*** This benign fungal skin infection typically produces macular hypopigmented, fawn-colored, or brown patches of varying sizes and shapes. All are slightly scaly. Lesions commonly affect the upper trunk, arms, and lower abdomen, sometimes the neck and, rarely, the face.

Other causes

◆ ***Drugs.*** Many drugs—including penicillins, sulfonamides, barbiturates, quinidine, diazepam, phenytoin, and isoniazid—can produce scaling patches.

Special considerations

If scaling results from corticosteroid therapy, withhold the drug. Prepare the patient for such diagnostic tests as a Wood's light examination, skin scraping, and skin biopsy.

Pediatric pointers

In children, scaly skin may stem from infantile eczema, pityriasis rosea, epidermolytic hyperkeratosis, psoriasis, various forms of ichthyosis, atopic dermatitis, a viral infection (especially hepatitis B virus, which can cause Gianotti-Crosti syndrome), seborrhea capitis (cradle cap), or an acute transient dermatitis. Desquamation may follow a febrile illness.

Patient counseling

Teach the patient proper skin care, and suggest lubricating baths and emollients. Instruct him not to use hot water to bathe or shower.

Skin turgor, decreased

Skin turgor—the skin's elasticity—is determined by observing the time required for the skin to return to its normal position after being stretched or pinched. With decreased turgor, pinched skin "holds" for up to 30 seconds, then slowly returns to its normal contour. Skin turgor is commonly assessed over the hand, arm or sternum, areas normally free from wrinkles and wide variations in tissue thickness. (See *Evaluating skin turgor*.)

Decreased skin turgor results from dehydration, or volume depletion, which moves interstitial fluid into the vascular bed to maintain circulating blood volume, leading to slackness in the skin's dermal layer. It's a normal finding in elderly patients and in people who have lost weight rapidly; it also occurs with disorders affecting the GI, renal, endocrine, and other systems.

History and physical examination

If your examination reveals decreased skin turgor, ask the patient about food and fluid intake and fluid loss. Has he recently experienced prolonged fluid loss from vomiting, diarrhea, draining wounds, or increased urination? Has he recently had a fever with sweating? Is the patient taking a diuretic? If so, how often? Does he frequently use alcohol?

Next, take the patient's vital signs. Note if his systolic blood pressure is abnormally low (90 mm Hg or less) when he's in a supine position, if it drops 15 to 20 mm Hg or more when he stands, or if his pulse increases by 10 beats/minute when he sits or stands. If you detect these signs of orthostatic hypotension or resting tachycardia, start an I.V. catheter for fluids.

Evaluate the patient's level of consciousness for confusion, disorientation, and signs of profound dehydration. Inspect his oral mucosa, the furrows of his tongue (especially under the tongue), and his axillae for dryness. Check his neck veins for flatness and monitor his urine output.

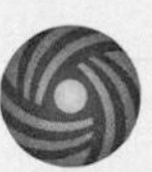

EXAMINATION TIP

Evaluating skin turgor

To evaluate skin turgor in an adult, pick up a fold of skin over the sternum or the arm, as shown at top. (In an infant, roll a fold of loosely adherent skin on the abdomen between your thumb and forefinger.) Then release it. Normal skin will immediately return to its previous contour. In decreased skin turgor, the skin fold will "hold," or "tent," as shown at bottom, for up to 30 seconds.

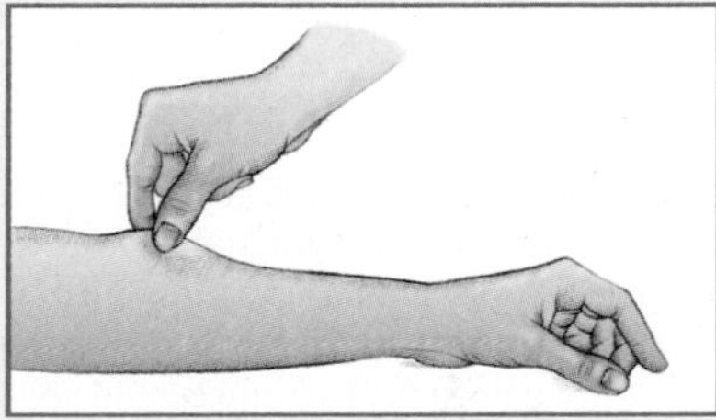

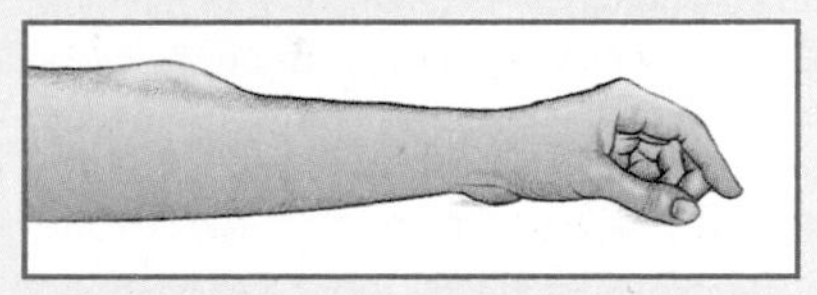

Medical causes

◆ ***Cholera.*** This infection is characterized by abrupt watery diarrhea and vomiting, which leads to severe water and electrolyte loss. These imbalances cause the following symptoms: decreased skin turgor, thirst, weakness, muscle cramps, oliguria, tachycardia, and hypotension. Without treatment, death can occur within hours.

◆ ***Dehydration.*** Decreased skin turgor commonly occurs with moderate to severe dehydration. Associated findings include dry oral mucosa, decreased perspiration, resting tachycardia, orthostatic hypotension, dry and furrowed tongue, increased thirst, weight loss, oliguria, fever, and fatigue. As dehydration worsens, other findings include enophthalmos, lethargy, weakness, confusion, delirium or obtundation, anuria, and shock. Hypotension persists even when the patient lies down.

Special considerations

Even a small deficit in body fluid may be critical in patients with diminished total body fluid—young children, elderly people, the obese, and people who have rapidly lost a large amount of weight.

To prevent skin breakdown in a dehydrated patient with poor skin turgor, decreased level of consciousness, and impaired peripheral circulation, turn the patient every 2 hours, and frequently massage his back and pressure points. Monitor his intake and output, administer I.V. fluid replacement, and frequently offer oral fluids. Weigh the patient daily at the same time on the same scale. Be alert for urine output that falls below 30 ml/hour and for continued weight loss. Closely monitor the patient for signs of electrolyte imbalance.

Pediatric pointers

Diarrhea secondary to gastroenteritis is the most common cause of dehydration in children, especially up to age 2.

Geriatric pointers

Because it's a natural part of the aging process, decreased skin turgor may be an unreliable physical finding in elderly patients. Other signs of volume depletion—such as dry oral mucosa, dry axillae, decreased urine output, or hypotension—must be carefully evaluated.

Patient counseling

Advise patients who experience fluid loss (for example, from vomiting or diarrhea) to drink enough fluids to replace their losses. Tell them to drink at least one glass of water (or, preferably, a beverage with higher electrolyte content such as a sports drink) after each loose bowel movement or episode of vomiting, to avoid dehydration. If the patient can't keep fluids down because of persistent vomiting, he may need an antiemetic or I.V. fluid replacement.

Spider angioma

[Arterial spider, spider nevus, spider telangiectasia, stellate angioma, vascular spider]

A spider angioma is a fiery red vascular lesion with an elevated central body, branching spiderlike legs, and a surrounding flush. A form of telangiectasia, this characteristic lesion ranges from a few millimeters to several centimeters in diameter and may occur singly or in multiples. Spider angiomas usually appear on the face and neck; less commonly, they occur on the shoulders, thorax, arms, backs of the hands and fingers, and mucous membranes of the lips and nose. They rarely appear below the waist or on the lips, ears, nail beds, or palms. (See *Recognizing a spider angioma*.)

In most cases, spider angiomas are associated with cirrhosis but are also found in hyperestrogenic states such as pregnancy or in those taking hormonal contraceptives. They may erupt in the second or third month of pregnancy, enlarge and multiply, then disappear about 6 weeks after delivery. Occasionally, a few lesions may persist. These lesions may also appear in elderly patients—but they're smaller and fewer in number (nine or fewer). They may persist indefinitely or spontaneously disappear.

History and physical examination

Begin your examination by asking the patient how long he has had the spider angiomas and where they're located. Then carefully examine him yourself, noting the size and location of the angiomas. On palpation, the angiomas may be slightly warmer than the surrounding skin and may have a pulsating central body. Also, check for other skin abnormalities, such as jaundice, dryness, and palmar erythema.

Recognizing a spider angioma

A hallmark sign of cirrhosis, spider angiomas are red vascular lesions with a raised central body and branching spiderlike legs.

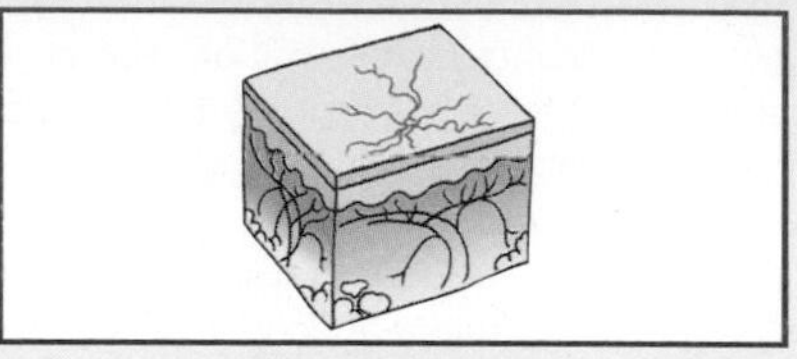

Medical causes

◆ ***Cirrhosis.*** Multiple spider angiomas are a hallmark of cirrhosis. They're typically a late sign, enlarging and multiplying as the disorder progresses. Associated signs and symptoms are widespread, varying with the degree of hepatic insufficiency and related portal hypertension. Splenomegaly and hematemesis, for example, point to portal hypertension.

Other skin effects include severe pruritus and dryness, palmar erythema, and decreased tissue turgor. Cardinal hepatic effects include jaundice, hepatomegaly, ascites, and leg edema. Right-upper-quadrant pain that worsens when the patient sits up or leans forward is common. The patient may also display key signs of hepatic encephalopathy, such as slurred speech, asterixis, fetor hepaticus, and decreased level of consciousness that progresses to coma. The male patient may develop testicular atrophy, gynecomastia, and loss of chest and axillary hair; the female patient may have menstrual irregularities.

Special considerations

Treatment isn't indicated for spider angiomas during pregnancy. However, cautery, electrodesiccation, or freezing may be used to treat them in the patient with cirrhosis.

Pediatric pointers

Occasionally, spider angiomas occur in normal children. Typically, they're small and few, appearing on the backs of the hands and forearms.

Geriatric pointers

Although spider angiomas may appear normally in elderly persons, they're usually associated with liver disorders.

PATIENT COUNSELING

Advise the patient that spider angiomas may recur and that vigorous electrodesiccation may cause pitting edema.

Splenomegaly

Because it occurs with various disorders and in up to 5% of normal adults, splenomegaly—an enlarged spleen—isn't a diagnostic sign by itself. Usually, however, it points to infection, trauma, or a hepatic, autoimmune, neoplastic, or hematologic disorder.

Because the spleen functions as the body's largest lymph node, splenomegaly can result from any process that triggers lymphadenopathy. For example, it may reflect reactive hyperplasia (a response to infection or inflammation), proliferation or infiltration of neoplastic cells, extramedullary hemopoiesis, phagocytic cell proliferation, increased blood cell destruction, or vascular congestion associated with portal hypertension.

Splenomegaly may be detected by light palpation under the left costal margin. (See *How to palpate for splenomegaly*, page 636.) However, because this technique isn't always advisable or effective, splenomegaly may need to be confirmed by a computed tomography or radionuclide scan.

EMERGENCY INTERVENTIONS *If the patient has a history of abdominal or thoracic trauma, don't palpate the abdomen because this may aggravate internal bleeding. Instead, examine the patient for left-upper-quadrant pain and signs of shock, such as tachycardia and tachypnea. If you detect these signs, suspect splenic rupture. Insert an I.V. catheter for emergency fluid and blood replacement, and administer oxygen. Catheterize the patient to evaluate urine output, and begin cardiac monitoring. Prepare the patient for possible surgery.*

HISTORY AND PHYSICAL EXAMINATION

If you detect splenomegaly during a routine physical examination, begin by exploring associated signs and symptoms. Ask the patient if he has been unusually tired lately. Does he frequently have colds, sore throats, or other infections? Does he bruise easily? Ask about left-upper-quadrant pain, abdominal fullness, and early satiety. Finally, examine the patient's skin for pallor and ecchymoses, and palpate his axillae, groin, and neck for lymphadenopathy.

MEDICAL CAUSES

◆ ***Amyloidosis.*** Marked splenomegaly may occur with this disorder from excessive protein deposits in the spleen. Associated signs and symptoms vary, depending on which other organs are involved. The patient may display signs of renal failure, such as oliguria and anuria, and signs of heart failure, such as dyspnea, crackles, and tachycardia. GI effects may include constipation or diarrhea and a stiff, enlarged tongue, resulting in dysarthria.

◆ ***Brucellosis.*** With severe cases of this rare infection, splenomegaly is a major sign. Typically, brucellosis begins insidiously with fatigue, headache, backache, anorexia, arthralgia, fever, chills, sweating, and malaise. Later, it may cause hepatomegaly, lymphadenopathy, weight loss, and vertebral or peripheral nerve pain on pressure.

◆ ***Cirrhosis.*** About one-third of patients with advanced cirrhosis develop moderate to marked splenomegaly. Among other late findings are jaundice, hepatomegaly, leg edema, hematemesis, and ascites. Signs of hepatic encephalopathy—such as asterixis, fetor hepaticus, slurred speech, and decreased level of consciousness that may progress to coma—are also common. Besides jaundice, skin effects may include severe pruritus, poor tissue turgor, spider angiomas, palmar erythema, pallor, and signs of bleeding tendencies. Endocrine effects may include menstrual irregularities or testicular atrophy, gynecomastia, and loss of chest and axillary hair. The patient may also develop fever and right-upper-abdominal pain that's aggravated by sitting up or leaning forward.

◆ ***Endocarditis (subacute infective).*** This infection usually causes an enlarged, but nontender, spleen. Its classic sign, however, is a suddenly changing murmur or the discovery of a new murmur in the presence of fever. Other features include anorexia, pallor, weakness, fever, night sweats, fatigue, tachycardia, weight loss, arthralgia, petechiae, hematuria and, in chronic cases, clubbing. If embolization occurs, the patient may develop chest, abdominal, or limb pain; paralysis; hematuria; and blindness. Endocarditis may produce Osler's nodes (tender, raised, subcutaneous lesions on the fingers or toes), Roth's spots (hemorrhagic areas with white centers on the retina), and Janeway lesions (purplish macules on the palms or soles).

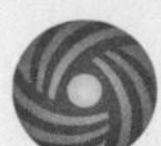

EXAMINATION TIP

How to palpate for splenomegaly

Detecting splenomegaly requires skillful and gentle palpation to avoid rupturing the enlarged spleen. Follow these steps carefully:

◆ Place the patient in the supine position and stand at his right side. Place your left hand under the left costovertebral angle and push lightly to move the spleen forward. Then press your right hand gently under the left front costal margin.

◆ Have the patient take a deep breath and then exhale. As he exhales, move your right hand along the tissue contours under the border of the ribs, feeling for the spleen's edge. The enlarged spleen should feel like a firm mass that bumps against your fingers. Remember to begin palpation low enough in the abdomen to catch the edge of a massive spleen.

◆ Grade the splenomegaly as slight (½″ to 1½″ [1 to 4 cm] below the costal margin), moderate (1½″ to 3″ [4 to 8 cm] below the costal margin), or great (greater than or equal to 3″ [8 cm] below the costal margin).

◆ Reposition the patient on his right side with his hips and knees flexed slightly to move the spleen forward. Then repeat the palpation procedure.

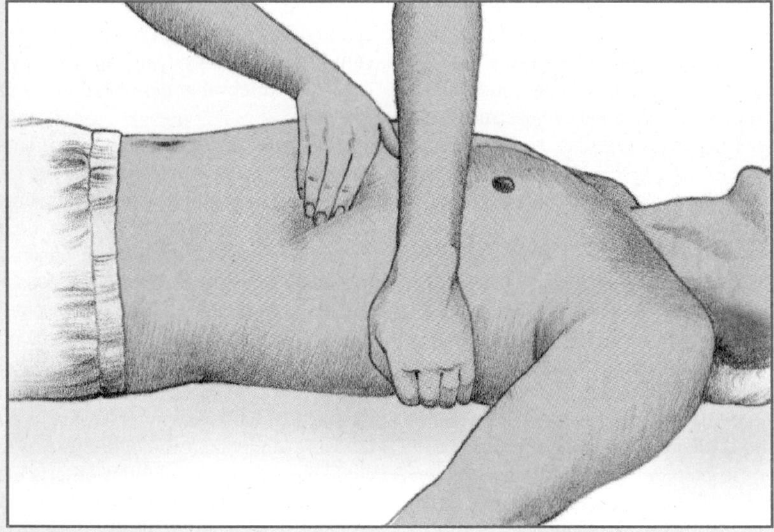

◆ ***Felty's syndrome.*** Splenomegaly is characteristic in this syndrome that occurs with chronic rheumatoid arthritis. Associated findings are joint pain and deformity, sensory or motor loss, rheumatoid nodules, palmar erythema, lymphadenopathy, and leg ulcers.

◆ ***Hepatitis.*** Splenomegaly may occur with this disorder. More characteristic findings include hepatomegaly, vomiting, jaundice, and fatigue.

◆ ***Histoplasmosis.*** Acute disseminated histoplasmosis commonly produces splenomegaly and hepatomegaly. It may also cause lymphadenopathy, jaundice, fever, anorexia, emaciation, and signs and symptoms of anemia, such as weakness, fatigue, pallor, and malaise. Occasionally, the patient's tongue, palate, epiglottis, and larynx become ulcerated, resulting in pain, hoarseness, and dysphagia.

◆ ***Hypersplenism (primary).*** With this syndrome, splenomegaly accompanies signs of pancytopenia—anemia, neutropenia, or thrombocytopenia. If the patient has anemia, findings may include weakness, fatigue, malaise, and pallor. If he has severe neutropenia, frequent bacterial infections are likely. If he has severe thrombocytopenia, easy bruising or spontaneous, widespread hemorrhage may occur. The patient also experiences left-sided abdominal pain, and a feeling of fullness after eating a small amount of food.

◆ ***Leukemia.*** Moderate to severe splenomegaly is an early sign of both acute and chronic leukemia. With chronic granulocytic leukemia, splenomegaly is sometimes painful. Accompanying it may be hepatomegaly, lymphadenopathy, fatigue, malaise, pallor, fever, gum swelling, bleeding tendencies, weight loss, anorexia, and abdominal, bone, and joint pain. At times, acute leukemia also causes dyspnea, tachycardia, and palpitations. With advanced disease, the patient may display confusion, headache, vomiting, seizures, papilledema, and nuchal rigidity.

◆ ***Lymphoma.*** Moderate to massive splenomegaly is a late sign and may be accompanied by hepatomegaly, painless lymphadenopathy, scaly dermatitis with pruritus, fever, fatigue, weight loss, and malaise.

◆ ***Malaria.*** A common sign of malaria, splenomegaly is typically preceded by the malarial paroxysm of chills, followed by high fever and then diaphoresis. Related effects include headache, muscle pain, and hepatomegaly. With benign malaria, these paroxysms alternate with periods of well-being. With severe malaria, however, the patient may develop a persistent high fever, orthostatic hypotension, seizures, delirium, coma, coughing (with possible hemoptysis), vomiting, abdominal pain, diarrhea, melena, oliguria or anuria and, possibly, hemiplegia.

◆ ***Mononucleosis (infectious).*** A common sign of this disorder, splenomegaly is most pronounced during the second and third weeks of illness. Typically, it's accompanied by a triad of signs and symptoms: sore throat, cervical lymphadenopathy, and fluctuating temperature with an evening peak of 101° to 102° F (38.3° to 38.9° C). Occasionally, hepatomegaly, jaundice, and a maculopapular rash may also occur.

◆ ***Pancreatic cancer.*** This cancer may cause moderate to severe splenomegaly if tumor growth compresses the splenic vein. Other characteristic findings include abdominal or back pain, anorexia, nausea and vomiting, weight loss, GI bleeding, jaundice, pruritus, skin lesions, emotional lability, weakness, and fatigue. Palpation may reveal a tender abdominal mass and hepatomegaly; auscultation reveals a bruit in the periumbilical area and left upper quadrant.

◆ ***Polycythemia vera.*** Late in this disorder, the spleen may become markedly enlarged, resulting in easy satiety, abdominal fullness, and left-upper-quadrant or pleuritic chest pain. Signs and symptoms accompanying splenomegaly are widespread and numerous. The patient may exhibit deep, purplish red oral mucous membranes, headache, dyspnea, dizziness, vertigo, weakness, and fatigue. He may also develop finger and toe paresthesia, impaired mentation, tinnitus, blurred or double vision, scotoma, increased blood pressure, and intermittent claudication. Other signs and symptoms include pruritus, urticaria, ruddy cyanosis, epigastric distress, weight loss, hepatomegaly, and bleeding tendencies.

◆ ***Sarcoidosis.*** This granulomatous disorder may produce splenomegaly and hepatomegaly, possibly accompanied by vague abdominal discomfort. Its other signs and symptoms vary with the affected body system but may include nonproductive cough, dyspnea, malaise, fatigue, arthralgia, myalgia, weight loss, skin lesions, lymphadenopathy, irregular pulse, impaired vision, dysphagia, and seizures.

◆ ***Splenic rupture.*** Splenomegaly may result from massive hemorrhage with this disorder. The patient may also experience left-upper-quadrant pain, abdominal rigidity, and Kehr's sign.

◆ ***Thrombotic thrombocytopenic purpura.*** This disorder may produce splenomegaly and hepatomegaly accompanied by fever, generalized purpura, jaundice, pallor, vaginal bleeding, and hematuria. Other effects include fatigue, weakness, headache, pallor, abdominal pain, and arthralgias. Eventually, the patient develops signs of neurologic deterioration and of renal failure.

SPECIAL CONSIDERATIONS

Prepare the patient for diagnostic studies, such as a complete blood count, blood cultures, and radionuclide and computed tomography scans of the spleen.

PEDIATRIC POINTERS

Besides the causes of splenomegaly described above, children may develop splenomegaly in histiocytic disorders, congenital hemolytic anemia, Gaucher's disease, Niemann-Pick disease, hereditary spherocytosis, sickle cell disease, or beta-thalassemia (Cooley's anemia). Splenic abscess is the most common cause of splenomegaly in immunocompromised children.

Stools, clay-colored

Pale, putty-colored stools usually result from hepatic, gallbladder, or pancreatic disorders. Normally, bile pigments give the stool its characteristic brown color. However, hepatocellular degeneration or biliary obstruction may interfere with the formation or release of these pigments into the intestine, resulting in clay-colored stools. These stools are commonly associated with jaundice and dark "cola-colored" urine.

HISTORY AND PHYSICAL EXAMINATION

After documenting when the patient first noticed clay-colored stools, explore associated signs and symptoms, such as abdominal pain, nausea and vomiting, fatigue, anorexia, weight loss, and dark urine. Does the patient have trouble digesting fatty foods or heavy meals? Does he bruise easily?

Next, review the patient's medical history for gallbladder, hepatic, or pancreatic disorders. Has he ever had biliary surgery? Has he recently undergone barium studies? (Barium lightens stool color for several days.) Ask about antacid use because large amounts may lighten stool color. Note a history of alcoholism or exposure to other hepatotoxic substances.

After assessing the patient's general appearance, take his vital signs and check his skin and eyes for jaundice. Then examine the abdomen; inspect for distention, ascites, and auscultate for hypoactive bowel sounds. Percuss and palpate for masses and rebound tenderness. Finally, obtain urine and stool specimens for laboratory analysis.

MEDICAL CAUSES

◆ ***Bile duct cancer.*** Commonly a presenting sign of this cancer, clay-colored stools may be accompanied by jaundice, pruritus, anorexia and weight loss, upper abdominal pain, bleeding tendencies, and a palpable mass.

◆ ***Biliary cirrhosis.*** Clay-colored stools typically follow unexplained pruritus that worsens at bedtime, weakness, fatigue, weight loss, and vague abdominal pain; these features may be present for years. Associated findings include jaundice, hyperpigmentation, and signs of malabsorption, such as nocturnal diarrhea, steatorrhea, purpura, and bone and back pain due to osteomalacia. The patient may also develop firm, nontender hepatomegaly, hematemesis, ascites, edema, and xanthomas on his palms, soles, and elbows.

◆ ***Cholangitis (sclerosing).*** Characterized by fibrosis of the bile ducts, this chronic inflammatory disorder may cause clay-colored stools, chronic or intermittent jaundice, pruritus, right-upper-quadrant pain, chills, and fever.

◆ ***Cholelithiasis.*** Stones in the biliary tract may cause clay-colored stools when they obstruct the common bile duct (choledocholithiasis). However, if the obstruction is intermittent, the stools may alternate between normal and clay color. Associated symptoms include dyspepsia and—in sudden, severe obstruction—characteristic biliary colic. This right-upper-quadrant pain intensifies over several hours, may radiate to the epigastrium or shoulder blades, and is unrelieved by antacids. The pain is accompanied by tachycardia, restlessness, nausea, intolerance to certain foods, vomiting, upper abdominal tenderness, fever, chills, and jaundice.

◆ ***Hepatic cancer.*** Before clay-colored stools develop, the patient usually experiences weight loss, weakness, and anorexia. Later, he may develop nodular, firm hepatomegaly, jaundice, right-upper-quadrant pain, ascites, dependent edema, and fever. A bruit, hum, or rubbing sound may be heard on auscultation if the cancer involves a large part of the liver.

◆ ***Hepatitis.*** With viral hepatitis, clay-colored stools signal the start of the icteric phase and are typically followed by jaundice within 1 to 5 days. Associated signs include mild weight loss and dark urine as well as continuation of some preicteric findings, such as anorexia and tender hepatomegaly. During the icteric phase, the patient may become irritable and develop right-upper-quadrant pain, splenomegaly, enlarged cervical lymph nodes, and severe pruritus. After jaundice disappears, the patient continues to experience fatigue, flatulence, abdominal pain or tenderness, and dyspepsia, although his appetite usually returns and hepatomegaly subsides. The posticteric phase generally lasts from 2 to 6 weeks, with full recovery in 6 months.

With cholestatic nonviral hepatitis, clay-colored stools occur with other signs of viral hepatitis.

◆ ***Pancreatic cancer.*** Common bile duct obstruction associated with this insidious cancer may cause clay-colored stools. Classic associated features include abdominal or back pain, jaundice, pruritus, nausea and vomiting, anorexia, weight loss, fatigue, weakness, and fever. Other possible effects include diarrhea, skin lesions (especially on the legs), emotional lability, splenomegaly, and signs of GI bleeding. Auscultation may reveal a bruit in the periumbilical area and left upper quadrant.

◆ ***Pancreatitis (acute).*** This inflammatory disorder may cause clay-colored stools, dark urine, and jaundice. Typically, it also causes severe epigastric pain that radiates to the back and is aggravated by lying down. Associated findings include nausea and vomiting, fever, abdominal rigidity and tenderness, hypoactive bowel sounds, and crackles at the lung bases. With severe pancreatitis, findings include marked restlessness, tachycardia, mottled skin, and cold, sweaty extremities.

Other causes

◆ ***Biliary surgery.*** This surgery may cause bile duct stricture, resulting in clay-colored stools.

Special considerations

Prepare the patient for diagnostic tests, such as liver enzyme and serum bilirubin levels, hepatitis panels, sonograms, computed tomography, endoscope, retrograde cholangiopancreatography, and stool analysis.

Pediatric pointers

Clay-colored stools may occur in infants with biliary atresia.

Geriatric pointers

Because elderly patients with cholelithiasis have a greater risk of developing complications if the condition isn't treated, surgery should be considered early on for treatment of persistent systems.

Stridor

A loud, harsh, musical respiratory sound, stridor results from an obstruction in the trachea or larynx. Usually heard during inspiration, this sign may also occur during expiration in severe upper airway obstruction. It may begin as low-pitched "croaking" and progress to high-pitched "crowing" as respirations become more vigorous.

Life-threatening upper airway obstruction can stem from foreign-body aspiration, increased secretions, intraluminal tumor, localized edema or muscle spasms, and external compression by a tumor or aneurysm.

EMERGENCY INTERVENTIONS *If you hear stridor, quickly check the patient's vital signs including oxygen saturation and examine him for other signs of partial airway obstruction—choking or gagging, tachypnea, dyspnea, shallow respirations, intercostal retractions, nasal flaring, tachycardia, cyanosis, and diaphoresis. (Be aware that abrupt cessation of stridor signals complete obstruction in which the patient has inspiratory chest movement but absent breath sounds. Unable to talk, he quickly becomes lethargic and loses consciousness.)*

If you detect any signs of airway obstruction, try to clear the airway with back blows or abdominal thrusts (Heimlich maneuver). Next, administer oxygen by nasal cannula or face mask, or prepare for emergency endotracheal intubation or tracheostomy and mechanical ventilation. *(See* Emergency endotracheal intubation, *page 640.)* *Have equipment ready to suction any aspirated vomitus or blood through the endotracheal or tracheostomy tube. Connect the patient to a cardiac monitor, and position him upright to ease his breathing.*

History and physical examination

When the patient's condition permits, obtain a patient history from him or a family member. First, find out when the stridor began. Has he had it before? Does he have an upper respiratory tract infection? If so, how long has he had it?

Ask about a history of allergies, tumors, and respiratory and vascular disorders. Note recent exposure to smoke or noxious fumes or gases. Next, explore associated signs and symptoms. Does stridor occur with pain or a cough?

Then examine the patient's mouth for excessive secretions, foreign matter, inflammation, and swelling. Assess his neck for swelling, masses, subcutaneous crepitation, and scars. Observe the patient's chest for delayed, decreased, or asymmetrical chest expansion. Auscultate for wheezes, rhonchi, crackles, rubs, and other abnormal breath sounds. Percuss for dullness, tympany, or flatness. Finally, note any burns or signs of trauma, such as ecchymoses and lacerations.

Medical causes

◆ ***Airway trauma.*** Local trauma to the upper airway commonly causes acute obstruction, resulting in the sudden onset of stridor. Accompanying this sign are dysphonia, dysphagia, hemoptysis, cyanosis, accessory muscle use, intercostal retractions, nasal flaring, tachypnea, progressive dyspnea, and shallow respirations. Palpation may reveal subcutaneous crepitation in the neck or upper chest.

◆ ***Anaphylaxis.*** With a severe allergic reaction, upper airway edema and laryngospasm cause stridor and other signs and symptoms of respiratory distress: nasal flaring, wheezing, accessory muscle use, intercostal retractions, and dyspnea. The patient may also develop nasal congestion and profuse, watery rhinorrhea. Typically, these respiratory effects are preceded by a feeling of impending doom or fear, weakness, diaphoresis, sneezing, nasal pruritus, urticaria, erythema, and angioedema. Common associated findings include chest or throat tightness,

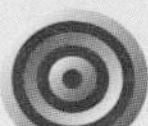

EMERGENCY INTERVENTION

Emergency endotracheal intubation

For a patient with stridor, you may have to perform emergency endotracheal (ET) intubation to establish a patent airway and administer mechanical ventilation. Just follow these essential steps:

- Gather the necessary equipment.
- Explain the procedure to the patient.
- Placc thc paticnt flat on his back with a small blanket or pillow under his head. This position aligns the axis of the oropharynx, posterior pharynx, and trachea.
- Check the cuff on the ET tube for leaks.
- After intubation, inflate the cuff, using the minimal leak technique.
- Check tube placement by auscultating for bilateral breath sounds or using a capnometer; observe the patient for chest expansion and feel for warm exhalations at the ET tube's opening.
- Insert an oral airway or bite block.
- Secure the tube and airway with tape applied to skin treated with compound benzoin tincture or a commercial securement device.
- Suction secretions from the patient's mouth and the ET tube as needed.
- Administer oxygen or initiate mechanical ventilation (or both).

After the patient has been intubated, suction secretions as needed and check cuff pressure once every shift (correcting any air leaks with the minimal leak technique). Provide mouth care every 2 to 3 hours and as needed. Prepare the patient for chest X-rays to check tube placement, and reassure him as needed.

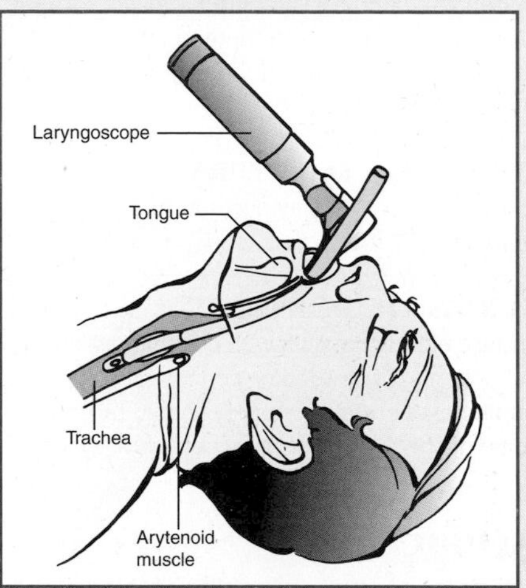

dysphagia and, possibly, signs of shock, such as hypotension, tachycardia, and cool, clammy skin.

- ***Anthrax, inhalation.*** Initial signs and symptoms are flulike and include fever, chills, weakness, cough, and chest pain. The disease generally occurs in two stages with a period of recovery after the initial symptoms. The second stage develops abruptly with rapid deterioration marked by stridor, fever, dyspnea, and hypotension generally leading to death within 24 hours. Radiologic findings include mediastinitis and symmetric mediastinal widening.
- ***Aspiration of a foreign body.*** Sudden stridor is characteristic in this life-threatening situation. Related findings include abrupt onset of dry, paroxysmal coughing, gagging or choking, hoarseness, tachycardia, wheezing, dyspnea, tachypnea, intercostal muscle retractions, diminished breath sounds, cyanosis, and shallow respirations. The patient typically appears anxious and distressed.
- ***Epiglottiditis.*** With this inflammatory condition, stridor is caused by an erythematous, edematous epiglottis that obstructs the upper airway. Stridor occurs along with fever, sore throat, and a croupy cough.
- ***Hypocalcemia.*** With this disorder, laryngospasm can cause stridor. Other findings include paresthesia, carpopedal spasm, and positive Chvostek's and Trousseau's signs.
- ***Inhalation injury.*** Within 48 hours after inhalation of smoke or noxious fumes, the patient may develop laryngeal edema and bronchospasms, resulting in stridor. Associated signs and symptoms include singed nasal hairs, orofacial burns, coughing, hoarseness, sooty sputum, crackles, rhonchi, wheezes, and other signs and symptoms of respiratory distress, such as dyspnea, accessory muscle use, intercostal retractions, and nasal flaring.
- ***Laryngeal tumor.*** Stridor is a late sign and may be accompanied by dysphagia, dyspnea, enlarged cervical nodes, and pain that radiates to the ear. Typically, stridor is preceded by hoarseness, minor throat pain, and a mild, dry cough.
- ***Laryngitis (acute).*** This disorder may cause severe laryngeal edema, resulting in stridor and dyspnea. Its chief sign, however, is mild to

severe hoarseness, perhaps with transient voice loss. Other findings include sore throat, dysphagia, dry cough, malaise, and fever.

◆ ***Mediastinal tumor.*** Commonly producing no symptoms at first, this type of tumor may eventually compress the trachea and bronchi, resulting in stridor. Its other effects include hoarseness, brassy cough, tracheal shift or tug, dilated neck veins, swelling of the face and neck, stertorous respirations, and suprasternal retractions on inspiration. The patient may also report dyspnea, dysphagia, and pain in the chest, shoulder, or arm.

◆ ***Retrosternal thyroid.*** This anatomic abnormality causes stridor, dysphagia, cough, hoarseness, and tracheal deviation. It can also cause signs of thyrotoxicosis.

◆ ***Thoracic aortic aneurysm.*** If this aneurysm compresses the trachea, it may cause stridor accompanied by dyspnea, wheezing, and a brassy cough. Other findings include hoarseness or complete voice loss, dysphagia, jugular vein distention, prominent chest veins, tracheal tug, paresthesia or neuralgia, and edema of the face, neck, and arms. The patient may also complain of substernal, lower back, abdominal, or shoulder pain.

Other causes

◆ ***Diagnostic tests.*** Bronchoscopy or laryngoscopy may precipitate laryngospasm and stridor.

◆ ***Treatments.*** After prolonged intubation, the patient may exhibit laryngeal edema and stridor when the tube is removed. Aerosol therapy with epinephrine may reduce stridor. Reintubation may be necessary in some cases. Neck surgery, such as thyroidectomy, may cause laryngeal paralysis and stridor.

Special considerations

Continue to monitor the patient's vital signs closely. Prepare him for diagnostic tests, such as arterial blood gas analysis and chest X-rays.

Pediatric pointers

Stridor is a major sign of airway obstruction in children. When you hear this sign, you must intervene quickly to prevent total airway obstruction. This emergency can happen more rapidly in a child because his airway is narrower than an adult's.

Causes of stridor include foreign-body aspiration, croup syndrome, laryngeal diphtheria, pertussis, retropharyngeal abscess, and congenital abnormalities of the larynx.

Therapy for partial airway obstruction typically involves hot or cold steam in a mist tent or hood, parenteral fluids and electrolytes, and plenty of rest.

Syncope

A common neurologic sign, syncope (or fainting) refers to transient loss of consciousness associated with impaired cerebral blood supply or cerebral hypoxia. It usually occurs abruptly and lasts for seconds to minutes. An episode of syncope usually starts as a feeling of light-headedness. A patient can usually prevent an episode of syncope by lying down or sitting with his head between his knees. Typically, the patient lies motionless with his skeletal muscles relaxed but sphincter muscles controlled. However, the depth of unconsciousness varies—some patients can hear voices or see blurred outlines; others are unaware of their surroundings.

In many ways, syncope simulates death: The patient is strikingly pale with a slow, weak pulse, hypotension, and almost imperceptible breathing. If severe hypotension lasts for 20 seconds or longer, the patient may also develop convulsive, tonic-clonic movements.

Syncope may result from cardiac and cerebrovascular disorders, hypoxemia, and postural changes in the presence of autonomic dysfunction. It may also follow vigorous coughing (tussive syncope) and emotional stress, injury, shock, or pain (vasovagal syncope, or common fainting). Hysterical syncope may also follow emotional stress but isn't accompanied by other vasodepressor effects.

EMERGENCY INTERVENTIONS *If you see a patient faint, ensure a patent airway, patient safety, and take vital signs. Then place the patient in a supine position, elevate his legs, and loosen any tight clothing. Be alert for tachycardia, bradycardia, or an irregular pulse. Meanwhile, place him on a cardiac monitor to detect arrhythmias. If an arrhythmia appears, give oxygen and insert an I.V. catheter for drugs or fluids. Be ready to begin cardiopulmonary resuscitation. Cardioversion, defibrillation, or insertion of a temporary pacemaker may be required.*

History and physical examination

If the patient reports a fainting episode, gather information about the episode from him and his family. Did he feel weak, light-headed, nauseous, or sweaty just before he fainted? Did he get up quickly from a chair or from lying down? During the fainting episode, did he have muscle spasms or incontinence? How long was he unconscious? When he regained consciousness, was he alert or confused? Did he have a headache? Has he fainted before? If so, how often does it occur?

Next, take the patient's vital signs and examine him for any injuries that may have occurred during his fall.

MEDICAL CAUSES

◆ ***Aortic arch syndrome.*** With this syndrome, the patient experiences syncope and may exhibit weak or abruptly absent carotid pulses and unequal or absent radial pulses. Early signs and symptoms include night sweats, pallor, nausea, anorexia, weight loss, arthralgia, and Raynaud's phenomenon. He may also develop hypotension in the arms; neck, shoulder, and chest pain; paresthesia; intermittent claudication; bruits; vision disturbances; and dizziness.

◆ ***Aortic stenosis.*** A cardinal late sign, syncope is accompanied by exertional dyspnea and angina. Related findings include marked fatigue, orthopnea, paroxysmal nocturnal dyspnea, palpitations, and diminished carotid pulses. Typically, auscultation reveals atrial and ventricular gallops as well as a harsh, crescendo-decrescendo systolic ejection murmur that's loudest at the right sternal border of the second intercostal space.

◆ ***Cardiac arrhythmias.*** Any arrhythmia that decreases cardiac output and impairs cerebral circulation may cause syncope. Other effects—such as palpitations, pallor, confusion, diaphoresis, dyspnea, and hypotension—usually develop first. However, with Adams-Stokes syndrome, syncope may occur without warning. During syncope, the patient develops asystole, which may precipitate spasm and myoclonic jerks if prolonged. He also displays an ashen pallor that progresses to cyanosis, incontinence, bilateral Babinski's reflex, and fixed pupils.

◆ ***Carotid sinus hypersensitivity.*** Syncope is triggered by compression of the carotid sinus, which may be caused by turning the head to one side or by wearing a tight collar. The fainting episode is usually of short duration.

◆ ***Hypoxemia.*** Regardless of its cause, severe hypoxemia may produce syncope. Common related effects include confusion, tachycardia, restlessness, and incoordination.

◆ ***Orthostatic hypotension.*** Syncope occurs when the patient rises quickly from a recumbent position. Look for a drop of 10 to 20 mm Hg or more in systolic or diastolic blood pressure as well as tachycardia, pallor, dizziness, blurred vision, nausea, and diaphoresis.

◆ ***Transient ischemic attacks.*** Marked by transient neurologic deficits, these attacks may produce syncope and decreased level of consciousness. Other findings vary with the affected artery but may include vision loss, nystagmus, aphasia, dysarthria, unilateral numbness, hemiparesis or hemiplegia, tinnitus, facial weakness, dysphagia, and staggering or uncoordinated gait.

◆ ***Vagal glossopharyngeal neuralgia.*** With this disorder, localized pressure may trigger pain in the base of the tongue, pharynx, larynx, tonsils, and ear, resulting in syncope that lasts for several minutes.

OTHER CAUSES

◆ ***Drugs.*** Quinidine may cause syncope—and possibly sudden death—associated with ventricular fibrillation. Prazosin may cause severe orthostatic hypotension and syncope, usually after the first dose. Occasionally, griseofulvin, levodopa, and indomethacin can produce syncope.

SPECIAL CONSIDERATIONS

Continue to monitor the patient's vital signs closely. Prepare the patient for an electrocardiogram, Holter monitor, carotid duplex, carotid Doppler, and electrophysiology studies.

PEDIATRIC POINTERS

Syncope is much less common in children than in adults. It may result from a cardiac or neurologic disorder, allergies, or emotional stress.

PATIENT COUNSELING

Advise the patient to pace his activities, to rise slowly from a recumbent position, to avoid standing still for a prolonged time, and to sit or lie down as soon as he feels faint.

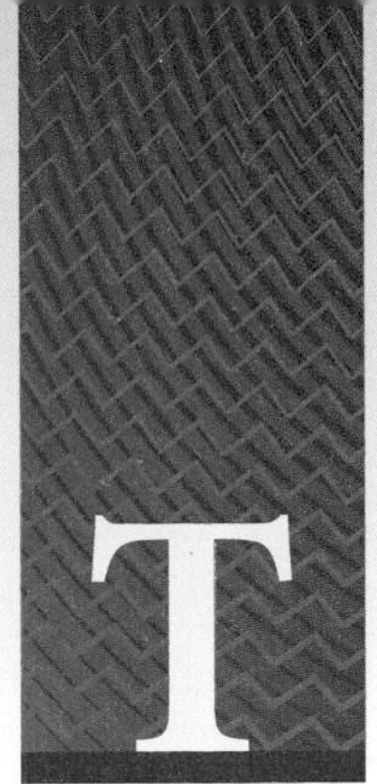

Tachycardia

Easily detected by counting the apical, carotid, or radial pulse rate, tachycardia is a heart rate greater than 100 beats/minute. The patient with tachycardia usually complains of palpitations or a "racing" heart. This common sign normally occurs in response to emotional or physical stress, such as excitement, exercise, pain, anxiety, and fever. It may also result from the use of stimulants, such as caffeine and tobacco. However, tachycardia may be an early sign of a life-threatening disorder, such as cardiogenic, hypovolemic, or septic shock. It may also result from a cardiovascular, respiratory, or metabolic disorder or from the effects of certain drugs, tests, or treatments. (See *What happens in tachycardia*, page 644.)

EMERGENCY INTERVENTIONS *If you detect tachycardia, first perform an electrocardiogram (ECG) to check for reduced cardiac output, which may initiate or result from tachycardia. Take the patient's other vital signs and determine his level of consciousness (LOC). If the patient has increased or decreased blood pressure and is drowsy or confused, administer oxygen and begin cardiac monitoring. Insert an I.V. catheter for fluid, blood product, and drug administration, and gather emergency resuscitation equipment.*

History and physical examination

If the patient's condition permits, take a focused history. Find out if he has had palpitations before. If so, how were they treated? Explore associated symptoms. Is the patient dizzy or short of breath? Is he weak or fatigued? Is he experiencing episodes of syncope or chest pain? Next, ask about a history of trauma, diabetes, or cardiac, pulmonary, or thyroid disorders. Also, obtain an alcohol and drug history, including prescription, over-the-counter, and illicit drugs.

Inspect the patient's skin for pallor or cyanosis. Assess pulses, noting peripheral edema. Finally, auscultate the heart and lungs for abnormal sounds or rhythms.

Medical causes

◆ ***Acute respiratory distress syndrome.*** Besides tachycardia, this syndrome causes crackles, rhonchi, dyspnea, tachypnea, nasal flaring, and grunting respirations. Other findings include cyanosis, anxiety, decreased LOC, and abnormal chest X-ray findings.

◆ ***Adrenocortical insufficiency.*** In this disorder, tachycardia is commonly accompanied by a weak pulse as well as progressive weakness and fatigue, which may become so severe that the patient requires bed rest. Other signs and symptoms include abdominal pain, nausea and vomiting, altered bowel habits, weight loss, orthostatic hypotension, irritability, bronze skin, decreased libido, and syncope. Some patients report an enhanced sense of taste, smell, and hearing.

◆ ***Alcohol withdrawal syndrome.*** Tachycardia can occur with tachypnea, profuse diaphoresis, fever, insomnia, anorexia, and anxiety. The patient is characteristically anxious,

What happens in tachycardia

Tachycardia represents the heart's effort to deliver more oxygen to body tissues by increasing the rate at which blood passes through the vessels. This sign can reflect overstimulation within the sinoatrial node, the atrium, the atrioventricular node, or the ventricles.

Because heart rate affects cardiac output (cardiac output = heart rate × stroke volume), tachycardia can lower cardiac output by reducing ventricular filling time and stroke volume (the output of each ventricle at every contraction). As cardiac output plummets, arterial pressure and peripheral perfusion decrease. Tachycardia further aggravates myocardial ischemia by increasing the heart's demand for oxygen while reducing the duration of diastole—the period of greatest coronary blood flow.

irritable, and prone to visual and tactile hallucinations.

◆ ***Anaphylactic shock.*** In life-threatening anaphylactic shock, tachycardia and hypotension develop within minutes after exposure to an allergen, such as penicillin or an insect sting. Typically, the patient is visibly anxious and has severe pruritus, perhaps with urticaria and a pounding headache. Other findings may include flushed and clammy skin, a cough, dyspnea, nausea, abdominal cramps, seizures, stridor, change or loss of voice associated with laryngeal edema, and urinary urgency and incontinence.

◆ ***Anemia.*** Tachycardia and bounding pulse are characteristic signs of anemia. Associated signs and symptoms include fatigue, pallor, dyspnea and, possibly, bleeding tendencies. Auscultation may reveal an atrial gallop, a systolic bruit over the carotid arteries, and crackles.

◆ ***Anxiety.*** A fight-or-flight response produces tachycardia, tachypnea, chest pain, nausea, and light-headedness. The symptoms dissipate as anxiety resolves.

◆ ***Aortic insufficiency.*** Accompanying tachycardia in this disorder are a "water-hammer" bounding pulse and a large, diffuse apical heave. Severe insufficiency also produces widened pulse pressure. Auscultation reveals a hallmark decrescendo, high-pitched, and blowing diastolic murmur that starts with the second heart sound and is heard best at the left sternal border of the second and third intercostal spaces. An atrial or ventricular gallop, an early systolic murmur, an Austin Flint murmur (apical diastolic rumble), or Duroziez's sign (a murmur over the femoral artery during systole and diastole) may also be heard. Other findings include angina, dyspnea, palpitations, strong and abrupt carotid pulsations, pallor, and signs of heart failure, such as crackles and neck vein distention.

◆ ***Aortic stenosis.*** Typically, this valvular disorder causes tachycardia, an atrial gallop, and a weak, thready pulse. Its chief features, however, are exertional dyspnea, angina, dizziness, and syncope. Aortic stenosis also causes a harsh, crescendo-decrescendo systolic ejection murmur that's loudest at the right sternal border of the second intercostal space. Other findings include palpitations, crackles, and fatigue.

◆ ***Cardiac arrhythmias.*** Tachycardia may occur with an irregular heart rhythm. The patient may be hypotensive and report dizziness, palpitations, weakness, and fatigue. Depending on his heart rate, he may also exhibit tachypnea, decreased LOC, and pale, cool, clammy skin.

◆ ***Cardiac contusion.*** The result of blunt chest trauma, a cardiac contusion may cause tachycardia, substernal pain, dyspnea, and palpitations. Assessment may detect sternal ecchymoses and a pericardial friction rub.

◆ ***Cardiac tamponade.*** In life-threatening cardiac tamponade, tachycardia is commonly accompanied by paradoxical pulse, dyspnea, and tachypnea. The patient is visibly anxious and restless and has cyanotic, clammy skin and distended jugular veins. He may develop muffled heart sounds, a pericardial friction rub, chest pain, hypotension, narrowed pulse pressure, and hepatomegaly.

◆ ***Cardiogenic shock.*** Although many features of cardiogenic shock appear in other types of shock, they're usually more profound in this type. Accompanying tachycardia are a weak, thready pulse; narrowed pulse pressure; hypotension; tachypnea; cold, pale, clammy, and cyanotic skin; oliguria; restlessness; and altered LOC.

◆ ***Cholera.*** This infectious disease is marked by abrupt watery diarrhea and vomiting. Severe fluid and electrolyte loss leads to tachycardia, thirst, weakness, muscle cramps, decreased skin turgor, oliguria, and hypotension. Without treatment, death can occur within hours.

◆ ***Chronic obstructive pulmonary disease.*** Although clinical findings vary widely in this disorder, tachycardia is a common sign. Other characteristic findings include cough, tachypnea, dyspnea, pursed-lip breathing, accessory muscle use, cyanosis, diminished breath sounds, rhonchi, crackles, and wheezing. Clubbing and barrel chest are usually late findings.

◆ ***Diabetic ketoacidosis.*** This life-threatening disorder commonly produces tachycardia and a thready pulse. Its cardinal sign, however, is Kussmaul's respirations—abnormally rapid, deep breathing. Other signs and symptoms of ketoacidosis include fruity breath odor, orthostatic hypotension, generalized weakness, anorexia, nausea, vomiting, and abdominal pain. The patient's LOC may vary from lethargy to coma.

◆ ***Febrile illness.*** Fever can cause tachycardia. Related findings reflect the specific disorder.

◆ ***Heart failure.*** Especially common in left-sided heart failure, tachycardia may be accompanied by a ventricular gallop, fatigue, dyspnea (exertional and paroxysmal nocturnal), orthopnea, and leg edema. Eventually, the patient develops widespread signs and symptoms, such as palpitations, narrowed pulse pressure, hypotension, tachypnea, crackles, dependent edema, weight gain, slowed mental response, diaphoresis, pallor and, possibly, oliguria. Late signs include hemoptysis, cyanosis, marked hepatomegaly, and pitting edema.

◆ ***Hyperosmolar hyperglycemic nonketotic syndrome.*** A rapidly deteriorating LOC is commonly accompanied by tachycardia, hypotension, tachypnea, seizures, oliguria, and severe dehydration marked by poor skin turgor and dry mucous membranes.

◆ ***Hypertensive crisis.*** A life-threatening hypertensive crisis is characterized by tachycardia, tachypnea, diastolic blood pressure that exceeds 120 mm Hg, and systolic blood pressure that may exceed 200 mm Hg. Typically, the patient develops pulmonary edema with jugular vein distention, dyspnea, and pink, frothy sputum. Related findings include chest pain, severe headache, drowsiness, confusion, anxiety, tinnitus, epistaxis, muscle twitching, seizures, nausea and vomiting and, possibly, focal neurologic signs such as paresthesia.

◆ ***Hypoglycemia.*** A common sign of hypoglycemia, tachycardia is accompanied by hypothermia, nervousness, trembling, fatigue, malaise, weakness, headache, hunger, nausea, diaphoresis, and moist, clammy skin. Central nervous system effects include blurred or double vision, motor weakness, hemiplegia, seizures, and decreased LOC.

◆ ***Hyponatremia.*** Tachycardia is a rare effect of this electrolyte imbalance. Other findings include orthostatic hypotension, headache, muscle twitching and weakness, fatigue, oliguria or anuria, poor skin turgor, thirst, irritability, seizures, nausea and vomiting, and decreased LOC that may progress to coma. Severe hyponatremia may cause cyanosis and signs of vasomotor collapse such as thready pulse.

◆ ***Hypovolemia.*** Tachycardia may occur with this disorder along with hypotension, decreased skin turgor, sunken eyeballs, thirst, syncope, and dry skin and tongue.

◆ ***Hypovolemic shock.*** Mild tachycardia, an early sign of life-threatening hypovolemic shock, may be accompanied by tachypnea, restlessness, thirst, and pale, cool skin. As shock progresses, the patient's skin becomes clammy and his pulse, increasingly rapid and thready. He may also develop hypotension, narrowed pulse pressure, oliguria, subnormal body temperature, and decreased LOC.

◆ ***Hypoxemia.*** Tachycardia may be accompanied by tachypnea, dyspnea, cyanosis, confusion, syncope, and incoordination.

◆ ***Myocardial infarction (MI).*** A life-threatening MI may cause tachycardia or bradycardia. Its classic symptom, however, is crushing substernal chest pain that may radiate to the left arm, jaw, neck, or shoulder. Auscultation may reveal an atrial gallop, a new murmur, and crackles. Other signs and symptoms include dyspnea, diaphoresis, nausea and vomiting, anxiety, restlessness, increased or decreased blood pressure, and pale, clammy skin.

◆ ***Neurogenic shock.*** Tachycardia or bradycardia may accompany tachypnea, apprehension, oliguria, variable body temperature, decreased LOC, and warm, dry skin.

◆ ***Orthostatic hypotension.*** Tachycardia accompanies the characteristic signs and symptoms of this condition, which include dizziness, syncope, pallor, blurred vision, diaphoresis, and nausea.

◆ ***Pheochromocytoma.*** Characterized by sustained or paroxysmal hypertension, this rare tumor may also cause tachycardia and palpitations. Other findings include headache, chest and abdominal pain, diaphoresis, paresthesia, tremors, nausea and vomiting, insomnia, extreme anxiety (possibly even panic), and pale or flushed, warm skin.

◆ ***Pneumothorax.*** Life-threatening pneumothorax causes tachycardia and other signs and symptoms of distress, such as severe dyspnea

Normal pediatric vital signs

This chart lists the normal resting respiratory rate, blood pressure, and pulse rate for girls and boys up to age 16.

Vital signs	Neonate	2 years	4 years	6 years	8 years	10 years
Respiratory rate (breaths/minute)						
Girls	28	26	25	24	24	22
Boys	30	28	25	24	22	23
Blood pressure (mm Hg)						
Girls	—	98/60	98/60	98/64	104/68	110/72
Boys	—	96/60	98/60	98/62	102/68	110/72
Pulse rate (beats/minute)						
Girls	130	110	100	100	90	90
Boys	130	110	100	100	90	90

and chest pain, tachypnea, and cyanosis. Related findings include dry cough, subcutaneous crepitation, absent or decreased breath sounds, cessation of normal chest movement on the affected side, and decreased vocal fremitus.

◆ ***Pulmonary embolism.*** In this disorder, tachycardia is usually preceded by sudden dyspnea, angina, or pleuritic chest pain. Common associated signs and symptoms include weak peripheral pulses, cyanosis, tachypnea, low-grade fever, restlessness, diaphoresis, and a dry cough or a cough producing blood-tinged sputum.

◆ ***Septic shock.*** Initially, septic shock produces chills, sudden fever, tachycardia, tachypnea and, possibly, nausea, vomiting, and diarrhea. The patient's skin is flushed, warm, and dry; his blood pressure is normal or slightly decreased. Eventually, he may display anxiety; restlessness; thirst; oliguria or anuria; cool, clammy, cyanotic skin; rapid, thready pulse; and severe hypotension. His LOC may decrease progressively, perhaps culminating in a coma.

◆ ***Thyrotoxicosis.*** Tachycardia is a classic feature of this thyroid disorder. Others include an enlarged thyroid gland, nervousness, heat intolerance, weight loss despite increased appetite, diaphoresis, diarrhea, tremors, palpitations, and sometimes exophthalmos.

Because thyrotoxicosis affects virtually every body system, its associated features are diverse and numerous. Some examples include full and bounding pulse, widened pulse pressure, dyspnea, anorexia, nausea, vomiting, altered bowel habits, hepatomegaly, and muscle weakness, fatigue, and atrophy. The patient's skin is smooth, warm, and flushed; his hair is fine and soft and may gray prematurely or fall out. The female patient may have a reduced libido and oligomenorrhea or amenorrhea; the male patient may exhibit a reduced libido and gynecomastia.

Other causes

◆ ***Diagnostic tests.*** Cardiac catheterization and electrophysiologic studies may induce transient tachycardia.

◆ ***Drugs and alcohol.*** Various drugs affect the nervous system, circulatory system, or heart muscle, resulting in tachycardia. Examples of these include sympathomimetics; phenothiazines; anticholinergics such as atropine; thyroid drugs; vasodilators, such as hydralazine and nifedipine; acetylcholinesterase inhibitors such as captopril; nitrates such as nitroglycerin; alpha-adrenergic blockers such as phentolamine; and beta-adrenergic bronchodilators such as albuterol. Excessive caffeine intake and alcohol intoxication may also cause tachycardia.

◆ ***Surgery and pacemakers.*** Cardiac surgery and pacemaker malfunction or wire irritation may cause tachycardia.

Special considerations

Continue to monitor the patient closely. Explain ordered diagnostic tests, such as a thyroid panel,

12 years	14 years	16 years
20	18	16
20	16	16
114/74	118/76	120/78
112/74	120/76	124/78
90	85	80
85	80	75

electrolyte and hemoglobin levels, hematocrit, pulmonary function studies, and 12-lead ECG. If appropriate, prepare him for an ambulatory ECG.

Teach the patient that tachycardia may recur. Explain that an antiarrhythmic and an internal defibrillator or ablation therapy may be indicated for symptomatic tachycardia.

Pediatric pointers

When assessing a child for tachycardia, be aware that normal heart rates for children are higher than those for adults. (See *Normal pediatric vital signs*.) Many of the adult causes described above may also cause tachycardia in children.

Tachypnea

A common sign of cardiopulmonary disorders, tachypnea is an abnormally fast respiratory rate—20 or more breaths/minute. Tachypnea may reflect the need to increase minute volume—the amount of air breathed each minute. Under these circumstances, it may be accompanied by an increase in tidal volume—the volume of air inhaled or exhaled per breath—resulting in hyperventilation. Tachypnea, however, may also reflect stiff lungs or overloaded ventilatory muscles, in which case tidal volume may actually be reduced.

Tachypnea may result from reduced arterial oxygen tension or arterial oxygen content, decreased perfusion, or increased oxygen demand. Increased oxygen demand may result from fever, exertion, anxiety, or pain. It may also occur as a compensatory response to metabolic acidosis or may result from pulmonary irritation, stretch receptor stimulation, or a neurologic disorder that upsets medullary respiratory control. Generally, the respiratory rate increases by 4 breaths/minute for every 1° F (0.5° C) increase in body temperature.

EMERGENCY INTERVENTIONS *If you detect tachypnea, quickly evaluate the patient's cardiopulmonary status; obtain vital signs including oxygen saturation; and check for cyanosis, chest pain, dyspnea, tachycardia, and hypotension. If the patient has paradoxical chest movement, suspect flail chest and immediately splint his chest with your hands or with sandbags. Then administer supplemental oxygen by nasal cannula or face mask and, if possible, place the patient in semi-Fowler's position to help ease his breathing. Intubation and mechanical ventilation may be necessary if respiratory failure occurs. Also, insert an I.V. catheter for fluid and drug administration and begin cardiac monitoring.*

History and physical examination

If the patient's condition permits, obtain a medical history. Find out when the tachypnea began. Did it follow activity? Has he had it before? Does the patient have a history of asthma, chronic obstructive pulmonary disease (COPD), or any other pulmonary or cardiac conditions? Then have him describe associated signs and symptoms, such as diaphoresis, chest pain, and recent weight loss. Is he anxious about anything or does he have a history of anxiety attacks? Note whether he takes any drugs for pain relief. If so, how effective are they?

Begin the physical examination by taking the patient's vital signs, including oxygen saturation, if you haven't already done so, and observing his overall behavior. (See *Differential diagnosis: Tachypnea*, pages 648 and 649.) Does he seem restless, confused, or fatigued? Then auscultate the chest for abnormal heart and breath sounds. If the patient has a productive cough, record the color, amount, and consistency of sputum. Finally, check for jugular vein distention, and examine the skin for pallor, cyanosis, edema, and warmth or coolness.

(Text continues on page 650.)

Differential diagnosis: Tachypnea

History of present illness

Focused physical examination: Skin, cardiovascular and respiratory systems

Common signs and symptoms
- Tachycardia
- Dyspnea
- Cyanosis

Pulmonary embolism

Additional signs and symptoms
- Acute dyspnea
- Sudden pleuritic chest pain
- Low-grade fever
- Nonproductive cough or productive cough with blood-tinged sputum
- Pleural friction rub
- Crackles
- Hemoptysis (possibly)
- Wheezing
- Dullness on percussion
- Decreased breath sounds
- Diaphoresis
- Restlessness
- Anxiety
- Signs of shock (possibly)

Diagnosis: Imaging studies (chest X-rays, pulmonary $\dot{V}/\dot{Q}$ scan, spiral chest computed tomography scan, pulmonary angiography), electrocardiogram (ECG)
Treatment: Oxygen therapy, medication (anticoagulants, thrombolytic therapy)
Follow-up: Return visit within first week after hospitalization

Pneumothorax

Additional signs and symptoms
- Severe, sharp, and usually unilateral chest pain that's aggravated by chest wall movement
- Accessory muscle use
- Dry cough
- Anxiety
- Restlessness

Diagnosis: Physical examination, arterial blood gas (ABG) analysis, chest X-rays
Treatment: Chest tube insertion, analgesics, oxygen therapy
Follow-up: Referral to pulmonologist

Pneumonia

Additional signs and symptoms
- Hacking, dry cough that progresses to a productive cough
- High-grade fever
- Shaking chills
- Headache
- Pleuritic chest pain
- Fatigue
- Nasal flaring

Diagnosis: Chest X-rays, sputum specimens, bronchoscopy if necessary
Treatment: Medication (antibiotics, expectorants), oxygen if necessary, intubation if warranted
Follow-up: Referral to pulmonologist, hospitalization if necessary

Asthma

Signs and symptoms
- Acute dyspneic attacks
- Audible or auscultated wheezing
- Dry cough
- Hyperpnea
- Chest tightness
- Accessory muscle use
- Nasal flaring
- Intercostal and supraclavicular retractions
- Tachycardia
- Diaphoresis
- Prolonged expiration
- Flushing or cyanosis
- Apprehension

Diagnosis: Laboratory tests (complete blood count [CBC], ABG analysis, allergy skin testing), chest X-rays, pulmonary function tests
Treatment: Avoidance of allergens, tobacco, and beta-adrenergic blockers; medication (inhaled $beta_2$-agonists, inhaled corticosteroids, leukotriene receptor agonists [possibly], systemic corticosteroids during infections and exacerbations), peak expiratory flow monitoring
Follow-up: For acute exacerbations, return visit within 24 hours, then every 3 to 5 days, and then every 1 to 3 months; referral to pulmonologist if treatment is ineffective

Common signs and symptoms
- Gradually developing dyspnea
- Chronic paroxysmal nocturnal dyspnea
- Orthopnea
- Tachycardia
- Palpitations
- S_3
- Fatigue
- Dependent peripheral edema
- Hepatomegaly
- Dry cough
- Anorexia
- Weight gain
- Loss of mental acuity
- Hemoptysis

Heart failure

Acute onset heart failure

Additional signs and symptoms
- Distended jugular veins
- Bibasilar crackles
- Oliguria
- Hypotension

Diagnosis: Laboratory tests (CBC, cardiac enzymes, troponin), imaging studies (chest X-rays, echocardiogram), ECG
Treatment: Medication (angiotensin-converting enzyme inhibitors, diuretics, possibly carvedilol, possibly digoxin)
Follow-up: Return visit within 1 week after discharge, at 4 weeks, and then every 3 months; referral to cardiologist if condition is chronic

Additional differential diagnoses: abdominal pain ◆ anaphylactic shock ◆ anemia ◆ ARDS ◆ ascites ◆ bronchiectasis ◆ bronchitis (chronic) ◆ cardiac arrhythmias ◆ cardiac tamponade ◆ cardiogenic shock ◆ chest trauma ◆ COPD ◆ emphysema ◆ febrile illness ◆ flail chest ◆ foreign body aspiration ◆ head trauma ◆ hepatic failure ◆ HHNS ◆ hypovolemic shock ◆ hypoxia ◆ interstital fibrosis ◆ lung abscess ◆ lung, pleural, or mediastinal tumor ◆ mesothelioma (malignant) ◆ neurogenic shock ◆ pancreatis ◆ pleural effusion ◆ pulmonary edema ◆ pulmonary hypertension ◆ septic shock
Other cause: salicylates

MEDICAL CAUSES

◆ ***Acute respiratory distress syndrome (ARDS).*** Tachypnea and apprehension may be the earliest features of this life-threatening disorder. Tachypnea gradually worsens as fluid accumulates in the patient's lungs, causing them to stiffen. It's accompanied by accessory muscle use, grunting expirations, suprasternal and intercostal retractions, crackles, and rhonchi. Eventually, ARDS produces hypoxemia, resulting in tachycardia, dyspnea, cyanosis, respiratory failure, and shock.

◆ ***Alcohol withdrawal syndrome.*** A late sign in the acute phase of this syndrome, tachypnea typically accompanies anorexia, insomnia, tachycardia, fever, and diaphoresis. The patient may also experience anxiety, irritability, and bizarre visual or tactile hallucinations.

◆ ***Anaphylactic shock.*** In this life-threatening type of shock, tachypnea develops within minutes after exposure to an allergen, such as penicillin or insect venom. Accompanying signs and symptoms include anxiety, pounding headache, skin flushing, intense pruritus and, possibly, diffuse urticaria. The patient may exhibit widespread edema of the eyelids, lips, tongue, hands, feet, and genitalia. Other findings include cool, clammy skin; rapid, thready pulse; cough; dyspnea; stridor; and change or loss of voice associated with laryngeal edema.

◆ ***Anemia.*** Tachypnea may occur in this disorder, depending on the duration and severity of anemia. Associated signs and symptoms include fatigue, pallor, dyspnea, tachycardia, orthostatic hypotension, bounding pulse, an atrial gallop, and a systolic bruit over the carotid arteries.

◆ ***Anxiety.*** Tachypnea may occur during high-anxiety states because of the "fight-or-flight" response. Associated signs and symptoms include tachycardia, restlessness, chest pain, nausea, and light-headedness, all of which dissipate as the anxiety state resolves.

◆ ***Aspiration of a foreign body***. A life-threatening upper airway obstruction may result from aspiration of a foreign body. In a partial obstruction, the patient abruptly develops a paroxysmal dry cough with rapid, shallow respirations. Other signs and symptoms include dyspnea, gagging or choking, intercostal retractions, nasal flaring, cyanosis, decreased or absent breath sounds, hoarseness, and stridor or coarse wheezing. Typically, the patient appears frightened and distressed. A complete obstruction may rapidly cause asphyxia and death.

◆ ***Asthma.*** Tachypnea is common in life-threatening asthma exacerbations, which commonly occur at night. These exacerbations usually begin with mild wheezing and a dry cough that progresses to mucus expectoration. Eventually, the patient becomes apprehensive and develops prolonged expirations, intercostal and supraclavicular retractions on inspiration, accessory muscle use, severe audible wheezing, rhonchi, flaring nostrils, tachycardia, diaphoresis, and flushing or cyanosis.

◆ ***Bronchiectasis.*** Although this disorder may produce tachypnea, its classic sign is a chronic productive cough that produces copious amounts of mucopurulent, foul-smelling sputum and, occasionally, hemoptysis. Related findings include coarse crackles on inspiration, exertional dyspnea, rhonchi, and halitosis. The patient may also exhibit fever, malaise, weight loss, fatigue, and weakness. Clubbing is a common late sign.

◆ ***Bronchitis (chronic).*** Mild tachypnea may occur in this form of COPD, but it isn't typically a characteristic sign. Chronic bronchitis usually begins with a dry, hacking cough, which later produces copious amounts of sputum. Other characteristic findings include dyspnea, prolonged expirations, wheezing, scattered rhonchi, accessory muscle use, and cyanosis. Clubbing and barrel chest are late signs.

◆ ***Cardiac arrhythmias.*** Depending on the patient's heart rate, tachypnea may occur along with hypotension, dizziness, palpitations, weakness, and fatigue. The patient's level of consciousness (LOC) may be decreased.

◆ ***Cardiac tamponade.*** In life-threatening cardiac tamponade, tachypnea may accompany tachycardia, dyspnea, and paradoxical pulse. Related findings include muffled heart sounds, pericardial friction rub, chest pain, hypotension, narrowed pulse pressure, and hepatomegaly. The patient is noticeably anxious and restless. His skin is clammy and cyanotic, and his jugular veins are distended.

◆ ***Cardiogenic shock.*** Although many signs of cardiogenic shock appear in other types of shock, they're usually more severe in this type. Besides tachypnea, the patient commonly displays cold, pale, clammy, cyanotic skin; hypotension; tachycardia; narrowed pulse pressure; a ventricular gallop; oliguria; decreased LOC; and jugular vein distention.

◆ ***Emphysema.*** This form of COPD commonly produces tachypnea accompanied by exertional dyspnea. It may also cause anorexia, malaise, peripheral cyanosis, pursed-lip breathing, accessory muscle use, and a chronic productive cough. Percussion yields a hyperresonant tone;

auscultation reveals wheezing, crackles, and diminished breath sounds. Clubbing and barrel chest are late signs.

◆ ***Febrile illness.*** Fever can cause tachypnea, tachycardia, and other signs.

◆ ***Flail chest.*** Tachypnea usually appears early in this life-threatening disorder. Other findings include paradoxical chest wall movement, rib bruises and palpable fractures, localized chest pain, hypotension, and diminished breath sounds. The patient may also develop signs of respiratory distress, such as dyspnea and accessory muscle use.

◆ ***Head trauma.*** When trauma affects the brain stem, the patient may display central neurogenic hyperventilation, a form of tachypnea marked by rapid, even, and deep respirations. The tachypnea may be accompanied by other signs of life-threatening neurogenic dysfunction, such as coma, unequal and nonreactive pupils, seizures, hemiplegia, flaccidity, and hypoactive or absent deep tendon reflexes.

◆ ***Hyperosmolar hyperglycemic nonketotic syndrome.*** Rapidly deteriorating LOC occurs along with tachypnea, tachycardia, hypotension, seizures, oliguria, and signs of dehydration.

◆ ***Hypovolemic shock.*** An early sign of life-threatening hypovolemic shock, tachypnea is accompanied by cool, pale skin; restlessness; thirst; and mild tachycardia. As shock progresses, the patient develops clammy skin and an increasingly rapid and thready pulse. Other findings include hypotension, narrowed pulse pressure, oliguria, subnormal body temperature, and decreased LOC.

◆ ***Hypoxia.*** Lack of oxygen from any cause increases the rate (and often the depth) of breathing. Associated symptoms are related to the cause of the hypoxia.

◆ ***Interstitial fibrosis.*** In this disorder, tachypnea develops gradually and may become severe. Associated features include exertional dyspnea, pleuritic chest pain, a paroxysmal dry cough, crackles, late inspiratory wheezing, cyanosis, fatigue, and weight loss. Clubbing is a late sign.

◆ ***Lung abscess.*** In this type of abscess, tachypnea is usually paired with dyspnea and accentuated by fever. However, the chief sign is a productive cough with copious amounts of purulent, foul-smelling, usually bloody sputum. Other findings include chest pain, halitosis, diaphoresis, chills, fatigue, weakness, anorexia, weight loss, and clubbing.

◆ ***Lung, pleural, or mediastinal tumor.*** These types of tumors may cause tachypnea along with exertional dyspnea, cough, hemoptysis, and pleuritic chest pain. Other effects include anorexia, weight loss, and fatigue.

◆ ***Mesothelioma (malignant).*** Commonly related to asbestos exposure, this pleural mass initially produces tachypnea and dyspnea on mild exertion. Other classic symptoms are persistent dull chest pain and aching shoulder pain that progresses to arm weakness and paresthesia. Later signs and symptoms include a cough, insomnia associated with pain, clubbing, and dullness over the malignant mesothelioma.

◆ ***Neurogenic shock.*** Tachypnea is characteristic in this life-threatening type of shock. It's commonly accompanied by apprehension, bradycardia or tachycardia, oliguria, fluctuating body temperature, and decreased LOC that may progress to coma. The patient's skin is warm, dry, and perhaps flushed. He may experience nausea and vomiting.

◆ ***Plague.*** The onset of the pneumonic form of this virulent bacterial infection is usually sudden and marked by chills, fever, headache, and myalgia. Pulmonary signs and symptoms include tachypnea, a productive cough, chest pain, dyspnea, hemoptysis, increasing respiratory distress, and cardiopulmonary insufficiency. The pneumonic form may be contracted by inhaling respiratory droplets from an infected person. It could also be contracted from aerosolization and inhalation of the organism in biological warfare.

◆ ***Pneumonia (bacterial).*** A common sign in this infection, tachypnea is usually preceded by a painful, hacking, dry cough that rapidly becomes productive. Other signs and symptoms quickly follow, including high fever, shaking chills, headache, dyspnea, pleuritic chest pain, tachycardia, grunting respirations, nasal flaring, and cyanosis. Auscultation reveals diminished breath sounds and fine crackles; percussion yields a dull tone.

◆ ***Pneumothorax.*** Tachypnea, a common sign of life-threatening pneumothorax, is typically accompanied by severe, sharp, and commonly unilateral chest pain that's aggravated by chest movement. Associated signs and symptoms include dyspnea, tachycardia, accessory muscle use, asymmetrical chest expansion, a dry cough, cyanosis, anxiety, and restlessness. Examination of the affected lung reveals hyperresonance or tympany, subcutaneous crepitation, decreased vocal fremitus, and diminished or absent breath sounds. The patient with tension pneumothorax also develops a deviated trachea.

◆ ***Pulmonary edema.*** An early sign of this life-threatening disorder, tachypnea is accompanied by exertional dyspnea, paroxysmal nocturnal dyspnea and, later, orthopnea. Other features include a dry cough, crackles, tachycardia, and a ventricular gallop. In severe pulmonary edema, respirations become increasingly rapid and labored, tachycardia worsens, crackles become more diffuse, and. the cough produces frothy, bloody sputum. Signs of shock—such as hypotension, thready pulse, and cold, clammy skin—may also occur.

◆ ***Pulmonary embolism (acute).*** In pulmonary embolism, tachypnea occurs suddenly and is usually accompanied by dyspnea. The patient may complain of angina or pleuritic chest pain. Other characteristic findings include tachycardia, a dry or productive cough with blood-tinged sputum, low-grade fever, restlessness, and diaphoresis. Less common signs include massive hemoptysis, chest splinting, leg edema, and—with a large embolus—jugular vein distention and syncope. Other findings include pleural friction rub, crackles, diffuse wheezing, dullness on percussion, diminished breath sounds, and signs of shock, such as hypotension and a weak, rapid pulse.

◆ ***Pulmonary hypertension (primary).*** In this rare disorder, tachypnea is usually a late sign that's accompanied by exertional dyspnea, general fatigue, weakness, and episodes of syncope. The patient may complain of angina on exertion, which may radiate to the neck. Other effects include a cough, hemoptysis, and hoarseness.

◆ ***Septic shock.*** Early in septic shock, the patient usually experiences tachypnea; sudden fever; chills; flushed, warm, yet dry skin; and possibly nausea, vomiting, and diarrhea. He may also develop tachycardia and normal or slightly decreased blood pressure. As this life-threatening type of shock progresses, the patient may display anxiety; restlessness; decreased LOC; hypotension; cool, clammy, and cyanotic skin; rapid, thready pulse; thirst; and oliguria that may progress to anuria.

OTHER CAUSES

◆ ***Salicylates.*** Tachypnea may result from an overdose of these drugs.

SPECIAL CONSIDERATIONS

Continue to monitor the patient's vital signs closely. Be sure to keep suction and emergency equipment nearby. Prepare to intubate the patient and to provide mechanical ventilation if necessary. Prepare the patient for diagnostic studies, such as arterial blood gas analysis, blood cultures, chest X-rays, pulmonary function tests, and an electrocardiogram.

PEDIATRIC POINTERS

When assessing a child for tachypnea, be aware that the normal respiratory rate varies with the child's age. (See *Normal pediatric vital signs,* pages 646 and 647.) If you detect tachypnea, first rule out the causes listed above. Then consider these pediatric causes: congenital heart defects, meningitis, metabolic acidosis, and cystic fibrosis. Keep in mind, however, that hunger and anxiety may also cause tachypnea.

GERIATRIC POINTERS

Tachypnea may have a variety of causes in elderly patients, such as pneumonia, heart failure, COPD, anxiety, or failure to take cardiac and respiratory medications appropriately; mild increases in respiratory rate may be unnoticed.

PATIENT COUNSELING

Reassure the patient that slight increases in respiratory rate may be normal.

Taste abnormalities

There are several types of taste impairment. Ageusia is complete loss of taste; hypogeusia, partial loss of taste; and dysgeusia, a distorted sense of taste. In cacogeusia, food may taste unpleasant or even revolting.

The sensory receptors for taste are the taste buds, which are concentrated over the tongue's surface and scattered over the palate, pharynx, and larynx. These buds can differentiate among sweet, salty, sour, and bitter stimuli. More complex flavors are perceived by taste and olfactory receptors together. In fact, much of what people call taste is actually smell; food odors typically stimulate the olfactory system more strongly than food tastes stimulate the taste buds.

Any factor that interrupts transmission of taste stimuli to the brain may cause taste abnormalities. (See *Tracing taste pathways to the brain.*) Such factors include trauma, infection, vitamin and mineral deficiencies, neurologic and oral disorders, and drug effects. In addition, because tastes are most accurately perceived in a fluid medium, mouth dryness may interfere with taste.

Tracing taste pathways to the brain

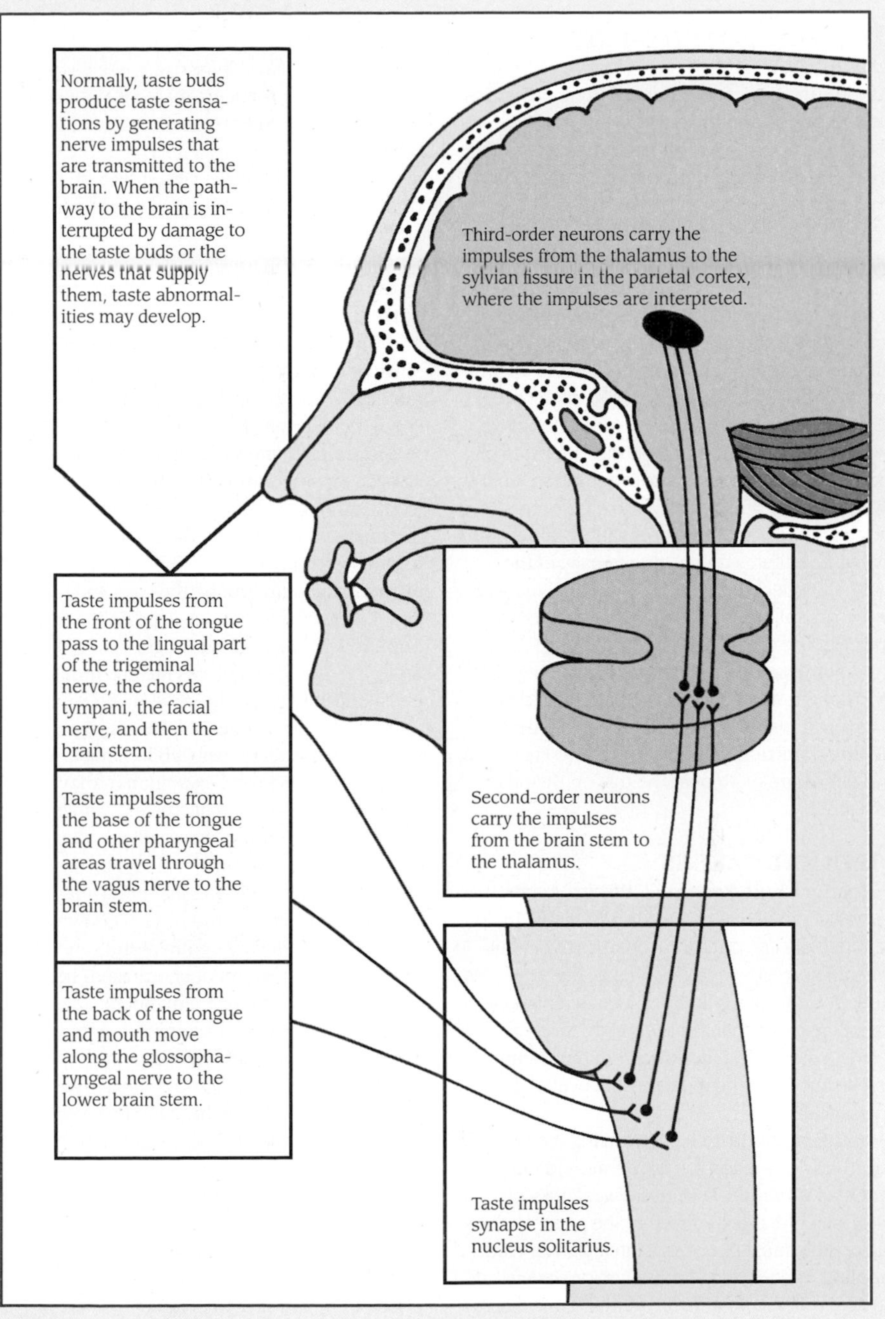

Normally, taste buds produce taste sensations by generating nerve impulses that are transmitted to the brain. When the pathway to the brain is interrupted by damage to the taste buds or the nerves that supply them, taste abnormalities may develop.
Third-order neurons carry the impulses from the thalamus to the sylvian fissure in the parietal cortex, where the impulses are interpreted.
Taste impulses from the front of the tongue pass to the lingual part of the trigeminal nerve, the chorda tympani, the facial nerve, and then the brain stem.
Taste impulses from the base of the tongue and other pharyngeal areas travel through the vagus nerve to the brain stem.
Taste impulses from the back of the tongue and mouth move along the glossopharyngeal nerve to the lower brain stem.
Second-order neurons carry the impulses from the brain stem to the thalamus.
Taste impulses synapse in the nucleus solitarius.

Two major nonpathologic causes of impaired taste are aging, which normally reduces the number of taste buds, and heavy smoking (especially pipe smoking), which dries the tongue.

History and physical examination

After noting the patient's age, find out when his taste abnormality began and then search for possible causes. Does the patient have a history of oral or other disorders? Has he recently had the flu or suffered head trauma? Does he smoke? Is he receiving radiation treatments? Is he currently taking any medications?

Next, thoroughly evaluate the patient's sense of taste. Gently withdraw his tongue slightly with a gauze sponge. Then use a moistened applicator to place a few crystals of salt or sugar on one side of the tongue. Ask the patient to identify the taste sensation while his tongue is protruded. Repeat the test on the other side of the tongue. To test bitter taste sensation, apply a tiny amount of quinine to the base of the tongue. To test sour taste sensation, apply a tiny amount of dilute vinegar on the base of the tongue. Inspect the oral cavity for lesions, sores, and mucosal abnormalities. Observe the taste buds for any obvious abnormalities.

Finally, evaluate the patient's sense of smell. Pinch one nostril and ask the patient to close his eyes and sniff through the open nostril to identify nonirritating odors, such as coffee, lime, and wintergreen. Repeat the test on the other nostril.

Medical causes

◆ ***Basilar skull fracture.*** If the first cranial nerve is involved in this traumatic injury, the patient usually can't detect aromatic flavors but can still correctly identify sweet, salty, sour, and bitter stimuli. Other findings include epistaxis, rhinorrhea, otorrhea, Battle's sign, raccoon eyes, headache, nausea and vomiting, hearing and vision loss, and a decreased level of consciousness.

◆ ***Bell's palsy.*** Taste loss involving the anterior two-thirds of the tongue is common in this disorder, as is hemifacial muscle weakness or paralysis. The affected side of the patient's face sags and is masklike. Associated signs include drooling and tearing, diminished or absent corneal reflex, and difficulty blinking the affected eye.

◆ ***Common cold.*** Although impaired taste sense is a common complaint, it's usually secondary to loss of smell. Other common features include rhinorrhea with nasal congestion, sore throat, headache, fatigue, myalgia, arthralgia, malaise, and a dry, hacking cough.

◆ ***Geographic tongue.*** Taste abnormalities occur along with many areas of loss and regrowth of filiform papillae. These areas are continually changing and produce a maplike appearance with denuded red patches surrounded by thick white borders.

◆ ***Influenza.*** After this viral infection, the patient may have hypogeusia, dysgeusia, or both. Typically, he also reports an impaired sense of smell.

◆ ***Oral cancer.*** About half of all oral tumors involve the tongue, especially the posterior portion and the lateral borders. These tumors may destroy or damage taste buds, resulting in impaired taste. The patient also has difficulty chewing and speaking and may develop halitosis.

◆ ***Sjögren's syndrome.*** In this autosomal recessive disorder, impaired sense of taste results from extreme mouth dryness associated with inadequate production of saliva. Ocular dryness, another characteristic finding, initially causes burning and pain around the eyes and under the lids. Later, the patient develops photosensitivity, impaired vision, and eye fatigue and redness. Other signs and symptoms include mouth soreness; difficulty chewing, swallowing, and talking; a dry cough; hoarseness; epistaxis; dry, scaly skin; decreased sweating; abdominal distress; and polyuria. Physical examination may reveal corneal ulceration, nasal crusting, and enlarged lacrimal, parotid, and submaxillary glands.

◆ ***Thalamic syndrome.*** This syndrome, caused by a lesion in the thalamus, may produce a distorted sense of taste. This symptom is typically preceded by contralateral sensory loss (both deep and cutaneous), transient hemiparesis, and homonymous hemianopia. Later, the patient gradually regains sensation and may then experience pain or hyperpathia.

◆ ***Thrush.*** Cream-colored or bluish-white patches of exudate on the tongue, mouth, or pharynx cause altered taste, pain, and a burning sensation. Thrush may cause respiratory distress in infants.

◆ ***Viral hepatitis (acute).*** Hypogeusia commonly precedes jaundice by 1 to 2 weeks. Associated signs and symptoms in the preicteric phase of hepatitis include altered sense of smell, anorexia, nausea and vomiting, fatigue, malaise, headache, photophobia, sore throat, and a cough. The patient may also experience muscle and joint aches.

◆ ***Vitamin B_{12} deficiency.*** In this vitamin deficiency, hypogeusia is accompanied by an impaired sense of smell, anorexia, weight loss, abdominal discomfort, and glossitis. The patient may also exhibit yellow skin, peripheral neuropathy, dyspnea, ataxic gait, and dementia.

◆ ***Zinc deficiency.*** This mineral deficiency is common in patients with idiopathic hypogeusia, suggesting that zinc plays an important role in normal taste sensation. Common associated findings include cacogeusia, an altered sense of smell, anorexia, soft and misshapen nails, and sparse hair growth. Palpation may reveal an enlarged liver and spleen.

OTHER CAUSES

◆ ***Drugs.*** Drugs that may distort the sense of taste include penicillamine, captopril, griseofulvin, lithium, rifampin, antithyroid preparations, procarbazine, vincristine, and vinblastine.

◆ ***Radiation therapy.*** Irradiation of the head or neck may cause excessive dryness of the mouth, resulting in impaired taste sensation.

SPECIAL CONSIDERATIONS

Modify the patient's diet, if necessary, so that he can distinguish and enjoy as many tastes as possible.

PEDIATRIC POINTERS

Recognize that young children are frequently unable to differentiate between an abnormal taste sensation and a simple taste dislike.

Tearing, increased

[Epiphora]

Tears normally bathe the eyes, keeping the epithelium moist and flushing away foreign bodies. Excessive lacrimation (tear production) usually results from inadequate tear drainage due to obstruction of the lacrimal drainage system or malposition of the lower lid. Reflex tearing occurs with any disturbance of the corneal epithelium.

Lacrimation may be classified as psychic or neurogenic. Psychic lacrimation normally occurs in response to emotional or physical stress, such as pain, and is the most common cause of increased tearing. Neurogenic lacrimation is triggered by reflex stimulation associated with ocular trauma or inflammation or with exposure to environmental irritants, such as strong light, dry or hot wind, or airborne allergens. This type of lacrimation may also accompany eyestrain, yawning, vomiting, and laughing.

Decreased tearing can be caused by aging, vitamin A deficiency, eye trauma, and the use of certain drugs. (See *Causes of decreased tearing*.)

Causes of decreased tearing

Decreased tearing makes the patient's eyes uncomfortably dry. This symptom is usually associated with aging, but it may also result from the following:

Anticholinergic use. Decreased tearing commonly follows administration of an anticholinergic (mydriatic), such as atropine, scopolamine, cyclopentolate, or tropicamide.

Keratoconjunctivitis sicca (dry eye syndrome). In this syndrome, atrophy of the lacrimal glands curtails tear production.

Ocular trauma. Decreased tearing may accompany healing and scar formation after acute ocular trauma.

Sarcoidosis. Decreased tearing results from inflammation of the lacrimal and salivary glands in this syndrome.

Stevens-Johnson syndrome. In this syndrome, decreased tearing is accompanied by purulent conjunctivitis and severe eye pain.

Turner's syndrome (Bonnevie-Ullrich syndrome). Characterized by congenital absence of the lacrimal gland, this syndrome causes decreased tearing.

Vitamin A deficiency. Typically, this vitamin deficiency causes decreased tearing and poor night vision.

Nontraumatic decreased tearing is usually treated with artificial tear drops or ointment.

HISTORY AND PHYSICAL EXAMINATION

If the patient complains of increased tearing, begin by fully exploring this sign. When did it begin? Is it constant or intermittent? Minimal or extensive? Is increased tearing accompanied by pain, irritation, or any other eye drainage or discharge? Next, ask about recent eye trauma and about ocular and systemic disorders. Then record which drugs the patient is taking. Note his occupation and the nature of his work. For example, does he read extensively, look at a computer screen frequently, or work with small or fine objects? Is he exposed to any chemicals or dust in the workplace?

After taking vital signs, examine both eyes—unless the history suggests a perforating or penetrating injury. Carefully inspect the external structures. Do the eyelashes contain debris? Examine the eyelids for lesions and edema. Ask the patient to look straight ahead at a fixed object while you check for ptosis. Are the lid margins turned inward or outward? Examine the eyeballs. Do they appear sunken or bulging? Examine the conjunctivae for redness and abnormal drainage. Also, note the color of the sclera. Hold a flashlight at the side of each eye and examine the cornea and iris for scars, irregularities, and foreign bodies. Evaluate extraocular muscle function by testing the six cardinal fields of gaze. (See *Testing extraocular muscles,* page 217.) Finally, test the patient's visual acuity.

Medical causes

◆ ***Blepharophimosis.*** Increased tearing and exposure keratitis—corneal inflammation with incomplete lid closure—are common signs of this disorder. Examination also reveals ectropion; a small, expressionless face with deep-set eyes and pursed lips; and a high-arched palate.

◆ ***Conjunctival foreign body or abrasion.*** Increased tearing may accompany localized conjunctival injection, severe eye pain, and photophobia. A foreign-body sensation may be present.

◆ ***Conjunctivitis.*** Typically, increased tearing is accompanied by conjunctival injection and itching in this disorder. *Allergic conjunctivitis* also causes a stringy discharge. *Bacterial conjunctivitis* also causes a copious purulent discharge, burning, a foreign-body sensation and, possibly, eye pain if the cornea is involved. Associated signs of *fungal conjunctivitis* include lid edema, burning, and a copious thick, purulent discharge that may form sticky crusts on the lids. The patient complains of photophobia and pain if the cornea is involved. Highly contagious viral conjunctivitis also causes a foreign-body sensation, slight exudate, and lid edema.

◆ ***Corneal abrasion.*** Marked by severe corneal pain that's aggravated by blinking, this injury also causes increased tearing. Associated features are a foreign-body sensation, blurred vision, conjunctival injection, and photophobia, which makes opening the lids difficult.

◆ ***Corneal foreign body.*** When a foreign body lodges in the cornea, the patient experiences increased tearing, blurred vision, a foreign-body sensation, photophobia, eye pain, miosis, and conjunctival injection. A dark speck may also be visible in the cornea.

◆ ***Corneal ulcer.*** In this vision-threatening disorder, increased tearing is accompanied by severe photophobia and eye pain. Typically, the disorder begins with pain that's aggravated by blinking. Ulcers also cause blurred vision, conjunctival injection, and a white opaque cornea. Bacterial ulcers also produce a copious purulent discharge that may form sticky crusts on the lids.

◆ ***Dacryocystitis.*** Increased tearing and a purulent discharge are the chief complaints in this disorder, which usually affects only one eye. Associated signs and symptoms include pain and tenderness around the tear sac with marked eyelid edema and redness near the lacrimal punctum. Pressure on the tear sac expresses a thick, purulent discharge or, in chronic cases, a mucoid discharge.

◆ ***Dry eye syndrome.*** Excessive dryness of the cornea and conjunctiva can cause reflex stimulation of the lacrimal gland and excess tearing.

◆ ***Episcleritis.*** Commonly unilateral, this disorder causes increased tearing, photophobia, and—if the sclera is inflamed—eye pain and tenderness on palpation. Inspection reveals conjunctival injection and edema, a purplish pink sclera, and episcleral edema.

◆ ***Eyelid contractions.*** In this disorder, increased tearing usually results from stricture of the canaliculi. Because eyelid contractions are caused by burns or chemical or mechanical trauma, eyelid scars are also commonly visible.

◆ ***Herpes zoster.*** Increased tearing usually occurs when herpes zoster affects the trigeminal nerve. It's accompanied by severe unilateral facial and eye pain that's followed in several days by the eruption of vesicles. The patient's eyelids are red and swollen with scanty serous discharge. Other common findings include a white, cloudy cornea and conjunctival injection.

◆ ***Psoriasis vulgaris.*** When these psoriatic lesions affect the eyelids and extend into the conjunctivae, they may cause irritation, increased tearing, and a foreign-body sensation. The lesions are typically preceded by signs of chronic conjunctivitis, such as a copious mucoid discharge and conjunctival injection.

◆ ***Punctum misplacement.*** Increased tearing is characteristic when ectropion involves the punctum, causing misplacement. It may be accompanied by exposure keratitis.

◆ ***Raeder's syndrome.*** This syndrome is characterized by periodic attacks of unilateral paroxysmal neuralgic pain in the face lasting 5 minutes or longer. The patient may exhibit increased tearing, ptosis, diplopia, enophthalmos, abnormal pupillary response, ipsilateral headache, and anhidrosis of the face and neck.

◆ ***Scleritis.*** This rare chronic disorder causes increased tearing, photophobia, and severe eye pain with tenderness on palpation. Examination reveals conjunctival injection and a bluish purple sclera.

◆ ***Thyrotoxicosis.*** This disorder may cause increased tearing, usually in both eyes. Other ocular effects include ptosis, lid edema, photophobia, a foreign-body sensation, conjunctival injection, chemosis, diplopia and, at times, exophthalmos. Common associated features are heat intolerance, weight loss despite increased appetite, nervousness, diaphoresis, diarrhea, tremors, tachycardia, palpitations, and an enlarged thyroid gland.

◆ ***Trachoma.*** An early sign of trachoma, increased tearing is accompanied by visible conjunctival follicles, red and edematous eyelids, pain, photophobia, and exudation. If the infection is untreated, conjunctival follicles enlarge into inflamed papillae that later become yellow or gray and small blood vessels invade the cornea under the upper lid.

Other causes

◆ ***Cholinergics.*** Miotics, such as pilocarpine, may increase tearing.

Special considerations

Obtain a tear specimen for culture, and isolate the patient until a definitive diagnosis is made. Also, prepare him for irrigation of the lacrimal drainage system and for Schirmer's test to measure tear production and secretion.

Pediatric pointers

The most common causes of increased tearing in children are allergies, conjunctivitis, and the common cold.

Patient counseling

Instruct the patient not to touch the unaffected eye to avoid possible cross-contamination. Teach the patient not to share eye makeup or pillowcases and to practice good hand-washing techniques.

Throat pain

Throat pain—commonly known as a sore throat—refers to discomfort in any part of the pharynx: the nasopharynx, the oropharynx, or the hypopharynx. This common symptom ranges from a sensation of scratchiness to severe pain. It's commonly accompanied by ear pain because cranial nerves IX and X innervate the pharynx as well as the middle and external ear. (See *Anatomy of the throat*, page 658.)

Throat pain may result from infection, trauma, allergy, cancer, or a systemic disorder. It may also follow surgery and endotracheal intubation. Nonpathologic causes include dry mucous membranes associated with mouth breathing and laryngeal irritation associated with vocal strain, alcohol consumption, and inhalation of smoke or chemicals such as ammonia.

History and physical examination

Ask the patient when he first noticed the pain and have him describe it. Has he had throat pain before? Is it accompanied by fever, ear pain, or dysphagia? Review the patient's medical history for throat problems, allergies, and systemic disorders.

Next, carefully examine the pharynx, noting redness, exudate, or swelling. Examine the oropharynx, using a warmed metal spatula or tongue blade, and the nasopharynx, using a warmed laryngeal mirror or a fiber-optic nasopharyngoscope. Laryngoscopic examination of the hypopharynx may be required. (If necessary, spray the soft palate and pharyngeal wall with a local anesthetic to prevent gagging.) Observe the tonsils for redness, swelling, or exudate; if exudate is present, obtain a specimen for culture. Then examine the nose, using a nasal speculum. Also, check the patient's ears, especially if he reports ear pain. Finally, palpate the neck and oropharynx for nodules or lymph node enlargement.

Medical causes

◆ ***Agranulocytosis.*** In this disorder, sore throat may accompany other signs and symptoms of infection, such as fever, chills, and headache. Typically, it follows progressive fatigue and weakness. Other findings include nausea and

Anatomy of the throat

The throat, or pharynx, is divided into three areas: the nasopharynx (the soft palate and the posterior nasal cavity), the oropharynx (the area between the soft palate and the upper edge of the epiglottis), and the hypopharynx (the area between the epiglottis and the level of the cricoid cartilage). A disorder affecting any of these areas may cause throat pain. Pinpointing the causative disorder begins with accurate assessment of the throat structures illustrated here.

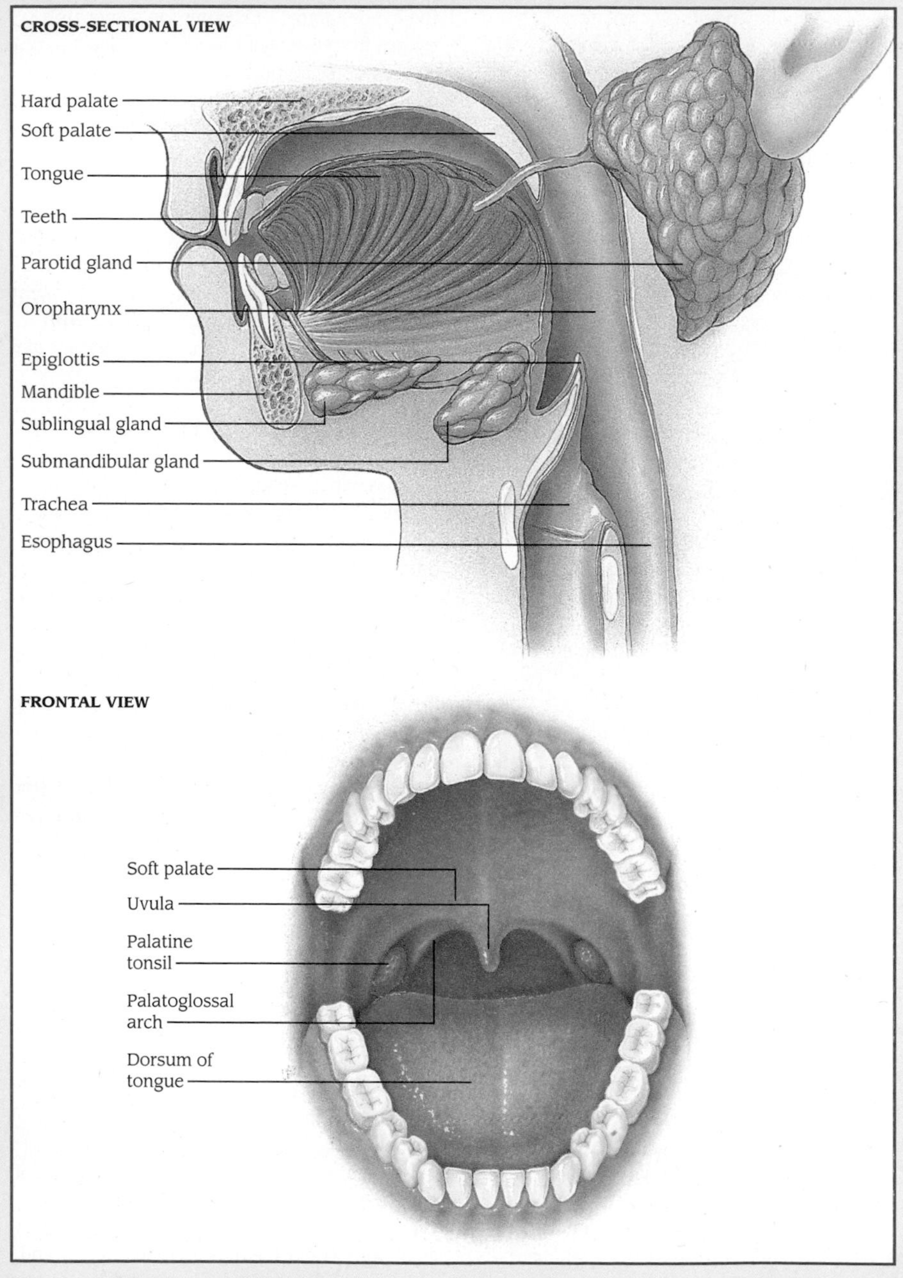

vomiting, anorexia, and bleeding tendencies. Rough-edged ulcers with gray or black membranes may appear on the gums, palate, or perianal area.

◆ ***Allergic rhinitis.*** Occurring seasonally or year-round, this disorder may produce sore throat as well as nasal congestion with a thin nasal discharge, postnasal drip, paroxysmal sneezing, decreased sense of smell, frontal or temporal headache, and itchy eyes, nose, and throat. Examination reveals pale and glistening nasal mucosa with edematous nasal turbinates, watery eyes, reddened conjunctivae and eyelids and, possibly, swollen eyelids.

◆ ***Avian influenza.*** Throat pain, muscle aches, cough, and fever are common early symptoms of avian influenza. The most virulent of these viruses, avian influenza A (H5N1), may also cause pneumonia, acute respiratory distress, and other life-threatening complications. A recent outbreak of the H5N1 virus among domesticated birds (chickens, turkeys, geese) in Asian countries has caused human sickness and death in those who contracted the virus from infected poultry and contaminated surfaces. Studies are underway to investigate the effectiveness of antiviral medications and vaccines.

◆ ***Bronchitis (acute).*** This disorder may produce lower throat pain, fever, chills, cough, and muscle and back pain. Auscultation reveals rhonchi, wheezing, and sometimes crackles.

◆ ***Chronic fatigue syndrome.*** This nonspecific symptom complex is characterized by incapacitating fatigue. Associated findings include sore throat, myalgia, and cognitive dysfunction.

◆ ***Common cold.*** Sore throat may accompany cough, sneezing, nasal congestion, rhinorrhea, fatigue, headache, myalgia, and arthralgia.

◆ ***Contact ulcers.*** Common in men with stressful jobs, contact ulcers appear symmetrically on the posterior vocal cords, resulting in sore throat. The pain is aggravated by talking and may be accompanied by referred ear pain and occasionally hemoptysis. Typically, the patient also has a history of chronic throat clearing or acid reflux.

◆ ***Foreign body.*** A foreign body lodged in the palatine or lingual tonsil and pyriform sinus may produce localized throat pain. The pain may persist after the foreign body is dislodged until mucosal irritation resolves.

◆ ***Gastroesophageal reflux disease.*** In this disorder, an incompetent gastroesophageal sphincter allows gastric juices to enter the hypopharynx and irritate the larynx, causing chronic sore throat and hoarseness. The arytenoid cartilage may also appear red and swollen, resulting in a sensation of a lump in the throat.

◆ ***Glossopharyngeal neuralgia.*** Triggered by a specific pharyngeal movement, such as yawning or swallowing, this condition causes unilateral, knifelike throat pain in the tonsillar fossa that may radiate to the ear.

◆ ***Herpes simplex virus.*** Sore throat may result from lesions on the oral mucosa, especially the tongue, gingivae, and cheeks. After causing brief prodromal discomfort, lesions erupt into erythematous vesicles that eventually rupture and leave a painful ulcer, followed by a yellowish crust. In generalized infection, the vesicles accompany submaxillary lymphadenopathy, halitosis, increased salivation, anorexia, and fever of up to 105° F (40.6° C).

◆ ***Influenza.*** Patients with the flu commonly complain of sore throat, fever with chills, headache, weakness, malaise, myalgia, cough and, occasionally, hoarseness and rhinorrhea.

◆ ***Laryngeal cancer.*** In extrinsic laryngeal cancer, the chief symptom is pain or burning in the throat when drinking citrus juice or hot liquids, or a lump in the throat; in intrinsic laryngeal cancer, it's hoarseness that persists for longer than 3 weeks. Later signs and symptoms of metastasis include dysphagia, dyspnea, a cough, enlarged cervical lymph nodes, and pain that radiates to the ear.

◆ ***Laryngitis (acute).*** This disorder produces sore throat, but its cardinal sign is mild to severe hoarseness, perhaps with temporary loss of voice. Other findings are malaise, low-grade fever, dysphagia, dry cough, and tender, enlarged cervical lymph nodes.

◆ ***Monkeypox.*** Early symptoms of this rare viral disease include sore throat, fever, lymphadenopathy, chills, myalgia, and rash. The virus exhibits some similarities to smallpox, but its symptoms tend to be milder. Monkeypox is spread primarily through contact with lesions or body fluids of infected animals. Although it occurs primarily in central and western Africa, the virus has also been reported in the United States since 2003. There's no specific treatment for monkeypox, which typically lasts 2 to 4 weeks.

◆ ***Mononucleosis (infectious).*** Sore throat is one of the three classic findings in this infection. The other two classic signs are cervical lymphadenopathy and fluctuating temperature with an evening peak of 101° to 102° F (38.3° to 38.9° C). Splenomegaly and hepatomegaly may also develop.

◆ ***Necrotizing ulcerative gingivitis (acute).*** Also known as trench mouth, this disorder usually begins abruptly with sore throat and tender gums that ulcerate and bleed. A gray exudate may cover the gums and pharyngeal tonsils. Related signs and symptoms include a foul taste in the mouth, halitosis, cervical lymphadenopathy, headache, malaise, and fever.

◆ ***Peritonsillar abscess.*** A complication of bacterial tonsillitis, this abscess typically causes severe throat pain that radiates to the ear. Accompanying the pain may be dysphagia, drooling, dysarthria, halitosis, fever with chills, malaise, and nausea. The patient usually tilts his head toward the side of the abscess. Examination may also reveal a deviated uvula, trismus, and tender, enlarged cervical lymph nodes.

◆ ***Pharyngeal burns.*** First- or second-degree burns of the posterior pharynx may cause throat pain and dysphagia.

◆ ***Pharyngitis.*** Whether bacterial, fungal, or viral, pharyngitis may cause sore throat and localized erythema and edema. *Bacterial pharyngitis* begins abruptly with a unilateral sore throat. Associated signs and symptoms include dysphagia, fever, malaise, headache, abdominal pain, myalgia, and arthralgia. Inspection reveals an exudate on the tonsil or tonsillar fossa, uvular edema, soft palate erythema, and tender cervical lymph nodes.

Also known as thrush, *fungal pharyngitis* causes diffuse sore throat—commonly described as a burning sensation—accompanied by pharyngeal erythema and edema. White plaques mark the pharynx, tonsil, tonsillar pillars, base of the tongue, and oral mucosa; scraping these plaques uncovers a hemorrhagic base.

Viral pharyngitis produces a diffuse sore throat, malaise, fever, and mild erythema and edema of the posterior oropharyngeal wall. Tonsil enlargement and anterior cervical lymphadenopathy may be present.

◆ ***Pharyngomaxillary space abscess.*** A complication of untreated pharyngeal or tonsillar infection or tooth extraction, pharyngomaxillary space abscess causes mild throat pain. Inspection reveals a bulge in the medial wall of the pharynx accompanied by swelling of the neck and at the jaw angle on the affected side. Other signs and symptoms include fever, dysphagia, trismus and, possibly, signs of respiratory distress or toxemia.

◆ ***Sinusitis (acute).*** This disorder may cause sore throat with a purulent nasal discharge and postnasal drip, resulting in halitosis. Other effects include headache, malaise, cough, fever, and facial pain and swelling associated with nasal congestion.

◆ ***Tongue cancer.*** The patient with tongue cancer experiences localized throat pain that may occur around a raised white lesion or ulcer. The pain may radiate to the ear and be accompanied by dysphagia.

◆ ***Tonsillar cancer.*** Sore throat is the presenting symptom in tonsillar cancer. Unfortunately, the cancer is usually quite advanced before this symptom appears. The pain may radiate to the ear and is accompanied by a superficial ulcer on the tonsil or one that extends to the base of the tongue.

◆ ***Tonsillitis.*** Mild to severe sore throat is usually the first symptom of acute tonsillitis. The pain may radiate to the ears and be accompanied by dysphagia and headache. Related findings include malaise, fever with chills, halitosis, myalgia, arthralgia, and tender cervical lymph nodes. Examination reveals edematous, reddened tonsils with a purulent exudate.

Chronic tonsillitis causes a mild sore throat, malaise, and tender cervical lymph nodes. The tonsils appear smooth, pink and, possibly, enlarged, with purulent debris in the crypts. Halitosis and a foul taste in the mouth are other common findings.

Unilateral or bilateral throat pain occurs just above the hyoid bone in lingual tonsillitis. The lingual tonsils appear red and swollen and are covered with exudate. Other findings include a muffled voice, dysphagia, and tender cervical lymph nodes on the affected side.

◆ ***Uvulitis.*** This inflammation may cause throat pain or a sensation of something in the throat. The uvula is usually swollen and red but, in allergic uvulitis, it's pale.

Other causes

◆ ***Treatments.*** Endotracheal intubation and local surgery, such as tonsillectomy and adenoidectomy, commonly cause sore throat.

Special considerations

Provide analgesic sprays or lozenges to relieve throat pain. Also, prepare the patient for a throat culture, a complete blood count, and a mononucleosis spot test.

Pediatric pointers

Sore throat is a common complaint in children and may result from many of the same disorders that affect adults. Other pediatric causes of sore throat include acute epiglottiditis, herpangina, scarlet fever, acute follicular tonsillitis, and retropharyngeal abscess.

Patient counseling

If the patient is taking antibiotics, stress the importance of completing the 10-day course of treatment, even if symptoms improve after only a few days. Tell the patient that he's presumed noninfectious after 24 hours of antibiotic coverage. Suggest gargling with salt water to soothe the throat.

Thyroid enlargement

An enlarged thyroid can result from inflammation, physiologic changes, iodine deficiency, and thyroid tumors. Depending on the medical cause, hyperfunction or hypofunction may occur with resulting excess or deficiency, respectively, of the hormone thyroxine. If no infection is present, enlargement is usually slow and progressive. An enlarged thyroid that causes visible swelling in the front of the neck is called a *goiter*.

History and physical examination

The patient's history commonly reveals the cause of thyroid enlargement. Important data include a family history of thyroid disease, when the thyroid enlargement began, any previous irradiation of the thyroid or the neck, recent infections, and the use of thyroid replacement drugs.

Begin the physical examination by inspecting the patient's trachea for midline deviation. Although you can usually see the enlarged gland, you should always palpate it. To palpate the thyroid gland, you'll need to stand behind the patient. Give the patient a cup of water, and have him extend his neck slightly. Place the fingers of both hands on the patient's neck, just below the cricoid cartilage and just lateral to the trachea. Tell the patient to take a sip of water and swallow. The thyroid gland should rise as he swallows. Use your fingers to palpate laterally and downward to feel the whole thyroid gland. Palpate over the midline to feel the isthmus of the thyroid.

During palpation, be sure to note the size, shape, and consistency of the gland as well as the presence or absence of nodules. Using the bell of a stethoscope, listen over the lateral lobes for a bruit, which is commonly continuous.

Medical causes

- ***Hypothyroidism.*** This disorder, which is most prevalent in women, usually results from a dysfunction of the thyroid gland caused by surgery, irradiation therapy, chronic autoimmune thyroiditis (Hashimoto's disease), or inflammatory conditions, such as amyloidosis and sarcoidosis. Besides an enlarged thyroid, signs and symptoms include weight gain despite anorexia; fatigue; cold intolerance; constipation; menorrhagia; slowed intellectual and motor activity; dry, pale, cool skin; dry, sparse hair; and thick, brittle nails. Eventually, the face assumes a dull expression with periorbital edema.
- ***Iodine deficiency.*** A goiter may result from a lack of iodine in the diet. A goiter that arises from a deficiency of iodine in the food or water of a particular area is called an *endemic goiter*. Associated signs and symptoms of an endemic goiter include dysphagia, dyspnea, and tracheal deviation. This condition is uncommon in developed countries with iodized salt.
- ***Thyroiditis.*** Thyroiditis, an inflammation of the thyroid gland, may be classified as acute or subacute. It may be due to bacterial or viral infections, in which case associated features include fever and thyroid tenderness. The most prevalent cause of spontaneous hypothyroidism, however, is an autoimmune reaction, as occurs in Hashimoto's thyroiditis. Autoimmune thyroiditis usually produces no symptoms other than thyroid enlargement.
- ***Thyrotoxicosis.*** Overproduction of thyroid hormone causes thyrotoxicosis. The most common form is Graves' disease, which may result from genetic or immunologic factors. Associated signs and symptoms include nervousness; heat intolerance; fatigue; weight loss despite increased appetite; diarrhea; diaphoresis; palpitations; tremors; smooth, warm, flushed skin; fine, soft hair; exophthalmos; nausea and vomiting due to increased GI motility and peristalsis; and, in females, oligomenorrhea or amenorrhea.
- ***Tumors.*** An enlarged thyroid may result from a malignant tumor or a nonmalignant tumor (such as an adenoma). A malignant tumor usually appears as a single nodule in the neck; a nonmalignant tumor may appear as multiple nodules in the neck. Associated signs and symptoms include hoarseness, loss of voice, and dysphagia.

Thyroid tissue contained in ovarian dermoid tumors can function autonomously or in combination with thyrotoxicosis. Pituitary tumors that secrete thyroid-stimulating hormone (TSH), a rare type, are the only cause of normal or high TSH levels in association with thyrotoxicosis. Finally, high levels of human chorionic gonadotropin, as seen in trophoblastic tumors and pregnant women, can cause thyrotoxicosis.

Other causes

◆ ***Goitrogens.*** Goitrogens are drugs and substances in foods that decrease thyroxine production. Drugs containing goitrogens include lithium, sulfonamides, and para-aminosalicylic acid. Foods containing goitrogens include peanuts, cabbage, soybeans, strawberries, spinach, rutabagas, and radishes.

Special considerations

Prepare the patient with an enlarged thyroid for scheduled tests, which may include needle aspiration, ultrasound, and radioactive thyroid scanning. Also prepare him for surgery or radiation therapy, if necessary. If the patient has a goiter, support him as he expresses his feelings about his appearance.

The hypothyroid patient will need a warm room and moisturizing lotion for his skin. A gentle laxative and stool softener may help with constipation. Provide a high-fiber, low-calorie diet, and encourage activity to promote weight loss. Warn the patient to report any infection immediately; if he develops a fever, monitor his temperature until it's stable. After thyroid replacement therapy begins, watch for signs and symptoms of hyperthyroidism, such as restlessness, diaphoresis, and excessive weight loss. Avoid administering a sedative, if possible, or reduce the dosage because hypothyroidism delays metabolism of many drugs. Check arterial blood gas levels for indications of hypoxia and respiratory acidosis to determine whether the patient needs ventilatory assistance.

Give patients with thyroiditis an antibiotic and watch for elevations in temperature, which may indicate developing resistance to the antibiotic. Check vital signs, and examine the patient's neck for unusual swelling or redness. Provide a liquid diet if the patient has difficulty swallowing. Check for signs of hyperthyroidism, such as nervousness, tremor, and weakness, which are common in subacute thyroiditis. If the patient has severe hyperthyroidism (thyroid storm), closely monitor his temperature, volume status, heart rate, and blood pressure.

After thyroidectomy, check vital signs every 15 to 30 minutes until the patient's condition stabilizes. Be alert for signs of tetany secondary to parathyroid injury during surgery. Monitor postoperative serum calcium levels, and keep 10% calcium gluconate available for I.V. use as needed. Evaluate dressings frequently for excessive bleeding, and watch for signs of airway obstruction, such as difficulty talking, increased swallowing, or stridor. Keep tracheotomy equipment handy.

Pediatric pointers

Congenital goiter occurs in infantile myxedema (cretinism), a syndrome characterized by mental retardation, growth failure, and other signs and symptoms of hypothyroidism. Early treatment can prevent mental retardation. Advise the parents to obtain genetic counseling because their subsequent children are also at risk for this disorder.

Patient counseling

Instruct the patient to watch for signs and symptoms of hypothyroidism, such as lethargy, restlessness, dry skin, and sensitivity to cold. Advise the patient with Graves' disease to use artificial tears frequently if proptosis causes his eyes to become dry. If the hyperthyroid patient is receiving therapy with radioactive iodine, tell him not to expectorate or cough freely after treatment because his saliva is radioactive for 24 hours.

Inform the patient that lifelong thyroid hormone replacement therapy is necessary after thyroidectomy or radioactive destruction of the thyroid gland. Tell him to watch for signs of an overdose, such as nervousness and palpitations.

Tics

A tic is an involuntary, repetitive movement of a specific group of muscles—usually those of the face, neck, shoulders, trunk, and hands. This sign typically occurs suddenly and intermittently. It may involve a single isolated movement—such as lip smacking, grimacing, blinking, sniffing, tongue thrusting, throat clearing, hitching up one shoulder, or protruding the chin—or a complex set of movements. Mild tics, such as twitching of an eyelid, are especially common. Tics differ from minor seizures in that tics aren't associated with transient loss of consciousness or amnesia. (See *Classifying tics*.)

Tics are usually psychogenic and may be aggravated by stress or anxiety. Psychogenic tics typically begin between ages 5 and 10 as voluntary, coordinated, and purposeful actions that

Classifying tics

According to the *Diagnostic and Statistical Manual of Mental Disorders,* Fourth Edition, Text Revision, motor and vocal tics are classified as simple or complex; however, category boundaries remain unclear. Also, combinations of tics may occur simultaneously.

Motor tics

Simple motor tics include eye blinking, neck jerking, shoulder shrugging, head banging, head turning, tongue protrusion, lip or tongue biting, nail biting, hair pulling, and facial grimacing.

Some examples of complex motor tics are facial gestures, grooming behaviors, hitting or biting oneself, jumping, hopping, touching, squatting, deep knee bends, retracing steps, twirling when walking, stamping, smelling an object, and imitating the movements of someone who is being observed (echopraxia).

Vocal tics

Simple vocal tics include coughing, throat clearing, grunting, sniffing, snorting, hissing, clicking, yelping, and barking.

Complex vocal tics may involve repeating words out of context; using socially unacceptable words, many of which are obscene (coprolalia); or repeating the last-heard sound, word, or phrase of another person (echolalia).

the child feels compelled to perform to decrease anxiety. Unless the tics are severe, the child may be unaware of them. The tics may subside as the child matures, or they may persist into adulthood. However, tics are also associated with one rare affliction—Tourette syndrome, which typically begins during childhood.

HISTORY AND PHYSICAL EXAMINATION

Begin by asking the parents how long the child has had the tic and how often he experiences it. Can they identify any precipitating or exacerbating factors? Can the patient control the tics with conscious effort? Ask about stressors in the child's life, such as difficult school work. Next, carefully observe the tic. Is it a purposeful or involuntary movement? Note whether it's localized or generalized, and describe it in detail.

MEDICAL CAUSES

◆ ***Tourette syndrome.*** This syndrome, which is thought to be largely a genetic disorder, typically begins between ages 2 and 15 with a tic that involves the face or neck. It may include both motor and vocal tics that may involve the muscles of the shoulders, arms, trunk, and legs. The tics may be associated with violent movements and outbursts of obscenities (coprolalia). The patient snorts, barks, and grunts and may emit explosive sounds, such as hissing, when he speaks. He may involuntarily repeat another person's words (echolalia) or movements (echopraxia). Tourette syndrome sometimes subsides spontaneously or undergoes a prolonged remission, but it may persist throughout life.

SPECIAL CONSIDERATIONS

Psychotherapy and administration of a tranquilizer may provide relief. Many patients with Tourette syndrome receive haloperidol, pimozide, or another antipsychotic to control tics. Help the patient identify and eliminate any avoidable stressors and learn positive ways to deal with anxiety. Offer emotional support to the patient and family.

Tinnitus

Tinnitus literally means ringing in the ears, but many other abnormal sounds fall under this term. For example, tinnitus may be described as the sound of escaping air, running water, or the inside of a seashell or as a sizzling, buzzing, or humming noise. Occasionally, it's described as a roaring or musical sound. This common symptom may be unilateral or bilateral and constant or intermittent. Although the brain may adjust to or suppress constant tinnitus, some patients are so disturbed by the sounds that they contemplate suicide as their only source of relief.

Tinnitus can be classified in several ways. Subjective tinnitus is heard only by the patient; objective tinnitus is also heard by the observer who places a stethoscope near the patient's affected ear. Tinnitus aurium refers to noise that the patient hears in his ears; tinnitus cerebri, to noise that he hears in his head.

Tinnitus is usually associated with neural injury in the auditory pathway, resulting in spontaneous altered firing of sensory auditory neurons. It may stem from an ear disorder, a cardiovascular or systemic disorder, or the effects of certain drugs. Nonpathologic causes of

Common causes of tinnitus

Tinnitus usually results from a disorder that affects the external, middle, or inner ear. Below are some of its more common causes and their locations.

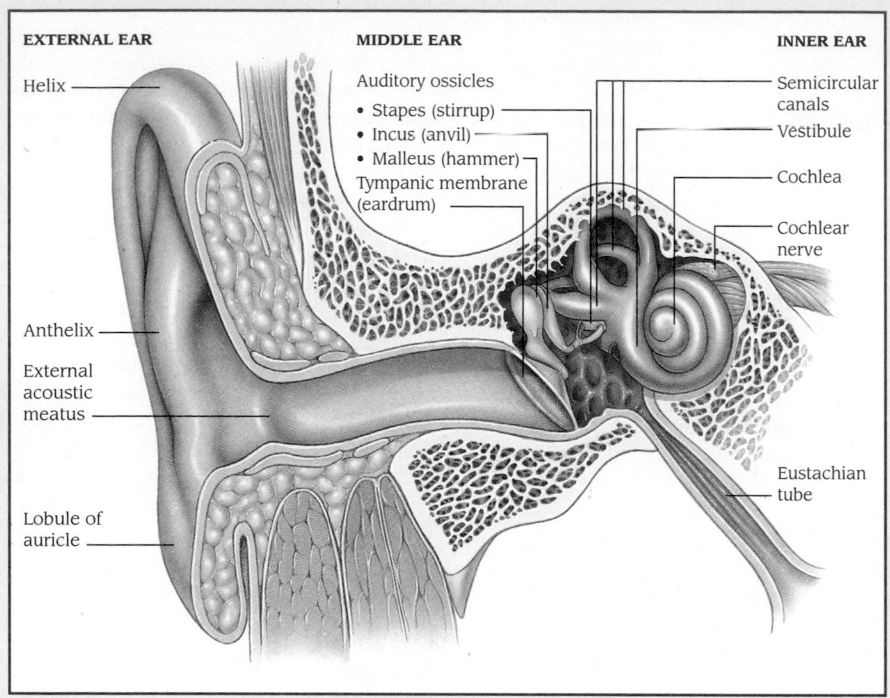

External ear
- ◆ Ear canal obstruction by cerumen or a foreign body
- ◆ Otitis externa
- ◆ Tympanic membrane perforation

Middle ear
- ◆ Ossicle dislocation
- ◆ Otitis media
- ◆ Otosclerosis

Inner ear
- ◆ Acoustic neuroma
- ◆ Atherosclerosis of carotid artery
- ◆ Labyrinthitis
- ◆ Ménière's disease

tinnitus include acute anxiety and presbycusis. (See *Common causes of tinnitus*.)

History and physical examination

Ask the patient to describe the sound he hears, including its onset, pattern, pitch, location, and intensity. Ask whether it's accompanied by other symptoms, such as vertigo, headache, or hearing loss. Next, take a health history, including a complete drug history.

Using an otoscope, inspect the patient's ears and examine the tympanic membrane. To check for hearing loss, perform the Weber and Rinne tuning fork tests. (See *Differentiating conductive from sensorineural hearing loss,* page 350.)

Also, auscultate for bruits in the neck. Then compress the jugular vein or carotid artery to see if this affects the tinnitus. Finally, examine the nasopharynx for masses that might cause eustachian tube dysfunction and tinnitus.

Medical causes

◆ ***Acoustic neuroma.*** An early symptom of this eighth cranial nerve tumor, unilateral tinnitus precedes unilateral sensorineural hearing loss and vertigo. Facial paralysis, headache, nausea, vomiting, and papilledema may also occur.

◆ ***Anemia.*** Severe anemia may produce mild, reversible tinnitus. Other common effects include pallor, weakness, fatigue, exertional dyspnea, tachycardia, bounding pulse, atrial gallop, and a systolic bruit over the carotid arteries.
◆ ***Atherosclerosis of the carotid artery.*** In this disorder, the patient has constant tinnitus that can be stopped by applying pressure over the carotid artery. Auscultation over the upper part of the neck, on the auricle, or near the ear on the affected side may detect a bruit. Palpation may reveal a weak carotid pulse.
◆ ***Cervical spondylosis.*** In this degenerative disorder, osteophytic growths may compress the vertebral arteries, resulting in tinnitus. Typically, a stiff neck and pain aggravated by activity accompany tinnitus. Other features include brief vertigo, nystagmus, hearing loss, paresthesia, weakness, and pain that radiates down the arms.
◆ ***Ear canal obstruction.*** When cerumen or a foreign body blocks the ear canal, the patient may experience tinnitus, conductive hearing loss, itching, and a feeling of fullness or pain in the ear.
◆ ***Eustachian tube patency.*** Normally, the eustachian tube remains closed, except during swallowing. However, persistent patency of this tube can cause tinnitus, audible breath sounds, loud and distorted voice sounds, and a sense of fullness in the ear. Examination with a pneumatic otoscope reveals movement of the tympanic membrane with respirations. At times, breath sounds can be heard with a stethoscope placed over the auricle.
◆ ***Glomus jugulare or glomus tympanicum tumor.*** A pulsating sound is usually the first symptom of these tumors. Other early features include a reddish blue mass behind the tympanic membrane and progressive conductive hearing loss. Later, total unilateral deafness is accompanied by ear pain and dizziness. Otorrhagia may also occur if the tumor breaks through the tympanic membrane.
◆ ***Hypertension.*** Severe hypertension (diastolic blood pressure exceeding 120 mm Hg) may cause bilateral high-pitched tinnitus, a severe throbbing headache, restlessness, nausea, vomiting, blurred vision, seizures, and decreased level of consciousness.
◆ ***Intracranial arteriovenous malformation.*** A large malformation may cause pulsating tinnitus accompanied by a bruit over the mastoid process.
◆ ***Labyrinthitis (suppurative).*** In this disorder, tinnitus may accompany sudden, severe attacks of vertigo, unilateral or bilateral sensorineural hearing loss, nystagmus, dizziness, nausea, and vomiting.
◆ ***Ménière's disease.*** Most common in adults—especially in men between ages 30 and 60—this labyrinthine disease is characterized by attacks of tinnitus, vertigo, a feeling of fullness or blockage in the ear, and fluctuating sensorineural hearing loss. These attacks last from 10 minutes to several hours; they occur over a few days or weeks and are followed by a remission. Severe nausea, vomiting, diaphoresis, and nystagmus may also occur during attacks.
◆ ***Ossicle dislocation.*** Acoustic trauma, such as a slap on the ear, may dislocate the ossicle, resulting in tinnitus and sensorineural hearing loss. Bleeding from the middle ear may also occur.
◆ ***Otitis externa (acute).*** Although not a major complaint in this disorder, tinnitus may result if debris in the external ear canal impinges on the tympanic membrane. More typical findings include pruritus, a foul-smelling purulent discharge, and severe ear pain that's aggravated by manipulation of the tragus or auricle, teeth clenching, mouth opening, and chewing. The external ear canal typically appears red and edematous and may be occluded by debris, causing partial hearing loss.
◆ ***Otitis media.*** This infection may cause tinnitus and conductive hearing loss. However, its more typical features include ear pain, a red and bulging tympanic membrane, high fever, chills, and dizziness.
◆ ***Otosclerosis.*** In this disorder, the patient may describe ringing, roaring, or whistling tinnitus or a combination of these sounds. He may also report progressive hearing loss, which may lead to bilateral deafness, and vertigo.
◆ ***Palatal myoclonus.*** In this disorder, muscles of the palate contract rhythmically, either intermittently or continuously, causing a clicking sound in the ear and vibratory tinnitus. The contractions are visible with a nasopharyngeal mirror.
◆ ***Presbycusis.*** This otologic effect of aging produces tinnitus and progressive, symmetrical, bilateral sensorineural hearing loss, usually of high-frequency tones.
◆ ***Tympanic membrane perforation.*** Tinnitus and hearing loss go hand-in-hand in this disorder. Tinnitus is usually the chief complaint in a small perforation; hearing loss, in a larger perforation. These symptoms typically develop suddenly and may be accompanied by pain, vertigo, and a feeling of fullness in the ear.

Other causes

◆ ***Drugs and alcohol.*** An overdose of salicylates commonly causes reversible tinnitus.

Quinine, alcohol, and indomethacin may also cause reversible tinnitus. Common drugs that may cause irreversible tinnitus include the aminoglycoside antibiotics (especially kanamycin, streptomycin, and gentamicin) and vancomycin.

◆ ***Noise.*** Chronic exposure to noise, especially high-pitched sounds, can damage the ear's hair cells, causing tinnitus and bilateral hearing loss. These symptoms may be temporary or permanent.

Special considerations

Tinnitus is typically difficult to treat successfully. If reversible causes have been ruled out, educate the patient about strategies for adapting to the tinnitus, including biofeedback and masking devices. In addition, a hearing aid may be prescribed to amplify environmental sounds, thereby obscuring tinnitus. For some patients, a device that combines the features of a masker and a hearing aid may be used to block out tinnitus.

Pediatric pointers

An expectant mother's use of ototoxic drugs during the third trimester of pregnancy can cause labyrinthine damage in the fetus, resulting in tinnitus. Many of the disorders described above can also cause tinnitus in children.

Patient counseling

Advise the patient to avoid exposure to excessive noise, ototoxic agents, and other factors that may cause cochlear damage. Inform him that even people with normal hearing may experience intermittent periods of mild, high-pitched tinnitus that can last for several minutes.

Tracheal deviation

Normally, the trachea is located at the midline of the neck—except at the bifurcation, where it shifts slightly toward the right. Visible deviation from its normal position signals an underlying condition that can compromise pulmonary function and possibly cause respiratory distress. A hallmark of life-threatening tension pneumothorax, tracheal deviation occurs in disorders that produce a mediastinal shift due to asymmetrical thoracic volume or pressure. (See *Detecting slight tracheal deviation*.)

EMERGENCY INTERVENTIONS *If you detect tracheal deviation, be alert for signs and symptoms of respiratory distress (tachypnea, dyspnea, decreased or absent breath sounds, stridor, nasal flaring, accessory muscle use, asymmetrical chest expansion, restlessness, and anxiety). If possible, place the patient in semi-Fowler's position to aid respiratory excursion and improve oxygenation. Give supplemental oxygen, and intubate the patient if necessary. Insert an I.V. catheter for fluid and drug administration. In addition, palpate the neck and chest for subcutaneous crepitation, a sign of tension pneumothorax. Chest tube insertion may be necessary to release trapped air or fluid and to restore normal intrapleural and intrathoracic pressure gradients.*

History and physical examination

If the patient doesn't display signs of distress, ask about a history of pulmonary or cardiac disorders, surgery, trauma, or infection. If he smokes, determine how much. Ask about associated signs and symptoms, especially breathing difficulty, pain, and cough.

Medical causes

◆ ***Atelectasis.*** Extensive lung collapse can produce tracheal deviation toward the affected side. Respiratory findings include dyspnea, tachypnea, pleuritic chest pain, a dry cough, dullness on percussion, decreased vocal fremitus and breath sounds, inspiratory lag, and substernal or intercostal retraction.

◆ ***Hiatal hernia.*** Intrusion of abdominal viscera into the pleural space causes tracheal deviation toward the unaffected side. The degree of attendant respiratory distress depends on the extent of herniation. Other effects include pyrosis, regurgitation or vomiting, and chest or abdominal pain.

◆ ***Kyphoscoliosis.*** This disorder can cause rib cage distortion and mediastinal shift, producing tracheal deviation toward the compressed lung. Respiratory effects include a dry cough, dyspnea, asymmetrical chest expansion and, possibly, asymmetrical breath sounds. Backache and fatigue are also common.

◆ ***Mediastinal tumor.*** This type of tumor commonly produces no symptoms in its early stages; however, a large mediastinal tumor can press against the trachea and nearby structures, causing tracheal deviation and dysphagia. Other late findings include stridor, dyspnea, a brassy cough, hoarseness, and stertorous respirations with suprasternal retraction. The patient may experience shoulder, arm, or chest pain as well as edema of the neck, face, or arm. His neck and chest wall veins may be dilated.

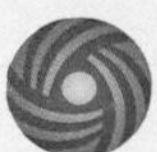

EXAMINATION TIP

Detecting slight tracheal deviation

Although gross tracheal deviation is visible, slight deviation can only be detected by palpation or sometimes an X-ray. Try palpation first.

With the tip of your index finger, locate the patient's trachea by palpating between the sternocleidomastoid muscles. Then compare the trachea's position to an imaginary line drawn vertically through the suprasternal notch. Any deviation from midline is usually considered abnormal.

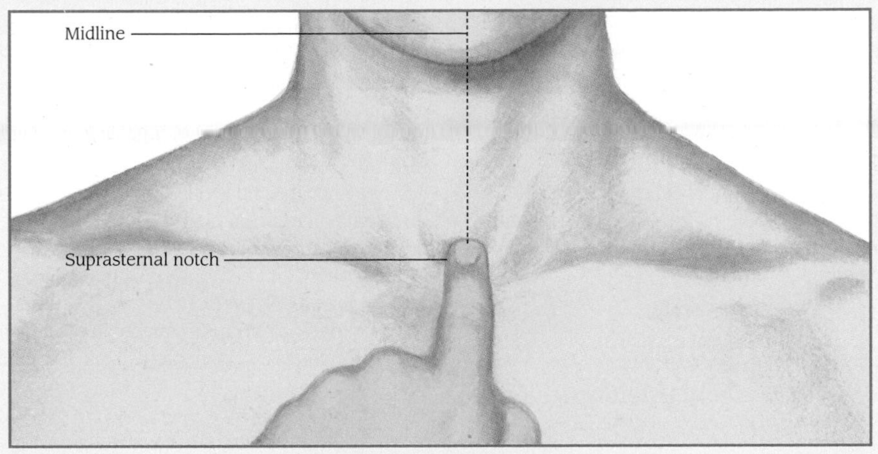

◆ ***Pleural effusion.*** A large pleural effusion can shift the mediastinum to the contralateral side, producing tracheal deviation. Related effects include a dry cough, dyspnea, pleuritic chest pain, pleural friction rub, tachypnea, decreased chest motion, decreased or absent breath sounds, egophony, flatness on percussion, decreased tactile fremitus, fever, and weight loss.

◆ ***Pulmonary fibrosis.*** Asymmetrical fibrosis can cause tracheal deviation as the mediastinum shifts toward the affected side. Associated findings reflect the underlying condition and pattern of fibrosis. Dyspnea, cough, clubbing, malaise, and fever commonly occur.

◆ ***Pulmonary tuberculosis.*** In a large cavitation, tracheal deviation toward the affected side accompanies asymmetrical chest excursion, dullness on percussion, increased tactile fremitus, amphoric breath sounds, and inspiratory crackles. Insidious early effects include fatigue, anorexia, weight loss, fever, chills, and night sweats. A productive cough, hemoptysis, pleuritic chest pain, and dyspnea develop as the disease progresses.

◆ ***Retrosternal thyroid.*** This anatomic abnormality can displace the trachea. The gland is felt as a movable neck mass above the suprasternal notch. Dysphagia, cough, hoarseness, and stridor are common. Signs of thyrotoxicosis may be present.

◆ ***Tension pneumothorax.*** This acute, life-threatening condition produces tracheal deviation toward the unaffected side. It's marked by a sudden onset of respiratory distress with sharp chest pain, a dry cough, severe dyspnea, tachycardia, wheezing, cyanosis, accessory muscle use, nasal flaring, air hunger, and asymmetrical chest movement. Restless and anxious, the patient may also develop subcutaneous crepitation in the neck and upper chest, decreased vocal fremitus, decreased or absent breath sounds on the affected side, jugular vein distention, and hypotension.

◆ ***Thoracic aortic aneurysm.*** This disorder usually causes the trachea to deviate to the right. Highly variable associated findings may include stridor, dyspnea, wheezing, a brassy cough, hoarseness, and dysphagia. Edema of the face, neck, or arm may occur with distended chest wall and jugular veins. The patient may also experience substernal, neck, shoulder, or low back pain as well as paresthesia or neuralgia.

Special considerations

Because tracheal deviation usually signals a severe underlying disorder that can cause respiratory distress at any time, monitor the patient's respiratory and cardiac status constantly, and make sure that emergency equipment is readily available. Prepare the patient for diagnostic tests, such as chest X-rays, bronchoscopy, an electrocardiogram, and arterial blood gas analysis.

Pediatric pointers

Keep in mind that respiratory distress typically develops more rapidly in children than in adults.

Geriatric pointers

In elderly patients, tracheal deviation to the right commonly stems from an elongated, atherosclerotic aortic arch, but this deviation isn't considered abnormal.

Tracheal tugging

[Cardarelli's sign, Castellino's sign, Oliver's sign]

A visible recession of the larynx and trachea that occurs in synchrony with cardiac systole, tracheal tugging commonly results from an aneurysm or a tumor near the aortic arch and may signal dangerous compression or obstruction of major airways. The tugging movement, best observed with the patient's neck hyperextended, reflects abnormal transmission of aortic pulsations due to compression and distortion of the heart, esophagus, great vessels, airways, and nerves.

EMERGENCY INTERVENTIONS *If you observe tracheal tugging, examine the patient for signs of respiratory distress, such as tachypnea, stridor, accessory muscle use, cyanosis, and agitation. If the patient is in distress, check airway patency. Administer oxygen and prepare to intubate the patient if necessary. Insert an I.V. catheter for fluid and drug access, and begin cardiac monitoring.*

History and physical examination

If the patient isn't in distress, obtain a pertinent history. Ask about associated symptoms, especially pain, and about a history of cardiovascular disease, cancer, chest surgery, or trauma.

Then examine the patient's neck and chest for abnormalities. Palpate the neck for masses, enlarged lymph nodes, abnormal arterial pulsations, and tracheal deviation. Percuss and auscultate the lung fields for abnormal sounds, and auscultate the heart for murmurs.

Medical causes

◆ ***Aortic arch aneurysm.*** A large aneurysm can distort and compress surrounding tissues and structures, producing tracheal tugging. The cardinal sign of this aneurysm is severe pain in the substernal area, sometimes radiating to the back or side of the chest. A sudden increase in pain may herald impending rupture—a medical emergency. Depending on the aneurysm's site and size, associated findings may include a visible pulsatile mass in the first or second intercostal space or suprasternal notch, a diastolic murmur of aortic insufficiency, and an aortic systolic murmur and thrill without any peripheral signs of aortic stenosis. Dyspnea and stridor may occur with hoarseness, dysphagia, a brassy cough, and hemoptysis. Jugular vein distention may also develop along with edema of the face, neck, or arm. Compression of the left main bronchus can cause atelectasis of the left lung.

◆ ***Hodgkin's disease.*** A tumor that develops adjacent to the aortic arch can cause tracheal tugging. Initial signs and symptoms include usually painless cervical lymphadenopathy, sustained or remittent fever, fatigue, malaise, pruritus, night sweats, and weight loss. Swollen lymph nodes may become tender and painful. Later findings include dyspnea and stridor; dry cough; dysphagia; jugular vein distention; edema of the face, neck, or arm; hepatosplenomegaly; hyperpigmentation, jaundice, or pallor; and neuralgia.

◆ ***Malignant lymphoma.*** Tracheal tugging may reflect anterior mediastinal lymphadenopathy or tumor development next to the aortic arch. The most common initial sign, however, is painless peripheral lymphadenopathy. Other early findings include fever, fatigue, malaise, night sweats, and weight loss. Later findings include a crowing cough, dyspnea, stridor, dysphagia, jugular vein distention, neck edema, hepatomegaly, and splenomegaly.

◆ ***Thymoma.*** This rare tumor can cause tracheal tugging if it develops in the anterior mediastinum. Cough, chest pain, dysphagia, dyspnea, hoarseness, a palpable neck mass, jugular vein distention, and edema of the face, neck, or upper arm are common findings.

Special considerations

Place the patient in semi-Fowler's position to ease respiration. Administer a cough suppressant and prescribed pain medications, but be alert for signs of respiratory depression.

Prepare the patient for diagnostic procedures, which may include chest X-rays, computed tomography scan, lymphangiography, aortography, bone marrow biopsy, liver biopsy, echocardiography, and a complete blood count.

PEDIATRIC POINTERS

In infants and children, tracheal tugging may indicate a mediastinal tumor, as occurs in Hodgkin's disease and malignant lymphoma. This sign may also occur in Marfan syndrome.

Tremors

The most common type of involuntary muscle movement, tremors are regular rhythmic oscillations that result from alternating contraction of opposing muscle groups. They're typical signs of extrapyramidal or cerebellar disorders and can also result from the use of certain drugs.

Tremors can be characterized by their location, amplitude, and frequency. They're classified as resting, intention, or postural. *Resting tremors* occur when an extremity is at rest and subside with movement. They include the classic pill-rolling tremor of Parkinson's disease. Conversely, *intention tremors* occur only with movement and subside with rest. *Postural (or action) tremors* appear when an extremity or the trunk is actively held in a particular posture or position. A common type of postural tremor is called an essential tremor.

Tremorlike movements may also be elicited—for example, asterixis, the characteristic flapping tremor seen in hepatic failure. (See "Asterixis," page 68.)

Stress or emotional upset tends to aggravate tremors. Alcohol commonly diminishes postural tremors.

HISTORY AND PHYSICAL EXAMINATION

Begin the patient history by asking the patient about the tremor's onset (sudden or gradual) and about its duration, progression, and any aggravating or alleviating factors. Does the tremor interfere with the patient's normal activities? Does he have other symptoms? Has he noticed any behavioral changes or memory loss? (The patient's family or friends may provide more accurate information on this.)

Explore the patient's personal and family medical history for a neurologic (especially seizures), endocrine, or metabolic disorder. Obtain a complete drug history, noting especially the use of phenothiazines. Also, ask about alcohol use.

Assess the patient's overall appearance and demeanor, noting mental status. Test range of motion and strength in all major muscle groups while observing for chorea, athetosis, dystonia, and other involuntary movements. Check deep tendon reflexes and, if possible, observe the patient's gait.

MEDICAL CAUSES

◆ ***Alcohol withdrawal syndrome.*** Acute alcohol withdrawal after long-term dependence may first be manifested by resting and intention tremors that appear as soon as 7 hours after the last drink and progressively worsen. Other early signs and symptoms include diaphoresis, tachycardia, elevated blood pressure, anxiety, restlessness, irritability, insomnia, headache, nausea, and vomiting. Severe withdrawal may produce profound tremors, agitation, confusion, hallucinations, and seizures.

◆ ***Alkalosis.*** Severe alkalosis may produce a severe intention tremor along with twitching, carpopedal spasms, agitation, diaphoresis, and hyperventilation. The patient may complain of dizziness, tinnitus, palpitations, and peripheral and circumoral paresthesia.

◆ ***Benign familial essential tremor.*** This disorder of early adulthood produces a bilateral essential tremor that typically begins in the fingers and hands and may spread to the head, jaw, lips, and tongue. Laryngeal involvement may result in a quavering voice.

◆ ***Cerebellar tumor.*** An intention tremor is a cardinal sign of this disorder; related findings may include ataxia, nystagmus, incoordination, muscle weakness and atrophy, and hypoactive or absent deep tendon reflexes.

◆ ***General paresis.*** This effect of neurosyphilis may cause an intention tremor accompanied by clonus, a positive Babinski's sign, ataxia, Argyll Robertson pupils, and a diffuse, dull headache.

◆ ***Graves' disease.*** Fine tremors of the hand, nervousness, weight loss, fatigue, palpitations, dyspnea, and increased heat intolerance are typical signs and symptoms of this disorder. An enlarged thyroid gland (goiter) and exophthalmos are also characteristic.

◆ ***Hypercapnia.*** Elevated partial pressure of carbon dioxide may result in a rapid, fine intention tremor. Other common findings include headache, fatigue, blurred vision, weakness, lethargy, and decreasing level of consciousness (LOC).

◆ ***Hypoglycemia.*** Acute hypoglycemia may produce a rapid, fine intention tremor accompanied by confusion, weakness, tachycardia, diaphoresis, and cold, clammy skin. Early patient complaints typically include a mild generalized headache, profound hunger, nervousness, and blurred or double vision. The tremor may disappear as hypoglycemia worsens and hypotonia and decreased LOC become evident.

◆ ***Kwashiorkor.*** Coarse intention and resting tremors may occur in the advanced stages of this disease. Examination reveals myoclonus, rigidity of all extremities, hyperreflexia, hepatomegaly, and pitting edema in the hands, feet, and sacral area. Other signs include a flat affect, pronounced hair loss, and dry, peeling skin.

◆ ***Multiple sclerosis (MS).*** An intention tremor that waxes and wanes may be an early sign of MS, but visual and sensory impairments are usually the earliest findings. Associated effects vary greatly and may include nystagmus, muscle weakness, paralysis, spasticity, hyperreflexia, ataxic gait, dysphagia, and dysarthria. Constipation, urinary frequency and urgency, incontinence, impotence, and emotional lability may also occur.

◆ ***Parkinson's disease.*** Tremors, a classic early sign of this degenerative disease, usually begin in the fingers and may eventually affect the foot, eyelids, jaw, lips, and tongue. The slow, regular, rhythmic resting tremor takes the form of flexion-extension or abduction-adduction of the fingers or hand, or pronation-supination of the hand. Flexion-extension of the fingers combined with abduction-adduction of the thumb is known as the characteristic pill-rolling tremor.

Leg involvement produces flexion-extension foot movement. Lightly closing the eyelids causes them to flutter. The jaw may move up and down, and the lips may purse. The tongue, when protruded, may move in and out of the mouth in tempo with tremors elsewhere in the body. The rate of the tremor remains constant over time, but its amplitude varies.

Other characteristic findings include cogwheel or lead-pipe rigidity, bradykinesia, propulsive gait with forward-leaning posture, monotone voice, masklike facies, drooling, dysphagia, dysarthria, and occasionally oculogyric crisis (eyes fix upward, with involuntary tonic movements) or blepharospasm (eyelids close completely).

◆ ***Porphyria.*** Involvement of the basal ganglia in porphyria can produce a resting tremor with rigidity accompanied by chorea and athetosis. As the disease progresses, generalized seizures may appear along with aphasia and hemiplegia.

◆ ***Thalamic syndrome.*** Central midbrain syndromes are heralded by contralateral ataxic tremors and other abnormal movements along with Weber's syndrome (oculomotor palsy with contralateral hemiplegia), paralysis of vertical gaze, and stupor or coma.

Anteromedial-inferior thalamic syndrome produces varying combinations of tremor, deep sensory loss, and hemiataxia. However, the main effect of this syndrome may be an extrapyramidal dysfunction, such as hemiballismus or hemichoreoathetosis.

◆ ***Thyrotoxicosis.*** Neuromuscular effects of this disorder include a rapid, fine intention tremor of the hands and tongue, along with clonus, hyperreflexia, and Babinski's reflex. Other common signs and symptoms include tachycardia, cardiac arrhythmias, palpitations, anxiety, dyspnea, diaphoresis, heat intolerance, weight loss despite increased appetite, diarrhea, an enlarged thyroid and, possibly, exophthalmos.

◆ ***Wernicke's encephalopathy.*** An intention tremor is an early sign of this thiamine deficiency. Other features include ocular abnormalities (such as gaze paralysis and nystagmus), ataxia, apathy, and confusion. Orthostatic hypotension and tachycardia may also develop.

◆ ***West Nile encephalitis.*** This brain infection is caused by West Nile virus, a mosquito-borne flavivirus endemic in Africa, the Middle East, western Asia, and the United States. Mild infections are common and include fever, headache, and body aches, commonly accompanied by rash and swollen lymph glands. More severe infections are marked by headache, high fever, neck stiffness, stupor, disorientation, coma, tremors, occasional seizures, and paralysis. Death rarely occurs.

◆ ***Wilson's disease.*** This disorder of abnormal copper metabolism produces slow "wing-flapping" tremors in the arms and pill-rolling tremors in the hands; these tremors appear early in the disease and progressively worsen. The most characteristic sign, however, is Kayser-Fleischer rings—rusty brown rings around the corneas. Other signs and symptoms include incoordination, dysarthrial chorea, ataxia, muscle spasms and rigidity, abdominal distress, fatigue, personality changes, hypotension, syncope, and seizures. Liver and spleen enlargement, ascites, jaundice, and hyperpigmentation may also occur.

Other causes

◆ ***Drugs.*** Phenothiazines (particularly piperazine derivatives such as fluphenazine) and other antipsychotics may cause resting and pill-rolling tremors. Metoclopramide and metyrosine also cause these tremors occasionally. Lithium toxicity, sympathomimetics (such as terbutaline and pseudoephedrine), amphetamines, and phenytoin can all cause tremors that disappear when the dosage is decreased.

HERB ALERT *Herbal products, such as ephedra (ma huang), have been known to cause serious adverse reactions, which may include tremors. (Note: The FDA has banned the sale of dietary supplements containing ephedra because they pose an unreasonable risk of injury or illness.)*

◆ ***Manganese toxicity.*** Early signs of manganese poisoning include resting tremor, chorea, propulsive gait, cogwheel rigidity, personality changes, amnesia, and masklike facies.

◆ ***Mercury poisoning.*** The chronic form of mercury poisoning is characterized by irritability, copious amounts of saliva, loose teeth, gum disease, slurred speech, and tremors.

Special considerations

Severe intention tremors may interfere with the patient's ability to perform activities of daily living. Assist the patient with these activities as necessary, and take precautions against possible injury during such activities as walking and eating.

Pediatric pointers

A normal neonate may display coarse tremors with stiffening—an exaggerated hypocalcemic startle reflex—in response to noises and chills. Pediatric-specific causes of pathologic tremors include cerebral palsy, fetal alcohol syndrome, and maternal drug addiction.

Trismus

Commonly known as "lockjaw," trismus is a prolonged and painful tonic spasm of the masticatory jaw muscles. This characteristic early sign of tetanus is produced by the neuromuscular effects of tetanospasmin, a potentially lethal exotoxin. It can also result from drug therapy; occasionally, a milder form may accompany neuromuscular involvement in other disorders, or infection or disease of the jaw, teeth, parotid glands, or tonsils.

History and physical examination

Ask the patient if he experienced a recent injury (even a slight wound), infection, or animal bite. Does he have a history of epilepsy, neuromuscular disease, or endocrine or metabolic disorders? Obtain a complete drug history, including self-injected drugs because the use of a contaminated needle may produce tetanus. Also, ask about paresthesia or pain in the throat, jaw, neck, or shoulders.

Examination of the oral cavity may be difficult or impossible to perform. If possible, examine the pharynx, tonsils, oral mucosa, gingivae, and teeth. Perform a neurologic assessment, evaluating cranial nerve, motor, and sensory function and deep tendon reflexes. Also, check the jaw jerk reflex. An extremely hyperactive response and a careful patient history usually establish the diagnosis. (See *Performing the jaw jerk test*, page 672.)

Medical causes

◆ ***Hypocalcemia.*** Severe hypocalcemia can produce trismus and cramping spasms in virtually all muscle groups, except those of the eye. It also causes fatigue, weakness, chorea, and palpitations. Chvostek's and Trousseau's signs may be elicited.

◆ ***Peritonsillar abscess.*** This disorder occurs after an episode of acute tonsillitis when infection penetrates the tonsillar capsule and surrounding deeper tissues. Symptoms include severe sore throat, trismus, odynophagia, deviation of the uvula, and fever.

◆ ***Rabies.*** Trismus commonly develops after a prodromal period of fever, headache, photophobia, hyperesthesia, and increasing restlessness and agitation. Other neuromuscular effects include excessive salivation, painful laryngeal and pharyngeal muscle spasms and, possibly, respiratory distress.

◆ ***Seizure disorders.*** Trismus commonly occurs during a generalized tonic-clonic seizure along with spasms of other facial muscles, the limbs, and the trunk.

◆ ***Temporomandibular joint syndrome.*** This syndrome causes trismus, mandibular dysfunc-

EXAMINATION TIP

Performing the jaw jerk test

If your patient reports difficulty in opening her mouth, perform the jaw jerk test because even slight trismus may indicate an otherwise asymptomatic mild localized tetanus.

Here's how to elicit and interpret this important reflex: Ask the patient to relax her jaw and open her mouth slightly. Then place your index finger over the middle of her chin, and firmly tap it with a reflex hammer.

Normally, this tap produces sudden jaw closing; then an inhibitory mechanism abruptly halts motor nerve activity, and the mouth remains closed. In trismus, however, this inhibitory mechanism fails and motor activity increases, causing immediate spasm of jaw muscles.

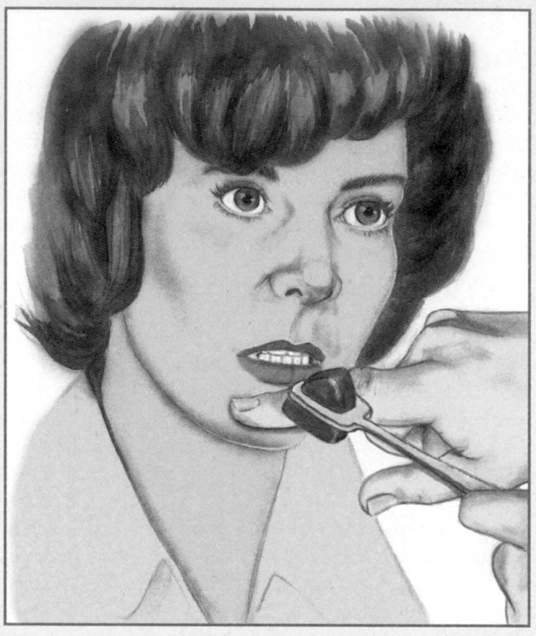

tion, and facial pain. The pain may range from a severe dull ache to an intense spasm that radiates to the cheek, temple, lower jaw, ear, mastoid area, neck, or shoulders. Earache occurs without involvement of the tympanic membrane or external auditory canal.

◆ ***Tetanus.*** This acute, life-threatening infection is heralded by trismus, which typically appears within 14 days of the initial infection. The painful spasms increase in frequency and intensity during the initial disease stage, then gradually subside. Although trismus is commonly the first sign of tetanus, it occasionally follows a short prodromal period of headache, restlessness, irritability, slight fever, chills, swelling at the wound site, and dysphagia. As the disease progresses, painful involuntary muscle spasms spread to other areas, such as the abdomen, producing boardlike rigidity; the back, resulting in opisthotonos; the face, producing a characteristic grotesque grin (risus sardonicus); or possibly the laryngeal or chest wall muscles. Tachycardia, diaphoresis, hyperactive deep tendon reflexes, and seizures may also develop.

Other causes

◆ ***Drugs.*** Phenothiazines (particularly the piperazine derivatives such as fluphenazine) and other antipsychotics may produce an acute dystonic reaction marked by trismus, involuntary facial movements, and tonic spasms in the limbs. These complications usually occur early in drug therapy, sometimes after the initial dose.

◆ ***Strychnine poisoning.*** In this potentially fatal condition, tonic seizures characterized by trismus, leg muscle rigidity, and respiratory muscle spasm follow early symptoms of irritability and twitching.

Special considerations

Maintain a quiet environment for the patient with trismus; darken his room and keep all stimulation to a minimum. Administer a sedative as needed.

Because inadequate ventilation from laryngeal or respiratory muscle spasm is a constant threat during the acute phase of tetanus, constantly assess the patient's respiratory status and make sure that oxygen and emergency airway equipment are readily available. To treat tetanus, expect to administer human tetanus immune globulin, which neutralizes unbound toxin.

Administer I.V. fluids to prevent dehydration if the patient can't drink fluids. If trismus is prolonged enough to affect his nutritional status, the patient may require parenteral nutrition. If the patient can't speak, make sure that he has a pen and paper and that his call bell is within reach at all times.

Pediatric pointers

Trismus in a neonate can result from tetanus neonatorum, which occurs when the tetanus toxin is introduced through the umbilical cord. Trismus usually develops within 10 days of birth.

Patient counseling

Teach the patient with tetanus about the importance of annual booster injections to ensure immunization.

Tunnel vision

[Gun barrel vision, tubular vision]

Resulting from severe constriction of the visual field that leaves only a small central area of sight, tunnel vision is typically described as the sensation of looking through a tunnel or gun barrel. It may be unilateral or bilateral and usually develops gradually. (See *Comparing tunnel vision with normal vision*, page 674.) This abnormality results from chronic open-angle glaucoma and advanced retinal degeneration. Tunnel vision also can result from laser photocoagulation therapy, which aims to correct retinal detachment. Also a common complaint of malingerers, tunnel vision can be verified or discounted by visual field examination performed by an ophthalmologist.

History and physical examination

Ask the patient when he first noticed a loss of peripheral vision, and have him describe the progression of vision loss. Ask him to describe in detail exactly what and how far he can see peripherally. Explore the patient's personal and family history for ocular problems, especially progressive blindness that began at an early age.

To rule out malingering, observe the patient as he walks. A patient with severely limited peripheral vision typically bumps into objects (and may even have bruises), whereas a malingerer manages to avoid them.

If your examination findings suggest tunnel vision, refer the patient to an ophthalmologist for further evaluation.

Medical causes

- ***Glaucoma, chronic open-angle.*** Bilateral tunnel vision occurs late in this insidious disorder and slowly progresses to complete blindness. Other late findings include mild eye pain, halo vision, and reduced visual acuity (especially at night) that isn't correctable with glasses.
- ***Retinal pigmentary degeneration.*** This group of hereditary disorders, such as retinitis pigmentosa, produces an annular scotoma that progresses concentrically, causing tunnel vision and eventually complete blindness, usually by age 50. Impaired night vision, the earliest symptom, typically appears during the first or second decade of life. An ophthalmoscopic examination may reveal narrowed retinal blood vessels and a pale optic disk.

Special considerations

To protect the patient from injury, be sure to remove all potentially dangerous objects and orient him to his surroundings. Because visual impairment is frightening, reassure the patient and clearly explain diagnostic procedures, such as tonometry, perimeter examination, and visual field testing.

Pediatric pointers

In children with retinitis pigmentosa, night blindness foreshadows tunnel vision, which usually doesn't develop until later in the disease process.

Patient counseling

If tunnel vision is permanent, teach the patient to move his eyes from side to side when he walks to avoid bumping into objects.

Comparing tunnel vision with normal vision

The patient with tunnel vision experiences drastic constriction of his peripheral visual field. The illustrations here convey the extent of this constriction, comparing test findings for normal and tunnel vision.

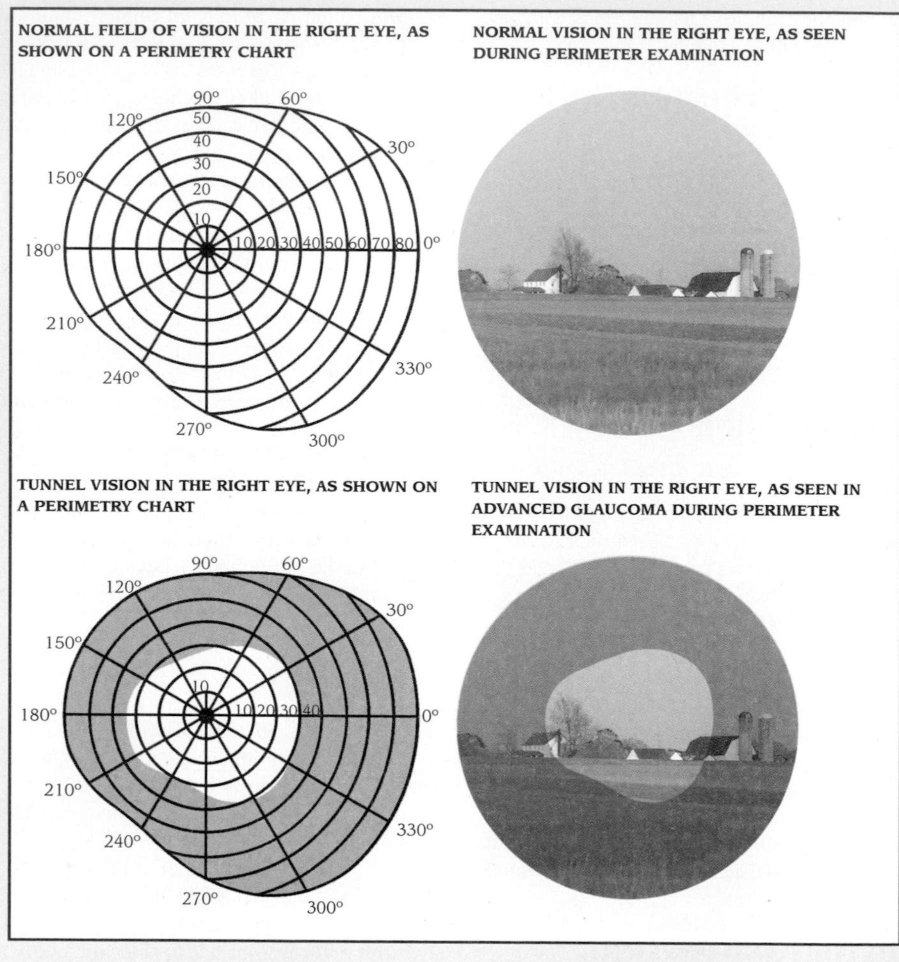

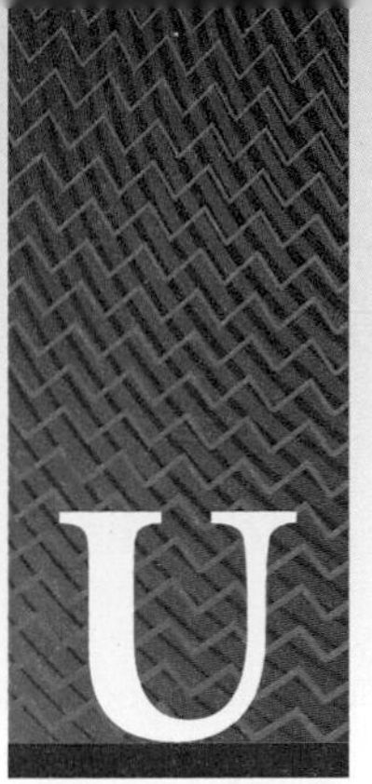

Uremic frost

Uremic frost—a fine white powder, believed to be urate crystals, that covers the skin—is a characteristic sign of end-stage renal failure, or uremia. Urea compounds and other waste substances that can't be excreted by the kidneys in urine are excreted through small superficial capillaries on the skin and remain as powdery deposits. The frost typically appears on the face, neck, axillae, groin, and genitalia.

Because of advances in managing renal failure, uremic frost is now relatively rare. However, it does occur in patients with chronic renal failure who—because of their advanced age, the severity of their accompanying illnesses (such as extensive neurologic deterioration), or personal preference—are unable or unwilling to undergo dialysis.

Physical examination

Uremic frost usually appears well after a diagnosis of chronic renal failure has been established. As a result, your examination will be limited to inspecting the skin to determine the extent of uremic frost.

Medical causes

◆ ***End-stage chronic renal failure.*** Uremic frost heralds the preterminal stage of chronic renal failure. The patient may also have pruritus, hypertension, lassitude, fatigue, irritability, and decreased level of consciousness. Additional findings include muscle cramps, gross myoclonus, peripheral neuropathies, and seizures. Anorexia, nausea and vomiting, constipation or diarrhea, and oliguria or anuria may occur along with GI bleeding, petechiae, and ecchymosis. Integumentary effects may include mouth and gum ulceration, skin pigment changes and excoriation, and brown arcs under nail margins. Acidosis results in Kussmaul's respirations; the patient may also have ammonia breath odor (uremic fetor). Laboratory test results reveal increased blood urea nitrogen and serum creatinine levels and decreased creatinine clearance.

Special considerations

Because a patient with end-stage renal failure is prone to seizures from uremic encephalopathy, take seizure precautions. Monitor his vital signs frequently, pad the bed's side rails, and keep artificial airway and suction equipment at hand.

Because the patient is also prone to respiratory or cardiac arrest from metabolic acidosis or hyperkalemia, constantly monitor his respiratory and cardiac status. As necessary, administer supplemental oxygen. Intubation and mechanical ventilation may be required. Establish an I.V. catheter for medication administration. Also, begin cardiac monitoring, and be prepared to initiate cardiopulmonary resuscitation, if indicated.

Enhance patient comfort by regularly changing the patient's position to prevent skin breakdown and by bathing him often with tepid water and minimal soap to remove the frost. Moisturize the patient's skin with alcohol-free lotion. Trim his fingernails to prevent scratching.

Because the appearance of uremic frost invariably signals impending death, prepare the patient and his family for this eventuality, and provide emotional support. Death from uremia is generally peaceful, following a deep coma.

Pediatric pointers

Uremic frost is rare in children because most undergo dialysis or kidney transplantation before renal failure reaches the end stage.

Geriatric pointers

Elderly patients with end-stage renal disease usually have other complicating medical illnesses that further reduce their life expectancy. However, maintenance dialysis can still offer such patients an improved quality of life.

Urethral discharge

Urethral discharge from the urinary meatus may be purulent, mucoid, or thin; sanguineous or clear; and scant or profuse. It usually develops suddenly, most commonly in men with a prostate infection.

History and physical examination

Ask the patient when he first noticed the discharge, and have him describe its color, consistency, and quantity. Does he experience pain or burning on urination? Does he have difficulty initiating a urine stream? Does he experience urinary frequency? Ask the patient about other associated signs and symptoms, such as fever, chills, and perineal fullness. Explore his history for prostate problems, sexually transmitted disease, or urinary tract infection. Ask the patient if he has had recent sexual contacts or a new sexual partner.

Inspect the patient's urethral meatus for inflammation and swelling. Using proper technique, obtain a culture specimen. (See *Collecting a urethral discharge specimen*.) Then obtain a urine specimen for urinalysis and culture and sensitivity. Palpation of the male patient's prostate gland may be necessary.

Collecting a urethral discharge specimen

To obtain a urethral specimen from a male patient, follow these steps:

Instruct the patient not to void for 1 hour before specimen collection to prevent flushing of secretions from the urethra.

▼

Provide privacy for the patient. Help him onto an examination table and into a supine position, and expose his penis. Have him grasp and raise his penis to allow visualization of the urethra.

▼

Wash your hands, and put on sterile gloves. Then insert a thin, sterile urogenital alginate swab no more than 3/4" (2 cm) into the urethra. Rotate the swab, and leave it in place for 10 to 30 seconds to absorb organisms.

▼

Remove the swab, allow it to dry, and then send it to the laboratory. Help the patient off of the examination table, and tell him to dress.

Medical causes

◆ ***Prostatitis.*** Acute prostatitis is characterized by a purulent urethral discharge. Initial signs and symptoms include sudden fever, chills, low back pain, perineal fullness, myalgia, and arthralgia. Urination becomes increasingly frequent and urgent, and the urine may appear cloudy. Dysuria, nocturia, and some degree of urinary obstruction may also occur. The prostate may be tense, boggy, tender, and warm. Prostate massage to obtain prostatic fluid is contraindicated.

Chronic prostatitis commonly produces no symptoms, but it may produce a persistent urethral discharge that's thin, milky or clear, and sometimes sticky. The discharge appears at the meatus after a long interval between voidings—for example, in the morning. Associated effects include a dull ache in the prostate or rectum, sexual dysfunction such as ejaculatory pain, and urinary disturbances, such as frequency, urgency, and dysuria.

◆ ***Reiter's syndrome.*** In this self-limiting syndrome that usually affects males, a urethral discharge and other signs of acute urethritis occur 1 to 2 weeks after sexual contact. Asymmetrical arthritis, conjunctivitis of one or both eyes, and ulcerations on the oral mucosa, glans penis, palms, and soles may also occur.

◆ ***Urethral neoplasm.*** This rare cancer is sometimes heralded by a painless urethral discharge that's initially opaque and gray and later yellowish and blood-tinged. Dysuria progresses to anuria as the urethra becomes blocked.

◆ ***Urethritis.*** This inflammatory disorder, which is often sexually transmitted (as in gonorrhea), commonly produces a scant or profuse urethral discharge that's either thin and clear, mucoid, or thick and purulent. Other effects include urinary hesitancy, urgency, and frequency; dysuria; and itching and burning around the meatus.

SPECIAL CONSIDERATIONS

Advise the patient with acute prostatitis to discontinue sexual activity until acute symptoms subside. However, encourage the patient with chronic prostatitis to regularly engage in sexual activity because ejaculation may relieve pain. To help this patient relieve symptoms, suggest that he take hot sitz baths several times daily, increase his fluid intake, void frequently, and avoid caffeine, tea, and alcohol. Monitor him for urine retention.

PEDIATRIC POINTERS

Carefully evaluate a child with a urethral discharge for evidence of sexual and physical abuse.

GERIATRIC POINTERS

Urethral discharge in elderly males isn't usually related to a sexually transmitted disease.

Urinary frequency

Urinary frequency refers to an increased urge to void without an increase in the total volume of urine produced. Usually resulting from decreased bladder capacity, urinary frequency is a cardinal sign of urinary tract infection (UTI). However, it can also stem from another urologic disorder, neurologic dysfunction, or pressure on the bladder from a nearby tumor or from organ enlargement (as occurs in pregnancy).

HISTORY AND PHYSICAL EXAMINATION

Ask the patient how many times a day he voids and how this compares to his previous pattern of voiding. Also ask about the onset and duration of the increased frequency and about any associated urinary signs or symptoms, such as dysuria, urgency, incontinence, hematuria, discharge, or lower abdominal pain during urination.

Also ask about neurologic symptoms, such as muscle weakness, numbness, and tingling. Explore the patient's medical history for UTIs or other urologic problems, recent urologic procedures, and neurologic disorders. Ask a male patient about a history of prostatic enlargement. Ask a female patient of childbearing age whether she is or could be pregnant.

Obtain a clean-catch midstream urine specimen for urinalysis and culture and sensitivity tests. Then palpate the patient's suprapubic area, abdomen, and flanks, noting any tenderness. Examine the urethral meatus for redness, discharge, or swelling. The physician may palpate the prostate gland of a male patient.

If the patient's history or symptoms suggest a neurologic disorder, perform a neurologic examination.

MEDICAL CAUSES

◆ ***Anxiety neurosis.*** Morbid anxiety produces urinary frequency and other types of genitourinary dysfunction, such as dysuria, impotence, and frigidity. Other findings may include headache, diaphoresis, hyperventilation, palpitations, muscle spasm, generalized motor weakness, dizziness, polyphagia, and constipation or other GI complaints.

◆ ***Benign prostatic hyperplasia.*** Prostatic enlargement causes urinary frequency along with nocturia and possibly incontinence and hematuria. Initial effects are those of prostatism: reduced caliber and force of the urine stream, urinary hesitancy and tenesmus, inability to stop the urine stream, a feeling of incomplete voiding, and occasionally urine retention. Assessment reveals bladder distention.

◆ ***Bladder calculus.*** Bladder irritation from a calculus may lead to urinary frequency and urgency, dysuria, terminal hematuria, and suprapubic pain from bladder spasms. If the calculus lodges in the bladder neck, the patient may have overflow incontinence and referred pain to the lower back or heel.

◆ ***Bladder cancer.*** Urinary frequency, urgency, dribbling, and nocturia may develop from bladder irritation. The first sign of bladder cancer commonly is intermittent gross, painless hematuria (often with clots). Patients with invasive lesions commonly have suprapubic or pelvic pain from bladder spasms.

◆ ***Multiple sclerosis (MS).*** Urinary frequency, urgency, and incontinence are common urologic findings in patients with MS, but these effects widely vary and tend to wax and wane. Visual problems (such as diplopia and blurred vision) and sensory impairment (such as paresthesia) are usually the earliest symptoms. Other findings may include constipation, muscle weakness, paralysis, spasticity, hyperreflexia, intention tremor, ataxic gait, dysarthria, impotence, and emotional lability.

◆ ***Prostate cancer.*** In advanced prostate cancer, urinary frequency may occur along with hesitancy, dribbling, nocturia, dysuria, bladder distention, perineal pain, constipation, and a hard, irregularly shaped prostate.

◆ ***Prostatitis.*** Acute prostatitis commonly produces urinary frequency and urgency, dysuria, nocturia, and a purulent urethral discharge. Other findings include fever, chills, low back pain, myalgia, arthralgia, and perineal fullness. The prostate may be tense, boggy, tender, and warm. Prostate massage to obtain prostatic fluid is contraindicated. Signs and symptoms of chronic prostatitis are usually the same as those of the acute form, but to a lesser degree. The patient may also experience pain on ejaculation.

◆ ***Rectal tumor.*** The pressure that this tumor exerts on the bladder may cause urinary frequency. Early findings include altered bowel elimination habits, commonly starting with an urgent need to defecate on arising or obstipation alternating with diarrhea; blood or mucus in the stool; and a sense of incomplete evacuation.

◆ ***Reiter's syndrome.*** In this self-limiting syndrome, urinary frequency and other symptoms of acute urethritis occur 1 to 2 weeks after sexual contact. Other symptoms of Reiter's syndrome include asymmetrical arthritis of the knees, ankles, and metatarsophalangeal joints; unilateral or bilateral conjunctivitis; and small painless ulcers on the mouth, tongue, glans penis, palms, and soles.

◆ ***Reproductive tract tumor.*** A tumor in the female reproductive tract may compress the bladder, causing urinary frequency. Other findings vary but may include abdominal distention, menstrual disturbances, vaginal bleeding, weight loss, pelvic pain, and fatigue.

◆ ***Spinal cord lesion.*** Incomplete cord transection results in urinary frequency, continuous overflow, dribbling, urgency when voluntary control of sphincter function weakens, urinary hesitancy, and bladder distention. Other effects occur below the level of the lesion and include weakness, paralysis, sensory disturbances, hyperreflexia, and impotence.

◆ ***Urethral stricture.*** Bladder decompensation produces urinary frequency, urgency, and nocturia. Early signs include hesitancy, tenesmus, and reduced caliber and force of the urine stream. Eventually, overflow incontinence, urinoma, and urosepsis may develop.

◆ ***UTI.*** Affecting the urethra, the bladder, or the kidneys, this common cause of urinary frequency may also produce urgency, dysuria, hematuria, cloudy urine and, in males, a urethral discharge. The patient may report a fever and bladder spasms or a feeling of warmth during urination. Women may experience suprapubic or pelvic pain. In young adult males, a UTI is usually related to sexual contact.

Other causes

◆ ***Diuretics.*** These substances, which include caffeine, reduce the body's total volume of water and salt by increasing urine excretion. Excessive intake of coffee, tea, and other caffeinated beverages leads to urinary frequency.

◆ ***Treatments.*** Radiation therapy may cause bladder inflammation, leading to urinary frequency.

Special considerations

Prepare the patient for diagnostic tests, such as urinalysis, culture and sensitivity tests, imaging tests, ultrasonography, cystoscopy, cystometry, postvoid residual tests, and a complete neurologic workup. If the patient's mobility is impaired, keep a bedpan or commode near his bed. Carefully and accurately document the patient's daily intake and output.

Pediatric pointers

UTIs are a common cause of urinary frequency in children, especially girls. Congenital anomalies that can cause UTIs include a duplicated ureter, congenital bladder diverticulum, and an ectopic ureteral orifice.

Geriatric pointers

Men older than age 50 are prone to frequent UTIs that aren't related to sexual contact. Decreased estrogen levels in postmenopausal women cause urinary frequency, urgency, and nocturia.

Patient counseling

Instruct sexually active male patients in safe sex practices. Advise girls to clean the genital area from front to back to reduce contamination by *Escherichia coli.* Encourage women to increase intake of fluids, especially water; to void frequently throughout the day; and to clean themselves in the same manner as girls.

Urinary hesitancy

Urinary hesitancy—difficulty starting a urine stream generally followed by a decrease in the force of the stream—can result from a urinary tract infection (UTI), a partial lower urinary tract obstruction, a neuromuscular disorder, or use of certain drugs. Occurring at all ages and in both sexes, it's most common in older men with prostatic enlargement. It also occurs in women with gravid uterus, tumors in the reproductive system (such as uterine fibroids), or ovarian, uterine, or vaginal cancer. Hesitancy usually arises gradually, commonly going unnoticed until urine retention causes bladder distention and discomfort.

History and physical examination

Ask the patient when he first noticed hesitancy and if he has ever had the problem before. Ask about other urinary problems, especially reduced force or interruption of the urine stream. Ask if he has ever been treated for a prostate problem, a UTI, or a urinary tract obstruction. Obtain a drug history.

Inspect the patient's urethral meatus for inflammation, discharge, and other abnormalities. Examine the anal sphincter and test sensation in the perineum. Obtain a clean-catch urine specimen for urinalysis and culture and sensitivity tests. A male patient requires prostate gland palpation. A female patient requires a gynecologic examination.

Medical causes

◆ ***Benign prostatic hyperplasia.*** Signs and symptoms of this disorder depend on the extent of prostatic enlargement and the lobes affected. Characteristic early findings include urinary hesitancy, reduced caliber and force of the urine stream, perineal pain, a feeling of incomplete voiding, inability to stop the urine stream, and occasionally urine retention. As the obstruction increases, the patient may develop urinary frequency, nocturia, urinary overflow, incontinence, bladder distention and, possibly, hematuria.

◆ ***Prostate cancer.*** In advanced cancer, urinary hesitancy may occur along with frequency, dribbling, nocturia, dysuria, bladder distention, perineal pain, and constipation. Digital rectal examination commonly reveals a hard, nodular prostate.

◆ ***Spinal cord lesion.*** A lesion below the micturition center that has destroyed the sacral nerve roots causes urinary hesitancy, tenesmus, and constant dribbling from urine retention and overflow incontinence. Associated findings are urinary frequency and urgency, dysuria, and nocturia.

◆ ***Urethral stricture.*** Partial obstruction of the lower urinary tract secondary to trauma or infection produces urinary hesitancy, tenesmus, and decreased force and caliber of the urine stream. Urinary frequency and urgency, nocturia, and eventually overflow incontinence may develop. Pyuria usually indicates accompanying infection. Increased obstruction may lead to urine extravasation and formation of urinomas.

◆ ***UTI.*** Urinary hesitancy may be associated with UTIs. Characteristic urinary changes include frequency, dysuria, nocturia, cloudy urine and, possibly, hematuria. Associated findings include bladder spasms; costovertebral angle tenderness; suprapubic, low back, pelvic, or flank pain; urethral discharge in males; fever; chills; malaise; nausea; and vomiting.

Other causes

◆ ***Drugs.*** Anticholinergics and drugs with anticholinergic properties (such as tricyclic antidepressants and some nasal decongestants and cold remedies) may cause urinary hesitancy. Hesitancy also may occur in patients recovering from general anesthesia.

Special considerations

Monitor the patient's voiding pattern, and palpate the abdomen frequently for bladder distention. Apply local heat to the perineum or the abdomen to enhance muscle relaxation and aid urination. Also, teach the patient how to perform a clean, intermittent self-catheterization. (See *How to catheterize yourself,* page 680.) Prepare the patient for tests, such as cystometrography or cystourethrography.

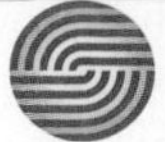

PATIENT-TEACHING AID

How to catheterize yourself

Dear Patient:
Follow the steps below to perform catheterization:

- Gather the necessary equipment: clean catheter, water-soluble lubricant, basin for collecting urine, clean washcloth, soap and water, paper towels, and a plastic bag.
- Wash your hands thoroughly; during the procedure, touch only the catheter equipment to avoid spreading germs.
- If you're a male, wash your penis and surrounding area with soap and water. If you're a female, separate the folds of your vulva with one hand and, with the other hand, wash the surrounding area using a downward (front to back) motion. Then pat the area dry.
- Open the container of lubricant and squeeze a generous amount onto a paper towel; then roll the first 7" to 10" (18 to 25.5 cm) of the catheter (or 3" [7.5 cm] for a female) in the lubricant.
- Put the open end of the catheter in the basin or toilet. If you're a male, hold your penis at a right angle to your body, grasp the catheter like a pencil, and slowly insert it into the urethra. If you're a female, spread the lips of the vulva with one hand and, with your other hand, insert the catheter in an upward and backward direction. Then inhale as you advance the catheter 7" to 10" if male, or 3" if female, until urine begins to flow. Allow urine to drain into the basin or toilet.
- When the catheter stops draining, pinch it closed and slowly remove it.
- Wash the catheter in warm soapy water, rinse it inside and out, dry it with a clean towel, and store it in a plastic bag.
- After you've used the catheter a few times, boil it in water for 20 minutes to keep it germ-free.

PEDIATRIC POINTERS

The most common cause of urinary obstruction in male infants is posterior strictures. Infants with this problem may have a less forceful urine stream and may also exhibit a fever due to UTI, failure to thrive, and a palpable bladder.

Urinary incontinence

Incontinence, the uncontrollable passage of urine, can result from a bladder abnormality, a neurologic disorder, or an alteration in pelvic muscle strength. A common urologic sign, incontinence may be transient or permanent and may involve large volumes of urine or scant dribbling. It can be classified as stress, overflow, urge, or total incontinence. *Stress incontinence* refers to intermittent leakage resulting from a sudden physical strain, such as a cough, sneeze, laugh, or quick movement. *Overflow incontinence* is a dribble resulting from urine retention, which fills the bladder and prevents it from contracting with sufficient force to expel a urine stream. *Urge incontinence* refers to the inability to suppress a sudden urge to urinate. *Total incontinence* is continuous leakage resulting from the bladder's inability to retain urine.

HISTORY AND PHYSICAL EXAMINATION

Ask the patient when he first noticed the incontinence and whether it began suddenly or gradually. Have him describe his typical urinary pattern: Does incontinence usually occur during the day or at night? Does he have any urinary control, or is he totally incontinent? If can control urination occasionally, ask him the usual times and amounts voided. Determine his normal fluid intake. Ask about other urinary problems, such as hesitancy, frequency, urgency, nocturia, and decreased force or interruption of the urine stream. Also ask if he's ever sought treatment for incontinence or found a way to deal with it himself.

Obtain a medical history, especially noting urinary tract infection (UTI), prostate conditions, spinal injury or tumor, stroke, or surgery involving the bladder, prostate, or pelvic floor. Ask a woman how many pregnancies and childbirths she has had.

After completing the history, have the patient empty his bladder. Inspect the urethral meatus for obvious signs of inflammation or an anatomic defect. Have female patients bear down, and note any urine leakage. Gently palpate the abdomen for bladder distention, which signals urine retention. Perform a complete neurologic assessment, noting motor and sensory function and obvious muscle atrophy.

MEDICAL CAUSES

◆ ***Benign prostatic hyperplasia (BPH).*** Overflow incontinence is common in this disorder as a result of urethral obstruction and urine retention. BPH begins with a group of signs and symptoms known as prostatism: reduced caliber and force of the urine stream, urinary hesitancy, and a feeling of incomplete voiding. As the obstruction increases, the patient may develop urinary frequency, nocturia and, possibly, hematuria. Examination reveals bladder distention and an enlarged prostate.

◆ ***Bladder calculus.*** Overflow incontinence may occur if the calculus lodges in the bladder neck. Associated findings vary but may include those of an irritable bladder: urinary frequency and urgency, dysuria, hematuria, and suprapubic pain from bladder spasms. Pelvic pain may be referred to the tip of the penis, vulva, low back, or heel and may be exacerbated by movement.

◆ ***Bladder cancer.*** Urge incontinence and hematuria are common findings in bladder cancer; obstruction by a tumor may produce overflow incontinence. The early stages can be asymptomatic. Other urinary signs and symptoms include frequency, dysuria, nocturia, dribbling, and suprapubic pain from bladder spasms after voiding. A mass may be palpable on bimanual examination.

◆ ***Diabetic neuropathy.*** Autonomic neuropathy may cause painless bladder distention with overflow incontinence. Related findings include episodic constipation or diarrhea (which is commonly nocturnal), impotence and retrograde ejaculation, orthostatic hypotension, syncope, and dysphagia.

◆ ***Guillain-Barré syndrome.*** Urinary incontinence may occur early in this disorder as a result of peripheral and autonomic nerve dysfunction. The cardinal sign is progressive, profound muscle weakness, which typically starts in the legs and extends to the arms and facial nerves within 24 to 72 hours. Associated findings include paresthesia, dysarthria, nasal speech, dysphagia, orthostatic hypotension, tachycardia, fecal incontinence, diaphoresis, drooling, and pain in the shoulders, thighs, or lumbar region.

◆ ***Multiple sclerosis (MS).*** Urinary incontinence, urgency, and frequency are common urologic findings in MS. Visual problems and sensory impairment are usually the first symptoms. Other findings include constipation, muscle weakness, paralysis, spasticity, hyperreflexia, intention tremor, ataxic gait, dysarthria, impotence, and emotional lability.

◆ ***Prostate cancer.*** Urinary incontinence usually occurs only in the advanced stages of prostate cancer. Urinary frequency and hesitancy, nocturia, dysuria, bladder distention, perineal pain, constipation, and a hard, irregularly shaped, nodular prostate are other common late findings.

◆ ***Prostatitis (chronic).*** Urinary incontinence may occur as a result of urethral obstruction from an enlarged prostate. Other findings include urinary frequency and urgency, dysuria, hematuria, bladder distention, a persistent urethral discharge, dull perineal pain that may radiate to other areas, ejaculatory pain, and decreased libido.

◆ ***Spinal cord injury.*** Complete cord transection above the sacral level causes flaccid paralysis of the bladder. Overflow incontinence follows rapid bladder distention. Other findings include paraplegia, sexual dysfunction, sensory loss, muscle atrophy, anhidrosis, and loss of reflexes distal to the injury.

◆ ***Stroke.*** Urinary incontinence may be transient or permanent in a stroke patient. Associated findings reflect the site and extent of the lesion and may include impaired mentation, emotional lability, behavioral changes, altered level of consciousness, and seizures. Sensorimotor effects may include contralateral hemiplegia, dysarthria, dysphagia, ataxia, apraxia, agnosia, aphasia, and unilateral sensory loss. Headache, vomiting, visual deficits, and decreased visual acuity may also occur.

◆ ***Urethral stricture.*** Partial obstruction of the lower urinary tract due to trauma or infection produces urinary hesitancy, tenesmus, and decreased force and caliber of the urine stream. Urinary frequency and urgency, nocturia, and eventually overflow incontinence may also occur. As the obstruction increases, urine extravasation may lead to formation of urinomas and urosepsis.

◆ ***UTI.*** Besides incontinence, a UTI may produce urinary urgency, dysuria, hematuria, cloudy urine and, in males, a urethral discharge. Bladder spasms or a feeling of warmth during urination may occur.

OTHER CAUSES

◆ ***Surgery.*** Urinary incontinence may occur after prostatectomy as a result of urethral sphincter damage.

Correcting incontinence with bladder retraining

The incontinent patient typically feels frustrated, embarrassed, and sometimes hopeless. Fortunately, though, his problem may be be corrected by bladder retraining—a program that aims to establish a regular voiding pattern. Here are some guidelines for establishing such a program:

◆ Before you start the program, assess the patient's intake pattern, voiding pattern, and behavior (for example, restlessness or talkativeness) before each voiding episode.
◆ Encourage the patient to use the toilet 30 minutes before he's usually incontinent. If this isn't successful, readjust the schedule. Once he's able to stay dry for 2 hours, increase the time between voidings by 30 minutes each day until he achieves a 3- to 4-hour voiding schedule.
◆ When your patient voids, make sure that the sequence of conditioning stimuli is always the same.
◆ Make sure that the patient has privacy while voiding; any inhibiting stimuli should be avoided.
◆ Keep a record of continence and incontinence for 5 days; this may reinforce your patient's efforts to remain continent.

Tips for success

Remember that both you and your patient need a positive attitude to ensure his successful bladder retraining. Here are some additional tips that may help your patient succeed:
◆ Make sure the patient is close to a bathroom or portable toilet. Leave a light on at night and ensure that the pathway to the bathroom is clear.
◆ If your patient needs assistance getting out of his bed or chair, promptly answer his call for help.
◆ Encourage the patient to wear his usual clothing as an indication that you're confident he can remain continent. Acceptable alternatives to diapers include condoms for the male patient and incontinence pads or panties for the female patient.
◆ Encourage the patient to drink 2 to 2½ qt (2 to 2.5 L) of fluid each day. Less fluid doesn't prevent incontinence but does promote bladder infection. Limiting his intake after 5 p.m., however, will help him remain continent during the night.
◆ Reassure your patient that episodes of incontinence don't signal a failure of the program. Encourage him to maintain a positive attitude.

SPECIAL CONSIDERATIONS

Prepare the patient for diagnostic tests, such as cystoscopy, cystometry, and a complete neurologic workup. Obtain a urine specimen.

Begin management of incontinence by implementing a bladder retraining program. (See *Correcting incontinence with bladder retraining*.) To prevent stress incontinence, teach the patient Kegel exercises to help strengthen the pelvic floor muscles. (See *Strengthening pelvic floor muscles*.)

If the patient's incontinence has a neurologic cause, monitor him for urine retention, which may require periodic catheterizations. If appropriate, teach the patient self-catheterization techniques. (See *How to catheterize yourself*, page 680.) A patient with permanent urinary incontinence may require surgical creation of a urinary diversion.

PEDIATRIC POINTERS

Incontinence in children may be caused by infrequent or incomplete voiding, which may also lead to a UTI. Ectopic ureteral orifice is an uncommon congenital anomaly associated with incontinence. A complete diagnostic evaluation usually is necessary to rule out organic disease.

GERIATRIC POINTERS

Diagnosing a UTI in elderly patients can be problematic because they may complain only of urinary incontinence or a seemingly unrelated symptom, such as altered mental status, anorexia, or malaise. Also, many elderly patients with dysuria, frequency, urgency, or incontinence don't have a UTI.

Urinary urgency

A sudden compelling urge to urinate accompanied by bladder pain is a classic symptom of urinary tract infection (UTI). As inflammation decreases bladder capacity, discomfort results from the accumulation of even small amounts of urine. Frequent voiding in an effort to alleviate this discomfort produces urine output of only a few milliliters at each voiding.

Urgency without bladder pain may point to an upper-motor-neuron lesion that has disrupted bladder control.

History and physical examination

Ask the patient about the onset of urinary urgency and whether he's ever experienced it before. Ask about other urologic symptoms, such as dysuria and cloudy urine. Also ask about neurologic symptoms such as paresthesia. Explore his medical history for recurrent or chronic UTIs and for surgery or procedures involving the urinary tract.

Obtain a clean-catch urine specimen for urinalysis and culture and sensitivity tests. Note urine character, color, and odor, and use a reagent strip to test for pH, glucose, and blood. Then palpate the suprapubic area and both flanks for distention and tenderness. If the patient's history or symptoms suggest neurologic dysfunction, perform a neurologic examination.

Medical causes

◆ ***Amyotrophic lateral sclerosis (ALS).*** ALS occasionally produces urinary urgency. More common findings include muscle weakness, cramping, atrophy, and coarse fasciculations in the forearms and hands. Brain stem involvement causes difficulty speaking, chewing, swallowing, and breathing. Cognitive function is usually unaffected.

◆ ***Bladder calculus.*** Bladder irritation can lead to urinary urgency and frequency, dysuria, terminal hematuria, and suprapubic pain from bladder spasms. Pain may be referred to the penis, vulva, lower back, or heel.

◆ ***Multiple sclerosis (MS).*** Urinary urgency, frequency, and incontinence are common urologic findings in MS. Like other symptoms of MS, these effects may wax and wane. Visual and sensory impairments are usually the earliest findings. Others include constipation, muscle weakness, paralysis, spasticity, intention tremor, hyperreflexia, ataxic gait, dysphagia, dysarthria, impotence, and emotional lability.

◆ ***Reiter's syndrome.*** In this self-limiting syndrome that primarily affects males, urinary urgency and other symptoms of acute urethritis occur 1 to 2 weeks after sexual contact. Other symptoms include asymmetrical arthritis of the knees, ankles, or metatarsal phalangeal joints; conjunctivitis in one or both eyes; and ulcers on the penis, mouth, tongue, palms, or soles.

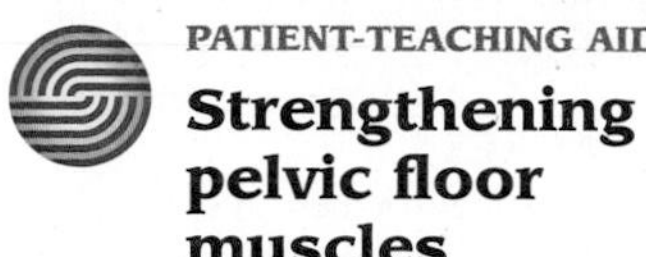

PATIENT-TEACHING AID

Strengthening pelvic floor muscles

Dear Patient:

Many women suffer from stress incontinence—urine leakage during a sudden physical strain, such as a cough, sneeze, or laugh. You can prevent or minimize this problem by doing simple exercises to strengthen your pelvic floor muscles. You can perform them sitting or standing and during various activities, such as reading, watching TV, waiting in a line, and especially while urinating.

Here's how to do the exercises:

◆ Tense the muscles around your anus. This tightens the posterior muscles of the pelvic floor.

◆ While urinating, stop the flow of urine and then restart it. This tightens the anterior muscles of the pelvic floor.

◆ Now that you've identified these muscles, you can exercise them anywhere and anytime. As you perform the exercises, slowly tighten each group of muscles and then release them.

◆ ***Spinal cord lesion.*** Urinary urgency can result from incomplete cord transection when voluntary control of sphincter function weakens. Urinary frequency, difficulty initiating and inhibiting a urine stream, and bladder distention and discomfort may also occur. Neuromuscular effects distal to the lesion include weakness, paralysis, hyperreflexia, sensory disturbances, and impotence.

◆ ***Urethral stricture.*** Bladder decompensation produces urinary urgency, frequency, and nocturia. Early signs and symptoms include hesitancy, tenesmus, and reduced caliber and force of the urine stream. Eventually, overflow incontinence may occur.

◆ ***UTI.*** Urinary urgency is commonly associated with UTIs. Other characteristic urinary changes include frequency, hematuria, dysuria, nocturia, cloudy urine, and sometimes urinary hesitancy. Associated findings include bladder spasms; costovertebral angle tenderness; suprapubic, low back, or flank pain; urethral discharge in males; fever; chills; malaise; nausea; and vomiting.

Other causes

◆ ***Treatments.*** Radiation therapy may irritate and inflame the bladder, causing urinary urgency.

Special considerations

Prepare the patient for the diagnostic workup, including a complete urinalysis, culture and sensitivity studies and, possibly, neurologic tests.

Increase the patient's intake of fluids, especially water, if not contraindicated, to dilute the urine and diminish the feeling of urgency. Administer an antibiotic and a urinary anesthetic such as phenazopyridine.

Pediatric pointers

In young children, urinary urgency may appear as a change in toilet habits, such as a sudden onset of bed-wetting or daytime accidents in a toilet-trained child. Urgency may also result from urethral irritation by bubble bath salts.

Patient counseling

Instruct sexually active patients in safer sex practices. Teach women and girls about proper genital hygiene such as cleaning from front to back to reduce contamination from fecal bacteria. Instruct women to maintain adequate fluid intake to promote frequent urination.

Urine cloudiness

Cloudy, murky, or turbid urine reflects the presence of bacteria, mucus, leukocytes or erythrocytes, epithelial cells, fat, or phosphates (in alkaline urine). It's characteristic of urinary tract infection (UTI), but it can also result from prolonged storage of a urine specimen at room temperature.

History and physical examination

Ask about symptoms of UTI, such as dysuria; urinary urgency or frequency; and pain in the flank, lower back, or suprapubic area. Also ask the patient if he has had recurrent UTIs or recent surgery or treatment involving the urinary tract.

Obtain a urine specimen to check for pus or mucus. Using a reagent strip, test for blood, glucose, and pH. Palpate the suprapubic area and flanks for tenderness.

If you note cloudy urine in a patient with an indwelling urinary catheter, especially if he also has a fever, remove the catheter immediately (or change it if the patient must have one in place).

Medical causes

◆ ***UTI.*** Cloudy urine is common in UTIs. Other urinary findings include urgency, frequency, hesitancy, hematuria, dysuria, nocturia and, in males, a urethral discharge. Other effects include fever, chills, malaise, nausea and vomiting, bladder spasms, costovertebral angle tenderness, and suprapubic, low back, or flank pain.

Special considerations

Collect urine specimens for urinalysis and culture and sensitivity tests. Increase the patient's fluid intake, and administer an antibiotic and a urinary anesthetic (such as phenazopyridine). Continue checking the appearance of the patient's urine to monitor the effectiveness of therapy.

Pediatric pointers

Cloudy urine in children also points to a UTI.

Urticaria

[Hives]

Urticaria is a vascular skin reaction characterized by the eruption of transient pruritic wheals—smooth, slightly elevated patches with well-defined erythematous margins and pale centers of various shapes and sizes. This reaction is caused by the local release of histamine or other vasoactive substances as part of a hypersensitivity reaction. (See *Recognizing common skin lesions,* pages 518 and 519.)

Acute urticaria evolves rapidly and usually has a detectable cause, such as hypersensitivity to certain drugs, foods, insect bites, inhalants, or contactants; emotional stress; or environmental factors. Although individual lesions usually subside within 12 to 24 hours, new crops of lesions may erupt continuously, thus prolonging the attack.

Urticaria lasting longer than 6 weeks is classified as chronic. The lesions may recur for months or years, and the underlying cause is usually unknown. Occasionally, a diagnosis of psychogenic urticaria is made.

Angioedema, or giant urticaria, is characterized by the acute eruption of wheals involving the mucous membranes and occasionally the arms, legs, or genitalia.

EMERGENCY INTERVENTIONS *In a patient with acute urticaria, quickly evaluate his respiratory status and take his vital signs. Ensure patent I.V. access if you note respiratory difficulty or signs of impending anaphylactic shock. Also, as appropriate, give local epinephrine or apply ice to the affected site to decrease absorption of the irritating agent through vasoconstriction. Clear and maintain the airway, give oxygen as needed, and institute cardiac monitoring. Have resuscitation equipment at hand, and be prepared to begin cardiopulmonary resuscitation. Intubation or a tracheostomy may be required.*

History and physical examination

If the patient isn't in distress, obtain a complete history. Does he have any known allergies? Does the urticaria follow a seasonal pattern? Do certain foods or drugs seem to aggravate it? Is it related to physical exertion? Is the patient routinely exposed to chemicals on the job or at home? Has he recently used new skin products? Obtain a detailed drug history, including prescription and over-the-counter drugs. Note any history of chronic or parasitic infection, skin disease, or a GI disorder.

Medical causes

◆ ***Anaphylaxis.*** This life-threatening reaction is marked by the rapid eruption of diffuse urticaria and angioedema, with wheals ranging from pinpoint to palm-size or larger. Lesions are usually pruritic and stinging and preceded by paresthesia. Other acute findings include profound anxiety, weakness, diaphoresis, sneezing, shortness of breath, profuse rhinorrhea, nasal congestion, dysphagia, and warm, moist skin.

◆ ***Lyme disease.*** Urticaria may result from the characteristic skin lesion (erythema chronicum migrans) produced by this tick-borne disease. Later effects include constant malaise and fatigue, intermittent headache, fever, chills, lymphadenopathy, neurologic and cardiac abnormalities, and arthritis.

Other causes

◆ ***Drugs.*** Many drugs can produce urticaria. Among the most common are aspirin, atropine, codeine, dextrans, immune serums, insulin, morphine, penicillin, quinine, sulfonamides, and vaccines. In addition, radiographic contrast media commonly produce urticaria, especially when administered I.V.

Special considerations

To help relieve the patient's discomfort, apply a bland skin emollient or one containing menthol and phenol. Expect to give an antihistamine, a systemic corticosteroid or, if stress is a suspected contributing factor, a tranquilizer. Tepid baths and cool compresses may also enhance vasoconstriction and decrease pruritus. Advise the patient to avoid the causative stimulus if it's identified.

Pediatric pointers

Pediatric forms of urticaria include acute papular urticaria (usually after insect bites) and urticaria pigmentosa (rare).

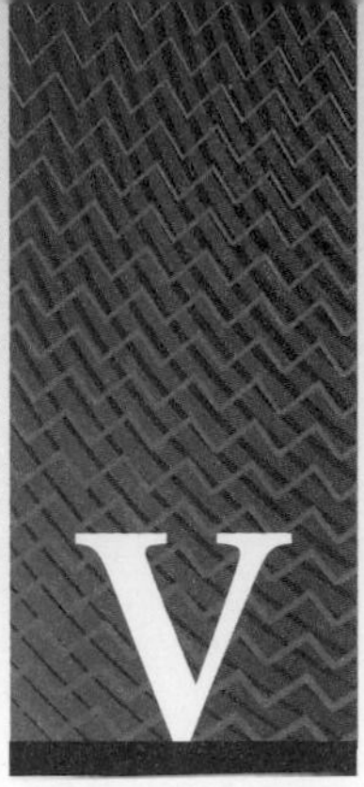

Vaginal bleeding, postmenopausal

Postmenopausal vaginal bleeding—bleeding that occurs 6 or more months after menopause—is an important indicator of gynecologic cancer. But it can also result from infection, a local pelvic disorder, estrogenic stimulation, atrophy of the endometrium, and physiologic thinning and drying of the vaginal mucous membranes. Sometimes, what appears to be bleeding from the vagina is actually bleeding from another gynecologic location—such as the ovaries, fallopian tubes, uterus, or cervix—that exits the body through the vagina. Vaginal bleeding usually occurs as brown or red spotting that either develops spontaneously or follows coitus or douching, but it may also occur as oozing of fresh blood or bright red hemorrhaging. Many patients—especially those with a history of heavy menstrual flow—minimize the importance of vaginal bleeding, thus delaying diagnosis.

History and physical examination

Determine the patient's age and her age at menopause. Ask when she first noticed the abnormal bleeding. Then obtain a thorough obstetric and gynecologic history. When did she begin menstruating? Were her periods regular? If not, ask her to describe any menstrual irregularities. How old was she when she first had intercourse? How many sexual partners has she had? Has she had any children? Has she had fertility problems? If possible, obtain an obstetric and gynecologic history of the patient's mother, and ask about a family history of gynecologic cancer. Determine if the patient has any associated symptoms and if she's taking estrogen.

Observe the external genitalia, noting the character of any vaginal discharge and the appearance of the labia, vaginal rugae, and clitoris. Carefully palpate the patient's breasts and lymph nodes for nodules or enlargement. The patient will require pelvic and rectal examinations.

Medical causes

◆ ***Atrophic vaginitis.*** When bloody staining occurs in this disorder, it usually follows coitus or douching. The characteristic watery white vaginal discharge may be accompanied by pruritus, dyspareunia, and a burning sensation in the vagina and labia. Sparse pubic hair, a pale vagina with decreased rugae and small hemorrhagic spots, clitoral atrophy, and shrinking of the labia minora may also occur.

◆ ***Cervical cancer.*** Early invasive cervical cancer causes vaginal spotting or heavier bleeding, usually after coitus or douching but occasionally spontaneously. Related findings include a persistent, pink-tinged, and foul-smelling vaginal discharge and postcoital pain. As the cancer spreads, back and sciatic pain, leg swelling, anorexia, weight loss, hematuria, dysuria, rectal bleeding, and weakness may occur.

◆ ***Cervical or endometrial polyps.*** These small, pedunculated growths may cause spotting (possibly as a mucopurulent pink discharge) after coitus, douching, or straining at defecation. However, many endometrial polyps produce no symptoms.

◆ ***Endometrial hyperplasia or cancer.*** Bleeding occurs early in these disorders; it can be brownish and scant or bright red and profuse, and usually follows coitus or douching. Bleeding later becomes heavier and more frequent, leading to clotting and anemia. It may be accompanied by pelvic, rectal, low back, and leg pain and an enlarged uterus.

◆ ***Ovarian tumors (feminizing).*** Estrogen-producing ovarian tumors can stimulate endometrial shedding and cause heavy bleeding that isn't associated with coitus or douching. A palpable pelvic mass, increased cervical mucus, breast enlargement, and spider angiomas may be present.

◆ ***Vaginal cancer.*** Characteristic spotting or bleeding may be preceded by a thin, watery vaginal discharge. Bleeding may be spontaneous but usually follows coitus or douching. A firm, ulcerated vaginal lesion may be present; dyspareunia, urinary frequency, bladder and pelvic pain, rectal bleeding, and vulvar lesions may develop later.

Other causes

◆ ***Drugs.*** Unopposed estrogen replacement therapy is a common cause of abnormal vaginal bleeding. This can usually be reduced by adding progesterone (in women who haven't had a hysterectomy) and by adjusting the patient's estrogen dosage.

Special considerations

Prepare the patient for diagnostic tests, such as ultrasonography to outline a cervical or uterine tumor; endometrial biopsy, colposcopy, or dilatation and curettage with hysteroscopy to obtain tissue specimens for histologic examination; testing for occult blood in the stool; and vaginal and cervical cultures to detect infection. Discontinue estrogen until a diagnosis is made.

Geriatric pointers

About 80% of cases of postmenopausal vaginal bleeding are benign, caused primarily by endometrial atrophy. However, malignancy should still be ruled out.

Patient counseling

Reassure the patient that most cases of postmenopausal vaginal bleeding are benign and not cancer related.

Vaginal discharge

Common in women of childbearing age, a physiologic vaginal discharge is mucoid, clear or white, nonbloody, and odorless. Produced by the cervical mucosa and, to a lesser degree, by the vulvar glands, this discharge may occasionally be scant or profuse because of estrogenic stimulation and changes during the patient's menstrual cycle. However, a marked increase in discharge or a change in discharge color, odor, or consistency can signal disease and may result from infection, sexually transmitted disease, reproductive tract disease, fistulas, and the use of certain drugs. In addition, the prolonged presence of a foreign body, such as a tampon or diaphragm, in the patient's vagina can cause irritation and an inflammatory exudate, as can frequent douching and the use of feminine hygiene products, contraceptive products, bubble baths, and colored or perfumed toilet papers.

History and physical examination

Ask the patient to describe the onset, color, consistency, odor, and texture of her vaginal discharge. How does the discharge differ from her usual vaginal secretions? Is the onset related to her menstrual cycle? Also, ask about associated symptoms, such as dysuria and perineal pruritus and burning. Does she have spotting after coitus or douching? Ask about recent changes in her sexual habits and hygiene practices. Is she or could she be pregnant? Next, ask if she has had a vaginal discharge before or has ever been treated for a vaginal infection. What treatment did she receive? Did she complete the course of medication? Ask about her current use of medications, especially antibiotics, oral estrogens, and hormonal contraceptives.

Examine the external genitalia and note the character of the discharge. (See *Identifying causes of vaginal discharge*, page 688.) Observe vulvar and vaginal tissues for redness, edema, and excoriation. Palpate the inguinal lymph nodes to detect tenderness or enlargement, and palpate the abdomen for tenderness. A pelvic examination may be required. Obtain vaginal discharge specimens for testing.

Medical causes

◆ ***Atrophic vaginitis.*** In this disorder, a scant, watery white vaginal discharge may be accompanied by pruritus, burning, tenderness, and bloody spotting after coitus or douching. Sparse

Identifying causes of vaginal discharge

The color, consistency, amount, and odor of your patient's vaginal discharge provide important clues about the underlying disorder. For quick reference, use this chart to match common characteristics of vaginal discharge and their possible causes.

Characteristics	Possible causes
Scant thin, watery white discharge	Atrophic vaginitis
Thin, green or gray-white, foul-smelling discharge	Bacterial vaginosis
Profuse white curdlike discharge with yeasty, sweet odor	Candidiasis
Mucopurulent, foul-smelling discharge	Chancroid
Yellow, mucopurulent, odorless or acrid discharge	Chlamydial infection
Scant serosanguineous or purulent discharge with foul odor	Endometritis
Copious mucoid discharge	Genital herpes
Profuse mucopurulent discharge, possibly foul smelling	Genital warts
Yellow or green, foul-smelling discharge from the cervix or occasionally from Bartholin's or Skene's ducts	Gonorrhea
Chronic, watery, bloody or purulent discharge, possibly foul smelling	Gynecologic cancer
Frothy, green-yellow, and profuse (or thin, white, and scant) foul-smelling discharge	Trichomoniasis

pubic hair, a pale vagina with decreased rugae and small hemorrhagic spots, clitoral atrophy, and shrinking of the labia minora may also occur.

◆ ***Bacterial vaginosis.*** This infection, caused by *Gardnerella vaginalis*, results from an ecozogic disturbance of the vaginal flora. It produces a thin, foul-smelling, green or gray-white discharge that adheres to the vaginal walls and can be easily wiped away, leaving healthy-looking tissue. Pruritus, redness, and other mild signs of vaginal irritation may also occur.

◆ ***Candidiasis.*** Infection with *Candida albicans* causes a profuse, white, curdlike discharge with a yeasty, sweet odor. Onset is abrupt, usually just before menses or during a course of antibiotics. Exudate may be lightly attached to the labia and vaginal walls and is commonly accompanied by vulvar redness and edema. The inner thighs may be covered with a fine red dermatitis and weeping erosions. Intense labial itching and burning may also occur. Some patients experience external dysuria.

◆ ***Chancroid.*** This rare but highly contagious sexually transmitted disease produces a mucopurulent, foul-smelling discharge and vulvar lesions that are initially erythematous and later ulcerated. Within 2 to 3 weeks, inguinal lymph nodes (usually unilateral) may become tender and enlarged, with pruritus, suppuration, and spontaneous drainage of nodes. Headache, malaise, and a fever as high as 102.2° F (39° C) are common.

◆ ***Chlamydial infection.*** This infection causes a yellow, mucopurulent, odorless or acrid vaginal discharge. Other findings include dysuria, dyspareunia, and vaginal bleeding after douching or coitus, especially after menses. Many women, however, remain asymptomatic.

◆ ***Endometritis.*** A scant serosanguineous discharge with a foul odor can result from bacterial invasion of the endometrium. Associated findings include fever, low back and abdominal pain, abdominal muscle spasm, malaise, dysmenorrhea, and an enlarged uterus.

◆ ***Genital warts.*** These mosaic, papular vulvar lesions can cause a profuse mucopurulent vaginal discharge, which may be foul smelling if the warts are infected. Patients commonly complain of burning or paresthesia in the vaginal introitus.
◆ ***Gonorrhea.*** Although 80% of women with gonorrhea are asymptomatic, others have a foul-smelling yellow or green discharge that can be expressed from Bartholin's or Skene's ducts. Other findings include dysuria, urinary frequency and incontinence, bleeding, and vaginal redness and swelling. Severe pelvic and lower abdominal pain and fever may develop.
◆ ***Gynecologic cancer.*** Endometrial or cervical cancer produces a chronic, watery, bloody or purulent vaginal discharge that may be foul smelling. Other findings include abnormal vaginal bleeding and, later, weight loss; pelvic, back, and leg pain; fatigue; urinary frequency; and abdominal distention.
◆ ***Herpes simplex (genital).*** A copious mucoid discharge results from this disorder, but the initial complaint is painful, indurated vesicles and ulcerations on the labia, vagina, cervix, anus, thighs, or mouth. Erythema, marked edema, and tender inguinal lymph nodes may occur with fever, malaise, and dysuria.
◆ ***Trichomoniasis.*** This infection can cause a foul-smelling discharge, which may be frothy, green-yellow, and profuse or thin, white, and scant. Other findings include pruritus; an inflamed, erythematous vagina with tiny petechiae; dysuria and urinary frequency; dyspareunia; postcoital spotting; and menorrhagia or dysmenorrhea. About 70% of patients are asymptomatic.

OTHER CAUSES

◆ ***Contraceptive creams and jellies.*** These products can increase vaginal secretions.
◆ ***Drugs.*** Drugs that contain estrogen, including hormonal contraceptives, can cause a mucoid vaginal discharge. Antibiotics such as tetracycline may increase the risk of a candidal vaginal infection and associated discharge.
◆ ***Radiation therapy.*** Irradiation of the reproductive tract can cause a watery, odorless vaginal discharge.

SPECIAL CONSIDERATIONS

Teach the patient to keep her perineum clean and dry. Also, tell her to avoid wearing tight-fitting clothing and nylon underwear and to instead wear cotton-crotched underwear and pantyhose. If appropriate, suggest that the patient douche with a solution of 5 tbsp of white vinegar in 2 qt (2 L) of warm water to help relieve her discomfort.

If the patient has a vaginal infection, tell her to continue taking the prescribed medication even if her symptoms clear or she menstruates. Also, advise her to avoid intercourse until her symptoms clear and then to have her partner use condoms until she completes her course of medication. If her condition is sexually transmitted, teach her about safer sex methods.

PEDIATRIC POINTERS

Female neonates who have been exposed to maternal estrogens in utero may have a white mucous vaginal discharge for the first month after birth; a yellow mucous discharge indicates a pathologic condition. In an older child, a purulent, foul-smelling and, possibly, bloody vaginal discharge commonly results from a foreign object placed in the vagina; in such cases, consider the possibility of sexual abuse.

GERIATRIC POINTERS

The vaginal mucosa becomes thin in postmenopausal women because of their decreased estrogen levels. This mucosal thinning combined with a rise in vaginal pH results in decreased resistance to infectious agents and an increased incidence of vaginitis.

Venous hum

A venous hum is a functional or innocent murmur heard above the clavicles throughout the cardiac cycle. Loudest during diastole, it may be low pitched, rough, or noisy. The hum commonly accompanies a thrill or, possibly, a high-pitched whine. It's best heard by applying the bell of the stethoscope to the medial aspect of the right supraclavicular area with the patient seated upright, or by placing the stethoscope bell in the second or third parasternal interspace with the patient standing upright. (See *Detecting a venous hum,* page 690.)

A venous hum is a common, normal finding in children and pregnant women. However, it also occurs in hyperdynamic states, such as anemia and thyrotoxicosis. The hum results from increased blood flow through the internal jugular veins, especially on the right side, which causes audible vibrations in the tissues.

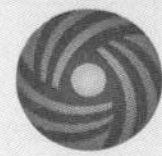

EXAMINATION TIP

Detecting a venous hum

To detect a venous hum, have your patient sit upright and then place the bell of the stethoscope over his right supraclavicular area. Gently lift his chin and turn his head toward the left, which increases the loudness of the hum (top). If you still can't hear the hum, press his jugular vein with your thumb (bottom). The hum will disappear with pressure but will suddenly return, temporarily louder than before, when you release your thumb—a result of the turbulence created by pressure changes.

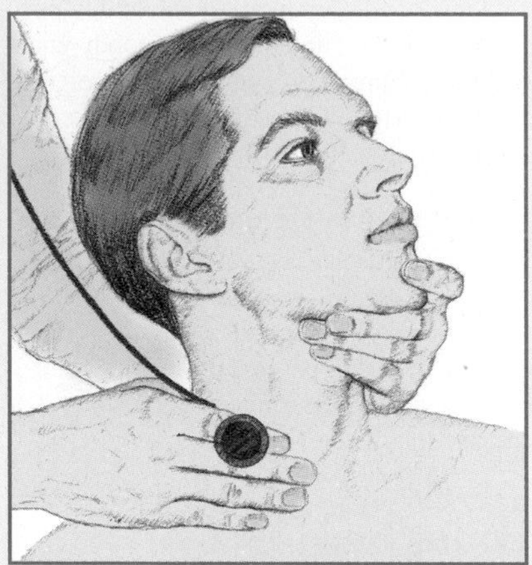

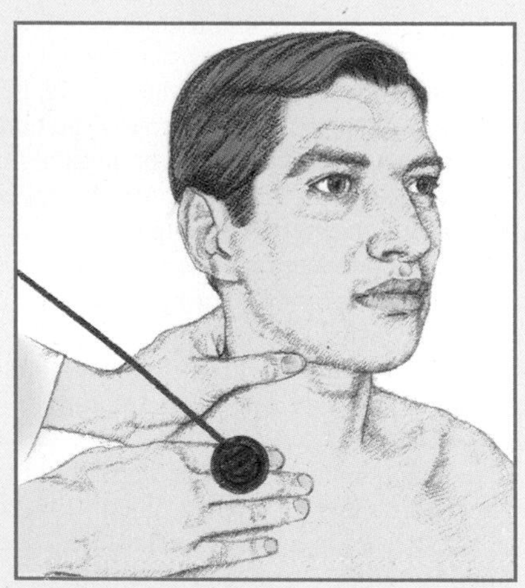

Occasionally, a venous hum may be mistaken for an intracardiac murmur or a thyroid bruit. However, a venous hum disappears with jugular vein compression and waxes and wanes with head turning. In contrast, an intracardiac murmur and a thyroid bruit persist despite jugular vein compression and head turning.

History and physical examination

Determine if the patient has a history of anemia or thyroid disorders. If he does, ask which medications or other treatments he has received. If he doesn't, ask if he has had associated signs and symptoms, such as palpitations, dyspnea, nervousness, tremors, heat intolerance, weight loss, fatigue, or malaise.

Take the patient's vital signs, noting especially tachycardia, hypertension, a bounding pulse, and widened pulse pressure. Auscultate his heart for gallops or murmurs. Examine his skin and mucous membranes for pallor.

Medical causes

◆ ***Anemia.*** A venous hum is common in severe anemia (hemoglobin level below 7 g/dl). Additional findings include pale skin and mucous membranes, dyspnea, crackles, tachycardia, bounding pulse, atrial gallop, systolic bruits over both carotid arteries, bleeding tendencies, weakness, fatigue, and malaise.

◆ ***Thyrotoxicosis.*** This disorder may cause a loud venous hum, audible whether the patient is sitting or in a supine position. Auscultation may also reveal an atrial or ventricular gallop. Additional findings include tachycardia, palpitations, weight loss despite increased appetite, diarrhea, an enlarged thyroid gland, dyspnea, nervousness, difficulty concentrating, tremors, diaphoresis, heat intolerance, and exophthalmos. Women may have oligomenorrhea or amenhorrhea; men, gynecomastia. Both sexes may have a decreased libido.

Special considerations

Prepare the patient for diagnostic tests, which may include an electrocardiogram, a complete blood count, and thyroid hormone (triiodothyronine and thyroxine) assays.

Pediatric pointers

A cervical venous hum occurs normally in more than two-thirds of children ages 5 to 15.

Vertigo

Vertigo is an illusion of movement in which the patient feels that he's revolving in space (subjective vertigo) or that his surroundings are revolving around him (objective vertigo). He may complain of feeling pulled sideways, as though drawn by a magnet.

A common symptom, vertigo usually begins abruptly and may be temporary or permanent and mild or severe. It may worsen when the patient moves and subside when he lies down. It's commonly confused with dizziness—a sensation of imbalance and light-headedness that is nonspecific. However, unlike dizziness, vertigo is commonly accompanied by nausea, vomiting, nystagmus, and tinnitus or hearing loss. Although the patient's limb coordination is unaffected, he may exhibit a vertiginous gait.

Vertigo may result from a neurologic or otologic disorder that affects the equilibratory apparatus (the vestibule, semicircular canals, eighth cranial nerve, vestibular nuclei in the brain stem and their temporal lobe connections, and eyes). However, this symptom may also result from alcohol intoxication, hyperventilation, postural changes (benign postural vertigo), and the effects of certain drugs, tests, or procedures.

History and physical examination

Ask your patient to describe the onset and duration of his vertigo, being careful to distinguish this symptom from dizziness. Does he feel that he's moving or that his surroundings are moving around him? How often do the attacks occur? Do they follow position changes, or are they unpredictable? Find out if the patient can walk during an attack, if he leans to one side, and if he's ever fallen. Ask if he experiences motion sickness and if he prefers one position during an attack. Obtain a recent drug history, and note any evidence of alcohol abuse.

Perform a neurologic assessment, focusing particularly on eighth cranial nerve function. Observe the patient's gait and posture for abnormalities.

Medical causes

◆ ***Acoustic neuroma.*** This tumor of the eighth cranial nerve causes mild, intermittent vertigo and unilateral sensorineural hearing loss. Other findings include tinnitus, postauricular or suboccipital pain, and—with cranial nerve compression—facial paralysis.

◆ ***Benign positional vertigo.*** In this disorder, debris in a semicircular canal produces vertigo lasting a few minutes when the patient changes head position. This type of vertigo is usually temporary and can be effectively treated with positional maneuvers.

◆ ***Brain stem ischemia.*** This condition produces sudden, severe vertigo that may become episodic and later persistent. Associated findings include ataxia, nausea, vomiting, increased blood pressure, tachycardia, nystagmus, and lateral deviation of the eyes toward the side of the lesion. Hemiparesis and paresthesia may also occur.

◆ ***Head trauma.*** Persistent vertigo, occurring soon after a head injury, accompanies spontaneous or positional nystagmus and, if the temporal bone is fractured, hearing loss. Associated findings include headache, nausea, vomiting, and decreased level of consciousness. Behavioral changes, diplopia or visual blurring, seizures, motor or sensory deficits, and signs of increased intracranial pressure may also occur.

◆ ***Herpes zoster.*** Infection of the eighth cranial nerve produces sudden onset of vertigo accompanied by facial paralysis, hearing loss in the affected ear, and herpetic vesicular lesions in the auditory canal.

◆ ***Labyrinthitis.*** Severe vertigo begins abruptly in this inner ear infection. Vertigo may occur in a single episode or may recur over months or years. Associated findings include nausea, vomiting, progressive sensorineural hearing loss, and nystagmus.

◆ ***Ménière's disease.*** In this disease, labyrinthine dysfunction causes abrupt onset of vertigo, lasting minutes, hours, or days. Unpredictable episodes of severe vertigo and unsteady gait may cause the patient to fall. During an attack, any sudden motion of the head or eyes can precipitate nausea and vomiting.

◆ ***Motion sickness.*** This condition is characterized by vertigo, nausea, vomiting, and headache in response to rhythmic or erratic motions.

◆ ***Multiple sclerosis (MS).*** Episodic vertigo may occur early and become persistent in MS. Other early findings include diplopia, visual blurring, and paresthesia. MS may also produce nystagmus, constipation, muscle weakness, paralysis, spasticity, hyperreflexia, intention tremor, and ataxia.

◆ ***Posterior fossa tumor.*** This type of tumor may produce positional vertigo that lasts for a few seconds as well as papilledema, headache, memory loss, nausea, vomiting, nystagmus, apneustic or ataxic respirations, and increased blood pressure. The patient may also fall sideways.

◆ ***Seizures.*** Temporal lobe seizures may produce vertigo, usually associated with other symptoms of partial complex seizures.

◆ ***Vestibular neuritis.*** In this disorder, severe vertigo usually begins abruptly, lasts several days, and isn't accompanied by tinnitus or hearing loss. Other findings include nausea, vomiting, and nystagmus.

Other causes

◆ ***Diagnostic tests.*** Caloric testing (irrigating the ears with warm or cold water) can induce vertigo.

◆ ***Drugs and alcohol.*** High or toxic doses of certain drugs or alcohol may produce vertigo. These drugs include salicylates, aminoglycosides, antibiotics, quinine, and hormonal contraceptives.

◆ ***Surgery and other procedures.*** Ear surgery may cause vertigo that lasts for several days. Administration of overly warm or cold eardrops or irrigating solutions can also cause vertigo.

Special considerations

Place the patient in a comfortable position, and monitor his vital signs and level of consciousness. Keep the side rails up if he's in bed, or help him to a chair if he's standing when vertigo occurs. Darken the room and keep him calm. Administer drugs to control nausea and vomiting and meclizine or dimenhydrinate to decrease labyrinthine irritability.

Prepare the patient for diagnostic tests, such as electronystagmography, EEG, and X-rays of the middle and inner ears.

Pediatric pointers

Ear infection is a common cause of vertigo in children. Vestibular neuritis may also cause this symptom.

Vesicular rash

A vesicular rash is a scattered or linear distribution of blisterlike lesions that are sharply circumscribed and filled with clear, cloudy, or bloody fluid. The lesions, which are usually less than 0.5 cm in diameter, may occur singly or in groups. (See *Recognizing common skin lesions,* pages 518 and 519.) They sometimes occur with bullae—fluid-filled lesions larger than 0.5 cm in diameter.

A vesicular rash may be mild or severe and temporary or permanent. It can result from infection, inflammation, or allergic reactions.

History and physical examination

Ask your patient when the rash began, how it spread, and whether it has appeared before. Did other skin lesions precede eruption of the vesicles? Obtain a thorough drug history. If the patient has treated the rash with a topical medication, what type did he use and when did he last apply it? Also, ask about associated signs and symptoms. Find out if he has a family history of skin disorders, and ask about allergies and recent infections, insect bites, or exposure to allergens.

Examine the patient's skin, noting if it's dry, oily, or moist. Observe the general distribution of the lesions and record their exact location. Note the color, shape, and size of the lesions, and check for crusts, scales, scars, macules, papules, or wheals. Palpate the vesicles or bullae to determine if they're flaccid or tense. Slide your finger across the skin to see if the outer layer of epidermis separates easily from the basal layer (Nikolsky's sign).

Medical causes

◆ ***Burns (second-degree).*** Thermal burns that affect the epidermis and part of the dermis cause vesicles and bullae along with erythema, swelling, pain, and moistness.

◆ ***Dermatitis.*** In *contact dermatitis,* a hypersensitivity reaction produces an eruption of small vesicles surrounded by redness and marked edema. The vesicles may ooze, scale, and cause severe pruritus.

Dermatitis herpetiformis, a skin disease that is most common in men between ages 20 and 50 (and is occasionally associated with celiac disease, organ malignancy, or immunoglobulin A immunotherapy), produces a chronic inflammatory eruption marked by vesicular, papular, bullous, pustular, or erythematous lesions. The rash is usually distributed symmetrically on the buttocks, shoulders, and extensor surfaces of the elbows and knees, but it may sometimes appear on the face, scalp, and neck. Other symptoms include severe pruritus, burning, and stinging.

In *nummular dermatitis,* groups of pinpoint vesicles and papules appear on erythematous or pustular lesions that are nummular (coinlike) or annular (ringlike). The pustular lesions commonly ooze a purulent exudate, itch severely, and rapidly become crusted and scaly. Two or three lesions may develop on the hands, but the lesions typically develop on the extensor surfaces of the limbs and on the buttocks and posterior trunk.

◆ ***Dermatophytid.*** This allergic reaction to a fungal infection produces vesicular lesions on the hands, usually in response to tinea pedis. The lesions are extremely pruritic and tender and may be accompanied by fever, anorexia, generalized adenopathy, and splenomegaly.

◆ ***Erythema multiforme.*** This acute inflammatory skin disease is heralded by a sudden eruption of erythematous macules, papules and, occasionally, vesicles and bullae. The characteristic rash appears symmetrically over the hands, arms, feet, legs, face, and neck and tends to reappear. Although vesicles and bullae may also erupt on the eyes and genitalia, vesiculobullous lesions usually appear on the mucous membranes—especially the lips and buccal mucosa—where they rupture and ulcerate, producing a thick, yellow or white exudate. Bloody, painful crusts, a foul-smelling oral discharge, and difficulty chewing may develop. Lymphadenopathy may also occur.

◆ ***Herpes simplex.*** This common viral infection produces groups of vesicles on an inflamed base, most commonly on the lips and lower face. In about 25% of cases, the genital region is involved. Vesicles are preceded by itching, tingling, burning, or pain; develop singly or in groups; are 2 to 3 mm in diameter; and don't coalesce. Eventually, they rupture, forming a painful ulcer followed by a yellowish crust.

◆ ***Herpes zoster.*** A vesicular rash is preceded by erythema and, occasionally, by a nodular skin eruption and unilateral, sharp pain along a dermatome. About 5 days later, the lesions erupt and the pain becomes burning. Vesicles dry and scab about 10 days after eruption. Associated findings include fever, malaise, pruritus, and paresthesia or hyperesthesia of the involved area. Herpes zoster involving the cranial nerves produces facial palsy, hearing loss, dizziness, loss of taste, eye pain, and impaired vision.

◆ ***Pemphigoid (bullous).*** Generalized pruritus or an urticarial or eczematous eruption may precede the classic bullous rash. Bullae are large, thick walled, tense, and irregular, typically forming on an erythematous base. They usually appear on the lower abdomen, groin, inner thighs, and forearms.

◆ ***Pemphigus.*** In *chronic familial pemphigus,* groups of tiny vesicles erupt on normal skin or mucous membranes. The vesicles are thin walled, flaccid, and easily broken, producing small denuded areas that become covered with crust and typically itch and burn. The eruption remits spontaneously but recurs.

Pemphigus foliaceus usually develops slowly and may begin with bullous lesions, commonly on the head and trunk. As these lesions spread to other areas, they become moist, scaly, and foul smelling. Nikolsky's sign is present, and denudation of lesions results in extensive erythema, with large, loose scales and crusts. Pruritus and burning are common.

Pemphigus vulgaris may be acute and rapidly progressive or chronic. The typically flaccid bullae may be tender or painful and large or small. When they rupture, denuded skin exudes a clear, bloody, or purulent discharge. Commonly, the bullae first erupt in a specific location, such as the mouth or scalp, and eventually become widespread. Nikolsky's sign and pruritus may be present.

◆ ***Pompholyx (dyshidrosis or dyshidrotic eczema).*** This common, recurrent disorder produces symmetrical vesicular lesions that can become pustular. The pruritic lesions are more common on the palms than on the soles and may be accompanied by minimal erythema.

◆ ***Porphyria cutanea tarda.*** This disorder, resulting from abnormal porphyrin metabolism, produces bullae—especially on areas exposed to sun, friction, trauma, or heat—and photosensitivity. Papulovesicular lesions may evolve into erosions or ulcers and scars. Chronic skin changes include hyperpigmentation or hypopigmentation, hypertrichosis, and sclerodermoid lesions. Urine is pink to brown.

◆ ***Scabies.*** In this disorder, mites that burrow under the skin cause small vesicles to erupt on the webs of the fingers, wrists, elbows, axillae, and waistline; the glans, shaft, and scrotum in males; and the nipples in females. The lesions are a few millimeters long, with a swollen nodule or red papule that contains the mite. Pustules and excoriations may also occur. Associated pruritus worsens at night and with inactivity and warmth.

◆ ***Smallpox (variola major).*** Initial signs and symptoms include high fever, malaise, prostration, severe headache, backache, and abdominal pain. A maculopapular rash develops on the mucosa of the mouth, pharynx, face, and forearms and then spreads to the trunk and

Drugs that cause toxic epidermal necrolysis

Various drugs can trigger toxic epidermal necrolysis, a rare but potentially fatal immune reaction characterized by a vesicular rash. This type of necrolysis produces large, flaccid bullae that rupture easily, exposing extensive areas of denuded skin. The resulting loss of fluid and electrolytes—along with widespread systemic involvement—can lead to such life-threatening complications as pulmonary edema, shock, renal failure, sepsis, and disseminated intravascular coagulation.

Here's a list of some drugs that can cause toxic epidermal necrolysis:

- allopurinol
- aspirin
- barbiturates
- chloramphenicol
- chlorpropamide
- gold salts
- nitrofurantoin
- penicillin
- phenytoin
- primidone
- sulfonamides
- tetracycline.

legs. Within 2 days, the rash becomes vesicular and later pustular. The lesions develop at the same time, appear identical, and are more prominent on the face and extremities. The pustules are round, firm, and deeply embedded in the skin. After 8 to 9 days, the pustules form a crust, which later separates from the skin leaving a pitted scar. Death may result from encephalitis, extensive bleeding, or secondary infection.

◆ ***Tinea pedis.*** This fungal infection causes vesicles and scaling between the toes and possibly scaling over the entire sole. Severe infection causes inflammation, pruritus, and difficulty walking.

◆ ***Toxic epidermal necrolysis.*** In this immune reaction to drugs or other toxins, vesicles and bullae are preceded by a diffuse, erythematous rash and followed by large-scale epidermal necrolysis and desquamation. Large, flaccid bullae develop after mucous membrane inflammation, a burning sensation in the conjunctivae, malaise, fever, and generalized skin tenderness. The bullae rupture easily, exposing extensive areas of denuded skin. (See *Drugs that cause toxic epidermal necrolysis.*)

Other causes

◆ ***Insect bites.*** Vesicles appear on red hivelike papules and may become hemorrhagic.

Special considerations

Any skin eruption that covers a large area may cause substantial fluid loss through the vesicles, bullae, or other weeping lesions. If necessary, start an I.V. catheter to replace fluids and electrolytes. Keep the patient's environment warm and free from drafts, cover him with sheets or blankets as necessary, and take his rectal temperature every 4 hours because increased fluid loss and increased blood flow to inflamed skin may lead to hyperthermia.

Obtain cultures to determine the causative organism. Use precautions until infection is ruled out. Tell the patient to wash his hands often and not to touch the lesions. Be alert for signs of secondary infection. Give the patient an antibiotic and apply corticosteroid or antimicrobial ointment to the lesions.

Pediatric pointers

Vesicular rashes in children are caused by staphylococcal infections (such as staphylococcal scalded skin syndrome, a life-threatening infection occurring in infants), varicella, hand-foot-and-mouth disease, contact dermatitis, and miliaria rubra.

Violent behavior

Marked by sudden loss of self-control, violent behavior refers to the use of physical force to violate, injure, or abuse an object or person. This behavior may also be self-directed. It may result from an organic or psychiatric disorder or from the use of certain drugs.

History and physical examination

During your evaluation, determine if the patient has a history of violent behavior. Is he intoxicated or suffering symptoms of alcohol or drug withdrawal? Does he have a history of family violence, including corporal punishment and child or spouse abuse? (See *Understanding family violence.*)

Watch for clues indicating that the patient is losing control and may become violent. Has he

Understanding family violence

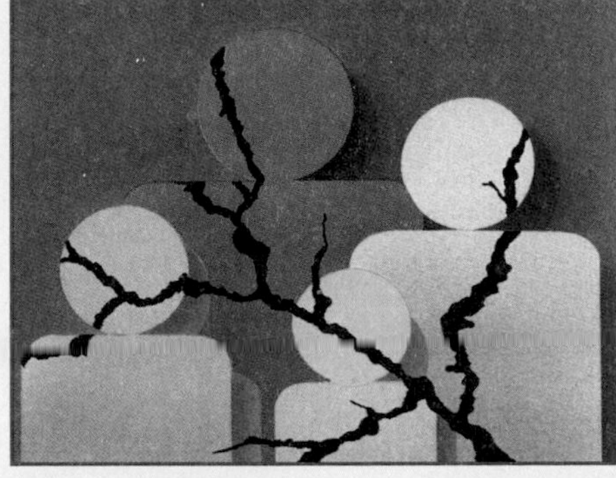

Effectively managing a violent patient requires an understanding of the roots of his behavior. For example, violent behavior may be spawned by a family history of corporal punishment or child or spouse abuse. It may also be associated with drug or alcohol abuse and fixed family roles that stifle growth and individuality.

What causes family violence? Social scientists suggest that it stems from cultural attitudes fostering violence and from the frustration and stress associated with overcrowded living conditions and poverty. Albert Bandura, a social learning theorist, believes that individuals learn violent behavior by observing and imitating other family members who vent their aggressive feelings through verbal abuse and physical force. (They also learn from television and movies, especially those in which the violent hero gains power and recognition.) Members of families with these characteristics may have an increased potential for violent behavior, thus initiating a cycle of violence that passes from generation to generation.

exhibited abrupt behavioral changes? Is he unable to sit still? Increased activity may indicate an attempt to discharge aggression. Does he suddenly cease activity (suggesting the calm before the storm)? Does he make verbal threats or angry gestures? Is he jumpy, extremely tense, or laughing? Such intensifying of emotion may herald loss of control.

If your patient's violent behavior is a new development, he may have an organic disorder. Obtain a medical history, and perform a physical examination. Watch for a sudden change in his level of consciousness. Disorientation, failure to recall recent events, and a display of tics, jerks, tremors, and asterixis all suggest an organic disorder.

Medical causes

◆ ***Organic disorders.*** Disorders resulting from metabolic or neurologic dysfunction can cause violent behavior. These include epilepsy, brain tumor, encephalitis, endocrine disorders, and metabolic disorders (such as uremia and calcium imbalance). Severe physical trauma, such as a head injury, can also cause violent behavior.

◆ ***Psychiatric disorders.*** Violent behavior occurs as a protective mechanism in response to a perceived threat in psychotic disorders such as schizophrenia. A similar response may occur in personality disorders, such as antisocial or borderline personality.

Other causes

◆ ***Drugs and alcohol.*** Violent behavior is an adverse effect of some drugs, such as lidocaine, penicillin G, hallucinogens, and amphetamines. Alcohol abuse or withdrawal and barbiturate withdrawal may also cause violent behavior.

Special considerations

Violent behavior is most prevalent in emergency departments, intensive care units, and crisis and acute psychiatric units. Natural disasters and accidents also increase the potential for violent behavior, so be on guard in these situations.

If your patient becomes violent or potentially violent, your goal is to remain composed and to establish environmental control. First, protect yourself. Remain at a distance from the patient, call for assistance, and don't overreact. Remain calm and make sure you have enough personnel to subdue or restrain the patient if necessary. Encourage the patient to move to a quiet location—free from noise, activity, and people—to avoid frightening or stimulating him further. Reassure him, explain what's happening, and tell him that he's safe.

If the patient makes violent threats, take them seriously, and inform those at whom the threats are directed. If ordered, administer a psychotropic medication.

Remember that your own attitudes can affect your ability to care for a violent patient. If you feel fearful or judgmental, ask another staff member for help.

PEDIATRIC POINTERS

Adolescents and younger children sometimes make threats resulting from violent dreams or fantasies or unmet needs. Adolescents who come from families with a history of physical or psychological abuse may display violent behavior toward their peers, siblings, and pets.

Vision loss

Vision loss—the inability to perceive visual stimuli—can be sudden or gradual and temporary or permanent. The deficit can range from a slight impairment of vision to total blindness. It can result from an ocular, a neurologic, or a systemic disorder or from trauma or the use of certain drugs. The ultimate visual outcome may depend on early, accurate diagnosis and treatment.

HISTORY AND PHYSICAL EXAMINATION

Sudden vision loss can signal an ocular emergency. Don't touch the eye if the patient has a perforating or penetrating ocular trauma. (See *Managing sudden vision loss*.)

If the patient's vision loss occurred gradually, ask him if it affects one eye or both and all or only part of the visual field. Is the vision loss transient or persistent? Did it occur abruptly or develop over hours, days, or weeks? What is the patient's age? Ask the patient if he has experienced photosensitivity, and ask about the location, intensity, and duration of any eye pain. Also, obtain an ocular history and a family history of eye problems or systemic diseases that may lead to eye problems, such as hypertension; diabetes mellitus; thyroid, rheumatic, or vascular disease; infections; and cancer.

The first step in performing the eye examination is to assess visual acuity with the best available correction in each eye. (See *Testing visual acuity,* page 698.)

Carefully inspect both eyes, noting edema, foreign bodies, drainage, or conjunctival or scleral redness. Observe whether lid closure is complete or incomplete, and check for ptosis. Using a flashlight, examine the cornea and iris for scars, irregularities, and foreign bodies. Observe the size, shape, and color of the pupils, and test the direct and consensual light reflex (see "Pupils, nonreactive," page 573) and the effect of accommodation. Evaluate extraocular muscle function by testing the six cardinal fields of gaze. (See *Testing extraocular muscles,* page 217.)

MEDICAL CAUSES

◆ ***Amaurosis fugax.*** In this disorder, recurrent attacks of unilateral vision loss may last from a few seconds to a few minutes. Vision is normal at other times. Other findings may include transient unilateral weakness, hypertension, and elevated intraocular pressure (IOP) in the affected eye.

◆ ***Cataract.*** Typically, painless and gradual visual blurring precedes vision loss. As the cataract progresses, the pupil turns milky white.

◆ ***Concussion.*** Immediately or shortly after blunt head trauma, the patient may develop blurred, double, or lost vision. Vision loss is usually temporary. Other findings include headache, anterograde and retrograde amnesia, transient loss of consciousness, nausea, vomiting, dizziness, irritability, confusion, lethargy, and aphasia.

◆ ***Corneal dystrophies, hereditary.*** Some corneal dystrophies cause vision loss with associated pain, photophobia, tearing, and corneal opacities.

◆ ***Diabetic retinopathy.*** Retinal edema and hemorrhage lead to visual blurring, which may progress to blindness.

◆ ***Endophthalmitis.*** Typically, this intraocular inflammation follows penetrating trauma, I.V. drug use, or intraocular surgery, causing unilateral vision loss that may be permanent; a sympathetic inflammation may affect the other eye.

◆ ***Glaucoma.*** This disorder produces gradual visual blurring that may progress to total blindness. *Acute angle-closure glaucoma* is an ocular emergency that may produce blindness within 3 to 5 days. It's characterized by rapid onset of unilateral inflammation and pain, pressure over the eye, moderate pupil dilation, nonreactive pupillary response, a cloudy cornea, reduced visual acuity, photophobia, and perception of blue or red halos around lights. Nausea and vomiting may also occur.

Chronic angle-closure glaucoma has a gradual onset and usually produces no symptoms,

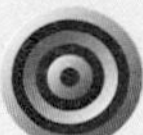

EMERGENCY INTERVENTION

Managing sudden vision loss

Sudden vision loss can signal central retinal artery occlusion or acute angle-closure glaucoma—ocular emergencies that require immediate intervention. If your patient reports sudden vision loss, immediately notify an ophthalmologist for an emergency examination, and perform the following interventions.

For a patient with suspected central retinal artery occlusion, perform light massage over his closed eyelid. Increase his carbon dioxide level by administering a set flow of oxygen and carbon dioxide through a Venturi mask, or have the patient rebreathe in a paper bag to retain exhaled carbon dioxide. These steps will dilate the artery and may restore blood flow to the retina.

For a patient with suspected acute angle-closure glaucoma, measure intraocular pressure (IOP) with a tonometer. (You can also estimate IOP without a tonometer by placing your fingers over the patient's closed eyelid. A rock-hard eyeball usually indicates increased IOP.) Expect to instill timolol drops and to administer I.V. acetazolamide to help decrease IOP.

SUSPECTED CENTRAL RETINAL ARTERY OCCLUSION

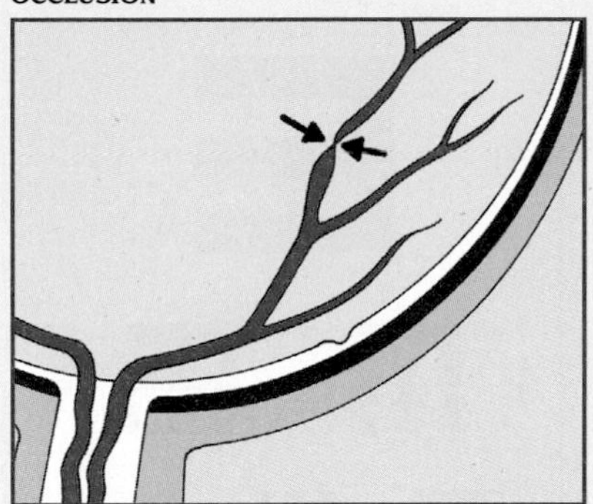

SUSPECTED ACUTE ANGLE-CLOSURE GLAUCOMA

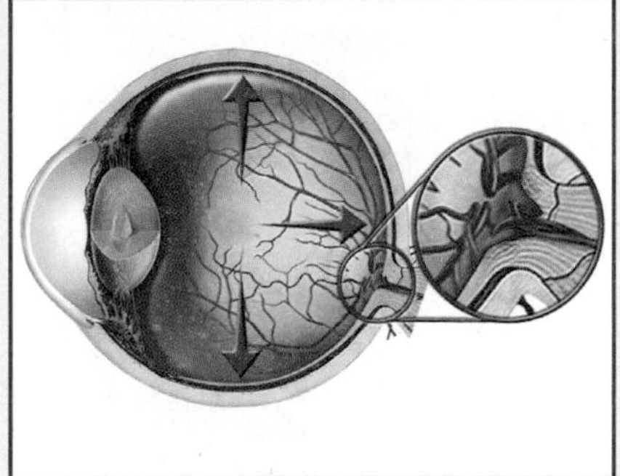

although blurred or halo vision may occur. If untreated, it progresses to blindness and extreme pain.

Chronic open-angle glaucoma usually has an insidious onset, progresses slowly, and affects both eyes. It causes peripheral vision loss, aching eyes, halo vision, and reduced visual acuity (especially at night).

- ***Herpes zoster.*** When this disorder affects the nasociliary nerve, bilateral vision loss is accompanied by eyelid lesions, conjunctivitis, skin lesions (usually on the nose), and ocular muscle palsies.
- ***Hyphema.*** Blood in the anterior chamber can reduce vision to light perception only. Most hyphemas are the direct result of blunt trauma to the normal eye.
- ***Keratitis.*** This inflammation of the cornea may lead to complete unilateral vision loss. Other findings include an opaque cornea, increased tearing, irritation, and photophobia.
- ***Ocular trauma.*** Sudden unilateral or bilateral vision loss may occur after an eye injury. Vision loss may be total or partial and permanent or temporary. The eyelids may be reddened, edematous, and lacerated; intraocular contents may be extruded.
- ***Optic atrophy.*** Degeneration of the optic nerve, optic atrophy can develop spontaneously or follow inflammation or edema of the nerve head, causing irreversible loss of the visual field with changes in color vision. Pupillary reactions are sluggish, and optic disk pallor is evident.
- ***Optic neuritis.*** An umbrella term for inflammation, degeneration, or demyelinization of the optic nerve, optic neuritis usually produces temporary but severe unilateral vision loss, pain around the eye (especially with movement of the globe), a sluggish pupillary response to light and, possibly, visual field defects. Ophthalmoscopic examination commonly reveals hyperemia of the optic disk, blurred disk margins, and filling of the physiologic cup.

Testing visual acuity

Use a Snellen letter chart to test visual acuity in a literate patient older than age 6. Have the patient sit or stand 20′ (6 m) from the chart. Then tell him to cover his left eye and read aloud the smallest line of letters that he can see. Record the fraction assigned to that line on the chart (the numerator indicates the distance from the chart; the denominator indicates the distance at which a normal eye can read the chart). Normal vision is 20/20. Repeat the test with the patient's right eye covered.

If your patient can't read the largest letter from a distance of 20′ (6 m), have him approach the chart until he can read it. Then record the distance between him and the chart as the numerator of the fraction. For example, if he can see the top line of the chart at a distance of 3′ (1 m), record the test result as 3/200.

Use a Snellen symbol chart to test children ages 3 to 6 and illiterate patients. Follow the same procedure as for the Snellen letter chart, but ask the patient to indicate the direction of the E's fingers as you point to each symbol.

SNELLEN LETTER CHART

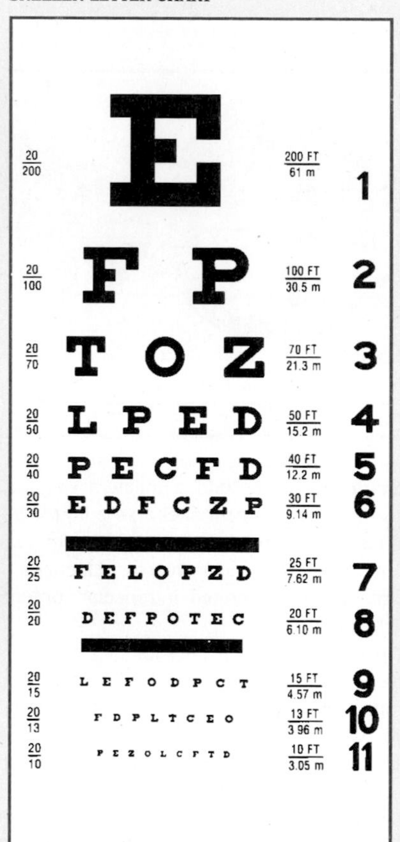

SNELLEN SYMBOL CHART

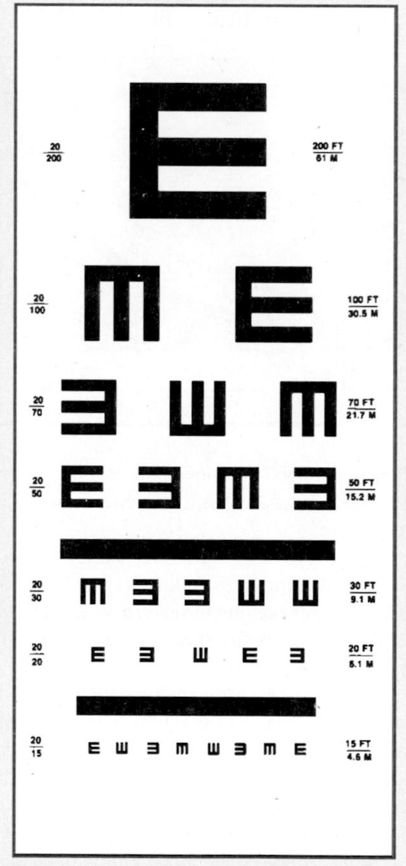

◆ ***Paget's disease.*** In this disorder, bony impingements on the cranial nerves may cause bilateral vision loss, which may be accompanied by hearing loss, tinnitus, vertigo, and severe, persistent bone pain. Cranial enlargement may be noticeable frontally and occipitally, and headaches may occur. Sites of bone involvement are warm and tender, and impaired mobility and pathologic fractures are common.

◆ ***Papilledema.*** Papilledema is characterized by swelling of both optic disks from increased intracranial pressure. Acute papilledema may lead to momentary blurring or transiently obscured vision, whereas chronic papilledema may lead to vision loss.

◆ ***Pituitary tumor.*** As a pituitary adenoma grows, blurred vision progresses to hemianopia and, possibly, unilateral blindness. Double vision, nystagmus, ptosis, limited eye movement, and headaches may also occur.

◆ ***Retinal artery occlusion (central).*** This painless ocular emergency causes sudden unilateral vision loss, which may be partial or complete. Pupil examination reveals a sluggish direct pupillary response and a normal consensual response. Permanent blindness may occur within hours.

◆ ***Retinal detachment.*** Depending on the degree and location of detachment, painless vision loss may be gradual or sudden and total or partial. Macular involvement causes total blindness. Other effects include visual floaters, light flashes, and a sensation of a shadow or curtain over the visual field.

◆ ***Retinal vein occlusion (central).*** Most common in geriatric patients, this painless disorder causes a unilateral decrease in visual acuity with variable vision loss. IOP may be elevated in both eyes.

◆ ***Rift Valley fever.*** Inflammation of the retina is a complication of this viral disease that may result in some degree of permanent vision loss. Typical signs and symptoms include fever, myalgia, weakness, dizziness, and back pain. A small percentage of patients may develop encephalitis or hemorrhagic fever that can lead to shock and hemorrhage.

◆ ***Senile macular degeneration.*** Occurring in elderly patients, this disorder causes painless blurring or loss of central vision. Vision loss may proceed slowly or rapidly, eventually affecting both eyes. Visual acuity may be worse at night.

◆ ***Stevens-Johnson syndrome.*** Corneal scarring from associated conjunctival lesions produces marked vision loss, which may be accompanied by purulent conjunctivitis, eye pain, and difficulty opening the eyes. Additional findings include widespread bullae, fever, malaise, cough, drooling, inability to eat, sore throat, chest pain, vomiting, diarrhea, myalgia, arthralgia, hematuria, and signs of renal failure.

◆ ***Temporal arteritis.*** Vision loss and visual blurring with a throbbing, unilateral headache characterize this disorder. Other findings include malaise, anorexia, weight loss, weakness, low-grade fever, generalized muscle aches, and confusion.

◆ ***Trachoma.*** This rare disorder may initially produce varying degrees of vision loss and a mild infection resembling bacterial conjunctivitis. Conjunctival follicles, red and edematous eyelids, pain, photophobia, tearing, and exudation also occur. After about 1 month, conjunctival follicles enlarge into inflamed yellow or gray papillae.

◆ ***Uveitis.*** Inflammation of the uveal tract may result in unilateral vision loss. Anterior uveitis produces moderate to severe eye pain, severe conjunctival injection, photophobia, and a small, nonreactive pupil. Posterior uveitis may produce insidious onset of blurred vision, conjunctival injection, visual floaters, pain, and photophobia. Associated posterior scar formation distorts the shape of the pupil.

◆ ***Vitreous hemorrhage.*** This condition, which may result from intraocular trauma, ocular tumors, or systemic disease (especially diabetes, hypertension, sickle cell anemia, or leukemia), can cause sudden unilateral vision loss, visual floaters, and a reddish haze. The vision loss may be permanent.

Other causes

◆ ***Drugs.*** Chloroquine therapy may cause patchy retinal pigmentation that typically leads to blindness. Digoxin derivatives, indomethacin, ethambutol, quinine sulfate, and methanol toxicity may also cause vision loss.

Special considerations

Any degree of vision loss can be extremely frightening to your patient. To ease his fears, orient him to his environment and make sure it's safe, and announce your presence each time you approach him. If the patient reports photophobia, darken the room and suggest that he wear sunglasses during the day. Obtain cultures of any drainage, and instruct him not to touch the unaffected eye with anything that has come in contact with the affected eye. Instruct him to wash his hands often and to avoid rubbing his eyes. If necessary, prepare him for surgery.

Pediatric pointers

Children who complain of slowly progressive vision loss may have an optic nerve glioma (a slow-growing, usually benign tumor) or retinoblastoma (a malignant tumor of the retina). Congenital rubella and syphilis may cause vision loss in infants. Retrolental fibroplasia may cause vision loss in premature infants. Other congenital causes of vision loss include Marfan syndrome, retinitis pigmentosa, and amblyopia.

GERIATRIC POINTERS

In elderly patients, reduced visual acuity may be caused by morphologic changes in the choroid, pigment epithelium, or retina or by decreased function of the rods, cones, or other neural elements.

Visual blurring

Visual blurring is a common symptom that refers to the loss of visual acuity with indistinct visual details. It may result from an eye injury, a neurologic or eye disorder, or a disorder with vascular complications, such as diabetes mellitus. Visual blurring may also result from mucus passing over the cornea, a refractive error, improperly fitted contact lenses, or the use of certain drugs.

HISTORY AND PHYSICAL EXAMINATION

If your patient has visual blurring accompanied by sudden, severe eye pain, a history of trauma, or sudden vision loss, order an ophthalmologic examination. If he has a penetrating or perforating eye injury, don't touch the eye. (See *Managing sudden vision loss,* page 697.)

If the patient isn't in distress, ask him how long he has had the visual blurring. Does it occur only at certain times? Ask about associated signs and symptoms, such as pain or discharge. If visual blurring followed injury, obtain details of the accident, and ask if vision was impaired immediately after the injury. Obtain a medical and drug history.

Inspect the patient's eye, noting lid edema, drainage, or conjunctival or scleral redness. Also note an irregularly shaped iris, which may indicate previous trauma, and excessive blinking, which may indicate corneal damage. Assess the patient for pupillary changes, and test visual acuity in both eyes. (See *Testing visual acuity,* page 698.)

MEDICAL CAUSES

- ***Brain tumor.*** A brain tumor may cause visual blurring, decreased level of consciousness (LOC), headache, apathy, behavioral changes, memory loss, decreased attention span, dizziness, confusion, aphasia, seizures, ataxia, and signs of hormonal imbalance. Its later effects may include papilledema, vomiting, increased systolic blood pressure, widened pulse pressure, and decorticate posture.
- ***Cataract.*** This painless disorder causes gradual visual blurring. Other effects include halo vision (an early sign), visual glare in bright light, progressive vision loss, and a gray pupil that later turns milky white.
- ***Concussion.*** Immediately or shortly after blunt head trauma, the patient may develop blurred, double, or temporarily lost vision. Other findings include changes in LOC and behavior.
- ***Conjunctivitis.*** Visual blurring may be accompanied by photophobia, pain, burning, tearing, itching, and a feeling of fullness around the eyes. Other findings include redness near the fornices (brilliant red suggests a bacterial cause; milky red, an allergic cause) and drainage (copious, mucopurulent, and flaky in bacterial conjunctivitis; stringy in allergic conjunctivitis). Copious tearing, minimal exudate, and an enlarged preauricular lymph node occur in viral conjunctivitis.
- ***Corneal abrasions.*** Visual blurring may occur with severe eye pain, photophobia, redness, and excessive tearing.
- ***Corneal dystrophies, hereditary.*** Visual blurring may remain stable or may progressively worsen throughout life in this disorder. Some corneal dystrophies cause associated pain, vision loss, photophobia, tearing, and corneal opacities.
- ***Corneal foreign bodies.*** Visual blurring may accompany a foreign-body sensation, excessive tearing, photophobia, intense eye pain, miosis, conjunctival injection, and a dark corneal speck.
- ***Diabetic retinopathy.*** Retinal edema and hemorrhage produce gradual blurring, which may progress to blindness.
- ***Dislocated lens.*** Dislocation of the lens, especially beyond the line of vision, causes visual blurring and (with trauma) redness.
- ***Eye tumor.*** If the tumor involves the macula, visual blurring may be the presenting symptom. Related findings include varying visual field losses.
- ***Glaucoma.*** In *acute angle-closure glaucoma,* an ocular emergency, unilateral visual blurring and severe pain begin suddenly. Other findings include halo vision; a moderately dilated,

nonreactive pupil; conjunctival injection; a cloudy cornea; and decreased visual acuity. Severely elevated intraocular pressure may cause nausea and vomiting.

In *chronic angle-closure glaucoma,* transient visual blurring and halo vision may precede pain and blindness.

◆ ***Hypertension.*** This disorder may cause visual blurring and a throbbing morning headache that decreases in severity during the day. However, if diastolic blood pressure exceeds 120 mm Hg, the headache may persist. Associated findings include restlessness, confusion, nausea, vomiting, seizures, and decreased LOC.

◆ ***Hyphema.*** Blunt eye trauma with hemorrhage into the anterior chamber causes visual blurring. Other effects include moderate pain, diffuse conjunctival injection, visible blood in the anterior chamber, ecchymosis, eyelid edema, and a hard eye.

◆ ***Iritis.*** Acute iritis causes sudden visual blurring, moderate to severe eye pain, photophobia, conjunctival injection, and a constricted pupil.

◆ ***Migraine headache.*** This disorder may cause visual blurring and paroxysmal attacks of severe, throbbing, unilateral or bilateral headache. Other effects include nausea, vomiting, sensitivity to light and noise, and sensory or visual auras.

◆ ***Multiple sclerosis (MS).*** Blurred vision, diplopia, and paresthesia may occur in the early stages of MS. Later effects vary and may include nystagmus, muscle weakness, paralysis, spasticity, hyperreflexia, intention tremor, and ataxic gait. Urinary frequency, urgency, and incontinence may also occur.

◆ ***Optic neuritis.*** Inflammation, degeneration, or demyelinization of the optic nerve usually causes an acute attack of visual blurring and vision loss. Related findings include scotomas and eye pain. Ophthalmoscopic examination reveals hyperemia of the optic disk, large vein distention, blurred disk margins, and filling of the physiologic cup.

◆ ***Retinal detachment.*** Sudden visual blurring may be the initial symptom of a detached retina. Other effects include visual floaters and recurring flashes of light. As the detachment progresses, the patient experiences gradual vision loss, likened to a curtain covering the visual field.

◆ ***Retinal vein occlusion (central).*** This disorder causes gradual unilateral visual blurring and varying degrees of vision loss.

◆ ***Senile macular degeneration.*** This retinal disorder may cause visual blurring (initially worse at night) and slowly or rapidly progressive vision loss.

◆ ***Serous retinopathy (central).*** Visual blurring may accompany darkened vision in the affected eye.

◆ ***Stroke.*** Brief attacks of bilateral visual blurring may precede or accompany a stroke. Associated findings include a decreased LOC, contralateral hemiplegia, dysarthria, dysphagia, ataxia, unilateral sensory loss, and apraxia. Stroke may also cause agnosia, aphasia, homonymous hemianopia, diplopia, disorientation, memory loss, and poor judgment. Other features include urine retention or urinary incontinence, constipation, personality changes, emotional lability, headache, vomiting, and seizures.

◆ ***Temporal arteritis.*** Most common in women older than age 60, this disorder causes sudden blurred vision accompanied by vision loss and a throbbing unilateral headache in the temporal or frontotemporal region. Prodromal signs and symptoms include malaise, anorexia, weight loss, weakness, low-grade fever, and generalized muscle aches. Other findings include confusion; disorientation; swollen, nodular, tender temporal arteries; and erythema of overlying skin.

◆ ***Uveitis (posterior).*** This disorder may produce insidious onset of blurred vision, conjunctival injection, visual floaters, pain, and photophobia.

◆ ***Vitreous hemorrhage.*** This condition may cause sudden unilateral visual blurring, varying degrees of vision loss, visual floaters, or dark streaks.

Other causes

◆ ***Drugs.*** Visual blurring may stem from the effects of cycloplegics, reserpine, clomiphene, thiazide diuretics, antihistamines, anticholinergics, and phenothiazines.

Special considerations

Prepare the patient for diagnostic tests, such as tonometry, slit-lamp examination, X-rays of the skull and orbit and, if a neurologic lesion is suspected, a computed tomography scan. As necessary, teach him how to instill ophthalmic medication. If visual blurring leads to permanent vision loss, provide emotional support, orient him to his surroundings, and provide for his safety. If necessary, prepare him for surgery.

Pediatric pointers

Visual blurring in children may stem from congenital syphilis, congenital cataracts, refractive errors, eye injuries or infections, or increased intracranial pressure. Refer the child to an ophthalmologist if appropriate.

Test vision in school-age children as you would in adults; test children ages 3 to 6 with the Snellen symbol chart. (See *Testing visual acuity,* page 698.) Test toddlers with Allen cards, each illustrated with a familiar object such as an animal. Ask the child to cover one eye and identify the objects as you flash them. Then ask him to identify them as you gradually back away. Record the maximum distance at which he can identify at least three pictures.

Visual floaters

Visual floaters are particles of blood or cellular debris that move about in the vitreous. As they enter the visual field, they appear as spots or dots. Chronic floaters may occur normally in elderly or myopic patients. However, the sudden onset of visual floaters commonly signals retinal detachment, an ocular emergency.

EMERGENCY INTERVENTIONS *Sudden onset of visual floaters may signal retinal detachment. Ask the patient if he also sees flashing lights or spots in the affected eye. Is he experiencing a curtainlike loss of vision? If so, notify an ophthalmologist immediately and restrict his eye movements until the diagnosis is made.*

History and physical examination

If the patient's condition permits, obtain a drug and allergy history. Ask about nearsightedness (a predisposing factor), use of corrective lenses, eye trauma, or other eye disorders. Also ask about a history of granulomatous disease, diabetes mellitus, or hypertension, which may have predisposed him to retinal detachment, vitreous hemorrhage, or uveitis. If appropriate, inspect his eyes for signs of injury, such as bruising or edema, and determine his visual acuity. (See *Testing visual acuity,* page 698.)

Medical causes

◆ ***Retinal detachment.*** Floaters and light flashes appear suddenly in the portion of the visual field where the retina is detached from the choroid. As the retina detaches further (a painless process), the patient develops gradual vision loss, likened to a cloud or curtain falling in front of the eyes. Ophthalmoscopic examination reveals a gray, opaque, detached retina with an indefinite margin. Retinal vessels appear almost black.

◆ ***Uveitis (posterior).*** This disorder may cause visual floaters accompanied by gradual eye pain, photophobia, blurred vision, and conjunctival injection.

◆ ***Vitreous hemorrhage.*** Rupture of the retinal vessels produces a shower of red or black dots or a red haze across the visual field. Vision suddenly becomes blurred in the affected eye, and visual acuity may be greatly reduced.

Special considerations

Encourage bed rest and provide a calm environment. Depending on the cause of the floaters, the patient may require eye patches, surgery, or a corticosteroid or other drug therapy. If bilateral eye patches are necessary—as in retinal detachment—ensure the patient's safety. Identify yourself when you approach the patient, and orient him to time frequently. Provide sensory stimulation, such as a radio or tape player. Place pillows or towels behind the patient's head to maintain the appropriate patient position. Warn him not to touch or rub his eyes and to avoid straining or sudden movements.

Pediatric pointers

Visual floaters in children usually follow a traumatic injury that causes retinal detachment or vitreous hemorrhage. However, they may also result from vitreous debris, a benign congenital condition with no other signs or symptoms.

Geriatric pointers

Elderly patients may experience increased myopia caused by lens changes. In elderly or myopic patients, chronic floaters may occur normally.

Vomiting

Vomiting is the forceful expulsion of gastric contents through the mouth. Characteristically preceded by nausea, vomiting results from a coordinated sequence of abdominal muscle contractions and reverse esophageal peristalsis.

A common sign of GI disorders, vomiting also occurs with fluid and electrolyte imbalances; infections; and metabolic, endocrine, labyrinthine, central nervous system (CNS), and cardiac disorders. It can also result from drug therapy, surgery, or radiation.

Vomiting occurs normally during the first trimester of pregnancy, but its subsequent development may signal complications. It can also result from stress, anxiety, pain, alcohol intoxication, overeating, or ingestion of distasteful foods or liquids.

History and physical examination

Ask your patient to describe the onset, duration, and intensity of his vomiting. What started it? What makes it subside? If possible, collect, measure, and inspect the character of the vomitus. (See *Vomitus: Characteristics and causes.*) Explore any associated complaints, particularly nausea, abdominal pain, anorexia and weight loss, changes in bowel elimination patterns or the appearance of stools, excessive belching or flatus, and bloating or fullness.

Obtain a medical history, noting GI, endocrine, and metabolic disorders; recent infections; and cancer, including chemotherapy or radiation therapy. Ask about current medication use and alcohol consumption. If the patient is a female of childbearing age, ask if she is or could be pregnant and which contraceptive method she uses.

Inspect the abdomen for distention, and auscultate for bowel sounds and bruits. Palpate for rigidity and tenderness, and test for rebound tenderness. Next, palpate and percuss the liver for enlargement. Assess other body systems as appropriate.

During the examination, keep in mind that projectile vomiting *unaccompanied by nausea* may indicate increased intracranial pressure, a life-threatening emergency. If this occurs in a patient with a CNS injury, quickly check his vital signs. Be alert for widened pulse pressure or bradycardia.

Vomitus: Characteristics and causes

When you collect a specimen of the patient's vomitus, observe it carefully for clues to the underlying disorder.

Bile-stained (greenish) vomitus
Obstruction below the pylorus, as from a duodenal lesion

Bloody vomitus
Upper GI bleeding (if bright red, may result from gastritis or a peptic ulcer; if dark red, from esophageal or gastric varices)

Brown vomitus with a fecal odor
Intestinal obstruction or infarction

Burning, bitter-tasting vomitus
Excessive hydrochloric acid in gastric contents

Coffee-ground vomitus
Digested blood from a slowly bleeding gastric or duodenal lesion

Undigested food
Gastric outlet obstruction, as from a gastric tumor or ulcer

Medical causes

◆ ***Adrenal insufficiency.*** Common GI findings in the disorder include nausea and vomiting, anorexia, and diarrhea. Other findings include weakness, fatigue, weight loss, bronze skin, orthostatic hypotension, and a weak, irregular pulse.

◆ ***Anthrax, GI.*** Initial signs and symptoms after ingestion of contaminated meat from an infected animal include nausea and vomiting, anorexia, and fever. Later, abdominal pain, severe bloody diarrhea, and hematemesis may occur.

◆ ***Appendicitis.*** Nausea and vomiting may follow or accompany abdominal pain. Pain typically begins as vague epigastric or periumbilical discomfort and rapidly progresses to severe, stabbing pain in the right lower quadrant. The patient generally has a positive McBurney's sign—severe pain and tenderness at a point two-thirds the distance from the umbilicus to the right anterior superior spine of the ilium. Associated findings usually include abdominal rigidity and tenderness, anorexia, constipation or diarrhea, cutaneous hyperalgesia, fever, tachycardia, and malaise.

◆ ***Bulimia.*** Most common in women ages 18 to 29, bulimia is characterized by polyphagia that alternates with self-induced vomiting, fasting, or diarrhea. It's commonly accompanied by anorexia. The patient typically weighs less than normal but has a morbid fear of obesity. Self-induced vomiting may be evidenced by calloused knuckles and changes in teeth (enamel loss).

◆ ***Cholecystitis (acute).*** With this disorder, nausea and mild vomiting commonly follow severe right-upper-quadrant pain that may radiate to the back or shoulders. Associated findings include abdominal tenderness and, possibly, rigidity and distention, fever, and diaphoresis.
◆ ***Cholelithiasis.*** Nausea and vomiting accompany severe unlocalized right-upper-quadrant or epigastric pain after ingestion of fatty foods. Other findings include abdominal tenderness and guarding, flatulence, belching, epigastric burning, pyrosis, tachycardia, and restlessness.
◆ ***Cholera.*** Signs and symptoms of cholera include vomiting and abrupt watery diarrhea. Severe water and electrolyte loss leads to thirst, weakness, muscle cramps, decreased skin turgor, oliguria, tachycardia, and hypotension. Without treatment, death can occur within hours.
◆ ***Cirrhosis.*** Insidious early signs and symptoms of cirrhosis typically include nausea and vomiting, anorexia, aching abdominal pain, and constipation or diarrhea. Later findings include jaundice, hepatomegaly, and abdominal distention.
◆ ***Ectopic pregnancy.*** Nausea, vomiting, vaginal bleeding, and lower abdominal pain occur in this potentially life-threatening disorder.
◆ ***Electrolyte imbalances.*** Such disturbances as hyponatremia, hypernatremia, hypokalemia, and hypercalcemia commonly cause nausea and vomiting. Other effects include arrhythmias, tremors, seizures, anorexia, malaise, and weakness.
◆ **Escherichia coli *O157:H7.*** The signs and symptoms of this infection include nausea and vomiting, watery or bloody diarrhea, fever, and abdominal cramps. Children younger than age 5 and elderly people may develop hemolytic uremic syndrome, which causes red blood cell destruction and may eventually lead to acute renal failure.
◆ ***Food poisoning.*** Vomiting, diarrhea, and fever are common findings in food poisoning, which is caused by ingestion of preformed toxins produced by bacteria typically found in foods, such as *Bacillus cereus*, *Clostridium*, and *Staphylococcus*.
◆ ***Gastric cancer.*** This rare type of cancer may produce mild nausea, vomiting (possibly of mucus or blood), anorexia, upper abdominal discomfort, and chronic dyspepsia. Fatigue, weight loss, melena, and altered bowel elimination habits are also common.
◆ ***Gastritis.*** Nausea and vomiting of mucus or blood are common in gastritis, especially after ingestion of alcohol, aspirin, spicy foods, or caffeine. Epigastric pain, belching, and fever may also occur.
◆ ***Gastroenteritis.*** This disorder causes nausea, vomiting (often of undigested food), diarrhea, and abdominal cramping. Fever, malaise, hyperactive bowel sounds, and abdominal pain and tenderness may also occur.
◆ ***Heart failure.*** Nausea and vomiting may occur, especially in right-sided heart failure. Associated findings include tachycardia, ventricular gallop, fatigue, dyspnea, crackles, peripheral edema, and jugular vein distention.
◆ ***Hepatitis.*** Vomiting commonly follows nausea as an early sign of viral hepatitis. Other early findings include fatigue, myalgia, arthralgia, headache, photophobia, anorexia, pharyngitis, cough, and fever.
◆ ***Hyperemesis gravidarum.*** Unremitting nausea and vomiting that last beyond the first trimester characterize this disorder of pregnancy. Vomitus contains undigested food, mucus, and small amounts of bile early in the disorder; later, it has a coffee-ground appearance. Associated findings include weight loss, headache, delirium and, possibly, thyroid dysfunction.
◆ ***Increased intracranial pressure.*** Projectile vomiting that isn't preceded by nausea is a sign of increased intracranial pressure. The patient may exhibit a decreased level of consciousness (LOC) and Cushing's triad (bradycardia, hypertension, and respiratory pattern changes). He may also have a headache, widened pulse pressure, impaired movement, visual disturbances, pupillary changes, and papilledema.
◆ ***Infection.*** Acute localized or systemic infection may cause vomiting and nausea. Other common findings include fever, headache, malaise, and fatigue.
◆ ***Influenza type A H1N1 virus (swine flu).*** Influenza type A H1N1, or swine flu, is a respiratory disease of pigs caused by type A influenza virus. Swine flu viruses cause high levels of illness and low death rates in pigs. Swine flu viruses normally don't infect humans. However, sporadic human infections with swine flu have occurred. Most commonly, these cases occur in persons with direct exposure to pigs. The virus has changed slightly and is known as H1N1 flu. Recent outbreaks of H1N1 flu have shown that the virus can be transmitted from person to person, causing transmission across the globe. The H1N1 flu is similar to influenza, and causes illness and in some cases death. The symptoms of swine flu include vomiting, nonproductive cough, fatigue, headache, chills,

fever, and myalgia. The use of antiviral drugs is recommended to treat H1N1 flu.

◆ ***Intestinal obstruction.*** Nausea and vomiting (bilious or fecal) are common in this type of obstruction, especially of the upper small intestine. Abdominal pain is usually episodic and colicky but can become severe and steady. Constipation occurs early in large intestinal obstruction and late in small intestinal obstruction. Obstipation, however, may signal complete obstruction. In partial obstruction, bowel sounds are typically high pitched and hyperactive; in complete obstruction, hypoactive or absent. Abdominal distention and tenderness also occur, possibly with visible peristaltic waves and a palpable abdominal mass.

◆ ***Labyrinthitis.*** Nausea and vomiting commonly occur in this acute inner ear inflammation. Other findings include severe vertigo, progressive hearing loss, nystagmus and, possibly, otorrhea.

◆ ***Listeriosis.*** After ingesting food contaminated with the bacterium *Listeria monocytogenes*, the patient develops nausea, vomiting, abdominal pain, diarrhea, fever, and myalgia. If the infection spreads to the nervous system, he may develop meningitis. Signs and symptoms may include fever, headache, nuchal rigidity, and altered LOC. This food-borne illness primarily affects pregnant women, newborns, and those with weakened immune systems.

GENDER CUE *Listeriosis that occurs during pregnancy may lead to premature delivery, infection of the neonate, or stillbirth.*

◆ ***Ménière's disease.*** This disorder results in sudden, brief, recurrent attacks of nausea and vomiting, dizziness, vertigo, hearing loss, tinnitus, diaphoresis, and nystagmus.

◆ ***Mesenteric artery ischemia.*** This life-threatening disorder may cause nausea and vomiting and severe, cramping abdominal pain, especially after meals. Other findings include diarrhea or constipation, abdominal tenderness and bloating, anorexia, weight loss, and abdominal bruits.

◆ ***Mesenteric venous thrombosis.*** Insidious or acute onset of nausea, vomiting, and abdominal pain occurs along with diarrhea or constipation, abdominal distention, hematemesis, and melena.

◆ ***Metabolic acidosis.*** This imbalance may produce nausea, vomiting, anorexia, diarrhea, Kussmaul's respirations, and decreased LOC.

◆ ***Migraine headache.*** Prodromal signs and symptoms of migraine include nausea and vomiting, fatigue, photophobia, light flashes, increased noise sensitivity and, possibly, partial vision loss and paresthesia.

◆ ***Motion sickness.*** Nausea and vomiting may be accompanied by headache, vertigo, dizziness, fatigue, diaphoresis, and dyspnea.

◆ ***Myocardial infarction.*** Nausea and vomiting may occur, but the cardinal symptom is severe substernal chest pain, which may radiate to the left arm, jaw, or neck. Dyspnea, pallor, clammy skin, diaphoresis, and restlessness also occur.

◆ ***Norovirus infection.*** Violent vomiting may occur frequently and without warning in this infection. Children infected with noroviruses tend to experience acute-onset vomiting more often than adults. Additional symptoms include nausea, diarrhea, and abdominal pain or cramping. There are no drugs or vaccines for noroviruses, but symptomatic therapy may be necessary to replace fluids and correct electrolyte disturbances resulting from frequent vomiting and diarrhea. Young children, elderly people, and those who are otherwise ill are at increased risk for dehydration.

◆ ***Pancreatitis (acute).*** Vomiting, usually preceded by nausea, is an early sign of pancreatitis. Associated findings include steady, severe epigastric or left-upper-quadrant pain that may radiate to the back; abdominal tenderness and rigidity; hypoactive bowel sounds; anorexia; vomiting; and fever. Severe pancreatitis may result in tachycardia, restlessness, hypotension, skin mottling, and cold, sweaty extremities.

◆ ***Peptic ulcer***. Nausea and vomiting may follow sharp, burning or gnawing epigastric pain, especially when the stomach is empty or after ingestion of alcohol, caffeine, or aspirin. Attacks are relieved by eating or taking antacids. Hematemesis or melena may also occur.

◆ ***Peritonitis.*** Nausea and vomiting usually accompany acute abdominal pain in the area of inflammation. Other findings include high fever with chills; tachycardia; hypoactive or absent bowel sounds; abdominal distention, rigidity, and tenderness; weakness; pale, cold skin; diaphoresis; hypotension; signs of dehydration; and shallow respirations.

◆ ***Preeclampsia.*** Nausea and vomiting are common in this disorder of pregnancy. Rapid weight gain, epigastric pain, generalized edema, elevated blood pressure, oliguria, a severe frontal headache, and blurred or double vision also occur.

◆ ***Q fever.*** Signs and symptoms of this rickettsial infection include nausea and vomiting, fever, chills, severe headache, malaise, chest pain, and diarrhea. Fever may last up to 2 weeks. In severe cases, the patient may develop hepatitis or pneumonia.
◆ ***Renal and urologic disorders.*** Cystitis, pyelonephritis, calculi, and other renal and urologic disorders can cause vomiting. Accompanying findings reflect the specific disorder. Persistent nausea and vomiting are typical findings in patients with acute or worsening chronic renal failure.
◆ ***Rhabdomyolysis.*** Signs and symptoms of this disorder include nausea and vomiting, muscle weakness or pain, fever, malaise, and dark urine. Acute renal failure, the most commonly reported complication of rhabdomyolysis, results from renal structure obstruction and injury during the kidneys' attempt to filter the myoglobin from the bloodstream.
◆ ***Thyrotoxicosis.*** Nausea and vomiting may accompany the classic findings of severe anxiety, heat intolerance, weight loss despite increased appetite, diaphoresis, diarrhea, tremors, tachycardia, and palpitations. Other findings include exophthalmos, ventricular or atrial gallop, and an enlarged thyroid gland.
◆ ***Typhus.*** Typhus is a rickettsial disease transmitted to humans by fleas, mites, or body louse. Initial symptoms include headache, myalgia, arthralgia, and malaise, followed by an abrupt onset of nausea, vomiting, chills, and fever. A maculopapular rash may be present in some cases.
◆ ***Ulcerative colitis.*** Nausea, vomiting, and anorexia may occur, but the most common sign is recurrent diarrhea with blood, pus, and mucus. Fever, chills, and weight loss are other common signs and symptoms.

Other causes

◆ ***Drugs.*** Drugs that commonly cause vomiting include antineoplastics, opiates, ferrous sulfate, levodopa, oral potassium, chloride replacements, estrogens, sulfasalazine, antibiotics, quinidine, anesthetics, and overdoses of cardiac glycosides and theophylline.
◆ ***Radiation and surgery.*** Radiation therapy may cause nausea and vomiting if it disrupts the gastric mucosa. Postoperative nausea and vomiting are common, especially after abdominal surgery.

Special considerations

Draw blood to determine fluid, electrolyte, and acid-base balance because prolonged vomiting can cause dehydration, electrolyte imbalances, and metabolic alkalosis. Have the patient breathe deeply to ease his nausea and help prevent further vomiting. Keep his room fresh and clean smelling by removing bedpans and emesis basins promptly after use. Elevate his head or position him on his side to prevent aspiration of vomitus. Continuously monitor vital signs and intake and output (including vomitus and liquid stools). If necessary, administer I.V. fluids or have the patient sip clear liquids to maintain hydration.

Because pain can precipitate or intensify nausea and vomiting, administer pain medications promptly. If possible, give them by injection or suppository to prevent exacerbating associated nausea. If an opioid is used to treat pain, monitor bowel sounds, flatus, and bowel movements carefully because they may slow GI motility and exacerbate vomiting. If you administer an antiemetic, be alert for abdominal distention and hypoactive bowel sounds, which may indicate gastric retention. If this occurs, insert a nasogastric tube.

Pediatric pointers

In a neonate, pyloric obstruction may cause projectile vomiting, and Hirschsprung's disease may cause fecal vomiting. Intussusception may lead to vomiting of bile and fecal matter in an infant or toddler. Because an infant may aspirate vomitus as a result of his immature cough and gag reflexes, position him on his side or abdomen and clear any vomitus immediately.

Geriatric pointers

Although elderly patients can develop several of the disorders mentioned earlier, always rule out intestinal ischemia first—it's especially common in this age-group and has a high mortality.

Patient counseling

Advise patients to replace fluid losses to avoid dehydration. If vomiting is persistent, administer an antiemetic; consider hospitalizing the patient for I.V. fluid replacement or parenteral nutrition therapy. Advise patients suffering from migraine headaches that vomiting may be a prodromal symptom and that they should take antimigraine medication.

Vulvar lesions

Vulvar lesions are cutaneous lumps, nodules, papules, vesicles, or ulcers that result from benign or malignant tumors, dystrophies, dermatoses, or infection. They can appear anywhere on the vulva and may go undetected until a gynecologic examination. Usually, however, the patient notices the lesions because of associated symptoms, such as pruritus, dysuria, or dyspareunia.

History and physical examination

Ask the patient when she first noticed a vulvar lesion, and find out about associated features, such as swelling, pain, tenderness, itching, or discharge. Does she have lesions elsewhere on her body? Ask about signs and symptoms of systemic illness, such as malaise, fever, or a rash on other body areas. Is the patient sexually active? Could she have been exposed to a sexually transmitted disease?

Also, examine the lesion, do a pelvic examination, and obtain cultures. (See *Recognizing common vulvar lesions,* page 708.)

Medical causes

◆ ***Basal cell carcinoma.*** Most common in postmenopausal women, this nodular tumor has a central ulcer and a raised, poorly rolled border. Although it typically produces no symptoms, basal cell carcinoma occasionally causes pruritus, bleeding, discharge, and a burning sensation.

◆ ***Benign cysts.*** Epidermal inclusion cysts, the most common vulvar cysts, appear primarily on the labia majora. They're usually round and cause no symptoms; occasionally, they become erythematous and tender.

Bartholin's duct cysts are usually unilateral, tense, nontender, and palpable; they appear on the posterior labia minora and may cause minor discomfort during intercourse or, when large, difficulty with intercourse or even walking. Bartholin's abscess, an infected Bartholin's duct cyst, causes gradual pain and tenderness and possibly vulvar swelling, redness, and deformity.

◆ ***Benign vulvar tumors.*** Cystic or solid benign vulvar tumors usually produce no symptoms.

◆ ***Chancroid.*** This rare sexually transmitted disease causes painful vulvar lesions. Other findings may include headache, malaise, fever up to 102.2° F (39° C), and enlarged, tender inguinal lymph nodes.

◆ ***Dermatoses (systemic).*** Psoriasis, seborrheic dermatitis, and other skin conditions may produce vulvar lesions that resemble the causative lesions found in other body areas.

◆ ***Genital warts.*** This sexually transmitted condition is characterized by painless warts on the vulva, vagina, and cervix. The warts start as tiny red or pink swellings that grow and become pedunculated. Multiple swellings with a cauliflower-like appearance are common. Other findings include pruritus, erythema, burning or paresthesia in the vaginal introitus, and a profuse mucopurulent vaginal discharge.

◆ ***Gonorrhea.*** Although most women with gonorrhea are asymptomatic, some develop vulvar lesions, which are usually confined to Bartholin's glands and may be accompanied by pruritus, a burning sensation, pain, and a green-yellow vaginal discharge. Other findings include dysuria and urinary incontinence; vaginal redness, swelling, bleeding, and engorgement; and severe pelvic and lower abdominal pain.

◆ ***Granuloma inguinale.*** This rare, chronic venereal infection begins with a single painless macule or papule on the vulva that ulcerates into a raised, beefy-red lesion with a granulated, friable border. Later, other painless and possibly foul-smelling lesions may erupt on the labia, vagina, or cervix. Eventually, they become infected and painful and may be accompanied by enlarged and tender regional lymph nodes, fever, weight loss, and malaise.

◆ ***Herpes simplex (genital).*** In this disorder, fluid-filled vesicles appear on the cervix and, possibly, on the vulva, labia, perianal skin, vagina, or mouth. The vesicles, initially painless, may rupture and develop into extensive shallow, painful ulcers, with redness, marked edema, and tender inguinal lymph nodes. Other findings include fever, malaise, and dysuria.

◆ ***Herpes zoster.*** This viral infection may produce vulvar lesions, although other areas are more commonly affected. Small, red nodular lesions erupt on painful erythematous areas. The lesions quickly evolve into vesicles or pustules, which dry and form scabs about 10 days later. Other findings include fever, malaise, paresthesia or hyperesthesia, and pain.

◆ ***Lymphogranuloma venereum.*** Most patients with this bacterial infection initially exhibit a single painless papule or ulcer on the posterior vulva that heals in a few days. Painful, swollen lymph nodes, usually unilateral, develop 2 to 6 weeks later. Other findings include fever, chills, headache, anorexia, myalgia, arthralgia, weight loss, and perineal edema.

◆ ***Malignant melanoma.*** This type of skin cancer may cause irregular, pigmented vulvar

Recognizing common vulvar lesions

Various disorders can cause vulvar lesions. For example, sexually transmitted diseases account for most vulvar lesions in premenopausal women, whereas vulvar tumors and cysts account for most lesions in women ages 50 to 70. The illustrations below will help you recognize some of the most common lesions.

Primary genital herpes produces multiple ulcerated lesions surrounded by red halos.

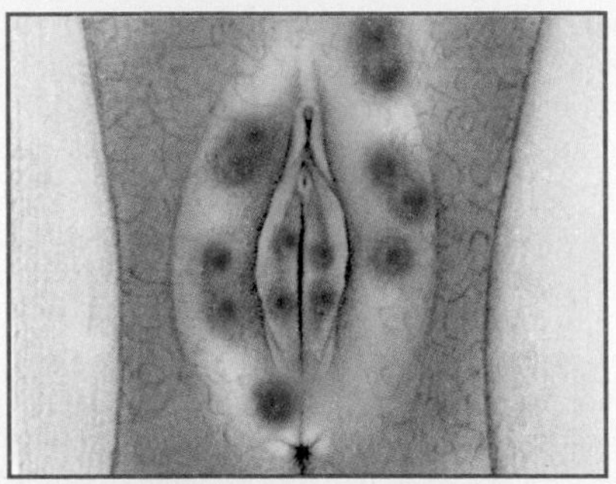

Basal cell carcinoma can produce an ulcerated lesion with raised, poorly rolled edges.

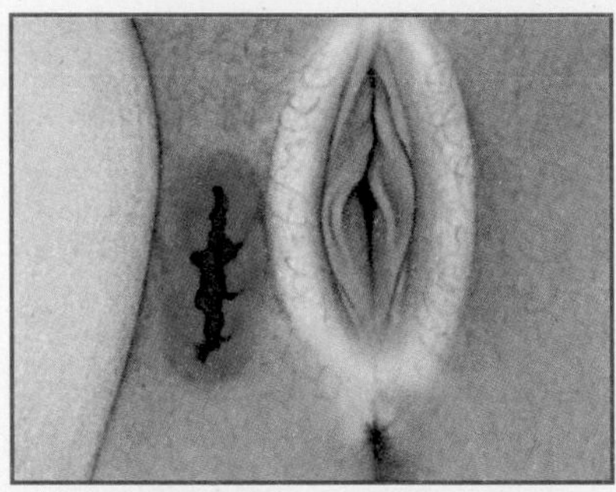

Primary syphilis produces chancres that appear as ulcerated lesions with raised borders.

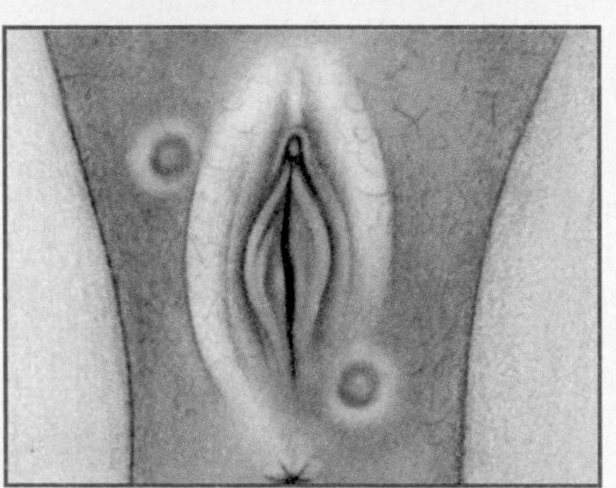

Epidermal inclusion cysts produce a round lump that usually appears on the labia majora.

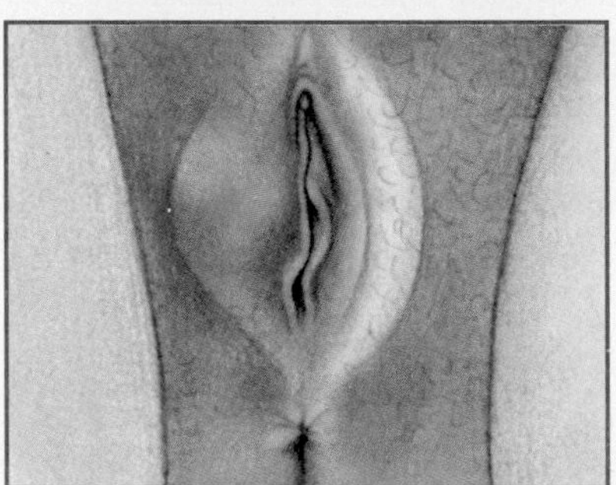

Squamous cell carcinoma can produce a large, granulomatous-appearing ulcer.

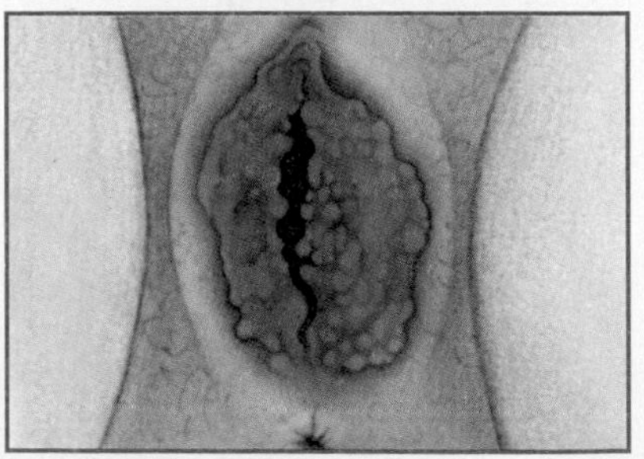

Bartholin's duct cysts produce a tense, nontender, palpable lump that usually appears on the labia minora.

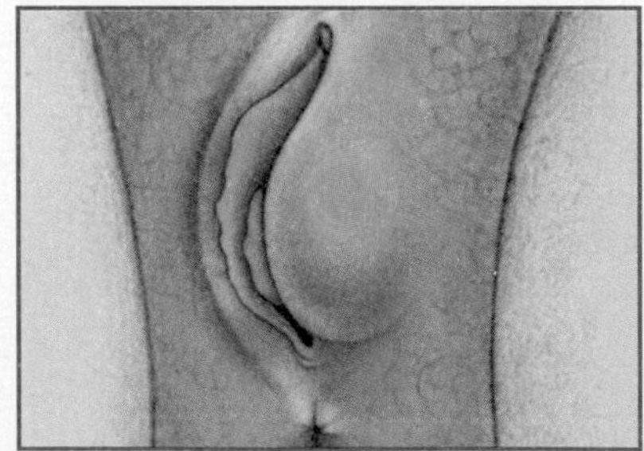

or clitoral lesions that enlarge rapidly and may ulcerate and bleed.

◆ ***Molluscum contagiosum.*** This viral infection produces raised, umbilicated, pearly or flesh-colored vulvar papules that are 1 to 2 mm in diameter and have a white core. Pruritic lesions may also appear on the face, eyelids, breasts, and inner thighs.

◆ ***Pediculosis pubis.*** This parasitic infection produces erythematous vulvar papules with pruritus and skin irritation. Adult pubic lice and nits are visible on pubic hair with magnification.

◆ ***Squamous cell carcinoma.*** Invasive carcinoma occurs primarily in postmenopausal women and may produce a painful, pruritic vulvar tumor. As the tumor enlarges, it may encroach on the vagina, anus, and urethra, causing bleeding, discharge, or dysuria. Carcinoma in situ is most common in premenopausal women and produces a vulvar lesion that may be white or red, raised, well defined, moist, crusted, and isolated.

◆ ***Squamous cell hyperplasia.*** Formerly known as hyperplastic dystrophy, this disorder produces vulvar lesions that may be well delineated or poorly defined; localized or extensive; and red, brown, white, or red and white. However, its cardinal symptom is intense pruritus, possibly with vulvar pain, intense burning, and dyspareunia. In lichen sclerosis, a type of vulvar dystrophy, vulvar skin has a parchmentlike appearance. Fissures may develop between the clitoris and urethra or other vulvar areas.

◆ ***Syphilis.*** In this sexually transmitted disease, chancres may appear on the vulva, vagina, or cervix 10 to 90 days after initial contact. They usually start as painless papules and then erode to form indurated ulcers with raised edges and clear bases. Condylomata lata develop after these ulcers clear up. These highly contagious secondary vulvar lesions are raised, gray, flat topped, and commonly ulcerated. Other findings include a maculopapular, pustular, or nodular rash; headache; malaise; anorexia; weight loss; fever; nausea and vomiting; generalized lymphadenopathy; and sore throat.

◆ ***Viral diseases (systemic).*** Varicella, measles, and other systemic viral diseases may produce vulvar lesions.

Special considerations

Expect to administer a systemic antibiotic, an antiviral, a topical corticosteroid, topical testosterone, or an antipruritic.

Pediatric pointers

Vulvar lesions in children may result from congenital syphilis or gonorrhea. Evaluate for sexual abuse.

Geriatric pointers

Vulvar dystrophies and neoplasia become more common with advancing age. All vulvar lesions should be considered malignant until proven otherwise. Many women remain sexually active well into their older years, so be sure to question them about sexual activities and teach them safer sex practices.

Patient counseling

Show the patient how to give herself a sitz bath to promote healing and comfort. If she has a sexually transmitted disease, encourage her to inform her sexual partners and persuade them to be treated. Advise her to avoid sexual contact until the lesions are no longer contagious. Provide information about safer sex practices.

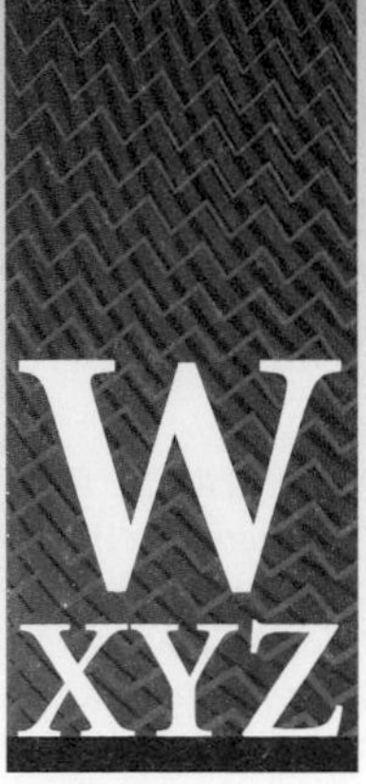

Weight gain, excessive

Weight gain occurs when ingested calories exceed body requirements for energy, causing increased adipose tissue storage. It can also occur when fluid retention causes edema. When weight gain results from overeating, emotional factors—most commonly anxiety, guilt, and depression—and social factors may be the primary causes.

Among elderly people, weight gain commonly reflects a sustained food intake in the presence of the normal, progressive fall in basal metabolic rate. Among women, progressive weight gain occurs in pregnancy, whereas periodic weight gain usually occurs with menstruation.

Weight gain, a primary sign of many endocrine disorders, also occurs in conditions that limit activity, especially cardiovascular and pulmonary disorders. It can also result from drug therapy that increases appetite or causes fluid retention or from cardiovascular, hepatic, and renal disorders that cause edema.

History and physical examination

Determine your patient's previous patterns of weight gain and loss. Does he have a family history of obesity, thyroid disease, or diabetes mellitus? Assess his eating and activity patterns. Has his appetite increased? Does he exercise regularly or at all? Next, ask about associated symptoms. Has he experienced visual disturbances, hoarseness, paresthesia, or increased urination and thirst? Has he become impotent? If the patient is female, has she had menstrual irregularities or experienced weight gain during menstruation?

Form an impression of the patient's mental status. Is he anxious or depressed? Does he respond slowly? Is his memory poor? What medications is he using?

During your physical examination, measure skin-fold thickness to estimate fat reserves. (See *Evaluating nutritional status*, pages 712 and 713.) Note fat distribution, the presence of localized or generalized edema, and overall nutritional status. Examine the patient for other abnormalities, such as abnormal body hair distribution or hair loss and dry skin. Take and record the patient's vital signs.

Evaluate the patient's weight distribution by measuring his waist circumference around his abdomen at the level of the iliac crest. If the measurement is greater than 35" (89 cm) for a woman or 40" (102 cm) for a man (with a normal body mass index), the patient is at greater risk for health problems. People with a high distribution of fat around their waists, as opposed to their hips and thighs, are at greater risk for such diseases as type 2 diabetes, dyslipidemia, hypertension, and cardiovascular disease.

Medical causes

◆ ***Acromegaly.*** This disorder causes moderate weight gain. Other findings include coarsened facial features, prognathism, enlarged hands and feet, increased sweating, oily skin, deep voice, back and joint pain, lethargy, sleepiness, heat intolerance and, occasionally, hirsutism.

◆ ***Cushing's syndrome (hypercortisolism).*** Excessive weight gain, usually over the trunk and the back of the neck (buffalo hump), characteristically occurs in this disorder. Other cushingoid features include slender extremities, moon face, weakness, purple striae, emotional lability, and increased susceptibility to infection. Gynecomastia may occur in men; hirsutism, acne, and menstrual irregularities may occur in women.

◆ ***Diabetes mellitus.*** The increased appetite associated with this disorder may lead to weight gain, although weight loss sometimes occurs instead. Other findings include fatigue, polydipsia, polyuria, nocturia, weakness, polyphagia, and somnolence.

◆ ***Heart failure.*** Despite anorexia, weight gain may result from edema. Other typical findings include paroxysmal nocturnal dyspnea, orthopnea, and fatigue.

◆ ***Hyperinsulinism.*** This disorder increases appetite, leading to weight gain. Emotional lability, indigestion, weakness, diaphoresis, tachycardia, visual disturbances, and syncope also occur.

◆ ***Hypogonadism.*** Weight gain is common in this disorder. Prepubertal hypogonadism causes eunuchoid body proportions with relatively sparse facial and body hair and a high-pitched voice. Postpubertal hypogonadism causes loss of libido, impotence, and infertility.

◆ ***Hypothalamic dysfunction.*** Conditions such as Laurence-Moon-Biedl syndrome cause a voracious appetite and subsequent weight gain along with altered body temperature and sleep rhythms.

◆ ***Hypothyroidism.*** In this disorder, weight gain occurs despite anorexia. Related signs and symptoms include fatigue; cold intolerance; constipation; menorrhagia; slowed intellectual and motor activity; dry, pale, cool skin; dry, sparse hair; and thick, brittle nails. Myalgia, hoarseness, hypoactive deep tendon reflexes, bradycardia, and abdominal distention may occur. Eventually, the face assumes a dull expression with periorbital edema.

◆ ***Metabolic syndrome.*** This syndrome, previously called *syndrome X*, consists of a group of disorders that affect metabolism, including excessive weight gain (usually in the central abdomen), hypertension (blood pressure greater than 135/85 mm Hg), abnormal cholesterol levels (high low-density lipoprotein and triglyceride levels, low high-density lipoprotein level), and high insulin levels. Inefficient use of insulin in the body is thought to be a major contributor to metabolic syndrome, as are physical inactivity, poor diet, and genetic factors. Individuals with metabolic syndrome are at a significantly increased risk for heart disease, stroke, and diabetes. Treatment typically involves exercising, following a heart-healthy diet, and refraining from smoking; medical therapy may be prescribed to treat the individual disorders.

◆ ***Nephrotic syndrome.*** In this syndrome, weight gain results from edema. Severe edema (anasarca) can increase body weight by up to 50%. Related effects include abdominal distention, orthostatic hypotension, and lethargy.

◆ ***Pancreatic islet cell tumor.*** This type of tumor causes excessive hunger, which leads to weight gain. Other findings include emotional lability, weakness, malaise, fatigue, restlessness, diaphoresis, palpitations, tachycardia, visual disturbances, and syncope.

◆ ***Preeclampsia.*** In this disorder, rapid weight gain (exceeding the normal weight gain of pregnancy) may accompany nausea and vomiting, epigastric pain, elevated blood pressure, and blurred or double vision.

◆ ***Sheehan's syndrome.*** Most common in women who experience severe obstetric hemorrhage, this syndrome may cause weight gain caused by impaired pituitary gland function.

Other causes

◆ ***Drugs.*** Corticosteroids, phenothiazines, and tricyclic antidepressants cause weight gain from fluid retention and increased appetite. Other drugs that can lead to weight gain include hormonal contraceptives, which cause fluid retention; cyproheptadine, which increases appetite; and lithium, which can induce hypothyroidism.

Special considerations

Psychological counseling may be needed for patients with excessive weight gain, particularly when it's caused by emotional problems or alters body image. If the patient is obese or has a cardiopulmonary disorder, any exercise should be monitored closely. Further study to rule out possible secondary causes should include thyroid-stimulating hormone determination and dexamethasone suppression testing. Laboratory test results of all patients ideally include cardiac risk factors: cholesterol, triglyceride, and glucose levels.

Evaluating nutritional status

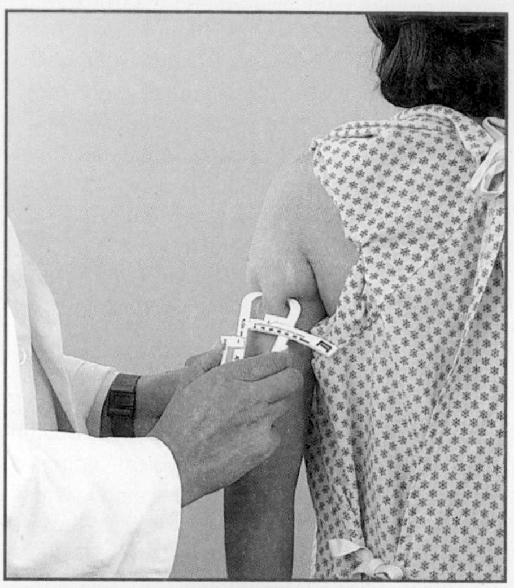

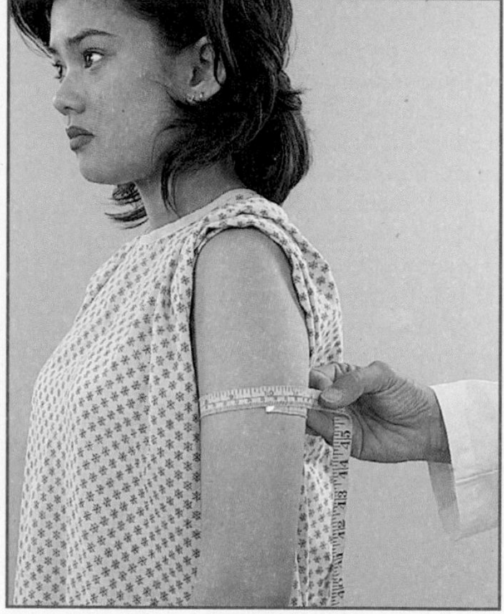

If your patient gains or loses excessive weight, you can help assess her nutritional status by measuring her skin-fold thickness and midarm circumference and by calculating her midarm muscle circumference. Skin-fold measurement reflects adipose tissue mass (subcutaneous fat accounts for about 50% of the body's adipose tissue). Midarm measurement reflects both skeletal muscle and adipose tissue mass.

Use the steps described here to gather these measurements. Then express them as a percentage of standard measurements by using this formula:

$$\frac{\text{actual measurement}}{\text{standard measurement}} \times 100 = \_\_\_\_\_\_\%$$

Standard anthropometric measurements vary according to the patient's age and sex and can be found in a chart of normal anthropometric values. The abridged chart below lists standard arm measurements for adult men and women.

Test	Standard	
Triceps skin fold	Men	12.5 mm
	Women	16.5 mm
Midarm circumference	Men	29.3 mm
	Women	28.5 mm
Midarm muscle circumference	Men	25.3 mm
	Women	23.2 mm

A triceps or subscapular skin-fold measurement below 60% of the standard value indicates severe depletion of fat reserves; measurement between 60% and 90% indicates moderate to mild depletion; and above 90% indicates significant fat reserves. A midarm circumference of less than 90% of the standard value indicates caloric deprivation; greater than 90% indicates adequate or ample muscle and fat. A midarm muscle circumference of less than 90% indicates protein depletion; greater than 90% indicates adequate or ample protein reserves.

To measure the triceps skin fold, locate the midpoint of the patient's upper arm, using a nonstretch tape measure, and mark it with a felt-tip pen. Then grasp the skin with your thumb and forefinger about 1 cm above the midpoint. Place the calipers at the midpoint and squeeze them for about 3 seconds. Record the measurement registered on the handle gauge to the nearest 0.5 mm. Take two more readings and average all three to compensate for any measurement error.

To measure midarm circumference, return to the midpoint you marked on the patient's upper arm. Then use a tape measure to determine the arm circumference at this point. This measurement reflects both skeletal muscle and adipose tissue mass and helps evaluate protein and calorie reserves. To calculate midarm muscle circumference, multiply the triceps skin-fold thickness (in centimeters) by 3.143, and subtract this figure from the midarm circumference. Midarm muscle circumference reflects muscle mass alone, providing a more sensitive index of protein reserves.

Pediatric pointers

Weight gain in children can result from an endocrine disorder such as Cushing's syndrome or from disorders that cause inactivity, such as Prader-Willi syndrome, Down syndrome, Werdnig-Hoffmann disease, late stages of muscular dystrophy, and severe cerebral palsy.

The incidence of obesity is increasing among children. Nonpathologic causes include poor eating habits, sedentary recreation, and emotional problems, especially among adolescents. Regardless of the cause, discourage fad diets and provide a balanced weight loss program.

Geriatric pointers

Desired weights (associated with lowest mortality rates) increase with age.

Patient counseling

Educating the patient about weight control is extremely important. Stress the benefits of behavior modification and dietary compliance. Help the patient plan an appropriate exercise routine.

Weight loss, excessive

Weight loss can reflect decreased food intake, decreased food absorption, increased metabolic requirements, or a combination of the three. It may be caused by endocrine, neoplastic, GI, and psychiatric disorders; nutritional deficiencies; infections; or neurologic lesions that cause paralysis and dysphagia. Weight loss may also result from conditions that prevent sufficient food intake, such as painful oral lesions, ill-fitting dentures, and loss of teeth, or from the metabolic effects of poverty, fad diets, excessive exercise, or certain drugs.

Weight loss may be a late sign in such chronic diseases as heart failure and renal disease, usually as the result of anorexia (see "Anorexia," page 46).

History and physical examination

Begin with a thorough diet history because weight loss is almost always caused by inadequate caloric intake. If the patient hasn't been eating properly, try to determine why. Ask about his previous weight and whether the recent loss was intentional. Be alert for lifestyle or occupational changes that may be causing anxiety or depression. For example, has he gotten separated or divorced? Has he recently changed jobs?

Inquire about recent changes in bowel habits, such as diarrhea or bulky, floating stools. Has the patient had nausea, vomiting, or abdominal pain, which may indicate a GI disorder? Has he had excessive thirst, excessive urination, or heat intolerance, which may signal an endocrine disorder? Take a careful drug history, noting especially the use of diet pills or laxatives.

Carefully check the patient's height and weight, and ask about exact weight changes with approximate dates. Take his vital signs and note his general appearance: Is he well nourished? Do his clothes fit? Is muscle wasting evident?

Next, examine the patient's skin for turgor and abnormal pigmentation, especially around the joints. Does he have pallor or jaundice? Examine his mouth, including the condition of his teeth or dentures. Look for signs of infection or irritation on the roof of the mouth, and note any hyperpigmentation of the buccal mucosa. Also, check the patient's eyes for exophthalmos and his neck for swelling; auscultate his lungs for adventitious sounds. Inspect his abdomen for signs of wasting, and palpate for masses, tenderness, and an enlarged liver.

Conventional laboratory and radiologic tests, such as complete blood count, serum albumin levels, urinalysis, chest X-rays, and upper GI series, usually reveal the cause. Almost all physical causes are clinically evident during the initial evaluation. Cancer, GI disorders, and depression are the most common pathologic causes.

Medical causes

◆ ***Adrenal insufficiency.*** Weight loss occurs in this disorder along with anorexia, weakness, fatigue, irritability, syncope, nausea, vomiting, abdominal pain, and diarrhea or constipation. Hyperpigmentation may occur at the joints, belt line, palmar creases, lips, gums, tongue, and buccal mucosa.

◆ ***Anorexia nervosa.*** This psychogenic disorder, most common in young women, is characterized by a severe, self-imposed weight loss ranging from 10% to 50% of premorbid weight, which typically was normal or no more than 5 lb (2.3 kg) over ideal weight. Related findings include skeletal muscle atrophy, loss of fatty tissue, hypotension, constipation, dental caries, susceptibility to infection, blotchy or sallow skin, cold intolerance, hairiness on the face and body, dryness or loss of scalp hair, and amenorrhea. The patient usually demonstrates restless activity and vigor and may have a morbid fear of becoming fat. Self-induced vomiting or use of laxatives or diuretics may lead to dehydration or to metabolic alkalosis or acidosis.

◆ ***Cancer.*** Weight loss can be a sign of many types of cancer. Other findings reflect the type, location, and stage of the tumor and can include fatigue, pain, nausea, vomiting, anorexia, abnormal bleeding, and a palpable mass.

◆ ***Crohn's disease.*** Weight loss occurs with chronic cramping, abdominal pain, and anorexia. Other signs and symptoms include diarrhea, nausea, fever, tachycardia, hyperactive bowel sounds, and abdominal distention, tenderness, and guarding. Perianal lesions and a palpable mass in the right or left lower quadrant may also be present.

◆ ***Cryptosporidiosis.*** This opportunistic protozoan infection may cause weight loss, profuse watery diarrhea, abdominal cramping, flatulence, anorexia, nausea, vomiting, malaise, fever, and myalgia.

◆ ***Depression.*** Severe depression may cause weight loss or weight gain along with insomnia or hypersomnia, anorexia, apathy, fatigue, and feelings of worthlessness. Indecisiveness, incoherence, and suicidal thoughts or behavior may also occur.

◆ ***Diabetes mellitus.*** In this disorder, weight loss may occur despite increased appetite. Other findings include polydipsia, weakness, fatigue, and polyuria with nocturia.

◆ ***Esophagitis.*** Painful inflammation of the esophagus leads to temporary avoidance of eating and subsequent weight loss. Intense pain in the mouth and anterior chest is accompanied by hypersalivation, dysphagia, tachypnea, and hematemesis. If a stricture develops, dysphagia and weight loss will recur.

◆ ***Gastroenteritis.*** Malabsorption and dehydration cause weight loss in this disorder. The weight loss may be sudden in acute viral infections or reactions or gradual in parasitic infection. Other findings include poor skin turgor, dry mucous membranes, tachycardia, hypotension, diarrhea, abdominal pain and tenderness, hyperactive bowel sounds, nausea, vomiting, fever, and malaise.

◆ ***Herpes simplex type 1.*** Painful fluid-filled blisters in and around the mouth make eating painful, causing decreased food intake and weight loss.

◆ ***Leukemia.*** Acute leukemia causes progressive weight loss accompanied by severe prostration; high fever; swollen, bleeding gums; and other bleeding tendencies. Dyspnea, tachycardia, palpitations, and abdominal or bone pain may occur. As the disease progresses, neurologic symptoms may eventually develop.

Chronic leukemia, which occurs insidiously in adults, causes progressive weight loss with malaise, fatigue, pallor, enlarged spleen, bleeding tendencies, anemia, skin eruptions, anorexia, and fever.

◆ ***Lymphomas.*** Hodgkin's disease and malignant lymphoma cause gradual weight loss. Associated findings include fever, fatigue, night sweats, malaise, hepatosplenomegaly, and lymphadenopathy. Scaly rashes and pruritus may develop.

◆ ***Popcorn lung disease.*** Popcorn lung disease occurs in factory workers who experience respiratory symptoms after inhaling butter flavoring chemicals such as diacetyl, used in the manufacture of microwave popcorn. The patient typically complains of gradual onset of a nonproductive cough that worsens over time, progressive shortness of breath, and unusual fatigue. Clinical findings include wheezing, chest pain, fever, night sweats, and weight loss. Bronchiolitis fibrosa obliterans, an irreversible fixed airway obstructive lung disorder, is the most severe condition reported.

◆ ***Pulmonary tuberculosis.*** This disorder causes gradual weight loss along with fatigue, weakness, anorexia, night sweats, and low-grade fever. Other clinical effects include a cough with bloody or mucopurulent sputum, dyspnea, and pleuritic chest pain. Examination may reveal dullness on percussion, crackles after coughing, increased tactile fremitus, and amphoric breath sounds.

◆ ***Stomatitis.*** Inflammation of the oral mucosa (which are usually red, swollen, and ulcerated) in this disorder causes weight loss due to decreased eating. Associated findings include fever, increased salivation, malaise, mouth pain, anorexia, and swollen, bleeding gums.

◆ ***Thyrotoxicosis.*** In this disorder, increased metabolism causes weight loss. Other characteristic signs and symptoms include nervousness, heat intolerance, diarrhea, increased appetite, palpitations, tachycardia, diaphoresis, a fine tremor, and possibly an enlarged thyroid gland and exophthalmos. A ventricular or atrial gallop may be heard.

◆ ***Ulcerative colitis.*** Weight loss is a late sign of this disorder, which is initially characterized by bloody diarrhea with pus or mucus. Other findings include weakness, crampy lower abdominal pain, hyperactive bowel sounds, tenesmus, anorexia, low-grade fever and, occasionally, nausea and vomiting. Constipation may occur late. Fulminant colitis causes severe and steady abdominal pain and diarrhea, high fever, and tachycardia.

◆ ***Whipple's disease.*** This rare disease causes progressive weight loss along with abdominal pain, diarrhea, steatorrhea, arthralgia, fever, hyperpigmentation, lymphadenopathy, and splenomegaly.

Other causes

◆ ***Drugs.*** Amphetamines and inappropriate dosage of thyroid preparations commonly lead to weight loss. Laxative abuse may cause a malabsorptive state that leads to weight loss. Chemotherapeutic agents may result in weight loss from severe stomatitis.

Special considerations

Refer your patient for psychological counseling if weight loss negatively affects his body image. If the patient has a chronic disease, administer total parenteral nutrition or tube feedings to maintain adequate nutrition and to prevent edema, poor healing, and muscle wasting. Count his caloric intake daily and weigh him weekly. Consult a nutritionist to determine an appropriate diet with adequate calories.

Pediatric pointers

In infants, weight loss may be caused by failure-to-thrive syndrome. In children, severe weight loss may be the first indication of diabetes mellitus. Chronic, gradual weight loss occurs in children with marasmus—nonedematous protein-calorie malnutrition.

Weight loss may also result from child abuse or neglect; an infection causing high fevers; hand-foot-and-mouth disease, which causes painful oral sores; a GI disorder causing vomiting or diarrhea; or celiac disease.

Geriatric pointers

Some elderly patients experience mild, gradual weight loss due to changes in body composition (such as loss of height and lean body mass) and lower basal metabolic rate, leading to decreased energy requirements. Rapid, unintentional weight loss, however, is highly predictive of morbidity and mortality in the elderly. Other nonpathologic causes of weight loss in this age-group include tooth loss, difficulty chewing, social isolation, and alcoholism.

Wheezing

[Sibilant rhonchi]

Wheezes are adventitious breath sounds with a high-pitched, musical, squealing, creaking, or groaning quality. They're caused by air flowing at a high velocity through a narrowed airway. When they originate in the large airways, they can be heard by placing an unaided ear over the chest wall or at the mouth. When they originate in smaller airways, they can be heard by placing a stethoscope over the anterior or posterior chest. Unlike crackles and rhonchi, wheezes can't be cleared by coughing.

Usually, prolonged wheezing occurs during expiration when bronchi are shortened and narrowed. Causes of airway narrowing include bronchospasm; mucosal thickening or edema; partial obstruction from a tumor, a foreign body, or secretions; and extrinsic pressure, as in tension pneumothorax or goiter. In airway obstruction, wheezing occurs during inspiration.

EMERGENCY INTERVENTIONS *Assess whether the patient is in respiratory distress. Is he responsive? Is he restless, confused, anxious, or afraid? Are his respirations abnormally fast, slow, shallow, or deep? Are they irregular? Can you hear wheezing through his mouth? Does he exhibit increased use of accessory muscles; increased chest wall motion; intercostal, suprasternal, or supraclavicular retractions; stridor; or nasal flaring? Take his other vital signs, noting hypotension or hypertension, decreased oxygen saturation, and an irregular, weak, rapid, or slow pulse.*

Help the patient relax. Administer humidified oxygen by face mask, and encourage slow, deep breathing. Have endotracheal intubation and emergency resuscitation equipment readily available. Call the respiratory therapy department to supply intermittent positive-pressure breathing and nebulization treatments with bronchodilators. Insert an I.V. catheter for administration of drugs, such as diuretics, steroids, bronchodilators, and sedatives. Perform the abdominal thrust maneuver, as indicated, for airway obstruction.

HISTORY AND PHYSICAL EXAMINATION

If the patient isn't in respiratory distress, obtain a history. What provokes his wheezing? Does he have asthma or allergies? Does he smoke or have a history of a pulmonary, cardiac, or circulatory disorder? Does he have cancer? Ask about recent surgery, illness, or trauma and recent changes in appetite, weight, exercise tolerance, or sleep patterns. Obtain a drug history. Ask about exposure to toxic fumes or any respiratory irritants. If he has a cough, ask how it sounds, when it starts, and how often it occurs. Does he have paroxysms of coughing? Is his cough dry, sputum producing, or bloody?

Ask the patient about chest pain. If he reports pain, determine its quality, onset, duration, intensity, and radiation. Does it increase with breathing, coughing, or certain positions?

Examine the patient's nose and mouth for congestion, drainage, or signs of infection such as halitosis. If he produces sputum, obtain a specimen for examination. Check for cyanosis, pallor, clamminess, masses, tenderness, swelling, distended jugular veins, and enlarged lymph nodes. Inspect his chest for abnormal configuration and asymmetrical motion, and determine if the trachea is midline. (See *Detecting slight tracheal deviation,* page 667.) Percuss for dullness or hyperresonance, and auscultate for crackles, rhonchi, or pleural friction rub. Note absent or hypoactive breath sounds, abnormal heart sounds, gallops, or murmurs. Also note arrhythmias, bradycardia, or tachycardia. (See *Evaluating breath sounds.* See also *Differential diagnosis: Wheezing,* pages 718 and 719.)

MEDICAL CAUSES

◆ ***Anaphylaxis.*** This allergic reaction can cause tracheal edema or bronchospasm, resulting in severe wheezing and stridor. Initial signs and symptoms include apprehension, weakness, sneezing, dyspnea, nasal pruritus, urticaria, erythema, and angioedema. Respiratory distress occurs with nasal flaring, accessory muscle use, and intercostal retractions. Other findings include nasal edema and congestion, profuse watery rhinorrhea, chest or throat tightness, and dysphagia. Cardiac effects include arrhythmias and hypotension.

◆ ***Aspiration of a foreign body.*** Partial obstruction by a foreign body produces sudden onset of wheezing and possibly stridor; a dry, paroxysmal cough; gagging; and hoarseness. Other findings include tachycardia, dyspnea, decreased breath sounds, and possibly cyanosis. A retained foreign body may cause inflammation leading to fever, pain, and swelling.

Evaluating breath sounds

Diminished or absent breath sounds indicate some interference with airflow. If pus, fluid, or air fills the pleural space, breath sounds will be quieter than normal. If a foreign body or secretions obstruct a bronchus, breath sounds will be diminished or absent over distal lung tissue. Increased thickness of the chest wall, as occurs in a patient who is obese or extremely muscular, may cause breath sounds to be decreased, distant, or inaudible. Absent breath sounds typically indicate loss of ventilation power.

When air passes through narrowed airways or through moisture, or when the membranes lining the chest cavity become inflamed, adventitious breath sounds will be heard. These include crackles, rhonchi, wheezes, and pleural friction rubs. Usually, these sounds indicate pulmonary disease.

Follow the auscultation sequences shown to assess the patient's breath sounds. Have the patient take full, deep breaths, and compare sound variations from one side to the other. Note the location, timing, and character of any abnormal breath sounds.

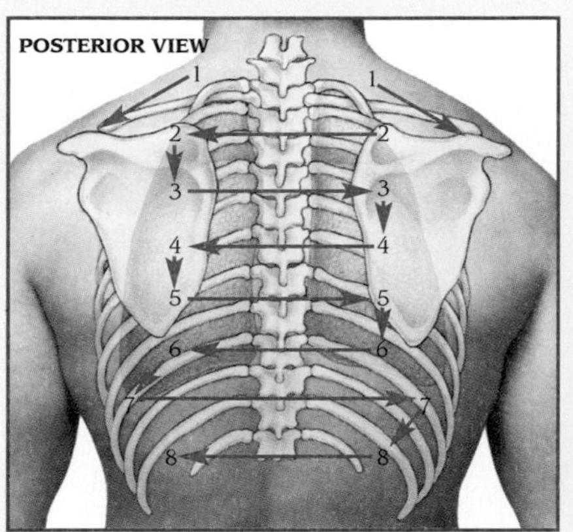

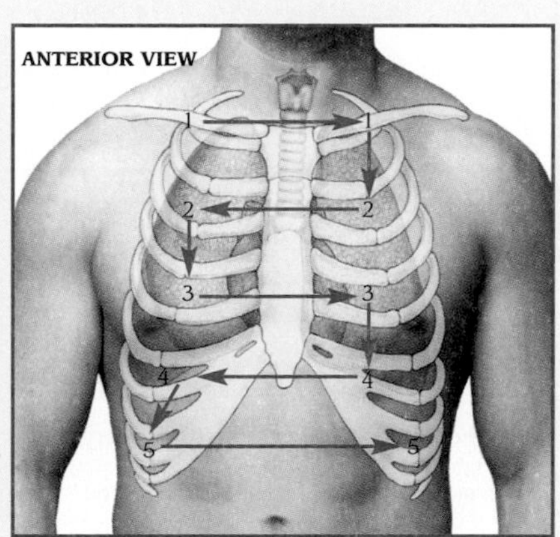

◆ ***Aspiration pneumonitis.*** In this disorder, wheezing may accompany tachypnea, marked dyspnea, cyanosis, tachycardia, fever, a productive (eventually purulent) cough, and frothy pink sputum.

◆ ***Asthma.*** Wheezing is an initial and cardinal sign of asthma. It's heard at the mouth during expiration. An initially dry cough later becomes productive with thick mucus. Other findings include apprehension, prolonged expiration, intercostal and supraclavicular retractions, rhonchi, accessory muscle use, nasal flaring, and tachypnea. Asthma also produces tachycardia, diaphoresis, and flushing or cyanosis.

◆ ***Blast lung injury.*** Wheezing is a common symptom of this condition, which is characterized by hypoxia and respiratory difficulty. The forceful blast wave that follows an explosive detonation can cause serious lung injury, including hemorrhage, contusion, edema, and tearing. In addition to wheezing, patients may exhibit chest pain, dyspnea, cyanosis, and hemoptysis. The diagnosis is confirmed by chest X-rays that show a classic "butterfly" pattern.

◆ ***Bronchial adenoma.*** This insidious disorder produces unilateral, possibly severe wheezing. Common features are a chronic cough and recurring hemoptysis. Symptoms of airway obstruction may occur later.

◆ ***Bronchiectasis.*** In this disorder, excessive mucus commonly causes intermittent and localized or diffuse wheezing. Characteristic findings include a chronic cough that produces copious amounts of foul-smelling, mucopurulent sputum; hemoptysis; rhonchi; and coarse crackles. Weight loss, fatigue, weakness, exertional dyspnea, fever, malaise, halitosis, and late-stage clubbing may also occur.

◆ ***Bronchitis (chronic).*** This disorder causes wheezing that varies in severity, location, and

(Text continues on page 720.)

Differential diagnosis: Wheezing

History of present illness

Focused physical examination: Head, eyes, ears, nose, and throat; respiratory and cardiovascular systems

Common signs and symptoms
- Audible or auscultated wheezing
- Dyspnea
- Chest tightness
- Apprehension
- Tachypnea
- Tachycardia
- Diaphoresis
- Nasal flaring
- Accessory muscle use

Asthma

Additional signs and symptoms
- Dry or productive cough
- Prolonged expiration
- Intercostal and supraclavicular retractions
- Rhonchi

Diagnosis: Allergy skin testing, pulmonary function tests (PFTs), laboratory tests (complete blood count [CBC], arterial blood gas [AGB] analysis), chest X-rays

Treatment: Avoidance of allergens, tobacco, and beta-adrenergic blockers; medication (inhaled $beta_2$ agonists, inhaled corticosteroids, leukotriene receptor agonists, systemic steroids [during infections and exacerbations]), peak expiratory flow monitoring

Follow-up: Reevaluation in 24 hours; then every 3 to 5 days; then every 1 to 3 months

Anaphylaxis

Additional signs and symptoms
- Stridor
- Weakness
- Angioedema
- Intercostal retractions
- Nasal edema and congestion
- Watery rhinorrhea

Diagnosis: Physical examination, history of allergen exposure

Treatment: Symptomatic treatment, airway and oxygenation maintenance, allergy testing (after treatment), medication (I.V. or subcutaneous epinephrine, antihistamines, nebulized albuterol)

Follow-up: Reevaluation within 24 hours

Chronic bronchitis

Signs and symptoms
- Wheezing that varies in severity, location, and intensity
- Prolonged expiration
- Coarse crackles
- Scattered rhonchi
- Hacking, productive cough
- Dyspnea
- Clubbing
- Accessory muscle use
- Cyanosis
- Edema

Diagnosis: PFTs, laboratory tests (CBC, ABG analysis), chest X-rays
Treatment: Smoking cessation, medication (pneumococcal and influenza vaccines, $beta_2$ agonist, bronchodilator, corticosteroids), avoidance of environmental irritants, avoidance of beta-adrenergic blockers and antihistamines, early treatment of infections, oxygen therapy
Follow-up: Return visit within 48 hours after acute exacerbation; then every 3 months

Gastroesophageal reflux disease

Signs and symptoms
- Hematemesis
- Abdominal pain
- Pyrosis
- Flatulence
- Dyspepsia
- Postural regurgitation

Diagnosis: Laboratory tests (electrolyte levels, CBC, stool guaiac), imaging studies (barium swallow, upper GI series, endoscopy), biopsy
Treatment: Diet and lifestyle modification, medication ($histamine_2$ blockers, antacids, proton pump inhibitors), blood transfusion (if indicated)
Follow-up: Reevaluation every 6 months unless the condition worsens; then referral to a gastroenterologist

Additional differential diagnosis: aspiration of a foreign body ◆ aspiration pneumonitis ◆ bronchial adenoma ◆ bronchiectasis ◆ bronchogenic carcinoma ◆ chemical pneumonitis (acute) ◆ emphysema ◆ inhalation injury ◆ pneumothorax (tension) ◆ pulmonary coccidioidomycosis ◆ pulmonary edema ◆ pulmonary embolus ◆ pulmonary tuberculosis ◆ thyroid goiter ◆ tracheobronchitis ◆ Wegener's granulomatosis

intensity. Associated findings include prolonged expiration, coarse crackles, scattered rhonchi, and a hacking cough that later becomes productive. Other effects include dyspnea, accessory muscle use, barrel chest, tachypnea, clubbing, edema, weight gain, and cyanosis.

◆ ***Bronchogenic carcinoma.*** Obstruction may cause localized wheezing. Typical findings include a productive cough, dyspnea, hemoptysis (initially blood-tinged sputum, possibly leading to massive hemorrhage), anorexia, and weight loss. Upper extremity edema and chest pain may also occur.

◆ ***Chemical pneumonitis (acute).*** Mucosal injury causes increased secretions and edema, leading to wheezing, dyspnea, orthopnea, crackles, malaise, fever, and a productive cough with purulent sputum. The patient may also have signs of conjunctivitis, pharyngitis, laryngitis, and rhinitis.

◆ ***Emphysema.*** Mild to moderate wheezing may occur in this form of chronic obstructive pulmonary disease. Related findings include dyspnea, tachypnea, diminished breath sounds, peripheral cyanosis, pursed-lip breathing, anorexia, and malaise. Accessory muscle use, barrel chest, a chronic productive cough, and clubbing may also occur.

◆ ***Inhalation injury.*** Early findings include hoarseness and coughing, singed nasal hairs, orofacial burns, and soot-stained sputum. Later effects may include wheezing, crackles, rhonchi, and respiratory distress.

◆ ***Pneumothorax (tension).*** This life-threatening disorder causes respiratory distress with possible wheezing, dyspnea, tachycardia, tachypnea, and sudden, severe, sharp chest pain (often unilateral). Other findings include a dry cough, cyanosis, accessory muscle use, asymmetrical chest wall movement, anxiety, and restlessness. Examination reveals hyperresonance or tympany and diminished or absent breath sounds on the affected side, subcutaneous crepitation, decreased vocal fremitus, and tracheal deviation.

◆ ***Popcorn lung disease.*** Popcorn lung disease occurs in factory workers who experience respiratory symptoms after inhaling butter flavoring chemicals such as diacetyl, used in the manufacture of microwave popcorn. The patient typically complains of gradual onset of a nonproductive cough that worsens over time, progressive shortness of breath, and unusual fatigue. Clinical findings include wheezing, chest pain, fever, night sweats, and weight loss. Bronchiolitis fibrosa obliterans, an irreversible fixed airway obstructive lung disorder, is the most severe condition reported.

◆ ***Pulmonary coccidioidomycosis.*** This disorder may cause wheezing and rhonchi along with cough, fever, chills, pleuritic chest pain, headache, weakness, malaise, anorexia, and macular rash.

◆ ***Pulmonary edema.*** This life-threatening disorder may cause wheezing, coughing, exertional and paroxysmal nocturnal dyspnea and, later, orthopnea. Examination reveals tachycardia, tachypnea, dependent crackles, and a diastolic gallop. Severe pulmonary edema produces rapid, labored respirations; diffuse crackles; a productive cough with frothy, bloody sputum; arrhythmias; cold, clammy, cyanotic skin; hypotension; and a thready pulse.

◆ ***Pulmonary embolus.*** Diffuse, mild wheezing rarely occurs in this disorder, which is characterized by dyspnea, chest pain, and cyanosis.

◆ ***Pulmonary tuberculosis.*** In late stages, fibrosis causes wheezing. Common findings include a mild to severe productive cough with pleuritic chest pain and fine crackles, night sweats, anorexia, weight loss, fever, malaise, dyspnea, and fatigue. Examination reveals dullness on percussion, increased tactile fremitus, and amphoric breath sounds.

◆ ***Respiratory syncytial virus (RSV).*** Infected individuals commonly develop wheezing and other symptoms within 4 to 6 days of exposure to this virus. Healthy adults and children older than age 3 usually have mild cases of RSV and experience wheezing along with other common cold-like symptoms of runny nose, cough, and low-grade fever. In children ages 3 and younger, high-pitched expiratory wheezing can accompany a severe cough, rapid breathing, and high-grade fever. RSV is the primary cause of lower respiratory tract infection in infants, who may develop pneumonia or bronchiolitis. Infection-control practices help prevent the spread of this virus, which can be inactivated by disinfectants or soap and water. A vaccine is being researched for this common condition that affects most children by age 2.

◆ ***Thyroid goiter.*** This disorder may produce no symptoms, or it may cause wheezing, dysphagia, and respiratory difficulty related to a compressed airway.

◆ ***Tracheobronchitis.*** Auscultation may detect wheezing, rhonchi, and crackles. The patient also has a cough, a slight fever, sudden chills, muscle and back pain, and substernal tightness.

◆ ***Wegener's granulomatosis.*** This disorder may cause mild to moderate wheezing if it compresses major airways. Other findings include a cough (possibly bloody), dyspnea, pleuritic chest pain, hemorrhagic skin lesions, and progressive renal failure. Epistaxis and severe sinusitis are common.

SPECIAL CONSIDERATIONS

Prepare the patient for diagnostic tests, such as chest X-rays, arterial blood gas analysis, pulmonary function tests, and sputum culture. Ease the patient's breathing by placing him in semi-Fowler's position and repositioning him frequently. Perform pulmonary physiotherapy as necessary.

Administer an antibiotic to treat infection, a bronchodilator to relieve bronchospasm and maintain patent airways, a steroid to reduce inflammation, and a mucolytic or an expectorant to increase the flow of secretions. Provide humidification to thin secretions.

PEDIATRIC POINTERS

Children are especially susceptible to wheezing because their small airways allow rapid obstruction. Primary causes of wheezing include bronchospasm, mucosal edema, and accumulation of secretions. These may occur with such disorders as cystic fibrosis, aspiration of a foreign body, acute bronchiolitis, and pulmonary hemosiderosis.

PATIENT COUNSELING

If appropriate, encourage increased activity to promote drainage and prevent pooling of secretions. Encourage regular deep breathing and coughing. Also encourage the patient to drink fluids to liquefy secretions and prevent dehydration.

Wristdrop

In wristdrop, the hand remains in a flexed position from paresis of the extensor muscles of the hand, wrist, and fingers. This weakness may be slight or severe and temporary or permanent. Wristdrop may occur unilaterally and suddenly after a radial nerve injury, or bilaterally and gradually in a neurologic disorder, such as myasthenia gravis, Guillain-Barré syndrome, or multiple sclerosis.

HISTORY AND PHYSICAL EXAMINATION

Begin by asking the patient when wristdrop began and if he can extend his hand at all. Also ask about associated signs and symptoms, such as muscle weakness, vision disturbances, difficulty swallowing or chewing, and urinary incontinence. Has he recently injured his arm or axilla? Test the extent of his wristdrop by asking him to make a fist. Try to pull the fist down. If he can't resist your pull, his extensor muscles are weak. Test complete range of motion in the arm to detect radial nerve injury. Is there an area of numbness over the "snuffbox" areas of the hand—a sign of radial nerve damage?

If the patient reports leg or arm weakness or vision disturbances, proceed with a complete neurologic examination. Assess his level of consciousness; cranial nerve, motor, and sensory function; and reflexes. Are other areas weak? If so, does the weakness increase with fatigue and decrease with rest, as in myasthenia gravis? Does the patient have exacerbations and remissions of signs and symptoms, suggesting multiple sclerosis, or rapidly ascending weakness, indicating Guillain-Barré syndrome?

MEDICAL CAUSES

◆ ***Guillain-Barré syndrome.*** Wristdrop may occur in this syndrome, but the primary neurologic sign is diffuse muscle weakness that typically begins in the legs and ascends to the arms and facial nerves within 24 to 72 hours. Associated findings include paresthesia, diminished or absent corneal reflexes, dysarthria, hypernasality, dysphagia, respiratory insufficiency, and possibly respiratory paralysis. Sympathetic nerve dysfunction—such as orthostatic hypotension, loss of bladder and bowel control, diaphoresis, and tachycardia—may also occur.

◆ ***Multiple sclerosis.*** This disorder may cause wristdrop, but the earliest symptoms are usually diplopia, visual blurring, and paresthesia. Other findings include nystagmus, constipation, muscle weakness, paralysis, spasticity, hyperreflexia, intention tremor, gait ataxia, dysphagia, dysarthria, urinary dysfunction, impotence, and emotional lability.

◆ ***Myasthenia gravis.*** In this disorder, weakness causes wristdrop. Associated findings vary with the muscle group affected and may include weak eye closure, ptosis, diplopia, masklike facies, difficulty chewing and swallowing, nasal regurgitation of fluids, and hypernasality. Weakened neck muscles may lead to head bobbing.

Respiratory muscle weakness produces myasthenic crisis.

◆ ***Radial nerve injury.*** Compression, severance, or inflammation of the radial nerve causes a loss of motor and sensory function in the involved area. This may result in wristdrop, which may be temporary if the injury is incomplete. Other findings in radial nerve injury include loss of finger and elbow extension, forearm supination, and thumb abduction; paresthesia and numbness; and hand muscle atrophy.

Other causes

◆ ***Lead poisoning.*** Inorganic lead poisoning may cause a motor neuropathy that typically involves the radial nerve.

Special considerations

Help the patient with wristdrop perform routine tasks of eating and maintaining personal hygiene. If his wristdrop is permanent, contact a physical therapist to teach him range-of-motion exercises to strengthen weakened muscles. Contact an occupational therapist to provide assistive devices, such as a swivel spoon with a cuff that enables the patient to feed himself. Apply splints to help prevent contractures. Remind the patient to avoid holding hot objects in the affected hand. Also, teach the family to assist with routine activities.

Pediatric pointers

Radial nerve injury is the most common cause of wristdrop in children.

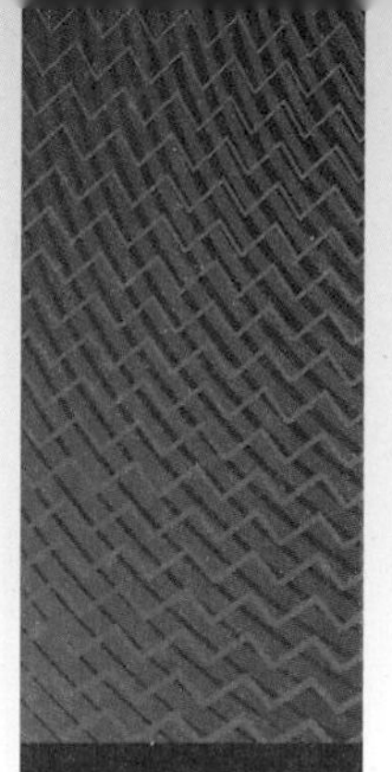

APPENDICES

SELECTED SIGNS & SYMPTOMS

POTENTIAL AGENTS OF BIOTERRORISM

ADVERSE EFFECTS ASSOCIATED WITH HERBS

OBTAINING A HEALTH HISTORY

GUIDE TO LABORATORY TEST RESULTS

SELECTED REFERENCES

INDEX

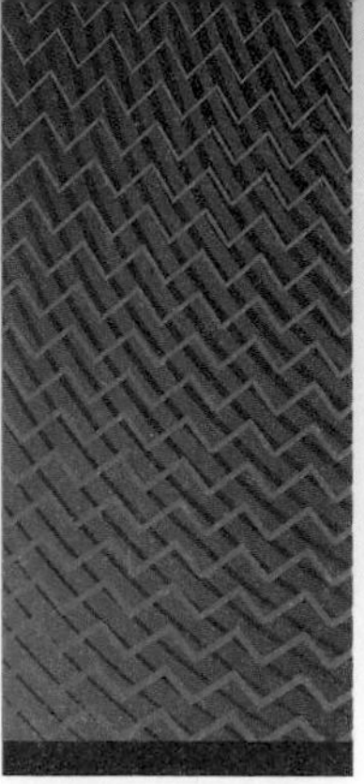

Selected signs & symptoms

This appendix supplements the main text of *Professional Guide to Signs & Symptoms,* Sixth Edition, which provides detailed coverage of about 300 signs and symptoms that are familiar, diagnostically significant, or indicative of an emergency. The appendix, in contrast, provides the definition and common causes of about 250 less familiar, accessory, or nonspecific signs and symptoms. For an elicited sign, such as Chaddock's sign, it also includes the technique for evoking the patient's response.

The appendix also covers selected pediatric signs, such as low-set ears and Allis' sign; psychiatric symptoms, such as delusions and hallucinations; and nail and tongue signs, such as nail plate hypertrophy and tongue discoloration.

A

Aaron's sign Pain in the chest or abdominal (precordial or epigastric) area that's elicited by applying gentle but steadily increasing pressure over McBurney's point. A positive sign indicates appendicitis.

Abadie's sign Spasm of the levator muscle of the upper eyelid. This sign may be slight or pronounced and may affect one eye or both eyes. It reflects an exophthalmic goiter in Graves' disease.

adipsia Abnormal absence of thirst. This symptom commonly occurs in hypothalamic injury or tumor, head injury, bronchial tumor, and cirrhosis.

agnosia Inability to recognize and interpret sensory stimuli, even though the principal sensation of the stimulus is known. Auditory agnosia refers to the inability to recognize familiar sounds. Astereognosis, or tactile agnosia, is the inability to recognize objects by touch or feel. Anosmia is the inability to recognize familiar smells; gustatory agnosia, the inability to recognize familiar tastes. Visual agnosia refers to the inability to recognize familiar objects by sight. Autotopagnosia is the inability to recognize body parts. Anosognosia refers to the denial or unawareness of a disease or defect (especially paralysis).

Agnosias stem from lesions that affect the association areas of the parietal sensory cortex. They're a common sequelae of stroke.

agraphia Inability to express thoughts in writing. Aphasic agraphia is associated with spelling and grammatical errors, whereas constructional agraphia refers to the reversal or incorrect ordering of correctly spelled words. Apraxic agraphia refers to the inability to form letters in the absence of significant motor impairment.

Agraphia commonly results from a stroke.

Allis' sign In an adult: relaxation of the fascia lata between the iliac crest and greater trochanter due to fracture of the neck of the femur. To detect this sign, place a finger over the area between the iliac crest and greater trochanter and press firmly. If your finger sinks deeply into this area, you've detected Allis' sign.

In an infant: unequal leg lengths due to hip dislocation. To detect this sign, place the infant on his back with his pelvis flat. Then flex both legs at the knee and hip with the feet even. Next, compare the height of the knees. If they differ, suspect hip dislocation in the shorter leg.

ALLIS' SIGN

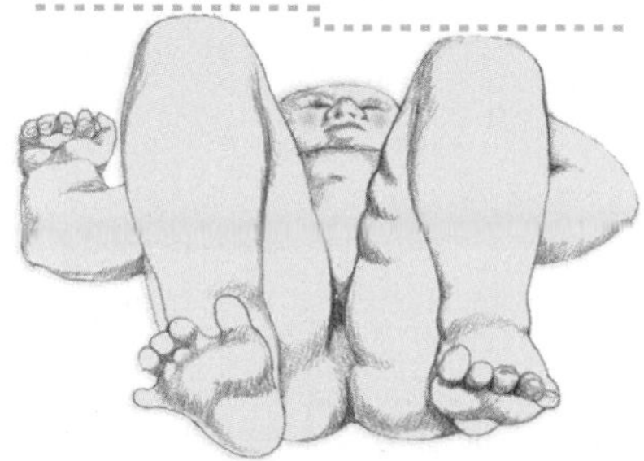

ambivalence Simultaneous conflicting feelings (such as both love and hate) about a person, idea, or object. It causes uncertainty or indecisiveness about which course to follow. Severe, debilitating ambivalence can occur in schizophrenia.

Amoss' sign A sparing maneuver to avoid pain upon flexion of the spine. To detect this sign, ask the patient to rise from a supine to a sitting position. If he supports himself by placing his hands far behind him on the examining table, you've observed this sign.

anesthesia Absence of cutaneous sensation of touch, temperature, and pain. This sensory loss may be partial or total, and unilateral or bilateral. To detect anesthesia, ask the patient to close his eyes. Then touch him and ask him to specify the location. If the patient's verbal skills are immature or poor, watch for movement or changes in facial expression in response to your touch.

anisocoria A difference of 0.5 to 2 mm in pupil size. Anisocoria occurs normally in about 2% of people, in whom the pupillary inequality remains constant over time and despite changes in light. However, if anisocoria results from fixed dilation or constriction of one pupil or from slowed or impaired constriction of one pupil in response to light, it may indicate neurologic disease. Determining whether the abnormal pupil is dilated or constricted aids diagnosis.

apathy Absence or suppression of emotion or interest in the external environment and personal affairs. This indifference can result from many disorders, chiefly neurologic, psychological, respiratory, and renal, as well as from alcohol and drug use and abuse. It's associated with many chronic disorders that cause personality changes and depression. In fact, apathy may be an early indicator of a severe disorder, such as a brain tumor or schizophrenia.

aphonia Inability to produce speech sounds. This sign may result from overuse of the vocal cords, disorders of the larynx or laryngeal nerves, psychological disorders, or muscle spasm.

Argyll Robertson pupil A small, irregular pupil that constricts normally in accommodation for near vision but poorly or not at all in response to light. Response to mydriatics is also poor or absent. This condition may be unilateral or bilateral, or the degree of involvement in the eyes may be asymmetrical. Chronic syphilitic meningitis or other forms of late syphilis are the most common causes.

arthralgia Joint pain. This symptom may have no pathologic importance or may indicate such disorders as arthritis or systemic lupus erythematosus.

asthenocoria Slow dilation or constriction of the pupils in response to light changes. Photophobia may be present if constriction occurs slowly. Asthenocoria occurs in adrenal insufficiency. Also known as Arroyo's sign.

asynergy Impaired coordination of muscles or organs that normally function harmoniously. This extrapyramidal symptom stems from disorders of the basal ganglia and cerebellum.

atrophy Shrinkage or wasting away of a tissue or organ due to a reduction in the size or number of its cells. Its etiology may be physiologic, as in ovary, brain, and skin atrophy, or pathologic, such as atrophy commonly associated with neurologic disorders or spleen, liver, and thyroid abnormalities. This symptom is normally observed using inspection and palpation techniques.

attention span decrease Inability to focus selectively on a task while ignoring extraneous stimuli. Anxiety, emotional upset, and any dysfunction of the central nervous system may decrease the attention span.

autistic behavior Exaggerated self-centered behavior marked by a lack of responsiveness to other people. It's characterized by highly personalized speech and actions that are not meaningful to an observer. For example, the patient may rock his body or repeatedly bang his head against the floor or wall. Autistic behavior may occur in schizophrenic children and adults.

B

Ballance's sign A fixed mass or area of dullness found by palpation and percussion of the left upper quadrant of the abdomen. It may indicate subcapsular or extracapsular hematoma following splenic rupture.

Ballet's sign Ophthalmoplegia, or paralysis of the external ocular muscles. The patient displays no control of voluntary eye movement but has normal reflexive movement and pupillary light reflexes. This sign is an indicator of thyrotoxicosis.

Bárány's sign With warm water irrigation of the ear, rotary nystagmus toward the irrigated side; with cold water irrigation, rotary nystagmus away from the irrigated side. Absence of this symptom indicates labyrinthine dysfunction. Also called the caloric test.

Barlow's sign An indicator of congenital dislocation of the hip, detected during the first 6 weeks of life. To elicit this sign, place the infant supine with the hips flexed 90 degrees and the knees fully flexed. Place your palm over the infant's knee, your thumb in the femoral triangle opposite the lesser trochanter, and your index finger over the greater trochanter. Bring the hip into midabduction while gently exerting posterior and lateral pressure with your thumb, and posterior and medial pressure with your palm. If you detect a click of the femoral head as it dislocates across the posterior lip of the acetabular socket, you've elicited this sign.

Barré's pyramidal sign Inability to hold the lower legs still with the knees flexed. To detect this sign, help the patient into a prone position and flex his knees 90 degrees. Then ask him to hold his lower legs still. If he can't maintain this position, you've observed this sign of pyramidal tract or prefrontal brain disease.

Barré's sign Delayed contraction of the iris, seen in mental deterioration.

Beau's lines Transverse white linear depressions on the fingernails. These lines may develop after any severe illness or toxic reaction. Other common causes include malnutrition, nail bed trauma, and coronary artery occlusion.

BEAU'S LINES

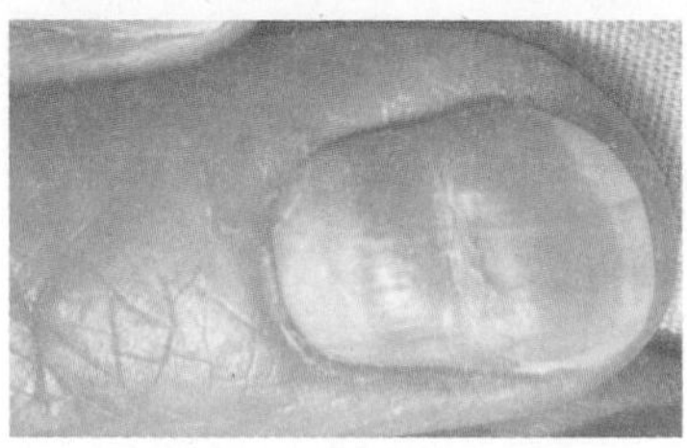

Beevor's sign Upward movement of the umbilicus upon contraction of the abdominal muscles. To detect this sign, help the patient into a supine position and then ask him to sit up. If the umbilicus moves upward, you've observed this sign—an indicator of paralysis of the lower rectus abdominis muscles associated with lesions at T10.

Bell's sign Reflexive upward and outward deviation of the eyes that occurs when the patient attempts to close his eyelid. It occurs on the affected side in Bell's palsy and indicates that the defect is supranuclear. Also known as Bell's phenomenon.

Bezold's sign Swelling and tenderness of the mastoid area. Resulting from formation of an abscess beneath the sternocleidomastoid muscle, Bezold's sign indicates mastoiditis.

BEZOLD'S SIGN

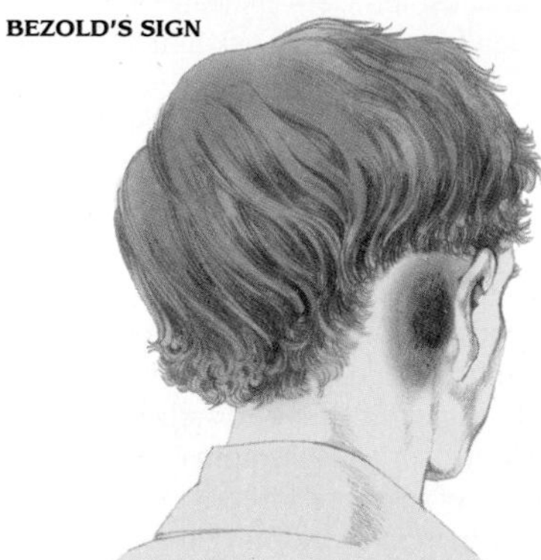

Bitot's spots Triangular white or foamy gray spots, varying from a few bubbles to a frothy white coating, that appear on the conjunctiva at the lateral margin of the cornea. They're associated with vitamin A deficiency.

blepharoclonus Excessive blinking of the eyes. This extrapyramidal sign occurs in disorders of the basal ganglia and cerebellum.

blocking A cognitive disturbance resulting in interruption of a stream of speech or thought. It usually occurs in midsentence or before completion of a thought. In most cases, the patient can't explain the interruption. Blocking may occur in normal individuals but usually occurs in schizophrenic patients.

Bonnet's sign Pain on adduction of the thigh, seen in sciatica.

Bozzolo's sign Pulsation of arteries in the nasal mucous membrane, seen occasionally in thoracic aortic aneurysms. To detect this sign, examine both nostrils, using a speculum and light.

bradykinesia Slowness of all voluntary movement and speech, believed to be due to a reduced level of dopamine in the neurons in the brain stem region. Bradykinesia can be a symptom of inhibited central nervous system functioning and is usually associated with parkinsonism or extrapyramidal or cerebellar disorders. It can also result from the use of certain drugs. Bradykinesia usually affects patients older than age 50, but it may also occur in children who have suffered hypoxic accidents. Associated findings include tremor and muscle rigidity.

Braunwald sign Occurrence of a weak pulse rather than a strong pulse immediately after a premature ventricular contraction (PVC). To detect this sign, watch for a PVC during cardiac monitoring and check the quality of the pulse after it. Braunwald sign may indicate hypertrophic cardiomyopathy.

breath sounds, absent or decreased Diminished loudness of breath sounds—or their absence—detected by auscultation. This may reflect reduced airflow to a lung segment caused by a tumor, a foreign body, a mucus plug, or mucosal edema. It may also reflect hyperinflation of the lungs in emphysema or an asthma attack. Or, it may indicate air or fluid in the pleural cavity from pneumothorax, hemothorax, pleural effusion, atelectasis, or empyema. In an obese or extremely muscular patient, breath sounds may be diminished or inaudible because of increased thickness of the chest wall.

Broadbent's inverted sign Pulsations in the left posterolateral chest wall during ventricular systole. To detect this sign, palpate the patient's chest with your fingers and palm over areas of visible pulsation while auscultating for ventricular systole. When you feel pulsations, note their rate, rhythm, and intensity. This sign may indicate gross dilation of the left atrium.

Broadbent's sign Visible retraction of the left posterior chest wall (back) near the 11th and 12th ribs, occurring during systole. To detect this sign, inspect the chest wall while standing at the patient's right side. Position a strong light so that it casts rays tangential to the skin. While auscultating the heart, watch for retraction of the skin and muscles and determine its timing in the cardiac cycle. Broadbent's sign may occur in extensive adhesive pericarditis.

C

catatonia Marked inhibition or excitation in motor behavior, occurring in psychotic disorders. Catatonic stupor refers to extreme inhibition of spontaneous activity or movement. Catatonic excitement refers to extreme psychomotor agitation.

Chaddock's sign Chaddock's toe sign: extension (dorsiflexion) of the great toe and fanning of the other toes. To elicit this sign, firmly stroke the side of the patient's foot just distal to the lateral malleolus. A positive sign indicates pyramidal tract disorders.

Chaddock's wrist sign: flexion of the wrist and extension of the fingers. To elicit this sign, stroke the ulnar surface of the patient's forearm near the wrist. A positive sign occurs on the affected side in hemiplegia. Although Chaddock's sign signals pathology in children and adults, it's a normal finding in infants up to age 7 months.

CHADDOCK'S SIGN

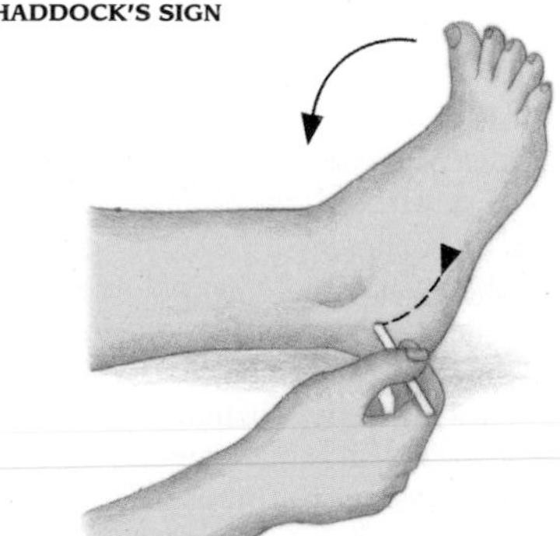

cherry-red spot The choroid appearing as a red circular area surrounded by an abnormal gray-white retina. It's viewed through the fovea centralis of the eye with an ophthalmoscope. A cherry-red spot appears in infantile cerebral sphingolipidosis; for example, this spot is detected in more than 90% of patients with Tay-Sachs disease.

circumstantiality Speech in which the main point is obscured by minute detail. Although the speaker may recognize his main point and return to it after many digressions, the listener may fail to recognize it. Circumstantiality commonly occurs in compulsive disorders, organic brain disorders, and schizophrenia.

Claude's hyperkinesis sign Increased reflex activity of paretic muscles, elicited by painful stimuli.

clavicular sign Swelling, puffiness, or edema at the medial third of the right clavicle; usually seen in congenital syphilis.

Cleeman's sign Slight linear depression or wrinkling of the skin superior to the patella. It usually indicates a femoral fracture with overriding bone fragments.

clenched fist sign The patient's placement of a clenched fist against his chest. This gesture may be performed by patients with angina pectoris when they're asked to indicate the location of their pain. The patient's gesture conveys the constricting, oppressive quality of substernal pain.

clicks Extra, brief, high-frequency heart sounds auscultated during systole or diastole. Ejection clicks occur soon after the first heart sound. They're believed to result from sudden distention of a dilated pulmonary artery or the aorta, or from forceful opening of the pulmonic or aortic valves. Associated with increased pulmonary resistance and hypertension, they usually occur in septal defects or patent ductus arteriosus. To detect ejection clicks best, have the patient sit upright or lie down, and then auscultate the heart with the diaphragm of the stethoscope.

Systolic clicks usually occur in mid-to-late systole and are characteristic of mitral valve prolapse. They're heard most distinctly at or medial to the heart's apex but may also be heard at the lower left sternal border. These clicks are heard best using the diaphragm of the stethoscope.

clonus Abnormal response of a muscle to stretching. It's a sign of damage to nerve fibers that carry impulses to a particular muscle from the motor cortex. Usually, a muscle that is stretched responds by contracting once and then relaxing. In clonus, stretching sets off a series of muscle contractions in rapid succession. Clonuslike, or clonic, muscle contractions are also a feature of generalized tonic-clonic seizures.

Codman's sign Pain resulting from rupture of the supraspinatus tendon. To elicit this sign, have the patient relax the arm on the affected side while you abduct it. If the patient reports no pain until you remove your support and the deltoid muscle contracts, you've detected Codman's sign.

cognitive dysfunction Inability to perceive, organize, and interpret sensory stimuli and to think and solve problems. It may arise from various causes, including central nervous system disturbances, extrapyramidal conditions, systemic illness, endocrine diseases, and deficiency states, or from unknown causes, as in chronic fatigue syndrome.

Comolli's sign Triangular swelling over the scapula that matches its shape. This sign indicates a scapular fracture.

complementary opposition sign Increased effort in lifting a paretic leg, demonstrated in the opposite leg. To elicit this sign, help the patient into a supine position, and place your hand under the heel of the unaffected leg. Then ask the patient to lift the paretic leg. If his effort produces marked downward pressure on your hand, you've detected this sign. Also known as Grasset-Gaussel-Hoover sign.

compulsion Stereotyped, repetitive behavior in which the individual recognizes the irrationality of his actions but is unable to stop them. An example is constant hand washing. Compulsion occurs in obsessive-compulsive disorders and occasionally in schizophrenia.

confabulation Fabrication of facts and experiences to cover gaps in memory. The fabrications are generally plausible and detailed. Confabulation is most often seen in alcoholism, Korsakoff's syndrome, dementia, lead poisoning, and head injuries.

conjunctival paleness Lack of color in the tissues inside the eyelid. Although the conjunctiva is a transparent mucous membrane, the portion lining the eyelids normally appears pink or red because it overlies the vasculature of the inner lid. Pale conjunctiva indicates anemia. To detect this sign, separate the eyelids widely by applying gentle pressure against the orbit of the eye. Then ask the patient to look up, down, and to each side.

conversion An alteration in physical activity or function that resembles an organic disorder but lacks an organic cause. Occurring without voluntary control, conversion is generally considered symbolic of psychological conflict and usually occurs in conversion disorders.

Coopernail's sign Ecchymoses on the perineum, scrotum, or labia. This sign indicates pelvic fracture.

Corrigan's pulse A jerky pulse in which a strong surge precedes an abrupt collapse. To detect this sign, hold the patient's hand above his head and palpate the carotid artery. Corrigan's pulse occurs in aortic insufficiency. It may also occur in severe anemia, patent ductus arteriosus, coarctation of the aorta, and systemic arteriosclerosis.

Cowen's sign A jerky, consensual pupillary light reflex that occurs in Graves' disease. To detect this sign, observe for constriction and dilation of one pupil while the other is stimulated by increased and decreased light.

crossed extensor reflex Extension of one leg in response to stimulation of the opposite leg; a normal reflex in neonates. It's mediated at the spinal cord level and should disappear after age 6 months. To elicit this sign, place the infant in a supine position with his legs extended. Tap the medial aspect of the thigh just above the patella. The infant should respond by extending and adducting the opposite leg and fanning the toes of that foot. Persistence of this reflex beyond age 6 months indicates anoxic brain damage. Its appearance in a child signals a central nervous system lesion or injury.

crowing respirations Slow, deep inspirations accompanied by a high-pitched crowing sound—the characteristic whoop of the paroxysmal stage of pertussis.

Cruveilhier's sign Swelling in the groin associated with inguinal hernia. To detect this sign, ask the patient to flex one knee slightly while you insert your index finger in the inguinal canal on the same side. When your finger is inserted as deeply as possible, ask the patient to cough. If a hernia is present, you'll feel a mass of tissue that meets your finger and then withdraws.

Cullen's sign Irregular, bluish hemorrhagic patches on the skin around the umbilicus and occasionally around abdominal scars. Cullen's sign indicates massive hemorrhage after trauma or rupture in such disorders as duodenal ulcer, ectopic pregnancy, abdominal aneurysm, gallbladder or common bile duct obstruction, or acute hemorrhagic pancreatitis. Usually, Cullen's sign appears gradually as blood travels from a retroperitoneal organ or structure to the periumbilical area, where it diffuses through subcutaneous tissues. It may be difficult to detect in a dark-skinned patient. The extent of discoloration depends on the extent of bleeding. In time, the bluish discoloration fades to greenish yellow and then yellow before disappearing.

D

Dalrymple's sign Abnormally wide palpebral fissures associated with retraction of the upper eyelids. To detect this sign of thyrotoxicosis, observe the eyes while the patient focuses on a fixed point, or ask him to close his eyes. You may detect infrequent blinking and noticeable restriction of lid movement. The patient may not be able to close his eyes completely.

Darier's sign Wheals and itching of the skin upon rubbing the macular lesions of urticaria pigmentosa (mastocytosis). To elicit this sign, vigorously rub the pigmented macules with the blunt end of a pen or a similar blunt object. The appearance of pruritic, red, palpable wheals around the macules—a positive Darier's sign—follows the release of histamine when mast cells are irritated.

Dawbarn's sign Pain on palpation of the acromial process in acute subacromial bursitis. To elicit this sign, palpate the patient's shoulder while his arm hangs at his side and as he abducts it. If palpation causes pain that disappears on abduction, you've detected Dawbarn's sign.

Delbet's sign Adequate collateral circulation to the distal portion of a limb associated with aneurysmal occlusion of the main artery. To detect this sign, check the pulses, color, and temperature in the affected limb. If you find absent pulses but normal color and temperature, you've detected Delbet's sign.

delirium Acute confusion characterized by restlessness, agitation, incoherence, and often hallucinations. Typically, delirium develops suddenly and lasts for a short period. It's a common effect of drug and alcohol abuse, metabolic disorders, and high fever. Delirium may also follow head trauma or seizures.

delusion A persistent false belief held despite invalidating evidence. A delusion of grandeur, which may occur in schizophrenia and bipolar disorder, refers to an exaggerated belief in one's importance, wealth, or talent. The patient may take a powerful figure, such as Napoleon, as his persona. In a paranoid delusion, which may occur in schizophrenia and paranoid disorders, the patient believes that he or someone close to him is the victim of an attack, harassment, or conspiracy. In a somatic delusion, which may occur in psychotic disorders, the patient believes that his body is diseased or distorted.

Demianoff's sign Lumbar pain caused by stretching the sacrolumbalis muscle. To elicit this sign, help the patient into a supine position on the examining table and raise his extended leg. Lumbar pain that prevents lifting the leg high enough to form a 10-degree angle to the table—a positive Demianoff's sign—occurs in lumbago.

denial An unconscious defense mechanism used to ward off distressing feelings, thoughts, wishes, or needs. Denial occurs in normal and pathologic mental states. In terminally ill patients, denial is the first of five stages of grief, as described by Elisabeth Kübler-Ross.

depersonalization Perception of the self as strange or unreal. For example, a person may report feeling as if he's observing himself from a distance. This symptom occurs in patients with schizophrenia or depersonalization disorder and in normal individuals during periods of great stress, fatigue, or anxiety.

Desault's sign Alteration of the arc made by the greater trochanter on rotation of the femur; seen in fracture of the intracapsular region of the femur. In this fracture, the greater trochanter rotates only on the axis of the femur, making a much smaller arc than it does upon normal rotation of the femur in the capsule of the hip joint, which normally describes the arc of a circle.

disorientation Inaccurate perception of time, place, or identity. Disorientation may occur in organic brain disorders, cerebral anoxia, and drug and alcohol intoxication. It occurs occasionally after prolonged, severe stress.

Dorendorf's sign Fullness at the supraclavicular groove. This sign may occur in an aneurysm of the aortic arch.

DORENDORF'S SIGN

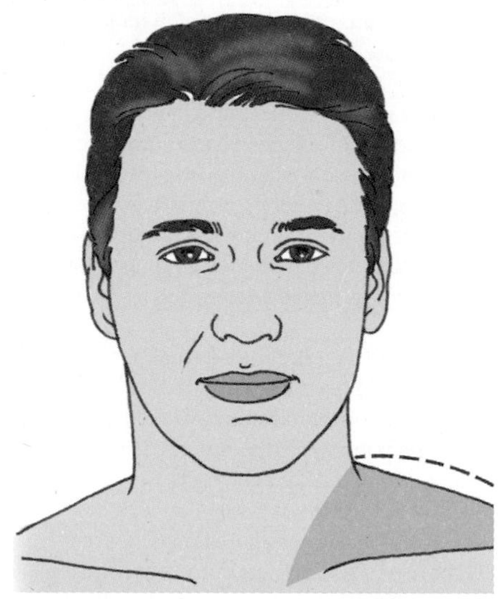

Duchenne's sign Inward movement of the epigastrium during inspiration. This may indicate diaphragmatic paralysis or accumulation of fluid in the pericardium.

Dugas' sign An indicator of a dislocated shoulder. To detect this sign, ask the patient to place the hand of the affected side on his opposite shoulder and to move his elbow toward his chest. The inability to perform this maneuver—a positive Dugas' sign—indicates dislocation.

Duroziez's sign A double murmur heard over a large peripheral artery. To detect this sign, auscultate over the femoral artery, alternately compressing the vessel proximally and then distally. If you hear a systolic murmur with proximal compression and a diastolic murmur with distal compression, you've detected Duroziez's sign—an indicator of aortic insufficiency. It's also known as Duroziez's murmur.

dysdiadochokinesia Difficulty performing rapidly alternating movements. This extrapyramidal sign occurs in disorders of the basal ganglia and cerebellum.

dysphonia Hoarseness or difficulty producing voice sounds. This sign may reflect disorders of the larynx or laryngeal nerves, overuse or spasm of the vocal cords, or central nervous system disorders such as Parkinson's disease. Pubertal voice changes are termed dysphonia puberum.

E

echolalia In an adult: repetition of another's words or phrases with no comprehension of their meaning. This sign occurs in schizophrenia and frontal lobe disorders.

In a child: an imitation of sounds or words produced by others.

echopraxia Repetition of another's movements with no comprehension of their meaning. This sign may occur in catatonic schizophrenia and certain neurologic disorders.

ectropion Eversion of the eyelid. It may affect the lower eyelid or both lids, exposing the palpebral conjunctiva. If the lacrimal puncta are everted, the eye can't drain properly, and tearing occurs. Ectropion may occur gradually as part of aging, or it may result from injury or paralysis of the facial nerve.

ECTROPION

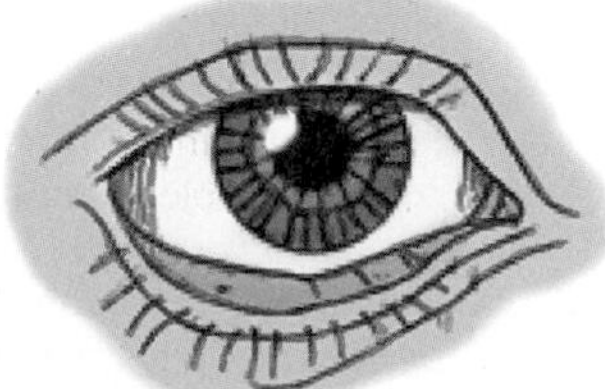

entropion Inversion of the eyelid. It typically affects the lower lid but may also affect the upper lid. The eyelashes may touch and irritate the cornea. Usually associated with aging, entropion may also stem from chemical burns, mechanical injuries, spasm of the orbicularis muscle, pemphigoid, Stevens-Johnson syndrome, or trachoma.

ENTROPION

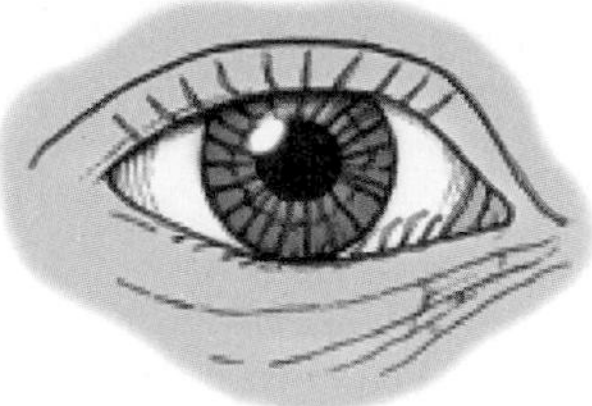

epicanthal folds Vertical skin folds that partially or fully obscure the inner canthus of the eye. These folds may make the eyes appear crossed because the pupil lies closer to the inner canthus than to the outer canthus. Epicanthal folds are a normal characteristic in many young children and Asian people. They also occur as a familial trait in other ethnic groups and as an acquired trait in aging. However, the presence of epicanthal folds along with oblique palpebral fissures in non-Asian children indicates Down syndrome.

Erben's reflex Slowing of the pulse when the head and trunk are forcibly bent forward. It may indicate vagal excitability.

Erb's sign In tetany, increased irritability of motor nerves, detected by electromyography. Erb's sign also refers to dullness on percussion over the sternum's manubrium in acromegaly.

Escherich's sign In tetany, contraction of the lips, tongue, and masseters on percussion of the inner surface of the lips or the tongue.

euphoria A feeling of great happiness or well-being. When euphoria occurs for no apparent reason, it may reflect bipolar disorder, organic brain disease, or use of such drugs as heroin, cocaine, and amphetamines.

Ewart's sign Bronchial breathing heard on auscultation of the lungs and dullness heard on percussion below the angle of the left scapula. These compression signs commonly occur in pericardial effusion. They also occur beneath the prominence of the sternal end of the first rib in some cases of pericardial effusion.

extensor thrust reflex In neonates, extension of the leg upon stimulation of the sole. This normal reflex is mediated at the spinal cord level and should disappear after age 6 months.

To elicit the extensor thrust reflex, place the infant in a supine position with the leg flexed; then stimulate the sole of the foot. If the extensor thrust reflex is present, the leg will slowly extend. In premature infants, this reflex may be weak. Its persistence beyond age 6 months indicates anoxic brain damage. Its recurrence in a child signals a central nervous system lesion or injury.

extinction In neurology: inability to perceive one of two stimuli presented simultaneously. To detect this sign, simultaneously stimulate two corresponding areas on opposite sides of the body. Extinction is present if the patient fails to perceive one sensation.

In neurophysiology: loss of excitability of a nerve, synapse, or nervous tissue in response to stimuli that were previously adequate.

In psychology: disappearance of a conditioned reflex resulting from lack of reinforcement.

extrapyramidal signs and symptoms Movement and posture disturbances characteristically resulting from disorders of the basal ganglia and cerebellum. These disturbances include asynergy, ataxia, athetosis, blepharoclonus, chorea, dysarthria, dysdiadochokinesia, dystonia, muscle rigidity and spasticity, myoclonus, spasmodic torticollis, and tremors.

F

fabere sign Pain produced by maneuvers used in Patrick's test. It indicates an arthritic hip. The name is an acronym for maneuvers used to elicit the sign: flexion, abduction, external rotation, and extension. Begin by helping the patient into a supine position and asking him to flex the thigh and knee of the leg being examined. Then have him externally rotate the leg and place the lateral malleolus on the patella of the opposite leg. Depress the knee. If he experiences pain, you've detected the fabere sign.

Fajersztajn's crossed sciatic sign In sciatica, pain on the affected side caused by lifting the extended opposite leg. To elicit this sign, place the patient supine and have him flex his unaffected hip, keeping his knee extended. Flexion at the hip will produce pain on the affected side caused by stretching of the irritated sciatic nerve.

fan sign Spreading apart of the toes after the patient's foot is firmly stroked; a component of Babinski's reflex.

flexor withdrawal reflex In neonates, flexion of the knee upon stimulation of the sole. This normal reflex is mediated at the spinal cord level and should disappear after age 6 months.

To elicit this reflex, place the infant in a supine position, extend his legs, and pinch the sole of his foot. Normally, an infant younger than age 6 months will respond with slow, uncontrolled flexion of the knee. This reflex may be weak in premature infants. Its persistence beyond age 6 months may indicate anoxic brain damage. Its recurrence signals a central nervous system lesion or injury.

flight of ideas A speech pattern characterized by incessant talking and abrupt changes of topic. In contrast to loose association, a listener can discern the connection between topics based on word similarities or sounds. This sign characteristically occurs in the manic phase of bipolar disorder.

foot malposition, congenital Anomalous positioning of the foot, present at birth in roughly 0.4% of infants. It may reflect the fetal position of comfort, neuromuscular disease, or malformation of a joint or connective tissue. To assess this sign, observe the resting infant's foot to determine the position of comfort. Then observe the foot during spontaneous activity. Using gentle passive maneuvers, determine the full range of motion of the foot and ankle.

Fränkel's sign In tabes dorsalis, the excessive range of passive motion at the hip joint. This excessive motion stems from decreased tone in the surrounding muscles.

G

Galant's reflex Movement of the pelvis toward the stimulated side when the back is stroked laterally to the spinal column. Normally present at birth, this reflex disappears by age 2 months. To elicit this reflex, place the infant in a prone position on the examining table or on your hand. Then, using a pin or your finger, stroke the back laterally to the midline. Normally, the infant responds by moving the pelvis toward the stimulated side, indicating integrity of the spinal cord from T1 to S1. The absence, irregularity, or asymmetry of this reflex may indicate a spinal cord lesion.

GALANT'S REFLEX

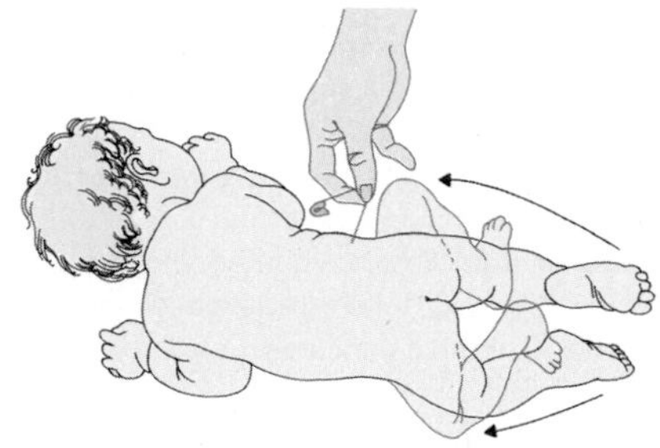

Galeazzi sign Unequal leg lengths in an infant, seen in congenital dislocation of the hip. To detect this sign, place the infant in a supine position on a flat, hard surface. Flex the knees and hips 90 degrees and compare the heights of the knees. In dislocation of the hip, the knee will be lower and the femur will appear shortened on the affected side.

Gifford's sign Resistance to everting the upper eyelid, seen in thyrotoxicosis. To detect this sign, attempt to raise the eyelid and evert it over a blunt object.

glabella tap reflex Persistent blinking in response to repeated light tapping on the forehead between the eyebrows. This reflex occurs in Parkinson's disease, presenile dementia, and diffuse tumors of the frontal lobes.

Goldthwait's sign Pain elicited by maneuvers of the leg, pelvis, and lower back to differentiate irritation of the sacroiliac joint from irritation of the lumbosacral or sacroiliac articulation. To elicit this sign, help the patient into a supine position and place one hand under the small of his back. With your other hand, raise the patient's leg. If the patient reports pain, suspect sacroiliac joint irritation. If he reports no pain, place your hand under his lower back and apply pressure. If the patient reports pain, suspect irritation of the lumbosacral or sacroiliac articulation.

Gowers' sign In an adult: irregular contraction of the iris when the eye is illuminated. This sign can be detected in certain stages of tabes dorsalis.

In a child: the characteristic maneuver used to rise from the floor or a low sitting position to compensate for proximal muscle weakness in Duchenne's or Becker's muscular dystrophy. See "Gait, waddling," page 321.

grasp reflex In infants, flexion of the fingers when the palmar surface is touched, and of the toes when the plantar surface is touched. This normal reflex develops at 26 to 28 weeks' gestation but may be weak until term. The absence, weakness, or asymmetry of this reflex during the neonatal period may indicate paralysis, central nervous system depression, or injury. To elicit this reflex, place a finger in each of the infant's palms. His reflexive grasping should be symmetrical and strong enough at term to allow him to be lifted. Elicit flexion of the toes by gently touching the ball of the foot.

The grasp reflex is an *abnormal* finding in adults, indicating a disorder of the premotor cortex.

Grasset's phenomenon Inability to raise both legs simultaneously, even though each can be raised separately; a normal finding in infants until age 5 to 7 months.

In adults, this phenomenon occurs in complete organic hemiplegia. To elicit it, help the patient into a supine position, lift and support the affected leg, and then try to lift the opposite leg. In Grasset's phenomenon, the unaffected leg will drop—the result of an upper-motor-neuron lesion.

grief Deep anguish or sorrow typically felt upon separation, bereavement, or loss. In patients with terminal illness, grief may precede acceptance of dying. Unlike depression, grief proceeds in stages and often resolves with the passage of time.

Griffith's sign Lagging motion of the lower eyelids during upward rotation of the eyes, seen in thyrotoxicosis. To detect this sign, ask the patient to focus on a steadily rising point, such as your moving finger. If the lower lid doesn't follow eye motion smoothly, you've observed this sign.

Guilland's sign Quick, energetic flexion of the hip and knee in response to pinching of the contralateral quadriceps muscle. This sign indicates meningeal irritation.

H

hallucination A sensory perception without corresponding external stimuli that occurs while awake. Hallucinations may occur in depression, schizophrenia, bipolar disorder, organic brain disorders, and drug-induced and toxic conditions.

An *auditory hallucination* refers to the perception of nonexistent sounds—typically voices but occasionally music or other sounds. Occurring in schizophrenia, this is the most common type of hallucination.

An *olfactory hallucination*—a perception of nonexistent odors from the patient's own body or from some other person or object—is typically associated with somatic delusions. It occurs most often in temporal lobe lesions and sometimes in schizophrenia.

A *tactile hallucination* refers to the perception of nonexistent tactile stimuli, generally described as something crawling on or under the skin. It occurs mainly in toxic conditions and addiction to certain drugs. Formication—the sensation of insects crawling on the skin—usually occurs in alcohol withdrawal syndrome and cocaine abuse.

A *visual hallucination* is a perception of images of nonexistent people, flashes of light, or other scenes. It usually occurs in acute, reversible organic brain disorders but may also occur in drug and alcohol intoxication, schizophrenia, febrile illness, and encephalopathy.

A *gustatory hallucination* refers to the perception of nonexistent, usually unpleasant tastes.

Hamman's sign A loud, crushing, crunching sound synchronous with the heartbeat. Auscultated over the precordium, it reflects mediastinal emphysema, which occurs in such life-threatening conditions as pneumothorax and rupture of the trachea or bronchi. To detect this sign, help the patient into a left lateral recumbent position and gently auscultate over the precordium.

harlequin sign A benign, erythematous color change occurring primarily in low-birth-weight infants. This reddening of one longitudinal half of the body appears when the infant is placed on either side for a few minutes. When he's placed on his back, the sign usually disappears immediately but may persist for up to 20 minutes.

hemorrhage, subungual Bleeding under the nail plate. Hemorrhagic lines, called splinter hemorrhages, run proximally from the distal edge and serve as an indicator of subacute bacterial endocarditis and trichinosis. Large hemorrhagic areas generally reflect nail bed injury.

SUBUNGUAL HEMORRHAGE

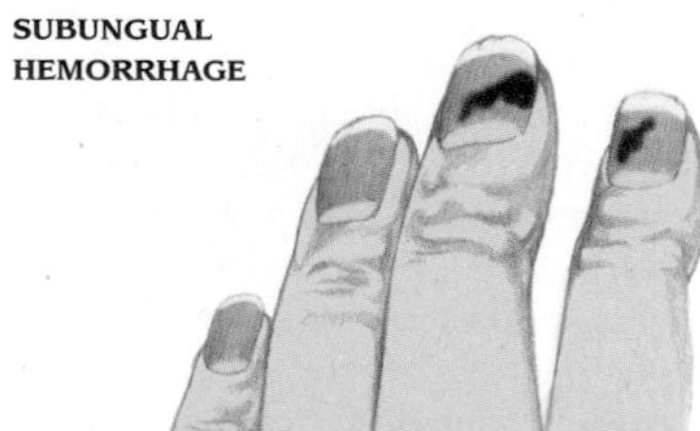

Hill's sign A femoral systolic pulse pressure that's 60 to 100 mm Hg higher in the right leg than in the right arm. Hill's sign may indicate severe aortic insufficiency. To detect this sign, help the patient into a supine position and take blood pressure readings, first in the right arm and then in the right leg, noting the difference.

Hoehne's sign Absence of uterine contractions during delivery, despite repeated doses of oxytocic drugs. This sign indicates a ruptured uterus.

Hoffmann's sign Flexion of the terminal phalanx of the thumb and the second and third phalanges of another finger when the nail of the index, middle, or ring finger is snapped or flicked. A bilateral or strongly unilateral response suggests a pyramidal tract disorder, such as spastic hemiparesis. To elicit this sign, dorsiflex the patient's wrist, have him flex his fingers, and then snap the nail of his index, middle, or ring finger.

Hoffmann's sign also refers to increased sensitivity of sensory nerves to electrical stimulation, as in tetany.

Hoover's sign Inward movement of one or both costal margins on inspiration. Bilateral movement occurs in emphysema with acute respiratory distress. Unilateral movement occurs in intrathoracic disorders that cause flattening of one-half of the diaphragm. A contralateral leg-lifting movement occurs when a patient is directed to press a leg against the examination table. This movement is absent in hysteria and malingering.

hyperacusis Abnormally acute hearing caused by increased irritability of the auditory neural mechanism. It results in an unusually low hearing threshold.

hyperesthesia Increased or altered cutaneous sensitivity to touch, temperature, or pain.

hypernasality A voice quality reflecting excessive expiration of air through the nose during speech. It's commonly associated with symptoms of dysarthria and possibly with swallowing defects. The sudden onset of hypernasality may indicate a neuromuscular disorder. This sign may also accompany cleft palate, a short soft and hard palate, abnormal nasopharyngeal size, and partial or complete velar paralysis. To detect this sign, ask the patient to extend vowel sounds first with the nostrils open, then closed (pinched). A significant shift in tone may indicate hypernasality.

hypoesthesia Decreased cutaneous sensitivity to touch, temperature, or pain.

I

idea of reference A delusion that statements, actions, events, or other people have a meaning specific to oneself. This delusion occurs in schizophrenia and paranoid states. Also known as delusion of reference.

Illusion A misperception of external stimuli—usually visual or auditory—for example, the sound of the wind being perceived as a voice. Illusions occur normally as well as in schizophrenia and toxic states.

J

Jellinek's sign In Graves' disease, brownish pigmentation on the eyelids, usually more prominent on the upper lid than on the lower one. Also known as Rasin's sign.

Joffroy's sign Immobility of the facial muscles with upward rotation of the eyes; associated with exophthalmos in Graves' disease. To detect this sign, observe the patient's forehead as he quickly rotates his eyes upward.

Joffroy's sign also refers to the inability to perform simple mathematics, a possible early sign of organic brain disorder.

K

Kanavel's sign An area of tenderness in the palm, caused by inflammation of the tendon sheath of the little finger. To detect this sign, apply pressure to the palm proximal to the metacarpophalangeal joint of the little finger.

Keen's sign Increased ankle circumference in Pott's fracture of the fibula. To detect this sign, measure the ankles at the malleoli and compare their circumferences.

Kleist's sign Flexion, or hooking, of the fingers when passively raised; associated with frontal lobe and thalamic lesions. To elicit this sign, have the patient turn his palms down; then gently raise his fingers. If his fingers hook onto yours, you've detected Kleist's sign.

Koplik's spots Small red spots with bluish white centers on the lingual and buccal mucosa; characteristic of measles. The measles rash usually erupts 1 to 2 days after these spots appear. Also known as Koplik's sign.

KOPLIK'S SPOTS

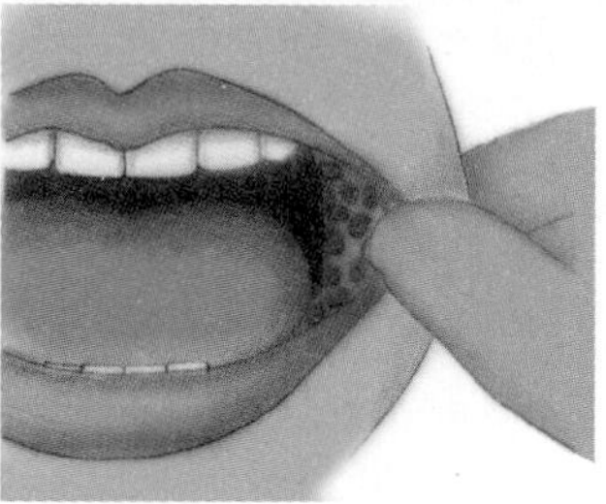

Kussmaul's respirations An abnormal breathing pattern characterized by deep, rapid sighing respirations, generally associated with diabetic ketaoacidosis.

Kussmaul's sign Distention of the jugular veins on inspiration, occurring in constrictive pericarditis and mediastinal tumor.

Kussmaul's sign also refers to a paradoxical pulse and to seizures and coma that result from absorption of toxins.

L

Langoria's sign Relaxation of the extensor muscles of the thigh and hip joint, resulting from intracapsular fracture of the femur. To elicit this sign, help the patient into a prone position; then press firmly on the gluteus maximus and hamstring muscles on both sides, noting greater muscle relaxation on the affected side. (The muscles are soft and spongy.)

large for gestational age Neonatal weight that exceeds the 90th percentile for the gestational age of the infant. The high-birth-weight neonate is at increased risk for birth trauma, respiratory distress, hypocalcemia, hypoglycemia, and polycythemia.

Lasègue's sign Pain upon passive movement of the leg, distinguishing hip joint disease from sciatica. To elicit this sign, help the patient into a supine position, raise one of his legs, and bend the knee to flex the hip joint. Pain with this movement indicates hip joint disease. With the hip still flexed, slowly extend the knee. Pain with this movement results from stretching an irritated sciatic nerve, indicating sciatica.

Laugier's sign An abnormal spatial relationship of the radial and ulnar styloid processes, resulting from fracture of the distal radius. To detect this sign, compare the patient's wrists. Normally more distal than the ulnar process, the radial process may migrate proximally in a fracture of the distal radius so that it's level with the ulnar process.

lead-pipe rigidity Diffuse muscle stiffness occurring, for example, in Parkinson's disease.

Leichtenstern's sign Pain upon gentle tapping of the bones of an extremity. This sign occurs in cerebrospinal meningitis. The patient may wince, draw back suddenly, or cry out loudly.

Lhermitte's sign Sensations of sudden, transient, electric-like shocks spreading down the back and into the extremities, precipitated by forward flexion of the head. This sign occurs in multiple sclerosis, spinal cord degeneration, and cervical spinal cord injury.

Lichtheim's sign An inability to speak that's associated with subcortical aphasia. However, the patient can indicate with his fingers the number of syllables in the word he wants to say.

Linder's sign Pain upon neck flexion, indicating sciatica. To elicit this sign, help the patient into a supine or sitting position with his legs fully extended. Then passively flex his neck, noting whether he experiences pain in the lower back or the affected leg from stretching of the irritated sciatic nerve.

Lloyd's sign Referred loin pain elicited by deep percussion over the kidney. This sign is associated with renal calculi.

loose association A cognitive disturbance marked by absence of a logical link between spoken statements. It occurs in schizophrenia, bipolar disorder, and other psychotic disorders.

low-set ears A position of the ears in which the superior helix lies lower than the eyes. This sign appears in several genetic disorders, including Down, Apert's, Turner's, Noonan's, and Potter's syndromes, and in other congenital abnormalities.

Ludloff's sign Inability to raise the thigh while sitting, along with edema and ecchymosis at the base of Scarpa's triangle (the depressed area just below the fold of the groin). Occurring in children, this sign indicates traumatic separation of the epiphyseal growth plate of the greater trochanter.

lumbosacral hair tuft Abnormal growth of hair over the lower spine, possibly accompanied by skin depression or discoloration. This may mark the site of spina bifida occulta or spina bifida cystica.

LUMBOSACRAL HAIR TUFT

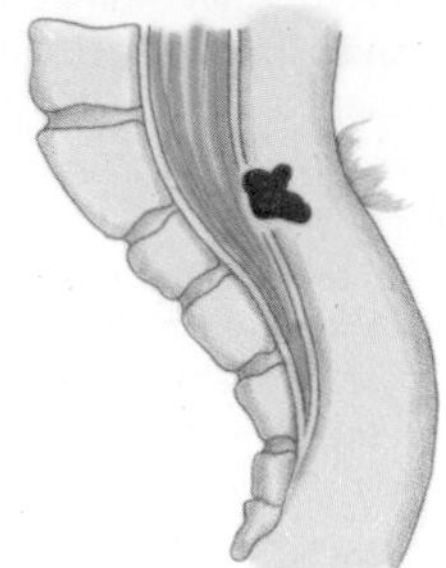

M

Macewen's sign A "cracked pot" sound heard on light percussion with one finger over an infant's or young child's anterior fontanel. An early indicator of hydrocephalus, this sign may also occur in cerebral abscess.

Maisonneuve's sign Hyperextension of the wrist in Colles' fracture. Hyperextension results when a fracture of the lower radius causes posterior displacement of the distal fragment.

malaise Listlessness, weariness, or absence of the sense of well-being. This nonspecific symptom may begin suddenly or gradually and may precede characteristic signs of an illness by several days or weeks. Malaise may reflect the metabolic alterations that precede or accompany infectious, endocrine, or neurologic disorders.

malingering Exaggeration or simulation of symptoms to avoid an unpleasant situation or to gain attention or some other goal.

mania An alteration in mood characterized by increased psychomotor activity, euphoria, flight of ideas, and pressured speech. It usually occurs in the manic phase of bipolar disorder.

Mannkopf's sign Elevated pulse rate when pressure is applied over a painful area. This sign can help distinguish real pain from simulated pain because it doesn't occur in the latter.

Marcus Gunn's phenomenon Unilateral reflexive elevation of an upper ptotic eyelid, associated with movement of the lower jaw. This occurs in misdirectional syndrome, involving the oculomotor and trigeminal nerves (cranial nerves III and V). To elicit this sign, ask the patient to open his mouth and move his lower jaw from side to side.

Marcus Gunn's pupillary sign Paradoxical dilation of a pupil in response to afferent visual stimuli. This sign results from an optic nerve lesion or severe retinal dysfunction. However, vision loss in the affected eye is minimal. To detect this pupillary sign, darken the room and instruct the patient to focus on a distant object. Shine a bright beam of light into the unaffected eye, and observe for bilateral pupillary constriction. Then shine the light into the affected eye; you'll observe brief bilateral dilation. Next, return the light beam to the unaffected eye; you'll observe prompt and persistent bilateral pupillary constriction.

Mean's sign Lagging eye motion when the patient looks upward. In this sign of Graves' disease, the globe of the eye moves more slowly than the upper lid.

meconium staining of amniotic fluid The presence of greenish brown or yellow meconium in the amniotic fluid during labor. Although not necessarily indicative of distress, this sign signals the need for close fetal monitoring to detect decreased variability, or deceleration, of the heart rate. It may also signal the need for infant intubation and resuscitation at delivery to prevent meconium aspiration into the lungs.

menorrhagia Abnormally heavy menstrual flow occurring at the normal time but abnormally prolonged, saturating a pad or tampon in less than an hour.

metrorrhagia Vaginal bleeding or spotting between menses.

Möbius' sign Inability to maintain convergence of the eyes. To detect this sign of Graves' disease, observe the patient's attempt to focus on any small object, such as a pencil, as you move it toward him in line with his nose.

Moro's reflex An infant's generalized response to a loud noise or sudden movement. Usually, this reflex disappears by about age 3 months. Its persistence after age 6 months may indicate brain damage. To elicit this reflex, make a sudden loud noise near the infant, or carefully hold his body with one hand while allowing his head to drop a few centimeters with the other hand. In a complete response, the infant's arms extend and abduct, and his fingers open; then his arms adduct and flex over his chest in a grasping motion. The infant may also extend his hips and legs and cry briefly. A bilaterally equal response is normal; an asymmetrical response may indicate a fractured clavicle or brachial nerve damage. The absence of a response may indicate hearing loss or severe central nervous system depression. Also called the startle reflex.

Murphy's sign The arrest of inspiratory effort when gentle finger pressure beneath the right subcostal arch and below the margin of the liver causes pain during deep inspiration. This classic (but not always present) sign of acute cholecystitis may also occur in hepatitis.

muscle rigidity Muscle tension, stiffness, and resistance to passive movement. This extrapyramidal symptom occurs in disorders affecting the basal ganglia and cerebellum, such as Parkinson's disease, Wilson's disease, Hallervorden-Spatz disease in adults, and kernicterus in infants.

myalgia Diffuse muscle pain, usually accompanied by malaise, occurring in many infectious diseases. These diseases include brucellosis, dengue, influenza, leptospirosis, measles, and poliomyelitis. Myalgia also occurs in arteriosclerosis obliterans, fibrositis, fibromyositis, Guillain-Barré syndrome, hyperparathyroidism, hypoglycemia, hypothyroidism, muscle tumor, myoglobinuria, myositis, and renal tubular acidosis. In addition, various drugs may cause myalgia, including amphotericin B, chloroquine, clofibrate, and corticosteroids.

N

nail dystrophy Changes in the nail plate, such as pitting, furrowing, splitting, or fraying. It usually results from injury, chronic nail infection, neurovascular disorders affecting the extremities, or collagen disorders. It also occurs secondary to repeated wetting and drying of the nails associated with frequent immersion in water.

nail plate discoloration A change in the color of the nail plate resulting from infection or drugs. Blue-green discoloration may occur with Pseudomonas infection; brown or black, with fungal infection or fluorosis; and bluish gray, with excessive use of silver salts.

nail plate hypertrophy Thickening of the nail plate resulting from the accumulation of irregular keratin layers. This condition is commonly associated with fungal infection of the nails, although it can be hereditary.

nail separation The separation of the nail plate from the nail bed. This occurs primarily in injury or infection of the nail and in thyrotoxicosis.

neologism A new word or condensation of several words with special meaning for the patient but not readily understood by others. This coining occurs in schizophrenia and organic brain disorders.

neuralgia Severe, paroxysmal pain over an area innervated by specific nerve fibers. Neuralgia may be precipitated by pressure, cold, movement, or stimulation of a trigger zon; however, in many cases, the cause is unknown. Usually brief, neuralgia may be accompanied by vasomotor symptoms, such as sweating or tearing.

Nicoladoni's sign Bradycardia resulting from finger pressure on an artery proximal to an arteriovenous fistula. Also known as Branham's sign.

nodules Small, solid, circumscribed masses of differentiated tissue, detected on palpation.

O

obsession A persistent, usually disturbing thought or image that can't be eliminated by reason or logic. It's associated with an obsessive-compulsive disorder and, occasionally, schizophrenia.

obturator sign Pain in the right hypogastric region, occurring with flexion of the right leg at the hip with the knee bent and internally rotated. It indicates irritation of the obturator muscle.

In children, this sign may signal acute appendicitis because the appendix lies rectocecally over the obturator muscle.

oculocardiac reflex Bradycardia that occurs in response to vagal stimulation when pressure is applied to the eyeball or carotid sinus. This reflex can aid in the diagnosis of angina or it can relieve it. *Caution:* Repeated application of pressure to the eye to elicit this response may precipitate retinal detachment. Also known as Aschner's phenomenon.

orbicularis sign Inability to close one eye at a time, occurring in hemiplegia.

orgasmic disorders Transient or persistent inhibition of the orgasmic phase of sexual excitement.

In the female: delayed or absent orgasm following a phase of sexual excitement. It usually results from psychological or interpersonal problems but may also stem from chronic disorders, congenital anomalies, and chronic vaginal or pelvic infections.

In the male: delayed or absent ejaculation following a phase of sexual excitement. Its causes include psychological problems, neurologic disorders, and the effects of antihypertensives. See "Impotence," page 393.

orthotonos A form of tetanic spasm producing a rigid, straight line of the neck, limbs, and body.

ostealgia Bone pain associated with such disorders as osteomyelitis.

otorrhagia Bleeding from the ear occurring with a tumor, severe infection, or injury affecting the auricle, external canal, tympanic membrane, or temporal bone.

PQ

palmar crease abnormalities An abnormal line pattern on the palms, resulting from faulty embryonic development during the second and fourth months of gestation. This pattern may occur normally but usually appears in Down syndrome as a single transverse crease (called the simian crease) formed by fusion of the proximal and distal palmar creases. It also appears in Turner's syndrome and congenital rubella syndrome.

paradoxical respirations An abnormal breathing pattern marked by paradoxical movement of an injured portion of the chest wall—it contracts on inspiration and bulges on expiration. This ominous sign is characteristic of flail chest, a thoracic injury involving multiple free-floating, fractured ribs.

paranoia Extreme suspiciousness related to delusions of persecution by another person, a group, or an institution. This may occur in schizophrenia, drug-induced or toxic states, or paranoid disorders.

Pastia's sign Petechiae or hemorrhagic lines appearing along skin creases in such areas as the antecubital fossa, the groin, and the wrists. They accompany the rash of scarlet fever as a response to the erythrogenic toxin produced by scarlatinal strains of group A streptococci.

Pel-Ebstein fever A cyclic fever pattern characterized by several days of high fever alternating with afebrile periods that last for days or weeks. Typically, the fever becomes progressively higher and continuous. Pel-Ebstein fever occasionally occurs in Hodgkin's disease or malignant lymphoma. Also known as Pel-Ebstein symptom or Pel-Ebstein pyrexia.

Perez's sign Crackles or friction sounds auscultated over the lungs when a seated patient raises and lowers his arms. This sign commonly occurs in fibrous mediastinitis and may also occur in aortic arch aneurysm.

peroneal sign Dorsiflexion and abduction of the foot upon tapping over the common peroneal nerve. To elicit this sign of latent tetany, tap over the lateral neck of the fibula with the patient's knee relaxed and slightly flexed.

phobia An irrational and persistent fear of an object, situation, or activity. Occurring in phobic disorders, it may interfere with normal functioning. Typical manifestations include faintness, fatigue, palpitations, diaphoresis, nausea, tremor, and panic.

Piotrowski's sign Dorsiflexion and supination of the foot on percussion of the anterior tibial muscle. Excessive flexion may indicate a central nervous system disorder.

Pitres' sign In tabes dorsalis, hyperesthesia of the scrotum and testes. This sign also refers to the anterior deviation of the sternum in pleural effusion.

Plummer's sign Inability to ascend stairs or step up onto a chair. This sign can be demonstrated in Graves' disease.

pneumaturia The passage of gas in the urine while voiding. Causes include a fistula between the bowel and bladder, sigmoid diverticulitis, rectosigmoid cancer and, rarely, gas-forming urinary tract infections.

Pool-Schlesinger sign In tetany, muscle spasm of the forearm, hand, and fingers or of the leg and foot. To detect this sign, forcefully abduct and elevate the patient's arm with his forearm extended. Or, forcefully flex the patient's extended leg at the hip. Spasm results from tension on the brachial plexus or the sciatic nerve. Also known as Pool's phenomenon and Schlesinger's sign.

Potain's sign Dullness on percussion over the aortic arch, extending from the manubrium to the third costal cartilage on the right. This occurs in aortic dilation.

Prehn's sign Relief of pain with elevation and support of the scrotum, occurring in epididymitis. This sign differentiates epididymitis from testicular torsion. Both disorders produce severe pain, tenderness, and scrotal swelling.

pressured speech Speech that's accelerated, difficult to interrupt, and at times unintelligible. This may accompany flight of ideas in the manic phase of bipolar disorder.

Prévost's sign Conjugate deviation of the head and eyes in hemiplegia. Typically, the eyes gaze toward the affected hemisphere.

prognathism An enlarged, protuberant jaw associated with normal mandible condyles and temporomandibular joints. This sign usually appears in acromegaly.

R

rectal tenesmus Spasmodic contraction of the anal sphincter with a persistent urge to defecate and involuntary, ineffective straining. This occurs in inflammatory bowel disorders, such as ulcerative colitis and Crohn's disease, and in rectal tumors. Often painful, rectal tenesmus usually accompanies passage of small amounts of blood, pus, or mucus.

regression Return to a behavioral level appropriate to an earlier developmental age. This defense mechanism may occur in various psychiatric and organic disorders. It may also result from worsening of symptoms or of a disease process.

repression The unconscious retreat or thrusting back from awareness of unacceptable ideas or impulses. This defense mechanism may occur normally or may accompany psychiatric disorders.

Rosenbach's sign Absence of the abdominal skin reflex, associated with intestinal inflammation and hemiplegia. This sign also refers to the fine, rapid tremor of gently closed eyelids in Graves' disease and to the inability to close the eyes immediately on command, as occurs in neurasthenia.

Rotch's sign Dullness on percussion over the right lung at the fifth intercostal space. This sign occurs in pericardial effusion.

Rovsing's sign Pain in the right lower quadrant on palpation and quick withdrawal of the fingers in the left lower quadrant. This referred rebound tenderness suggests appendicitis.

Rumpel-Leede sign Extensive petechiae distal to a tourniquet placed around the upper arm, indicating capillary fragility in scarlet fever and in severe thrombocytopenia. To elicit this sign, place a tourniquet around the upper arm for 5 to 10 minutes and observe for distal petechiae. Also known as Rumpel-Leede phenomenon.

S

Seeligmüller's sign In facial neuralgia, pupillary dilation on the affected side.

Siegert's sign Short, inwardly curved little fingers, typically appearing in Down syndrome.

SIEGERT'S SIGN

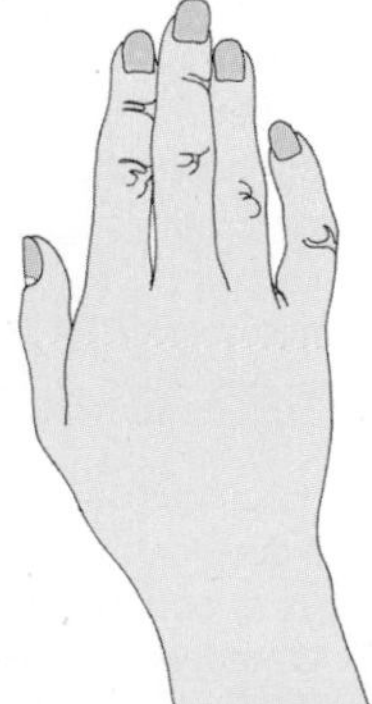

Simon's sign Incoordination of the movements of the diaphragm and thorax, occurring early in meningitis. This sign also refers to retraction or fixation of the umbilicus during inspiration.

Soto-Hall sign Pain in the area of a lesion, occurring on passive flexion of the spine. To elicit this sign, help the patient into a supine position and progressively flex his spine from the neck downward. The patient will complain of pain in the area of the lesion.

spasmodic torticollis Intermittent or continuous spasms of the shoulder and neck muscles that turn the head to one side. Often transient and idiopathic, this sign can occur in paients with extrapyramidal disorders or shortened neck muscles. See "Dystonia," page 248.

spine sign Resistance to anterior flexion of the spine, resulting from pain in poliomyelitis.

spoon nails Malformation of the nails characterized by a concave instead of the normal convex outer surface. The nail is also abnormally thin. This sign commonly occurs in severe hypochromic anemia but occasionally may be hereditary.

Stellwag's sign Incomplete and infrequent blinking, usually related to exophthalmos in Graves' disease.

stepping reflex In neonates, spontaneous stepping movements that simulate walking. This reciprocal flexion and extension of the legs disappears after about age 4 weeks. To elicit this sign, hold the infant erect with the soles of his feet touching a hard surface. Although the stepping reflex is normal, scissoring movements with persistent extension and crossing of the legs or asymmetrical stepping is abnormal, possibly indicating central nervous system damage.

STEPPING REFLEX

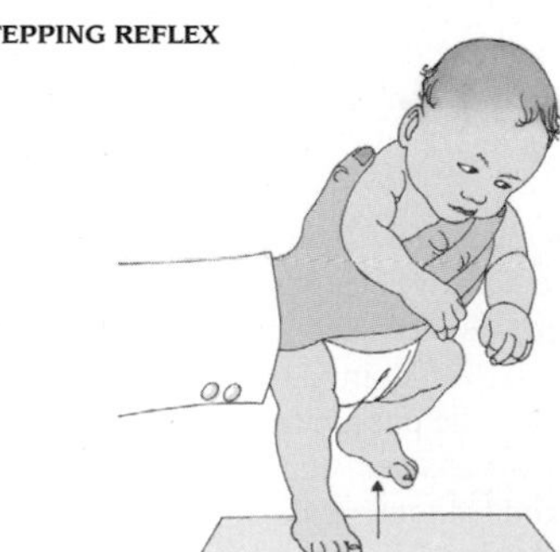

Strunsky's sign Pain on plantar flexion of the toes and forefoot, caused by inflammatory disorders of the anterior arch. To detect this sign, have the patient assume a relaxed position with his foot exposed; then grasp his toes and quickly plantarflex his toes and forefoot.

succussion splash A splashing sound heard over a hollow organ or body cavity, such as the stomach or thorax, after rocking or shaking the patient's body. Indicating the presence of fluid or air and gas, this sound may be auscultated in a pyloric or intestinal obstruction, a large hiatal hernia, or hydropneumothorax. However, it may also be auscultated over a normal empty stomach.

sucking reflex Involuntary circumoral sucking movements in response to stimulation. Present at about 26 weeks' gestation, this reflex is initially weak and isn't synchronized with swallowing. It persists through infancy, becoming more discriminating during the first few months and disappearing by age 1. To elicit this response, place your finger in the infant's mouth. Rhythmic sucking movements are normal. Weak or absent sucking movements may indicate elevated intracranial pressure.

T

tangentiality Speech characterized by tedious detail that never gets to the point. This occurs in schizophrenia and organic brain disorders.

Terry's nails A white, opaque surface over more than 80% of the nail and a normal pink distal edge. This sign is commonly associated with cirrhosis.

testicular pain Unilateral or bilateral pain localized in or around the testicle and possibly radiating along the spermatic cord and into the lower abdomen. It usually results from trauma, infection, or testicular torsion. Typically, its onset is sudden and severe; however, its intensity can vary from sharp pain accompanied by nausea and vomiting to a chronic dull ache. In a child, sudden onset of severe testicular pain is a urologic emergency. Assume torsion is the cause until disproven. If a young male complains of abdominal pain, always carefully examine the scrotum because abdominal pain commonly precedes testicular pain in testicular torsion.

Thornton's sign Severe flank pain resulting from nephrolithiasis.

thrill A palpable sensation resulting from the vibration of a loud murmur or from turbulent blood flow in an aneurysm. Thrills are associated with heart murmurs of grades IV to VI and may be palpable over major arteries. See "Bruits," page 126, and "Murmurs," page 450.

tibialis sign Involuntary dorsiflexion and inversion of the foot upon brisk, voluntary flexion of the patient's knee and hip, occurring in spastic paralysis of the lower limb. Also known as Strümpell's sign.

To detect this sign, help the patient into a supine position and have him flex his leg at the hip and knee so that the thigh touches the abdomen. Or, help the patient into a prone position, and have him flex his leg at the knee so that the calf touches the thigh. If this sign is present, you may observe dorsiflexion of the great toe, or of all the toes, as the foot dorsiflexes and inverts. Normally, plantar flexion of the foot occurs with this action.

Tinel's sign Distal paresthesia on percussion over an injured nerve in an extremity, as in carpal tunnel syndrome. To elicit this sign in the patient's wrist, tap over the median nerve on the wrist's flexor surface. This sign indicates a partial lesion or the early regeneration of the nerve.

tongue, hairy Hypertrophy and elongation of the tongue's filiform papillae. Normally white, the papillae may turn yellow, brown, or black from bacteria, food, tobacco, coffee, or dyes in drugs and food. Hairy tongue may also result from antibiotic therapy, irradiation of the head and neck, chronic debilitating disorders, and habitual use of mouthwashes containing oxidizing or astringent agents.

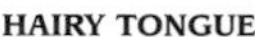

HAIRY TONGUE

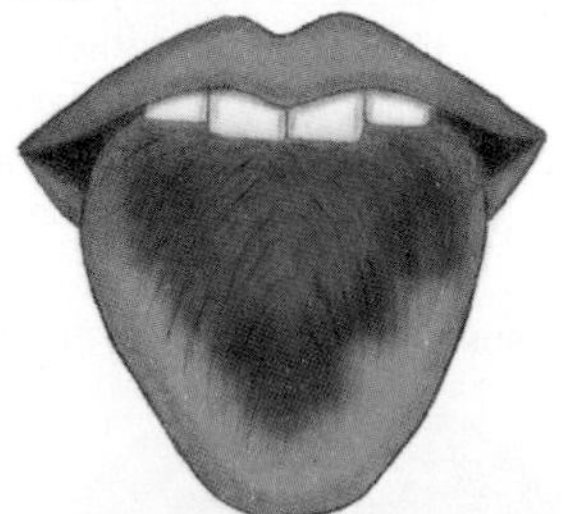

tongue, magenta, cobblestone Swelling and hyperemia of the tongue, forming rows of elevated fungiform and filiform papillae that give the tongue a magenta-colored or cobblestone appearance. It's usually a sign of vitamin B_2 (riboflavin) deficiency.

tongue, red Patchy or uniform redness (ranging from pink to magenta) of the tongue, which may be swollen and smooth, rough, or fissured. It usually indicates glossitis, resulting from emotional stress or nutritional disorders, such as pernicious anemia, Plummer-Vinson syndrome, pellagra, sprue, and folic acid or vitamin B deficiency.

tongue, smooth Absence or atrophy of the filiform papillae, causing a smooth (patchy or uniform), glossy red tongue. This primary sign of malnutrition results from anemia and vitamin B deficiency.

tongue, white A uniform white coating or plaques on the tongue. Lesions associated with a white tongue may be premalignant or malignant and may require a biopsy. Necrotic white lesions—collections of cells, bacteria, and debris—are painful and can be scraped from the tongue. They commonly appear in children, usually resulting from candidiasis or thermal burns. Keratotic white lesions—thick, keratinized patches—are usually asymptomatic and can't be scraped from the tongue. These lesions commonly result from alcohol use and local irritation from tobacco smoke or other substances.

tongue enlargement An increase in the tongue's size, causing it to protrude from the mouth. Its causes include Down syndrome, acromegaly, lymphangioma, Beckwith's syndrome, and congenital micrognathia. An enlarged tongue can also result from cancer of the tongue, amyloidosis, and neurofibromatosis.

tongue fissures Shallow or deep grooving of the dorsum of the tongue. Usually a congenital defect, tongue fissures occur normally in about 10% of the population. However, deep fissures may promote collection of food particles, leading to chronic inflammation and tenderness.

TONGUE FISSURES

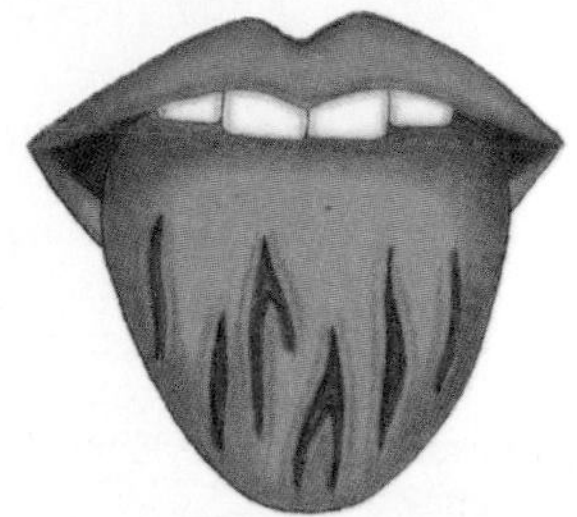

tongue swelling Edema of the tongue, usually associated with pernicious anemia, pellagra, hypothyroidism, or allergic angioneurotic edema.

tongue ulcers Circumscribed necrotic lesions of the dorsum, margin, tip, and inferior surface of the tongue. Ulcers usually result from biting, chewing, or burning of the tongue. They may also stem from herpes simplex virus type 1, tuberculosis, histoplasmosis, or cancer of the tongue.

tonic neck reflex Extension of the limbs on the side to which the head is turned and flexion of the opposite limbs. In the neonate, this normal reflex appears between 28 and 32 weeks' gestation, diminishes as voluntary muscle control increases, and disappears by age 3 to 4 months. The absence or persistence of this reflex may indicate central nervous system damage. To elicit this response, place the infant in a supine position, and then turn his head to one side.

tooth discoloration Bluish yellow or gray teeth may result from hypoplasia of the dentin and pulp, nerve damage, or caries. Yellow teeth may indicate caries. Mottling and staining suggest excessive fluorine and may also be associated with the effects of certain drugs such as tetracycline. Tooth discoloration (and small tooth size) may occur in osteogenesis imperfecta.

tophi Deposit of sodium urate crystals in cartilage, soft tissue, synovial membranes, and tendon sheaths, producing painless nodular swellings, a classic symptom of gout. Tophi commonly appear on the ears, hands, and feet. They may erode the skin, producing open lesions, and cause gross deformity, limiting joint mobility. Inflammatory flare-ups may occur.

TOPHI

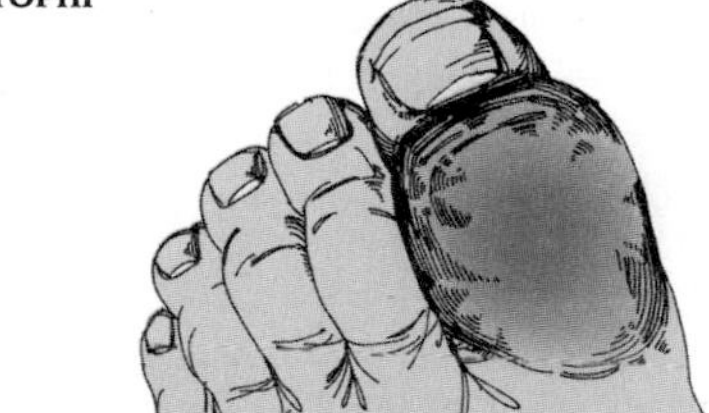

transference The unconscious transferring of feelings and attitudes originally associated with important figures, such as parents, to another.

Used therapeutically in psychoanalysis, transference can also occur in other settings and relationships.

Trendelenburg's test A demonstration of valvular incompetence of the saphenous vein and inefficiency of the communicating veins at different levels. To perform this test, raise the patient's legs above the heart level until the veins empty; then rapidly lower his legs. If the valves are incompetent, the veins immediately distend.

If the patient has poliomyelitis, an unlimited femoral neck fracture, coxa vara, or a congenital dislocation, have him disrobe with his back to the examiner. Tell the patient to lift first one foot and then the other. Note the position and movements of the gluteal fold: When the patient is standing on the affected limb, the gluteal fold on the sound side falls instead of rising.

Troisier's sign Enlargement of a single lymph node, usually in the left supraclavicular group. It indicates metastasis from a primary carcinoma in the upper abdomen, commonly the stomach. To detect this sign, have the patient sit erect facing you. Palpate the region behind the sternocleidomastoid muscle as the patient performs Valsalva's maneuver. Although the enlarged node usually lies so deep that it escapes detection, it may rise and become palpable with this maneuver.

Trousseau's sign In tetany, carpal spasm upon ischemic compression of the upper arm. To elicit this sign, apply a blood pressure cuff to the patient's arm; then inflate the cuff to a pressure between the patient's diastolic and systolic readings, and maintain it for 4 minutes. The patient's hand and fingers assume the "obstetrical hand" position, with wrist and metacarpophalangeal joints flexed, interphalangeal joints extended, and fingers and thumb adducted. Also known as Trousseau's phenomenon. See also "Carpopedal spasm," page 135.

Turner's sign A bruiselike discoloration of the skin of the flanks. This sign appears 6 to 24 hours after onset of retroperitoneal hemorrhage in acute pancreatitis.

twitching Nonspecific intermittent contraction of muscles or muscle bundles. See also "Fasciculations," page 289, and "Tics," page 662.

urinary tenesmus Persistent, ineffective, painful straining to empty the bladder. This results from irritation of nerve endings in the bladder mucosa, caused by infection or an indwelling catheter.

V

vaginal bleeding abnormalities Passage of blood from the vagina at times other than menses. It may indicate abnormalities of the uterus, cervix, ovaries, fallopian tubes, or vagina. It may also indicate an abnormal pregnancy. See also "Menorrhagia," page 442, "Metrorrhagia," page 443, and "Vaginal bleeding, postmenopausal," page 686.

vein sign A palpable, bluish, cordlike swelling along the line formed in the axilla by the junction of the thoracic and superficial epigastric veins. This sign appears in tuberculosis and obstruction of the superior vena cava.

WX

Weill's sign In infantile pneumonia, absence of expansion in the subclavicular area of the affected side on inspiration.

Westphal's sign Absence of the knee jerk reflex, occurring in tabes dorsalis.

Wilder's sign Subtle twitching of the eyeball on medial or lateral gaze. This early sign of Graves' disease is discernible as a slight jerk of the eyeball when the patient changes his direction of gaze.

YZ

yawning, excessive Persistent involuntary opening of the mouth, accompanied by attempted deep inspiration. In the absence of sleepiness, excessive yawning may indicate cerebral hypoxia.

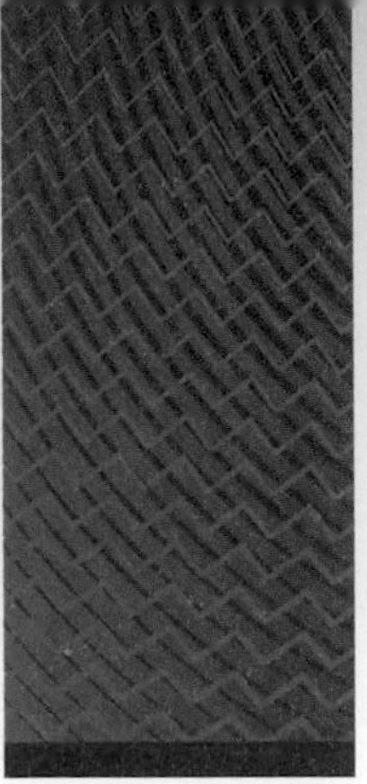

POTENTIAL AGENTS OF BIOTERRORISM

Listed below are examples of biological agents that may be used as biological weapons and the major signs and symptoms that each one may produce.

Major associated signs and symptoms

Potential agents	Abdominal pain	Back pain	Blood pressure, decreased	Chest pain	Chills	Cough	Diarrhea, bloody	Diarrhea, watery	Diplopia	Dysarthria	Dysphagia	Dyspnea	Fever	Headache
Anthrax (cutaneous)													●	●
Anthrax (GI)	●						●						●	
Anthrax (inhalation)			●	●	●	●						●	●	
Botulism									●	●	●	●		
Cholera			●					●						
Plague (bubonic and septicemic)					●								●	
Plague (pneumonic)				●	●	●						●	●	●
Smallpox	●	●											●	●
Tularemia				●	●	●						●	●	●

	Hematemesis	Hemoptysis	Lymphadenopathy	Malaise	Muscle spasms (muscle cramps)	Myalgia	Nausea	Oliguria	Papular rash (skin lesions)	Ptosis	Skin turgor, decreased	Stridor	Tachycardia	Tachypnea	Vomiting	Weakness
			●	●					●							
	●						●								●	
												●				●
										●						●
					●			●			●		●		●	●
			●													
		●				●								●		
				●					●							
						●										

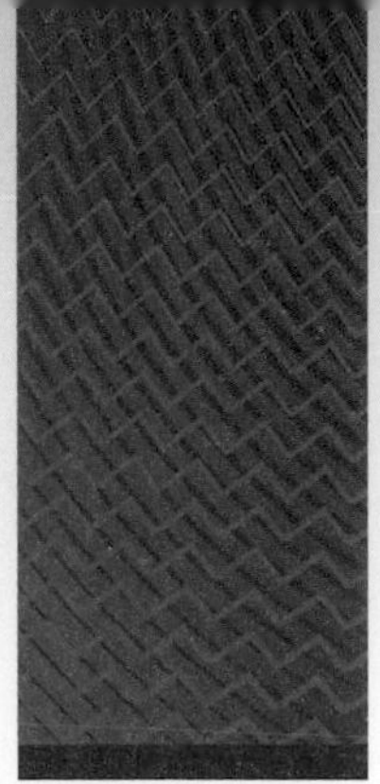

ADVERSE EFFECTS ASSOCIATED WITH HERBS

Listed below are commonly used herbs and their most common adverse effects.

Common adverse effects

Common herbs	Bleeding	Blood pressure, decreased	Blood pressure, increased	Confusion	Diarrhea	Dizziness	Dyspnea	Edema, generalized
Aloe					●			●
Capsicum	●				●		●	
Chamomile								
Echinacea								
Ephedra		●	●	●		●		
Evening primrose oil					●			
Fennel							●	
Feverfew	●					●		
Garlic	●				●		●	
Ginger	●							
Ginkgo	●				●	●		
Ginseng (Asian, Siberian)		●	●		●	●		●

	Erythema	Fatigue	Flatulence	Headache	Insomnia	Level of consciousness, decreased	Nausea	Palpitations	Pulse rhythm abnormalities	Seizure	Tachycardia	Vomiting
									●			
	●											
	●						●					●
							●					●
	●			●	●		●	●	●	●	●	
			●	●			●					●
	●						●			●		●
	●						●				●	
	●	●	●	●	●		●				●	●
						●			●			
			●	●			●	●				●
				●	●						●	●

(continued)

Common adverse effects

Common herbs	Bleeding	Blood pressure, decreased	Blood pressure, increased	Confusion	Diarrhea	Dizziness	Dyspnea	Edema, generalized
Goldenseal		●	●		●			
Kava	●							
Milk thistle					●			
Passion flower		●		●			●	
St. John's wort					●			
SAM-e					●			
Saw palmetto			●		●			
Valerian					●			

	Erythema	Fatigue	Flatulence	Headache	Insomnia	Level of consciousness, decreased	Nausea	Palpitations	Pulse rhythm abnormalities	Seizure	Tachycardia	Vomiting
	●					●	●		●			●
		●				●						
							●					●
				●			●		●		●	●
		●		●			●					
				●			●					
				●			●					
	●	●		●	●		●		●			●

OBTAINING A HEALTH HISTORY

Use a health history to gather subjective data about your patient and explore his previous and current health problems. The information you obtain combined with the results of the physical examination and diagnostic testing will assist you in making an accurate diagnosis.

Start the history by asking the patient about his general physical and emotional health, and then ask him questions about the specific body systems.

Make the patient comfortable

Before asking your first question, make sure you establish a good rapport with the patient. The following tips may help:

- Choose a quiet, private, well-lit interview setting away from distractions.
- Introduce yourself; then ask the patient to sit down. Make sure he's comfortably seated.
- Explain to the patient that the purpose of the health history and assessment is to identify his problem and provide information for planning care.
- Speak slowly and clearly. Avoid using medical terms and jargon.
- Listen attentively and use reassuring gestures to encourage the patient to talk.
- Watch for nonverbal cues that indicate the patient is uncomfortable or unsure about how to answer a question. Make sure that he understands each question.

Ask specific questions

Asking the right question is a critical part of any interview. To obtain a complete health history, gather information from each of the following categories, in sequence:

- Biographical data: name, address, phone number, date of birth, birthplace, sex, marital status, ethnic origin, occupation
- Source of history: patient, family member, friend
- Chief complaint: a brief statement by the patient describing the reason for seeking care
- History of present illness: a chronological description of the present illness from the time of symptom onset
- Current medications: prescribed and over-the-counter medications, herbal remedies, and supplements
- Past medical history: childhood illnesses, accidents, injuries, hospitalizations, surgeries, blood transfusions, serious or chronic illnesses, obstetric history in females, immunizations, and allergies (drug, food, environmental, and latex)
- Family history: health status or cause of death of immediate relatives
- Psychosocial history: how the patient feels about himself, his place in society, and his relationships with others; his coping strategies; his feelings of safety, which may refer to physical, psychological, emotional, or sexual abuse issues
- Activities of daily living: diet and elimination patterns; exercise and sleeping patterns; work and leisure activities; alcohol, tobacco, or illicit drug use; religious observances; and use of safety measures, such as seat belts, bike helmets, and sunscreen

- Health maintenance: date of last examination or office visit with family physician, dentist, and optometrist; also, screening procedures and immunizations.

Review of systems

The last part of the health history is a systematic review of each body system to make sure that important symptoms weren't missed. The systems are reviewed from head to toe.

- General health
- Skin and hair
- Head
- Eyes, ears, and nose
- Mouth and throat
- Neck
- Respiratory system
- Cardiovascular system
- Breasts
- Gastrointestinal system
- Urinary system
- Reproductive system
- Musculoskeletal system
- Neurologic system
- Endocrine system
- Hematologic system
- Emotional status

GUIDE TO LABORATORY TEST RESULTS

This chart provides normal values for common laboratory tests, including chemistry, hematology, and coagulation tests. Where indicated, conventional and SI units are given.

Laboratory test	Conventional	SI Units
Comprehensive metabolic panel		
Albumin	3.5-5 g/dl	35-50 g/L
Alanine aminotransferase	Male: 10-40 U/L Female: 7-35 U/L	0.17-0.68 µkat/L 0.12-0.60 µkat/L
Alkaline phosphatase	45-115 U/L	45-115 U/L
Aspartate aminotransferase	10-36 U/L	0.17-0.60 µkat/L
Bilirubin, total	0.3-1 mg/dl	5-17 µmol/L
Blood urea nitrogen	6-20 mg/dl	2.1-7.5 mmol/L
Calcium	8.8-10.4 mg/dl	2.2-2.6 mmol/L
Carbon dioxide	22-26 mEq/L	22-26 mmol/L
Chloride	100-108 mEq/L	100-108 mmol/L
Creatinine	Male: 0.8-1.3 mg/dl Female: 0.6-0.9 mg/dl	62-115 µmol/L 53-97 µmol/L
Glucose	70-100 mg/dl	3.9-6.1 mmol/L
Potassium	3.5-5.2 mEq/L	3.5-5.2 mmol/L
Protein, total	6.3-8.3 g/dl	64-83 g/L
Sodium	136-145 mEq/L	136-145 mmol/L

Laboratory test	Conventional	SI Units
Lipid panel		
Total cholesterol	< 200 mg/dl	< 5.05 mmol/L
High-density lipoprotein cholesterol	> 60 mg/dl	> 1.55 mmol/L
Low-density lipoprotein cholesterol	< 130 mg/dl	< 3.36 mmol/L
Very-low-density lipoprotein cholesterol	< 130 mg/dl	< 3.4 mmol/L
Triglycerides	< 150 mg/dl	< 1.7 mmol/L
Thyroid panel		
Thyroid-stimulating hormone	0.4-4.2 mIU/L	0.4-4.2 mIU/L
Thyroxine, free	0.9-2.3 ng/dl	10-30 nmol/L
Thyroxine, total	5-13.5 mcg/dl	60-165 mmol/L
Triiodothyronine	80-200 ng/dl	1.2-3 nmol/L
Other chemistry tests		
Albumin/globulin ratio	3.4-4.8 g/dl	34-38 g/dl
Ammonia	< 50 ng/dl	< 36 μmol/L
Amylase	25-125 U/L	0.4-2.1 μkat/L
Anion gap	8-14 mEq/L	8-14 mmol/L
Bilirubin, direct	< 0.5 mg/dl	< 6.8 μmol/L
Calcitonin	Male: < 16 pg/ml Female: < 8 pg/ml	< 16 ng/L < 8 ng/L
Calcium, ionized	4.65-5.28 mg/dl	1.1-1.25 mmol/L
Cortisol	a.m.: 7-25 mcg/dl p.m.: 2-14 mcg/dl	0.2-0.7 μmol/L 0.06-0.39 μmol/L
C-reactive protein	< 0.8 mg/dl	< 8 mg/L
Ferritin	Male: 20-300 ng/ml Female: 20-120 ng/ml	20-300 mcg/L 20-120 mcg/L
Folate	1.8-20 ng/ml	4.5-45.3 nmol/L
Gamma glutamyl transferase	Male: 7-47 U/L Female: 5-25 U/L	0.12-1.80 μkat/L 0.08-0.42 μkat/L

(continued)

Laboratory test	Conventional	SI Units
Other chemistry tests *(continued)*		
Glycosylated hemoglobin	4%-7%	0.04-0.07
Homocysteine	< 12 μmol/L	< 12 μmol/L
Iron	Male: 65-175 mcg/dl Female: 50-170 mcg/dl	11.6-31.3 μmol/L 9-30.4 μmol/L
Iron-binding capacity	250-400 mcg/dl	45-72 μmol/L
Lactic acid	0.5-2.2 mEq/L	0.5-2.2 mmol/L
Lipase	Adults over 60: 10-140 U/L Adults under 60: 18-180 U/L	0.17-2.3 μkat/L 0.30-3 μkat/L
Magnesium	1.8-2.6 mg/dl	0.74-1.07 mmol/L
Osmolality	275-295 mOsm/kg	275-295 mOsm/kg
Phosphate	2.7-4.5 mg/dl	0.87-1.45 mmol/L
Prealbumin	19-38 mg/dl	190-380 mg/L
Uric acid	Male: 3.4-7 mg/dl Female: 2.3-6 mg/dl	202-416 μmol/L 143-357 μmol/L
Hematology tests		
Hemoglobin	Male: 14-17.4 g/dl Female: 12-16 g/dl	140-174 g/L 120-160 g/L
Hematocrit	Male: 42%-52% Female: 36%-48%	0.42-0.52 0.36-0.48
Red blood cell	Male: 4.2-5.4 million/mm^3 Female: 3.6-5 million/mm^3	4.2-5.4 × 10^{12}/L 3.6-5 × 10^{12}/L

Laboratory test	Conventional	SI Units
Hematology tests *(continued)*		
Leukocytes	4,000-10,000/mm^3	4-10 × 10^9/L
• Bands	0%-5%	0.03-0.08
• Basophils	0%-1%	0-0.01
• Eosinophils	1%-3%	0.01-0.03
• Lymphocytes	25%-40%	0.25-0.40
– B lymphocytes	270-640/mm^3	—
– T lymphocytes	1,400-2,700/mm^3	—
• Monocytes	2%-7%	0.02-0.07
• Neutrophils	54%-75%	0.54-0.75
Platelets	140,000-400,000/mm^3	140-400 × 10^9/L
Coagulation tests		
Activated clotting time	107 sec ± 13 sec	107 sec ± 13 sec
Bleeding time	3-6 min	3-6 min
D-dimer	< 250 mcg/L	< 1.37 nmol/L
Fibrinogen	200-400 mg/dl	2-4 g/L
International Normalized Ratio (therapeutic target)	2.0-3.0	2.0-3.0
Partial thromboplastin time	21-35 sec	21-35 sec
Prothrombin time	10-13 sec	10-13 sec

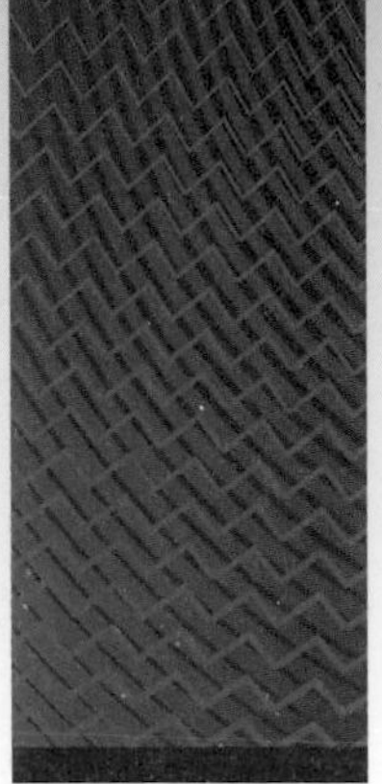

Selected References

American Heart Association. "Guidelines 2005 for Cardiopulmonary Resuscitation and Emergency Cardiovascular Care," *Circulation* 112 (24 Suppl), December 2005.

Baronski, S., and Ayello, E.A. *Wound Care Essentials: Practice Principles,* 2nd ed. Philadelphia: Lippincott Williams & Wilkins, 2008.

Berger, E., et al. "Sickle Cell Disease in Children: Differentiating Osteomyelitis from Vaso-occlusive Crisis," *Archives of Pediatric and Adolescent Medicine* 163(3):251-55, March 2009.

Bickley, L.S., and Szilagyi, P.G. *Bates' Guide to Physical Examination and History Taking,* 10th ed. Philadelphia: Lippincott Williams & Wilkins, 2010.

Eliopoulos, C. *Gerontological Nursing*, 6th ed. Philadelphia: Lippincott Williams & Wilkins, 2005.

Fauci, A. *Harrison's Principles of Internal Medicine*, 17th ed. New York: McGraw-Hill, 2009.

Hadley, A.C., et al. "The Prevalence of Resistant Bacterial Colonization in Chronic Hemodialysis Patients," *American Journal of Nephrology* 27(4):352-59, May 2007.

Hockenberry, M.J., and Wilson, D. *Wong's Nursing Care of Infants and Children,* 8th ed. St. Louis: Mosby-Year Book, Inc., 2007.

Kanwal, R., et al. "Evaluation of Flavorings-Related Lung Disease Risk at Six Microwave Popcorn Plants," *Journal of Occupational and Environmental Medicine* 48(2):149-57, February 2006.

Karasz, A. "Cultural Differences in the Experience of Everyday Symptoms: A Comparative Study of South Asian and European American Women," *Culture, Medicine, and Psychiatry* 31(4):473-97, December 2007.

Kasper, D.L., et al., eds. *Harrison's Principles of Internal Medicine*, 17th ed. New York: McGraw-Hill, 2008.

Kenner, C., and Wright Lott, J. *Comprehensive Neonatal Care: An Interdisciplinary Approach*, 4th ed. Philadelphia: Elsevier, 2008.

Kittisupamongkol, W. "Testing for Celiac Disease in Patients with Symptoms of Irritable Bowel Syndrome," *JAMA* 301(11):1126; author reply 1126, March 2009.

Nursing 2010 Drug Handbook, 30th ed. Philadelphia: Lippincott Williams & Wilkins, 2010.

Pillitteri, A. *Maternal and Child Health Nursing: Care of the Childbearing and Childrearing Family,* 5th ed. Philadelphia: Lippincott Williams & Wilkins, 2006.

Porth, C.M. *Pathophysiology: Concepts of Altered Health States*, 8th ed. Philadelphia: Lippincott Williams & Wilkins, 2008.

Professional Guide to Diseases, 9th ed. Philadelphia: Lippincott Williams & Wilkins, 2009.

Relman, D.A. "Bioterrorism—Preparing to Fight the Next War," *The New England Journal of Medicine* 354(2):113-15, January 2006.

Schulmeister, L., and Holmes, G.B., "Symptom Management Issues in Oncology Nursing," *Nursing Clinics of North America* 43(2):205-20, June 2008.

Selwyn, A.P. "Weight Reduction and Cardiovascular and Metabolic Disease Prevention: Clinical Trial Update," *American Journal of Cardiology* 100(12A):33P-37P, December 2007.

Spector, N., et al. "Dyspnea: Applying Research to Bedside Practice," *AACN Advanced Critical Care* 18(1):45-58, January-March 2007.

Stevens, W.W., et al. "RSV 2007: Recent Advances in Respiratory Syncytial Virus Research," *Viral Immunology* 21(2):133-40, June 2008.

Williams, M., et al. "The Language of Breathlessness Differentiates Between Patients with Chronic Obstructive Pulmonary Disease and Age-Matched Adults," *Chest* 134(3):489-96, September 2008.

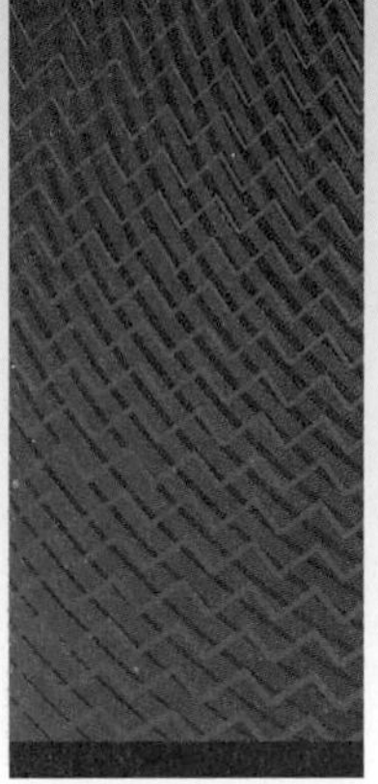

INDEX

A

i refers to an illustration; t refers to a table.

i refers to an illustration; t refers to a table.

i refers to an illustration; t refers to a table.

i refers to an illustration; t refers to a table.

i refers to an illustration; t refers to a table.

B

i refers to an illustration; t refers to a table.

i refers to an illustration; t refers to a table.

C

i refers to an illustration; t refers to a table.

i refers to an illustration; t refers to a table.

i refers to an illustration; t refers to a table.

i refers to an illustration; t refers to a table.

D

i refers to an illustration; t refers to a table.

i refers to an illustration; t refers to a table.

E

i refers to an illustration; t refers to a table.

i refers to an illustration; t refers to a table.

F

i refers to an illustration; t refers to a table.

G

i refers to an illustration; t refers to a table.

i refers to an illustration; t refers to a table.

i refers to an illustration; t refers to a table.

i refers to an illustration; t refers to a table.

i refers to an illustration; t refers to a table.

I

i refers to an illustration; t refers to a table.

J

K

i refers to an illustration; t refers to a table.

L

i refers to an illustration; t refers to a table.

i refers to an illustration; t refers to a table.

M

i refers to an illustration; t refers to a table.

i refers to an illustration; t refers to a table.

N

i refers to an illustration; t refers to a table.

O

i refers to an illustration; t refers to a table.

P

i refers to an illustration; t refers to a table.

i refers to an illustration; t refers to a table.

i refers to an illustration; t refers to a table.

i refers to an illustration; t refers to a table.

i refers to an illustration; t refers to a table.

i refers to an illustration; t refers to a table.

Q

R

i refers to an illustration; t refers to a table.

i refers to an illustration; t refers to a table.

i refers to an illustration; t refers to a table.

i refers to an illustration; t refers to a table.

i refers to an illustration; t refers to a table.

T

i refers to an illustration; t refers to a table.

i refers to an illustration; t refers to a table.

U

i refers to an illustration; t refers to a table.

i refers to an illustration; t refers to a table.

W

X

Y

Z

i refers to an illustration; t refers to a table.

Signs & symptoms in English and Spanish *(continued from inside front cover)*

Genitourinary system

amenorrhea / not getting a menstrual period
bladder distention / bladder fullness
breast dimpling
breast nodules
breast pain
breast ulcers
dysmenorrhea / painful menstrual periods
dyspareunia / painful intercourse
dysuria / painful urination / burning on urination
enuresis / nighttime urination
flank pain
genital lesions in the male
gynecomastia / breast enlargement in men
hematuria / urinating blood
impotence / inability to have intercourse
menorrhagia / profuse or extended menstrual bleeding
metrorrhagia / menstrual bleeding that occurs between menstrual periods
nipple discharge
nipple retraction / a nipple that turns inward
nocturia / excessive urination at night
oligomenorrhea / abnormally infrequent menstrual bleeding
oliguria / abnormally decreased urination
peau d'orange / orange-peel skin
polyuria / excessive urination
priapism / persistent, painful erection
scrotal swelling
urethral discharge / discharge from the penis
urinary frequency / having to urinate frequently
urinary hesitancy / difficulty starting to urinate
urinary incontinence / uncontrollable passage of urine
urinary urgency / sudden compelling urge to urinate
urine cloudiness / cloudy urine
vaginal bleeding, postmenopausal / bleeding that occurs after a woman has stopped menstruating
vaginal discharge (*color:* yellow, green, colorless, or bloody; *odor:* fish, foul, or yeast; *consistency:* cheesy, thin, or thick)

Sistema genitourinario

amenorrea / no tener un periodo menstrual
distensión de la vejiga / plenitud en la vejiga
pequeñas depresiones en la mama
nódulos en la mama
dolor de la mama
úlcera en la mama
dismenorrea / menstruación dolorosa
dispareunia / dolor al tener relaciones sexuales
disuria / dolor al orinar / sencasión ardiente al orinar
enuresis / orinar durante la noche
dolor de costado
lesiones genitales del hombre
ginecomastia / desarrollo excesivo de la mama en el hombre
hematuria / orinar sangre
impotencia / incapacidade de mantener relaciones sexuales
menorrea / flujo menstrual profuso o prolongado
metrorragia / flujo menstrual que ocurre entre períodos
excreción del pezón
retracción del pezón / pezón invertido
nocturia / orinar excesivamente durante la noche
oligomenorrea / períodos menstruales anormales poco frecuentes
oliguria / secreción disminuida deorina
piel como cáscara de naranja
poliuria / orinar con mucha frecuencia
priapismo / erección persistente y dolorosa del pene
hinchazón escrotal
excreción de la uretra / excreción del pene
orinar con frecuencia / tener que orinar frecuentemente
vacilación urinaria / dificultad al empezar a orinar
incontinencia urinaria / pasaje incontrolable de la orina
urgencia urinaria / repentina urgencia de orinar
orina turbia
sangrado vaginal posmenopáusico / sangrado que ocurre después de dejar de tener periodos menstruales
excreción vaginal (*color:* amarillo, verde, sin color, o con sangre; *color:* a pez, fétido, o levadura; *consistencia:* de queso, aguada, o espesa)

Nervous system

amnesia / memory loss
aura
cat's cry / high-pitched cry
dizziness
drooling
fasciculation / wavelike twitching of the skin
fontanel bulging / bulging soft spots on a baby's head
fontanel depression / sunken soft spots on a baby's head
footdrop
gag reflex abnormalities
gait, bizarre
gait, propulsive
gait, scissors
gait, spastic
gait, steppage
gait, waddling
headache
insomnia / difficulty sleeping or falling asleep
level of consciousness, decreased
masklike facies / loss of facial expression
myoclonus / sudden shocklike contractions of a single muscle
neck pain
nuchal rigidity / neck stiffness
orofacial dyskinesia / abnormal involuntary movements of the face, mouth, tongue, eyes, and neck
paralysis / total loss of voluntary movement
paresthesia / numbness, prickling, or tingling
ptosis / excessive drooping of the upper eyelid
raccoon eyes / dark circles under the eyes, like those of a raccoon, that don't result from head trauma
seizure
syncope / fainting
taste abnormalities / loss of taste / partial loss of taste / distorted sense of taste
tics / involuntary twitches in the face, shoulders, neck, trunk, or hands
tremors / shaking / shakiness
trismus / spasm of the jaw muscles / inability to open the mouth
vertigo / feeling of being pulled sideways / feeling as if the world is revolving around you or you are spinning despite being still